SECOND EDITION

Basic & Clinical Endocrinology

Edited By

Francis S. Greenspan, MD

*Clinical Professor of Medicine and Radiology
Department of Medicine, and Chief, Thyroid Clinic
University of California, San Francisco*

Peter H. Forsham, MD

*Professor of Medicine and Pediatrics
Former Chief of Endocrinology, and
Former Director of Metabolic Research Unit
University of California, San Francisco*

LMP **LANGE Medical Publications/Los Altos, California**

APPLETON-CENTURY-CROFTS/East Norwalk, Connecticut A̅C̅C̅

Notice: Our knowledge in clinical sciences is constantly changing. As new information becomes available, changes in treatment and in the use of drugs become necessary. The author(s) and the publisher of this volume have taken care to make certain that the doses of drugs and schedules of treatment are correct and compatible with the standards generally accepted at the time of publication. The reader is advised to consult carefully the instruction and information material included in the package insert of each drug or therapeutic agent before administration. This advice is especially important when using new or infrequently used drugs.

Prentice-Hall of Australia, Pty. Ltd., Sydney
Prentice-Hall Canada, Inc.
Prentice-Hall Hispanoamericana, S.A., Mexico
Prentice-Hall of India Private Limited, New Delhi
Prentice-Hall International (UK) Limited, London
Prentice-Hall of Japan, Inc., Tokyo
Prentice-Hall of Southeast Asia (Pte.) Ltd., Singapore
Whitehall Books Ltd., Wellington, New Zealand
Editora Prentice-Hall do Brasil Ltda., Rio de Janeiro

ISBN: 0 – 8385 – 0547 – 3

PRINTED IN THE UNITED STATES OF AMERICA

Table of Contents

The Authors

Claude D. Arnaud, MD
Professor of Medicine and Physiology, University of California, San Francisco, and Chief of Endocrinology, Veterans Administration Medical Center, San Francisco.

John D. Baxter, MD
Professor of Medicine and Biochemistry and Biophysics, Director of the Metabolic Research Unit, and Chief of the Division of Endocrinology, Moffitt Hospital and University of California, San Francisco.

Christopher C. Benz, MD
Assistant Professor of Medicine, Cancer Research Institute, University of California, San Francisco.

Edward G. Biglieri, MD
Chief of Endocrinology, San Francisco General Hospital, and Professor of Medicine, University of California, San Francisco.

Glenn D. Braunstein, MD
Director, Division of Endocrinology, Cedars-Sinai Medical Center, Los Angeles, and Professor of Medicine, University of California, Los Angeles.

Bayard D. Catherwood, MD
Assistant Professor of Medicine in Residence, University of California, San Diego, and Clinical Investigator, Veterans Administration Medical Center, San Diego.

Felix A. Conte, MD
Professor of Pediatrics, University of California, San Francisco.

Leonard J. Deftos, MD
Professor of Medicine in Residence, University of California, San Diego, and Chief, Endocrine Section, Veterans Administration Medical Center, San Diego.

Clifford W. Deveney, MD
Associate Professor of Surgery, University of Pennsylvania, Philadelphia; Adjunct Associate Professor of Surgery, Medical College of Pennsylvania, Philadelphia; and Chief, Surgical Service, Veterans Administration Medical Center, Philadelphia.

James W. Findling, MD
Academic Chairman, Department of Internal Medicine, St. Luke's Hospital, Milwaukee, and Associate Professor of Clinical Medicine, Medical College of Wisconsin, Milwaukee.

Peter H. Forsham, MD
Professor of Medicine and Pediatrics, Former Chief of Endocrinology, and Former Director of Metabolic Research Unit, University of California, San Francisco.

William F. Ganong, MD
Lange Professor and Chairman, Department of Physiology, University of California, San Francisco.

Barry J. Gertz, MD, PhD
Assistant Professor of Medicine, University of California, San Francisco.

Alan Goldfien, MD
Professor of Medicine, Departments of Medicine and Obstetrics, Gynecology, and Reproductive Sciences and the Cardiovascular Research Institute, University of California, San Francisco.

Marc E. Goldyne, MD, PhD
Associate Professor in Residence, Dermatology and Medicine, Departments of Dermatology and Medicine, University of California, San Francisco, and Assistant Chief, Department of Dermatology, Veterans Administration Medical Center, San Francisco.

Gilbert S. Gordan, MD, PhD
Associate Chief of Staff for Education, Veterans Administration Medical Center, Martinez, and Professor of Medicine Emeritus, University of California, San Francisco and Davis.

Francis S. Greenspan, MD
Clinical Professor of Medicine and Radiology, Department of Medicine, and Chief, Thyroid Clinic, University of California, San Francisco.

Melvin M. Grumbach, MD
Edward B. Shaw Professor and Chairman, Department of Pediatrics, University of California, San Francisco.

Philip G. Hoffman, Jr., MD, PhD
Associate Clinical Professor of Obstetrics, Gynecology, and Reproductive Sciences, University of California, San Francisco, and Associate Clinical Director, Reproductive Medicine, Syntex Research, Palo Alto.

John P. Kane, MD, PhD
Professor of Medicine and Biochemistry and Biophysics, University of California, San Francisco.

John H. Karam, MD
Professor of Medicine, Co-Director of Diabetes Clinic, and Associate Director of Metabolic Research Unit, University of California, San Francisco.

Claudio E. Kater, MD
Associate Professor of Medicine, Endocrinology Service, Escola Paulista de Medicina, São Paulo, Brazil.

John L. Kitzmiller, MD
Associate Professor of Obstetrics, Gynecology, and Reproductive Sciences, University of California, San Francisco, and Chief, Perinatal Service, Children's Hospital, San Francisco.

Felix O. Kolb, MD
Clinical Professor of Medicine, University of California, San Francisco.

Brian J. Lewis, MD
Clinical Professor of Medicine, Cancer Research Institute, University of California, San Francisco.

Mary J. Malloy, MD
Associate Clinical Professor of Pediatrics and Medicine, University of California, San Francisco.

Mary C. Martin, MD
Assistant Professor of Obstetrics, Gynecology, and Reproductive Sciences, University of California, San Francisco.

Scott E. Monroe, MD
Adjunct Associate Professor of Obstetrics, Gynecology, and Reproductive Sciences, University of California, San Francisco.

David J. Ramsay, DM, DPhil
Professor of Physiology, University of California, San Francisco.

Basil Rapoport, MB, ChB
Professor of Medicine, University of California, San Francisco, and Staff Physician, Veterans Administration Medical Center, San Francisco.

Betty S. Roof, MD
Professor of Medicine, Medical University of South Carolina, Charleston.

Patricia R. Salber, MD
Clinical Instructor of Medicine, University of California, San Francisco, and Staff Physician, Kaiser Permanente Medical Group, San Francisco.

E. Martin Spencer, MD, PhD
Associate Clinical Professor of Medicine, University of California, San Francisco, and Director, Laboratory of Growth and Development, Children's Hospital, San Francisco.

Dennis M. Styne, MD
Associate Professor of Pediatrics, University of California, Davis.

J. Blake Tyrrell, MD
Associate Clinical Professor of Medicine, Metabolic Research Unit, University of California, San Francisco.

Lawrence W. Way, MD
Professor of Surgery, University of California, San Francisco, and Chief of Surgical Service, Veterans Administration Medical Center, San Francisco.

John A. Williams, MD, PhD
Professor of Physiology and Medicine, University of California, San Francisco.

Clinton W. Young, MD
Assistant Clinical Professor of Medicine, University of California, San Francisco.

Preface

Endocrinology is a rapidly expanding field with changing concepts of pathophysiology and hormone action. The purpose of this book is to provide an authoritative, current, and concise review of the field. The text includes the basic anatomy, physiology, and biochemistry of the endocrine system as well as the pathology, diagnosis, and management of the clinical syndromes. Thus, it will provide both the student and the practitioner with a clear and practical guide to the field of endocrinology.

In the second edition of *Basic & Clinical Endocrinology,* all of the chapters have been revised and updated. The following are of particular interest:

- A new chapter on the applications of gene expression and recombinant DNA methodology to endocrinology.
- A totally rewritten chapter on hormones and cancer.
- A completely revised chapter on syndromes involving multiple endocrine glands.
- Descriptions of new diagnostic tests with corticotropin-releasing hormone and growth hormone–releasing hormone and a discussion of the application of thin needle aspiration cytology to the diagnosis of thyroid nodules and thyroid cancer.
- A reevaluation of the current status of insulin therapy for diabetes mellitus, emphasizing the use of self-monitoring of blood glucose levels, indications for intensive multiple-dose insulin therapy, the role of insulin pump therapy, current information on second-generation hypoglycemic agents, and management of diabetes in pregnancy.
- New and easy-to-use growth charts to aid in the diagnosis and management of growth problems.

The special feature of this book is that it provides comprehensive coverage of the endocrine system (the pancreas and the pituitary, adrenal, thyroid, and parathyroid glands) as well as coverage of the neuroendocrine, renal, gonadal, gastrointestinal, and other organ systems. Carefully chosen illustrations add clarity to the discussions. In each subject area, the clinical aspects of each endocrine problem are discussed by experienced clinicians, with emphasis on the practical management of clinical problems. Current references for further reading are appended to each chapter.

This book will serve equally well the initial educational needs of students and residents and the lifelong learning needs of practicing physicians. The former should benefit from the comprehensive, current, and well-organized discussions. The practicing physician should find the authoritative yet concise summary of the basic and clinical aspects of endocrinology of particular value.

Francis S. Greenspan, MD
Peter H. Forsham, MD

San Francisco
July, 1986

Mechanisms in Hormone Secretion, Action, & Response

John A. Williams, MD, PhD

Hormones are molecules that are synthesized and secreted by specialized cells, released into the blood, and exert biochemical effects on target cells at a distance from their site of origin. Some hormones such as thyroid-stimulating hormone act exclusively on one target tissue (in this case the thyroid gland); other hormones such as insulin and thyroid hormone act on many cell types, including (in this example) liver, brain, and skin. The specificity of hormone action is determined by the presence of specific hormone receptors on or in these target cells. The cellular response, however, is determined by the genetic programming of the particular cell. Thus, the same hormone may have different actions on different tissues. For example, adrenal glucocorticoids cause cytolysis of lymphocytes but induce enzymes necessary for the production of glucose in the liver.

Classes of Hormones
(Table 1–1)

Hormones have diverse molecular structures ranging from single modified amino acids (epinephrine)

Acronyms Used in This Chapter

ACTH	Adrenocorticotropic hormone
ADP	Adenosine diphosphate
AMP	Adenosine monophosphate
ATP	Adenosine triphosphate
AUG	Adenine-uridine-guanine
cAMP	Cyclic adenosine monophosphate
cGMP	Cyclic guanosine monophosphate
DNA	Deoxyribonucleic acid
FSH	Follicle-stimulating hormone
GDP	Guanosine diphosphate
GMP	Guanosine monophosphate
GTP	Guanosine triphosphate
hCG	Human chorionic gonadotropin
LH	Luteinizing hormone
mRNA	Messenger ribonucleic acid
MSH	Melanocyte-stimulating hormone
PNMT	Phenylethanolamine-N-methyltransferase
RNA	Ribonucleic acid
SRP	Signal recognition particle
TSH	Thyroid-stimulating hormone (thyrotropin)

Table 1–1. Classes of hormones based on structure.

Peptides and Proteins		Steroids	Amines
Glycoprotein	**Polypeptides**	**Steroids**	**Amines**
Follicle-stimulating hormone (FSH)	Adrenocorticotropic hormone (ACTH)	Aldosterone	Epinephrine
Human chorionic gonadotropin (hCG)	Angiotensin	Cortisol	Norepinephrine
Luteinizing hormone (LH)	Calcitonin	Estradiol	Thyroxine (T_4)
Thyroid-stimulating hormone (TSH)	Cholecystokinin	Progesterone	Triiodothyronine (T_3)
	Erythropoietin	Testosterone	
	Gastrin	Vitamin D	
	Glucagon		
	Growth hormone		
	Insulin		
	Insulinlike growth peptides (somatomedins)		
	Melanocyte-stimulating hormone (MSH)		
	Nerve growth factor		
	Oxytocin		
	Parathyroid hormone		
	Prolactin		
	Relaxin		
	Secretin		
	Somatostatin		
	Vasopressin (ADH)		

through lipids (estrogen, cortisol) to proteins (glucagon, insulin, growth hormone). In correlating properties of hormones with physiologic actions, it is generally useful to categorize them as (1) peptides and proteins, (2) steroids, and (3) amines or amino acid derivatives (Table 1–1). This listing is representative and not complete, since new molecules with hormonal activity are continually being discovered. For example, an area of investigation that is particularly active at present is the identification of new gastrointestinal hormones.

Hormones as Regulatory Molecules

Hormones are one class of regulatory molecules and act in somewhat the same ways as other regulatory molecules such as the neurotransmitters, paracrine agents, and metabolites. In general, the mechanism of intercellular regulation consists of perception of a stimulus by a cell by means of a specialized cell receptor, followed by the cellular response. In the case of hormone action, the stimulating hormone becomes bound to its specific receptor on the cell, and the result is a cascade of intracellular events including integration of several stimuli and amplification of the original bound stimulus, culminating in the cellular response. The stimulus may consist of only a few molecules of hormone per target cell. Intracellular amplification generally involves either intracellular messengers such as cAMP and Ca^{2+} or the synthesis of new RNA and protein. Cellular regulation by hormones, then, follows the same general pattern of **cell activation** observed in the control of other biologic processes; examples are the development of an egg following fertilization, the contraction of muscle following electrical excitation, and the activation, following exposure to antigen, of a quiescent lymphocyte into one that actively synthesizes specific antibody.

Hormone Specificity Through Unique Receptors

Binding sites for peptide hormones and catecholamines are generally large glycoproteins on or in cellular membranes, including the plasma membrane, Golgi complex, and (in some cases) nuclear membrane. Hormones initially bind to receptors present on the cell surface membrane (plasma membrane) that is exposed to the cell's environment. It is not clear whether binding sites in intracellular membranes, such as those on the Golgi complex, endoplasmic reticulum, and nuclear membrane, play a role in hormone action or are merely being transported to or from the plasma membrane as part of a general turnover of membrane proteins. In contrast to polypeptide hormones, the known receptors for steroids and thyroid hormones are located chiefly within the cell. Steroid receptors are located in the cytoplasm; thyroid receptors are located in the plasma membrane, nucleus, and mitochondria. Steroid and thyroid hormones are small lipophilic molecules that are assumed to be taken up through the cell membranes; the mechanism of cellular penetration by these molecules is not known, but evidence exists for mechanisms other than simple diffusion. Once inside the cell, these hormones interact with their intracellular receptors. In some cases, the action of these hormones may be initiated by their initial interactions with plasma membrane receptors at the cell membrane.

While receptors (as distinct from binding proteins) must have the potential to be coupled to a biologic response, the receptor itself is a separate unit involved with recognition. In general, hormone-receptor interactions are noncovalent; they are reversible, involving hydrogen bonding and hydrophobic and electrostatic forces. Both membrane and intracellular receptors can be solubilized and isolated and their properties studied. In the case of membrane receptors, which are normally coupled to an effector protein (adenylate cyclase, Ca^{2+} channel), addition of a new receptor by cell fusion or reimplantation of a solubilized receptor to a previously unresponsive cell possessing the effector system will allow that cell to respond to that hormone.

Abnormalities in receptors or absences of specific receptors are now known to underlie some pathologic states, including insulin resistance, testicular feminization, and certain types of dwarfism, diabetes insipidus, and pseudohypoparathyroidism.

Figure 1–1. Electron micrograph of a portion of a pancreatic B cell, showing the features of cells secreting polypeptide hormones. N, nucleus; PM, plasma membrane; G, Golgi complex; arrows, granules. (Courtesy of EP Reaven.)

SYNTHESIS & SECRETION OF HORMONES

POLYPEPTIDE & AMINE HORMONES

The cells that secrete polypeptide hormones have many common structural features (Fig 1–1) related to the synthesis, packaging, and release of these molecules. Polypeptide hormones, along with other proteins destined for export from the cell, are synthesized on membrane-bound ribosomes and then sequestered in the cisternae of the endoplasmic reticulum. By contrast, proteins destined to remain in the cell are synthesized on free ribosomes.

Initially, the messenger RNA (mRNA) specific for the polypeptide hormone attaches to a free ribosome, and this is followed by initiation of translation at an adenine-uridine-guanine (AUG) initiation codon (Fig 1–2). The initial amino acid sequence of the nascent protein, termed the signal peptide, is bound by a cytoplasmic ribonucleoprotein termed the signal recognition particle (SRP). SRP then attaches to a "docking protein" in the endoplasmic reticulum membrane, thus serving a targeting function. The nascent polypeptide is then extruded, signal peptide first, through the membrane of the endoplasmic reticulum and into its lumen. While the signal peptide usually contains a number of hydrophobic amino acids, there is no common sequence between secretory proteins, and the mechanism of passage across the membrane remains largely unknown.

The complete molecule, including the signal peptide, is referred to as a **prehormone;** its lifetime is very short, however, as the signal peptide is rapidly cleaved off by a trypsinlike enzyme present in the endoplasmic reticulum.

In many cases, further modifications of the hormone are required before its secretion, such as the addition of sugars to the glycoprotein hormones hCG, TSH, LH, and FSH. If extra amino acids are still present following cleavage of the signal peptide, this form of the molecule is referred to as a **prohormone.** In the case of insulin, the prohormone proinsulin is a single chain, which allows folding and apposition of the 2 ends of the molecule so that interchain disulfide bonds can be correctly formed. When the middle sequence of proinsulin, the connecting (C) peptide, is removed, the mature 2-chain form of insulin remains.

In some cases, the prohormone may be the precursor for multiple peptides and is referred to as a **polyprotein.** The best-studied example is pro-opiomelanocortin, which in different portions of the pituitary and brain is cleaved to yield different peptides, including ACTH, MSH, and β-endorphin.

Following synthesis and sequestration within the lumen of the endoplasmic reticulum, the newly synthesized hormone moves to the Golgi region by vesicular transport and is there packaged into granules or vesicles (Fig 1–3). This intracellular transport is guided by microtubules and can be blocked by drugs such as colchicine that disrupt microtubules. It is in the Golgi

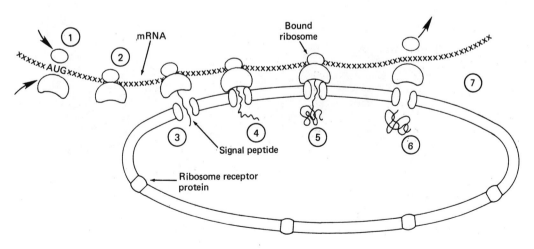

Figure 1–2. Synthesis and sequestration of polypeptide hormones. Synthesis begins at the left as ribosomal subunits aggregate ① and begin to read the mRNA specific for the hormones ②. Subsequent steps shown include (from left to right) synthesis of the initial signal peptide that interacts with ribosome receptor protein ③; extrusion of the nascent peptide into the lumen of the endoplasmic reticulum ④ and ⑤; release of the protein into the cisternae of the endoplasmic reticulum ⑥; and dissociation of the ribosomal subunits from the mRNA ⑦. (Reproduced, with permission, from Scheele GA: *Am J Physiol* 1980;**238**:G467.)

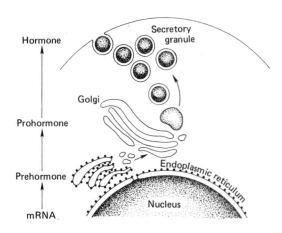

Figure 1–3. Intracellular transport of protein from the endoplasmic reticulum to the Golgi complex, packaging of newly synthesized polypeptide hormone into secretory granules, and release of hormone by exocytosis. At left are listed the molecular forms of the hormone (or information coding for the hormone) present in that portion of the cell.

region that terminal glycosylation occurs as well as conversion of prohormones to mature hormones. In some cases, substances such as proteins, amines (eg, dopamine), ATP, and Ca^{2+} are packaged along with the hormone into secretory granules. It is in this form that the hormone is stored within the cell until its secretion is required.

Thyroid Hormones
(See also Chapter 7.)

The synthesis of thyroid hormones proceeds in part by the steps of synthesis and packaging discussed above in that thyroid hormones are first synthesized within the matrix of a large glycoprotein, thyroglobulin (Fig 1–4). Newly synthesized thyroglobulin is packaged in the Golgi region into vesicles and secreted into a specialized compartment, the follicular lumen. During this process of secretion, iodide that has been transported into the thyroid is oxidized by a peroxidase located on the apical plasma membrane. Oxidized iodine combines covalently with tyrosine residues of the protein to form mono- and diiodotyrosine. Two iodotyrosine residues then undergo a coupling reaction

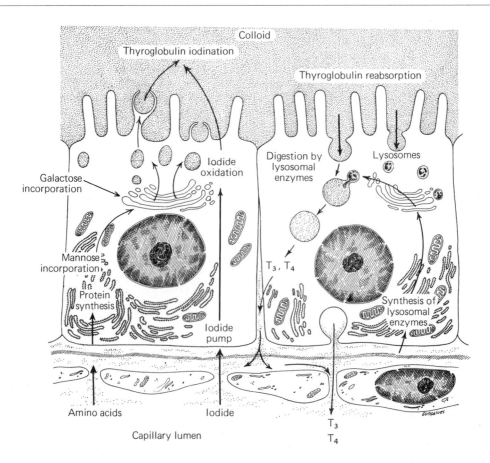

Figure 1–4. Processes of synthesis and iodination of thyroglobulin *(left)* and its reabsorption and digestion *(right)*. These events occur in the same cell. (Reproduced, with permission, from Junqueira LC, Carneiro J: *Basic Histology,* 4th ed. Lange, 1983.)

to form iodothyronine while still within the thyroglobulin matrix. The mature thyroglobulin in the follicular lumen thus can be considered a prohormone, since it contains a number of potential thyroid hormone molecules within its structure.

Conversion of the prohormone thyroglobulin to thyroid hormone requires phagocytosis or pinocytosis of colloid from the thyroid follicular lumen followed by lysosomal digestion. The released thyroid hormone then leaves the cell by an unknown avenue. The supply of thyroid hormone stored within follicular lumens may be sufficient to maintain normal secretory rates for several months.

Catecholamines

Cells secreting the catecholamine hormones epinephrine and norepinephrine appear similar to cells secreting polypeptide hormones in that they contain prominent secretory granules. The process of hormone synthesis and packaging is different, however, in that catecholamines are synthesized from the amino acid tyrosine by a series of enzymatic steps occurring in the cytoplasm (see Chapter 11). Dopamine is then taken up and concentrated within secretory granules by a transport process localized in the granule membrane. The enzyme dopamine β-hydroxylase, which is localized chiefly in the granule, catalyzes the conversion of dopamine to norepinephrine (Fig 1–5). Cells of the adrenal medulla also contain an enzyme called phenylethanolamine-N-methyltransferase (PNMT) that catalyzes the conversion of norepinephrine to epinephrine. The cytoplasmic localization of PNMT suggests that norepinephrine and epinephrine can also be transported across the granule membrane. Within the granules, catecholamines exist in a complex with ATP along with proteins of unknown function called **chromogranins.** All of the granule contents are released together when the granule fuses with the plasma membrane.

Stimulus-Secretion Coupling (Protein & Amine Hormones)

Amounts of polypeptide and catecholamine hormones sufficient to maintain normal secretory rates for hours to days are stored in secretory granules. Variations in the rate of hormone secretion into the blood are acutely brought about by control of the rate at which secretory granule contents are released from the cell by exocytosis. In this process, the membrane surrounding the secretory granule fuses with the cell membrane, the intervening membrane breaks down, and the contents of the granule are released into the extracellular space. Calcium ions (Ca^{2+}) are necessary for fusion to occur, and secretion is controlled by the level of intracellular Ca^{2+}. In this process of stimulus-secretion coupling, the agent inducing secretion (sometimes referred to as a secretagogue) acts at a receptor on the endocrine cell to open channels in the cell membrane selective for Ca^{2+}; Ca^{2+} then enters the cell down its electrochemical gradient (Ca^{2+} outside = 10^{-3} mol/L; Ca^{2+} inside = 10^{-7} mol/L), and the rise in cytoplasmic Ca^{2+} triggers secretion. These events are accompanied by changes in the electrical potential across the cell membrane. Endocrine cells, related to nerve cells by virtue of their origin from neuroectodermal tissue, may also show action potentials similar to those of neurons when stimulated to release hormones.

Endocrine cells are now known to contain contractile proteins such as actin and myosin. There is

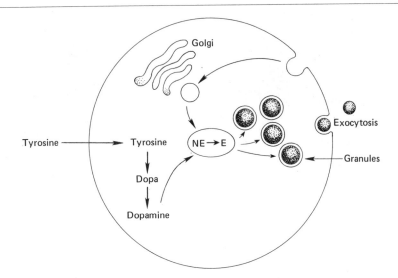

Figure 1–5. Synthesis and packaging of norepinephrine (NE) and epinephrine (E). Tyrosine is converted in the cytoplasm to dopamine, which is concentrated within secretory granules and converted to NE and E. Following release of the granule contents, the empty vesicles or their membranes are recycled through the Golgi complex and then refilled.

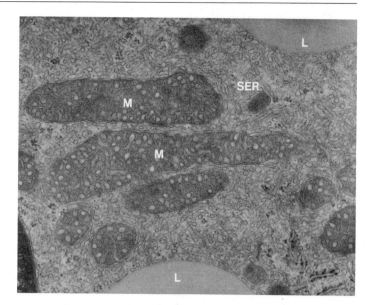

Figure 1–6. Electron micrograph of a portion of a cell from human adrenal cortex showing the common features of steroid-secreting cells. M, mitochondrion; L, lipid droplet; SER, smooth endoplasmic reticulum. (Courtesy of JA Long.)

increasing evidence that these proteins may be important both in moving secretory granules to the plasma membrane and bringing about their subsequent fusion. Along with Ca^{2+} in some secretory cells, cAMP may also play an ancillary role in the control of hormone secretion. Specific Ca^{2+}- and cAMP-activated protein kinases are probably involved, as discussed later in the section on hormone action.

SYNTHESIS & SECRETION OF STEROID HORMONES

In contrast to polypeptide hormones, appreciable amounts of steroid hormones are not stored within the

cells that produce them. Steroid hormones are able to pass through membranes and leave the cell rapidly after synthesis. As a result, the rate of secretion of most steroid hormones is controlled by the rate of synthesis. Steroid synthesis begins with cholesterol, and the various steps (primarily oxidative) in synthesis take place within the cytoplasm, smooth endoplasmic reticulum, and mitochondria. Cells secreting steroids generally contain an abundant supply of these organelles (Fig 1–6) plus prominent lipid droplets containing the cholesterol precursor.

Control of the rate of steroid synthesis (Fig 1–7) is by regulation of rate-limiting enzymes in the biosynthetic pathway—specifically, the initial hydroxylations and side-chain cleavage of cholesterol within

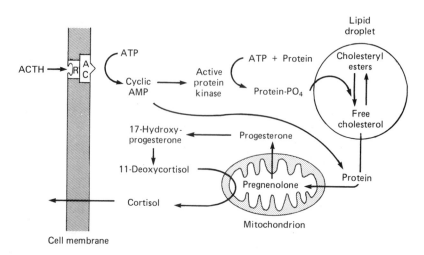

Figure 1–7. Synthesis and secretion of the steroid hormone cortisol from the adrenal cortex in response to stimulation by ACTH. ACTH binds to specific receptors on the cell membrane, activates adenylate cyclase, and increases the formation of cAMP. Cyclic AMP, by activating protein kinase, brings about increased synthesis of pregnenolone from cholesterol. Pregnenolone is subsequently converted through several intermediates to cortisol, leaves the cell, and enters the circulation.

the mitochondrion that result in the production of pregnenolone. In the case of adrenal and gonadal steroids, whose synthesis is controlled by tropic hormones, the stimulating hormone interacts with a specific receptor that leads to activation of adenylate cyclase and a rise in cAMP. Cyclic AMP then brings about a change in the activity of enzymes that are rate-limiting for steroid synthesis. This process also requires the synthesis of new protein that is rapidly turning over; the role of these proteins is as yet unknown.

Ca^{2+} also plays a role in the regulation of steroid synthesis. Ca^{2+} is necessary in the adrenal cortex both for ACTH to increase the level of cAMP and for the subsequent action of cAMP. In the mitochondria of kidney tubule cells, the level of Ca^{2+} appears to be an important regulator in the production of another steroid hormone, 1,25-dihydroxycholecalciferol, which is the active form of vitamin D.

COMMON MECHANISMS OF HORMONE ACTION

HORMONE RECEPTORS

Hormone receptors on or in cells have 2 distinct roles: to distinguish a particular hormone from other hormones and regulatory molecules and to translate the hormonal signal into an appropriate cellular response. A receptor must have an affinity for its hormone that is high enough in relation to the concentration of the hormone in the blood so that the amount of hormone-receptor complex will increase or decrease in response to a change in the level of hormone present in the cell's environment. To ensure specificity, the affinity of the receptor for its hormone must be much higher than its affinity for other hormones. In general, the concentration of hormones in blood is 10^{-11} to 10^{-9} mol/L.

Kinetics of Hormone Binding

Biochemical studies of the properties of hormone receptors are carried out employing radiolabeled hormone and either intact target cells or a subcellular fraction prepared from the target cell that contains the receptor. Initially, hormone-receptor binding occurs as a bimolecular reaction:

$$[H] + [R] \underset{k_2}{\overset{k_1}{\rightleftharpoons}} [HR] \qquad \ldots (1)$$

where [H] is the concentration of free hormone, [R] the concentration of free receptor, [HR] the concentration of the hormone-receptor complex, and k_1 and k_2 the rate constants for association and dissociation.

When such a system is at equilibrium, the rates of the forward and backward reactions are equal, and

$$\frac{[H] \, [R]}{[HR]} = \frac{k_2}{k_1} = K_d \qquad \ldots (2)$$

where K_d is the equilibrium dissociation constant, a measure of the receptor's affinity for the hormone. Since the biologic response to the hormone is controlled by a signal generated in proportion to the num-

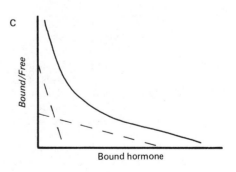

Figure 1–8. Binding of hormone to its specific receptor. *A:* Plot of bound versus free hormone over a range of free hormone concentrations. The dashed line indicates the asymptote; the value of free hormone at which half the receptors are saturated is the K_d or affinity constant. *B:* Scatchard transformation of the data in (A). The linear plot is indicative of a single binding site. *C:* Curvilinear Scatchard plot. The dashed lines indicate the contributions of 2 separate binding sites the sum of whose occupancy yields the curvilinear Scatchard plot.

ber of hormone-receptor complexes, the equation can be rearranged as

$$\text{Biologic response} \propto [HR] = [H][R]\frac{1}{K_d} \quad \ldots \text{(3)}$$

In addition to the concentration of the free hormone, the concentration of receptors ($[R]$) and their affinity (K_d) influence the biologic response. It is thus important to be able to determine these parameters.

For any value of K_d and with the total number of receptors ($[R_0]$) remaining constant, the number of hormone-receptor complexes, usually referred to as "bound hormone," shows a predictable hyperbolic relationship with regard to the concentration of free hormone (Fig 1-8). At high concentrations of hormone, $[HR]$ approaches a maximum equal to $[R_0]$, since all of the receptor sites are filled; at half-maximal occupancy, when $[R] = [HR]$, the free hormone concentration equals K_d. To make the data easier to interpret, various mathematical transformations are usually used of which the most common is the Scatchard plot. Since $[R_0] = [R] + [HR]$, we can substitute $[R_0] - [HR]$ for $[R]$ in equation (2) and rearrange to yield

$$\frac{[HR]}{[H]} = \frac{[R_0] - [HR]}{K_d} = \frac{[HR]}{K_d} + \frac{[R_0]}{K_d} \quad \ldots \text{(4)}$$

Since, in this equation, $[R_0]$ and K_d are constants, the equation describes a straight line when bound/free hormone ($[HR]/[H]$) is plotted against bound hormone ($[HR]$) (Fig 1-8B). The slope of this line yields the K_d (slope $= -1/K_d$), whereas the line cuts the x axis at $[R_0]$, the binding capacity.

In general, the binding of steroid and thyroid hormones (and some polypeptide hormones) to target cells or semipurified receptors results in linear Scatchard plots. The affinity (K_d) of most receptors is in the range of 10^{-10} to 10^{-8} mol/L, and the total number of receptors, $[R_0] = 4000-100,000$/cell.

In the case of certain polypeptide hormones, however, such as insulin, the binding data yield a curved rather than a linear Scatchard plot (Fig 1-8C). This curved plot may indicate 2 or more classes of specific receptors of differing binding affinity. The curvilinear Scatchard plot for hormone-receptor interaction could also result from negative cooperative interactions among a homogeneous class of receptors. It has been proposed that the binding of a hormone molecule to one receptor would decrease the affinity of the surrounding receptors for the same hormone. Evidence has been presented for negative cooperative interactions in the binding of insulin, although the issue is controversial.

Relation of Hormone-Receptor Occupancy to Biologic Response

The simplest relationship between receptor occupancy and the evoked biologic response is seen

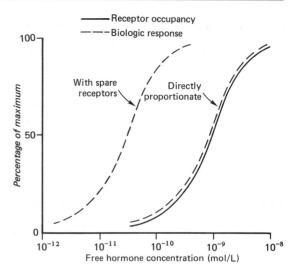

Figure 1-9. Relationship between receptor occupancy and induced biologic response as free hormone concentration is increased. Receptor occupancy is 50% of maximum when the free hormone concentration equals the K_d of the receptor.

when there is a close correlation between the concentration of hormone required to occupy the receptor and for induction of the biologic response (Fig 1-9). For example, the fractional occupancy of glucocorticoid receptors in cultured hepatoma cells parallels induction of the enzyme tyrosine aminotransferase. In other cases, only a small percentage of the hormone receptors must be occupied to generate a maximal response (Fig 1-9). These additional receptors, which are occupied when hormone concentration increases above that necessary to induce the maximal biologic response, are termed "spare" or reserve receptors. All the receptors are identical, potentially functional, and contribute to hormone sensitivity. An example is the stimulation of glucose transport in fat and muscle cells by insulin; in these cells, occupancy of only 2-10% of the insulin receptors leads to a maximal increase in the rate of glucose transport. This relationship increases the sensitivity of the system and in the case of the fat cell allows a receptor with a K_d of about 10^{-9} mol/L to respond to plasma concentrations of insulin that are approximately 100 times lower. Since "spare" receptors increase hormone sensitivity (equation [3]), a decrease in the number of spare receptors produced either by regulatory processes or by experimental manipulation leads to a decrease in hormone sensitivity (measured as the concentration of hormone necessary to elicit a half-maximal response). The maximal response of the tissue, however, is preserved if sufficient hormone is presented to the cell.

Regulation of Receptor Concentration

The number of receptors for polypeptide and catecholamine hormones is extensively regulated by the homologous hormone and in some cases by other hormones. Most commonly, there is negative regulation of the number of hormone receptors in response to changes in plasma hormone levels. In response to a high plasma concentration of the hormone, the number of receptors decreases—"down-regulation" or "densitization"—resulting in reduced sensitivity of the target cell. An example of this is seen in obesity, where high circulating levels of insulin are associated with a decreased number of functional insulin receptors. Regulation in the opposite direction ("up-regulation") is seen in the developing ovarian follicle, where increasing local concentrations of estrogen and FSH increase the number of receptors to luteinizing hormone (LH).

Regulation of the number of polypeptide receptors in the plasma membrane is believed to be due in part to the fact that receptors, like other membrane proteins, are not static but are being continually synthesized, inserted into the plasma membrane, removed, and degraded.

Removal of Receptors

The process of removal of receptor from the cell surface plasma membrane is related in part to the phenomenon of cellular entry of polypeptide hormones. Since hormones have been isolated, charac-terized, and radioactively labeled to high specific activity, more is known about hormones than about their receptors. Convincing ultrastructural and biochemical evidence is now available that polypeptide hormones and growth factors such as insulin, prolactin, and nerve growth factor rapidly penetrate target cells, with all or part of the molecules remaining structurally intact. Three models for the receptor-mediated entry of hormones and other proteins are shown in Fig 1–10. Model A is based on the entry of low-density lipoproteins and some polypeptide hormones into fibroblasts. The ligand binds to receptors located over specialized areas termed "coated pits," which are indentations in the membrane covered on the inside by a basketlike structure composed of the protein clathrin. The membrane containing the receptor and ligand is then endocytosed, forming a coated vesicle that rapidly loses its clathrin coat. The resulting smooth vesicle, termed an endosome or receptosome, is acidic; at this stage, the bound hormone may dissociate from the receptor. In different cells and for different ligands, the endosome may fuse with lysosomes, leading to degradation of both receptor and ligand; the receptor may remain intact and recycle back to the plasma membrane and be reutilized, or the hormone (ligand) may escape the vesicle to enter the cytoplasm.

Model A, however, does not account for the up-

Figure 1–10. Possible modes of internalization of polypeptide hormones (H) and receptors. In *A*, the hormone-receptor complexes are taken up by endocytosis from "coated pits," followed by fusion of the endocytotic vesicle with lysosomes. *B* and *C* are hypothetical mechanisms to allow the hormone receptor complex or hormone alone to be directly internalized. Free internalized hormone could then bind to intracellular receptors on target organelles such as endoplasmic reticulum, mitochondria, or nucleus (N).

take of hormones into cells such as those of the liver and pancreas, where coated vesicles are not prominent. Alternative models B and C (for which little direct evidence exists) involve nonpinocytotic mechanisms. In B, occupancy of the receptor triggers the entry of the hormone-receptor complex; whereas in C, occupancy of the receptor leads to internalization of the hormone but not the receptor. This last model has some similarity to the entry of nascent polypeptides into the cisternae of the endoplasmic reticulum in that binding leads to the opening of a previously hidden pore. Model B as well as A would lead to a depletion of membrane receptors while C would not, although there could be a time-dependent step in C before rebinding of a new hormone molecule could occur, thus accounting for down-regulation. At present, it is not clear what biologic activities of hormones initially binding to plasma (cell surface) membrane receptors are mediated either by the internalized hormone or its receptor. Other internalized proteins, however, such as nerve growth factor and diphtheria toxin, are established as having intracellular sites of action.

INTRACELLULAR MESSENGERS

Steroid and thyroid hormones are able either to interact with the plasma membrane or to penetrate intracellularly and combine with intracellular messengers that can directly mediate their actions. By contrast, some polypeptide hormones and catecholamines that interact with receptors on the cell membrane generally act through intracellular messengers to alter processes within the cell. The 2 major classes of intracellular messengers are cyclic nucleotides, primarily cAMP and the Ca^{2+}-phospholipid system (Table

Figure 1–11. Highly schematic model of 2 types of hormone receptors, R_1 and R_2, which selectively bind hormones H_1 and H_2 and are able to diffuse laterally and interact with a single type of effector, E, in a fluid mosaic membrane.

1–2). For many hormones, however, the primary intracellular messenger is unknown. In the case of insulin and epidermal growth factor, the receptor itself has been shown to possess protein kinase activity selectivity for tyrosine residues. Thus, receptor-mediated protein phosphorylation may be involved in intracellular signal transduction for these hormones.

Intracellular messengers ("second messengers") are generated by an effector protein such as adenylate cyclase or a Ca^{2+} channel protein that is an entity distinct from the hormone receptor itself. Both receptor and effector proteins are believed to be mobile within the plane of the membrane and are influenced by the state of fluidity of membrane lipids. In this "mobile receptor model," occupied receptors can move laterally within the membrane and make contact with and activate effectors (Fig 1–11). The phenomenon of spare receptors can be explained on the basis that there are more receptors than effectors. This model also explains the ability of multiple hormones, each acting on distinct receptors, to activate the same effector system. In fat cells, for example, at least 5 different hormones activate adenylate cyclase, whereas in liver 3 different hormones increase intracellular Ca^{2+}. It is unlikely that a single protein could contain 5 different receptor sites, whereas there could easily be a number of receptors clustered around and able to make contact with and activate a single effector protein.

The most convincing evidence for the separateness of receptors and effectors has been the demonstration that when receptors to a foreign hormone are added to a cell possessing adenylate cyclase, they confer responsiveness to the foreign hormone. This has been done both by fusion of 2 different types of cells—one containing receptors and the other only adenylate cyclase—and by adding an extract of solubilized receptor to the new cell. In both cases, the added proteins and lipids mix rapidly with those already present in the membrane, after which the previously unresponsive cell is able to respond to the hormone.

Genetic studies of clones from cultured cells have also shown that receptor and effector proteins are specified by different genes.

Table 1–2. Division of polypeptide hormones and other regulators according to intracellular messenger.

cAMP	Ca^{2+}	Unknown
Increase cAMP		
ACTH	Acetylcholine	Epidermal growth
Beta-adrenergic	Alpha-adrenergic	factor
catecholamines	catecholamines	Growth hormone
Calcitonin	Angiotensin	Insulin
FSH	Cholecystokinin	Insulinlike growth
Glucagon	Gastrin	peptides
LH	Oxytocin	Nerve growth factor
Parathyroid	Vasopressin	Prolactin
hormone		
Secretin		
TSH		
Vasopressin		
Decrease cAMP		
Acetylcholine		
Alpha-adrenergic		
catecholamines		
Dopamine		
Opiate peptides		
Somatostatin		

Cyclic AMP

The prototype intracellular messenger is cAMP, initially discovered and shown by Sutherland and his colleagues to be produced by the enzyme adenylate cyclase present in plasma membrane. After its activation by the hormone-receptor complex, adenylate cyclase catalyzes the conversion of ATP to cAMP (Fig 1–12). Mg^{2+} is required for this reaction, as the substrate is Mg^{2+}-ATP complex. Adenylate cyclase is a distinct protein that can be solubilized with detergent and is readily separable from the receptor. Adenylate cyclase has also been found to be activated by cholera toxin and guanine nucleotides, particularly GTP and its nonhydrolyzable analogs. Recent biochemical and genetic evidence indicates that these agents act on neither the receptor nor the adenylate cyclase but on a pair of homologous guanine nucleotide–binding proteins, or N proteins. One of these, N_s, mediates stimulation of adenylate cyclase, while the other, N_i, inhibits the cyclase. Hormone receptors that increase cAMP interact with N_s, while those that decrease cAMP (Table 1–2) interact with N_i. Both N_s and N_i are heterodimers with distinct alpha but common beta subunits. The alpha subunit in each case contains the guanine nucleotide–binding site and a site that can be ADP-ribosylated. N_s is ADP-ribosylated by cholera toxin, which brings about dissociation of the alpha and beta subunits and permanently activates the cyclase. N_i is ADP-ribosylated by pertussis toxin, which blocks the dissociation of the subunits and impairs the ability of inhibitory peptides to inhibit the cyclase.

Mutant cell lines without the regulatory protein N_s lack the ability to respond to either hormones or cholera toxin; addition of detergent-solubilized extract of normal membranes, however, restores their sensitivity. The N_s protein also mediates the action of guanine nucleotides that reduce the affinity of the receptor for the hormone. While the N proteins clearly serve as transducers or coupling proteins to link the receptor to the cyclase, the exact mechanism of this process is unknown. One possible model is that binding of the hormone to the receptor causes the regulatory protein N_s to bind GTP—a state that allows the N_s protein to activate the cyclase. The GTPase activity of the N protein would convert the bound GTP to GDP and terminate the action of the cyclase.

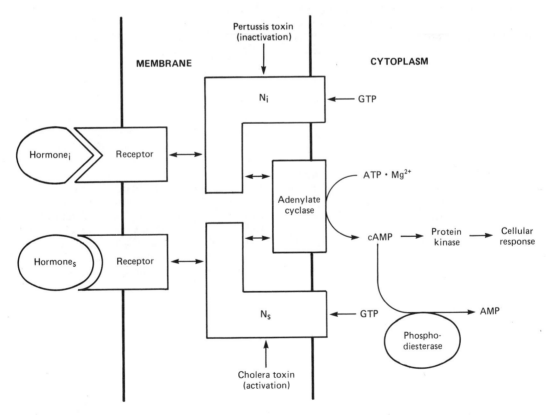

Figure 1–12. Model of receptor–adenylate cyclase coupling. The N_s (stimulating nucleotide) protein is shown coupling the hormone-receptor complex to its effector subunit (adenylate cyclase). The cAMP formed can either combine with protein kinase to initiate a cellular response or be metabolized (inactivated) by a specific phosphodiesterase. The N_i (inhibitory nucleotide) protein would inhibit adenylate cyclase. Hormone$_i$, inhibitory hormone; hormone$_s$, stimulating hormone; GTP, guanosine triphosphate; ATP, adenosine triphosphate; AMP, adenosine monophosphate.

The activity of adenylate cyclase may also be modulated by other factors. Ca^{2+} inhibits adenylate cyclase in a number of tissues, whereas the Ca^{2+}-calmodulin complex (see next section) is known to activate certain cyclases. The activity of adenylate cyclase is also affected in various cells by prostaglandins and adenosine (see Chapter 2).

Cyclic AMP normally exists at very low levels (10^{-8} to 10^{-6} mol/L) in all cells. It is continually being degraded by a specific enzyme, cAMP phosphodiesterase, such that a rise in cellular cAMP induced by hormone activation of adenylate cyclase is rapidly reversed when removal of the hormone stops the production of cAMP. This phosphodiesterase is inhibited by methylxanthines such as caffeine and theophylline.

All of the presently known actions of cAMP in eukaryotes involve phosphorylation of proteins catalyzed by cAMP-activated protein kinase. The mechanism of this activation is shown in Fig 1–13. Normally, this protein kinase is inactivated by binding to a regulatory subunit. When cAMP is elevated, it binds to this regulatory subunit, causing it to release the active catalytic subunit. The active kinase then catalyzes the phosphorylation from ATP of serine and threonine residues of target proteins. This phosphorylation brings about changes in the activity of these proteins. Examples are the phosphorylation of phosphorylase kinase in liver and muscle to activate glycogenolysis and of hormone-sensitive lipase in adipose tissue to activate lypolysis. A great many other structural and enzymatic proteins are phosphorylated in response to various hormones, but in most instances the physiologic effects are not yet known.

Calcium (Ca^{2+})

Ionic calcium (Ca^{2+}) is a well-established intracellular messenger important in coupling excitation to contraction in muscle, excitation to transmitter release in nerves, and secretagogue action to secretion in various exocrine and endocrine glands. The importance of Ca^{2+} as an intracellular messenger in the action of a number of hormones is becoming increasingly apparent (Table 1–2).

The free cytoplasmic Ca^{2+} concentration is highly regulated to maintain a very low intracellular concentration. In various cell types, a Ca^{2+}-activated

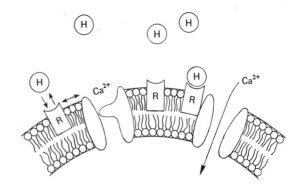

Figure 1–14. Hormone receptors (R) that bind hormone (H) and control the opening of selective Ca^{2+} channels in the cell membrane.

ATPase that directly uses ATP to transport Ca^{2+} out of the cell has been described. Ca^{2+} is also taken up (buffered) by intracellular organelles, including mitochondria and endoplasmic reticulum. At rest, the cytoplasmic concentration of Ca^{2+} is maintained at 10^{-7} mol/L or less. A rise in cytoplasmic Ca^{2+} can then be brought about either by the opening of Ca^{2+} channels in the membrane (Fig 1–14) or by release of Ca^{2+} from intracellular organelles such as endoplasmic reticulum. Analogous to the activation of adenylate cyclase, multiple hormones and neurotransmitters may activate the same Ca^{2+} channels, suggesting separate receptor and Ca^{2+} channel subunits.

Probably most actions of Ca^{2+} as an intracellular messenger result from its binding to Ca^{2+}-binding proteins. The major Ca^{2+}-binding protein involved in the action of hormones is **calmodulin,** a small, highly acidic protein that binds four Ca^{2+} per mole with an affinity (K_d) of about 10^{-6} mol/L. Calmodulin may exist as an integral subunit of an enzyme (Fig 1–15A) and confer Ca^{2+} sensitivity on the enzyme, as is the case with phosphorylase kinase. Alternatively, the Ca^{2+}-calmodulin complex may bind to other proteins and alter their activity (Fig 1–15B). An example is the activation of Ca^{2+}-regulated cyclic nucleotide phosphodiesterase by the Ca^{2+}-calmodulin complex

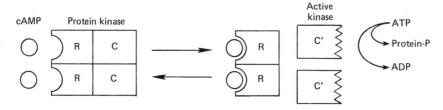

Figure 1–13. Activation of protein kinase by cAMP. R, regulatory subunit; C, repressed catalytic subunit; C', active catalytic subunit.

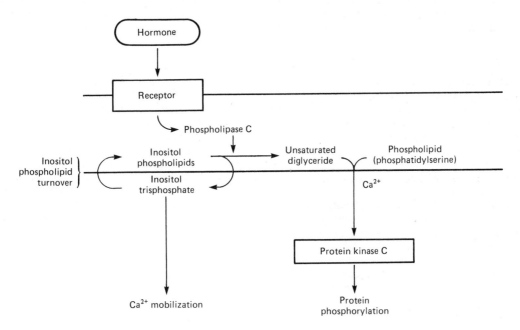

Figure 1–15. Mechanisms of enzyme activation by Ca^{2+} acting through binding to the Ca^{2+} receptor protein calmodulin. *A:* Ca^{2+} combines with calmodulin present as a subunit of phosphorylase kinase to activate the enzyme. *B:* Ca^{2+} combines with free calmodulin, and the Ca^{2+}-calmodulin complex then binds to and activates phosphodiesterase.

Figure 1–16. Schematic diagram of the mechanism by which a hormone or other signal acts via phospholipase C in the cell membrane to activate protein kinase C and increase inositol phospholipid turnover. One of the phosphorylated inositol derivatives, inositol trisphosphate, also acts to mobilize intracellular Ca^{2+}. (Modified and reproduced, with permission, from Nishizuka Y et al: Phospholipid turnover in hormone action. *Recent Prog Horm Res* 1984;**40**:301.)

in brain and other tissues. In the liver, where Ca^{2+} mediates the action of a number of hormones (ie, epinephrine, vasopressin, and angiotensin), a number of proteins (10–15) are phosphorylated following exposure of hepatocytes to these hormones. It seems likely, therefore, that many of the actions of Ca^{2+} will be found to be mediated by Ca^{2+}-activated kinases.

Related to the above Ca^{2+} system is the newly described phospholipid-activated, Ca^{2+}-dependent kinase system, the "C" kinase. An accelerated turnover of membrane phosphatidylinositol and its phosphorylated derivatives usually accompanies cell activation by calcium-dependent hormones. This activation (Fig 1–16), which is calcium-independent, involves the cleavage of phosphatidylinositides by phospholipase C to yield diglyceride and inositol phosphate. This diglyceride is rich in arachidonic acid and serves as a prostaglandin precursor; but in the presence of another membrane phospholipid (phosphatidylserine) and calcium, it activates a specific protein kinase, the C kinase. Moreover, one of the water-soluble inositol metabolites, inositol triphosphate, appears to act as an intracellular messenger to release stored intracellular Ca^{2+}. The C kinase may then work in concert with Ca^{2+}-calmodulin–regulated protein kinases to mediate hormone action.

Cyclic GMP

Ca^{2+} is also related to another cyclic nucleotide, cyclic guanosine monophosphate (cGMP). The formation of cGMP is catalyzed by guanylate cyclase, an enzyme present in both the plasma membrane and the cytoplasm. The cytoplasmic form is activated by Ca^{2+}. As a result, in almost all cases where there is a rise in cytoplasmic Ca^{2+}, there is a parallel rise in cGMP. While cGMP-activated protein kinases exist, there is at present no clear evidence for a role of cGMP in hormone action. It has been described as a second messenger in search of a hormone.

HORMONE ACTION

Membrane Permeability & Transport

Hormones regulate the cellular entry and exit of a large number of ions, metabolites, and biosynthetic precursors. Ions and small organic molecules frequently move across membranes by means of channels or carriers composed of specialized proteins whose purpose is to increase the rate of movement across the membrane. A molecule moving across a membrane down its electrochemical gradient is said to be undergoing **passive transport.** Passive transport may show kinetic characteristics of diffusion or, if mediated by a carrier, saturation kinetics analogous to enzyme activity. When cellular energy is used (usually by means of an ATPase enzyme) to move the transported molecule against its electrochemical gradient, it is undergoing **active transport.** Hormones affect all of these types of transport processes. These actions are important both in regulating the biosynthetic and metabolic activities of individual cells and in regulating the movement of ions and other molecules across cells such as in the intestine, kidney tubules, and bone.

Hormones regulate the movement of molecules across membranes by at least 4 different mechanisms: (1) alteration of the affinity of the transport mechanism for the molecule being transported; (2) activation of previously inactive transport mechanisms present in the plasma membrane; (3) insertion into the plasma membrane of preexisting transport mechanisms present inside the cell; and (4) synthesis of new transport proteins.

A. Glucose and Amino Acid Transport: The cellular uptake of glucose and amino acids is stimulated by hormones in a large number of target tissues. The earliest and best-studied example is the stimulation of glucose entry into fat and muscle cells by insulin. Glucose crosses the plasma membrane by means of a transport protein, the glucose carrier, that facilitates glucose entry into cells. Because the number of carriers is limited, this "facilitated diffusion" shows saturation kinetics that can be characterized by a K_m (the concentration at which transport is half-maximal) and a J_{max} (the maximal rate of transport). Insulin increases the J_{max} by bringing about the insertion of new carriers from the cell interior into the plasma membrane. This action of insulin is rapid (seconds to minutes) and does not require new protein synthesis. Other hormones also increase glucose uptake by their target cells; examples include TSH acting on thyroid cells and cholecystokinin acting on pancreatic acinar cells.

The cellular uptake of amino acids also involves a number of transport proteins that mediate amino acid entry by facilitated diffusion. In some cases, the entry of amino acids is driven by Na^+, which also binds to the carrier and, by moving down its electrochemical gradient, serves to concentrate the amino acid inside the cell. Acceleration of amino acid transport is brought about by a variety of hormones, including insulin, glucagon, growth hormone, and thyroid hormone. Thyroid hormone appears to act directly on the plasma membrane (Fig 1–21) independently of its effects on nuclear functions.

Other small molecules such as uridine and thymidine that are important as biosynthetic precursors enter cells by carrier-mediated facilitated diffusion. The transport of these molecules is stimulated by a number of polypeptide tropic hormones and by gonadal steroids acting on their respective target tissues.

B. Ion Transport: Cellular ionic balance is regulated to a great extent by the Na^+-K^+ ATPase that actively transports Na^+ out of and K^+ into cells. This active transport balances the passive entry of Na^+ and efflux of K^+ that occur by diffusion. Other ions either diffuse passively across the plasma membrane or their movements are coupled to Na^+ via carrier proteins. Two hormones that increase the activity of the Na^+-K^+ ATPase in a number of tissues are insulin and thyroid hormone. The effects of insulin are rapid and separate from its effects on glucose transport. The stimulation by thyroid hormone is slower, requiring the synthesis of new Na⁺-K⁺ ATPase molecules. The increased Na⁺ transport induced by thyroid hormone is the basis for part of the action of thyroid hormones to stimulate oxygen consumption and heat production (calorigenesis). Another specialized form of ion transport is the uptake of iodide by the thyroid, which is increased by TSH.

C. Epithelial Transport: Epithelia are specialized sheets or tubules of cells whose function is to separate 2 compartments and regulate the transport of water and other molecules. For example, in the distal tubule of the kidney (Fig 1–17), aldosterone acts to increase the reabsorption of Na^+. Na^+ enters the cell from the lumen of the tubule down its electrochemical gradient by means of a specialized transport protein and then is actively transported out of the cell into capillaries by means of Na^+-K^+ ATPase located in the basolateral membrane of the tubular cell. Aldosterone induces the synthesis of new Na^+ channel protein (see section on nuclear regulation) that facilitates the entry of Na^+ into the cell. It also induces the production of other proteins that increase mitochondrial ATP synthesis for the transport of Na^+ out of the cell.

In an analogous manner, vitamin D, a steroidlike substance, increases the transepithelial absorption of Ca^{2+} and PO_4^{3-} from the lumen of the small intestine. Growth hormone also increases Ca^{2+} and PO_4^{3-} absorption, while Ca^{2+} absorption is inhibited by adrenal glucocorticoids.

Other hormones regulating epithelial transport include parathyroid hormone in bone and kidney; gastrin, which increases the secretion of H^+-rich gastric juice by parietal cells of the stomach; and secretin, which increases the secretion of HCO_3^--rich pancreatic juice by the duct cells of the pancreas.

Enzyme Activation

Many effects of polypeptide and catecholamine hormones on intracellular enzymes involve alterations in the activity of preexisting enzymes rather than the synthesis of new enzymes. These effects are generally slower than those regulating membrane transport, occurring in minutes to hours, but are also independent of the synthesis of new protein. Insulin, for example, has well-established effects on the activity of various enzymes involved in the metabolism of glucose, amino acids, fatty acids, and nucleotides.

Major mechanisms by which hormones affect enzyme activity are phosphorylation and dephosphorylation. The first and best-studied example of phosphorylation is the regulation of glycogen metabolism in liver and muscle (Fig 1–18). The activity of both glycogen synthetase and phosphorylase is regulated by phosphorylation; in the case of phosphorylase, addition of phosphate activates the enzyme, whereas in

Figure 1–17. Mechanism by which aldosterone increases the resorption of Na⁺ by cells of the distal nephron. Aldosterone (A) enters the cell and binds to a cytoplasmic receptor (R). The aldosterone-receptor complexes then enter the nucleus and induce the synthesis of proteins, including the Na⁺ channel protein that mediates the entry of Na⁺ from the lumen into the cell and mitochondrial proteins necessary to synthesize more ATP used by the Na⁺-K⁺ ATPase to pump Na⁺ out of the cell and into the interstitial fluid.

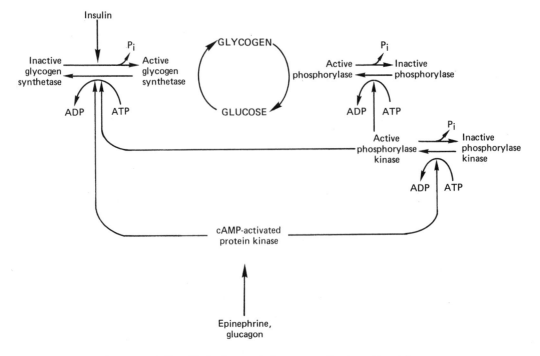

Figure 1-18. Simplified scheme of glycogen synthesis and breakdown.

the case of glycogen synthetase, it inhibits the enzyme. Thus, hormones such as epinephrine and glucagon, by increasing the activity of several kinases (including phosphorylase kinase), bring about the net conversion of glycogen to glucose. Insulin, possibly by activating a phosphatase, increases the activity of glycogen synthetase and accelerates the formation of glycogen.

Many other enzymes responsive to insulin have been shown to be regulated by phosphorylation and dephosphorylation independently of the cAMP activated protein kinases. A well-studied example is the regulation of pyruvate dehydrogenase, a mitochondrial enzyme complex that produces acetyl-CoA necessary for lipid synthesis. Exposure of adipose tissue to insulin rapidly increases pyruvate dehydrogenase activity as a result of dephosphorylation. Insulin also activates pyruvate kinase and hydroxymethylglutaryl-CoA reductase and inhibits hormone-sensitive lipase—all by dephosphorylation processes. It is not known in any of these cases whether insulin activates phosphatases or inhibits kinases.

Both of the second messengers (cAMP and Ca^{2+}) can act by phosphorylation mechanisms. An example where the 2 intracellular messengers act together is the regulation of phosphorylase kinase, the enzyme that phosphorylates phosphorylase. Phosphorylase kinase is a multisubunit enzyme and can be activated independently by cAMP-activated protein kinase, which phosphorylates its alpha and beta subunits, or by Ca^{2+}, which binds to the delta subunit, calmodulin. The 2 intracellular regulators potentiate each other in that cAMP-induced phosphorylation increases the

sensitivity of the enzyme to Ca^{2+}. Almost all hormones (including steroids) alter the state of phosphorylation of a small number of proteins in target cells. In most cases, however, the identity and functional role of the phosphorylated protein are unknown.

Besides phosphorylation, other enzymes can be directly activated by specialized binding proteins. Calmodulin, the protein that serves as the Ca^{2+} receptor for hormones utilizing Ca^{2+} as intracellular messenger, binds to and regulates a number of enzymes, including cyclic nucleotide phosphodiesterase, certain adenylate cyclases, and the Ca^{2+}-ATPase present in the cell membrane that acts to transport Ca^{2+} out of the cells.

Other ways in which enzyme activities can be regulated that may ultimately prove to be affected by hormones include aggregation of subunits, adenylation, methylation, and changes in the local concentration of ions or cofactors.

Nuclear Regulation

Certain actions of steroid, thyroid, and polypeptide hormones are brought about by increasing the number of a few specific types of mRNA. This effect on mRNA is caused by altering either the rate of synthesis and degradation of mRNA molecules or their processing from precursor RNAs and appearance in the cytoplasms. Hormone actions mediated by this mechanism are generally delayed in onset and blocked by inhibitors of RNA synthesis such as actinomycin D and cordycepin.

A. Steroid Hormones: The mechanism of nuclear regulation has been studied most extensively for steroid hormones. Furthermore, most of the known actions of steroids appear to follow this pathway. As previously mentioned, steroid hormones bind to receptors in the cytoplasm. Specific cytoplasmic receptor proteins have been found for all classes of steroids and bind biologically active steroids in relation to the steroid's potency. These steroid receptors are asymmetric proteins weighing 50,000–300,000 daltons.

Following the binding of steroid to its receptor (Fig 1–19), there is a reduction of the number of receptors in the cytosol and an increase in the nucleus (Fig 1–20). The steroid-receptor complex has the ability to bind to isolated nuclei, whereas neither the free steroid nor the receptor has this ability. Steroid hormone antagonists are structurally similar molecules that bind to the receptor in the cytoplasm but are unable to confer the ability to bind to the nucleus. The ability to enter the nucleus results from a change in the receptor (presumably allosteric in nature) termed "activation" that under physiologic conditions rapidly follows binding of agonist steroids. In cells responding to estrogens, activation appears to result in aggregation of 2 receptors to form a dimer.

Steroid-promoted nuclear binding is rapid and is usually maximal by 30 minutes. Nuclear binding sites termed "acceptors" are present in the chromatin fraction of nuclei. In studies of both isolated nuclei and chromatin, it has been impossible to saturate acceptor sites; it is generally concluded, therefore, that there are more nuclear acceptors than steroid receptors. Although steroid-receptor complexes bind to isolated DNA, there is no species or tissue specificity in this binding. It seems reasonable to conclude, therefore, that binding is also affected by chromatin proteins. In the case of the progesterone receptor, the receptor appears to be a dimer with one subunit that binds to DNA, while the other binds to a specific type of acidic protein present only in chromatin of target tissues. These observations suggest a model for steroid hormone action in which the protein-binding subunit localizes the receptor to a specific location in chromatin, while the DNA-binding subunit then acts as a nuclear regulator. Following removal of the steroid from the environment of the target cells, there is a relatively rapid dissociation of steroid from the receptor and a return of the unoccupied receptor to the cytosol.

It is generally believed that the actions of steroid hormones result from increased production of specific mRNA. In only a few cases, however, has this been convincingly demonstrated. A well-studied example is the increase in the protein ovalbumin that is induced in the chick oviduct by estrogen and progesterone. In parallel with the increase in ovalbumin, there is an increase in the number of ovalbumin mRNA molecules. These have been quantitated either by subsequent translation in a cell-free system or by binding

Figure 1–19. Proposed mechanism of steroid hormone action. The steroids enter target cells through diffusion or transport and in the cytoplasm bind to a receptor protein. The steroid-receptor complex is then able to bind to chromatin in the nucleus. New mRNA molecules are transcribed, leading to the synthesis of new protein.

Figure 1–20. Distribution of steroid receptors in the cell under conditions where it is exposed to no steroid, an agonist (dexamethasone), or an antagonist (progesterone). (Reproduced, with permission, from Baxter J: *Pharmacol Ther* [B] 1976;**2**:605.)

to complementary DNA. The latter approach indicates that there is an actual increase in the number of mRNA molecules. Similar studies of pituitary tumor cells have also shown that glucocorticoids induce an increase in the number of mRNA molecules coding for growth hormone.

Recently, progress has been made in research into the mechanism by which the nuclear steroid-receptor complex increases the transcription of specific genes. Studies on the ovalbumin gene have shown the importance of certain DNA sequences in its adjacent 5'-flanking region necessary for accurate and efficient expression. This "promoter region" preferentially binds the DNA-binding subunit of the steroid receptor. Moreover, when fused with a nonsteroid-regulated structural gene such as globin, the transcription of this protein becomes steroid-regulated. Thus, the linear sequence of the gene itself contains a regulatory sequence that determines which receptors bind and induce transcription of the structural sequence of the gene.

B. Thyroid Hormones: Thyroid hormones are now also known to regulate nuclear function (Fig 1–21). Thyroid hormones readily enter cells, but their uptake mechanism is unknown. They may either diffuse through the lipid bilayers of the cell membrane by virtue of their hydrophobicity or enter cells by means of a transport mechanism similar to that used by amino acids. After entry, thyroid hormones bind to cytoplasmic binding proteins that concentrate hormone intracellularly. In contrast to steroid hormone action, however, these cytoplasmic binding proteins do not translocate thyroid hormones. It is the free thyroid hormone in the cell that binds directly to receptors on or in the nucleus. Other receptors are present in mitochondria and may mediate certain effects of thyroid hormone on oxygen consumption.

Nuclear receptors for thyroid hormones are acidic proteins that can bind to DNA but are also influenced by the histone proteins present in chromatin. It is this interaction with histones that maintains the higher specificity for triiodothyronine (T_3) as compared to thyroxine (T_4) (see Chapter 7). The finding of thyroid hormone receptors associated with chromatin suggests that the hormone influences nuclear functions. It is possible that the binding of thyroid hormone to these receptor proteins may increase the content of cytoplasmic mRNA. Specific mRNAs known to be increased by thyroid hormones include those coding for growth hormone, liver $\alpha_{2\mu}$-globulin, and Na^+-K^+ ATPase. In general, these effects of thyroid hormones are slow, taking 1–2 days to reach a maximum.

C. Polypeptide Hormones: A number of polypeptide hormones—including growth hormone, prolactin, and insulin—also have prominent effects on nucleic acid and protein synthesis. Effects of insulin related to transcription have been reported in liver, adipose tissue, and mammary gland. Administration of insulin has been shown to increase both RNA polymerase activity and chromatin template activity in the liver in vivo. More recent studies have shown that in experimental diabetes, there is decreased production of mRNA for albumin in the liver and amylase in the pancreas. In both cases, the diminished level of mRNA can be restored by insulin administration, although the mechanism of this effect is unknown.

Other effects of polypeptide hormones on the ribosomal translation of preexisting mRNA are also known. In the muscle, fat, and liver of diabetic animals, there is decreased protein synthesis. Insulin increases the assembly of polysomes. Growth hormone administration in vivo also increases the rate of protein synthesis by subsequently isolated muscle ribosomes.

It is not presently known whether these effects of polypeptide hormones are primary or secondary ones. Polypeptide hormones stimulating protein and nucleic acid synthesis generally belong to the class of hormones with no known second messenger. Insulin and prolactin are known to be internalized, raising the possibility that they may act as their own intracellular messenger.

Figure 1–21. Proposed mechanism of thyroid hormone action. Thyroid hormone (in this case triiodothyronine, or T_3) binds to a receptor protein (R) on the cell surface and increases the uptake of glucose and amino acids. T_3 also enters the cell, where it reacts with cytoplasmic binding proteins (CBP) and receptors on chromatin and mitochondria. In the nucleus, the T_3-receptor complex leads to the synthesis of new protein.

SUMMARY & CONCLUSIONS

The action of hormones is initiated by interaction with receptors specific for the hormone. In the case of polypeptide and amine hormones, these receptors are localized on the plasma membranes. Occupancy of these membrane receptors directly regulates membrane functions. Effects on intracellular functions are mediated by intracellular messengers such as cAMP and Ca^{2+}. Steroid and thyroid hormones interact chiefly with intracellular receptors. Receptors for steroid hormones are present in the cytoplasm and, when oc-cupied, move to the nucleus to regulate nuclear function. Some receptors for thyroid hormone are present in the nucleus and regulate nuclear function; others present in mitochondria and plasma membrane regulate the responsiveness of these organelles. Many actions of steroid and thyroid hormones require the synthesis of new proteins and are relatively slow compared to those actions of polypeptide and amine hormones that do not require synthetic events. Lastly, we must be careful not to take rigid positions on the ways in which different classes of hormones act, since mechanisms of action are still being discovered.

REFERENCES

Baxter JD, Funder JW: Hormone receptors. *N Engl J Med* 1979; **301**:1149.

Czech MP: New perspectives on the mechanism of insulin action. *Recent Prog Horm Res* 1984;**40**:347.

DeLisle RC, Williams JA: Regulation of membrane fusion in secretory exocytosis. *Annu Rev Physiol* 1986;**48**:225.

Exton JH: Role of calcium and phosphoinositides in the action of certain hormones and neurotransmitters. *J Clin Invest* 1985;**75**:1753.

Gilman AG: Guanine nucleotide binding regulatory proteins and dual control of adenylate cyclase. *J Clin Invest* 1984;**73**:1.

Greengard P: Phosphorylated proteins as physiological effectors. *Science* 1978;**199**:146.

King AC, Cuatrecasas P: Peptide hormone–induced receptor mobility, aggregation, and internalization. *N Engl J Med* 1981;**305**:77.

Nishizuka Y: The role of protein kinase C in cell surface signal transduction and tumor promotion. *Nature* 1984;**308**:693.

O'Malley BW: Steroid hormone action in eukaryotic cells. *J Clin Invest* 1984;**74**:307.

Pastan I, Willingham MC: Receptor-mediated endocytosis: Coated pits, receptosomes and the Golgi. *Trends Biochem Sci* 1983;**8**:250.

Pollet RJ, Levey GS: Principles of membrane receptor physiology and their application to clinical medicine. *Ann Intern Med* 1980;**92**:663.

Rasmussen H, Barret PQ: Calcium messenger system: An integrated view. *Physiol Rev* 1984;**64**:938.

2 Prostaglandins & Cyclic Nucleotides

Marc E. Goldyne, MD, PhD

PROSTAGLANDINS AS LOCAL HORMONES

The prostaglandins—so named because of their initial isolation from human prostate—are now recognized as a widely distributed family of oxygenated, cyclized, 20-carbon (eicosanoic) fatty acids, all sharing structural similarities but often exhibiting individually distinct and sometimes frankly opposing biologic properties.

Synthesis, Site of Action, & Degradation

Prostaglandins are not stored within cells, as are classic hormones, but are synthesized from polyunsaturated fatty acid precursors within the cell membrane in response to various stimuli. Prostaglandins are produced by virtually every organ in the body, including those serving an endocrine function, although heterogeneity exists in the predominant types of prostaglandins or related lipids synthesized by various organs, tissues, or cells. Rapid degradation of prostaglandins within the systemic circulation suggests that their regulatory functions are performed within the same anatomic site at which they are produced rather than at anatomically distant sites, as is the case with classic hormones.

Autacoid Function

As local hormones, or **autacoids,** prostaglandins appear to perform different functions depending on the organ, tissue, or cell under consideration. Furthermore, classic hormones may in part accomplish some of their regulatory roles by inducing prostaglandin synthesis at target sites.

Eicosanoids

The realization that has emerged over the past 10 years that prostaglandins constitute just one family of a broader group of compounds derived from the same eicosanoic acids has given rise to the term **eicosanoids** to denote not only prostaglandins but also the thromboxanes and other biologically active metabolites described below.

Acronyms Used in This Chapter

ACTH	Adrenocorticotropic hormone
ATP	Adenosine triphosphate
cAMP	Cyclic adenosine monophosphate
cGMP	Cyclic guanosine monophosphate
FSH	Follicle-stimulating hormone
GH	Growth hormone
HETE	Hydroxyeicosatetraenoic acid
HHT	12L-Hydroxy-5,8,10-heptadecatrienoic acid
HPETE	Hydroperoxyeicosatetraenoic acid
LH	Luteinizing hormone
LT	Leukotriene (LTA, LTB, etc)
LX	Lipoxin (LXA, LXB, etc)
MDA	Malonyl dialdehyde
NDGA	Nordihydroguaiaretic acid
NSAID	Nonsteroidal anti-inflammatory drug
PG	Prostaglandin (PGE, PGF, etc)
SRS	Slow-reacting substance
TSH	Thyroid-stimulating hormone (thyrotropin)
TX	Thromboxane (TXA, TXB, etc)

NOMENCLATURE & BIOCHEMISTRY OF PROSTAGLANDINS & METABOLICALLY RELATED LIPIDS

Nomenclature of Eicosanoids

A. Prostaglandins: In the 1950s, the biologic activity originally attributed by the Swedish scientist von Euler to a single active principle—"prostaglandin"—was found by several of his colleagues to consist of at least 2 distinct though structurally related compounds. The activity that preferentially partitioned into ether was called prostaglandin (PGE) and that partitioning into *fosfat* (Swedish for phosphate) buffer was called PGF. Prostaglandins discovered subsequently were arbitrarily given letter names to combine the fortuitous alphabetic sequence started by the initial trivial nomenclature. To date, 9 prostaglandin groups are recognized (PGA–PGI), all sharing a 20-carbon molecular skeleton referred to as **prostanoic acid** (Fig 2–1A). These groups differ in the substitutions or location of a double bond within the pentane ring of prostanoic acid (Fig 2–1B). Two epimers of the F group exist and are designated with a subscript α or β (Fig 2–1B). PGG and PGH are

Figure 2–1. *A:* The molecular skeleton common to all prostaglandins is referred to as prostanoic acid. *B:* Prostaglandin groups are separated according to the substitutions made at carbon atoms 9 and 11 and, in the case of PGG, also at carbon 15. The 2 epimers of the F group are designated F_α and F_β according to the orientation of the hydroxyl group on carbon 9. *C:* Prostaglandins are given a numerical subscript series designation that not only identifies the total number of double bonds in the 2 aliphatic side chains of the molecule but also represents derivation from different fatty acid precursors (see text). (Reproduced, with permission, from Katzung BG [editor]: *Basic & Clinical Pharmacology,* 2nd ed. Lange, 1984.)

actually short-lived endoperoxide intermediates in the formation of all the remaining prostaglandins. Prostaglandin G (PGG) differs from all other prostaglandins in having a hydroperoxy rather than hydroxy group on carbon 15.

Each prostaglandin group can be further divided into one of 3 series (except for PGI) designated by a numerical subscript 1, 2, or 3 (Fig 2–1C). This series designation identifies the number of double bonds present in the prostanoic acid side chains (Fig 2–1C), which is a reflection of the degree of unsaturation of the fatty acid precursor of each series. (The 1- series derives from an eicosa*tri*enoic acid, the 2- series from

an eicosa*tetra*enoic acid [arachidonic acid], and the 3- series from an eicosa*penta*enoic acid.) Since the structure of PGI requires a $\Delta 5$ double bond (not present in eicosatrienoic acid), it exists only in the 2- and 3- series. PGI_2 is also referred to as **prostacyclin** or **epoprostenol.**

B. Other Eicosanoids: Other biologically active eicosanoids that derive from the same precursors as the prostaglandins but do not possess the prostanoic acid structure have been identified within the past 5 years. These include the thromboxanes, HETEs, and leukotrienes (Fig 2–2).

1. Thromboxanes–The thromboxanes were so

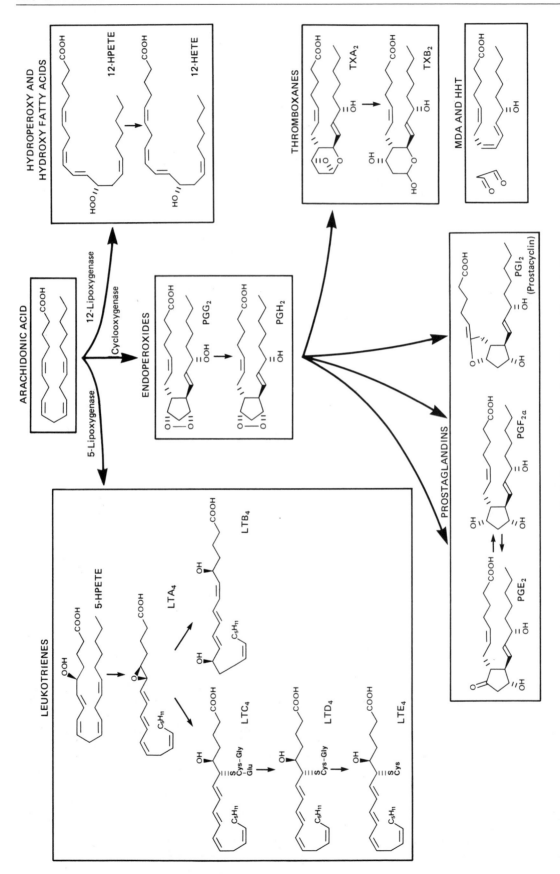

Figure 2–2. Major enzymatically derived products of arachidonic acid metabolism.

named because of their initial isolation from platelets (thrombocytes) and the presence of an oxane ring rather than a pentane ring. Thromboxane (TX) A_1, A_2, and A_3 are highly unstable and rapidly hydrate to TXB_1, B_2, or B_3. TXA_2 induces platelet aggregation as well as vasoconstriction. Other products that appear to derive from the TXA_2 biosynthetic pathway are malonyl dialdehyde (MDA) and 12L-hydroxy-5,8,10-heptadecatrienoic acid (HHT).

2. HETEs–The abbreviation HETE (for *h*ydroxy-*e*icosa*t*etra*e*noic acid) was initially assigned to a platelet-derived product of arachidonic acid having a hydroxy group on carbon 12. Subsequently, HETEs with the hydroxy group on other carbons (5, 8, 11, 15, etc) were recovered from leukocytes; thus, HETEs are individually identified by a numerical prefix designating the hydroxylation site (12-HETE, 5-HETE, etc). Some of these compounds are highly chemotactic for neutrophils and eosinophils.

3. Leukotrienes–The leukotrienes, so named because of their initial identification in leukocytes and the presence of a conjugated triene bonding (although the molecule is a tetraene), are also derivatives of the precursors for the prostaglandins (Fig 2–2). Among the leukotrienes are included the previously recognized but structurally undefined "slow-reacting substances" (SRS), some of which participate in anaphylactic responses (SRS-A). These specific leukotrienes differ from all of the other eicosanoids in being peptide-lipid conjugates. All leukotrienes derive from an unstable epoxide called LTA_4 that is generated through the action of 5-lipoxygenase on arachidonic acid. The subscript 4 signifies the total number of double bonds in the fatty acid chain. Conjugation of glutathione, a cysteine-containing tripeptide, to carbon 6 generates LTC_4. Enzymatically catalyzed loss of the glutamyl residue from LTC_4 generates LTD_4, and loss of the glycyl residue generates LTE_4. Readdition of glutamic acid to the cysteine on LTE_4 generates LTF_4. LTC_4, LTD_4, and, to a lesser extent, LTE_4 constitute the biologic activity formerly called SRS-A. LTB_4, which also derives from LTA_4, is not a peptide-lipid conjugate; it is a stereospecific 5,12-dihydroxyeicosatetraenoic acid that demonstrates a potent chemotactic effect on neutrophils.

4. Lipoxins–These recently identified eicosanoids were isolated following the incubation of human leukocytes with 15-HPETE. Lipoxin A (LXA) was found to be a 5,6,15L-trihydroxy-7,9,11,13-eicosatetraenoic acid. These compounds are structurally unique in having the 4 double bonds in a conjugated formation. Their possible biologic activities remain to be identified, although early studies suggest that they can affect the ability of natural killer cells to lyse tumor target cells.

5. Other novel compounds–In addition to the various derivatives of arachidonic acid described above, there are other products of both the cyclooxygenase and lipoxygenase pathways that have recently been discovered. One of these is an isomer of PGF. The other is a major metabolite generated from arachidonic acid by human monocytes; its synthesis is not blocked by nonsteroidal anti-inflammatory drugs (NSAIDs) but is susceptible to inhibition by nordihydroguaiaretic acid (NDGA), a known inhibitor of lipoxygenase enzymes. It therefore appears likely that further research will uncover other biologically active eicosanoids.

Biosynthesis of Eicosanoids

The biosynthesis of prostaglandins as well as of thromboxanes, HETEs, and leukotrienes occurs primarily at the cell membrane (Fig 2–3), although recent evidence suggests that some lipoxygenase enzymes may be cytosolic. In response to an appropriate stimulus for the cell in question, a phospholipase is activated that cleaves the fatty acid precursor (eg, arachidonic acid) from the phospholipids that comprise the lipid bilayer of the cell membrane. Once free, the precursor can activate several enzyme systems.

A. Pathways of Synthesis:

1. Cyclooxygenase pathway–One enzyme, cyclooxygenase, converts arachidonic acid, for example, into the unstable endoperoxide intermediate PGG_2, and this intermediate in turn is converted by a peroxidase to the unstable PGH_2. Depending on the cell type, the endoperoxide intermediate can be further metabolized into prostaglandins (including prostacyclin [PGI_2]) and thromboxanes.

2. Lipoxygenase pathway–Another group of enzymes, collectively referred to as lipoxygenases, can convert arachidonic acid into one of the HETE compounds and, in conjunction with yet other enzymes, into the leukotrienes. Various groups of cells synthesize different combinations of these eicosanoids; platelets synthesize chiefly thromboxanes and 12-HETE; vascular endothelium synthesizes chiefly PGI_2 and some 12-HETE; and epidermal cells synthesize chiefly PGD_2, PGE_2, $PGF_{2\alpha}$, and 12-HETE.

B. Inhibitors of Synthesis: Inhibition of prostaglandin synthesis can be accomplished with corticosteroids or nonsteroidal anti-inflammatory drugs such as aspirin, indomethacin, and ibuprofen. These 2 groups of drugs, however, inhibit biosynthesis of prostaglandins by different modes of action.

1. Corticosteroids–Corticosteroids block the initial release of the precursor fatty acid from the cellular phospholipids, so that none of the potential eicosanoids (prostaglandins, thromboxanes, HETEs, or leukotrienes) are synthesized. Corticosteroids appear to achieve this inhibition through preventing activation of the enzyme phospholipase A_2, which is responsible for liberating the esterified precursor; this effect is accomplished through a steroid-induced generation of an inhibitory protein called macrocortin or lipomodulin. However, at some sites, such as adipose tissue, free substrate can be derived not only from phospholipids but also from neutral lipid triglycerides, and this latter reaction appears to be enhanced rather than inhibited by corticosteroids. Therefore, the ability of corticosteroids to abolish prostaglandin synthesis may be tissue-specific.

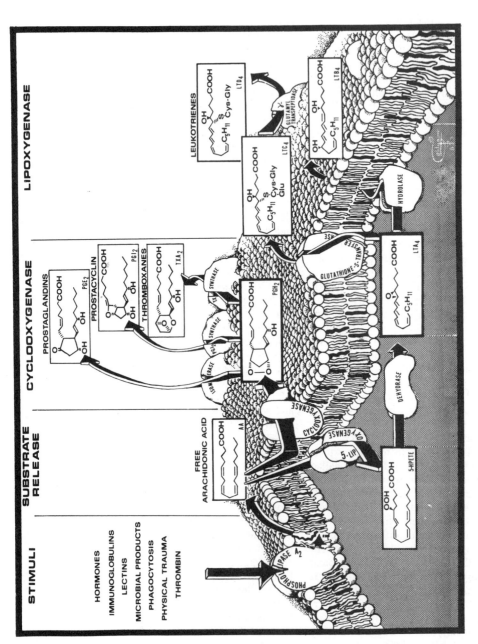

Figure 2–3. Biosynthesis of eicosanoids. The biosynthesis of prostaglandins and related lipids occurs for the most part at the cell membrane. However, the 5-lipoxygenase that catalyzes the generation of leukotrienes and 5-HETE appears to be a cytosolic enzyme. In response to an appropriate stimulus, a phospholipase is activated that cleaves arachidonic acid (a precursor of prostaglandins) from the phospholipids making up the lipid bilayer of the cell membranes. The stimuli that activate the phospholipases are often tissue- or cell-specific. The free arachidonic acid can activate several enzyme systems, depending on the enzymatic endowment of the cell(s) in question. One enzyme, cy-clooxygenase, converts arachidonic acid into an unstable endoperoxide intermediate that can be further converted, through appropriate enzymatic activity, to prostaglandins (including prostacyclin or epoprostenol) and thromboxanes. Another group of enzymes, the lipoxygenases, convert arachidonic acid to a series of hydroxy fatty acids (ie, HPETEs and HETEs) or, in conjunction with other enzymes, to the recently identified leukotrienes. (Reproduced, with permission, from Katzung BG [editor]: *Basic & Clinical Pharmacology,* 2nd ed. Lange, 1984.)

2. Nonsteroidal anti-inflammatory drugs (NSAIDs)–Aspirin, indomethacin, and some of the other nonsteroidal anti-inflammatory drugs do not block precursor release but rather inhibit the cyclooxygenase enzyme essential to prostaglandin and thromboxane synthesis. The lipoxygenase enzymes, on the other hand, are not inhibited by these drugs at low concentrations (10^{-8} to 10^{-6} mol/L), with the possible exception of benoxaprofen, which appears to block 5-lipoxygenase. Consequently, the synthesis of the biologically active HETEs and leukotrienes may be enhanced as a result of a drug-related increase in precursor availability.

RELATIONSHIPS BETWEEN EICOSANOIDS & CYCLIC NUCLEOTIDES

An intimate association exists between the effects—or absence of effects—of certain prostaglandins on various cellular responses and their ability to elevate intracellular levels of the cyclic nucleotides: cyclic adenosine $3',5'$-monophosphate (cAMP) and cyclic guanosine $3',5'$-monophosphate (cGMP). These cyclic nucleotides may act as intracellular "second messengers," translating the extracellular signal from the "first messenger" (prostaglandin or other appropriate stimulus) into a characteristic cellular response through their ability to activate a variety of protein kinases.

Adenylate Cyclase, Guanylate Cyclase, & Prostaglandin Receptors

Adenylate cyclase, the enzyme responsible for catalyzing the conversion of ATP to cAMP, has been shown in many tissues and cells to be linked to a specific prostaglandin receptor presumably on the cell surface. Among the prostaglandins, PGE_2 appears to be the most consistent stimulator of adenylate cyclase activity. However, there are exceptions. In adipocytes and gastric parietal cells, for example, PGE_2 inhibits cAMP generation. Another prostaglandin, $PFG_{2\alpha}$, which in general fails to activate adenylate cyclase, is able to activate guanylate cyclase in appropriate target cells.

Functional Antagonism Among Prostaglandins & Cyclic Nucleotides

Some of the observed antagonism between E and F prostaglandins may be explained on the basis of their mutually exclusive stimulation of these different cyclic nucleotides within the same cell or tissue. Thus, whereas PGE_2 and cAMP relax venular and bronchial smooth muscle and inhibit neutrophil chemotaxis, both $PGF_{2\alpha}$ and cGMP constrict vascular and respiratory smooth muscle and enhance chemotaxis. The control of cellular function via the opposing effects of cAMP and cGMP may explain certain aspects of prostaglandin as well as cyclic nucleotide interaction. However, available data disclose a more complex relationship between prostaglandins, cyclic nucleotides,

and the biologic responses elicited through their interaction. For example, both histamine and PGE_2 were found to elevate cAMP in isolated gastric mucosal preparations even though these 2 agents had antagonistic effects on gastric acid secretion. Further investigation reconciled these paradoxic observations by demonstrating that PGE_2 was affecting the cAMP in a population of mucosal cells different from that affected by histamine. Furthermore, the response to PGE_2 was probably occurring in only certain populations of gastric cells, since subsequent data from other laboratories have shown that in the specific case of isolated gastric parietal cells, PGE_2 inhibits adenylate cyclase activity. Additional studies have shown that while PGE_2 induced similar elevations of cAMP in 2 subpopulations of thymus-derived lymphocytes (T cells), it enhanced the proliferative response to mitogen in one subpopulation but suppressed it in the other; a cAMP analog, 8-bromo-cAMP, also induced diametrically opposed effects on the proliferative response of these subpopulations. These studies reveal that the function of a given prostaglandin or cyclic nucleotide can be specifically defined only in the context of a given cell type and that even within this context, its function may change according to the state of differentiation or activation of the responding cell. Such a qualified definition is an essential aspect of understanding the various physiologic or pathophysiologic roles of prostaglandins and related lipids as well as of the cyclic nucleotides they affect.

Effects of Cyclic Nucleotides on Prostaglandin Synthesis

In addition to the effect of prostaglandins on intracellular cyclic nucleotide levels, the cyclic nucleotides in their turn appear to be capable of affecting the biosynthesis of prostaglandins in the same cell. Stimulation of prostaglandin biosynthesis by cAMP has been demonstrated in thyroid cells, adrenocortical cells, adipocytes, graafian follicles, and a variety of cultured mammalian cells. The ability of E prostaglandins, for example, to activate adenylate cyclase and of cAMP to stimulate PGE synthesis suggests that a positive feedback may exist in some cells, and such a relationship naturally raises the question of how this positive feedback is controlled. Studies have demonstrated that a variety of cells exhibit a time-dependent agonist-specific desensitization of adenylate cyclase to stimulation by PGEs. Such desensitization would ensure that the mutual enhancement of prostaglandin and cyclic nucleotide synthesis would be limited. Furthermore, in some cells, cAMP does not enhance but rather inhibits prostaglandin synthesis. The heterogeneity among various cells in regard to this aspect of prostaglandin–cyclic nucleotide interaction further emphasizes the necessity of defining the functions of prostaglandins or cyclic nucleotides in the context of a specific cell or tissue type.

Other Eicosanoids & Cyclic Nucleotides

In addition, the other eicosanoids such as TXA_2,

the HETEs, and the leukotrienes also appear capable of affecting cyclic nucleotide levels. However, the data currently available do not permit more comprehensive evaluation at this time.

PROSTAGLANDINS, CYCLIC NUCLEOTIDES, & HORMONE FUNCTION

Hormonal Stimulation of Prostaglandin Synthesis

Since prostaglandins appear to function close to their site of synthesis, it is conceivable that they may in part regulate the response of such a site to a given hormonal stimulus. Studies have substantiated the ability of various hormones to stimulate prostaglandin or other eicosanoid synthesis in the appropriate target tissue. ACTH, for example, can stimulate prostaglandin synthesis in rat adrenocortical cells, whereas insulin, vasopressin, and luteinizing hormone (LH) do not. LH, on the other hand, stimulates prostaglandin synthesis in mature ovarian follicles. The ability of a hormone to stimulate prostaglandin biosynthesis may be direct, as with TSH, through a hormone-induced activation of phospholipase A_2 that releases the prostaglandin precursors. In the case of LH, prostaglandin synthesis appears to be indirectly stimulated by a hormone-induced rise in intracellular cAMP. However, there are data that suggest species specificity in the effects of a given hormone on the release of prostaglandins by a given tissue. For example, in human fetal adrenal tissue, ACTH inhibits prostaglandin generation, whereas the opposite effect is observed in rat adrenal tissue.

Additional examples of hormonal stimulation of prostaglandin synthesis are found in rat aortic smooth muscle cells in response to estradiol and in carbachol-stimulated rat gastric mucosa following exposure to somatostatin.

Hormonal Action of Prostaglandins

Whether or not hormone-induced synthesis of prostaglandins is essential to the expression of a given hormonal effect is not completely known. In vitro, PGE_2 can mimic the action of ACTH on adrenal cortex and stimulate aldosterone and corticosterone biosynthesis. There also is evidence that the ability of somatostatin to inhibit gastric acid secretion is mediated by PGE_2, since indomethacin blocks this inhibitory effect of the hormone. However, the current literature contains conflicting reports about the intermediary role of prostaglandins in hormone action, and further research is required to define the role of prostaglandins and other eicosanoids in the expression of hormonal function.

Prostaglandins & the Release of Hormones

Other data have accumulated implicating a role for certain prostaglandins in the regulation of hormone secretion. PGE_2 appears capable, for example, of causing the release of TSH, ACTH, GH, LH, and FSH from pituitary tissue. The effect of PGE_2 on GH release appears associated with a rise in tissue levels of cAMP. Conversely, somatostatin antagonizes the stimulatory effect of PGE_2 or of cAMP on GH synthesis; this antagonism appears to result from a somatostatin-induced rise in cGMP. While such studies suggest that prostaglandins and related eicosanoids may participate in the release of various hormones, this function is far from universally established. Other hormones whose release can be triggered by PGE_2 include aldosterone, renin, glucagon, and erythropoietin. In addition to the prostaglandins, other eicosanoids have been implicated in the release of specific hormones. For example, 5-HETE—but not PGE_2, $PGF_{2\alpha}$, or 12-HETE—can modulate insulin secretion from rat pancreas.

PROSTAGLANDINS & ENDOCRINOPATHIES

Since virtually all organs can synthesize some combination of prostaglandins or related eicosanoids, alterations in such synthesis could constitute a significant source of pathophysiology in a broad variety

Table 2–1. Disorders associated with alterations in prostaglandin or thromboxane synthesis.

Disorder	Alteration in Eicosanoid Synthesis	Effects Associated With Alteration
Bartter's syndrome	↑ PGE_2 in kidney ↑ PGI_2 in circulation	↑ Renin ↑ Aldosterone Antagonism of angiotensin II pressor response Hypokalemia
Primary dysmenorrhea	↑ $PGF_{2\alpha}$ in endometrium	↑ Myometrial contraction, cramping Headache Diarrhea
Diabetes mellitus	↑ TXA_2 ↓ PGI_2	↑ Coagulability of platelets Microvascular damage
Hypercalcemia of cancer	↑ PGE metabolite in urine (PGE-M)	PGE-mediated hypercalcemia (response to aspirin and indomethacin)

of diseases. In regard to endocrinopathies, prostaglandins, thromboxanes, HETEs, and leukotrienes may take on special significance in view of evidence supporting their potential roles as local regulators of hormone function (Table 2–1). In fact, a series of endocrinopathies have been investigated to determine whether their manifestations might be in part referable to alterations in the biosynthesis of prostaglandins or other eicosanoids. These include Bartter's syndrome, diabetes mellitus, primary dysmenorrhea, and the hypercalcemia accompanying some forms of cancer.

1. BARTTER'S SYNDROME

Bartter's syndrome is a rare disease characterized by hyperplasia of renal juxtaglomerular cells as well as renomedullary cells, the latter being a known source of E prostaglandins. Patients characteristically have increased urinary excretion of PGE_2, sometimes $PGF_{2\alpha}$, and—most recently demonstrated—6-keto $PGF_{1\alpha}$ (the principal metabolite of PGI_2). The important pathophysiologic markers of Bartter's syndrome, in addition to excess prostaglandin excretion, include hypokalemia, hyperreninemia, hyperaldosteronism, increased plasma bradykinin activity, and urinary kallikrein activity.

Clinical Findings

The presence of hypokalemia leads to diverse clinical presentations. These include generalized weakness, muscular cramping, spasms, and paralysis. Polyuria and salt craving may also occur. In children with this syndrome, growth retardation has been reported. Unlike individuals with primary hyperaldosteronism who are hypertensive, those having Bartter's syndrome are normotensive. Resistance is found to the angiotensin II–mediated pressor response. While the cause of the increased renal prostaglandin synthesis is presently unclear, it appears that excessive production of PGE_2 can account for virtually all of the physiologic aberrations that characterize this disease. As mentioned in the previous section, both PGE_2 and PGI_2 can directly stimulate renin and aldosterone release, renal sodium loss, and, indirectly, renal potassium loss. Furthermore, the vasodilator effect of excess PGE_2 or plasma bradykinin might antagonize the pressor effect of angiotensin II. The exact mechanism of increased plasma bradykinin activity is unclear. However, in dogs, it has been demonstrated that PGE_1 can increase urinary kallikrein excretion.

Treatment

Further evidence supporting excess PGE_2 or PGI_2 production as central to this disease comes from studies showing that this production can be blocked. Three structurally unrelated drugs (indomethacin, aspirin, and ibuprofen) known to block prostaglandin synthesis tend to reverse or completely normalize the alterations in renin, aldosterone, plasma bradykinin activity, and renal kallikrein excretion as well as promote a normal pressor response to angiotensin II. Hypokalemia is the one finding not completely corrected by inhibition of prostaglandin synthesis, although potassium levels do increase. Some studies suggest that hypokalemia can lead to increased prostaglandin synthesis and that it may be the most proximal abnormality in the pathogenesis of Bartter's syndrome.

2. DIABETES MELLITUS

An imbalance in the metabolism of arachidonic acid to TXA_2 and PGI_2 has been identified in diabetic rats and diabetic humans. TXA_2 and PGI_2 are mutually antagonistic metabolites of arachidonic acid. The former compound stimulates platelet aggregation and vasoconstriction; the latter elicits vasodilatation and prevents platelet aggregation or induces disaggregation. In diabetes, it appears that the synthesis of TXA_2 by platelets is increased, while the synthesis of PGI_2 by vascular endothelium is depressed. This latter observation may be explained by the recent demonstration in diabetics of increased release of a platelet protein, β-thromboglobulin, that can inhibit PGI_2 synthesis by vascular endothelium. Such alterations would be expected to lead to hypercoagulability of platelets and a tendency for increased vascular tone. It is conceivable that such changes would contribute to the microvascular complications associated with diabetes. The plausibility of this contribution is strengthened by the observation that insulin, which may ameliorate the severity and progression of vascular lesions, has been found to restore PGI_2 levels.

3. DYSMENORRHEA

Primary dysmenorrhea is a common gynecologic disorder. Since menstruation is under endocrine control, dysmenorrhea may be considered a form of endocrinopathy, although its origin is at present speculative. Nevertheless, current evidence strongly suggests that excessive $PGF_{2\alpha}$ production by the uterine endometrium is central to the pathogenesis of this disorder. Normally, under the influence of progesterone, the endometrial level of $PGF_{2\alpha}$ increases, reaching a maximum at the onset of menstruation. It has been hypothesized that the vasoconstrictive as well as smooth muscle–contracting properties of $PGF_{2\alpha}$ could be instrumental in inducing the endometrial slough characteristic of menstruation. In primary dysmenorrhea, significantly high levels of $PGF_{2\alpha}$ have been recovered from the menstrual fluid.

Clinical Findings

Many of the symptoms of dysmenorrhea can be induced in normal women by the intravenous administration of $PGF_{2\alpha}$; these include abdominal cramping, nausea, vomiting, headache, and diarrhea.

Treatment

Most significant in implicating $PGF_{2\alpha}$ in the pathogenesis of dysmenorrhea is the finding that several nonsteroidal anti-inflammatory drugs, such as indomethacin, ibuprofen, and mefenamic acid, which effectively block the synthesis of $PGF_{2\alpha}$ in the endometrium, are extremely effective in alleviating the symptoms of dysmenorrhea. Aspirin provides little benefit, because it is a markedly weaker inhibitor of endometrial cyclooxygenase than the other drugs, which can be used as specific therapy for this disorder.

4. HYPERCALCEMIA OF CANCER

Prostaglandins of the E group have been reported to be as potent as parathyroid hormone in effecting bone resorption in organ cultures. As with parathyroid hormone, the PGE_2-mediated resorption of bone is associated with elevation of bone cAMP. The concept that PGE_2 may be involved in the pathogenesis of certain hypercalcemic states is supported by a series of recent studies describing a population of patients with solid tumors, including renal cell carcinomas and squamous cell or undifferentiated carcinomas of lung, pancreas, or uterine cervix.

Clinical Findings

Common findings in all of these patients were (1) increased urinary excretion of a metabolite of PGE (referred to as PGE-M), (2) normal levels of parathyroid hormone, and (3) hypercalcemia.

Treatment

When these patients were treated with either indomethacin or aspirin, their serum calcium and urinary calcium excretion levels returned to normal if bone metastases were absent. In the presence of bone metastases, the elevated serum calcium was only partially reduced. Patients who had hypercalcemia in the absence of an elevated excretion of PGE-M received no benefit from therapy with these inhibitors of prostaglandin synthesis. This combination of findings suggests that a population of hypercalcemic cancer patients can be defined on the basis of an elevated excretion of PGE-M and will benefit from therapy with prostaglandin synthesis–inhibiting drugs.

5. EXCESSIVE PROSTAGLANDIN PRODUCTION BY TUMORS

The intravenous infusion of $PGF_{2\alpha}$ or PGI_2 can produce a variety of side effects when the circulating levels surpass the catabolic capacity of the pulmonary, hepatic, or renal sites of prostaglandin inactivation.

Clinical Findings

These symptoms include, in addition to the hypercalcemia reviewed above, flushing, hypotension, diarrhea, headache, nausea, and vomiting. A variety of tumors such as medullary carcinomas of the thyroid, carcinoid tumors, and non–B islet cell tumors of the pancreas (Verner-Morrison syndrome) can be associated with similar symptoms. Furthermore, some patients with these tumors have been found to have elevated levels of PGE_2 in the blood as well as in tumor tissue. This has created speculation that—for example—the diarrhea accompanying medullary carcinomas of the thyroid and pancreatic non–B islet cell tumors or the flushing associated with carcinoid syndrome may be due to excessive circulating PGE_2. However, since these tumors are able to secrete a variety of peptide or lipid substances having similar physiologic effects (kinins, vasoactive intestinal polypeptide, serotonin, etc), the role of prostaglandins in the pathogenesis of these symptoms is not clear. It has recently been reported that a group of patients suffering from systemic mastocytosis had increased circulating levels of PGD_2 during the characteristic and sometimes life-threatening hypotensive episodes associated with this disease. Since PGD_2 can be produced by mast cells and can induce hypotension when systemically administered, these patients were treated with indomethacin, and subsequently, while they were still receiving the medication, there was a cessation of hypotensive crises. Thus, the ability of prostaglandins to function in the manner of classic hormones, if there is an excessive secretion of these eicosanoids into the systemic circulation, appears definitely possible. However, this type of situation is obviously pathologic.

Treatment

The use of drugs such as indomethacin, aspirin, ibuprofen, and mefenamic acid may find new applications as various endocrine and other diseases are reevaluated to determine the possible contribution of prostaglandins to their pathogenesis.

PROSTAGLANDINS & NONSTEROIDAL ANTI-INFLAMMATORY DRUGS

The abilities of specific nonsteroidal anti-inflammatory drugs (NSAIDs), such as indomethacin, to alleviate dysmenorrhea in women and to induce ductal closure in neonates are directly related to their capacity to inhibit the generation of prostaglandins. However, whether all therapeutic benefits of NSAIDs derive solely from this shared pharmacologic property remains to be established. In fact, recent data indicate that indomethacin can inhibit the activation of human neutrophils in a manner unassociated with the inhibition of prostaglandin synthesis. These findings suggest that inhibition of prostaglandin synthesis by NSAIDs may not be the sole explanation for their antiphlogistic effects.

In some clinical situations, the concomitant inhibition by NSAIDs of prostaglandin generation in anatomic sites that are not the focus of therapy can account for some of the untoward effects associated with the use of NSAIDs. For example, attention has recently been given to renal syndromes associated with the use of NSAIDs for inflammatory conditions in patients who happen to have underlying renal disease. Although suppression of renal prostaglandin generation in individuals with normal renal function has no deleterious effect on the kidneys, similar suppression in patients who follow low-salt diets, take diuretics, or have impaired renal function may lead to acute renal failure. This problem seems to result from inhibition of synthesis of specific renal prostaglandins, especially prostacyclin (PGI_2, epoprostenol), which maintains normal renal blood flow and glomerular filtration. Under such circumstances, some investigators have found that sulindac (Clinoril) may be used because this NSAID appears to primarily affect extrarenal rather than renal prostaglandin generation.

REFERENCES

Prostaglandin Biochemistry

Borgeat P, Samuelsson B: Arachidonic acid metabolism in polymorphonuclear leukocytes: Unstable intermediate in formation of dihydroxy acids. *Proc Natl Acad Sci USA* 1979;**76**:3213.

Goldyne ME et al: A novel eicosanoid is the major arachidonic acid metabolite of cultured human monocytes. *Prostaglandins* 1985;**30**:77.

Liston TE, Roberts LJ II: Transformation of prostaglandin D_2 to $9\alpha,11\beta$-(15S)-trihydroxyprosta-(5Z,13E)-dien-1-oic acid ($9\alpha,11\beta$-prostaglandin F_2): A unique biologically active prostaglandin produced enzymatically in vivo in humans. *Proc Natl Acad Sci USA* 1985;**82**:6030.

Morris HR et al: Structure of slow-reacting substance of anaphylaxis from guinea pig lung. *Nature* 1980;**186**:104.

Murphy R et al: Leukotriene C: A slow reacting substance from murine mastocytoma cells. *Proc Natl Acad Sci USA* 1979;**76**:4725.

Samuelsson B: Leukotrienes: Mediators of immediate hypersensitivity reactions and inflammation. *Science* 1983;**220**:568.

Samuelsson B et al: Prostaglandins and thromboxanes. *Annu Rev Biochem* 1978;**47**:997.

Serhan CN et al: Lipoxins: Novel series of compounds formed from arachidonic acid in human leukocytes. *Proc Natl Acad Sci USA* 1984;**81**:5335.

Eicosanoids & Cyclic Nucleotides

Kuehl FA, Cirillo VJ, Oien HG: Prostaglandin–cyclic nucleotide interactions in mammalian tissues. Chap 5, pp 191–225, in: *Prostaglandins: Chemical and Biochemical Aspects.* Karim SMM (editor). University Park Press, 1976.

Stobo JD, Kennedy MS, Goldyne ME: Prostaglandin E modulation of the mitogenic response of human T cells: Differential response of T-cell subpopulations. *J Clin Invest* 1979;**64**:1188.

Prostaglandins, Cyclic Nucleotides, & Hormone Function

Ligumsky M et al: Prostaglandins mediate inhibition of gastric acid secretion by somatostatin in the rat. *Science* 1983;**219**:301.

Zor U, Lamprecht SA: Mechanism of prostaglandin action in endocrine glands. Chap 2, pp 85–133, in: *Biochemical Actions of Hormones.* Vol 4. Litwach G (editor). Academic Press, 1977.

Bartter's Syndrome

Gill JR et al: Bartter's syndrome: A disorder characterized by urinary prostaglandins and a dependence of hyperreninemia on prostaglandin synthesis. *Am J Med* 1976;**61**:43.

Gullner HG et al: Correction of increased prostacyclin synthesis in Bartter's syndrome by indomethacin treatment. *Prostaglandins Med* 1980;**4**:65.

Gullner HG et al: Hypokalemia stimulates prostacyclin synthesis in the rat. *Clin Sci* 1983;**65**:43.

Nasjletti A, Malik KU: Relationships between the kallikrein-kinin and prostaglandin systems. *Life Sci* 1979;**25**:99.

Norby L et al: Prostaglandins and aspirin therapy in Bartter's syndrome. *Lancet* 1976;**2**:604.

Patrono C et al: Evidence for a direct stimulatory effect of prostacyclin on renin release in man. *J Clin Invest* 1982;**69**:231.

Vinci JM et al: The kallikrein-kinin system in Bartter's syndrome and its response to prostaglandin synthetase inhibition. *J Clin Invest* 1978;**61**:1671.

Diabetes Mellitus

Johnson M, Reece AH, Harrison HE: An imbalance in arachidonic acid metabolism in diabetes. Pages 1283–1286 in: *Advances in Prostaglandin and Thromboxane Research.* Vol 6. Samuelsson B, Ramwell P, Paoletti R (editors). Raven Press, 1980.

Laychock SG: Effects of hydroxyeicosatetraenoic acids on fatty acid esterification in phospholipids and insulin secretion in pancreatic islets. *Endocrinology* 1985;**117**: 1011.

Robertson RP, Chen M: A role for prostaglandin E defective insulin secretion and carbohydrate intolerance in diabetes mellitus. *J Clin Invest* 1977;**60**:747.

Yamamoto S et al: Modulation of insulin secretion by lipoxygenase products of arachidonic acid. *J Biol Chem* 1983;**258**:12149.

Dysmenorrhea

Budoff PW: Mefenamic acid therapy in dysmenorrhea. Pages 1449–1453 in: *Advances in Prostaglandin and Thromboxane Research.* Vol 8. Samuelsson B, Ramwell P, Paoletti R (editors). Raven Press, 1980.

Chan WY, Dawood MY: Prostaglandin levels in menstrual fluid of nondysmenorrheic and of dysmenorrheic subjects with and without oral contraceptive or ibuprofen therapy. Pages 1443–1447 in: *Advances in Prostaglandin and Thromboxane Research.* Vol 8. Samuelsson B, Ramwell P, Paoletti R (editors). Raven Press, 1980.

Lundström V, Bygdeman M: Prostaglandin $F_{2\alpha}$ and E_2 in primary dysmenorrhea. Pages 1455–1458 in: *Advances in Prostaglandin and Thromboxane Research.* Vol 8. Samuelsson B, Ramwell P, Paoletti R (editors). Raven Press, 1980.

**Prostaglandins & Nonsteroidal
Anti-inflammatory Drugs**

Abramson S et al: Modes of action of aspirin-like drugs. *Proc Natl Acad Sci USA* 1985;**82:**7227.

Ciabattoni G et al: Effects of sulindac and ibuprofen in patients with chronic glomerular disease. *N Engl J Med* 1984; **310:**279.

Clive DM, Stoff JS: Renal syndromes associated with nonsteroidal anti-inflammatory drugs. *N Engl J Med* 1984; **310:**563.

Hypercalcemia of Cancer

Seyberth MW, Raisz LG, Oates JA: Prostaglandins and hypercalcemic states. *Annu Rev Med* 1978;**29:**23.

Excessive Prostaglandin Production by Tumors

Karmali RA: Review: Prostaglandins and cancer. *Prostaglandins Med* 1980;**5:**11.

Neuroendocrinology 3

William F. Ganong, MD

Research in the science of neuroendocrinology has demonstrated that the brain regulates the secretion of the endocrine glands and that hormones in turn act on the central nervous system to modify brain function. The brain-endocrine interactions are multiple, complex, and important, both in terms of normal physiology and in terms of the pathophysiology of disease. This chapter is a general review of neuroendocrine control mechanisms. Details of the neural regulation of individual hormones are presented in the chapters on those hormones.

Nerve cells and gland cells resemble each other in many ways. Both secrete chemical messengers that produce responses in target cells. Both have electrical activity, and this activity increases when the cells release their chemical messengers. Like gland cells, nerve cells secrete hormones that enter the circulation.

Acronyms Used in This Chapter

ACTH	Adrenocorticotropic hormone
cAMP	Cyclic adenosine monophosphate
CCK	Cholecystokinin
CRH	Corticotropin-releasing hormone
DNA	Deoxyribonucleic acid
FSH	Follicle-stimulating hormone
GH	Growth hormone
GnRH	Gonadotropin-releasing hormone
GRH	Growth hormone–releasing hormone
LH	Luteinizing hormone
LPH	Lipotropin
mRNA	Messenger ribonucleic acid
PIH	Prolactin-inhibiting hormone
PRH	Prolactin-releasing hormone
RNA	Ribonucleic acid
SIF	Small intensely fluorescent (cells)
TRH	Thyrotropin-releasing hormone
TSH	Thyroid-stimulating hormone (thyrotropin)
VIP	Vasoactive intestinal polypeptide

Table 3–1. Neuroendocrine messengers: Substances that function as neurotransmitters, neural hormones, and classic hormones.

	Neurotransmitter (Present in Nerve Endings)	Hormone Secreted by Neurons	Hormone Secreted by Endocrine Cells
Dopamine	+	+	+
Norepinephrine	+	+	+
Epinephrine	+		+
Somatostatin	+	+	+
Gonadotropin-releasing hormone (GnRH)	+	+	
Thyrotropin-releasing hormone (TRH)	+	+	
Oxytocin	+	+	
Vasopressin	+	+	
Vasoactive intestinal polypeptide (VIP)	+	+	
Cholecystokinin (CCK)	+		+
Glucagon	+		+
Enkephalins	+		+
Pro-opiomelanocortin derivatives	+		+
Other anterior pituitary hormones	+		+

In addition, nerve cells and gland cells often secrete the same substance, and the same peptide or amine can be secreted by neurons as a neurotransmitter, by neurons as a neural hormone, and by gland cells as a classic hormone. A partial list of substances known to perform these multiple functions is shown in Table 3–1.

Chemical messengers not only mediate cell-to-cell communication via synaptic junctions (neural communication) and via messengers in the circulating body fluids (endocrine communication), but some messengers may diffuse in the interstitial fluid to target cells without entering the bloodstream. This form of communication is called paracrine communication (Fig 3–1). It has been postulated to occur in the case of somatostatin in the pancreatic islets; in the case of catecholamines and serotonin, in the brain; and in the case of GnRH, in sympathetic ganglia. It may be an even more widespread phenomenon, but its existence is difficult to prove. A fourth form of communication involves transfer of substances between adjacent cells via gap junctions without extracellular release of chemical messengers.

	GAP JUNCTIONS	SYNAPTIC	PARACRINE	ENDOCRINE
	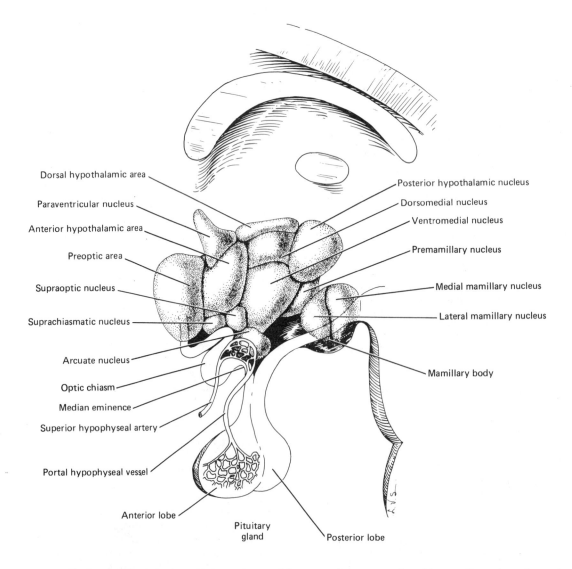			
Message transmission	Directly from cell to cell	Across synaptic cleft	By diffusion in interstitial fluid	By circulating body fluids
Local or general	Local	Local	Locally diffuse	General
Specificity depends on	Anatomic location	Anatomic location and receptors	Receptors	Receptors

Figure 3–1. Intercellular communication by chemical mediators.

Dorsal hypothalamic area
Paraventricular nucleus
Anterior hypothalamic area
Preoptic area
Supraoptic nucleus
Suprachiasmatic nucleus
Arcuate nucleus
Optic chiasm
Median eminence
Superior hypophyseal artery
Portal hypophyseal vessel
Anterior lobe
Pituitary gland

Posterior hypothalamic nucleus
Dorsomedial nucleus
Ventromedial nucleus
Premamillary nucleus
Medial mamillary nucleus
Lateral mamillary nucleus
Mamillary body
Posterior lobe

Figure 3–2. The human hypothalamus, with a superimposed diagrammatic representation of the portal hypophyseal vessels. (Reproduced, with permission, from Ganong WF: *Review of Medical Physiology,* 12th ed. Lange, 1985.)

BRAIN CONTROL OF ENDOCRINE FUNCTIONS

Neural regulation of endocrine function is achieved via input to neurons that secrete hypothalamic hormones, via the innervation of the intermediate lobe of the pituitary, and via the autonomic innervation of glands such as the pancreatic islets that are not directly controlled by tropic hormones from the pituitary gland. The posterior lobe of the pituitary gland is made up of the endings of neurons that secrete oxytocin and vasopressin into the general circulation, whereas the hormones of the anterior lobe of the pituitary are regulated by hypothalamic hypophyseotropic hormones reaching them in the portal hypophyseal vessels. These vessels provide a direct vascular path from the brain to the anterior pituitary. Humans and several other species of mammals have no intermediate lobe, but in the species that do, secretion is controlled in part by an inhibitory innervation from the hypothalamus. In addition, the secretion of the hormones of the adrenal medulla, pineal, kidney, parathyroid gland, and pancreatic islet cells is influenced by their autonomic innervation.

RELATION OF THE PITUITARY TO THE BRAIN

The main nuclei of the hypothalamus and the relationship of this part of the brain to the pituitary gland are shown in Fig 3–2. The posterior lobe of the pituitary arises embryologically as an evagination of the ventral hypothalamus, whereas the anterior and intermediate lobes of the pituitary are derived from Rathke's pouch, an evagination of the pharynx. The posterior lobe retains its neural character throughout life and is the site where the axons of neurons with their cell bodies in the supraoptic and paraventricular nuclei of the hypothalamus end on capillaries that drain via the posterior lobe veins and the cavernous sinuses to the general circulation. The anterior lobe receives no functionally important innervation from the hypothalamus, but its secretion is controlled by the hypothalamic hypophyseotropic hormones secreted into the portal hypophyseal vessels (Fig 3–3). This special system of blood vessels provides a short, direct connection between the ventral hypothalamus and the anterior lobe. It begins in a primary plexus of capillaries in the median eminence of the hypothalamus. Some of the capillaries lie on the ventral surface of the median eminence, and some form loops that penetrate the substance of the median eminence. The capillaries drain into the short sinusoidal portal hypophyseal vessels that pass down the pituitary stalk and break up into capillaries surrounding the cells of the adenohypophysis.

Dopamine-secreting neurons that have their cell

Figure 3–3. Secretion of hypothalamic hormones. The hormones of the posterior lobe (PL) are released into the general circulation from the endings of supraoptic and paraventricular neurons (SO and PV), whereas hypophyseotropic hormones are secreted into the portal hypophyseal circulation from the endings of arcuate (ARC) and other hypothalamic neurons. AL, anterior lobe; MB, mamillary bodies; OC, optic chiasm.

bodies in the arcuate nuclei and neighboring areas (see below) send axons to the posterior lobe and, in those species that have one, the intermediate lobe as well. The function of this tuberohypophyseal innervation is unknown in the case of the posterior lobe; in the case of the intermediate lobe, it inhibits the secretion of intermediate lobe hormones.

HYPOTHALAMIC HORMONES

The exact number of hormones secreted by neurons in the hypothalamus is unsettled, but there is good evidence for the existence of at least 9 (Table 3–2). The structures of 8 of the 9 are known. The remaining hormone is probably a peptide, but this has not been proved.

Posterior Pituitary Hormones

Oxytocin and arginine vasopressin are the 2 peptides known to be secreted from the posterior lobe of the pituitary in humans and most other mammals. Each peptide is synthesized as part of a preprohormone in the cell bodies of neurons in the supraoptic and paraventricular nuclei of the hypothalamus. The preprohormone includes the peptide and an associated protein or **neurophysin** specific for the peptide. Neurons

Table 3–2. Hypothalamic hormones.

Hormone	Structure
Posterior pituitary hormones	
Arginine vasopressin	┌─ S ──────── S ─┐ Cys-Tyr-Phe-Gln-Asn-Cys-Pro-Arg-Gly-NH$_2$
Oxytocin	┌─ S ──────── S ─┐ Cys-Tyr-Ile-Gln-Asn-Cys-Pro-Leu-Gly-NH$_2$
Hypophyseotropic hormones	
Thyrotropin-releasing hormone (TRH)	(pyro)Glu-His-Pro-NH$_2$
Gonadotropin-releasing hormone (GnRH)	(pyro)Glu-His-Trp-Ser-Tyr-Gly-Leu-Arg-Pro-Gly-NH$_2$
Somatostatin*	┌──────── S ──────── S ────────┐ Ala-Gly-Cys-Lys-Asn-Phe-Phe-Trp-Lys-Thr-Phe-Thr-Ser-Cys
Growth hormone–releasing hormone (GRH)	Tyr-Ala-Asp-Ala-Ile-Phe-Thr-Asn-Ser-Tyr-Arg-Lys-Val-Leu-Gly-Gln-Leu-Ser- Ala-Arg-Lys-Leu-Leu-Gln-Asp-Ile-Met-Ser-Arg-Gln-Gln-Gly-Glu-Ser-Asn-Gln- Glu-Arg-Gly-Ala-Arg-Ala-Arg-Leu-NH$_2$
Prolactin-inhibiting hormone (PIH, dopamine)	HO⟩ HO─⟨═⟩─CH$_2$CH$_2$NH$_2$
Prolactin-releasing hormone (PRH)	?
Corticotropin-releasing hormone (CRH)	Ser-Gln-Glu-Pro-Pro-Ile-Ser-Leu-Asp-Leu-Thr-Phe-His-Leu-Leu-Arg-Glu-Val- Leu-Glu-Met-Thr-Lys-Ala-Asp-Gln-Leu-Ala-Gln-Gln-Ala-His-Ser-Asn-Arg- Lys-Leu-Leu-Asp-Ile-Ala-NH$_2$

*In addition to the tetradecapeptide shown here (somatostatin 14), an N-terminal extended molecule (somatostatin 28) is found in most tissues.

synthesize one peptide or the other—not both—and there are oxytocin-synthesizing and vasopressin-synthesizing neurons in both nuclei. Synthesis occurs in the ribosomes, and the preprohormone enters the rough endoplasmic reticulum, where the leader sequence is promptly removed. The prohormone molecules are packaged into secretory granules in the Golgi apparatus, and the secretory granules migrate along the axons by axoplasmic flow to the endings in the posterior lobe. There is further processing in the granules as they move along the axons, and the bond between the peptide and its neurophysin is hydrolyzed before they are released from the endings. Secretion occurs by exocytosis, so that the octapeptides and neurophysins are released in equimolar amounts. Secretion

is initiated by action potentials reaching the endings along the hormone-secreting neurons; thus, the neurons not only function as gland cells that synthesize and secrete the peptides, but they have propagated action potentials like other neurons. The action potentials increase the Ca^{2+} influx at the endings, and this triggers exocytosis. Physiologic control of the secretion of vasopressin and oxytocin is considered in detail in Chapter 6.

Hypophyseotropic Hormones

Most of the hypophyseotropic hormones stimulate the secretion of anterior pituitary hormones, but growth hormone and prolactin are also regulated by inhibitory hypophyseotropic hormones (Fig 3–4). There is also

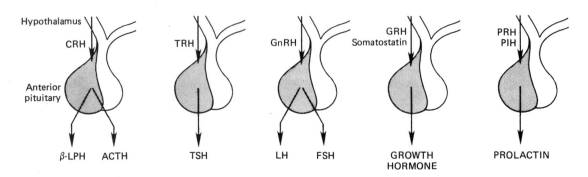

Figure 3–4. Effects of individual hypothalamic hypophyseotropic hormones on anterior pituitary secretion.

some overlap of function among the hypophyseotropic hormones.

TRH stimulates the secretion of TSH and prolactin. Its prolactin-stimulating activity is marked, but it is doubtful that it has a major physiologic role as a prolactin-releasing hormone, because in most situations in which prolactin secretion is stimulated, there is no concomitant increase in TSH secretion. The cell bodies of the TRH-secreting neurons are located in and around the dorsomedial nuclei of the hypothalamus, and their axonal endings are mainly located in the medial portion of the external layer of the median eminence.

GnRH, which is also known as LHRH, stimulates the secretion of FSH as well as LH, and it has not been possible to separate its LH- and FSH-releasing activities by changing the structure of the molecule. Some hypothalamic extracts have been reported to produce selective stimulation of FSH secretion, but efforts to purify an FSH-releasing hormone (FRH) have failed. Consequently, there is a good possibility that there is only one gonadotropin-releasing hormone (GnRH) and that this hypophyseotropic hormone regulates the secretion of both gonadotropins. Evidence indicating that LH and FSH come from the same anterior pituitary cell makes this hypothesis even more attractive. However, it is difficult to prove that a separate FRH does not exist.

The neurons that secrete GnRH have their cell bodies in the preoptic area, the arcuate nuclei, and a broad band of hypothalamic tissue between these 2 regions. Their axons converge on the median eminence and terminate primarily in the lateral portions of the external layer of the median eminence, especially near the pituitary stalk.

Somatostatin inhibits growth hormone secretion. It also inhibits TSH secretion, and administration of antisomatostatin antibodies causes a rise in circulating TSH. However, the physiologic role of somatostatin in the regulation of TSH secretion is unknown. The cells that secrete somatostatin into the portal hypophyseal blood have their cell bodies in the periventricular region immediately above the optic chiasm. Their axons terminate diffusely in all parts of the external layer of the median eminence.

GRH stimulates growth hormone secretion. The cell bodies of the GRH-secreting neurons are located in the arcuate nuclei, and the neuronal endings are in the external layer of the median eminence.

Dopamine is the principal and very possibly the only physiologically significant prolactin-inhibiting hormone. This catecholamine is secreted into the portal hypophyseal vessels by neurons of the tuberoinfundibular dopaminergic system (Fig 3– 5) that have their cell bodies in the arcuate nuclei and their endings in the external layer of the median eminence. The bulk of the endings are located laterally in the same area as the GnRH endings, but some dopaminergic neurons also end in the medial part of the external layer.

CRH stimulates the secretion of β-LPH as well

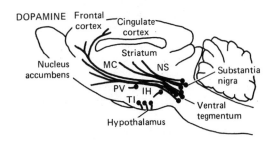

Figure 3–5. Dopaminergic neurons in the brain. The neurons are projected on a sagittal view of the rat brain. IH, incertohypothalamic system; MC, mesocortical system; NS, nigrostriatal system; PV, periventricular system; TI, tuberoinfundibular and tuberohypophyseal system. (Reproduced, with permission, from Ganong WF: *Review of Medical Physiology,* 12th ed. Lange, 1985.)

as ACTH. These pituitary hormones are formed in the same secretory granules from a large precursor molecule called **pro-opiomelanocortin** and are released in equimolar amounts by exocytosis (see Chapter 4). The CRH-secreting neurons are located in the anterior portion of the paraventricular nuclei, and their axons terminate in all parts of the external layer of the median eminence. Vasopressin has a moderate amount of CRH activity and may potentiate the activity of the CRH in the paraventricular neurons. In addition, angiotensin II and several other substances act directly on the pituitary to stimulate ACTH secretion, but their physiologic role in the regulation of ACTH secretion is unknown.

Hypophyseotropic Hormones Outside the Hypothalamus

All of the chemically identified hypothalamic hormones except the newly characterized GRH have also been found in other parts of the brain and in other organs of the body. Somatostatin is a neurotransmitter secreted in various parts of the brain, including primary afferent neurons conducting sensory impulses to the dorsal horn of the spinal cord. Somatostatin is also secreted by typical endocrine cells—the D cells—in the pancreatic islets and the gastrointestinal mucosa. From the latter location and possibly from the pancreas as well, somatostatin enters the general circulation and functions as a gastrointestinal hormone. TRH is also found in nerve endings in various parts of the brain and in the gastrointestinal tract. GnRH is found in neurons not only in the median eminence but also in other circumventricular organs (see below) and it appears to be the neurotransmitter responsible for a slow excitatory response in sympathetic ganglia. CRH-containing fibers project from the paraventricular nuclei to the brain stem. Dopamine is found in many parts of the nervous system and in interneurons called small intensely fluorescent (SIF) cells in sympathetic ganglia. Oxytocin and vasopressin are found in neurons projecting from the hypothalamus to the brain stem and spinal cord. They are also found in the gonads. In addition, posterior lobe–like peptides and TRH are found in invertebrates. Thus, it appears likely that when the pituitary evolved, existing neurotransmitters or neurohormones (or both) were preempted to become the hypothalamic hormones secreted by or involved in the regulation of the pituitary gland.

Other Hormones Common to the Brain, Pituitary, & Gastrointestinal Tract

In addition to somatostatin and TRH, a variety of gastrointestinal hormones are found in neurons in the brain as well as secretory cells or neurons in the gastric and intestinal mucosa. These hormones have no established function in the regulation of anterior pituitary secretion, although vasoactive intestinal polypeptide (VIP) has been found in high concentration in portal hypophyseal blood. In addition, ACTH, β-LPH, and the other derivatives of pro-opiomelanocortin are found not only in the anterior and intermediate lobes of the pituitary but also in neurons with their cell bodies in the arcuate nuclei of the hypothalamus. The function of these neurons is unknown. There is also evidence for the existence of prolactin and other anterior pituitary hormones in the brain.

NEUROTRANSMITTERS AFFECTING THE SECRETION OF HYPOTHALAMIC HORMONES

Afferent neural pathways converge from many different parts of the brain onto the neurons that secrete hypothalamic hormones. Not surprisingly, many different neurotransmitters are secreted by the neurons in these pathways, and drugs that modify the functions of neurotransmitters consequently affect the secretion of anterior and posterior pituitary hormones. Cholinergic discharge in the brain increases vasopressin secretion and may increase prolactin secretion. Discharge of gamma-aminobutyric acid–secreting neurons inhibits ACTH secretion, and histamine may be an excitatory mediator for ACTH. However, the transmitters that have received the most attention are the brain monoamines serotonin, dopamine, norepinephrine, and epinephrine. This is partly because the neurons secreting these substances can be identified by fluorescent or immunocytochemical techniques and partly because some diseases and various drugs used in the treatment of hypertension and psychiatric illness affect brain amine metabolism to the point that they alter pituitary function. Enkephalins and endorphins have also received considerable attention.

Dopamine

The dopaminergic neurons in the brain are summarized in Fig 3–5. As noted above, the tuberoinfundibular dopaminergic system is the source of the dopamine that inhibits prolactin secretion. The other dopaminergic systems include the nigrostriatal system, which is concerned with the regulation of movement and is disrupted in Parkinson's disease; the mesocortical dopaminergic system, which is probably concerned with mental functions and may discharge abnormally in schizophrenia; and several small systems in and near the hypothalamus. There is some evidence that in addition to its inhibitory effect on prolactin, dopamine stimulates growth hormone secretion in humans, but there is little convincing evidence that dopamine plays a role in regulation of secretion of any other anterior pituitary hormones.

Norepinephrine

The noradrenergic neurons in the brain are summarized in Fig 3–6. They are conveniently divided into 2 systems. The locus ceruleus system consists of neurons with cell bodies in the locus ceruleus that project to all parts of the central nervous system. However, hypothalamic innervation from the locus ceruleus is limited to the supraoptic and paraventricular nuclei and parts of the dorsal hypothalamus, and there is little evidence that this system is involved in the regulation of endocrine function. The lateral tegmental system is made up of neurons with cell bodies in several nuclei in the pons and medulla that project to the spinal cord and to all parts of the hypothalamus. This system includes many noradrenergic neurons projecting from sites in or near the nucleus of the tractus solitarius where afferent fibers from the arterial baroreceptors end. In experimental animals, central release of norepinephrine increases the secre-

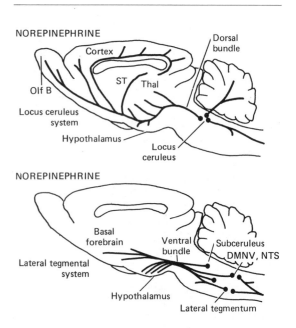

Figure 3–6. Noradrenergic neurons in the brain. Olf B, olfactory bulb; ST, stria terminalis; DMNV, dorsal motor nucleus of vagus; NTS, nucleus tractus solitarii. (Reproduced, with permission, from Ganong WF: *Review of Medical Physiology,* 12th ed. Lange, 1985.)

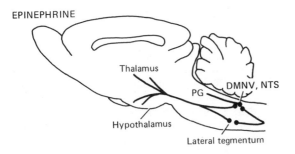

Figure 3–7. Epinephrine-secreting (adrenergic) neurons in the brain. See legend for Fig 3–6. PG, periaqueductal gray. (Reproduced, with permission, from Ganong WF: *Review of Medical Physiology,* 12th ed. Lange, 1985.)

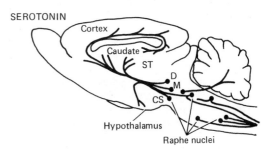

Figure 3–8. Serotoninergic neurons in the brain. CS, D, and M, central superior, dorsal, and medial raphe nuclei. ST, stria terminalis. See legend for Fig 3–6. (Reproduced, with permission, from Ganong WF: *Review of Medical Physiology,* 12th ed. Lange, 1985.)

tion of TSH, GH, LH, and FSH. It decreases the secretion of ACTH and apparently has a similar effect on oxytocin and vasopressin release, but it has no effect on prolactin secretion. Thus, norepinephrine plays an important role in regulating the secretion of hypophyseotropic hormones.

Epinephrine

Epinephrine-secreting neurons project from the medulla oblongata to the spinal cord and the hypothalamus (Fig 3–7). These neurons are involved in blood pressure regulation and are in a good position to exert effects on endocrine function. However, there is as yet little direct evidence that they play an important endocrine role.

Serotonin

Serotoninergic neurons have their cell bodies in the raphe nuclei in the midbrain, pons, and medulla and, like the dopaminergic and noradrenergic systems, project to the spinal cord and many different parts of the brain (Fig 3–8). Serotoninergic discharge increases prolactin secretion, probably by increasing the secretion of PRH. Serotoninergic neurons also project to the suprachiasmatic nuclei, and lesions of these

nuclei disrupt a variety of circadian rhythms, including the regular cycles in adrenocortical secretion and pineal secretion (see below). Drugs that decrease central secretion of serotonin abolish the circadian fluctuation in adrenocortical secretion, presumably via an effect on the suprachiasmatic nuclei.

Opioid Peptides

Many different opioid peptides have now been described. All are formed from 3 large precursor molecules (Table 3–3). All the precursors are found in the brain. They are also found outside the brain: **Proenkephalin** is found in the adrenal medulla; **proopiomelanocortin** is found in the anterior and intermediate lobes of the pituitary gland; and **prodynorphin** and proenkephalin are found in the gastrointestinal tract. The functions of these substances in peripheral tissues are considered in the chapters on the hormones of the adrenal medulla (Chapter 11), the anterior pituitary (Chapter 4), and the gastrointestinal tract (Chapter 18). In the brain, the opioid peptides produced from the precursors, particularly met-enkephalin and leu-enkephalin, are probably synaptic transmitters. There is considerable evidence that opioid peptides occur in the neural pathways involved in the

Table 3–3. Opioid peptides and their precursors.*

Precursor	Opioid Peptides	Structures
Proenkephalin	Met-enkephalin	Tyr-Gly-Gly-Phe-Met$_5$
	Leu-enkephalin	Tyr-Gly-Gly-Phe-Leu$_5$
	Octapeptide	Tyr-Gly-Gly-Phe-Met-Arg-Gly-Leu$_8$
	Heptapeptide	Tyr-Gly-Gly-Phe-Met-Arg-Phe$_7$
Pro-opiomelanocortin	β-Endorphin and other endorphins	See Chapter 4 and Fig 4–3.
Prodynorphin	Dynorphin 1–8	Tyr-Gly-Gly-Phe-Leu-Arg-Arg-Ile$_8$
	Dynorphin 1–17	Tyr-Gly-Gly-Phe-Leu-Arg-Arg-Ile-Arg-Pro-Lys-Leu-Lys-Trp-Asp-Asn-Gln$_{17}$
	α-Neoendorphin	Tyr-Gly-Gly-Phe-Leu-Arg-Lys-Tyr-Pro-Lys$_{10}$
	β-Neoendorphin	Tyr-Gly-Gly-Phe-Leu-Arg-Lys-Tyr-Pro$_9$

*Source of data: Rossier J: Opioid peptides have found their roots. *Nature* 1981;**298**:221. Reproduced, with permission, from Ganong WF: *Review of Medical Physiology,* 12th ed. Lange, 1985.

regulation of anterior and posterior pituitary secretion. In humans, the effects of opioids on growth hormone and TSH secretion are unsettled, but it appears that opioids in the brain inhibit the secretion of ACTH, LH, and vasopressin, whereas they increase the secretion of prolactin. However, the nature of the opioids involved, the location of the opioid-secreting neurons, and the exact role of the pathways in the regulation of pituitary secretion are still unknown.

BRAIN REGULATION OF OTHER ENDOCRINE GLANDS

Regulation of Pineal Secretion

The pineal gland secretes **melatonin,** an indole it produces by 5-methoxylation and N-acetylation of se-

Figure 3–9. Formation and metabolism of melatonin. HIOMT, hydroxyindole-O-methyltransferase. (Reproduced, with permission, from Ganong WF: *Review of Medical Physiology,* 12th ed. Lange, 1985.)

rotonin (Fig 3–9). There is some evidence that melatonin is also synthesized in the hypothalamus and in other parts of the body, but the melatonin in the circulation comes from the pineal. The pineal also appears to release melatonin into the cerebrospinal fluid, and cerebrospinal fluid levels are higher than those in plasma. The circulating melatonin level is markedly dependent on the incident light, with high levels in darkness (Fig 3–10). However, the function of melatonin is unknown. It has antigonadotropic activity in certain doses and under certain circumstances in experimental animals, but there is no good evidence for a physiologic antigonadotropic effect in humans.

The pineal is an excellent example of a gland that is under neural control. The light signals that regulate melatonin secretion are integrated in the suprachiasmatic nuclei, and disruption of these hypothalamic nuclei abolishes the light-dark fluctuations in circulating melatonin. From the suprachiasmatic nuclei, impulses descend to the spinal cord and on each side pass via preganglionic sympathetic fibers in the thoracic region to the superior cervical ganglion. From the superior cervical ganglion, postganglionic neurons pass to the pineal gland via the nervi conarii. Norepinephrine released at these endings acts via beta-adrenergic receptors and cAMP to increase the synthesis of the enzyme N-acetyltransferase in the pineal and thus increase melatonin synthesis. The beta receptors show fluctuations in sensitivity with variations in the amount of norepinephrine reaching them; they are more sensitive after decreased exposure to norepinephrine and less sensitive after increased exposure. The receptors have been extensively studied, because they provide an excellent example of the role of receptors in the regulation of an endocrine gland.

Regulation of Adrenal Medullary Secretion

The adrenal medulla is another endocrine gland under direct neural control. Its secretory cells are in effect postganglionic sympathetic neurons that have lost their axons and become endocrine cells. Consequently, they are innervated by preganglionic sympathetic neurons from the intermediolateral gray column of the spinal cord, and the transmitter that regulates adrenal medullary secretion is acetylcholine. The regulation of adrenal medullary secretion is discussed in detail in Chapter 11. It is worth noting that only a small part of the circulating norepinephrine comes from the adrenal medulla. The rest diffuses into the circulation from postganglionic noradrenergic endings in the viscera.

Autonomic Regulation of the Secretion of Other Endocrine Glands

Hormone secretion by the kidneys, the parathyroid glands, and the pancreatic islets is regulated in part by postganglionic sympathetic nerve fibers that secrete norepinephrine, and the islet cells also receive a parasympathetic cholinergic secretomotor innervation. In each of these instances, the neural components com-

Figure 3–10. Plasma melatonin (in melatonin equivalents per 10 mL) in 5 normal adult men. Hours and days are represented on the horizontal scale, with light and dark phases indicated by L and D, respectively. (Reproduced, with permission, from Pelham RW et al: Twenty-four-hour cycle of a melatonin-like substance in the plasma of human males. *J Clin Endocrinol Metab* 1973;**37**:341.)

plement nonneural factors that play a major role in the regulation of secretion.

Renin

The secretion of renin from the juxtaglomerular cells in the kidney is a good example of autonomic regulation. Renin secretion is increased by increased discharge of the sympathetic nerves to the kidneys, but it is also increased by a fall in intrarenal arterial pressure and a decrease in sodium and chloride crossing the macula densa in the distal tubules. The latter 2 effects are direct and independent of renal innervation. The effect of sympathetic discharge is exerted via β_1-adrenergic receptors probably situated directly on the juxtaglomerular cells. The sympathetic pathway provides a direct mechanism by which psychic stimuli can increase renin secretion. Renin secretion is considered in detail in Chapter 12.

Erythropoietin

The secretion of the renal factor erythropoietin, which stimulates red blood cell maturation, is also increased by sympathetic discharge via beta-adrenergic receptors, although the secretion of this factor is primarily regulated by the amount of oxygen supplied to the tissues.

Parathyroid Hormone

Parathyroid hormone is increased by increased sympathetic discharge via beta-adrenergic receptors, although the secretion of this hormone is primarily controlled by the amount of calcium ion (Ca^{2+}) in the blood perfusing the parathyroid glands. The regulation of parathyroid secretion is discussed in detail in Chapter 8.

Insulin

The secretion of insulin from the B cells and glucagon from the A cells of the pancreatic islets is increased by cholinergic mechanisms when the vagal nerve fibers innervating the pancreas are stimulated. Stimulation of the sympathetic innervation increases the secretion of insulin and glucagon via stimulation of beta-adrenergic receptors and inhibits the secretion of these hormones via alpha-adrenergic receptors. In the case of insulin, the alpha-inhibitory mechanism normally predominates, so that the net effect of sympathetic stimulation is inhibition of insulin secretion, whereas in the case of glucagon, the beta-excitatory mechanism predominates. There is evidence that the autonomic fibers also regulate the secretion of somatostatin and pancreatic polypeptide in the pancreatic islets. However, the secretion of insulin and glucagon is primarily regulated by glucose and other products of metabolism acting directly on the secretory cells. The regulation of islet cell secretion is considered in detail in Chapter 19.

EFFECTS OF HORMONES ON THE BRAIN

MECHANISMS OF HORMONE ACTION

Some of the multiple effects of hormones on the brain are indirect and are produced via hormone-induced changes in blood glucose, calcium, and the like. Others are direct and, in the case of hormones that penetrate the brain, may be due to direct actions of the hormone on neurons. In the case of hormones that do not penetrate the brain, the hormone-induced changes in brain function are mediated via the circumventricular organs, a unique group of brain structures that by their location outside the blood-brain barrier provide channels for chemical communication between the brain and the rest of the body.

Circumventricular Organs

The circumventricular organs are located in the midline portions of the brain that surround the third and fourth ventricles. Each has fenestrated capillaries, the type of highly permeable capillaries found in endocrine glands, the kidneys, and the intestinal epithelium. Each is readily penetrated by substances in the circulating blood, including peptides and other relatively large molecules. This is in marked contrast to the rest of the brain, where capillary endothelial junctions are tight and even small molecules penetrate brain tissue with great difficulty. Thus, the circumventricular organs are outside the blood-brain barrier. However, they have intimate neural connections with the rest of the brain.

The established circumventricular organs (Fig 3-11) are the **area postrema**, located at the caudal end of the fourth ventricle; the **subfornical organ**, located in the dorsal part of the third ventricle between the columns of the fornix; the **organum vasculosum of the lamina terminalis**, located over the optic chiasm in the thin layer of tissue that forms the rostral boundary of the third ventricle; and the **neurohypophysis** and adjacent **median eminence** of the hypothalamus, located below the third ventricle. The pineal gland has fenestrated capillaries, like other endocrine organs, but—except for its sympathetic innervation (see above)—it lacks direct neural connections with the brain. The subcommissural organ does not have fenestrated capillaries, and although it has some of the histologic characteristics of a circumventricular organ, it probably has some other function.

The circumventricular organs are in a position to permit transport of molecules from the brain to the circulation, and molecules in the blood can act on receptors in them. The neurohypophysis and median eminence function as **neurohemal organs,** sites where hypothalamic hormones secreted by neurons enter the general circulation (in the case of the posterior lobe

Figure 3–11. Circumventricular organs. The neurohypophysis (NH) and adjacent median eminence, the organum vasculosum of the lamina terminalis (OVLT), the subfornical organ (SFO), and the area postrema (AP) are shown projected on a sagittal section of the human brain. The pineal (PI) and the subcommissural organ (SCO) are also shown but probably do not function as circumventricular organs. (Reproduced, with permission, from Ganong WF: *Review of Medical Physiology,* 12th ed. Lange, 1985.)

hormones) and the portal hypophyseal circulation (in the case of the hypophyseotropic hormones). The circumventricular organs are also in an excellent position to function as **chemoreceptor trigger zones** where blood-borne chemicals can act on sensory cells to trigger changes in neural function without disruption of the blood-brain barrier. They carry out this function in particular for circulating peptides such as angiotensin II that affect brain function.

INDIRECT EFFECTS OF HORMONES ON THE BRAIN

Insulin produces changes in mental function, sweating, nervousness, convulsions, coma, and death by lowering blood glucose, the obligatory short-term substrate for brain metabolic processes. This is in contrast to the specific action of insulin on the glucoreceptor cells in the ventromedial nuclei of the hypothalamus to increase glucose utilization and thus produce satiety. Hypocalcemia due to parathyroid hormone deficiency causes the changes in neural function that produce tetany, and hypercalcemia due to hyperparathyroidism produces changes in mental function that on occasion can be severe. Indeed, patients with chronic hypoglycemia and patients with hyperparathyroidism have been admitted to mental hospitals because of psychotic behavior, and their behavioral symptoms were subsequently relieved by treatment of the endocrine disease. Hypothyroidism can also cause mental symptoms, but the pathophysiologic basis of these symptoms is uncertain. Patients with hyperthyroidism are alert, nervous, and hyperphagic, but the first 2 effects are probably secondary to increased sympathetic activity, whereas hyperphagia is secondary to loss of calories as a consequence of hypermetabolism.

EFFECTS OF HORMONES THAT PENETRATE BRAIN TISSUE

Steroids

Protein-bound steroids do not penetrate the brain, but free steroids enter with relative ease because of their high lipid solubility. Consequently, the brain level of active steroids is generally at least as high as the active, free fraction in plasma. The cells that take up the steroids have been identified as neurons by radioautography and are located throughout the central nervous system. Glucocorticoids, testosterone, estrogen, and progesterone all have effects on brain function.

Glucocorticoids increase the predominant frequency of the alpha rhythm of the EEG and produce mental symptoms that range from euphoria and bulimia to frank psychotic behavior. The mental symptoms associated with Cushing's syndrome are described in more detail in Chapter 9. Adrenal insufficiency is also associated with personality changes, although these are usually mild and subtle, and slowing of the basic frequency of the alpha rhythm is so characteristic that the EEG has been used as an aid in the diagnosis of Addison's disease. In rats, corticosterone binds to hippocampal neurons and stimulates DNA-dependent mRNA synthesis, but the physiologic significance of this action is unknown.

Progesterone in large doses stimulates sexual behavior in experimental animals, and smaller doses facilitate the effects of estrogens (see below). In addition, progesterone causes hyperthermia, probably by an action on the brain, and is believed to be responsible for the rise in basal body temperature at the time of ovulation in women.

Testosterone is responsible for male sexual behavior in many species of mammals, and sexual activity is reduced or abolished by castration. The site of this action of testosterone is the hypothalamus. In humans, male sex behavior is not dependent on testosterone and persists for long periods following castration. However, testosterone still acts on the brain to intensify sexual interest. Heterosexual drive in men is stimulated by estrogens as well as androgens, and increased libido can be a problem in men with cancer being treated with large doses of estrogens.

Estrogens are responsible for the period of heat at the time of ovulation in females of species that have

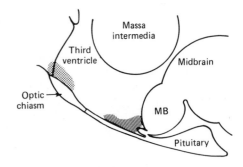

Figure 3–12. Loci where implantations of estrogens in the hypothalamus affect ovarian weight and sexual behavior in rats. The implants that stimulate sexual behavior are located anteriorly, above the optic chiasm (dotted area). They are separate from the posterior ventral sites (striped area), where implants inhibit LH secretion, causing ovarian atrophy. MB, mamillary body. (Reproduced, with permission, from Ganong WF: *Review of Medical Physiology,* 12th ed. Lange, 1985.)

an estrous rather than a menstrual cycle. During heat, the female seeks out the male and engages in copulation, whereas during the rest of the cycle she rebuffs sexual advances. Evidence from lesion experiments and local implantation of steroids (Fig 3–12) indicates that estrogens produce heat by an action on the anterior hypothalamus. Androgens also intensify female sexual behavior in adult females. Primates have a menstrual rather than an estrous cycle without a clearly defined period of heat, but in monkeys and apes, the rise in circulating estrogens at the time of ovulation is associated with increased sexual activity. A few studies suggest that a midcycle increase in sexual activity also occurs in women. Ovariectomized and postmenopausal women have little or no loss of libido. However, they still have circulating androgens and estrogens of adrenal origin, and it has been claimed that if the adrenals as well as the ovaries are removed, sexual activity is markedly reduced.

Effects of Gonadal Steroids During Development

In addition to its effects on adult sexual behavior, testosterone acts just after birth in rats to "masculinize" the brain. The transient rise in circulating testosterone at this time has no observable immediate effect on brain function, but it causes the animal to display the male pattern of sex behavior and the noncyclic male pattern of gonadotropin secretion when the animal becomes an adult. The same changes can be produced in female rats by a single injection of testosterone up to the fifth day of life. If male rats are castrated at birth, they develop the female pattern of sexual behavior and the female cyclic pattern of gonadotropin secretion in adulthood. The mechanism by which a brief exposure to testosterone produces lifelong changes in brain function is still unknown.

Changes similar to those occurring in rats can be

produced in other laboratory animals, although in species in which the young are born more mature than they are in the rat, the animals must be treated before rather than after birth by administering androgens to the mother. In monkeys, early exposure to androgen does not change the pattern of gonadotropin secretion in adulthood, but it does produce masculinization of behavior. In women with congenital adrenal hyperplasia and the adrenogenital syndrome, the androgens also fail to alter the pattern of gonadotropin secretion; these women menstruate regularly when treated with glucocorticoids. However, it has been claimed that there is measurable masculinization of behavior.

There is some evidence that the androgens that masculinize the brain are actually converted to estrogens by **aromatization** before exerting their effects. Aromatization occurs in various parts of the brain. Proponents of the view that aromatization is necessary for masculinization argue that estrogens do not masculinize normal females, because young females have an avid estrogen-binding protein in their blood and tissues. However, the concept of aromatization as a necessary step for masculinization is not yet proved.

Effects of Thyroid Hormones During Development

Thyroid hormones penetrate the brain and have marked effects on brain development in early life. If untreated, cretins with congenital hypothyroidism develop severe mental retardation. In animals that are hypothyroid from birth, neurons fail to develop to their normal size, there are fewer synaptic endings than normal, and dendritic trees are stunted. These morphologic changes are associated with abnormalities of brain enzyme concentrations and impaired RNA synthesis.

Peptides

Angiotensin II acts on the brain to produce several important effects. It increases water intake, blood pressure, and secretion of vasopressin. However, like most peptides, angiotensin II does not cross the blood-brain barrier; instead, it exerts its central effects by acting on the circumventricular organs. The increase in water intake is due primarily to the action of circulating angiotensin II on the subfornical organ, although the organum vasculosum of the lamina terminalis may have a secondary role in mediating this dipsogenic effect. In most but not all species studied, the blood pressure–raising effect is due to an action on the area postrema. The increase in vasopressin secretion appears to be due to an action on the subfornical organ. Angiotensin II also increases ACTH secretion, but it is uncertain how much, if any, of this effect is due to a direct action on the pituitary.

Insulin is also found in circumventricular organs in relatively large amounts, and there is evidence for retrograde transport of insulin to the cell bodies of the neurons innervating the circumventricular organs. However, the physiologic role of insulin at this site is unknown.

When administered systemically in small doses, posterior pituitary peptides have been reported to produce changes in the extinction of conditioned avoidance responses and other psychologic responses. It is difficult to see how these substances could penetrate the brain to produce the observed effects, but an effect mediated via the circumventricular organs is a possibility.

REFERENCES

Axelrod J: Pineal gland: A neurochemical transducer. *Science* 1974;**184:**1341.

Brownstein MJ, Russell JT, Gainer H: Synthesis, transport, and release of posterior pituitary hormones. *Science* 1980;**207:**373.

Cooper JR, Bloom FE, Roth RH: *The Biochemical Basis of Neuropharmacology,* 3rd ed. Oxford Univ Press, 1978.

Delitala G, Mota M, Serio M: *Opioid Modulation of Endocrine Function.* Raven Press, 1984.

Fitzimons JT: *The Physiology of Thirst and Sodium Appetite.* Cambridge Univ Press, 1979.

Ganong WF: *Review of Medical Physiology,* 12th ed. Lange, 1985.

Ganong WF: The role of catecholamines and acetylcholine in the regulation of endocrine function. *Life Sci* 1974;**15:**1401.

Ganong WF, Martini L (editors): *Frontiers in Neuroendocrinology.* Vol 9. Raven Press, 1986.

Guillemin R et al: Growth hormone–releasing factor: Chemistry and physiology. *Proc Soc Exp Biol Med* 1984;**175:**407.

Krieger DT, Liotta AS: Pituitary hormones in brain: Where, how and why? *Science* 1979;**205:**366.

Martin JB, Reichlin S, Brown GM: *Clinical Neuroendocrinology.* Davis, 1977.

Preslock JP: The pineal gland: Basic implications and clinical correlation. *Endocr Rev* 1984;**5:**282.

Weiner RI, Ganong WF: Role of brain monoamines and histamine in regulation of anterior pituitary secretion. *Physiol Rev* 1978;**58:**905.

Wood C, Porte DJR: Neural control of the endocrine pancreas. *Physiol Rev* 1974;**54:**596.

Anterior Pituitary & Somatomedins: I. Anterior Pituitary

4

James W. Findling, MD, & J. Blake Tyrrell, MD

Immunoassay techniques that measure the secretory products of the pituitary and advances in the neuroradiologic evaluation of the sella turcica have improved the diagnosis of pituitary disorders. Transsphenoidal microsurgery and bromocriptine now allow earlier and more effective therapy. This chapter describes the clinical evaluation of the anterior pituitary (adenohypophysis), including its anatomy, embryology, and histology; the physiologic action and secretion of its major hormones; and disorders of the gland with respect to neuroradiologic findings and secretory hypo- and hyperfunction.

EMBRYOLOGY

The human fetal pituitary anlage is initially recognizable at 4–5 weeks of gestation, and rapid cytologic differentiation leads to a mature hypothalamic-pituitary unit at 20 weeks. The adenohypophysis originates from Rathke's pouch, an ectodermal evagination of the oropharynx, and migrates to join the neurohypophysis (an outpouching of the third ventricle). The portion of Rathke's pouch in contact with the neurohypophysis develops less extensively and forms the intermediate lobe. This lobe remains intact in some species, but in humans its cells become interspersed with those of the anterior lobe. These cells do, however, develop the capacity to synthesize and secrete adrenocorticotropic hormone (ACTH) and its related peptide hormones.

Remnants of Rathke's pouch may persist at the boundary of the neurohypophysis, resulting in small colloid cysts. In addition, cells may persist in the lower portion of Rathke's pouch beneath the sphenoid bone, the pharyngeal pituitary. These cells have the potential to secrete hormones and have been reported to undergo adenomatous change.

ANATOMY
(Figs 4–1 and 4–2)

Gross Anatomy

The pituitary gland lies at the base of the skull in a portion of the sphenoid bone called the sella turcica ("Turkish saddle"). The anterior portion, the tuber-

Acronyms Used in This Chapter

ACTH	Adrenocorticotropic hormone
AVP	Arginine vasopressin
cAMP	Cyclic adenosine monophosphate
CLIP	Corticotropinlike intermediate lobe peptide
CRH	Corticotropin-releasing hormone
FSH	Follicle-stimulating hormone
GABA	Gamma-aminobutyric acid
GH	Growth hormone
GnRH	Gonadotropin-releasing hormone
GRH	Growth hormone-releasing hormone
hCG	Human chorionic gonadotropin
hGH	Human growth hormone
hMG	Human menopausal gonadotropin
hPL	Human placental lactogen
LH	Luteinizing hormone
LPH	Lipotropin
MEN	Multiple endocrine neoplasia
MRI	Magnetic resonance imaging
MSH	Melanocyte-stimulating hormone
PRL	Prolactin
SHBG	Sex hormone-binding globulin
SIADH	Syndrome of inappropriate secretion of vasopressin (antidiuretic hormone)
TRH	Thyrotropin-releasing hormone
TSH	Thyroid-stimulating hormone (thyrotropin)
VER	Visual evoked response
VIP	Vasoactive intestinal polypeptide

culum sellae turcicae, is flanked by posterior projections of the sphenoid wings, the anterior clinoid processes; the dorsum sellae form the posterior wall, and their upper corners project into the posterior clinoid processes. The gland is surrounded by dura, and the roof is formed by a reflection of the dura attached to the clinoid processes, the diaphragma sellae. In normal individuals, the arachnoid membrane and, therefore, cerebrospinal fluid are prevented from entering the sella turcica by the diaphragma sellae. The pituitary stalk and its blood vessels pass through an opening in this diaphragm. The lateral walls of the gland are in direct apposition to the cavernous sinuses and separated from them by dural membranes. The optic chiasm lies 5–10 mm above the diaphragma sellae and anterior to the stalk (Fig 4–1).

The size of the pituitary gland, of which the an-

Third ventricle

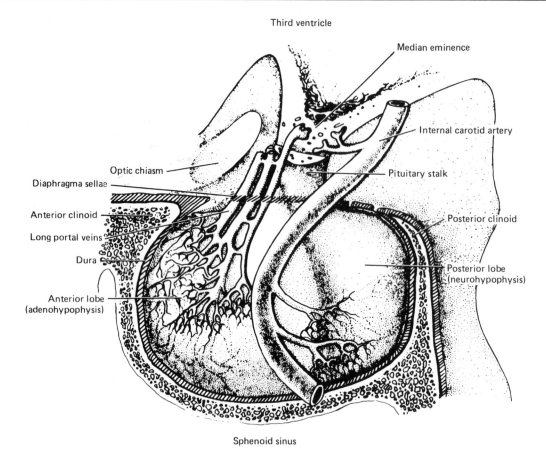

Median eminence

Internal carotid artery

Optic chiasm

Pituitary stalk

Diaphragma sellae

Anterior clinoid

Long portal veins

Dura

Posterior clinoid

Posterior lobe
(neurohypophysis)

Anterior lobe
(adenohypophysis)

Sphenoid sinus

Figure 4–1. Anatomic relationships and blood supply of the pituitary gland. (Reproduced, with permission, from Frohman LA: Diseases of the anterior pituitary. Chap 7, pp 151–231, in: *Endocrinology and Metabolism.* Felig P et al [editors]. McGraw-Hill, 1981.)

terior lobe constitutes two-thirds, varies considerably. It measures approximately 15 × 10 × 6 mm and weighs 500–900 mg; it may double in size during pregnancy. Since the sella turcica tends to conform to the shape and size of the gland, there is considerable variability in the contour of this bony structure.

Blood Supply

The anterior pituitary is the most richly vascularized of all mammalian tissues, receiving 0.8 mL/g/min from a portal circulation connecting the median eminence of the hypothalamus and the anterior pituitary. This arterial blood is supplied by the internal carotid arteries via middle and inferior hypophyseal arteries. The arteries form a capillary network in the median eminence of the hypothalamus that recombines in long portal veins draining down the pituitary stalk to the anterior lobe, where they break up into another capillary network and re-form into venous channels. The posterior pituitary is supplied directly from branches of the middle and inferior hypophyseal arteries (Fig 4–1).

Venous drainage of the pituitary, the route through

which anterior pituitary hormones reach the systemic circulation, is variable, but venous channels eventually drain via the cavernous sinus posteriorly into the superior and inferior petrosal sinuses to the jugular bulb and vein (Fig 4–2).

Recent evidence indicates that there is also retrograde blood flow between the pituitary and hypothalamus, providing a means of direct feedback between pituitary hormones and their neuroendocrine control.

Histology

The cells of the anterior pituitary were originally classified using techniques for staining intracellular granules as acidophils, basophils, and chromophobe cells. Immunocytochemical and electron microscopic techniques now permit classification of cells by their specific secretory products: somatotrophs (growth hormone [GH]–secreting cells), lactotrophs (prolactin [PRL]–secreting cells), thyrotrophs (cells secreting thyroid-stimulating hormone [thyrotropin; TSH]), corticotrophs (cells secreting adrenocorticotropic hormone [corticotropin; ACTH] and related

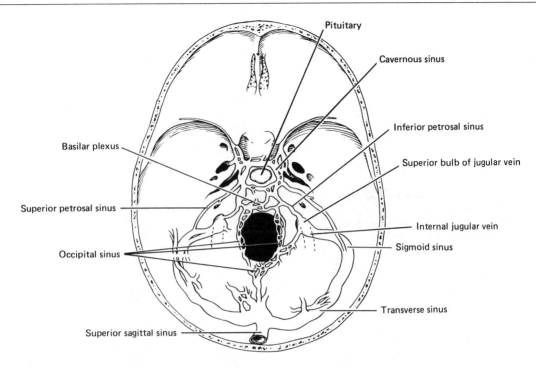

Figure 4–2. Venous drainage of the pituitary gland—the route by which adenohypophyseal hormones reach the systemic circulation. (Reproduced, with permission, from Findling JW et al: Selective venous sampling for ACTH in Cushing's syndrome: Differentiation between Cushing's disease and the ectopic ACTH syndrome. *Ann Intern Med* 1981;**94**:647.)

peptides), and gonadotrophs (luteinizing hormone [LH]– and follicle-stimulating hormone [FSH]–secreting cells). The specificity of the antibody used determines the ability of immunocytochemical techniques to differentiate the various cell types. Because the glycoprotein peptide hormones LH, FSH, and TSH share a common alpha subunit, an antiserum directed against this portion of these molecules would result in cross-reactivity; however, an antibody directed against the distinct beta subunit of these hormones provides clear differentiation.

A. Somatotrophs: The GH-secreting cells are identified as acidophilic in standard hematoxylin and eosin preparations and are usually located in the lateral portions of the anterior lobe. Granule size by electron microscopy is 300– 400 nm in diameter. These cells account for about 4– 10% of the net weight of the anterior pituitary.

B. Lactotrophs: A second but distinct acidophil-staining cell randomly distributed in the anterior pituitary is the PRL-secreting cell. Granule size averages approximately 550 nm on electron microscopy. These cells proliferate during pregnancy as a result of elevated estrogen levels and account for the 2-fold increase in gland size.

C. Thyrotrophs: These TSH-secreting cells, because of their glycoprotein product, are basophilic and also show a positive reaction with periodic acid–Schiff (PAS) stain. The thyrotroph granules are small (50– 100 nm); these cells are usually located in the anteromedial and anterolateral portions of the gland. During states of primary thyroid failure, the cells demonstrate marked hypertrophy, increasing overall gland size.

D. Corticotrophs: ACTH and its related peptides (see below), the lipotropins (LPH), and the endorphins are secreted by basophilic cells that are embryologically of intermediate lobe origin and usually located in the anteromedial portion of the gland. Electron microscopy shows that these secretory granules are about 360 nm in diameter. In states of glucocorticoid excess (both exogenous and endogenous), corticotrophs undergo degranulation and a microtubular hyalinization known as Crooke's hyaline degeneration.

E. Gonadotrophs: Both LH and FSH originate from these basophil-staining cells, whose secretory granules are about 200 nm in diameter. These cells are located in the lateral portion of the gland. They become hypertrophied and cause the gland to enlarge during states of primary gonadal failure such as Klinefelter's and Turner's syndromes.

F. Other Cell Types: Despite immunocytochemical staining with antibodies directed against all of the known anterior pituitary hormones, some cells remain unstained. These are chromophobes by conventional staining methods, but electron microscopy has identified secretory granules in many of them. It is not certain whether they represent undifferentiated primitive secretory cells or whether they produce as yet unidentified hormones, such as adrenal androgen–stimulating hormone, ovarian growth factor, or aldosterone-stimulating factor.

ANTERIOR PITUITARY HORMONES

There are 6 major anterior pituitary hormones whose biosynthesis, structure, function, and secretory control have been well characterized and which can be accurately measured in tissues and body fluids. These hormones—ACTH, GH, PRL, TSH, LH, and FSH—may be classified into 3 groups: corticotropin-related peptides (ACTH, LPH, melanocyte-stimulating hormone [MSH], and endorphins); the somatomammotropins (GH and PRL), which are also peptides; and the glycoproteins (LH, FSH, and TSH). The chemical features of these hormones are illustrated in Table 4–1.

ACTH & RELATED PEPTIDES

Biosynthesis

ACTH is a 39-amino-acid peptide hormone (MW 4500) processed from a large precursor molecule, pro-opiomelanocortin (MW 28,500). Within the corticotroph, a single mRNA directs the synthesis of this large precursor, which is then processed into smaller biologically active fragments (Fig 4–3). The function and importance of these related peptides (β-LPH, α-MSH, β-MSH, β-endorphin, N-terminal fragment) are an evolving and exciting area of endocrine research. Most of these peptides are glycosylated to some extent, resulting in various differences in the reporting of molecular weights. It is these carbohydrate moieties that are responsible for the basophilic staining of corticotrophs. Previous names for portions of the pro-opiomelanocortin precursor such as "big ACTH," "proACTH," and "preproACTH" were based on nonspecific techniques.

As depicted in Fig 4–3, 2 of these fragments are contained within the structure of ACTH: α-MSH is identical to $ACTH_{1-13}$, and corticotropinlike intermediate lobe peptide (CLIP) represents $ACTH_{18-39}$. Although these fragments are found in species with developed intermediate lobes (eg, the rat), they are not secreted as separate hormones in humans. β-Lipotropin, a fragment with 91 amino acids (1–91), is secreted by the corticotroph in equimolar quantities with ACTH. Within the β-LPH molecule exists the amino acid sequence for β-MSH (41–58), γ-LPH (1–58), and β-endorphin (61–91). There has been much controversy about the secretion and function of β-MSH, but current evidence suggests that it is not a distinct hormone in humans. On the other hand, β-endorphin appears to have importance in normal endocrine physiology and in disease. Despite the presence of the amino acid sequence for methionine-enkephalin (61–65) within β-LPH and β-endorphin, there is no evidence that it is secreted separately by the pituitary.

The N-terminal fragment (131 amino acids) of pro-opiomelanocortin has been isolated and sequenced. The first 76 amino acids of this N-terminal sequence appear to be the physiologically relevant form of this fragment. Plasma levels of this peptide increase in response to hypoglycemic stress. It may be an adrenal growth factor and may potentiate ACTH action on steroidogenesis.

Function

The primary effect of ACTH is to stimulate the secretion of glucocorticoids, mineralocorticoids, and androgenic steroids from the adrenal cortex (see Chap-

Table 4–1. Characteristics of anterior pituitary hormones.*

Pituitary Hormone	Molecular Weight	Amino Acids		Other Features
I. Corticotropin-lipotropin				
ACTH	4,500	39		
β-Lipotropin	11,200	91		All of these hormones are derived from a common precursor.
β-Endorphin	4,000	31		
II. Glycoprotein				
LH	29,000	Alpha subunit:	89	
		Beta subunit:	115	
FSH	29,000	Alpha subunit:	89	All have 2 subunits, with the alpha subunit being identical in
		Beta subunit:	115	each and the beta subunit conferring biologic specificity.
TSH	28,000	Alpha subunit:	89	
		Beta subunit:	112	
III. Somatomammotropin				
GH	21,500	191		Originated in evolution as a common hormone.
PRL	22,000	198		

*Adapted from Frohman LA: Diseases of the anterior pituitary. Chap 7, pp 151–231, in: *Endocrinology and Metabolism.* Felig P et al (editors). McGraw-Hill, 1981.

Figure 4–3. The processing of pro-opiomelanocortin (MW 28,500) into its biologically active peptide hormones. Abbreviations are expanded in the text.

ters 9 and 10). The amino-terminal end (residues 1–18) is responsible for this biologic activity. ACTH binds to receptors on the adrenal cortex and provokes steroidogenesis through the mediation of cyclic 3′,5′-adenosine monophosphate (cyclic AMP, cAMP).

The hyperpigmentation observed in states of ACTH hypersecretion (eg, Addison's disease, Nelson's syndrome) appears to be primarily due to ACTH. Because α- and β-MSH do not exist as separate hormones in humans, the exact cause of this increased pigmentation remains unclear.

The physiologic function of β-LPH and its family of peptide hormones, including β-endorphin, is not completely understood. However, it is known that both β-LPH and β-endorphin have the same secretory dynamics as ACTH; they increase in response to stress, hypoglycemia, and metyrapone and are suppressible with glucocorticoids. These hormones, including the N-terminal fragment, also parallel ACTH in disease states—eg, they are elevated in Addison's disease, Cushing's disease, and Nelson's syndrome. Furthermore, there is evidence that β-endorphin acts as an "endogenous opiate," suggesting a role in pain appreciation. It may affect the endocrine regulation of other pituitary hormones and perhaps also the neural control of breathing. A hyperendorphin syndrome reported in a child with necrotizing encephalomyelopathy suggests that it may be a causative factor in disease states.

Measurement

It is more difficult to measure plasma ACTH by radioimmunoassay than the other anterior pituitary hormones. Its low concentration, instability in human plasma, and structural homology within its family of peptides create technical difficulties. The basal morning concentration ranges from undetectable (usually 10–20 pg/mL) to 100 pg/mL. Its short plasma half-life (7–12 minutes) and episodic secretion cause wide and rapid fluctuations both in its plasma concentration and in that of cortisol. Because ACTH adheres avidly to glass (a phenomenon that is utilized for extraction in some radioimmunoassay procedures), specimens should be collected in chilled, heparinized plastic tubes. Plasma should be separated and frozen immediately after collection to avoid destruction by plasma peptidases.

Although β-LPH has a longer half-life than ACTH and is more stable in plasma, its measurement has not been extensively utilized. Current data suggest that the normal concentration of β-LPH is 10–40 pg/mL.

Various levels of β-endorphin have been reported, but limitations exist because of cross-reactivity of antisera with β-LPH. Because chromatographic procedures are essential to determine plasma levels accurately, this hormone's measurement remains investigational.

The normal level of the N-terminal fragment in human plasma appears to be less than 100 pg/mL; measurements are not clinically available.

Secretion

The physiologic secretion of ACTH is mediated through neural influences by means of a complex of hormones, the most important of which is corticotropin-releasing hormone (CRH) (Fig 4–4). Although CRH was the first recognized hypothalamic hormone, it was not isolated and identified until 1981. In that year, Vale et al isolated the 41-amino-acid peptide in ovine hypothalami. The structure of human CRH has more recently been identified and is identical to that of rat CRH. CRH has a long plasma half-life (approximately 60 minutes), and both arginine vasopressin (AVP) and angiotensin II potentiate the CRH-mediated

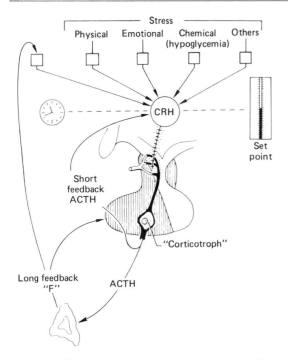

Figure 4–4. The hypothalamic-pituitary-adrenal axis, illustrating negative feedback by cortisol ("F") at the hypothalamic and pituitary levels. A short negative feedback loop of ACTH on the secretion of corticotropin-releasing hormone (CRH) also exists. (Reproduced, with permission, from Gwinup G, Johnson B: Clinical testing of the hypothalamic-pituitary-adrenocortical system in states of hypo- and hypercortisolism. *Metabolism* 1975;**24**:777.)

secretion of ACTH. In contrast, oxytocin inhibits CRH-mediated ACTH secretion.

The CRH complex stimulates ACTH in a pulsatile manner, with diurnal rhythmicity causing a peak before awakening and a decline as the day progresses. The diurnal rhythm is a reflection of neural control and provokes concordant diurnal secretion of cortisol from the adrenal cortex (Fig 4–5). This episodic release of ACTH is independent of circulating cortisol levels—ie, the magnitude of an ACTH impulse is not related to preceding plasma cortisol levels. An example is the persistence of diurnal rhythm in patients with primary adrenal failure (Addison's disease). ACTH secretion also increases in response to feeding in both humans and animals.

Many types of stresses stimulate ACTH, often superseding the normal diurnal rhythmicity. Physical, emotional, and chemical stresses such as pain, trauma, acute hypoglycemia, cold exposure, surgery, depression, and pyrogen and vasopressin administration have all been shown to stimulate ACTH and cortisol secretion. Although physiologic cortisol levels do not blunt the ACTH response to stress, exogenous corticosteroids in high doses suppress it.

Negative feedback of cortisol and synthetic glucocorticoids on ACTH secretion occurs at both the hypothalamic and pituitary levels and appears to act by 2 mechanisms: "Fast feedback" is sensitive to the rate of change in cortisol levels, while "slow feedback" is sensitive to the absolute cortisol level. The first mechanism is probably nonnuclear; ie, this phenomenon occurs too rapidly to be explained by the

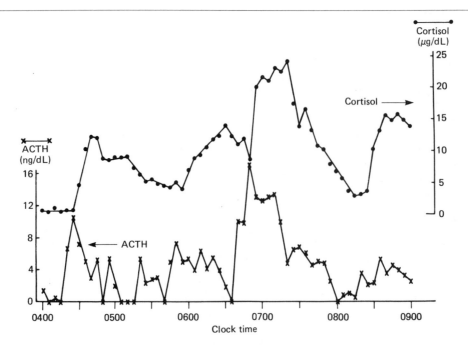

Figure 4–5. The episodic, pulsatile pattern of ACTH secretion and its concordance with cortisol secretion in a normal human subject during the early morning. (Reproduced, with permission, from Gallagher TF et al: ACTH and cortisol secretory patterns in man. *J Clin Endocrinol Metab* 1973;**36**:1058.)

influence of corticosteroids on nuclear transcription of the specific mRNA responsible for ACTH. ''Slow feedback,'' occurring later, may be explained by a nuclear-mediated mechanism and a subsequent decrease in synthesis of ACTH.

GROWTH HORMONE

Biosynthesis

Growth hormone (GH; somatotropin) is a 191-amino-acid polypeptide hormone (MW 21,500) synthesized and secreted by the somatotrophs of the anterior pituitary. It is derived from a larger precursor peptide, preGH (MW 28,000), which is also secreted but which has no physiologic significance. GH, PRL, and human placental lactogen (hPL) probably evolved as a single molecule; although they have subsequently diverged in both structure and functional importance, they continue to share intrinsic lactogenic and growth-promoting activity.

Function

As its name implies, the primary function of growth hormone (somatotropin) is promotion of linear growth. Its basic metabolic effects serve to achieve this result, but most of the growth-promoting effects are mediated by the somatomedins, a family of small peptides produced in the liver. These fascinating insulinlike growth factors are discussed in Chapter 4, Part II.

Growth hormone, via the somatomedins, increases protein synthesis by enhancing amino acid uptake and directly accelerating the transcription and translation of mRNA. In addition, GH tends to decrease protein catabolism by mobilizing fat as a more efficient fuel source: It directly causes the release of fatty acids from adipose tissue and enhances their conversion to acetyl-CoA, from which energy is derived. This protein-sparing effect may be the most important mechanism by which GH promotes growth and development.

GH also affects carbohydrate metabolism. In excess, it decreases carbohydrate utilization and impairs glucose uptake into cells. This GH-induced insulin resistance appears to be due to a postreceptor impairment in insulin action. These events result in glucose intolerance, which in turn stimulates insulin secretion.

Measurement

GH circulates unbound in plasma and has a half-life of 20–50 minutes. The normal adult secretes approximately 400 μg/d; in contrast, young adolescents secrete about 700 μg/d. The availability of specific antisera to GH allows measurement of serum levels and reproducibility in different laboratories. Because the structure of GH is similar to that of hPL, GH antiserum will cross-react, and determinations during pregnancy are therefore unreliable.

The early morning GH concentration in fasting adults is less than 5 ng/mL and usually less than 2 ng/mL. There are no significant sex differences.

Concentrations of somatomedins can now be determined by both radioreceptor assays and radioimmunoassays. Determining the levels of these mediators of GH action may result in more accurate assessment of the biologic activity of GH (see Chapter 4, Part II).

Secretion

The secretion of GH is mediated by 2 hypothalamic hormones: growth hormone–releasing hormone (GRH) and somatostatin (growth hormone–inhibiting hormone). These hypothalamic influences are tightly regulated by an integrated system of neural, meta-

Table 4–2. Factors affecting growth hormone secretion.*

Increase	Decrease†
Physiologic	
Sleep	Postprandial hyperglycemia
Exercise	Elevated free fatty acids
Stress (physical or psychologic)	
Postprandial:	
Hyperaminoacidemia	
Hypoglycemia (relative)	
Pharmacologic	
Hypoglycemia:	Hormones:
Absolute: insulin or 2-deoxyglucose	Somatostatin
Relative: postglucagon	Growth hormone
Hormones:	Progesterone
GRH	Glucocorticoids
Peptide (ACTH, α-MSH, vasopressin)	Neurotransmitters, etc:
Estrogen	Alpha-adrenergic antagonists (phentolamine)
Neurotransmitters, etc:	Beta-adrenergic agonists (isoproterenol)
Alpha-adrenergic agonists (clonidine)	Serotonin antagonists (methysergide)
Beta-adrenergic antagonists (propranolol)	Dopamine antagonists (phenothiazines)
Serotonin precursors	
Dopamine agonists (levodopa, apomorphine, bromocriptine)	
GABA agonists (muscimol)	
Pyrogens (*Pseudomonas* endotoxin)	
Pathologic	
Protein depletion and starvation	Obesity
Anorexia nervosa	Acromegaly: dopamine agonists
Ectopic production of GRH	Hypo- and hyperthyroidism
Chronic renal failure	
Acromegaly:	
TRH	
GnRH	

*Modified and reproduced, with permission, from Frohman LA: Diseases of the anterior pituitary. Chap 7, pp 151–231, in: *Endocrinology and Metabolism.* Felig P et al (editors). McGraw-Hill, 1981.

†Suppressive effects of some factors can be demonstrated only in the presence of a stimulus.

bolic, and hormonal factors. Because neither GRH nor somatostatin can be measured directly, the net result of any factor on GH secretion must be considered as the sum of its effects on these hypothalamic hormones. Table 4–2 summarizes the many factors that affect GH secretion in physiologic, pharmacologic, and pathologic states.

A. GRH: Two peptides (of 40 and 44 amino acids) with potent GH-releasing activity have been isolated from separate pancreatic tumors in patients with acromegaly. Full biologic activity of these releasing factors appears to reside in the 1 – 27 amino acid sequence of the N-terminal portion of the molecule. Human GRH is strikingly similar to many gastrointestinal peptides, including secretin, gastrin, vasoactive intestinal polypeptide (VIP), and gastric inhibitory peptide. Like CRH, GRH has a rather long half-life (50 minutes). The administration of GRH to humans appears to be a useful means of assessing GH secretory reserves and characterizing states of GH deficiency. GRH may also be useful therapeutically for treatment of GH deficiency.

Other peptide hormones such as vasopressin, ACTH, and α-MSH may act as GH-releasing factors when present in pharmacologic amounts. Even thyrotropin- and gonadotropin-releasing hormones (TRH and GnRH) often cause GH secretion in patients with acromegaly; however, it is not certain whether any of these effects are mediated by the hypothalamus or represent direct effects on the somatotroph.

B. Somatostatin: Somatostatin was isolated and characterized in 1973 by Brazeau et al while searching for GRH. Since then, this tetradecapeptide molecule has been found not only in the hypothalamus but also in the D cells of the pancreatic islets and the gastrointestinal mucosa. In addition to its profound inhibitory effect on GH secretion in spite of all provocative stimuli, somatostatin also has important inhibitory influences on many other hormones, including TSH, insulin, glucagon, gastrin, secretin, and VIP.

C. Neural Control: The neural control of basal GH secretion results in irregular and intermittent release associated with sleep and varying with age. Peak levels occur 1 – 4 hours after the onset of sleep (during stages 3 and 4) (Fig 4–6). These nocturnal sleep bursts, which account for nearly 70% of daily GH secretion, are greater in children and tend to decrease with age. Glucose infusion will not suppress this episodic release. Emotional, physical, and chemical stress, including surgery, trauma, exercise, electroshock therapy, and pyrogen administration, provoke GH release; and impairment of secretion, leading to growth failure, has been well documented in children with severe emotional deprivation.

D. Metabolic Control: The metabolic factors affecting GH secretion include all fuel substrates: carbohydrate, protein, and fat. Glucose administration, orally or intravenously, lowers GH in normal subjects and provides a simple physiologic maneuver useful in the diagnosis of acromegaly (see below). In contrast, hypoglycemia stimulates GH release. This effect depends on intracellular glycopenia, since the administration of 2-deoxyglucose (a glucose analog that causes intracellular glucose deficiency) also increases

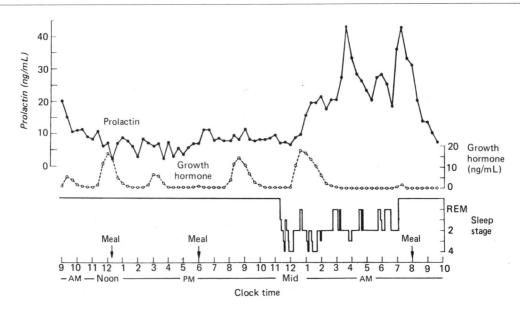

Figure 4–6. Sleep-associated changes in prolactin (PRL) and growth hormone (GH) secretion in humans. Peak levels of GH occur during sleep stages 3 or 4; the increase in PRL is observed 1 –2 hours after sleep begins and is not associated with a specific sleep phase. (Reproduced, with permission, from Sassin JF et al: Human prolactin: 24-hour pattern with increased release during sleep. *Science* 1972;**177**:1205.)

GH. This response to hypoglycemia depends on both the rate of change in blood glucose and the absolute level attained. GH increases have been noted during the recovery phase of a glucose tolerance test as blood glucose declines from the hyperglycemic to the euglycemic range.

A protein meal or intravenous infusion of amino acids (eg, arginine) causes GH release. Paradoxically, states of protein-calorie malnutrition also increase GH, possibly as a result of decreased somatomedin production and lack of inhibitory feedback.

Fatty acids suppress GH responses to certain stimuli, including arginine and hypoglycemia. Fasting stimulates GH secretion, possibly as a means of mobilizing fat as an energy source and preventing protein loss.

E. Effects of Other Hormones: Many hormones also influence GH secretion: Responses to stimuli are blunted in states of cortisol excess and during hypo- and hyperthyroidism; although estrogen enhances GH secretion in response to stimulation, estradiol has been used to treat acromegaly because it decreases somatomedin production.

F. Effects of Neuropharmacologic Agents: Many neurotransmitters and neuropharmacologic agents affect GH secretion. Biogenic amine agonists and antagonists act at the hypothalamic level and alter GRH or somatostatin release. Dopaminergic, alpha-adrenergic, and serotoninergic agents all stimulate GH release.

Dopamine agonists such as levodopa, apomorphine, and bromocriptine increase GH secretion, whereas dopaminergic antagonists such as phenothiazines inhibit GH. The effect of levodopa, a precursor of both norepinephrine and dopamine, may be mediated by its conversion to norepinephrine, since its effect is blocked by the alpha-adrenergic antagonist phentolamine. Moreover, phentolamine suppresses GH release in response to other stimuli such as hypoglycemia, exercise, and arginine, emphasizing the importance of alpha-adrenergic mechanisms in modulating GH secretion.

Beta-adrenergic agonists inhibit GH, and beta-adrenergic antagonists such as propranolol enhance secretion to provocative stimuli.

PROLACTIN

Biosynthesis

Prolactin (PRL) is a 198-amino-acid polypeptide hormone (MW 22,000) synthesized and secreted from the lactotrophs of the anterior pituitary. Despite evolution from an ancestral hormone common to GH and human placental lactogen (hPL), PRL shares only 16% of its residue with the former and 13% with hPL. A precursor molecule, prePRL (MW 40,000–50,000), is also secreted and may constitute 8–20% of the PRL plasma immunoreactivity in normal persons and in patients with PRL-secreting pituitary tumors.

Function

The primary effect of PRL is stimulation of lactation in the postpartum period (see Chapter 17). During pregnancy, PRL secretion increases and, in concert with many other hormones (estrogen, progesterone, hPL, insulin, and cortisol), promotes additional breast development in preparation for milk production. Despite its importance during pregnancy, PRL has not been demonstrated to play a role in the development of normal breast tissue in humans. During pregnancy, estrogen enhances breast development but blunts the effect of PRL on lactation; the decrease in both estrogen and progesterone after parturition allows initiation of lactation. Accordingly, galactorrhea may accompany the discontinuance of oral contraceptives. Although PRL secretion falls in the postpartum period, lactation is maintained by persistent breast suckling.

PRL levels are very high in the fetus and in newborn infants, declining during the first few months of life.

Although PRL does not appear to play a physiologic role in the regulation of gonadal function, hyperprolactinemia in humans leads to hypogonadism. In women, initially there is a shortening of the luteal phase; subsequently, anovulation, oligomenorrhea or amenorrhea, and infertility occur. In men, PRL excess leads to decreased testosterone synthesis and spermatogenesis, which clinically present as decreased libido, impotence, and infertility. The exact mechanisms of PRL inhibition of gonadal function are unclear, but the principal one appears to be alteration of hypothalamic-pituitary control of gonadotropin secretion. Basal LH and FSH levels are normal or subnormal; however, their pulsatile secretion is decreased and the midcycle LH surge is suppressed in women. Gonadotropin reserve, as assessed with GnRH, is usually normal or even exaggerated. PRL may also directly affect gonadal function by inhibiting the action of the gonadotropins on the ovary and testis, although the importance of this mechanism is less clear.

In addition, hyperprolactinemia in humans has been associated with glucose intolerance and hyperinsulinemia, and PRL may play a role as a diabetogenic factor during late pregnancy. Metabolic actions of PRL may occasionally mimic those of GH. Administration of ovine PRL to GH-deficient patients has resulted in positive nitrogen balance, lipolysis, and limited skeletal growth.

Prolactin also influences behavior patterns of numerous animal species. In humans, hyperprolactinemia has been associated with both anxiety and depression.

In several species, PRL is involved in the regulation of osmolality by influencing salt and water metabolism, although this effect has not been observed in humans. In salmon, it is critical for the adjustment from salt to fresh water.

Measurement

Reliable radioimmunoassay techniques for PRL

are available; with specific antisera, there is no cross-reactivity with either GH or hPL.

The PRL secretory rate is approximately 400 μg/d. The hormone is cleared by the liver (75%) and the kidney (25%), and its half-time of disappearance from plasma is about 50 minutes.

Basal levels of PRL in adults vary considerably, with a mean of 9 ng/mL in women and 5 ng/mL in men. The upper range of normal in most laboratories is 15–25 ng/mL. Because of variability in secretion, some authorities recommend collecting blood via an indwelling catheter and pooling 3 samples obtained at 20-minute intervals.

Secretion

The hypothalamic control of PRL secretion, unlike that of the other pituitary hormones, is predominantly inhibitory. Thus, disruption of the hypothalamic-pituitary connection by stalk section, hypothalamic lesions, or pituitary autotransplantation increases PRL secretion. Presently, dopamine is thought to be the primary factor inhibiting PRL release; it has been found in the portal circulation and binds to dopamine receptors in rat lactotrophs. The administration of dopamine or its precursor levodopa, either in vitro or in vivo, inhibits PRL release; drugs that block dopamine receptors (eg, phenothiazines, metoclopramide) or

cause hypothalamic dopamine depletion (reserpine, methyldopa) stimulate PRL release. The physiologic, pathologic, and pharmacologic factors influencing PRL secretion are listed in Table 4–3.

A. Prolactin-Releasing Factors: Hypothalamic extracts also contain fractions that stimulate release of PRL from the lactotroph. The best-studied of these PRL-releasing factors is TRH, which evokes release of PRL at a threshold dose similar to that which stimulates release of TSH. An exaggerated response of both TSH and PRL to TRH is observed in primary hypothyroidism, and their responses are blunted in hyperthyroidism. However, there are several discordant responses, suggesting that TRH is not the only PRL-releasing factor. The PRL increase associated with sleep, during stress, and after nipple stimulation or suckling is not accompanied by an increase in TSH.

Another hypothalamic peptide, VIP, stimulates PRL release in humans. Serotoninergic pathways may also stimulate PRL secretion, as demonstrated by the increased PRL secretion after the administration of serotonin precursors and by the reduction of secretion following treatment with serotonin antagonists. The neurotransmitter gamma-aminobutyric acid (GABA) and cholinergic pathways appear to inhibit PRL release.

B. Episodic and Sleep-Related Secretion: PRL secretion is episodic. An increase is observed 60–90 minutes after sleep begins but, in contrast to GH, is not associated with a specific sleep phase. Peak levels are usually attained between 4 and 7 AM (Fig 4–6). This sleep-associated augmentation of PRL release is not part of a circadian rhythm, like that of ACTH; it is related strictly to the sleeping period regardless of when it occurs during the day.

C. Other Stimuli: A variety of stresses, including surgery, exercise, hypoglycemia, and acute myocardial infarction, cause significant elevation of PRL levels. Nipple stimulation in nonpregnant women also increases PRL. This neurogenic reflex may also occur from chest wall injury such as mechanical trauma, burns, surgery, and herpes zoster of thoracic dermatomes. This reflex discharge of PRL is abolished by denervation of the nipple or by spinal cord or brain stem lesions.

D. Effects of Other Hormones: Many hormones influence PRL release. Estrogens increase the mitotic activity of lactotrophs, and their administration will augment basal and stimulated PRL secretion after 2–3 days of use (an effect that is of special clinical importance in patients with PRL-secreting pituitary adenomas); glucocorticoids tend to suppress TRH-induced PRL secretion; and thyroid hormone administration may blunt the PRL response to TRH.

E. Effects of Pharmacologic Agents: (Table 4–3.) Many pharmacologic agents alter PRL secretion. Dopamine agonists (eg, bromocriptine) decrease secretion, forming the basis for their use in states of PRL excess. Dopamine antagonists (eg, phenothiazines) may augment PRL release and serve as provocative agents in assessing PRL secretory capacity.

Table 4–3. Factors affecting prolactin secretion.

Increase	Decrease
Physiologic	
Pregnancy	
Nursing	
Nipple stimulation	
Exercise	
Stress (hypoglycemia)	
Sleep	
Neonatal	
Pharmacologic	
TRH	Dopamine agonists (levo-
Estrogen	dopa, apomorphine,
VIP	bromocriptine, pergolide)
Dopamine antagonists (pheno-	GABA
thiazines, haloperidol, meto-	
clopramide, reserpine, meth-	
yldopa, amoxapine, opiates)	
Opioids	
Monoamine oxidase inhibitors	
Cimetidine	
Verapamil	
Licorice	
Pathologic	
Pituitary tumors	Pseudohypoparathyroidism
Hypothalamic/pituitary stalk	Pituitary destruction or re-
lesions	moval
Chest wall lesions	
Spinal cord lesions	
Hypothyroidism	
Chronic renal failure	
Severe liver disease	

There is a good correlation between the antipsychotic potency of these drugs and their hyperprolactinemic response, perhaps related to the extent of dopamine antagonism. Serotonin agonists will enhance PRL secretion; serotonin receptor blockers suppress stress- and nursing-associated PRL release.

THYROTROPIN

Biosynthesis

Thyrotropin (thyroid-stimulating hormone, TSH) is a glycoprotein (MW 28,000) composed of 2 non-covalently linked subunits termed alpha and beta. The structure of the alpha subunit of TSH resembles that of the other glycoprotein molecules—FSH, LH, and human chorionic gonadotropin (hCG)—but the beta subunit differs in these glycoproteins and is responsible for their biologic and immunologic specificity. The peptides of these subunits appear to be synthesized separately and united before the carbohydrate groups are attached. The intact molecule is then secreted, as are small amounts of nonlinked subunits.

Function

The beta subunit of TSH attaches to high-affinity receptors in the thyroid, stimulating iodide uptake, hormonogenesis, and release of T_4 and T_3. This occurs through activation of adenylate cyclase and the generation of cAMP. TSH secretion also causes an increase in gland size and vascularity by promoting mRNA and protein synthesis. For a more detailed description of TSH action, see Chapter 7.

Measurement

TSH circulates unbound in the blood with a half-life of 50–60 minutes. Antibodies directed against the beta subunit allow specific measurement by radioimmunoassay. The normal range is usually 1–10 μU/mL; the upper range is lower in some laboratories, depending on the specificity of the antiserum. Since normal subjects may have an undetectable level of TSH, basal measurements may not indicate TSH secretory capacity.

Radioimmunoassay techniques have also been developed for determination of the alpha subunit and TSH-β. The alpha subunit can be detected in about 80% of normals, with a range of 0.5–2 ng/mL. Plasma alpha subunit levels increase after administration of TRH in normal subjects, and basal levels are elevated in primary hypothyroidism and in patients with pure alpha subunit–secreting pituitary adenomas. Free TSH-β is detectable only in primary hypothyroidism and increases in response to TRH in this condition. Since the TSH molecule does not spontaneously dissociate into the free subunits, these data represent secretion of subunits from the pituitary.

Secretion

The secretion of TSH is controlled by both stimulatory (TRH) and inhibitory (somatostatin) influ-

Figure 4–7. Diagram of the hypothalamic-pituitary-thyroid axis, illustrating the negative feedback of thyroid hormones (T_4, T_3) predominantly at the pituitary level. Hypothalamic factors may stimulate (TRH) or suppress (somatostatin) TSH secretion. Estrogen, GH, and glucocorticoids influence the effects of TRH on TSH secretion. (Reproduced, with permission, from Martin JB, Reichlin S, Brown GM: *Clinical Neuroendocrinology.* Davis, 1977.)

ences from the hypothalamus and in addition is modulated by the feedback inhibition of thyroid hormone on the hypothalamic-pituitary axis (Fig 4–7). Thyrotropin-releasing hormone (TRH), a tripeptide, is the major hypothalamic factor in TSH secretion. TRH has been found in the hypothalamus as well as the portal blood; perfusion of pituitary stalk vessels with TRH evokes TSH release, and interruption of the hypothalamic-pituitary portal vessels decreases TSH secretion. The availability of synthetic TRH has led to many studies involving its relationship with TSH secretion.

A. TRH: The response of TSH to TRH is modulated by the circulating concentration of thyroid hormones. Small changes in serum levels (even within the physiologic range) cause substantial alterations in the TSH response to TRH. As shown in Fig 4–8, the administration of T_3 (15 μg) and T_4 (60 μg) to normal persons for 3–4 weeks suppresses the TSH response to TRH despite only small increases in circulating T_3

Figure 4–8. Administration of small doses of T_3 (15 μg) and T_4 (60 μg) to normal subjects inhibits the TSH response to 2 doses (400 μg, left; 25 μg, right) of TRH (protirelin). (Reproduced, with permission, from Snyder PJ, Utiger RD: Inhibition of thyrotropin response to thyrotropin-releasing hormone by small quantities of thyroid hormones. *J Clin Invest* 1972;**51**:2077.)

and T_4 levels. Thus, the secretion of TSH is inversely proportionate to the concentration of thyroid hormone.

The set point (the level at which TSH secretion is maintained) is determined by TRH. Deviations from this set point result in appropriate changes in TSH release. Administration of TRH increases TSH within 2 minutes, and this response is blocked by previous T_3 administration; however, larger doses of TRH may overcome this blockade—suggesting that both T_3 and TRH act at the pituitary level to influence TSH secretion.

B. Somatostatin: This represents an inhibitory hypothalamic factor that may play a role in the physiologic secretion of TSH by augmenting the direct inhibitory effect of thyroid hormone on the thyrotrophs. Infusion of somatostatin blunts the early morning TSH surge and will suppress high levels of TSH in primary hypothyroidism. Hypothyroidism occasionally follows the treatment of GH-deficient children, perhaps because GH therapy would stimulate somatostatin and subsequently decrease TSH.

C. Neural Control: In addition to these hypothalamic influences on TSH secretion, neurally mediated factors may be important. Episodic or pulsatile TSH secretion has been demonstrated, with the highest levels during the early morning and lower levels in the late afternoon and early evening.

D. Temperature and Stress: Because thyroid hormone has such a critical role in the regulation of thermogenesis, the cold-induced increase of TSH in rats is not surprising. Nonetheless, neither acute nor chronic exposure to cold in adult humans has been shown to stimulate TSH release.

The effects of stress could affect TSH at various levels of the hypothalamic-pituitary-thyroid axis or by alteration of peripheral thyroid metabolism; however, except for insulin-induced hypoglycemia, stressful stimuli have not been demonstrated to have a direct influence on the secretion of TSH in humans.

E. Effects of Cortisol and Estrogens: Hormones such as cortisol and estrogens are also involved in TSH regulation. Glucocorticoid excess has been shown to impair the sensitivity of the pituitary to TRH. On the other hand, estrogens increase the sensitivity of the thyrotroph to TRH; women have a greater TSH response to TRH than men do, and pretreatment of men with estradiol will increase their TRH-induced TSH response. (See also Chapter 7.)

GONADOTROPINS: LUTEINIZING HORMONE, FOLLICLE-STIMULATING HORMONE

Biosynthesis

Luteinizing hormone (LH) and follicle-stimulating hormone (FSH) are glycoprotein gonadotropins composed of alpha and beta subunits and secreted by the same cell. The specific beta subunit confers on these hormones their unique biologic activity, as it does with TSH and hCG. The biologic activity of hCG, a placental glycoprotein, closely resembles that of LH. Human menopausal gonadotropin (hMG, menotropins)—an altered mixture of pituitary gonadotropins recovered from the urine of postmenopausal women—is a preparation with FSH-like activity. Menotropins and chorionic gonadotropin are used clinically for induction of spermatogenesis or ovulation (see Chapters 13 and 14).

Function

LH and FSH bind to receptors in the ovary and testis and regulate gonadal function by promoting sex steroid production and gametogenesis. These effects are mediated by the production of cyclic nucleotides.

In men, LH stimulates testosterone production from the interstitial cells of the testes (Leydig cells). For this reason, LH was formerly called interstitial cell–stimulating hormone (ICSH). Maturation of spermatozoa, however, requires both LH and FSH. FSH stimulates testicular growth and enhances the production of an androgen-binding protein by the Sertoli cells, which are a component of the testicular tubule necessary for sustaining the maturing sperm cell. This androgen-binding protein causes high local concentrations of testosterone near the sperm, an essential factor in the development of normal spermatogenesis (see Chapter 13).

In women, LH stimulates estrogen and progesterone production from the ovary. A surge of LH in the mid menstrual cycle is responsible for ovulation, and continued LH secretion subsequently stimulates the corpus luteum to produce progesterone by enhancing the conversion of cholesterol to pregnenolone. Development of the ovarian follicle is largely under FSH control, and the secretion of estrogen from this follicle is dependent on both FSH and LH.

Measurement

LH and FSH are measured by radioimmunoassay utilizing antisera specific for their individual beta subunits, and plasma determinations have made urinary gonadotropin excretion obsolete as an index of pituitary secretion. Despite the availability of radioimmunoassay, problems do exist: Standard and normal ranges vary; values vary markedly because of the episodic nature of secretion; and, because of the great similarities of LH and hCG, cross-reactivity may occur.

Presently, most laboratories utilize an International Reference Preparation (Second IRP/hMG) as a reference standard, and values for LH and FSH are expressed in mIU/mL.

The normal levels of LH and FSH vary with the age of the subject. They are low before puberty and elevated in postmenopausal women. A nocturnal rise of LH in boys and the cyclic secretion of FSH and LH in girls usually herald the onset of puberty before clinical signs are apparent. In women, LH and FSH vary during the menstrual cycle; during the initial phase of the cycle (follicular), LH steadily increases, with a midcycle surge that initiates ovulation. FSH, on the other hand, initially rises and then decreases during the later follicular phase until the midcycle surge, which is concordant with LH. Both LH and FSH levels fall steadily after ovulation (Fig 4–9).

LH and FSH levels in men are similar to those in women during the follicular phase before the ovulatory increase. The alpha subunit, shared by all the pituitary glycoprotein hormones, can also be measured (see TSH) and will rise following GnRH administration. The normal levels of LH and FSH are shown in Table 4–4.

Secretion

The secretion of LH and FSH is controlled by a single stimulatory hypothalamic hormone, gonadotropin-releasing hormone (GnRH). GnRH, isolated by Schally et al in 1972, is a linear decapeptide that stimulates only LH and FSH; it has no effect on other pituitary hormones except in some patients with acromegaly and Cushing's disease, in whom it may augment GH and ACTH secretion, respectively. GnRH maintains basal gonadotropin secretion, generates the phasic release of gonadotropins for ovulation, and determines the onset of puberty.

A. Episodic Secretion: In both males and females, secretion of LH and FSH is episodic, with secretory bursts that occur each hour and are mediated by a concordant episodic release of GnRH. The amplitude of these secretory surges is greater in patients with primary hypogonadism. The pulsatile nature of GnRH release is critical for sustaining gonadotropin secretion. A continuous, prolonged infusion of GnRH in women evokes an initial increase in LH and FSH followed by prolonged suppression of gonadotropin secretion. This phenomenon may be explained by

Table 4–4. Normal gonadotropin responses (± SD) to GnRH (100 μg).

	Mean Maximum Δ LH (mIU/mL)	Mean Maximum Δ FSH (mIU/mL)
Women		
Follicular phase	17 (± 3)	3 (± 1)
Around LH peak	162 (± 49)	8 (± 3)
Luteal phase	49 (± 8)	3 (± 0.4)
Men		
Age 18–40	32 (± 6)	3 (± 1)
Age > 65	23 (± 4)	3 (± 1)

Figure 4–9. The secretory pattern of gonadotropins (LH, FSH) and sex steroids (estradiol, progesterone) during the normal female menstrual cycle. A midcycle surge of LH and FSH, stimulated by the rise in estradiol during the follicular phase, results in ovulation. After ovulation, the luteinized follicle secretes progesterone. (Reproduced, with permission, from Odell WD, Moyer DL: *Physiology of Reproduction.* Mosby, 1971.)

down-regulation of GnRH receptors on the pituitary gonadotrophs. Consequently, long-acting synthetic analogs of GnRH may be used clinically to suppress LH and FSH secretion in conditions such as precocious puberty.

B. Positive Feedback: Circulating sex steroids affect GnRH secretion and thus LH and FSH secretion by both positive and negative (inhibitory) feedback mechanisms. During the menstrual cycle, estrogens provide a positive influence on GnRH effects on LH and FSH secretion, and the rise in estrogen during the follicular phase is the stimulus for the LH and FSH ovulatory surge. This phenomenon suggests that the secretion of estrogen is to some extent influenced by an intrinsic ovarian cycle. Following ovulation, progesterone secretion from the corpus luteum will, in the presence of estrogen, also enhance the GnRH release of LH, but it has an inhibitory effect at the hypothalamic level.

C. Negative Feedback: Negative feedback effects of sex steroids on gonadotropin secretion also occur. In women, primary gonadal failure or menopause results in elevations of LH and FSH, which can be suppressed with long-term, high-dose estrogen therapy. On the other hand, a shorter duration of low-dose estrogen may enhance the LH response to GnRH. In men, primary gonadal failure with low circulating testosterone levels is also associated with elevated

gonadotropins. However, testosterone is not the sole inhibitor of gonadotropin secretion in men, since selective destruction of the tubules (eg, by cyclophosphamide therapy) results in azoospermia and only an elevation of FSH. Inhibin, a polypeptide produced by the testicular tubule, is thought to be the major factor causing negative feedback of FSH secretion.

ENDOCRINOLOGIC EVALUATION OF THE HYPOTHALAMIC-PITUITARY AXIS

The precise assessment of the hypothalamic-pituitary axis has been made possible by radioimmunoassays of the major anterior pituitary hormones and by the introduction of 4 synthetic hypothalamic hormones: TRH (protirelin) and GnRH (gonadorelin), which are available commercially; and the newly synthesized ovine CRH and human GRH (GRH-40 and GRH-44), which are available investigationally. In addition, anterior pituitary function is also evaluated by measuring the specific target gland hormone secretion. Evaluation of the hypothalamic-pituitary axis should be performed carefully and the results interpreted critically, because the diagnosis of secretory abnormalities may indicate lifelong hormonal replacement in states of pituitary insufficiency or the necessity for surgical or radiation therapy in states of pituitary hypersecretion.

This section describes a practical approach to the evaluation of the hypothalamic-pituitary unit. The principles involved in testing each pituitary hormone are described, as well as special situations (eg, drugs, obesity) that may interfere with pituitary function or pituitary testing. Specific protocols for performing and interpreting diagnostic procedures are outlined at the end of this section. The clinical manifestations of either hypo- or hypersecretion of anterior pituitary hormones are discussed in subsequent sections.

EVALUATION OF ACTH

ACTH deficiency leads to adrenocortical insufficiency, characterized by decreased secretion of cortisol and the adrenal androgens; aldosterone secretion, controlled primarily by the renin-angiotensin axis, is usually maintained. Urine metabolites of adrenocorticosteroid secretion—17-hydroxycorticosteroids, 17-ketogenic steroids, and 17-ketosteroids—have long been used in the assessment of adrenal function; however, the development of specific plasma measurements of cortisol as well as other adrenal steroids has made these urine measurements largely obsolete (see Chapter 9).

Plasma ACTH Levels

Although ACTH can be directly determined in plasma, basal measurements are usually unreliable indicators of pituitary secretory reserve, since its short plasma half-life and episodic secretion result in wide fluctuations in plasma levels. Therefore, the interpretation of plasma ACTH levels requires the simultaneous assessment of cortisol secretion by the adrenal cortex. These measurements are of greatest utility in differentiating primary and secondary adrenocortical insufficiency and in establishing the etiology of Cushing's syndrome (see the later section on Cushing's disease and also Chapter 9).

Evaluation of ACTH Deficiency

In evaluating ACTH deficiency, measurement of basal cortisol levels is also unreliable. Although morning cortisol values are usually less than 10 μg/dL in states of diminished pituitary ACTH reserve, such low levels also occur in normal subjects because of the episodic nature of ACTH secretion. In addition, patients with ACTH deficiency following removal of ACTH-secreting pituitary adenomas or withdrawal of synthetic glucocorticoid therapy may have basal cortisol values exceeding 10 μg/dL that fail to increase in response to a stressful stimulus. Consequently, the diagnosis of ACTH hyposecretion (secondary adrenal insufficiency) must be established by provocative testing of the reserve capacity of the hypothalamic-pituitary axis.

Adrenal Stimulation

Since adrenal atrophy develops as a consequence of prolonged ACTH deficiency, the initial and most convenient approach to evaluation of the hypothalamic-pituitary-adrenal axis is assessment of the plasma cortisol response to synthetic ACTH (cosyntropin; Cortrosyn). In normal individuals, injection of cosyntropin (250 μg) causes a rapid increase (within 30 minutes) of cortisol to at least 16– 18 μg/dL, and this response usually correlates with the cortisol response to insulin-induced hypoglycemia and the 11-deoxycortisol rise after administration of metyrapone (discussed below). A subnormal cortisol response to ACTH confirms adrenocortical insufficiency. Although in most circumstances a normal ACTH stimulation test indicates adequate basal ACTH secretion, a normal response does not directly evaluate the ability of the hypothalamic-pituitary axis to respond to stress (see Chapter 9). Thus, patients withdrawn from long-term glucocorticoid therapy may have an adequate increase in cortisol following exogenous ACTH that precedes complete integrity of the hypothalamic-pituitary-adrenal axis. Therefore, such patients should receive glucocorticoids during periods of stress for at least 1 year after steroids are discontinued, unless the hypothalamic-pituitary axis is shown to be responsive to stress as described below.

Pituitary Stimulation

Direct evaluation of pituitary ACTH reserve can be performed by means of insulin-induced hypoglycemia, metyrapone administration, or CRH stimulation. These studies are unnecessary if the cortisol response to rapid ACTH stimulation is subnormal. The former 2 studies do not distinguish hypothalamic (CRH) from pituitary (ACTH) dysfunction; however, CRH stimulation (presently available only for investigational purposes) may be useful for this purpose.

A. Insulin-Induced Hypoglycemia: The stimulus of neuroglycopenia associated with hypoglycemia (blood glucose < 40 mg/dL) evokes a stress-mediated activation of the hypothalamic-pituitary-adrenal axis. Subjects should experience adrenergic symptoms (diaphoresis, tachycardia, weakness, headache) associated with the fall in blood sugar. In normal persons, plasma cortisol increases to more than 18 μg/dL following symptomatic hypoglycemia, indicating normal ACTH reserve. Although plasma ACTH also rises, its determination has not proved to be as useful, since pulsatile secretion requires frequent sampling, and the normal response is not well standardized. Although insulin-induced hypoglycemia most reliably predicts ACTH secretory capacity in times of stress, this procedure requires a physician's presence and is contraindicated in elderly patients, patients with cerebrovascular or cardiovascular disease, and those with seizure disorders. It should be used with caution in patients in whom diminished adrenal reserve is suspected, since severe hypoglycemia may occur and, in these patients, should be preceded by the rapid ACTH stimulation test.

B. Metyrapone Stimulation: Metyrapone administration is an alternative method for assessing ACTH secretory reserve. Metyrapone inhibits 11β-hydroxylase, the enzyme that catalyzes the final step in cortisol biosynthesis (see Chapter 9). The inhibition of cortisol secretion interrupts negative feedback on the hypothalamic-pituitary axis, resulting in a compensatory increase in ACTH. The increase in ACTH secretion stimulates increased steroid biosynthesis proximal to 11β-hydroxylase, and the increase can be detected as an increase in the precursor steroid (11-deoxycortisol) in plasma or by increases in urinary 17-hydroxycorticosteroids, which measure the urinary metabolite of 11-deoxycortisol. Two methods are available. The overnight test is preferred because of its simplicity; it is performed by administering 2–3 g of metyrapone orally at midnight. Plasma 11-deoxycortisol is determined the following morning and rises to greater than 7 μg/dL in normal individuals. Again, the test should be used cautiously in patients with suspected adrenal insufficiency and should be preceded by a rapid ACTH stimulation test (see above). Metyrapone may also be given in doses of 750 mg every 4 hours for 24 hours, with collection of urine for 17-hydroxycorticosteroid determination before, during, and for 24 hours after metyrapone. The urinary 17-hydroxycorticosteroid concentration doubles in normal individuals. The test is cumbersome because of the difficulty in collecting 24-hour urine samples, and there is a danger of provoking symptomatic adrenal insufficiency because of the large metyrapone doses.

C. CRH Stimulation: Ovine CRH has been administered intravenously as a means of assessing ACTH secretory dynamics. In normal subjects, CRH (1 μg/kg) provokes a peak ACTH response within 15 minutes and a peak cortisol response within 30–60 minutes. This dose may be associated with mild flushing, occasional shortness of breath, tachycardia, and hypotension. Patients with primary adrenal insufficiency have elevated basal ACTH levels and exaggerated responses to CRH. Secondary adrenal insufficiency results in an absent ACTH response to CRH in patients with pituitary corticotroph destruction; however, hypothalamic dysfunction causes a prolonged and augmented ACTH response to CRH with a delayed peak. This test may also be useful in the differential diagnosis of ACTH-dependent Cushing's syndrome (see below).

ACTH Hypersecretion

ACTH hypersecretion is manifested by adrenocortical hyperfunction (Cushing's syndrome). The evaluation of ACTH excess relies upon dexamethasone suppression of plasma cortisol and urine steroids. Basal urine free cortisol and plasma ACTH determinations are also helpful. The diagnosis and differential diagnosis of ACTH hypersecretion are outlined in a later section on Cushing's disease and also in Chapter 9.

EVALUATION OF GROWTH HORMONE

The evaluation of GH secretory reserve is important in the assessment of children with short stature and in adults with suspected hypopituitarism. Because basal levels of GH are usually low and do not distinguish between normal and GH-deficient conditions, it is necessary to perform provocative tests.

Insulin-Induced Hypoglycemia

The most reliable stimulus of GH secretion is insulin-induced hypoglycemia. In normal individuals, GH levels will increase to more than 10 ng/mL after adequate hypoglycemia is achieved. Since 10–20% of normal individuals fail to respond to hypoglycemia, other stimulatory tests may be necessary.

Tests With Levodopa, Arginine, Apomorphine, & Other Stimuli

GH will also rise after oral administration of 500 mg of levodopa, a precursor of dopamine and norepinephrine that readily crosses the blood-brain barrier. About 80% of normal subjects have a GH response greater than 6 ng/mL, and the mean maximal response is 28 ng/mL. This test is safer than insulin-induced hypoglycemia in older patients. An infusion of arginine (0.5 g/kg to a maximum of 30 g) will raise GH in 70% of normal individuals. Pretreatment with estrogen will enhance this response in many of the nonresponders, most of whom are men. Apomorphine, a derivative of morphine and a specific dopamine agonist, given subcutaneously in a subemetic dose (0.75 mg), will increase GH by more than 6 ng/mL in most patients and is preferred by some investigators over levodopa. Other stimuli, such as propranolol and glucagon, have also been utilized in considering GH secretory capacity.

GRH Test

Both forms of human pancreatic GRH (GRH-40 and GRH-44) have been used investigationally to evaluate GH secretory capacity. A dose of GRH (1 μg/kg) promptly stimulates GH; the mean peak is 10–15 ng/mL at 30–60 minutes in normal subjects. There is usually a small increase in somatomedin-C levels 24 hours after the administration of GRH. This test may be helpful in some patients in differentiating hypothalamic and pituitary causes of GH deficiency.

Exercise Test

In children with possible GH deficiency, an exercise test requiring 15 minutes of rapid stair-climbing is a convenient way to assess GH secretion. Hypogonadal or prepubertal children are usually pretreated for 3 days with estrogen, and an increment of greater than 5 ng/mL constitutes a normal response.

GH Hypersecretion

The evaluation of GH hypersecretion is discussed in the section on acromegaly and is most conveniently assessed by suppression testing with oral glucose.

Table 4–5. Normal responses of TSH and prolactin to TRH (500 µg).*

TSH (µU/mL)	
Maximum Δ TSH	
Women and men age < 40	≥ 6
Men age 40–79	≥ 2
Time of maximum Δ TSH (min)	≤ 45
Prolactin (ng/mL)	
Basal, men and women	< 15
Maximum Δ prolactin	
Men age 20–39	15–40
Men age 40–59	10–50
Men age 60–79	5–90
Women age 20–39	30–120
Women age 40–59	20–120
Women age 60–79	10–100

*Reproduced, with permission, from Snyder PJ et al: Diagnostic value of thyrotrophin-releasing hormone in pituitary and hypothalamic diseases: Assessment of thyrotrophin and prolactin secretion in 100 patients. *Ann Intern Med* 1974;81:751.

EVALUATION OF PROLACTIN

PRL secretion by the pituitary is the most resistant to local damage, and demonstration of decreased PRL secretory reserve indicates severe intrinsic pituitary disease. The evaluation of PRL secretion must also rely upon provocative testing, since basal PRL levels in normal individuals may be at the lower limits of assay detectability.

Prolactin Reserve

The administration of TRH (500 µg intravenously) is the simplest and most reliable means of assessing PRL reserve. Although the response of PRL to TRH varies somewhat according to sex and age (Table 4– 5), PRL levels usually increase 2-fold 15– 30 minutes after TRH administration. Chlorpromazine, a dopamine antagonist that abolishes the normal tonic inhibition of PRL secretion, is another agent that can be utilized to test PRL secretion. A 2- to 3-fold increase in PRL occurs in normal subjects after intramuscular administration of 25 mg of chlorpromazine. In addition, insulin-induced hypoglycemia will evoke a stress-related increase in PRL.

PRL Hypersecretion

PRL hypersecretion is a common endocrine problem, and differential diagnosis is often difficult. Clinical evaluation of hyperprolactinemia is discussed in the section on prolactinomas.

EVALUATION OF TSH

Basal Measurements

The laboratory evaluation of TSH secretory reserve begins with an assessment of target gland secretion; thyroid function tests (T$_4$RIA, T$_3$RIA, free thyroxine index [FT$_4$I]) should be performed. Normal thyroid function studies in a clinically euthyroid patient indicate adequate TSH secretion, and no further studies are warranted. Laboratory evidence of hypothyroidism requires a TSH level, and with primary thyroid gland failure, the TSH level will be elevated. Low or normal TSH suggests hypothalamic-pituitary dysfunction.

TRH Test

The introduction of synthetic TRH (protirelin) has made it possible to evaluate the complete hypothalamic-pituitary-thyroid axis. The TRH test has proved most useful in the evaluation of Graves' disease and thyrotoxicosis (see Chapter 7). In normal subjects, protirelin (500 µg intravenously) produces an increase of TSH of at least 6 µU/mL within 15– 30 minutes. In patients with primary hypothyroidism, an exaggerated TSH response to protirelin is observed; however, this test is helpful only in those few patients with primary hypothyroidism who have normal basal TSH levels. An impaired or absent TSH response in hypothyroid patients implicates hypothalamic-pituitary failure. Some investigators believe that the TRH test can distinguish a hypothalamic disorder (tertiary hypothyroidism) from intrinsic pituitary disease (secondary hypothyroidism). Patients with hypothalamic disease often show a delayed TSH response (60– 120 minutes) to TRH (Fig 4– 10) and, less commonly, an

Figure 4–10. The pattern of TSH secretion in response to intravenous TRH (protirelin) (500 µg) in patients with primary (thyroidal), secondary (pituitary), and tertiary (hypothalamic) hypothyroidism. Hatched area indicates normal range. (Reproduced, with permission, from Utiger RD: Thyrotropin releasing hormone: Physiology and clinical use. *Thyroid Today* [March] 1979;2:1.)

exaggerated TSH increase. Unlike gonadotropic function, prolonged TRH deficiency does not impair TSH responsiveness. An intrinsic pituitary disorder characteristically results in a subnormal or absent TSH response to TRH; however, many hypothyroid patients with documented pituitary disease have, in fact, normal responses to TRH or responses that resemble hypothalamic dysfunction. Accordingly, the TRH test is not a reliable means of differentiating pituitary from hypothalamic disease.

Responsiveness to TRH is often impaired in patients with hypothalamic pituitary disease (eg, acromegaly, Cushing's syndrome) who are euthyroid. Since GH or cortisol excess may decrease the TSH response to TRH, an absent response does not always indicate destruction of thyrotrophs. (See also Chapter 7.)

EVALUATION OF LH & FSH

Testosterone & Estrogen Levels

The evaluation of gonadotropin function also requires assessment of target gland secretory function, and measurement of gonadal steroids (testosterone in men, estradiol in women) is useful in the diagnosis of hypogonadism. In women, the presence of regular menstrual cycles is strong evidence that the hypothalamic-pituitary-gonadal axis is intact. Estradiol levels rarely fall below 50 pg/mL, even during the early follicular phase. A level of less than 30 pg/mL in the presence of oligomenorrhea or amenorrhea is indicative of gonadal failure. In men, serum testosterone (normal range, 3–9 ng/mL) is a sensitive index of gonadal function.

LH & FSH Levels

In the presence of gonadal insufficiency, high LH and FSH levels are a sign of primary gonadal disease; low or normal LH and FSH suggest hypothalamic-pituitary dysfunction (hypogonadotropic hypogonadism).

GnRH Test

LH and FSH secretory reserves may be assessed with the use of synthetic GnRH (gonadorelin, Factrel). Administration of GnRH (100 μg intravenously) causes a prompt increase in plasma LH and a lesser and slower increase in FSH (for normal responses, see Table 4–4). The LH response to GnRH is lowest during the follicular phase and greatest during the ovulatory surge. Normal subjects may occasionally have no FSH response to GnRH. On the other hand, in prepubertal children and in some patients with hyperprolactinemia, the FSH response is greater than that of LH.

A single GnRH test does not distinguish hypothalamic from pituitary disease in patients with hypogonadotropic hypogonadism. Patients with disturbances of the hypothalamus and pituitary may, in fact, have an absent, normal, or exaggerated gonadotropin response to GnRH. Hypothalamic disease with long-standing GnRH deficiency results in an absent LH response to GnRH, but normal responsiveness may be restored with more prolonged and intermittent stimulation. Such a return of responsiveness provides evidence for intact pituitary gonadotrophs.

Clomiphene Test

The hypothalamic-pituitary-gonadal axis can also be assessed by utilizing clomiphene citrate, an antiestrogen that blocks estrogen receptors, causing a state of functional estrogen deficiency resulting in GnRH and gonadotropin release. The occurrence of a normal menstrual period approximately 12 days after administration of the drug or evidence of ovulation by basal body temperature constitutes a normal response. Failure of LH levels to increase after 5–10 days of clomiphene in a patient with a normal GnRH test suggests hypothalamic disease.

PROBLEMS IN EVALUATION OF THE HYPOTHALAMIC-PITUITARY AXIS

Several metabolic abnormalities must be taken into account when assessing the hypothalamic-pituitary axis. This section briefly outlines some of the disorders that may cause confusion and lead to misinterpretation of pituitary function tests. The effects of drugs are described in the next section.

Obesity

GH dynamics are impaired in many obese patients; all provocative stimuli, including insulin-induced hypoglycemia, arginine, levodopa, and glucagon plus propranolol, often fail to provoke GH secretion. Obesity may increase urinary 17-hydroxycorticosteroid levels and the cortisol secretory rate, but plasma cortisol demonstrates normal diurnal variation and responds to hypoglycemia. In addition, obese patients occasionally fail to suppress plasma cortisol appropriately after the 1-mg overnight dexamethasone suppression test.

Diabetes

Although glucose normally suppresses GH secretion, most type I diabetics have normal or elevated GH levels that often do not rise in response to hypoglycemia or arginine. Levodopa will increase GH in some diabetic patients, and even a dopamine infusion (which produces no GH change in normal subjects, since it does not cross the blood-brain barrier) will stimulate GH in diabetics.

Uremia

Basal levels of GH, PRL, LH, FSH, TSH, and free cortisol tend to be elevated, for the most part owing to prolongation of their plasma half-life. GH may paradoxically increase following glucose administration and is often hyperresponsive to a hypoglycemic stimulus. Although the administration of TRH (protirelin) has no effect on GH secretion in normal subjects, the drug may increase GH in patients with chronic renal failure. The response of PRL to TRH is blunted and prolonged. Gonadotropin response to synthetic GnRH usually remains intact. Dexamethasone suppression of cortisol may be impaired.

Starvation/Anorexia Nervosa

GH secretion increases with fasting and malnutrition, and such conditions may cause a paradoxical increase in GH following glucose administration. Severe starvation, such as occurs in patients with anorexia nervosa, may result in low levels of gonadal steroids. LH and FSH responses to GnRH may be intact despite a state of functional hypogonadotropic hypogonadism. Cortisol levels may be increased and fail to suppress adequately with dexamethasone. PRL and TSH dynamics are usually normal despite a marked decrease in circulating total thyroid hormones (see Chapter 7).

Depression

Depression may alter the ability of dexamethasone to suppress plasma cortisol and may elevate cortisol secretion; the response to insulin-induced hypoglycemia usually remains intact. Some depressed patients also have abnormal GH dynamics: TRH may increase GH, and hypoglycemia or levodopa may fail to increase GH. These patients may also show blunted TSH responses to TRH.

EFFECTS OF PHARMACOLOGIC AGENTS ON HYPOTHALAMIC-PITUITARY FUNCTION

Glucocorticoid excess impairs the GH response to hypoglycemia, the TSH response to TRH, and the LH response to GnRH. Estrogens tend to augment GH dynamics as well as the PRL and TSH response to TRH. Estrogens increase plasma cortisol secondary to a rise in corticosteroid-binding globulin and may result in inadequate suppression with dexamethasone. Estrogens may also produce a subnormal response to metyrapone testing by accelerating the metabolism of metyrapone.

Phenytoin enhances the metabolism of metyrapone and dexamethasone, making studies with these agents difficult to interpret. Phenothiazines may blunt the GH response to hypoglycemia and levodopa and frequently cause hyperprolactinemia. The many other pharmacologic agents that increase PRL secretion are listed in Table 4–3.

Narcotics, including heroin, morphine, and methadone, may all raise PRL levels and suppress GH and cortisol responses to hypoglycemia.

In chronic alcoholics, alcohol excess or withdrawal may increase cortisol levels and cause inadequate dexamethasone suppression and an impaired cortisol increase after hypoglycemia.

Many drugs interfere with urine steroid collection (17-hydroxycorticosteroids and 17-ketosteroids), but since these measurements are no longer essential, such problems can be avoided.

ENDOCRINE TESTS OF HYPOTHALAMIC-PITUITARY FUNCTION

The methods for performing endocrine tests and the normal responses are described below. The indications for and the clinical utility of these procedures are described in the preceding section and will be mentioned again in the section on pituitary and hypothalamic disorders. Some of these procedures may be performed simultaneously; eg, the administration of insulin, TRH, and GnRH provides combined stimulation of the major anterior pituitary hormones. Alternatively, the rapid ACTH stimulation test may be combined with TRH and GnRH stimulation. When performed simultaneously, the methods, doses, sampling times, and interpretation of the various hormonal responses are identical with those described below for the individual procedures.

The CRH and GRH tests, which are also described below, are investigational at present but will be clinically relevant in the future.

Rapid ACTH Stimulation Test (Cortrosyn Test)

Method: Administer synthetic $ACTH_{1-24}$ (cosyntropin; Cortrosyn), 250 μg intravenously or intramuscularly.

Sample collection: Obtain samples for plasma cortisol at 0 and 30 minutes or at 0 and 60 minutes.

Possible side effects; contraindications: Rare allergic reactions have been reported.

Interpretation: A normal response is an increment in plasma cortisol of 7 μg/dL and a peak level of greater than 18 μg/dL when cortisol is measured fluorimetrically. When radioimmunoassays and protein-binding radioassays are utilized, the normal response is a peak cortisol level greater than 16 μg/dL.

Insulin Hypoglycemia Test

Method: Give nothing by mouth after midnight. Start an intravenous infusion with normal saline solution. Crystalline zinc (regular) insulin is given intravenously in a dose sufficient to cause adequate hypoglycemia (blood glucose < 40 mg/dL). The dose is 0.1–0.15 unit/kg (normal subjects); 0.2–0.3 unit/kg (obese subjects or those with Cushing's syndrome or acromegaly); 0.05 unit/kg (patients with suspected hypopituitarism).

Sample collection: Collect blood for glucose determinations every 15 minutes during the study. Samples for GH and cortisol are obtained at 0, 30, 45, 60, 75, and 90 minutes.

Possible side effects; contraindications: A physician must be in attendance. Symptomatic hypoglycemia (diaphoresis, headache, tachycardia, weakness) is necessary for adequate stimulation and occurs 20–35 minutes after insulin is administered in most patients. If severe central nervous system signs or symptoms occur, intravenous glucose (25–50 mL of 50% glucose) should be given immediately; otherwise, the test can be terminated with a meal or oral glucose. This test is contraindicated in the elderly or in patients with cardiovascular or cerebrovascular disease and seizure disorders.

Interpretation: Symptomatic hypoglycemia and a fall in blood glucose to less than 40 mg/dL will increase GH to a maximal level greater than 10 ng/mL; some investigators regard an increment of 6 ng/mL as normal. Plasma cortisol should increase to a peak level of at least 18 μg/dL.

Metyrapone Tests
Method:
Overnight test: Metyrapone is given orally between 11 and 12 PM with a snack to minimize gastrointestinal discomfort. The dose is 2 g for patients weighing less than 70 kg; 2.5 g for patients weighing 70–90 kg; and 3 g for patients weighing over 90 kg.
Three-day test: Twenty-four-hour urine collections are made for 3 consecutive days, and metyrapone, 750 mg, is given every 4 hours for 6 doses on the second day.
Sample Collection:
Overnight test: Blood for plasma 11-deoxycortisol and cortisol determinations is obtained at 8 AM the morning after metyrapone is given.
Three-day test: The 3 consecutive 24-hour urine samples are analyzed for 17-hydroxycorticosteroids and creatinine determinations.
Possible side effects; contraindications: Gastrointestinal upset may occur. Adrenal insufficiency may occur. Metyrapone should not be used in sick patients or those in whom primary adrenal insufficiency is suspected.
Interpretation:
Overnight test: Serum 11-deoxycortisol should increase to greater than 7 μg/dL. Cortisol should be less than 10 μg/dL in order to ensure adequate inhibition of 11β-hydroxylation.
Three-day test: Urine 17-hydroxycorticosteroids should double on day 2 or 3.

Levodopa Test
Method: The patient should be fasting and at bed rest after midnight. Levodopa, 500 mg, is given by mouth.
Sample collection: Blood samples for plasma GH determinations are obtained at 0, 30, and 60 minutes.
Possible side effects; contraindications: Nausea and vomiting may occur 45–60 minutes after levodopa is given. This test is safer than the insulin hypoglycemia test in older patients.

Interpretation: A normal response is a maximal level of GH greater than 6 ng/mL; however, the peak response is usually more than 20 ng/mL.

Arginine Infusion Test
Method: The patient should be fasting after midnight. Give arginine hydrochloride, 0.5 g/kg intravenously, up to a maximum of 30 g over 30 minutes. Pretreatment with estrogen in postmenopausal women and in men can also be done.
Sample collection: Blood for plasma GH determinations is collected at 0, 30, 60, 90, and 120 minutes. Arginine infusion also stimulates insulin and glucagon.
Possible side effects; contraindications: Nausea and vomiting may occur. This test is contraindicated in patients with severe liver disease, renal disease, or acidosis.
Interpretation: The response is greater in women than in men. The lower limit of normal for the peak GH response is 6 ng/mL in non–estrogen-treated patients and 10 ng/mL in estrogen-treated patients and premenopausal women.

Apomorphine Test
Method: The patient should be fasting. Give apomorphine, 0.75 mg subcutaneously.
Sample collection: Blood samples for GH determinations are obtained at 0, 30, 45, 60, and 90 minutes.
Possible side effects; contraindications: Nausea or vomiting occurs in 10–15% of patients.
Interpretation: An increase in GH to greater than 6 ng/mL is normal. The peak response usually occurs at 45–60 minutes during the test.

Glucose–Growth Hormone Suppression Test
Method: The patient should be fasting after midnight. Give glucose, 75–100 g orally.
Sample collection: GH and glucose should be determined at 0, 30, and 60 minutes after glucose administration.
Possible side effects; contraindications: Patients may complain of nausea after the large glucose load.
Interpretation: GH levels are suppressed to less than 5 ng/mL in normal subjects. Failure of adequate suppression or a paradoxical rise may be seen in acromegaly, starvation, protein-calorie malnutrition, and anorexia nervosa.

TRH Test
Method: Fasting is not required, but since nausea may occur, it is preferred. Give protirelin, 500 μg intravenously over 15–30 seconds. The patient should be kept supine, since slight hypertension or hypotension may occur. Protirelin (Thypinone, Relefact TRH) is supplied in vials of 500 μg, although 400 μg will evoke normal responses.

Sample collection: Blood for determinations of plasma TSH, PRL, or GH (in the case of suspected acromegaly) is obtained at 0, 30, and 60 minutes; a 90-minute sample for TSH may be necessary in cases of suspected tertiary hypothyroidism. An abbreviated test utilizes samples taken at 0 and 30 minutes only, but the additional 60-minute specimen is more reliable.

Possible side effects; contraindications: No serious complications have been reported. Most patients complain of a sensation of urinary urgency and a metallic taste in the mouth; other symptoms include flushing, palpitations, and nausea. These symptoms occur within 1–2 minutes of the injection and last 5 minutes at most.

Interpretation: Normal TSH and PRL responses to TRH are outlined in Table 4–5. GH should not increase in normal subjects.

Chlorpromazine Test

Method: Chlorpromazine, 25 mg, is given intramuscularly to a fasting, resting patient.

Sample collection: Blood for PRL determinations is taken at 0, 30, 60, and 90 minutes.

Possible side effects; contraindications: Drowsiness and mild hypotension occur in a few patients.

Interpretation: PRL levels increase 2–3 times above the basal level.

GnRH Test

Method: The patient should be at rest but need not be fasting. Give GnRH (gonadorelin), 100 μg intravenously, over 15 seconds.

Sample collection: Blood samples for LH and FSH determinations are taken at 0, 30, and 60 minutes. Since the FSH response is somewhat delayed, a 90-minute specimen may be necessary.

Possible side effects; contraindications: Side effects are rare, and no contraindications have been found.

Interpretation: This response is dependent on sex and time of the menstrual cycle. Table 4–4 illustrates the mean maximal change in LH and FSH after GnRH administration. An increase of LH of 10–20 mIU/mL is considered to be normal; FSH usually responds more slowly and less markedly. FSH may not increase even in normal subjects.

Clomiphene Test

Method: Clomiphene is administered orally. For women, give 100 mg daily for 5 days (begin on day 5 of the cycle if the patient is menstruating); for men, give 100 mg daily for 7–10 days.

Sample collection: Blood for LH and FSH determinations is drawn before and after clomiphene is given.

Possible side effects; contraindications: This drug may, of course, stimulate ovulation, and women should be warned accordingly.

Interpretation: In women, LH and FSH levels peak on the fifth day to a level above the normal range. After the fifth day, LH and FSH levels decline. In men, LH should double after 1 week; FSH will also increase, but to a lesser extent. (See Table 4–4 for normal values.)

CRH Test

Method: CRH (1μg/kg) is given intravenously as a bolus injection.

Sample collection: Blood samples for ACTH and cortisol are taken at 0, 15, 30, and 60 minutes.

Possible side effects; contraindications: Flushing often occurs. Transient tachycardia and hypotension have also been reported.

Interpretation: The ACTH response is dependent on the assay utilized and occurs 15 minutes after CRH is administered. The peak cortisol response occurs at 30–60 minutes and is usually greater than 10 μg/dL.

GRH Test

Method: GRH (1 μg/kg) is given intravenously as a bolus injection.

Sample collection: Blood samples for GH are drawn at 0, 30, and 60 minutes.

Possible side effects; contraindications: Mild flushing and a metallic taste or smell occur in a few patients.

Interpretation: The range of normal responses is wide. Most patients have a peak GH response of greater than 10 ng/mL at 30–60 minutes.

NEURORADIOLOGIC EVALUATION OF THE SELLA TURCICA

Intrasellar or parasellar disease is usually suspected on clinical grounds. Thus, symptoms of pituitary hormone excess or deficiency, headache, or visual disturbance may lead the clinician to consider a hypothalamic-pituitary disorder. Although accurate neuroradiologic assessment of the sella turcica is essential in confirming the existence and defining the extent of hypothalamic-pituitary lesions, the diagnosis of such lesions should be primarily endocrinologic and based on a thorough clinical and biochemical evaluation of pituitary function. This is because variability of sellar anatomy in the normal population may lead to false-positive interpretations. Furthermore, patients with pituitary microadenomas may have normal neuroradiologic studies. Roentgenographic studies of the sella must be interpreted in light of the fact that 10–20% of the general population harbor pituitary microadenomas.

This section describes current neuroradiologic procedures; however, the development of high-resolution computed tomography with thin-slice (1.5-mm collimation) techniques and the use of metrizamide cisternography have superseded other neuroradiologic tests in evaluation of the sella turcica.

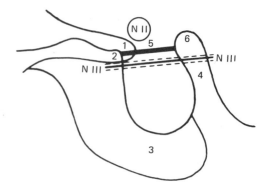

Figure 4–11. *Left:* Lateral radiograph of the normal sella turcica. (Reproduced, with permission, from Martin JB, Reichlin S, Brown GM: *Clinical Neuroendocrinology.* Davis, 1977.) *Right:* Diagram of the radiologic landmarks and relationships of the sella turcica and pituitary: (1) anterior clinoid process; (2) tuberculum sellae; (3) sphenoid sinus; (4) dorsum sellae; (5) diaphragma sellae; (6) posterior clinoid process; N II, optic chiasm; N III, oculomotor nerve lying lateral to the sella turcica. (Reproduced, with permission, from Bloch HJ, Joplin GF: Some aspects of the radiological anatomy of the pituitary gland and its relationship to surrounding structures. *Br J Radiol* 1959;**32**:527.)

Plain Films of the Sella Turcica

A. Radiologic Anatomy: The initial and most important radiographic examination of the sella is simply a coned-down lateral projection accompanied by a Caldwell frontal projection. These views provide the clinician with an impression of the size and shape of the sella. The tuberculum sellae, the anterior clinoid processes, the sphenoid sinus, the floor of the dorsum sellae, and the posterior clinoid processes can be easily identified (Fig 4–11). Although most neuroradiologists and endocrinologists rely on their overall impression of the sella, specific measurements can be made, and normal criteria have been established. The anteroposterior diameter (maximum distance from anterior concavity of the sella to the anterior rim of the dorsum) varies from 5 to 16 mm, with an average of 10 mm; the depth, measured as the greatest distance from the floor to a perpendicular line drawn between the tuberculum sellae and the top of the dorsum sellae, has an upper limit of normal of 13 mm; the width (determined from the frontal projection) is normally 10–15 mm.

The volume of the sella can be calculated using the DiChiro formula (anteroposterior diameter × depth × width ÷ 2). The mean volume of the normal sella is 600 mm³; a volume that exceeds 1100 mm³ is considered abnormal.

B. Variability of Sellar Shape: The normal sella may be oval, round, or flat. Pituitary tumors may produce focal erosion and distortion of the sella without increasing its volume; however, because of the variety of shapes seen in patients without clinical pituitary disease, such focal changes must be interpreted cautiously. Pituitary adenomas, which are predominantly lateral, may cause depression and expansion of only one side of the sellar floor, leading to a "double floor" appearance of the sella turcica on lateral projection.

C. Calcification: Calcification may also occur in the parasellar region. In older persons, the internal carotid artery may calcify, causing an arch of calcification in the center of the sella. Bridging calcification between the anterior and posterior clinoids occasionally occurs as a normal variant. Tumors such as craniopharyngiomas (70%) and parasellar meningiomas (30%) may calcify. In addition, pituitary adenomas that have undergone hemorrhagic necrosis may calcify, resulting in a "pituitary stone."

D. Tumors: Small pituitary tumors (microadenomas) do not increase the volume of the sella, and the size of the sella does not always correlate well with the pituitary size (eg, empty sella). Consequently, normal plain x-rays of the sella do not, by any means, prove or exclude a pituitary disorder. Nonetheless, the finding of an enlarged sella turcica on plain x-rays is a strong indication for further clinical investigation. The differential diagnosis of an enlarged sella turcica is discussed below.

High-Resolution Computed Tomography (Thin-Slice Technique)

The introduction of high-resolution computed to-

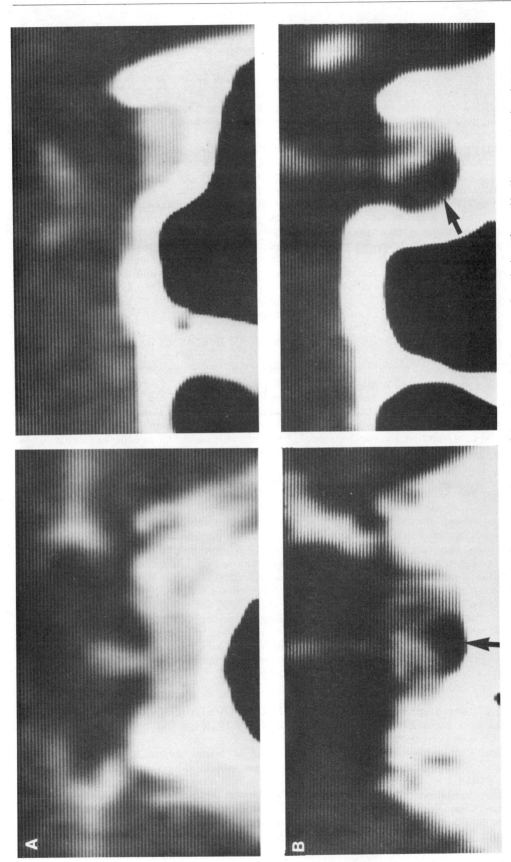

Figure 4–12. CT scans of normal and abnormal pituitary glands. The sections shown are computer re-formations derived from 1.5-mm axial sections through the sella turcica. Coronal re-formations are shown on the left and sagittal ones on the right. *A:* Normal pituitary gland. The upper border is flat; the pituitary stalk (seen on the coronal section) is midline; and the gland is relatively homogeneous in density. The lateral margins of the sella turcica (see coronal section) are formed by the contrast-enhancing cavernous sinuses. *B:* In a patient with Cushing's disease, a 3- to 4-mm pituitary adenoma is visualized as a low-density lesion in the anterior inferior portion of the anterior lobe (arrows).

mography with a thin-slice technique (1.5-mm collimation) using intravenous contrast media has altered the approach to parasellar disease. Invasive procedures such as arteriography or pneumoencephalography now have few, if any, applications in the diagnosis of pituitary disease. CT scanning now permits precise visualization of the pituitary gland itself and can define small hypothalamic and pituitary lesions. In addition, nonosseous structures such as the optic chiasm and pituitary stalk can be easily identified on CT scans reformatted in coronal and sagittal images (Fig 4–12).

A. Microadenomas and Empty Sella Syndrome: The superior margin of the normal pituitary gland is flat or concave, and the height of the gland ranges from 3 to 8 mm. The pituitary gland may occasionally be 10–12 mm in height in normal menstruating young women. The presence of a convex superior margin with increased height of the gland is one of 2 major criteria used to diagnose pituitary microadenomas. The second finding is a focal alteration in the enhancement of the gland with intravenous contrast. Most pituitary adenomas appear as "low-density" areas when compared with the surrounding normal pituitary tissue; less commonly, they are contrast-enhancing. High-resolution CT scanning is also a valuable tool in the diagnosis of empty sella syndrome, determination of extrasellar extension of pituitary adenomas, and diagnosis of hypothalamic tumors and other parasellar lesions.

B. Caution in Interpretation: Despite this technologic advance, high-resolution CT scans must be interpreted with caution. Nonhomogeneous enhancement of the gland is demonstrated in almost 20% of patients who have had incidental high-resolution scans but no clinical pituitary disease. These abnormalities may, of course, represent the clinically insignificant pituitary abnormalities present in 15–20% of the general population, and they may also be due to small intrapituitary cysts, which usually occur in the pars intermedia. Artifacts within the sella turcica associated with the bones of the skull base may also result in misinterpretation of CT scans. Finally, the authors have seen a number of patients with pituitary microadenomas who have had normal high-resolution CT scans. Therefore, despite increased accuracy of neuroradiologic diagnosis, the presence or absence of a small pituitary tumor and the decision concerning its treatment must be based on the entire clinical picture.

Metrizamide Cisternography

Metrizamide is a nonionic water-soluble compound with low neurotoxicity that can be injected into the cerebrospinal fluid and provides excellent anatomic delineation of the parasellar structures. Its use with high-resolution CT scanning has eliminated the need for pneumoencephalography because of its greater technical ease and safety. Headaches occur in 10–15% of patients and nausea in about 20% of patients following its use.

Since the newer high-resolution CT scanners can detect the presence of empty sella syndrome and pituitary adenomas with suprasellar extension, the use of metrizamide is required only in the minority of patients in whom CT scanning alone does not clearly establish a diagnosis, eg, patients with unexplained visual defects suggesting chiasmal compression or those in whom CT scanning cannot differentiate the empty sella syndrome from a low-density adenoma.

Sellar Polytomography

Complex motion tomography (hypocycloidal polytomography) of the sella turcica was formerly utilized as a means of detecting intrasellar abnormalities; however, many studies have demonstrated the poor sensitivity and low predictive value of this procedure. Even in patients in whom pituitary hypersecreting tumors are biochemically present, the degree and location of tomographic abnormalities do not correlate positively with the size or location of the tumors at surgery. Therefore, sellar polytomography has no place in the evaluation of pituitary disorders.

Magnetic Resonance Imaging (MRI)

Studies are now being performed to evaluate the role of magnetic resonance imaging in the evaluation of pituitary disorders. Current experience, although limited, suggests that use of MRI scans will soon supersede the use of CT scans for hypothalamic-pituitary lesions. Resolution is rapidly improving, and MRI allows better definition of the suprasellar cistern, cavernous sinuses, pituitary stalk, and optic chiasm.

Arteriography

Angiography of the internal carotid artery to characterize pituitary lesions has limited indications. Because of its significant risk of morbidity, including transient or permanent neurologic deficit or vascular occlusion, arteriography of the sellar region should be performed only to exclude a parasellar or suprasellar aneurysm as a cause of abnormal radiographic changes in the sella.

Pneumoencephalography

Pneumoencephalography has been replaced by high-resolution CT scanning and by metrizamide cisternography in the evaluation of pituitary and parasellar lesions.

NEURO-OPHTHALMOLOGIC EVALUATION

Although most patients with pituitary adenomas currently present with endocrine abnormalities, visual disturbances are a common feature of large pituitary tumors with suprasellar extension because of the close proximity of the pituitary to the optic chiasm, optic nerves, and optic tracts. Thus, the evaluation of any patient with a known pituitary tumor or an enlarged sella should include careful visual examination. Serial visual field testing is also a valuable method of following the clinical progression of a pituitary lesion.

Visual Field Examination

Visual field examination can be performed at the bedside by confrontation or in the neuro-ophthalmology laboratory with more precise equipment such as the Goldmann or Tubinger perimeter. The use of finger movements is not an adequate method for bedside evaluation. The employment of a small (2- to 3-mm diameter) object—preferably red—affords a more sensitive index of loss of vision. Visual field testing with the Goldmann perimeter may identify a compressive lesion earlier than confrontation. In chiasmal lesions, the most common among pituitary tumors, a central field (within 30 degrees of fixation) may be affected earlier than peripheral fields.

Visual Evoked Response (VER)

VER is a technique employed in the detection of compressive lesions of the optic chiasm and nerves. The functional integrity of the visual pathway can be assessed by determining the electrical response from the occipital cortex produced by photic stimulation. A distortion in wave form is a very sensitive index of compressive involvement of the visual pathways. VER improves with successful therapy of the compressive lesion and has been utilized intraoperatively to evaluate optic nerve and chiasmal function.

Lateral Tumor Extension

In addition to causing visual field defects, large pituitary lesions may occasionally extend laterally into the cavernous sinus, compromising the function of the third, fourth, or sixth cranial nerve, leading to diplopia.

PITUITARY & HYPOTHALAMIC DISORDERS

Approach to the Patient

Hypothalamic-pituitary lesions present with a variety of manifestations, including pituitary hormone hypersecretion and hyposecretion, sellar enlargement, and visual loss. The approach to evaluation should be designed to ensure early diagnosis at a stage when the lesions are amenable to therapy.

A. Etiology and Early Manifestations: In adults, the commonest cause of hypothalamic-pituitary dysfunction is a pituitary adenoma, of which the great majority are hypersecreting. Thus, the earliest symptoms of such tumors are due to endocrinologic abnormalities, and these precede sellar enlargement and local manifestations such as headache and visual loss, which are late manifestations seen only in patients with larger tumors or suprasellar extension.

In children, pituitary adenomas are uncommon; the most frequent structural lesions causing hypothalamic-pituitary dysfunction are craniopharyngiomas and other hypothalamic tumors. These also usually manifest as endocrine disturbances (low GH levels, delayed puberty, diabetes insipidus) prior to the development of headache, visual loss, or other central nervous system symptoms.

B. Pituitary Hypersecretion: Excessive secretion of anterior pituitary hormones by pituitary microadenomas is the most common early manifestation of hypothalamic-pituitary disorders. PRL is the hormone most commonly secreted in excess amounts by pituitary adenomas, and it is usually elevated in patients with hypothalamic disorders as well. Thus, PRL measurement is essential in evaluating patients with suspected pituitary disorders, and it should be obtained in patients presenting with galactorrhea, gonadal dysfunction, secondary gonadotropin deficiency, or enlargement of the sella turcica. Hypersecretion of GH or ACTH leads to the more characteristic syndromes of acromegaly and Cushing's disease (see below).

C. Pituitary Insufficiency: Although panhypopituitarism is a classic manifestation of pituitary adenomas, it is present in less than 20% of patients in current large series because of earlier diagnosis of these lesions.

At present, the earliest clinical manifestation of a pituitary adenoma in adults is hypogonadism secondary to elevated levels of PRL, GH, or ACTH and cortisol rather than to destruction of anterior pituitary tissue. Thus, patients with hypogonadism should first be screened with FSH/LH measurements to exclude primary gonadal failure (elevated FSH/LH) and those with hypogonadotropic hypogonadism should have serum PRL levels measured and be examined for clinical evidence of GH or ACTH and cortisol excess.

In children, short stature is the most frequent clinical presentation of hypothalamic-pituitary dysfunction; in these patients, GH deficiency should be considered.

TSH or ACTH deficiency is relatively unusual in current series of patients and usually indicates panhypopituitarism. Thus, in patients with hypothyroidism or hypoadrenalism, primary disorders of the thyroid or adrenal are excluded by the absence of elevated TSH or ACTH levels, and the patient should then undergo a complete assessment of pituitary function and neuroradiologic studies, since panhypopituitarism and large pituitary tumors are common in this setting. PRL measurement is again essential, since prolactinomas are the most frequent abnormalities in adults.

D. The Enlarged Sella Turcica: Patients may present with enlargement of the sella turcica, which may be noted on radiographs performed for head trauma or on sinus series. These patients usually have either a pituitary adenoma or empty sella syndrome. Evaluation should include clinical assessment of pituitary dysfunction and measurements of PRL and thyroid and adrenal function. If pituitary function is normal, empty sella syndrome is the most likely diagnosis, which should be confirmed by CT scanning. Patients with clinical or laboratory evidence of pituitary dysfunction usually have a pituitary adenoma.

E. Visual Field Defects: Patients presenting with unexplained visual field defects or visual loss should be considered to have a pituitary or hypothalamic disorder until proved otherwise. The initial step in evaluation should be by CT scanning, which will reveal the tumor if one is present. These patients should also have PRL measurements and be assessed for anterior pituitary insufficiency, which is especially common with large pituitary adenomas.

F. Diabetes Insipidus: Diabetes insipidus is a common manifestation of hypothalamic lesions but is rare in primary pituitary lesions. The diagnosis is established as described in Chapter 6. In addition, all patients should undergo CT scanning and assessment of anterior pituitary function.

EMPTY SELLA SYNDROME

Etiology & Incidence

The empty sella syndrome occurs when the subarachnoid space extends into the sella turcica, partially filling it with cerebrospinal fluid. This process causes remodeling and enlargement of the sella turcica and flattening of the pituitary gland. An empty sella may occur as a primary event resulting from congenital incompetence of the diaphragma sellae (Fig 4–13) or as a secondary phenomenon after radiation therapy, surgery, or pituitary infarction.

Primary empty sella syndrome is common, with an incidence in autopsy series ranging from 5 to 23%. It is the most frequent cause of enlarged sella turcica.

An empty sella is also commonly seen after pituitary surgery or radiation therapy and may also occur following postpartum pituitary infarction (Sheehan's syndrome). In addition, pituitary tumors may undergo subclinical hemorrhagic infarction and cause contraction of the overlying suprasellar cistern downward into the sella. This phenomenon has been described in both PRL-secreting and GH-secreting pituitary adenomas. Therefore, the presence of an empty sella does not exclude the possibility of a coexisting pituitary tumor.

Pathogenesis

The pathogenesis of primary empty sella syndrome is uncertain. It has been postulated that increased cerebrospinal fluid pressure leads to herniation of arachnoid through the diaphragma sellae. A mesenchymal defect may be present in some patients, resulting in hypoplasia of the sellar diaphragm. A kindred has been described in which both primary empty sella syndrome and Rieger's anomaly of the anterior chamber of the eye (a developmental abnormality of mesenchymal origin involving the iris) occurred in an autosomal dominant fashion.

Clinical Findings

A. Symptoms and Signs: Most patients are asymptomatic middle-aged obese women. Many have systemic hypertension; benign intracranial hypertension may also occur. Although 48% of patients complain of headache, this feature may have only initiated the evaluation (ie, skull x-rays), and its relationship with the empty sella is probably coincidental. Serious clinical manifestations are uncommon. Spontaneous

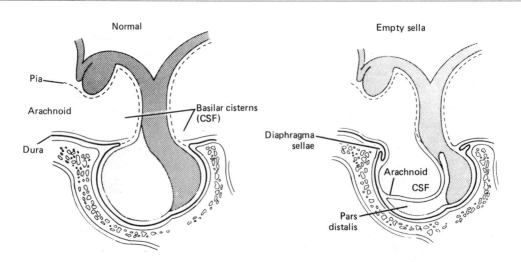

Figure 4–13. Representation of the normal relationship of the meninges to the pituitary gland *(left)* and the findings in the empty sella *(right)* as the arachnoid membrane herniates through the incompetent diaphragma sellae. (Reproduced, with permission, from Jordan RM, Kendall JW, Kerber CW: The primary empty sella syndrome: Analysis of the clinical characteristics, radiographic features, pituitary function, and cerebrospinal fluid adenohypophysial hormone concentrations. *Am J Med* 1977;**62**:569.)

cerebrospinal fluid rhinorrhea has been reported, and visual field impairment may rarely occur.

B. Laboratory Findings: Tests of anterior pituitary function are almost always normal. This observation correlates well with histologic immunocytochemical studies of the pituitary gland in patients with the syndrome. Such studies have demonstrated that the remodeled pituitary gland contains adequate amounts of all 6 adenohypophyseal hormones. TSH, GH, and gonadotropin secretory reserves have rarely been reported to be impaired; however, pituitary hypofunction in such cases may result from subclinical pituitary ischemic damage followed by contraction of glandular tissue and a secondary empty sella.

Endocrine function studies should be performed to exclude pituitary hormone insufficiency or a hypersecretory pituitary adenoma. The demonstration of normal diurnal variation in PRL secretion is another means of excluding pituitary tumor; the ratio of PRL drawn between 1 and 3 AM compared with 10 AM will be greater than 1.5 (normal) in patients with the empty sella and in normal subjects but less than 1.5 in patients with pituitary adenomas.

Diagnosis

The diagnosis of primary empty sella syndrome can be confirmed by radiographic studies. Plain x-rays often show a symmetrically enlarged sella, but all degrees of sellar deformity have been seen. The plain x-ray cannot distinguish an empty sella from a pituitary adenoma. High-resolution CT scanning (thin-slice technique) has provided a noninvasive means of establishing the presence of cerebrospinal fluid in the sellar contents. This technique has eliminated the need for pneumoencephalography. The newer CT scanners afford such good resolution (Fig 4–12) that metrizamide cisternography is rarely needed.

HYPOTHALAMIC TUMORS

Hypothalamic tumors are discussed below in the section on hypopituitarism. Craniopharyngioma is the most common tumor in children, adolescents, and young adults. In older adults, primary central nervous system tumors and those arising from hypothalamic (epidermoid and dermoid tumors) and pineal structures (pinealomas) are more common.

Clinical Findings

A. Craniopharyngioma: The initial symptoms of craniopharyngioma in children and adolescents are predominantly endocrinologic; however, these manifestations are frequently unrecognized, and at diagnosis over 80% of patients have hypothalamic-pituitary endocrine deficiencies. These endocrine abnormalities may precede presenting symptoms by months or years; GH deficiency is most common, with about 50% of patients having growth retardation and approximately 70% decreased GH responses to stimulation at diagnosis. Gonadotropin deficiency leading to absent or arrested puberty is usual in older children and adolescents of pubertal age; TSH and ACTH deficiency is less common, and diabetes insipidus is present in about 15%.

Symptoms leading to the diagnosis are, unfortunately, frequently neurologic and due to the mass effect of the expanding tumor. Symptoms of increased intracranial pressure such as headache and vomiting are present in about 42%; decreased visual acuity or visual field defects are the presenting symptoms in another 35%. Plain films of the skull reveal intrasellar or suprasellar calcification in 75% of these children. CT scans confirm the tumor in virtually all patients; in 95%, the tumor is suprasellar.

In adults, craniopharyngiomas have similar presentations; ie, the diagnosis is usually reached as a result of investigation of symptoms of increased intracranial pressure, headache, or visual loss. However, endocrine manifestations—especially hypogonadism, diabetes insipidus, or other deficiencies of anterior pituitary hormones—usually precede these late manifestations. Intrasellar or suprasellar calcification is less common in adults (for unknown reasons), but CT scans again readily demonstrate the tumors, which in adults are almost always both intrasellar and suprasellar.

B. Other Tumors: Other hypothalamic or pineal tumors and primary central nervous system tumors involving the hypothalamus have variable presentations in both children and adults. Thus, presentation is with headache, visual loss, symptoms of increased intracranial pressure, growth failure, various degrees of hypopituitarism, or diabetes insipidus. Endocrine deficiencies usually precede neurologic manifestations. Hypothalamic tumors in childhood may present with precocious puberty.

Diagnosis

Patients with suspected or proved hypothalamic tumors should have high-resolution CT scans to determine the extent and nature of the tumor. Complete assessment of anterior pituitary function is necessary in these patients, since deficiencies are present in the great majority (see section on hypopituitarism below) and the evaluation will establish the requirements for replacement therapy. PRL levels should also be determined, since most hypothalamic lesions cause hyperprolactinemia either by hypothalamic injury or by damage to the pituitary stalk.

Treatment

Treatment depends upon the type of tumor. Since complete resection of craniopharyngioma is usually not feasible, this tumor is best managed by limited neurosurgical removal of accessible tumor and decompression of cysts, followed by conventional radiotherapy. Patients treated by this method have a recurrence rate of approximately 20%; when surgery alone is used, the recurrence rate approximates 80%.

Other hypothalamic tumors are also usually not surgically resectable. Therapy is usually primarily surgical to obtain a histologic diagnosis followed by conventional radiotherapy.

HYPOPITUITARISM

Hypopituitarism is usually a subtle clinical event with diverse causes. It is manifested by diminished or absent secretion of one or more pituitary hormones. The development of signs and symptoms is often slow and insidious, depending on the rate of onset and the magnitude of hypothalamic-pituitary damage—factors that are influenced by the underlying pathogenesis. Hypopituitarism is either a primary event caused by destruction of the anterior pituitary gland or a secondary phenomenon resulting from deficiency of hypothalamic stimulatory (or inhibitory) factors normally acting on the pituitary. Although provocative endocrine testing is essential in evaluating anterior pituitary gland function, it is not always possible (even with the use of hypothalamic releasing hormones) to distinguish between a pituitary and a hypothalamic lesion. Treatment and prognosis depend on the extent of hypofunction, the underlying cause, and the location of the lesion in the hypothalamic-pituitary axis.

Etiology

The etiologic considerations in hypopituitarism are diverse. As shown below and in Table 4–6, a helpful mnemonic device is the phrase ''nine I's'': Invasive, Infarction, Infiltrative, Injury, Immunologic, Iatrogenic, Infectious, Idiopathic, and Isolated. Most of these lesions may cause pituitary or hypothalamic failure (or both). Although it is not always possible to do so, establishing the precise cause of hypopituitarism is helpful in determining treatment and prognosis.

A. Invasive: Space-occupying lesions cause hypopituitarism by destroying the pituitary gland or hypothalamic nuclei or by disrupting the hypothalamic-hypophyseal portal venous system. Large pituitary adenomas cause hypopituitarism by these mechanisms; however, small pituitary tumors—microadenomas (< 10 mm in diameter)—characteristically seen in the hypersecretory states (excess PRL, GH, ACTH) do not directly cause pituitary insufficiency. Craniopharyngioma, the most common tumor of the hypothalamic-pituitary region in children, may impair pituitary function by its compressive effects. Primary central nervous system tumors, including meningioma, chordoma, optic glioma, epidermoid tumors, and dermoid tumors, may decrease hypothalamic-pituitary secretion by their mass effects. Metastatic lesions to this area are common (especially breast carcinoma) but rarely result in clinically obvious hypopituitarism. Anatomic malformations such as basal encephalocele and parasellar aneurysms cause hypothalamic-pituitary dysfunction and may enlarge the sella turcica and mimic pituitary tumors.

B. Infarction: Ischemic damage to the pituitary has long been recognized as a cause of hypopituitarism. In 1914, Simmonds reported pituitary necrosis

Table 4–6. Hypopituitarism: Etiologic considerations. (The "nine I's.")

Invasive
  Large pituitary tumors
  Craniopharyngioma
  Primary central nervous system tumors (meningioma, chordoma, optic glioma; epidermoid, dermoid, pineal tumors)
  Carotid aneurysm
  Basal encephalocele
Infarction
  Postpartum necrosis (Sheehan's syndrome)
  Pituitary apoplexy
Infiltrative
  Sarcoidosis
  Hemochromatosis
  Histiocytosis X (Hand-Schüller-Christian disease, eosinophilic granuloma, Letterer-Siwe disease)
Injury
  Head trauma
  Child abuse
Immunologic
  Lymphocytic hypophysitis
Iatrogenic
  Surgery
  Radiation therapy
Infectious
  Mycoses, tuberculosis, syphilis
Idiopathic
  Familial
Isolated
  GH (dwarfism, emotional deprivation)
  LH, FSH (Kallmann's syndrome, weight loss, sickle cell anemia)
  TSH (chronic renal failure, pseudohypoparathyroidism)
  ACTH-LPH
  PRL (pseudohypoparathyroidism)

in a woman with severe puerperal sepsis, and in 1937 Sheehan published his classic description of its occurrence following postpartum hemorrhage and vascular collapse. The mechanism for the ischemia in such cases is not certain. Hypotension along with vasospasm of the hypophyseal arteries is currently believed to compromise arterial perfusion of the anterior pituitary. During pregnancy, the pituitary gland may be more sensitive to hypoxemia because of its increased metabolic needs or more susceptible to vasoconstrictive influences because of the hyperestrogenic state. Some degree of hypopituitarism has been reported in 32% of women with severe postpartum hemorrhage. Other investigators have noted that the hypopituitarism does not always correlate with the degree of hemorrhage but that there is good correlation between the pituitary lesion and severe disturbances of the clotting mechanism (as in patients with placenta previa). Ischemic pituitary necrosis has also been reported to occur with greater frequency in patients with diabetes mellitus.

The extent of pituitary damage determines the rapidity of onset as well as the magnitude of pituitary hypofunction. The gland has a great secretory reserve, and more than 75% must be destroyed before clinical manifestations are evident. The initial clinical feature in postpartum necrosis may be failure to lactate after parturition; failure to resume normal menstrual periods is another clue to the diagnosis. However, the clinical features of hypopituitarism are often subtle, and years may pass before pituitary insufficiency is recognized following an ischemic insult.

Spontaneous hemorrhagic infarction of a pituitary tumor (pituitary apoplexy) frequently results in partial or total pituitary insufficiency. Pituitary apoplexy is usually a fulminant clinical syndrome manifested by severe headache, visual impairment, ophthalmoplegias, meningismus, and an altered level of consciousness. Acute pituitary failure with hypotension may result, and rapid mental deterioration, coma, and death may ensue. Emergency treatment with corticosteroids (see Chapter 9) and transsphenoidal decompression of the intrasellar contents may be lifesaving and may prevent permanent visual loss. Most patients who have survived pituitary apoplexy have developed multiple adenohypophyseal deficits, but infarction of the tumor in some patients may cure the hypersecretory pituitary adenoma and its accompanying endocrinopathy. Pituitary infarction may also be a subclinical event (silent pituitary apoplexy), resulting in improvement of pituitary hormone hypersecretion without impairing the secretion of other anterior pituitary hormones.

C. Infiltrative: Hypopituitarism may be the initial clinical manifestation of infiltrative disease processes such as sarcoidosis, hemochromatosis, and histiocytosis X.

1. Sarcoidosis–The most common intracranial sites of involvement of sarcoidosis are the hypothalamus and pituitary gland. At one time, the most common endocrine abnormality in patients with sarcoidosis was thought to be diabetes insipidus; however, many of these patients actually have centrally mediated disordered control of thirst that results in polydipsia and polyuria, which in some cases explains the abnormal water metabolism. Deficiencies of multiple anterior pituitary hormones have been well documented in sarcoidosis and are usually secondary to hypothalamic insufficiency. Granulomatous involvement of the hypothalamic-pituitary unit is occasionally extensive, resulting in visual impairment, and therefore may simulate the clinical presentation of a pituitary tumor.

2. Hemochromatosis–Hypopituitarism, particularly hypogonadotropic hypogonadism, is a prominent manifestation of iron storage disease—either idiopathic hemochromatosis or transfusional iron overload. Hypogonadism occurs in most such cases and is often the initial clinical feature of iron excess; complete iron studies should be obtained in any male patient presenting with unexplained hypogonadotropic hypogonadism. Pituitary deficiencies of TSH, GH, and ACTH have also been documented but usually occur later in the course of the disease. The high incidence of hypothalamic-pituitary dysfunction in hemochromatosis requires careful documentation and

serial evaluation, so that treatment (such as with corticosteroids) during periods of stress can be employed when indicated. Iron chelation therapy does not reverse hypopituitarism in hemochromatosis.

3. Histiocytosis X–Histiocytosis X, the infiltration of multiple organs by well-differentiated histiocytes, is often heralded by the onset of diabetes insipidus and anterior pituitary hormone deficiencies. The disorders in this category include Hand-Schüller-Christian disease, Letterer-Siwe disease, and eosinophilic granuloma of bone (eosinophilic infiltration predominates). Most histologic and biochemical studies have indicated that this infiltrative process involves chiefly the hypothalamus, and hypopituitarism occurs only as a result of hypothalamic damage.

D. Injury: Severe head trauma is an often-overlooked cause of anterior pituitary insufficiency even though diabetes insipidus is a well-described complication of closed head injury in children and adults. Posttraumatic anterior hypopituitarism may be due to injury to the anterior pituitary, the pituitary stalk, or the hypothalamus. Pituitary insufficiency with growth retardation has been described in battered children who suffer closed head trauma with subdural hematoma. Since the onset of posttraumatic hypopituitarism may be insidious, patients with serious head injuries, regardless of cause, require long-term observation for signs of impaired pituitary function.

E. Immunologic: Lymphocytic hypophysitis resulting in anterior hypopituitarism is a distinct entity, occurring in women usually during pregnancy or in the postpartum period. It may present as a mass lesion of the sella turcica with visual field disturbances simulating pituitary adenoma. An autoimmune process with extensive infiltration of the gland by lymphocytes and plasma cells destroys the anterior pituitary cells. These morphologic features are similar to those of other autoimmune endocrinopathies, eg, thyroiditis, adrenalitis, oophoritis, and orchitis. About 50% of patients with lymphocytic hypophysitis have other endocrine autoimmune disease, and circulating pituitary autoantibodies have been found in several cases. It is presently uncertain how this disorder should be diagnosed and treated. It must be considered in the differential diagnosis of women with pituitary gland enlargement and hypopituitarism during pregnancy or the postpartum period.

F. Iatrogenic: Both surgical and radiation therapy to the pituitary gland may compromise its function. The anterior pituitary is quite resilient during transsphenoidal microsurgery, and despite extensive manipulation during the search for microadenomas, anterior pituitary function is usually preserved. The actual incidence of hypopituitarism following radiation therapy is unclear. The dose of conventional radiation therapy presently employed to treat pituitary tumors is 4500–5000 rads—considerably less than the 8000–10,000 rads required to ablate normal pituitary tissue. Nonetheless, follow-up studies of patients receiving radiation treatment for tumors disclose a high incidence of hypothalamic and pituitary insufficiency.

Hypopituitarism in such patients is frequently accompanied by modest hyperprolactinemia (PRL 30– 100 mg/mL). Heavy particle (proton beam) irradiation for pituitary tumors results in a 20– 50% incidence of hypopituitarism. In addition to radiotherapy directed at the pituitary or hypothalamus, irradiation of tumors of the head and neck (nasopharyngeal cancer, brain tumors) and prophylactic cranial irradiation in leukemia may also cause hypopituitarism. The clinical onset of pituitary failure in such patients is usually insidious and results from both pituitary and hypothalamic injury.

G. Infectious: Although many infectious diseases, including tuberculosis, syphilis, and mycotic infections, have been implicated as causative agents in pituitary hypofunction, anti-infective drugs have now made them rare causes of hypopituitarism.

H. Idiopathic: In some patients with hypopituitarism, no underlying cause is found. These may be isolated (see below) or multiple deficiencies. Familial forms of hypopituitarism characterized by a small, normal, or enlarged sella turcica have been described. Both autosomal recessive and X-linked recessive inheritance patterns have been reported. The pathogenesis of these familial disorders is uncertain.

I. Isolated: Isolated (monotropic) deficiencies of the anterior pituitary hormones have been described.

1. GH deficiency–In children, congenital monotropic GH deficiency may be sporadic or familial and must be considered in the differential diagnosis of short stature. These children, who may experience fasting hypoglycemia, have a gradual deceleration in growth velocity after 6– 12 months of age. Diagnosis must be based on failure of GH responsiveness to provocative stimuli and the demonstration of normal responsiveness of other anterior pituitary hormones. Monotropic GH deficiency and growth retardation have also been observed in children suffering severe emotional deprivation. This disorder is reversed by placing the child in a supportive psychosocial milieu. A more detailed description of GH deficiency and growth failure is provided in Chapter 5.

2. ACTH deficiency–Monotropic ACTH deficiency is rare and is manifested by the signs and symptoms of adrenocortical insufficiency. Lipotropin (LPH) deficiency has also been noted in such patients. The defect in these patients may be due to primary failure of the corticotrophs to release ACTH and its related peptide hormones or may be secondary to impaired secretion of CRH by the hypothalamus.

3. Gonadotropin deficiency–Isolated deficiency of gonadotropins is not uncommon. Kallman's syndrome, an X-linked dominant disorder with incomplete penetrance, is characterized by an isolated defect in GnRH secretion associated with maldevelopment of the olfactory center with hyposmia or anosmia. Sporadic cases occur, and other neurologic defects such as color blindness and nerve deafness have been seen. Since anterior pituitary function is otherwise intact, young men with isolated hypogonadotropic hypogonadism develop a eunuchoid appearance; this is because lack of testosterone results in excessive growth of the limbs owing to failure of epiphyseal closure. In women, a state of hypogonadotropic hypogonadism manifested by oligomenorrhea or amenorrhea often accompanies weight loss, emotional or physical stress, and athletic training. Anorexia nervosa and marked obesity both result in hypothalamic dysfunction and impaired gonadotropin secretion. Sickle cell anemia also causes hypogonadotropic hypogonadism due to hypothalamic dysfunction and results in delayed puberty. Clomiphene treatment has been effective in such cases. Other chronic illnesses, eg, poorly controlled diabetes and malnutrition, may result in gonadotropin deficiency. Isolated deficiencies of both LH and FSH without an obvious cause such as those described have been reported but are rare.

4. TSH deficiency–Monotropic TSH deficiency is rare and is caused by a reduction in hypothalamic TRH secretion (tertiary hypothyroidism). Some patients with chronic renal failure appear to have impaired TSH secretion.

5. Prolactin deficiency–PRL deficiency almost always indicates severe intrinsic pituitary damage, and panhypopituitarism is usually present. Deficiencies of TSH and PRL have been noted in patients with pseudohypoparathyroidism.

Clinical Findings

The onset of pituitary insufficiency is usually gradual, and clinical features are related to the lack of individual pituitary hormones and their specific target gland secretion. The classic course of progressive hypopituitarism is an initial loss of gonadotropins followed by deficiencies of TSH, then ACTH, and finally PRL. Impairment of GH secretion is actually the most common abnormality in hypopituitarism, but this is, of course, clinically occult in adult patients.

A. Symptoms: Hypogonadism, manifested by amenorrhea in women and decreased libido or impotence in men, may antedate the clinical appearance of a hypothalamic-pituitary lesion.

Hypothyroidism caused by TSH deficiency generally simulates the clinical changes observed in primary thyroid failure; however, it is usually less severe, and goiter is absent. Cold intolerance, dry skin, mental dullness, bradycardia, constipation, hoarseness, and anemia have all been observed; gross myxedematous changes are uncommon.

The lack of ACTH causes adrenocortical insufficiency, and its clinical features resemble those of primary adrenal failure. Weakness, nausea, vomiting, anorexia, fever, and postural hypotension may occur, although cardiovascular collapse as seen in Addison's disease is uncommon, since the renin-angiotensin system is usually intact. Again, these symptoms are less severe in secondary adrenal insufficiency and, because of their gradual onset, may go undetected for prolonged periods, becoming manifest only during periods of stress. Hypoglycemia aggravated by GH deficiency may occur with fasting and has been the initial presenting feature of some patients with isolated ACTH deficiency. Patients with type I (insulin-dependent) diabetes who develop hypopituitarism often have a reduction in their insulin requirements. In contrast to the hyperpigmentation that occurs during states of ACTH excess (Addison's disease, Nelson's syndrome), depigmentation and diminished tanning have been described as a result of ACTH insufficiency. In addition, lack of ACTH-stimulated adrenal androgen secretion will cause a decrease in body hair if gonadotropin deficiency is also present.

The only symptom of PRL deficiency is failure of postpartum lactation.

B. Signs: Abnormal findings on physical examination may be subtle and require careful observation. Patients with hypopituitarism are not cachectic. A photograph of a cachectic patient with "Simmonds' syndrome" that appeared in some older textbooks of endocrinology caused confusion. That particular patient probably suffered from anorexia nervosa and was found to have a normal pituitary gland at postmortem examination.

Patients with pituitary failure are usually slightly overweight. The skin is fine, pale, and smooth, with fine wrinkling of the face. Body and pubic hair may be deficient or absent, and atrophy of the genitalia may occur. Postural hypotension, bradycardia, decreased muscle strength, and delayed deep tendon reflexes occur in more severe cases. Neuro-ophthalmologic abnormalities depend on the presence of a large intrasellar or parasellar lesion.

C. Laboratory Findings: These may include anemia (related to thyroid and androgen deficiency), hypoglycemia, hyponatremia (related to hypothyroidism and inappropriate water retention, not sodium loss), and low-voltage bradycardia on ECG. Hyperkalemia, which is common in primary adrenal failure, is not present.

Diagnosis

The diagnosis of anterior pituitary insufficiency must be established with provocative endocrine testing. However, these procedures should be preceded by a thorough clinical history and physical examination. For example, the presence of a normal menstrual cycle in a euthyroid woman is strong evidence against pituitary dysfunction, and further studies in such cases are usually not warranted. A diagnostic strategy for the evaluation of hypopituitarism is presented in Fig 4–14.

A. Assessment of Target Gland Function: If endocrine hypofunction is suspected, pituitary hormone deficiencies must be distinguished from primary failure of the thyroid, adrenals, or gonads. Basal determinations of each anterior pituitary hormone are useful only if compared to target gland secretion. Baseline laboratory studies should include thyroid function tests (T$_4$RIA, RT$_3$U, FT$_4$I) and determination of serum testosterone levels. Testosterone is a sensitive indicator of hypopituitarism in women as well as in men. In women, a substantial decrease in testosterone is commonly observed in pituitary failure related to hy-

pofunction of the 2 endocrine glands responsible for its production—the ovary and the adrenal. Adrenocortical reserve should initially be evaluated by a rapid ACTH stimulation test.

B. Prolactin Evaluation: Since hyperprolactinemia (discussed later), regardless of its cause, leads to gonadal dysfunction, serum PRL should be measured early in the evaluation of hypogonadism.

C. Differentiation of Primary and Secondary Hypofunction: Subnormal thyroid function as shown by appropriate tests, a low serum testosterone level, or an impaired cortisol response to the rapid ACTH stimulation test requires measurement of basal levels of specific pituitary hormones. In primary target gland hypofunction (such as polyglandular failure syndrome), TSH, LH, FSH, or ACTH will be elevated. Low or normal values for these pituitary hormones suggest hypothalamic-pituitary dysfunction.

D. Stimulation Tests: Provocative endocrine testing should then be employed to confirm the diagnosis; to assess the extent of hypofunction; and, when possible, to determine whether the abnormality is at the level of the hypothalamus or pituitary. Evaluation of the secretory reserve of the pituitary hormones has been discussed earlier. For convenience, a triple stimulation test combining simultaneous insulin hypoglycemia, TRH, and GnRH can be utilized to test the secretory capacity of all 6 major anterior pituitary hormones. Some investigators have also successfully infused CRH, GRH, TRH, and GnRH simultaneously as a means of assessing complete adenohypophyseal function.

Treatment

Appropriate therapy for hypopituitarism must include consideration of individual hormonal deficiencies as well as the extent of the deficiencies. Except in the case of GH, replacement therapy is provided by use of synthetic target gland hormones.

A. ACTH: Treatment of secondary adrenal insufficiency, like that of primary adrenal failure, must include glucocorticoid support (see Chapter 9). Hydrocortisone (20–30 mg/d), cortisone acetate (25–35 mg/d), or prednisone (5–7.5 mg/d) orally in 2 or 3 divided doses provides adequate glucocorticoid replacement for most patients. The minimum effective dosage should be given in order to avoid iatrogenic hypercortisolism. Increased dosage is required during periods of stress such as illness, surgery, or trauma. Patients with only partial ACTH deficiency may need steroid treatment only during stress. A 2- or 3-fold increase in steroid dosage during the stressful situation should be recommended, followed by gradual tapering as the stress resolves. Unlike primary adrenal insufficiency, ACTH deficiency does not usually require mineralocorticoid therapy. Patients with adrenal insufficiency should wear medical alert bracelets so they may receive prompt treatment in case of emergency.

B. TSH: The decision to treat patients with secondary hypothyroidism must be based on clinical grounds and the circulating concentration of serum

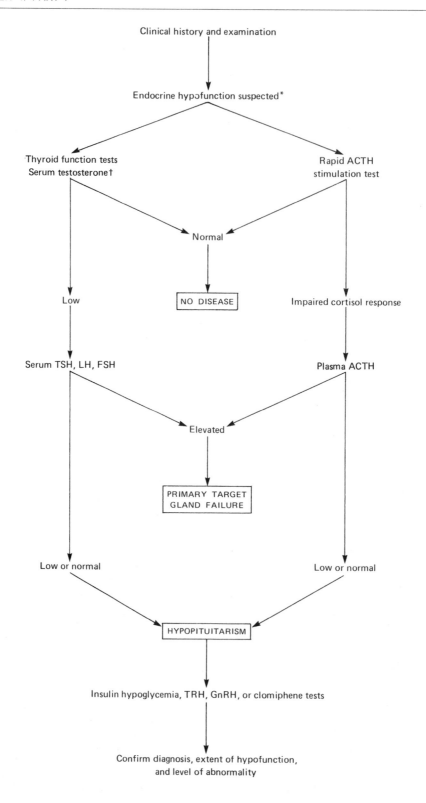

*Evaluate GH in children (see text).
†Measure prolactin if hypogonadism suspected.

Figure 4–14. Diagnostic evaluation of hypothalamic-pituitary–target gland hypofunction.

thyroxine (see Chapter 7). Since some patients with hypothyrotropic hypothyroidism have a normal TSH response to TRH, basal TSH levels and the TRH test should not be used as guidelines for thyroid replacement. The treatment of secondary and tertiary hypothyroidism is identical to that for primary thyroid failure. Levothyroxine sodium, 0.1–0.2 mg/d orally, is usually adequate. Response to therapy is monitored clinically and with measurement of serum thyroxine.

Caution must be urged in initiating thyroxine treatment in a patient with suspected hypoadrenalism. Since thyroid hormone replacement in patients with hypopituitarism may aggravate even partial adrenal insufficiency, the adrenal disorder should be treated first, followed by the judicious use of thyroxine.

C. Gonadotropins: The object of treatment of secondary hypogonadism is to replace sex steroids and restore gametogenesis (see Chapters 13 and 14).

1. Estrogens and progesterone–In women, estrogen replacement is essential. Adequate estrogen treatment will maintain secondary sex characteristics (eg, vulvar and vaginal lubrication), prevent osteoporosis, and abolish vasomotor symptoms, with an improvement in sense of well-being. Many estrogen preparations are available, but the optimal replacement dosage is unknown; the smallest dose that achieves the desired clinical effects should be used, eg, ethinyl estradiol, 0.02–0.05 mg orally daily, or conjugated estrogens, 0.3–1.25 mg orally daily. Since long-term therapy with estrogen compounds increases the risk of endometrial carcinoma, estrogens should be withheld during the last 5–7 days of each month, and a progestin compound (eg, medroxyprogesterone, 10 mg orally) should be given during days 15–25 of the cycle to induce withdrawal bleeding and prevent endometrial hyperplasia.

2. Androgens in women–Because of a deficiency of adrenal androgens, some women with hypopituitarism have diminished libido despite adequate estrogen therapy. Small doses of long-acting androgens (testosterone enanthate, 25–50 mg intramuscularly every 4–8 weeks) may be helpful in restoring sexual activity without causing hirsutism.

3. Ovulation induction–Ovulation can often be restored in women with hypothalamic-pituitary dysfunction (see Chapter 14). In patients with gonadal failure of hypothalamic origin, clomiphene citrate causes a surge of gonadotropin secretion resulting in ovulation. Multiple births are a risk with this form of treatment. Combined treatment with FSH (human menopausal gonadotropins; menotropins; Pergonal) and LH (chorionic gonadotropin) can be utilized to provoke ovulation in women with intrinsic pituitary failure. This form of therapy is expensive, and multiple births are a risk. Recently, pulsatile subcutaneous injections of GnRH with an infusion pump have induced ovulation and fertility in women with hypothalamic dysfunction.

4. Androgens in men–In men, testosterone replacement is essential to restore libido and potency, provide adequate beard growth and muscle strength,

prevent osteopenia, and improve the sense of well-being. Adequate treatment consists of a long-acting intramuscular preparation such as testosterone enanthate. Three dosage schedules have proved efficacy: 300 mg every 3 weeks, 200 mg every 2 weeks, or 100 mg every week. Side effects, including aggressive sexual behavior, acne, gynecomastia, and fluid retention, are unusual and can be managed by lowering the dosage. Therapy should be withheld in adolescents as long as possible in order to prevent premature epiphyseal closure and ensure maximum linear growth. Replacement therapy with oral androgenic preparations should be avoided, since inadequate absorption results in poor androgenization, and serious side effects such as peliosis hepatis (blood-filled cysts within the hepatic parenchyma) may occur.

5. Spermatogenesis–Spermatogenesis can be achieved in some patients with the combined use of chorionic gonadotropin and menotropins. If pituitary insufficiency is of recent onset, therapy with chorionic gonadotropin alone may restore both fertility and adequate gonadal steroid production.

D. Growth Hormone: (See Chapter 5.) The recent recognition of Creutzfeldt-Jakob disease, a transmissible subacute degeneration of the central nervous system, in young patients who had received growth hormone derived from human pituitary glands has resulted in a discontinuation of such therapy. Fortunately, production of human growth hormone (hGH) has been accomplished by recombinant DNA technology so that the hormone is again available for use in children with hypopituitarism. The identification of a subgroup of children with normal variant short stature (normal GH secretory capacity) who benefit from long-term administration of hGH may broaden the therapeutic horizons of biologically engineered growth hormone.

PITUITARY ADENOMAS

Advances in endocrinologic and neuroradiologic research in recent years have allowed earlier recognition and more successful therapy of pituitary adenomas. Prolactinomas are the most common type, accounting for about 60% of primary pituitary tumors; GH hypersecretion occurs in approximately 20% and ACTH excess in 10%. Hypersecretion of TSH, the gonadotropins, or alpha subunits is rare. Nonfunctional tumors currently represent only 10% of all pituitary adenomas, and some of these may in fact be alpha subunit–secreting adenomas.

Early clinical recognition of the endocrine effects of excessive pituitary secretion, especially the observation that PRL excess causes secondary hypogonadism, has led to early diagnosis of pituitary tumors before the appearance of late manifestations such as sellar enlargement, panhypopituitarism, and suprasellar extension with visual impairment.

Pituitary **microadenomas** are defined as intrasellar adenomas less than 1 cm in diameter that present with manifestations of hormonal excess without sellar enlargement or extrasellar extension. Panhypopituitarism is rare, and such tumors are very successfully treated.

Pituitary **macroadenomas** are those larger than 1 cm in diameter and cause generalized sellar enlargement. Tumors 1–2 cm in diameter confined to the sella turcica can usually be successfully treated; however, larger tumors—and especially those with suprasellar, sphenoid sinus, or lateral extensions—are much more difficult to manage. Panhypopituitarism and visual loss increase in frequency with tumor size and suprasellar extension.

Treatment

Pituitary adenomas are treated with surgery, irradiation, or drugs to suppress hypersecretion by the adenoma or its growth. Details are outlined in subsequent sections.

The aims of therapy are to correct hypersecretion of anterior pituitary hormones, to preserve normal pituitary tissue secreting other anterior pituitary hormones, and to remove or suppress the adenoma itself. These objectives are currently achievable in most patients with pituitary microadenomas; however, in the case of larger tumors, multiple therapies are frequently required and may be less successful.

A. Surgical Treatment: Pituitary surgery is the initial therapy of choice at many centers, and the transsphenoidal microsurgical approach to the sella turcica is the procedure of choice; transfrontal craniotomy is required only in the occasional patient with massive suprasellar extension of the adenoma. In the transsphenoidal procedure, the surgeon approaches the pituitary from the nasal cavity through the sphenoid sinus, removes the anterior-inferior sellar floor, and incises the dura. The adenoma is selectively removed; normal pituitary tissue is identified and preserved. Success rates approach 90% in patients with microadenomas. Major complications, including postoperative hemorrhage, cerebrospinal fluid leak, meningitis, and visual impairment, occur in less than 5% and are most frequent in patients with large or massive tumors. Transient diabetes insipidus lasting a few days to 1–2 weeks occurs in approximately 15%; permanent diabetes insipidus is rare. A transient form of the syndrome of inappropriate secretion of vasopressin (antidiuretic hormone) (SIADH) with symptomatic hyponatremia occurs in 10% of patients within 5–10 days of transsphenoidal pituitary microsurgery. Surgical hypopituitarism is rare in patients with microadenomas but approaches 5–10% in patients with larger tumors. The perioperative management of such patients should include glucocorticoid administration in stress doses (see Chapter 9) and postoperative assessment of daily weight, fluid balance, and electrolyte status. Mild diabetes insipidus is managed by giving fluids orally; in more severe cases—urine output greater than 5–6 L/24 h—aqueous vasopressin (Pitressin) should be administered (see Chapter 6). SIADH is managed by fluid restriction.

B. Radiation Therapy: Pituitary irradiation is usually reserved for patients with larger tumors who have had incomplete resection of large pituitary adenomas.

1. X-ray irradiation–Conventional irradiation using high energy sources, in total doses of 4000–5000 rads given in daily doses of 180–200 rads, is most commonly employed. The response to radiation therapy is slow, and 5–10 years may be required to achieve the full effect (see section on acromegaly). Treatment is ultimately successful in about 80% of acromegalics but only 15% of patients with Cushing's disease. The response rate in prolactinomas is not precisely known, but tumor progression is prevented in most patients. Morbidity during radiotherapy is minimal, though some patients experience malaise and nausea, and serous otitis media may occur. Rare late complications include damage to the optic nerves and chiasm, seizures, and radionecrosis of brain tissue. Hypopituitarism is common, and the incidence increases with time following radiotherapy—about 40–50% at 5–10 years.

2. Heavy particle irradiation–Heavy particle irradiation using alpha particles or protons is also used. Advantages of this technique are the ability to focus the radiation beam precisely; the smaller port allows larger doses (8000–12,000 rads) to be delivered to the sellar area and limits the radiation exposure of surrounding structures. Disadvantages are the limited availability, and the smaller radiation field precludes use of this technique in patients with tumors over 1.5 cm in diameter and in those with extrasellar extension. Responses to therapy are more rapid than with conventional irradiation and occur within 2 years in most patients. Successful responses are obtained in about 80% of patients with acromegaly or Cushing's disease. Experience with prolactinomas is limited. Neurologic damage and visual impairment are rare complications of heavy particle irradiation, but hypopituitarism occurs in 40–50% and will almost certainly increase with further follow-up.

C. Medical Treatment: Medical management of pituitary adenomas has become feasible with the availability of bromocriptine, a dopamine agonist. This drug is most successful in the treatment of hyperprolactinemia and is also useful in some patients with acromegaly or Cushing's disease. Specifics of the use of this and other medications are discussed below.

Posttreatment Follow-Up

Patients undergoing transsphenoidal microsurgery should be reevaluated 4–6 weeks postoperatively to document that complete removal of the adenoma and correction of endocrine hypersecretion have been achieved. Prolactinomas are assessed by basal PRL measurements, GH-secreting tumors by glucose suppression testing, and ACTH-secreting adenomas by measurement of urine free cortisol and the response to low-dose dexamethasone suppression (see below). Other anterior pituitary hormones—TSH, ACTH, and LH/FSH—should also be assessed as described above in the section on endocrine evaluation. In patients with successful responses, yearly evaluation should be done to watch for late recurrence; late hypopituitarism does not occur after microsurgery. CT scanning is not necessary in patients with normal postoperative pituitary function but should be utilized in patients with persisting or recurrent disease.

Follow-up of patients treated by pituitary irradiation is also essential, since the response to therapy may be delayed and the incidence of hypopituitarism increases with time. Yearly endocrinologic assessment of both the hypersecreted hormone and the other pituitary hormones is recommended.

1. PROLACTINOMAS

The clinical application of prolactin (PRL) assays has greatly expanded our understanding of pituitary disorders. Although the **galactorrhea-amenorrhea syndromes** were previously described, PRL measurement has greatly facilitated their early recognition and is a useful index of response to therapy.

PRL hypersecretion is the most common endocrine abnormality due to hypothalamic-pituitary disorders, and PRL is the hormone most commonly secreted in excess by pituitary adenomas. In addition, most chromophobe adenomas, which were previously classified as ''nonfunctional'' on the basis of routine histologic studies, have now been shown to be PRL-secreting adenomas.

The understanding that PRL hypersecretion causes not only galactorrhea but also gonadal dysfunction and the use of PRL measurements in screening such patients have permitted recognition of these PRL-secreting tumors before the development of sellar enlargement, hypopituitarism, or visual impairment.

Thus, plasma PRL should be measured in patients with galactorrhea, suspected hypothalamic-pituitary dysfunction, or sellar enlargement and in those with unexplained gonadal dysfunction, including amenorrhea, decreased libido, or impotence (Table 4–7).

Pathology

PRL-secreting pituitary adenomas arise most commonly from the lateral wings of the anterior pituitary, but with progression they fill the sella turcica and compress the normal anterior and posterior lobes. Tumor size varies greatly from microadenomas to large invasive tumors with extrasellar extension. Most patients have microadenomas, ie, tumors less than 1 cm in diameter at diagnosis. Prolactinomas frequently

Table 4–7. Indications for prolactin measurement.

Galactorrhea
Enlarged sella turcica
Suspected pituitary tumor
Hypogonadotropic hypogonadism
    Unexplained amenorrhea
    Unexplained male hypogonadism or infertility

undergo spontaneous partial necrosis, and thus a partially empty sella turcica accompanies the pituitary adenoma in 30–40% of patients.

Prolactinomas usually appear chromophobic on routine histologic study, reflecting the inadequacy of the techniques used. The cells are small and uniform, with round or oval nuclei and scanty cytoplasm, and secretory granules are usually not visible with routine stains. The stroma contains a diffuse capillary network.

Electron microscopic examination shows that prolactinoma cells characteristically contain secretory granules that usually range from 100 to 500 nm and are spherical. Larger granules (400–500 nm), which are irregular or crescent-shaped, are less commonly seen. The cells show evidence of secretory activity, with a large Golgi area, nucleolar enlargement, and a prominent endoplasmic reticulum. Immunocytochemical studies of these tumors have confirmed that the secretory granules indeed contain PRL.

Clinical Findings

The clinical manifestations of PRL excess are the same regardless of the cause (see below). The classic features are galactorrhea and amenorrhea in women and galactorrhea and decreased libido or impotence in men. Although the sex distribution of prolactinomas is approximately equal, microadenomas are much more common in females, presumably because of earlier recognition of the endocrine consequences of PRL excess.

A. Galactorrhea: Galactorrhea occurs in less than half of patients with prolactinomas and is less common in men than in women. It is usually not spontaneous, or may be present only transiently or intermittently; careful breast examination is required in most patients to demonstrate galactorrhea. The absence of galactorrhea despite markedly elevated PRL levels is probably due to concomitant deficiency of the gonadal hormones required to initiate lactation (see Chapter 17).

B. Gonadal Dysfunction in Women: Amenorrhea, oligomenorrhea with anovulation, or infertility is present in approximately 90% of women with prolactinomas. These menstrual disorders usually present concurrently with galactorrhea if it is present but may either precede or follow it. The amenorrhea is usually secondary and may follow pregnancy or oral contraceptive use. Primary amenorrhea occurs in the minority of patients who have onset of hyperprolactinemia during adolescence. The necessity of measuring PRL in patients with unexplained primary or secondary amenorrhea is emphasized by several studies showing that hyperprolactinemia occurs in as many as 20% of patients with neither galactorrhea nor other manifestations of pituitary dysfunction. A number of these patients have been shown to have prolactinomas.

Gonadal dysfunction in these women is due to interference with the hypothalamic-pituitary-gonadal axis by the hyperprolactinemia and except in patients with large or invasive adenomas is not due to destruction of the gonadotropin-secreting cells. This has been documented by the return of menstrual function following reduction of PRL levels to normal by drug treatment or surgical removal of the tumor. Although basal gonadotropin levels are frequently within the normal range despite reduction of sex steroid levels in hyperprolactinemic patients, PRL inhibits both the normal pulsatile secretion of LH and FSH and the midcycle LH surge, resulting in anovulation. The positive feedback effect of estrogen on gonadotropin secretion is also inhibited; in fact, patients with hyperprolactinemia are usually estrogen-deficient. PRL may also exert an effect directly on the ovary, although evidence suggests that its major influence is on the hypothalamic-pituitary axis by some mechanism not yet identified.

Estrogen deficiency in women with prolactinomas may be accompanied by decreased vaginal lubrication, other symptoms of estrogen deficiency, and osteopenia as assessed by bone densitometry. Other symptoms may include weight gain, fluid retention, and irritability. Hirsutism may also occur, accompanied by elevated plasma levels of dehydroepiandrosterone (DHEA) sulfate. Patients with hyperprolactinemia may also suffer from anxiety and depression. Treatment with bromocriptine has been shown to improve psychologic distress in such patients.

C. Gonadal Dysfunction in Men: In men, PRL excess may also occasionally cause galactorrhea; however, the usual manifestations are those of hypogonadism. The initial symptom is decreased libido, which may be dismissed by both the patient and physician as due to psychosocial factors; thus, the recognition of prolactinomas in men is frequently delayed, and marked hyperprolactinemia (PRL > 200 ng/mL) and sellar enlargement are usual. Unfortunately, prolactinomas in men are often not diagnosed until late manifestations such as headache, visual impairment, or hypopituitarism appear; virtually all such patients have a history of sexual or gonadal dysfunction. Serum testosterone levels are low, and in the presence of normal or subnormal gonadotropin levels, PRL excess should be suspected as well as other causes of hypothalamic-pituitary-gonadal dysfunction (see section on hypopituitarism). Impotence also occurs in hyperprolactinemic males, and its cause is unclear, since testosterone replacement may not reverse it, if hyperprolactinemia is not corrected. Male infertility occurs less commonly and is accompanied by reduction in sperm count.

D. Tumor Progression: In general, the growth of prolactinomas is slow, and although the natural history of microadenomas has not been well defined, they are presumed to be slowly progressive in most patients. With progression from micro- to macroadenomas, there is an increased incidence of sellar enlargement and extrasellar extension with hypopituitarism and visual impairment.

Differential Diagnosis

The many conditions associated with hyperprolac-

tinemia are listed in Table 4–3. Hypothalamic-pituitary disorders, hypothyroidism, and drug ingestion are the most common causes. Careful history and examination are essential in all cases in order to determine the origin of PRL excess.

Hypothalamic lesions frequently cause PRL hypersecretion by decreasing the secretion of factors that tonically inhibit PRL release (eg, dopamine); the lesions are usually accompanied by panhypopituitarism. Similarly, traumatic or surgical section of the pituitary stalk leads to hyperprolactinemia and hypopituitarism. The cause and clinical features of hypothalamic lesions are discussed in previous sections.

Pregnancy leads to a physiologic increase in PRL secretion; the levels increase as pregnancy continues and may reach 200 ng/mL during the third trimester. Following delivery, basal PRL levels gradually fall to normal over several weeks but increase in response to breast feeding. Hyperprolactinemia persisting for 6–12 months or longer following delivery is an indication for evaluation for prolactinoma. PRL levels are also high in normal neonates.

Several systemic disorders lead to hyperprolactinemia. Primary hypothyroidism is a common cause, and measurement of thyroid function, including TSH, should be part of the evaluation. The PRL response to TRH may be normal or exaggerated in these patients. PRL may also be increased in liver disease, particularly in patients with severe cirrhosis, and in patients with chronic renal failure.

PRL excess and galactorrhea may also be caused by breast disease, nipple stimulation, disease or injury to the chest wall, and spinal cord lesions. These disorders increase PRL secretion by stimulation of afferent neural pathways.

The most common cause of hyperprolactinemia is drug ingestion, and a careful history of drug intake must be obtained. Elevated PRL levels, galactorrhea, and amenorrhea may occur following estrogen therapy or oral contraceptive use, but their persistence should suggest prolactinoma. Many other drugs also cause increased PRL secretion and elevated plasma levels (Table 4–3). PRL levels are usually less than 100 ng/mL, and the evaluation of these patients is primarily by discontinuance of the drug or medication and reevaluation after several weeks. In patients in whom drug withdrawal is not feasible, neuroradiologic studies, if normal, will usually exclude prolactinoma.

Diagnosis

A. General Evaluation: The evaluation of patients with galactorrhea or unexplained gonadal dysfunction with normal or low plasma gonadotropin levels should first include a history regarding menstrual status, pregnancy, fertility, sexual function, and symptoms of hypothyroidism or hypopituitarism. Current or previous use of medication, drugs, or estrogen therapy should be documented. Basal PRL levels, gonadotropins, thyroid function tests, and TSH levels should be established, as well as serum testosterone in men. Liver and kidney function should be assessed. A pregnancy test should be performed in women with recent onset of amenorrhea or galactorrhea.

Patients with galactorrhea but normal menses usually do not have hyperprolactinemia or prolactinomas. If the PRL level is normal, they may be reassured and followed with sequential PRL measurements. Those with elevated levels require further evaluation as described below.

B. Specific Diagnosis: When other causes of hyperprolactinemia have been excluded, the most likely cause of persisting hyperprolactinemia is prolactinoma, especially if there is associated hypogonadism. Although the TRH stimulation test is useful in diagnosis (see below), other available suppression and stimulation tests do not clearly distinguish PRL-secreting tumors from other causes of hyperprolactinemia. Therefore, the diagnosis must be established primarily by the assessment of basal PRL levels and neuroradiologic studies of the pituitary and sella turcica. In our experience, both hyperprolactinemia and a radiologic abnormality are required to establish the diagnosis of prolactinoma with certainty. Patients with large tumors and marked hyperprolactinemia usually present little difficulty. With very rare exceptions, basal PRL levels greater than 200 ng/mL are virtually diagnostic of prolactinoma. In addition, since there is a general correlation between the PRL elevation and the size of the pituitary adenoma, these patients usually have sellar enlargement and obvious macroadenomas. Similarly, if the basal PRL level is between 100 and 200 ng/mL, the cause is usually prolactinoma. These patients may have either micro- or macroadenomas; however, with basal levels of PRL greater than 100 ng/mL, the PRL-secreting tumor is usually radiologically evident, and again the diagnosis is generally straightforward. Patients with mild to moderate hyperprolactinemia (20–100 ng/mL) present the greatest difficulty in diagnosis, since both PRL-secreting microadenomas and the many other conditions causing hyperprolactinemia (Table 4–3) cause PRL hypersecretion of this degree. In such patients, high-resolution CT scanning should be performed and will frequently demonstrate a definite pituitary microadenoma, thus establishing the diagnosis. CT scans showing only minor or equivocal abnormalities should be interpreted with caution, because of the high incidence of false-positive scans in the normal population (see neuroradiologic evaluation, above). Since the diagnosis cannot be either established or excluded in patients with normal or equivocal neuroradiologic studies, they require further evaluation or serial assessment (see below).

Although the clinical utility of TRH stimulation testing in patients with hyperprolactinemia is controversial, it gives useful information in patients with hyperprolactinemia but normal or equivocal radiologic studies. In patients with prolactinomas, there is subnormal PRL responsiveness to TRH stimulation, and in over 90% of patients the normal 2-fold increment in PRL levels is not achieved. Several studies have concluded that the test is not reliable in diagnosis because subnormal responses were also seen in patients considered to have "idiopathic" hyperprolactinemia. The difficulty with these studies is that the presence of radiologically occult PRL-secreting microadenomas cannot be ruled out in patients with so-called idiopathic hyperprolactinemia. Thus, in patients with hyperprolactinemia and radiologic evidence of a microadenoma, a subnormal PRL response to TRH gives further confirmation of the diagnosis. In patients with nondiagnostic neuroradiologic studies, the failure of PRL responsiveness to TRH supports the diagnosis of microadenoma. The frequency of normal PRL responsiveness to TRH in patients with very small microadenomas and only minimal hyperprolactinemia (20–50 ng/mL) is currently unknown, and thus a normal PRL response does not necessarily exclude the diagnosis of a PRL-secreting microadenoma.

Treatment

Satisfactory control of PRL hypersecretion, cessation of galactorrhea, and return of normal gonadal function can be achieved in most patients with PRL-secreting microadenomas, although the choice of primary therapy (surgical or medical) remains controversial. In patients with hyperprolactinemia, ovulation should not be induced without careful assessment of pituitary anatomy and sella turcica size, since pregnancy may cause further expansion of these tumors as discussed below. All patients with PRL-secreting macroadenomas should be treated, because of the risks of further tumor expansion, hypopituitarism, and visual impairment. Patients with larger prolactinomas—over 2 cm in diameter, or basal PRL levels over 200 ng/mL—may require combined therapy with surgery, radiation, and bromocriptine.

Treatment for all patients with microadenomas is recommended to prevent early osteoporosis secondary to persisting hypogonadism and to restore fertility. In addition, surgical or medical therapy is more successful in these patients than in those with larger tumors.

Patients with persisting hyperprolactinemia and hypogonadism and normal neuroradiologic studies—ie, those in whom prolactinoma cannot be definitely established—may be managed by observation if hypogonadism is of short duration. However, in patients whose hypogonadism has persisted for more than 1–2 years, bromocriptine should be used to suppress PRL secretion and restore normal gonadal function. In women with suspected or proved prolactinomas, replacement estrogen therapy is contraindicated because of the risk of tumor growth.

A. Surgical Treatment:

1. Transsphenoidal microsurgery–This is the surgical procedure of choice in patients with prolactinomas and is the preferred initial method of therapy in many institutions.

a. Microadenomas–In patients with microadenomas, success, as measured by restitution of normal PRL levels, normal menses, and cessation of galactorrhea, is achieved in 85–90% of cases. Success is most likely in patients with basal PRL levels under 200 ng/mL and a duration of amenorrhea of less than 5 years. In these patients, the incidence of surgical complications is less than 5%, and hypopituitarism is a rare complication. Thus, in this group of patients with PRL-secreting microadenomas, PRL hypersecretion can be corrected, gonadal function restored, and secretion of TSH and ACTH preserved. Recurrence rates vary considerably in reported series. In our experience, approximately 75% of patients have had long-term remissions, and 25% have had recurrences 5–10 years following surgery.

b. Macroadenomas–Transsphenoidal microsurgery is considerably less successful in restoring normal PRL secretion in patients with macroadenomas. The outcome is directly related to tumor size and the basal PRL level. Thus, in patients with tumors 1–2 cm in diameter without extrasellar extension and with basal PRL levels under 200 ng/mL, transsphenoidal surgery is successful in about 80% of cases. In patients with higher basal PRL levels and larger tumors, the success rate—defined as complete tumor resection and restoration of normal basal PRL secretion—is about 30–50%. Although surgical results are relatively poor in this latter group of patients, surgery is recommended at many centers as the primary therapy in order to reduce tumor bulk and PRL hypersecretion. Additional therapy with bromocriptine or radiotherapy is required in the subsequent management of these patients (see below).

2. Transfrontal craniotomy–This procedure should be used only in patients with major suprasellar extension of tumor not accessible via the transsphenoidal route. It must be followed by bromocriptine or radiation therapy, since residual tumor is virtually always present.

B. Medical Treatment:

1. Bromocriptine–Bromocriptine (Parlodel; 2-bromo-α-ergocryptine mesylate) is a potent dopamine agonist that has been used extensively in the treatment of hyperprolactinemia. Bromocriptine stimulates dopamine receptors and has effects at both the hypothalamic and pituitary levels. It is effective therapy for a PRL-secreting pituitary adenoma and directly inhibits PRL secretion by the tumor. The dosage is 2.5–10 mg/d orally in divided doses. Side effects consisting of dizziness, postural hypotension, nausea, and occasionally vomiting are common at onset of therapy but usually resolve with continuation of the medication. They can usually be avoided by starting with a low dose and gradually increasing the dose over days to weeks until the PRL level is suppressed to the normal range. An example would be to give 1.25 mg at bedtime for 2 or 3 days and then increase to 2.5 mg; if tolerated, an additional 2.5 mg can be added in the morning. PRL levels should then be assessed. If they remain elevated, the dosage is gradually increased to a total of 7.5–10 mg/d. With these dosages, hyperprolactinemia is controlled in most patients; further increases in dosage are usually not warranted and are usually accompanied by increased side effects. Most patients tolerate doses of 2.5–10 mg without difficulty; however, in a minority, persisting postural hypotension and gastrointestinal side effects necessitate discontinuance of therapy.

a. Microadenomas–In patients with microadenomas, bromocriptine successfully reduces PRL levels to normal in over 90% of cases. In addition, correction of hyperprolactinemia allows recovery of normal gonadal function; ovulation and fertility are restored, so that mechanical contraception should be advised if pregnancy is not desired. Bromocriptine induces ovulation in most female patients who wish to become pregnant. In these patients with microadenomas, the risk of major expansion of adenoma during the pregnancy appears to be less than 5%; however, both the patient and the physician must be aware of this potential complication. Current data do not indicate an increased risk of multiple pregnancy, abortion, or fetal malformations in pregnancies induced by bromocriptine; however, the patient should be instructed to discontinue bromocriptine at the first missed menstrual period and obtain a pregnancy test. At present, there is no evidence that bromocriptine causes permanent resolution of PRL-secreting microadenomas, and virtually all patients have resumption of hyperprolactinemia following discontinuation of therapy even when it has been continued for several years. Although no late toxicity has yet been reported other than the side effects noted above, questions about possible long-term risk and the indicated duration of therapy in such patients with microadenomas are currently unanswered.

b. Macroadenomas–Bromocriptine is effective in controlling hyperprolactinemia in patients with PRL-secreting macroadenomas even when basal PRL levels are markedly elevated. Bromocriptine may be used either as initial therapy or to control residual hyperprolactinemia in patients unsuccessfully treated with surgery or radiotherapy. Bromocriptine should not be used to induce ovulation and pregnancy in women with untreated macroadenomas, since the risk of tumor expansion and visual deficits in the later part of pregnancy is approximately 25%. These patients should be treated with surgery or radiotherapy prior to induction of ovulation with bromocriptine or by gonadotropin therapy.

Bromocriptine not only reduces PRL secretion in patients with macroadenomas but also reduces tumor size in about 70% of patients. Reduction of tumor size with bromocriptine may occur within days to weeks following institution of therapy. The drug has been used to restore vision in a few patients with major suprasellar extension and chiasmal compression. Tumor reduction in response to bromocriptine is sustained only as long as the medication is continued, and reexpansion of the tumor and recurrence of hyperprolactinemia may occur rapidly following discontinuation of therapy. The question of duration of therapy in patients with macroadenomas remains unanswered.

2. Pergolide–Pergolide mesylate is a long-acting ergot derivative with dopaminergic properties that has been shown to reduce hypersecretion and shrink most PRL-secreting macroadenomas. This new drug remains investigational. It is more potent than bromocriptine, requiring doses of $25-300$ $\mu g/d$ to treat hyperprolactinemia. The side effects of pergolide are similar to those of bromocriptine.

C. Radiation Therapy: Conventional radiation therapy is reserved for patients with PRL-secreting macroadenomas who have persisting hyperprolactinemia following surgical treatment. In this group of patients, radiotherapy with $4000-5000$ rads prevents further tumor expansion, though PRL levels usually do not fall into the normal range. Impairment of anterior pituitary function occurs in approximately $30-50\%$ of patients. Conventional radiation therapy has not been used as initial treatment for patients with microadenomas, since experience is limited and the radiation-induced damage to gonadotropin-secreting cells may further impair fertility.

Experience with heavy particle irradiation in prolactinomas is limited.

2. ACROMEGALY & GIGANTISM

GH-secreting pituitary adenomas are second in frequency to prolactinomas and the classic clinical syndromes of acromegaly and gigantism.

The characteristic clinical manifestations are the consequence of chronic GH hypersecretion, which in turn leads to excessive generation of the somatomedins, the mediators of most of the effects of GH (see Chapter 4, Part II). Although overgrowth of bone is the classic feature, GH excess causes a generalized systemic disorder with deleterious effects on many systems and an increased mortality rate, though deaths are rarely due to the space-occupying or destructive effects of pituitary adenoma per se.

Acromegaly and gigantism are virtually always secondary to pituitary adenoma. Ectopic GRH secretion has been identified as another cause of GH hypersecretion and acromegaly in a few patients with carcinoid or islet cell tumors. Reports of intrapituitary GRH-secreting gangliocytomas in direct contiguity with GH-secreting somatotroph adenomas and a report of a GRH-secreting hypothalamic hamartoma in a patient with acromegaly provide a link between ectopic and eutopic GRH production. Ectopic secretion of GH per se is very rare.

In adults, GH excess leads to acromegaly, the syndrome characterized by local overgrowth of bone, particularly of the skull and mandible. Linear growth does not occur, because of prior fusion of the epiphyses of long bones. In childhood and adolescence, the onset of chronic GH excess leads to gigantism. Many of these patients have associated hypogonadism, which further delays epiphyseal closure, and the combination of somatomedin excess and hypogonadism leads to a striking acceleration of linear growth. In addition,

most patients with gigantism also have features of acromegaly if GH hypersecretion persists through adolescence and into adulthood.

Pathology

Pituitary adenomas causing acromegaly are usually over 1 cm in diameter when the diagnosis is established. These tumors arise from the lateral wings of the anterior pituitary; less than 20% are diagnosed as microadenomas.

GH-secreting adenomas are of 2 histologic types: densely and sparsely granulated. However, there appears to be no difference in the degree of GH secretion or clinical manifestations in these patients. About 15% of GH-secreting tumors also contain lactotrophs, and these tumors thus hypersecrete both GH and PRL.

Densely granulated adenomas are acidophilic by light microscopy using routine stains and are usually strongly positive when stained for GH by immunocytochemical techniques. Electron microscopy demonstrates that the cells are similar to normal somatotrophs; ie, they are spherical or oval, with uniform features, round or oval centrally located nuclei, and abundant cytoplasm. The numerous spherical GH-containing granules are electron-dense, ranging in size from 300 to 600 nm, with the majority measuring $350-450$ nm.

The sparsely granulated adenomas are chromophobic by light microscopy, a feature that merely reflects the paucity of stainable secretory granules; they are indistinguishable from other chromophobe adenomas except by the demonstration of GH within them by immunocytochemistry. By electron microscopy, the cells do not resemble normal somatotrophs but have variable shape and size; pleomorphic, frequently crescent-shaped nuclei; and globular fibrous bodies within the cytoplasm. The secretory granules measure $100-250$ nm, and fewer are present than in normal somatotrophs or densely granulated adenomas.

Etiology & Pathogenesis

Excessive pituitary GH secretion may be secondary to abnormal hypothalamic function, but current evidence suggests that it is a primary pituitary disorder in most cases. Pituitary adenomas are present in virtually all patients and are usually greater than 1 cm in diameter; hyperplasia alone is rare, and nonadenomatous anterior pituitary tissue does not exhibit somatotroph hyperplasia when examined histologically. In addition, there is a return of normal GH levels and dynamic control of GH secretion following selective removal of the pituitary adenoma.

Indirect evidence that acromegaly may be a hypothalamic disorder consisting of either increased release of GRH or decreased secretion of somatostatin is based largely on the findings of abnormal GH dynamics in these patients.

Pathophysiology

In acromegaly, GH secretion is increased and its dynamic control is abnormal. Secretion remains episodic; however, the number, duration, and amplitude of secretory episodes are increased, and they occur randomly throughout the 24-hour period. The characteristic nocturnal surge is absent, and there are abnormal responses to suppression and stimulation. Thus, glucose suppressibility is lost (see diagnosis, below), and GH stimulation by hypoglycemia is usually absent. TRH and GnRH may cause GH release, whereas these substances do not normally stimulate GH secretion. Dopamine and dopamine agonists such as bromocriptine and apomorphine, which normally stimulate GH secretion, paradoxically cause GH suppression in about 70–80% of patients with acromegaly.

Most of the deleterious effects of chronic GH hypersecretion are caused by its stimulation of excessive amounts of the somatomedins (see Part II of this chapter), and plasma levels of these compounds are increased in acromegaly. The growth-promoting effects of the somatomedins (DNA, RNA, and protein synthesis) lead to the characteristic proliferation of bone, cartilage, and soft tissues and increase in size of other organs to produce the classic clinical manifestations of acromegaly. The insulin resistance and carbohydrate intolerance seen in acromegaly appear to be direct effects of GH and not due to somatomedin excess.

Clinical Findings

The sex incidence of acromegaly is approximately equal; the mean age at diagnosis is approximately 40 years; and the duration of symptoms is usually 5–10 years before the diagnosis is established.

Acromegaly is a chronic disabling and disfiguring disorder with increased late morbidity and mortality if untreated. Although spontaneous remissions have been described, the course is slowly progressive in the great majority of cases—patients once thought to be "burned out" can almost invariably be shown to have continuing clinical manifestations and GH hypersecretion.

A. Symptoms and Signs: Early manifestations (Table 4–8) include soft tissue proliferation, with enlargement of the hands and feet and coarsening of the facial features. This is usually accompanied by increased sweating, oiliness of the skin, fatigue, and weight gain.

At diagnosis, virtually all patients have classic manifestations; acral and soft tissue changes are always present. Bone and cartilage changes affect chiefly the face and skull (Fig 4–15). These changes include thickening of the calvarium; increased size of the frontal sinuses, which leads to prominence of the supraorbital ridges; enlargement of the nose; and downward and forward growth of the mandible, which leads to prognathism and widely spaced teeth. Soft tissue growth also contributes to the facial appearance, with coarsening of the features and facial and infraorbital puffiness. The hands and feet are predominantly affected by soft tissue growth; they are large, thickened, and bulky, with blunt, spadelike fingers (Fig 4–16)

Table 4–8. Clinical manifestations of acromegaly in 100 patients.*

Manifestations of GH excess	
Acral enlargement	100†
Soft tissue overgrowth	100
Hyperhidrosis	88
Lethargy or fatigue	87
Weight gain	73
Paresthesias	70
Joint pain	69
Photophobia	46
Papillomas	45
Hypertrichosis	33
Goiter	32
Acanthosis nigricans	29
Hypertension	24
Cardiomegaly	16
Renal calculi	11
Disturbance of other endocrine functions	
Hyperinsulinemia	70
Glucose intolerance	50
Irregular or absent menses	60
Decreased libido or impotence	46
Hypothyroidism	13
Galactorrhea	13
Gynecomastia	8
Hypoadrenalism	4
Local manifestations	
Enlarged sella	90
Headache	65
Visual deficit	20

*Adapted from Tyrrell JB, Wilson CB: Pituitary syndromes. In: *Surgical Endocrinology: Clinical Syndromes.* Friesen SR (editor). Lippincott, 1978.
†Percentage of patients in whom these features were present.

and toes. A bulky, sweaty handshake frequently suggests the diagnosis, and there are increases in ring, glove, and shoe sizes. There is generalized thickening of the skin, with increased oiliness and sweating. Acne, sebaceous cysts, and fibromata mollusca (skin tags and papillomas) are common, as is acanthosis nigricans of the axillae and neck and hypertrichosis in women.

These bony and soft tissue changes are accompanied by systemic manifestations, which include hyperhidrosis, heat intolerance, lethargy, fatigue, and increased sleep requirement. Moderate weight gain usually occurs. Paresthesias, usually due to carpal tunnel compression, occur in 70%; sensorimotor neuropathies occur uncommonly. Bone and cartilage overgrowth leads to arthralgias and in long-standing cases to degenerative arthritis of the spine, hips, and knees. Photophobia of unknown cause occurs in about half of cases and is most troublesome in bright sunlight and during night driving.

GH excess leads to generalized visceromegaly, clinically evident as thyromegaly and enlargement of the salivary glands. Enlargement of other organs is usually not clinically detectable.

Hypertension of unknown cause occurs in about

Figure 4–15. Serial photographs of an acromegalic patient at the ages indicated. Note the gradual increase in size of the nose, lips, and skin folds. (Reproduced, with permission, from Reichlin SR: Acromegaly. *Med Grand Rounds* 1982;**1**:9.)

Figure 4–16. Markedly increased soft tissue bulk and blunt fingers in a middle-aged man with acromegaly.

25% of patients and cardiomegaly in about 15%. Cardiac enlargement may be secondary to hypertension, atherosclerotic disease, or, rarely, to "acromegalic cardiomyopathy." Renal calculi occur in 11% secondary to the hypercalciuria induced by GH excess.

Other endocrine and metabolic abnormalities are common and may be due either to GH excess or to mechanical effects of the pituitary adenoma. Glucose intolerance and hyperinsulinism occur in 50% and 70%, respectively, owing to GH-induced insulin resistance. Overt clinical diabetes occurs in a minority, and diabetic ketoacidosis is rare. Hypogonadism occurs in 60% of female and 46% of male patients and is of multifactorial origin; tumor growth and compression may impair pituitary gonadotropin secretion, and associated hyperprolactinemia (see below) or the PRL-like effect of excessive GH secretion may impair gonadotropin and gonadal function. In men, low total plasma testosterone levels may be due to GH suppression of sex hormone–binding globulin (SHBG) levels; in these cases, plasma free testosterone levels may be normal, with normal gonadal function. With earlier diagnosis, hypothyroidism and hypoadrenalism due to destruction of the normal anterior pituitary are unusual and are present in only 13% and 4% of patients, respectively. Galactorrhea occurs in about 15% and is usually caused by hyperprolactinemia from a pituitary adenoma with a mixed cell population of somatotrophs and lactotrophs. Gynecomastia of unknown cause occurs in about 10% of men. Although acromegaly may be a component of multiple endocrine neoplasia (MEN) type I syndrome, it is distinctly unusual, and concomitant parathyroid hyperfunction or pancreatic islet cell tumors are rare.

When GH hypersecretion is present for many years, late complications occur, including progressive cosmetic deformity and disabling degenerative arthritis (which frequently requires operative treatment). In addition, the mortality rate is increased; after age 45, the death rate in acromegaly from cardiovascular and cerebrovascular atherosclerosis and respiratory diseases is twice that of the normal population. Death rates are highest in patients with hypertension or clinical diabetes mellitus.

Manifestations of the pituitary adenoma are also common in acromegaly; eg, 65% of patients have headache. Although visual impairment was usually present in older series, it now occurs in only 15–20%, since most patients are now diagnosed because of the manifestations of GH excess.

B. Laboratory Findings: Postprandial plasma glucose may be elevated, and serum insulin is increased in 70%. Elevated serum phosphorus (due to increased renal tubular resorption of phosphate) and hypercalciuria appear to be due to direct effects of GH or somatomedins.

C. X-Ray Findings: Plain films (Fig 4–17) show sellar enlargement in 90% of cases. Thickening of the calvarium, enlargement of the frontal and maxillary sinuses, and enlargement of the jaw can also be seen. Radiographs of the hand show increased soft tissue bulk, "arrowhead" tufting of the distal phalanges,

Figure 4–17. Radiologic signs in acromegaly: *Left:* Skull with enlarged sella turcica and frontal sinuses, thickening of the calvarium, and enlargement of the mandible. *Center:* Hand with enlarged sesamoid bone and increased soft tissue shadows. *Right:* Thickened heel pad. (Reproduced, with permission, from Levin SR: Manifestations and treatment of acromegaly. *Calif Med* [March] 1972;**116**:57.)

increased width of intra-articular cartilages, and cystic changes of the carpal bones. Radiographs of the feet show similar changes, and there is increased thickness of the heel pad (normal, < 22 mm).

Diagnosis

Acromegaly is usually clinically obvious and can be readily confirmed by assessment of GH secretion; basal fasting GH levels (normal, 1–5 ng/mL) are greater than 10 ng/mL in over 90% of patients and range from 5 ng/mL to over 500 ng/mL, with a mean of approximately 50 ng/mL. However, single measurements are not entirely reliable, because GH secretion is episodic in acromegaly and because other conditions may increase GH secretion (see below).

A. Glucose Suppression: Suppression with oral glucose is the simplest and most specific dynamic test for acromegaly. In normal subjects, oral administration of 100 g of glucose causes a reduction of the GH level to less than 5 ng/mL at 60 minutes. In acromegaly, GH levels may decrease, increase, or show no change; however, they do not decrease to less than 5 ng/mL, and this lack of response establishes the diagnosis.

B. Other Tests: Additional procedures that help establish or confirm the diagnosis are (1) GH stimulation with TRH; (2) the absence of a nocturnal GH surge; and (3) the paradoxical suppression of GH by levodopa, dopamine, bromocriptine, or apomorphine. These procedures are usually unnecessary except in patients with mild acromegaly who may have normal

or only mildly elevated GH levels and equivocal responses to glucose suppression.

C. Somatomedin Measurement: Measurement of somatomedin-C (see Part II of this chapter) is a useful means of establishing a diagnosis of GH hypersecretion, although at present many methods lack specificity and measurements may not be clinically available. Somatomedin levels are elevated in virtually all patients with acromegaly (normal ranges vary widely in different laboratories). Although they confirm the diagnosis, a clear-cut advantage over GH suppression with glucose has yet to be established. Further experience may elucidate the role of somatomedin measurements; however, direct measurement of GH secretion, the product of the pituitary adenoma, will continue to be necessary in diagnosis and follow-up.

D. Tumor Localization: Radiographic localization of the pituitary adenoma causing acromegaly is usually straightforward (see Neuroradiologic Evaluation, above). In virtually all patients, tumor location and size can be shown by high-resolution CT scanning; 90% have tumors over 1 cm in diameter that are readily visualized. In the rare patient with normal neuroradiologic studies, an extrapituitary ectopic source of GH or GRH should be considered.

Differential Diagnosis

A. Other Causes of GH Hypersecretion: The presence of clinical features of GH excess, elevated GH secretion, and abnormal GH dynamics, together with the demonstration of a pituitary tumor by neuroradiologic studies, is diagnostic of acromegaly. However, other conditions associated with GH hypersecretion must be considered in the differential diagnosis: anxiety, exercise, acute illness, chronic renal failure, cirrhosis, starvation, protein-calorie malnutrition, anorexia nervosa, and type I (insulin-dependent) diabetes mellitus. Estrogen therapy may increase GH responsiveness to various stimuli. These conditions may be associated with abnormal GH suppressibility by glucose and by abnormal GH responsiveness to TRH (protirelin); however, patients with these conditions do not have clinical manifestations of GH excess and are thus readily differentiated from patients with acromegaly.

B. Ectopic GH or GRH Secretion: There is a rare group of patients who have acromegaly due to ectopic secretion of GH or GRH and in whom clinical manifestations of acromegaly may be typical. This may occur in lung carcinoma, carcinoid tumors, and pancreatic islet cell tumors. These syndromes should be suspected in patients with a known extrapituitary tumor who have GH excess or in those with clinical and biochemical features of acromegaly who have no radiologically demonstrable pituitary adenoma.

Treatment

A. Objectives of Treatment: All patients with acromegaly should undergo therapy to halt progression of the disorder and to prevent late complications. The objectives of therapy are removal or destruction of the pituitary tumor, reversal of GH hypersecretion, and maintenance of normal anterior and posterior pituitary function. These objectives are currently attainable in most patients, especially those with smaller tumors and only moderate GH hypersecretion. In patients with large tumors who have marked GH hypersecretion, several therapies are usually required to achieve normal GH secretion.

Various criteria exist for what constitutes an adequate response to therapy. Most authors agree that basal GH values under 5 ng/mL indicate the return of normal GH secretion. The utility of somatomedin-C measurements is currently being evaluated, and preliminary results show that appropriate therapy lowers these values to normal.

B. Therapy: The choice of initial therapy is between transsphenoidal microsurgery, radiotherapy, and medical management. Microsurgery is preferred because of its high success rate, rapid reduction of GH levels, the low incidence of postoperative hypopituitarism, and the low surgical morbidity rate. Conventional radiotherapy (x-ray radiation) is also successful, although a much longer period is required to reduce GH levels to normal, and heavy particle irradiation has limited availability. Medical management with bromocriptine has the disadvantage of requiring chronic therapy to suppress GH secretion, and it is generally used in the minority of patients who have not responded to surgery or irradiation.

1. Surgical treatment–Transsphenoidal selective adenoma removal is the procedure of choice; craniotomy is necessary in the few patients in whom major suprasellar extension precludes the transsphenoidal approach. Successful reduction of GH levels is achieved in approximately 80% of patients. In those with small or moderate-sized tumors (< 2 cm), success is achieved in over 90%, whereas in those with larger tumors and basal GH levels greater than 50 ng/mL—and particularly in those with major extrasellar extension of the adenoma—successful responses occur in only 60–70%. Recurrence rates in those with a successful initial response are low (about 5% of patients at our institution). Surgical complications (discussed above) occur in less than 10%.

2. Radiation therapy–Conventional supervoltage irradiation in doses of 4500–5000 rads is successful in 60–80% of patients, although GH levels may not return to normal until several years after therapy. Thus, in one recent series, GH levels were under 10 ng/mL in only 38% of patients at 2 years posttreatment; however, at 5 and 10 years, 73% and 81% had achieved such levels. The incidence of hypopituitarism is appreciable, and in this series hypothyroidism occurred in 19%, hypoadrenalism in 38%, and hypogonadism in approximately 50–60% of patients as a consequence of radiotherapy. Because of the prolonged delay in achieving reduction in GH levels, conventional radiotherapy is generally reserved for patients with persisting GH secretion following pituitary microsurgery.

Heavy particle irradiation is more rapidly effective than conventional irradiation, but because of the limitations of the field size, it can be used only in patients with smaller tumors and those in whom no extrasellar extension is present. About 80% of patients have GH levels under 10 ng/mL at 5 years after irradiation, with most patients having a satisfactory response at 2 years. The incidence of hypopituitarism has been variously reported, but it appears to occur in approximately 40% of patients.

Therapy of acromegaly by radioactive implants within the sella turcica is limited to a few centers. Successful responses are achieved in about 70%; however, there is a significant incidence of hypopituitarism, cerebrospinal fluid rhinorrhea, and meningitis due to local radionecrosis. Because of these complications, the procedure has not gained wide acceptance.

3. Medical treatment–Bromocriptine, a long-acting dopamine agonist, reduces GH levels in 60–80% of patients; however, in only about 40% are the levels reduced to 10 ng/mL or less. In addition, although reduction in tumor size occurs in some patients, this therapy is suppressive only, and GH hypersecretion rapidly recurs upon discontinuation of the drug. For these reasons, bromocriptine is generally used in acromegalics in whom adequate reduction of GH levels has not been achieved with surgery or irradiation.

C. Response to Therapy: In patients with successful reduction in GH hypersecretion, there is cessation of bone overgrowth. In addition, these patients experience considerable clinical improvement, including reduction in soft tissue bulk of the extremities, decreased facial puffiness, increased energy, and cessation of hyperhidrosis, heat intolerance, and oily skin. Headache, carpal tunnel syndrome, arthralgias, and photophobia are also reversible with successful therapy. Glucose intolerance and hyperinsulinemia as well as hypercalciuria are also reversed in most cases.

In patients in whom operation is successful, reversal of clinical features is more rapid; decreased sweating and the onset of soft tissue regression may occur within a few days after surgery. The response to radiation therapy is much slower and occurs gradually over months to years.

Posttreatment Follow-Up

Patients undergoing surgery should be seen 4–6 weeks after the operation for assessment of GH secretion and pituitary function. Those with persisting GH hypersecretion should receive further therapy with radiation or bromocriptine. Patients with postoperative GH levels under 10 ng/mL should have follow-up GH determinations at 6-month intervals for 2 years and yearly thereafter. Late hypopituitarism after surgery alone does not occur.

Patients treated with radiotherapy either primarily or following unsuccessful surgery should have biannual assessment of GH secretion and annual assessment of anterior pituitary function, since the incidence of late hypopituitarism is appreciable and increases with time following irradiation.

3. ACTH-SECRETING PITUITARY ADENOMAS: CUSHING'S DISEASE

In 1932, Harvey Cushing documented the presence of small basophilic pituitary adenomas in 6 of 8 patients with clinical features of adrenocortical hyperfunction. Years later, ACTH hypersecretion was identified from such tumors and found to be the cause of bilateral adrenal hyperplasia. Pituitary ACTH hypersecretion (Cushing's disease) is now recognized as the most common cause of spontaneous hypercortisolism (Cushing's syndrome) and must be distinguished from the other forms of adrenocorticosteroid excess— ectopic ACTH syndrome and adrenal tumors (see Chapter 9).

Pathology

ACTH-secreting pituitary tumors exist in over 90% of patients with Cushing's disease. These tumors are usually benign microadenomas under 10 mm in diameter; 50% are 5 mm or less in diameter, and microadenomas as small as 1 mm have been described. These tumors in Cushing's disease are either basophilic or chromophobe adenomas and may be found anywhere within the anterior pituitary. Rarely, ACTH-secreting tumors are large, with invasive tendencies, and malignant tumors have occasionally been reported.

Histologically, the tumors are composed of compact sheets of uniform, well-granulated cells (granule size, 200–700 nm by electron microscopy) with a sinusoidal arrangement and a high content of ACTH and its related peptides (β-LPH, β-endorphin). A zone of perinuclear hyalinization (Crooke's changes) is frequently observed as a result of exposure of the corticotroph cells to prolonged hypercortisolism. A specific ultrastructural finding in these adenomas is the deposition of bundles of perinuclear microfilaments that encircle the nucleus; these are the ultrastructural equivalent of Crooke's hyaline changes seen on light microscopy. In contrast to the adenoma cells, ACTH content in the portion of the anterior pituitary not involved with the tumor is decreased.

Diffuse hyperplasia of anterior pituitary corticotrophs or adenomatous hyperplasia, presumed to result from hypersecretion of corticotropin-releasing hormone (CRH), occurs in a few patients.

The adrenal glands in Cushing's disease are enlarged, weighing 12–24 g (normal, 8–10 g). Microscopic examination shows a thickened cortex due to hyperplasia of both the zona reticularis and zona fasciculata; the zona glomerulosa is normal. In some cases, ACTH-secreting pituitary adenomas cause bilateral nodular hyperplasia; the adrenals show diffuse bilateral cortical hyperplasia and the presence of one or more nodules that vary from microscopic to several centimeters in diameter, with multiple small nodules being the most common. Occasionally, only a solitary nodule is observed on radiographic studies, and this entity may be confused with an autonomously functioning adrenal tumor (see Chapter 9).

Pathogenesis

The weight of current evidence is that Cushing's disease is a primary pituitary disorder and that hypothalamic abnormalities are secondary to hypercortisolism. Nonetheless, many authorities still believe that this disorder is the result of a primary central nervous system abnormality with excessive stimulation of anterior pituitary corticotrophs by CRH and secondary adenoma formation.

The endocrine abnormalities in Cushing's disease are as follows: (1) hypersecretion of ACTH, with bilateral adrenocortical hyperplasia and hypercortisolism; (2) absent circadian periodicity of ACTH and cortisol secretion; (3) absent responsiveness of ACTH and cortisol to stress (hypoglycemia or surgery); (4) abnormal negative feedback of ACTH secretion by glucocorticoids; and (5) subnormal responsiveness of GH, TSH, and gonadotropins to stimulation.

A primary central nervous system defect could explain these observed abnormalities in Cushing's disease as well as the occasional finding that certain pharmacologic agents such as cyproheptadine and bromocriptine inhibit ACTH release in some patients with Cushing's disease.

However, evidence that Cushing's disease is a primary pituitary disorder is based on the high frequency of pituitary adenomas, the response to their removal, and the interpretation of hypothalamic abnormalities as being secondary to hypercortisolism. These findings suggest that ACTH hypersecretion arises from a spontaneously developing pituitary adenoma and that the resulting hypercortisolism suppresses the normal hypothalamic-pituitary axis and CRH release and thereby abolishes the hypothalamic regulation of circadian variability and stress responsiveness. There is in vitro evidence that the negative feedback effects of glucocorticoids are exerted directly on the pituitary tumor and that other pharmacologic agents such as vasopressin, cyproheptadine, and bromocriptine directly inhibit the ACTH-secreting adenoma. In addition, the abnormalities of GH, TSH, and gonadotropin secretion are also observed in exogenous Cushing's syndrome and are due to the hypercortisolism per se and not to a primary hypothalamic disorder.

Analysis of the response to therapy by pituitary microsurgery sheds some light on the pathogenesis of Cushing's disease. Selective removal of pituitary microadenomas by transsphenoidal microsurgery corrects ACTH hypersecretion and hypercortisolism in most patients. This suggests that the adenoma—not corticotroph hyperplasia—is responsible for the ACTH excess. Postoperatively, these patients experience transient ACTH deficiency with secondary hypoadrenalism. The secretion of the other anterior pituitary hormones is not only preserved but enhanced once the microadenoma is removed. These findings, which suggest that the normal hypothalamic-pituitary axis is suppressed by the hypercortisolism, are supported by the in vitro demonstration of markedly decreased ACTH content in nonadenomatous pituitary tissue removed from patients with active Cushing's disease. After selective removal of the pituitary adenoma, the following return to normal: the circadian rhythmicity of ACTH and cortisol, the responsiveness of the hypothalamic-pituitary axis to hypoglycemic stress, and the dexamethasone suppressibility of cortisol secretion. Thus, in these patients, there is no evidence for a persisting hypothalamic abnormality.

Clinical Findings

Cushing's disease presents with the signs and symptoms of hypercortisolism and adrenal androgen excess (see Chapter 9). The onset of these features is usually insidious, developing over months or years. Obesity (with predominantly central fat distribution), hypertension, glucose intolerance, and gonadal dysfunction (amenorrhea or impotence) are common features. Other common manifestations include moon facies, plethora, osteopenia, proximal muscle weakness, easy bruisability, psychologic disturbances, violaceous striae, hirsutism, acne, poor wound healing, and superficial fungal infections. Unlike patients with the classic form of ectopic ACTH syndrome, patients with Cushing's disease rarely have hypokalemia, weight loss, anemia, or hyperpigmentation. Virilization, observed occasionally in patients with adrenal carcinoma, is unusual in Cushing's disease. Clinical symptoms related to the ACTH-secreting pituitary tu-

mor itself, such as headache or visual impairment, are rare because of early diagnosis and the small size of these adenomas.

The usual age range is 20–40 years, but Cushing's disease has been reported in infants and patients over 70. There is a female:male ratio of approximately 8:1. In contrast, the ectopic ACTH syndrome occurs more commonly in men (male:female ratio of 3:1).

Diagnosis

The initial step in the diagnosis of an ACTH-secreting pituitary adenoma is the documentation of endogenous hypercortisolism, which is confirmed by the presence of abnormal cortisol suppressibility to low-dose dexamethasone as well as an increased basal urine free cortisol or cortisol secretory rate. A more complete discussion of the diagnosis and differential diagnosis of Cushing's syndrome is presented in Chapter 9. The discussion here emphasizes the diagnosis of ACTH-secreting pituitary tumors.

The differentiation of an ACTH-secreting pituitary tumor from other causes of hypercortisolism must be based on biochemical studies, of which the measurement of basal plasma ACTH levels and the response to high-dose dexamethasone suppression testing are the most reliable.

A. ACTH Levels: Patients with Cushing's disease have normal or modestly elevated ACTH levels ranging from 50 to 200 pg/mL (normal, 20–100 pg/mL). Low levels (< 20–30 pg/mL) are indicative of an autonomously secreting adrenal tumor, and levels greater than 200 pg/mL suggest an ectopic ACTH-secreting neoplasm. Unfortunately, plasma ACTH levels do not adequately differentiate pituitary from ectopic sources of ACTH hypersecretion. Thus, 30–40% of patients with the ectopic ACTH syndrome have ACTH levels (100–200 pg/mL) that are in the range seen in Cushing's disease, and some patients actually have "normal" measurements (see Chapter 9).

B. Dexamethasone Suppression Tests: Although all patients with Cushing's syndrome have disordered regulation of glucocorticoid feedback at the hypothalamic-pituitary level (eg, failure of suppression with low-dose dexamethasone), some negative glucocorticoid feedback effect is maintained by ACTH-secreting pituitary tumors. Thus, administration of high-dose dexamethasone will suppress plasma or urine corticosteroids. The standard 2-day suppression test of Liddle requires administration of 2 mg of dexamethasone every 6 hours for 2 days. In patients with Cushing's disease, urine 17-hydroxycorticosteroids should fall to less than 50% of basal levels on the second day of dexamethasone therapy; failure of suppression indicates either an ectopic ACTH-secreting tumor or an adrenal neoplasm.

The rapid overnight high-dose dexamethasone test (see Chapter 9) is a reliable and simpler means of distinguishing ACTH-secreting pituitary tumors from other forms of endogenous hypercortisolism: The administration of 8 mg of dexamethasone at 11 PM will suppress plasma cortisol to less than 50% of baseline in Cushing's disease; failure of plasma cortisol to be suppressed indicates either ectopic ACTH syndrome or an adrenal tumor.

Caution must be urged in interpreting the results of these high-dose dexamethasone suppression tests, since they are not entirely specific. About 20–30% of patients with proved ACTH-secreting tumors fail to suppress basal urine steroids to less than 50% with the standard 2-day test, and some patients with ectopic ACTH syndrome (bronchial carcinoid; thymomas) do suppress with high-dose dexamethasone (see Chapter 9).

C. Problems in Diagnosis: Patients with ectopic ACTH syndrome may be clinically indistinguishable from those with Cushing's disease, and the tumor in each may be radiologically occult. With the advent of specific therapy directed at pituitary microadenomas, establishing the presence or absence of a pituitary source of ACTH hypersecretion is essential. Selective venous ACTH sampling from the inferior petrosal sinus (pituitary venous effluent) is a useful aid in differential diagnosis (see Chapter 9).

Problems in diagnosis may also result from intermittent Cushing's disease. In this unusual form of the disorder, ACTH-cortisol hypersecretion fluctuates with periods of normal secretion, during which laboratory studies will be misleading. Proper biochemical confirmation may require repeated studies in these patients.

D. CRH Testing: CRH stimulation testing has recently been employed as a means of differentiating pituitary from ectopic causes of Cushing's syndrome. In patients with Cushing's disease, the administration of CRH causes a further increase in ACTH and cortisol levels. In contrast, patients with ectopic ACTH syndrome usually have no ACTH or cortisol responses to CRH. However, several exceptions to these typical responses have been observed, and it seems unlikely that this new test will provide any major improvement in the differential diagnosis of ACTH-dependent Cushing's syndrome.

E. Radiologic Procedures: Neuroradiologic techniques are not particularly useful in the localization of ACTH-secreting pituitary adenomas. Since these tumors average only 5 mm in diameter and exceed 1 cm in diameter in only 10% of cases, findings on plain films of the sella turcica are almost always normal. Similarly, sellar polytomography is of little diagnostic utility in Cushing's disease.

High-resolution CT scanning of the sella turcica localizes pituitary adenomas in about 60% of cases of ACTH-secreting pituitary adenomas. However, both false-positive and false-negative findings occur—emphasizing again the importance of using clinical and biochemical techniques to establish the diagnosis of an ACTH-secreting microadenoma.

Roentgenographic studies of the adrenal glands in Cushing's disease must be interpreted with caution. CT scanning may demonstrate normal, enlarged, or asymmetric adrenal glands; and nodular adrenal hyperplasia secondary to an ACTH-secreting pituitary tumor may appear as a solitary adrenal mass and mimic an adrenal neoplasm. Radioactive iodocholesterol scanning of the adrenals is helpful in such cases, since it can usually differentiate between bilateral adrenocortical hyperfunction and a single adrenal tumor.

Treatment

The increasing clinical recognition of ACTH-secreting pituitary microadenomas and the clarification of their role in the pathogenesis of Cushing's disease have led to advances in treatment of this disorder. Sophisticated microsurgical techniques now permit removal of pituitary tumors by a transsphenoidal approach. A variety of other therapies—operative, radiologic, pharmacologic—are discussed below.

A. Surgical Treatment: Selective transsphenoidal resection of ACTH-secreting pituitary adenomas is the initial treatment of choice. Independent series from several centers have confirmed the efficacy of this procedure as well as its low morbidity rate and low incidence of surgical complications. The indication for this procedure is a secure biochemical diagnosis, as discussed earlier. Neuroradiologic procedures (CT scanning) are employed preoperatively, but findings may be normal because of the small size of these tumors.

At operation, meticulous exploration of the intrasellar contents by an experienced neurosurgeon is required. The tumor, which is often found within the anterior lobe tissue, is selectively removed, and normal gland is left intact. If the tumor is too small to locate at surgery, total hypophysectomy may be performed in adult patients who are past the age of reproduction and whose biochemical diagnosis has been confirmed with selective venous ACTH sampling.

In about 85% of patients with microadenomas, selective microsurgery is successful in correcting hypercortisolism. Surgical damage to anterior pituitary function is rare, but most patients develop transient secondary adrenocortical insufficiency requiring postoperative glucocorticoid support until the hypothalamic-pituitary-adrenal axis recovers, usually in 6–18 months. Total hypophysectomy is necessary to correct hypercortisolism in another 10% of patients. In the remaining 5% of patients with microadenomas, selective tumor removal is unsuccessful. By contrast, transsphenoidal surgery is successful in only 25% of the 10–15% of patients with Cushing's disease with pituitary macroadenomas or in those with extrasellar extension of tumor.

Transient diabetes insipidus occurs in about 20% of patients, but other surgical complications (eg, hemorrhage, cerebrospinal fluid rhinorrhea, infection, visual impairment, permanent diabetes insipidus) are rare. Hypopituitarism occurs only in patients who undergo total hypophysectomy.

Before the introduction of pituitary microsurgery, bilateral total adrenalectomy was the preferred treatment of Cushing's disease and may still be employed in patients in whom other therapies are unsuccessful. Total adrenalectomy usually corrects hypercortisolism but produces permanent hypoadrenalism, requiring lifelong glucocorticoid and mineralocorticoid therapy. Morbidity is high and relates to poor wound healing, postoperative infection, pancreatic injury, and thromboembolic phenomena. In addition, the ACTH-secreting pituitary adenoma persists and may progress, causing hyperpigmentation and invasive complications (Nelson's syndrome; see below). Persistent hypercortisolism may occasionally follow total adrenalectomy as ACTH hypersecretion stimulates adrenal remnants or congenital rests. Attempts to transplant adrenal tissue to a readily accessible location, such as the forearm, have been successful in only a few cases and may require several years before the transplant functions satisfactorily; recurrent hyperfunction may result.

B. Radiation Therapy: In Cushing's disease, conventional irradiation in doses of 4500– 5000 rads leads to biochemical and clinical improvement in only 15– 25% of adults—although it can lead to improvement in as many as 80% of children. Adjunctive antiadrenal drug therapy has been used with some success, but the ultimate response to radiation therapy is often unsatisfactory, and prolonged drug therapy is required. Because of these low response rates, we do not recommend conventional irradiation as initial therapy.

Heavy particle irradiation, also used as initial therapy in patients with no extrasellar tumor extension, is currently available at only one center in the USA. Alpha particle irradiation is effective in controlling hypercortisolism in 80% of patients, with an incidence of hypopituitarism of approximately one-third. Proton beam therapy is effective in 65% of patients, with a similar incidence of hypopituitarism. Neurologic complications of both forms of therapy include visual loss and oculomotor paralysis. With both of these techniques, there is a lag period of 6– 12 months or longer before cortisol secretion returns to normal.

Implantation of radioactive seeds (gold and yttrium) within the sella turcica has also been used in Cushing's disease. Such techniques have achieved a remission rate of 65%, with an additional 16% improved; however, the frequency of operative complications is high, and panhypopituitarism is common.

C. Medical Treatment: Drugs that inhibit adrenal cortisol secretion are useful in Cushing's disease, often as adjunctive therapy (see Chapter 9).

Metyrapone, an 11β-hydroxylase inhibitor, and **aminoglutethimide,** which inhibits conversion of cholesterol to pregnenolone, have both been utilized to reduce cortisol hypersecretion. These drugs are expensive; their use is accompanied by increased ACTH levels that may overcome the enzyme inhibition; and both agents cause gastrointestinal side effects that may limit their effectiveness. More effective control of hypercortisolism with fewer side effects is obtained by combined use of these agents. Adequate data are not available on the long-term use of these drugs as the sole treatment of Cushing's disease. Thus, metyrapone and aminoglutethimide ordinarily are used while awaiting a response to therapy or in the preparation of patients for surgery.

The adrenolytic drug **mitotane** (Lysodren; o,p'-DDD) results in adrenal atrophy predominantly of the zonae fasciculata and reticularis. Remission of hypercortisolism is achieved in approximately 80% of patients with Cushing's disease, but most relapse after therapy is discontinued. Mitotane therapy is limited by the delayed response, which may take weeks or months, and by the frequent side effects, including severe nausea, vomiting, diarrhea, somnolence, and skin rash.

Pharmacologic inhibition of ACTH secretion in Cushing's disease has also been attempted. **Cyproheptadine,** a drug with antiserotonin, antihistamine, and anticholinergic effects, has had the widest use. Although a few well-documented cases of clinical and biochemical remission of Cushing's disease have been reported with its use, cyproheptadine causes unpleasant side effects (sedation, increased appetite and weight gain) and is usually ineffective in treating ACTH-secreting pituitary adenomas. **Bromocriptine,** a dopamine agonist, has been reported to be effective in some cases and should probably be reserved for those few patients who have hyperprolactinemia associated with Cushing's disease.

Ketoconazole, an imidazole derivative used in clinical practice as a broad-spectrum antimycotic agent, has been found to be a potent inhibitor of adrenal steroid biosynthesis. Ketoconazole inhibits cytochrome P450 enzymes that are important in the synthetic pathway of glucocorticoids. This drug blocks the 14-demethylation of lanosterol to cholesterol as well as the cholesterol side-chain cleavage enzyme and the 11-hydroxylase enzyme. Recent reports have described its efficacy for treatment of patients with endogenous hypercortisolemia.

4. ACTH-SECRETING PITUITARY TUMORS FOLLOWING ADRENALECTOMY FOR CUSHING'S DISEASE: NELSON'S SYNDROME

The clinical appearance of an ACTH-secreting pituitary adenoma following bilateral adrenalectomy in patients with Cushing's disease was initially described by Nelson et al in 1958.

Pathogenesis

Based on current evidence, it now seems likely that Nelson's syndrome represents the clinical progression of a preexisting adenoma after the restraint of hypercortisolism on ACTH secretion and tumor growth is removed. That ACTH secretion in Cushing's disease is restrained by the circulating cortisol levels is demonstrated by its stimulation with metyrapone. Furthermore, the tumors in Nelson's syndrome are dexamethasone-suppressible, although larger doses may be required than with untreated Cushing's disease. Thus, following adrenalectomy, the suppressive effect of cortisol is no longer present, ACTH secretion increases, and the adenoma may progress.

Incidence

The incidence of Nelson's syndrome ranges from 10 to 78%, depending on what criteria are used for diagnosis (see Chapter 9). Pituitary irradiation before or after adrenalectomy does not prevent the development of this syndrome. Approximately 30% of patients adrenalectomized for Cushing's disease develop classic Nelson's syndrome with progressive hyperpigmentation and an obvious ACTH-secreting tumor; another 50% develop evidence of a microadenoma without marked progression; and about 20% never develop a progressive tumor. The reasons for these differences in clinical behavior are uncertain, and they cannot be predicted prior to adrenal surgery. Continued examination, including plasma ACTH levels, visual fields, and sellar radiology, is required following bilateral adrenalectomy in patients with Cushing's disease.

Clinical Findings

The pituitary tumors in patients with classic Nelson's syndrome are among the most aggressive and rapidly growing of all pituitary tumors. These patients present with hyperpigmentation and with manifestations of an expanding intrasellar mass lesion. Visual field defects, headache, cavernous sinus invasion with extraocular muscle palsies, and even malignant changes with local or distant metastases may occur. Pituitary apoplexy may also complicate the course of these tumors.

Diagnosis

Plasma ACTH levels are markedly elevated, usually over 1000 pg/mL and often as high as 10,000 pg/mL. The sella turcica is enlarged on routine radiographs; CT scanning defines the extent of the tumor.

Treatment

Pituitary surgery, either by the transsphenoidal approach or by transfrontal craniotomy, is the initial mode of treatment. Complete resection is usually not possible, because of the large size of these tumors. Conventional radiotherapy alone is satisfactory in a minority of patients but is often employed postoperatively in patients with extrasellar extension.

5. THYROTROPIN-SECRETING PITUITARY ADENOMAS

Thyrotropin-secreting pituitary adenomas have been the subject of isolated case reports. Clinically, these rare tumors are usually manifested by hyperthyroidism with goiter in the presence of elevated TSH. Patients with TSH-secreting tumors are often resistant to routine ablative thyroid therapy, requiring large, often multiple doses of ^{131}I and several oper-

ations for control of thyrotoxicosis. Histologically, the tumors are chromophobe adenomas. They are often very large and cause visual impairment, which alerts the physician to a pituitary abnormality. Although a patient has been described whose massive TSH-secreting adenoma invaded the orbit, causing unilateral exophthalmos, most patients with these tumors do not have extrathyroidal systemic manifestations of Graves' disease (ophthalmopathy, dermopathy). Pituitary TSH hypersecretion in the absence of a demonstrable pituitary tumor has also been reported to cause hyperthyroidism in a few patients.

TSH dynamics are variable; TRH (protirelin) administration rarely stimulates TSH secretion from these tumors, nor do levodopa and bromocriptine suppress TSH as they do the TSH hypersecretion of primary hypothyroidism. The diagnosis is based on findings of hyperthyroidism with elevated TSH and neuroradiologic studies consistent with pituitary tumor. Differential diagnosis includes those equally rare patients with primary hypothyroidism (thyroid failure) who develop major hyperplasia of pituitary thyrotrophs with sellar enlargement and occasional suprasellar extension.

Treatment should be directed initially at the adenoma, with surgery or radiation therapy. If TSH hypersecretion persists, ablative treatment of the thyroid with either ^{131}I or surgery is necessary to achieve clinical remission of the thyrotoxic state. (See Chapter 7.)

6. GONADOTROPIN-SECRETING PITUITARY ADENOMAS

Gonadotropin-secreting pituitary adenomas have been well documented in only a few patients. All reported cases have occurred in men; the majority hypersecrete only FSH, but tumors secreting both LH and FSH and a tumor secreting only LH have been described. Enlargement of the sella turcica has been noted in several patients with long-standing primary hypogonadism (eg, Klinefelter's syndrome). In most of these cases, a pituitary tumor was not proved histologically, and such sellar abnormalities probably reflect reactive pituitary enlargement and gonadotropin cell hyperplasia secondary to primary gonadal failure.

Gonadotropin-secreting pituitary adenomas are usually large chromophobe adenomas presenting with visual impairment and are often considered to be functionless before LH and FSH measurements are obtained. Testosterone levels may be low or elevated; in either case, the patients are frequently impotent or infertile. FSH and LH secretory dynamics are abnormal. GnRH may or may not stimulate gonadotropin release from these tumors, and testosterone administration results in subnormal or absent suppression. In addition, LH and FSH secretion in patients is often provoked by TRH, unlike the lack of stimulation observed in normal individuals. The alpha subunit of the glycoprotein hormones is also secreted in excess from these tumors.

Therapy for gonadotropin-secreting adenomas has been directed at surgical removal. Because of their large size, adequate control of LH/FSH hypersecretion has not been achieved.

7. ALPHA SUBUNIT–SECRETING PITUITARY ADENOMAS

Excessive quantities of the alpha subunit of the glycoprotein pituitary hormones have been observed in association with the hypersecretion of many anterior pituitary hormones (TSH, GH, PRL, LH, FSH). Recently, however, pure alpha subunit hypersecretion has been identified in 2 male patients with large invasive chromophobe adenomas and partial panhypopituitarism. Isolated alpha subunit–secreting tumors may become increasingly recognized, and the determination of the alpha subunit may be a useful marker in patients with presumed "nonfunctioning" pituitary adenomas.

8. NONFUNCTIONAL PITUITARY ADENOMAS

Until recently, "nonfunctional" chromophobe adenomas represented approximately 80% of all primary pituitary tumors; however, with clinical application of radioimmunoassay of anterior pituitary hormones, these tumors currently account for only about 10% of all pituitary adenomas. Thus, the great majority of these chromophobe adenomas have now been documented to be PRL-secreting; a smaller number secrete TSH or the gonadotropins. The incidence of alpha subunit hypersecretion is currently under investigation, and it is likely that the increasing applications of such assays will further decrease the percentage of pituitary adenomas which are truly "nonsecreting."

Nonfunctional tumors are usually large when the diagnosis is established; headache and visual field defects are the usual presenting symptoms. However, endocrine manifestations are usually present for months to years before the diagnosis is made, with gonadotropin deficiency being the most common initial symptom. Hypothyroidism and hypoadrenalism are also common, but the symptoms are subtle and may be missed.

Evaluation should include CT scans and visual field testing; endocrine studies should include assessment of pituitary hormones and end-organ function to determine whether the adenoma is hypersecreting or whether hormonal replacement is needed.

Since these tumors are generally large, both surgery and radiation therapy are usually required to prevent tumor progression or recurrence. In the absence of an endocrine index of tumor hypersecretion such as PRL excess, serial CT scans at yearly intervals are required to assess the response to therapy and to detect possible recurrence.

REFERENCES

General

Besser GM (editor): The hypothalamus and pituitary. *Clin Endocrinol Metab* 1977;**6**. [Entire issue.]

Daughaday WH: The adenohypophysis. Chap 3, pp 73– 116, in: *Textbook of Endocrinology*, 6th ed. Williams RH (editor). Saunders, 1981.

DeGroot LJ (editor): *Endocrinology*. 3 vols. Grune & Stratton, 1979.

Frohman LA: Diseases of the anterior pituitary. Chap 7, pp 151– 231, in: *Endocrinology and Metabolism*. Felig P et al (editors). McGraw-Hill, 1981. [Entire volume is of interest.]

Martin JB, Reichlin S, Brown GM: *Clinical Neuroendocrinology*. Davis, 1977.

Tolis G et al (editors): *Clinical Neuroendocrinology: A Pathophysiological Approach*. Raven Press, 1979.

Tyrrell JB, Wilson CB: Pituitary syndromes. Chap 19, pp 304– 328, in: *Surgical Endocrinology: Clinical Syndromes*. Friesen SR (editor). Lippincott, 1978.

ACTH: Cushing's Syndrome

Aron DC et al: Cushing's syndrome: Problems in diagnosis. *Medicine* 1981;**60**:25.

Aron DC et al: Cushing's syndrome: Problems in management. *Endocr Rev* 1982;**3**:229.

Borst GC et al: Discordant cortisol response to exogenous ACTH and insulin-induced hypoglycemia in patients with pituitary disease. *N Engl J Med* 1982;**306**:1462.

Carey RM et al: Ectopic secretion of corticotropin-releasing factor as a cause of Cushing's syndrome: A clinical, morphologic, and biochemical study. *N Engl J Med* 1984; **311**:13.

Chrousos GP et al: The corticotropin-releasing factor stimulation test. *N Engl J Med* 1984;**310**:622.

Crapo L: Cushing's syndrome: A review of diagnostic tests. *Metabolism* 1979;**28**:955.

Cunningham SK et al: Normal cortisol response to corticotropin in patients with secondary adrenal failure. *Arch Intern Med* 1983;**143**:2276.

Finding JW, Aron DC, Tyrrell JB: Cushing's disease. In: *The Pituitary*. Imura H (editor). Raven Press, 1985.

Ganong WF, Alpert LC, Lee TC: ACTH and the regulation of adrenocortical secretion. *N Engl J Med* 1974;**290**: 1066.

Gold EM: The Cushing's syndromes: Changing views of diagnosis and treatment. *Ann Intern Med* 1979;**90**:829.

Krieger DT: *Cushing's Syndrome*. Springer-Verlag, 1982.

Nelson DH, Meakin JW, Thorn GW: ACTH-producing pituitary tumors following adrenalectomy for Cushing's syndrome. *Ann Intern Med* 1960;**52**:560.

Nelson JC, Tindall DJ Jr: A comparison of the adrenal responses to hypoglycemia, metyrapone and ACTH. *Am J Med Sci* 1978;**275**:165.

Orth DN et al: Effects of synthetic ovine corticotropin-releasing factor: Dose response of plasma adrenocorticotropin and cortisol. *J Clin Invest* 1983;**71**:587.

Pont A et al: Ketoconazole blocks adrenal steroid synthesis. *Ann Intern Med* 1982;**97**:370.

Tyrrell JB et al: Cushing's disease: Selective transsphenoidal resection of pituitary microadenomas. *N Engl J Med* 1978;**298**:753.

Urbanic RC, George JM: Cushing's disease: Eighteen years' experience. *Medicine* 1981;**60**:14.

Vale W et al: Characterization of a 41-residue ovine hypothalamic peptide that stimulates secretion of corticotropin and β-endorphin. *Science* 1981;**213**:1394.

Yates FE et al: The pituitary adrenal cortical system: Stimulation and inhibition of secretion of corticotrophin. Pages 109–140 in: *Endocrine Physiology*. McCann SM (editor). Vol 5 of: *Physiology*. Butterworth, 1974.

GH: Acromegaly

Alford FP, Baker HWG, Burger HG: The secretion rate of human growth hormone. 1. Daily secretion rates: Effects of posture and sleep. *J Clin Endocrinol Metab* 1973;**37**:515.

Arafah BM et al: Transsphenoidal microsurgery in the treatment of acromegaly and gigantism. *J Clin Endocrinol Metab* 1980;**50**:578.

Brown P et al: Potential epidemic of Creutzfeldt-Jakob disease from human growth hormone therapy. *N Engl J Med* 1985;**313**:728.

Clemmons DR et al: Evaluation of acromegaly by radioimmunoassay of somatomedin-C. *N Engl J Med* 1979;**301**:1138.

Daughaday WH, Cryer PE: Growth hormone hypersecretion and acromegaly. *Hosp Pract* (Aug) 1978;**13**:75.

Eddy RL et al: Human growth hormone release: Comparison of provocative test procedures. *Am J Med* 1974;**56**:179.

Hanew K et al: The spectrum of pituitary growth hormone responses to pharmacological stimuli in acromegaly. *J Clin Endocrinol Metab* 1980;**51**:292.

Martin JB: Neural regulation of growth hormone secretion. *N Engl J Med* 1973;**288**:1384.

Melmed S et al: Pathophysiology of acromegaly. *Endocr Rev* 1983;**4**:271.

Mims RB, Behune JE: Acromegaly with normal fasting growth hormone concentrations but abnormal growth hormone regulation. *Ann Intern Med* 1974;**81**:781.

van Wyk JJ, Underwood LE: Growth hormone, somatomedins, and growth failure. *Hosp Pract* (Aug) 1978;**13**:57.

PRL: Prolactinoma

Carter JN et al: Prolactin-secreting tumors and hypogonadism in 22 men. *N Engl J Med* 1978;**299**:847.

Franz AG: Prolactin. *N Engl J Med* 1978;**298**:201.

Glickman SP et al: Multiple androgenic abnormalities, including elevated free testosterone, in hyperprolactinemic women. *J Clin Endocrinol Metab* 1982;**55**:251.

Johnston DG et al: Hyperprolactinemia: Long-term effects of bromocriptine. *Am J Med* 1983;**75**:868.

Keye WR Jr et al: Amenorrhea, hyperprolactinemia, and pituitary enlargement secondary to primary hypothyroidism: Successful treatment with thyroid replacement. *Obstet Gynecol* 1976;**48**:697.

Keye WR Jr et al: Prolactin-secreting pituitary adenomas. 3. Frequency and diagnosis in amenorrhea-galactorrhea. *JAMA* 1980;**244**:1329.

Kirby RW, Kotchen TA, Rees ED: Hyperprolactinemia: A review of recent clinical advances. *Arch Intern Med* 1979;**139**:1415.

Kleinberg DL, Noel GL, Franz AG: Galactorrhea: A study of 235 cases, including 48 with pituitary tumors. *N Engl J Med* 1977;**296**:589.

Kleinberg DL et al: Pergolide for the treatment of pituitary tumors secreting prolactin or growth hormone. *N Engl J Med* 1983;**309**:704.

Klibanski A et al: Decreased bone density in hyperprolactinemic women. *N Engl J Med* 1980;**303**:1511.

Molitch M: Hyperprolactinemia. *Med Grand Rounds* 1982;**1**:307.

Randall RV et al: Transsphenoidal microsurgical treatment of prolactin-producing pituitary adenomas: Results in 100 patients. *Mayo Clin Proc* 1983;**58**:108.

Serri O et al: Recurrence of hyperprolactinemia after selective transsphenoidal adenomectomy in women with prolactinoma. *N Engl J Med* 1983;**309**:280.

Spark RF et al: Bromocriptine reduces pituitary tumor size and hypersecretion. *JAMA* 1982;**247**:311.

Tolis G: Prolactin: Physiology and pathology. *Hosp Pract* (Feb) 1980;**15**:85.

Gonadotropins (LH/FSH)

Abraham GE et al: Simultaneous radioimmunoassay of plasma FSH, LH, progesterone, 17-hydroxyprogesterone, and estradiol-17β during the menstrual cycle. *J Clin Endocrinol Metab* 1972;**34**:312.

Beling CG et al: LH and FSH responses in normal males and females. Page 328 in: *The LH-Releasing Hormone*. Beling CG, Wentz AC (editors). Masson, 1980.

Hurley DM et al: Induction of ovulation and fertility in amenorrheic women by pulsatile low-dose gonadotropin-releasing hormone. *N Engl J Med* 1984;**310**:1069.

Jaffe RB, Monroe SE: Hormone interaction and regulation during the menstrual cycle. Chap 8, pp 219–247, in: *Frontiers in Neuroendocrinology*. Martini L, Ganong WF (editors). Raven Press, 1980.

McCann SM: Luteinizing hormone–releasing hormone. *N Engl J Med* 1977;**296**:797.

Ojeda SR et al: Recent advances in the endocrinology of puberty. *Endocr Rev* 1980;**1**:228.

Synder PJ, Sterling FH: Hypersecretion of LH and FSH by a pituitary adenoma. *J Clin Endocrinol Metab* 1976;**42**:544.

TSH

Jackson IMD: Thyrotropin-releasing hormone. *N Engl J Med* 1982;**306**:145.

Larsen PR: Thyroid-pituitary interaction: Feedback regulation of thyrotropin secretion by thyroid hormones. *N Engl J Med* 1982;**306**:23.

Synder PJ, Utiger RD: Inhibition of thyrotropin response to thyrotropin-releasing hormone by small quantities of thyroid hormones. *J Clin Invest* 1972;**51**:2077.

Vagenakis AG et al: Recovery of pituitary thyrotropic function after withdrawal of prolonged thyroid-suppression therapy. *N Engl J Med* 1975;**293**:681.

Weintraub BD (moderator): Inappropriate secretion of thyroid-stimulating hormone. *Ann Intern Med* 1981;**95**:339.

Pituitary Function Testing & Neuroradiology

Burrow GN et al: Microadenomas of the pituitary and abnormal sellar tomograms in an unselected autopsy series. *N Engl J Med* 1981;**304:**156.

Carroll BJ: Hypothalamic-pituitary function in depressive illness: Insensitivity to hypoglycaemia. *Br Med J* 1969;**3:**27.

Chambers EF et al: Regions of low density in the contrast-enhanced pituitary gland: Normal and pathologic processes. *Radiology* 1982;**144:**109.

Cohen KL: Metabolic, endocrine, and drug-induced interference with pituitary function tests: A review. *Metabolism* 1977;**26:**1165.

Feldman HA, Singer I: Endocrinology and metabolism in uremia and dialysis: A clinical review. *Medicine* 1974; **54:**345.

Glass AR et al: Endocrine function in human obesity. *Metabolism* 1981;**30:**89.

Gwinup G, Johnson B: Clinical testing of the hypothalamic-pituitary-adrenocortical system in states of hypo- and hypercortisolism. *Metabolism* 1975;**24:**777.

Lufkin EG et al: Combined testing of anterior pituitary gland with insulin, thyrotropin-releasing hormone, and luteinizing hormone–releasing hormone. *Am J Med* 1983;**75:**471.

Mortimer CH et al: Luteinizing hormone and follicle stimulating hormone–releasing hormone test in patients with hypothalamic-pituitary-gonadal dysfunction. *Br Med J* 1973;**4:**73.

Newton J, Dixon P: Site of action of clomiphene and its use as a test of pituitary function. *J Obstet Gynaecol Br Commonw* 1971;**78:**812.

Ontjes DA, Ney RL: Tests of anterior pituitary function. *Metabolism* 1972;**21:**159.

Snyder PJ et al: Diagnostic value of thyrotrophin-releasing hormone in pituitary and hypothalamic diseases: Assessment of thyrotrophin and prolactin secretion in 100 patients. *Ann Intern Med* 1974;**81:**751.

Syvertsen A et al: The computed tomographic appearance of the normal pituitary gland and pituitary microadenomas. *Radiology* 1979;**133:**385.

Valenta LJ et al: Diagnosis of pituitary tumors by hormone assays and computerized tomography. *Am J Med* 1982; **172:**861.

Pituitary Adenomas

Cook DM: Pituitary tumors: Current concepts of diagnosis and therapy. *West J Med* 1980;**133:**189.

Cusick JF, Hagen TC, Findling JW: Inappropriate secretion of antidiuretic hormone after transsphenoidal surgery for pituitary tumors. *N Engl J Med* 1984;**311:**36.

Lawrence JH et al: Treatment of pituitary tumors with heavy particles. Pages 253–262 in: *Diagnosis and Treatment of Pituitary Tumors.* Kohler PO, Ross GT (editors). Excerpta Medica, 1973.

Ridgway EC et al: Pure alpha-secreting pituitary adenomas. *N Engl J Med* 1981;**304:**1254.

Wass JAH et al: Reduction of pituitary tumor size in patients with prolactinomas and acromegaly treated with bromocriptine with or without radiotherapy. *Lancet* 1979;**2:**66.

Zervas NT, Martin JB: Management of hormone-secreting pituitary adenomas. *N Engl J Med* 1980;**302:**210.

Empty Sella Syndrome

Bergeron C, Kovacs K, Biilbao JM: Primary empty sella: A histologic and immunocytologic study. *Arch Intern Med* 1979;**139:**248.

Fleckman AM et al: Empty sella of normal size in Sheehan's syndrome. *Am J Med* 1983;**175:**585.

Jordan RM, Kendall JW, Kerber CW: The primary empty sella syndrome: Analysis of the clinical characteristics, radiographic features, pituitary function and cerebrospinal fluid adenohypophysial hormone concentrations. *Am J Med* 1977;**62:**569.

Malarkey WB, Goodenow TJ, Lanese RR: Diurnal variation of prolactin secretion differentiates pituitary tumors from the primary empty sella syndrome. *Am J Med* 1980; **69:**886.

Hypopituitarism

Asa SL et al: Lymphocytic hypophysitis of pregnancy resulting in hypopituitarism: A distinct clinicopathologic entity. *Ann Intern Med* 1981;**95:**166.

Braunstein GD, Kohler PO: Pituitary function in Hand-Schuller-Christian disease: Evidence for deficient growth-hormone release in patients with short stature. *N Engl J Med* 1972;**1286:**1225.

Kasper CS et al: Suprasellar germinoma: Unresolved problems in diagnosis, pathogenesis, and management. *Am J Med* 1983;**75:**705.

Males JL, Townsend JL, Schneider RA: Hypogonadotropic hypogonadism with anosmia—Kallmann's syndrome: A disorder of olfactory and hypothalamic function. *Arch Intern Med* 1973;**131:**501.

Miller WL, Kaplan SL, Grumbach MM: Child abuse as a cause of post-traumatic hypopituitarism. *N Engl J Med* 1980;**302:**724.

Purnell DC, Randall RV, Rynearson EH: Postpartum pituitary insufficiency (Sheehan's syndrome): Review of 18 cases. *Mayo Clin Proc* 1964;**139:**321.

Samaan NA et al: Hypopituitarism after external irradiation: Evidence of both hypothalamic and pituitary origin. *Ann Intern Med* 1975;**83:**771.

Schafer AL et al: Clinical consequences of acquired transfusional iron overload in adults. *N Engl J Med* 1981; **304:**319.

Schwabe AD (moderator): Anorexia nervosa. *Ann Intern Med* 1981;**94:**371.

Stuart CA, Neelon FA, Lebovitz HE: Hypothalamic insufficiency: The cause of hypopituitarism in sarcoidosis. *Ann Intern Med* 1978;**88:**589.

Thomsett MJ et al: Endocrine and neurologic outcome in childhood craniopharyngioma: Review of effect of treatment in 42 patients. *J Pediatr* 1980;**97:**728.

Veldhuis JD, Hammond JM: Endocrine function after spontaneous infarction of the human pituitary: Report, review, and reappraisal. *Endocr Rev* 1980;**1:**100.

Anterior Pituitary & Somatomedins: II. Somatomedins

4

E. Martin Spencer, MD, PhD

Somatomedins are a family of structurally related polypeptide cellular growth factors which mediate the growth-promoting action of growth hormone (GH). As a group, somatomedins share the following common properties: GH is the primary regulator of their plasma level; all have insulinlike activity; they are mitogenic for chondrocytes, osteoblasts, and a variety of cells derived from extraskeletal tissues; and they are transported in plasma bound to one or more large carrier proteins.

History

Our present understanding of somatomedins results from a convergence of knowledge from 3 different areas of research into (1) the mediators of the growth-promoting actions of GH, (2) the nature of the nonsuppressible insulinlike activity in serum, and (3) the identity of serum factors that stimulate cellular multiplication in vitro. Eventually it became apparent that each area concerned a different property of somatomedins.

Salmon and Daughaday found that while GH in vivo stimulated the incorporation of sulfate into cartilage cells, it was inactive in vitro. They presented evidence for an active factor in serum under the control of GH that stimulated in vitro sulfate incorporation into cartilage and called this mediator of GH action "sulfation factor." Clinical studies verified that the serum level of "sulfation factor" was elevated in GH excess and that the low level in GH deficiency rose to normal with GH treatment. Further research demonstrated that "sulfation factor" also stimulated the synthesis in chondrocytes of DNA, RNA, protein, and hydroxyproline; promoted the multiplication of cultured cells in serum-free media; and had insulinlike activity in all tissues. In recognition of these properties, the limiting term "sulfation factor" was replaced in 1972 by the name somatomedin to reflect what was thought to be its primary function, the mediation of the growth-promoting effect of GH. Later, human serum was found to contain at least 2 somatomedins, based on their isoionic points: A (neutral) and C (basic).

While the mediator of the action of GH was being studied, Froesch et al were investigating the nature of the insulinlike activity in serum detected by bioassay but not radioimmunoassay. The addition of excess insulin antibodies to serum revealed that about 90%

Acronyms Used in This Chapter

BRL-MSA	Multiplication-stimulating activity from cultured buffalo rat liver cell media
cAMP	Cyclic adenosine monophosphate
cGMP	Cyclic guanosine monophosphate
GH	Growth hormone
GRH	Growth hormone–releasing hormone
hPI	Human proinsulin
hPL	Human placental lactogen
hPM	Human placental membrane
IGF-I	Human insulinlike growth factor I (SM-C)
IGF-II	Human insulinlike growth factor II
MSA	Multiplication-stimulating activity
NSILA	Nonsuppressible insulinlike activity
NSILA-p	Nonsuppressible insulinlike activity precipitated by acid-ethanol
NSILA-s	Nonsuppressible insulinlike activity soluble in acid-ethanol
PRL	Prolactin
SM-A	Neutral human somatomedin (primarily IGF-II)
SM-C	Basic human somatomedin (IGF-I)
TRH	Thyrotropin-releasing hormone
TSH	Thyroid-stimulating hormone (thyrotropin)

of the total biologic insulinlike activity was unaffected. This activity was called nonsuppressible insulinlike activity (NSILA) and was found to consist of acid-ethanol–soluble (NSILA-s) and precipitable (NSILA-p) fractions. NSILA-s was later found to possess the same properties as somatomedins. Two polypeptides were purified from human serum and sequenced. They were renamed insulinlike growth factors I and II (IGF-I and IGF-II). The former appears to be identical with SM-C, and data now indicate that IGF-II is the major component of SM-A. (See Chemistry, below.)

Simultaneously with the research on somatomedins and NSILA, Pierson and Temin were studying the factor in serum that was responsible for the multiplication of cells in tissue cultures. The activity present in calf serum that stimulated the multiplication of chicken embryo fibroblasts was called multiplication-stimulating activity (MSA). Another MSA was found to be produced by continuous cultures of buffalo rat liver cells and named BRL-MSA. (This name is often shortened to the general term MSA, but the most appropriate name, based on structural homology, is now rat IGF-II. [See Chemistry, below.]) MSA from both sources has activity typical of somatomedins and is included in this family of polypeptides.

For simplicity, this chapter will employ the general term somatomedin or somatomedins to refer to what are probably common properties of all the peptides in the group: SM-A, SM-C, IGF-I, IGF-II, and BRL-MSA. The general term somatomedin will also be used in describing experiments conducted with preparations containing unknown proportions of more than one somatomedin, making it impossible to assign that effect to a unique somatomedin. When information is available, the name of the specific somatomedin will be used. The acidic glial cell growth factor previously referred to as SM-B is not one of the somatomedins.

Measurement of Somatomedin

Somatomedin levels can be measured by bioassays, competitive binding assays, and radioimmunoassays (Table 4–9). The most frequently used bioassay procedure measures the incorporation of labeled sulfate into the glycosaminoglycans of cartilage. The classic method uses hypophysectomized rat costal cartilage, but cartilage from different species or the

incorporation of ^{3}H-thymidine can be used. An improvement recently made in the embryonic chick cartilage bioassay has increased its usefulness. Somatomedins can also be bioassayed by their insulinlike activity in the rat epididymal fat pad. The disadvantages of bioassays lie in their laboriousness, imprecision, and lack of specificity, since inhibitors and in some cases other hormones may influence results. Bioassays that reflect the mitogenic activity of somatomedins for cultured cells, such as chicken embryo fibroblasts and GH$_3$ pituitary cells, considerably improve the precision and are less time-consuming.

The popularity of competitive binding assays stems from their substantial improvement in variability, ease of operation, and lack of influence by inhibitors. The most widely used competitive binding assays employ as receptors either human placental membrane (hPM) fractions or the plasma carrier protein of somatomedins. These assays, like the bioassay, measure all somatomedins. However, since individual somatomedins cross-react to different degrees, an accurate total somatomedin content cannot be determined. Exceptions appear to be the rat placental and hepatic membrane binding assays, which for practical purposes appear to measure IGF-II and give normal rather than increased serum values in acromegaly.

Radioimmunoassays have been developed for SM-C (IGF-I), IGF-II, and BRL-MSA (rat IGF-II). However, some problems still remain with their specificity. One SM-C radioimmunoassay cross-reacts with human placental lactogen (hPL), and Hall has reported an SM-A radioimmunoassay that is 10 times more sensitive to SM-C than SM-A and has the typical age dependency of SM-C rather than IGF-II. Because the specificity of the latter is questionable, it will not be mentioned further. In all likelihood, the somatomedin used for immunization was either a mixture or contained a modified form of SM-C.

The carrier protein complicates the measurement of the level of somatomedins in serum by hindering the access of bound somatomedin to the somatomedin receptor or antibody used in the assay and by competing for the labeled somatomedin. A probable exception to this is the rat cartilage sulfate uptake bioassay. Although some laboratories measure plasma or serum directly, others remove the carrier protein prior to assay either by gel filtration in acid media or by acid-ethanol extraction. Some radioimmunoassays are done under nonequilibrium assay conditions (delayed addition of the labeled antigen) or use samples that have first been acidified and then lyophilized or incubated to eliminate the effect of the serum binding protein. Radioimmunoassays that do not remove the carrier protein can still give qualitatively valid levels if high-affinity antibody is used. Free somatomedin cannot yet be measured.

Because of the scarcity of pure standards, the results of assays for somatomedins are usually expressed relative to a pool of normal sera arbitrarily assigned a value of 1 unit/mL. Normal values are established by each laboratory. For adults, our normal laboratory

Table 4—9. Tests for somatomedins.

	Measures	Specific For
Bioassays		
Hypophysectomized rat costal cartilage*	^{35}SO$_4$ uptake	All somatomedins
Embryonic chick pelvic cartilage	^{35}SO$_4$ uptake or or ^{3}H-thymidine uptake	All somatomedins
Rat epididymal fat pad*	^{14}C incorporation from ^{14}C-glucose (insulinlike activity)	All somatomedins
GH$_3$ cells	Cell multiplication	All somatomedins
Chicken embryonic fibroblasts*	^{3}H-thymidine uptake or cell multiplication	All somatomedins
Competitive binding assays		
Human placental membrane*	Displacement of ^{125}I-labeled somatomedins	All somatomedins
Plasma carrier protein	Displacement of ^{125}I-labeled somatomedins	All somatomedins
Rat placental membrane	Displacement of ^{125}I-IGF-II	?IGF-II
Radioimmunoassays		
SM-C* (IGF-I)	Displacement of ^{125}I-SM-C/IGF-I	SM-C (IGF-I)
IGF-II (SM-A)	Displacement of ^{125}I-IGF-II	IGF-II
BRL-MSA	Displacement of ^{125}I-BRL-MSA	BRL-MSA (rat IGF-II)

*Most commonly used.

Figure 4–18. Alignment of the amino acid sequences of insulinlike growth factors I and II (IGF-I and IGF-II) and human proinsulin (hPI). Symbols above hPI refer to the chain and residue number of insulin. The regions of the insulinlike molecules are listed in the column at right. A and B refer to the regions of hPI that give the classic A and B chains of insulin. C is the connecting peptide region, and D represents a C-terminal extension only in IGFs.

values range from 0.5 to 1.6 units/mL in the hPM-radioreceptor assay and 0.4–2 units/mL for the SM-C radioimmunoassay. Prepubertal children have lower values (see below). One unit of SM-C has been reported to average 200–250 ng by radioimmunoassay, and IGF-II has been found to be considerably higher—approximately 550 ng—by radioimmunoassay. However, the specific activity of the pure somatomedins has not been tested in many assay systems.

Chemistry

Two human somatomedins, IGF-I and IGF-II, have been sequenced, and both are structurally homologous with proinsulin. This undoubtedly explains the prominent insulinlike activity of somatomedins as well as the weak cellular proliferative action of insulin and suggests that the somatomedin and insulin genes evolved by duplication of and divergence from a common primitive gene. However, the primordial gene could have been the growth factor gene.

Like proinsulin, IGF-I and IGF-II are single polypeptide chains, cross-linked by 3 disulfide bonds. Fig 4–18 compares the sequence of the 3 peptides aligned for maximum homology with the common residues outlined. IGF-I and IGF-II consist of 70 and 67 residues, respectively, and have 62% homology. Twenty-six residues are identical between IGF-I and proinsulin and 25 between IGF-II and proinsulin. The 3 disulfide bonds occupy the same position in all 3 peptides. The IGFs have domains that correspond to the A and B "chain" regions and the C-peptide segment of proinsulin (Fig 4–18). The C-peptide regions of IGF-I and IGF-II are 12 and 8 residues, respectively, and have no sequence homology to the 35-residue C segment of proinsulin. The IGFs have an additional region, called the "D region," composed of a carboxy-terminal extension that is not found in proinsulin. This extension consists of 8 residues in IGF-I and 6 residues in IGF-II.

A theoretical model of the tertiary structure of IGF-I, constructed on the basis of its sequence homology with proinsulin, gave a 3-dimensional structure of IGF-I that corresponded closely to that for proinsulin (Fig 4–19). The shorter C-peptide region of IGF-I could be accommodated. When the model for IGF-I was compared to that for insulin, many of their similarities and differences could be explained. The cross-reaction of IGF-I with insulin receptors occurs because the area concerned with binding insulin to the insulin receptor appears to have been conserved during evolution. The nonreactivity of insulin antibodies with IGF-I can be explained by the C-peptide region and carboxy-terminal extension of IGF blocking one antigenic region which is exposed in insulin and by significant amino acid substitutions at the second antigenic region.

Recent chemical evidence by Spencer et al has established that SM-C and IGF-I are identical. These workers also found that the major component in the SM-A (neutral) peak on isoelectric focusing was IGF-

Figure 4–19. Three-dimensional representation of the structure of IGF-I based on model building and patterned after the known tertiary structure of insulin. *A, B, C,* and *D* represent different regions of the IGF-I molecule. Note the similarity of the *A* and *B* regions and the differences in the *C* and *D* areas in comparison with the insulin molecule. (Reproduced, with permission, from Blundell TL et al: Insulin-like growth factor: A model for tertiary structure accounting for immunoreactivity and receptor binding. *Proc Natl Acad Sci USA* 1978;**75**:180.)

II, with a modified form of SM-C being a minor component (see below). Two minor uncharacterized peaks with somatomedinlike activity are present on isoelectric focusing—one with an isoelectric point (pI) of 5.2 and the other with a pI of 9.5.

Two BRL-MSA peptides have been purified, with molecular weights of 8700 and 7500. The sequence of the latter shows 93% homology with human IGF-II, only 5 residues being different. Three of these residues are in the C-peptide region and one immediately adjacent. Immunologic evidence indicates that in fetal and neonatal rats, a similar peptide, rat IGF-II, is present. Rats also have another somatomedin, a basic peptide designated rat SM-C/IGF-I, because partial sequence analysis shows that 26 of the 29 N-terminal residues are identical to human SM-C.

Genetics

An analysis of the human genome indicates that there are only 2 somatomedin genes. The sequence of one corresponds to SM-C/IGF-I and the other to IGF-II. The SM-C–like material contaminating the SM-A peak on isoelectric focusing is either a genetic variant, a proform, or a modification of SM-C. The other peaks at pI 9.5 and 5.2 can also be explained by these possibilities. The SM-C/IGF-I gene has been localized to the short arm of chromosome 11 and the SM-A/IGF-II gene to the long arm of chromosome 12. Oncogenes have been identified in the proximity of the somatomedin genes.

Physiology

All vertebrate species tested have been shown to have somatomedin activity in serum. Contrary to GH, they show very little species specificity when tested in cartilage or receptor assays, in spite of their structural differences.

The liver is a site for production of SM-C, as

shown by perfusion and cell culture studies with GH. IGF-II synthesis has been demonstrated in fetal rat livers. These are the only hormones known to be produced by the liver. After synthesis, SM-C is not stored but is released into the plasma, which is the best source for isolation. Recent evidence suggests that certain tissues are capable of synthesizing somatomedins, and this local production may be physiologically more important than the amount of somatomedins in the circulation. Several types of malignant and fetal cells have also been found to synthesize peptides with somatomedinlike activity.

The somatomedins are transported in plasma bound to high-molecular-weight carrier proteins that are also synthesized in the liver and tissues. The serum level of the carrier protein is also GH-dependent and tightly coupled with the level of somatomedins, for little unsaturated carrier protein or free somatomedin is present in serum. (See section below on Somatomedin Carrier Protein.)

The major regulator of the SM-C (IGF-I) level in serum after birth is GH, while IGF-II is only weakly GH-dependent. GH administration to normal subjects causes a rise in the serum SM-C value after 4–6 hours. SM-C exerts a negative feedback on GH release by stimulating hypothalamic somatostatin release and by a direct effect on the pituitary that blocks the action of growth hormone–releasing hormone (GRH).

Several other hormones affect the somatomedin level, but not to the extent of GH (Table 4–10). The effects of most of these hormones on individual somatomedins is unknown, because in many cases assays measuring total somatomedins were used. Human placental lactogen (hPL) has a moderate and thyroxine a weak stimulatory effect. Estrogen administration decreases the serum somatomedin activity by bioassay and by SM-C radioimmunoassay in acromegalic subjects; this could result from decreased somatomedin synthesis, increased carrier protein synthesis, or increased catabolism. On the other hand, physiologic levels of estrogen appear to stimulate SM-C production. Adrenal corticosteroids increase the serum concentration of somatomedin when measured by hPM-radioreceptor assay and radioimmunoassay for SM-C, but decreased levels are observed with some bioassays. Insulin appears to stimulate somatomedin, but both low and elevated somatomedin serum levels have been reported in diabetes mellitus. The small increase in somatomedin release by hypophysectomized rat livers perfused with insulin could have resulted just from improved metabolism, since nutritional factors, especially dietary protein, can be involved in the regulation of the serum somatomedin level. In humans, an elevated prolactin (PRL) level has no effect on the serum somatomedin level measured by hPM-radioreceptor assay or SM-C radioimmunoassay. However, normal SM-C values have been reported in patients with hyperprolactinemia and GH deficiency due to pituitary tumors; thus, PRL may exert a weak effect on SM-C in GH deficiency. In rodents, the action of PRL is confusing. Its administration to hypophysectomized rats has been reported both to have no effect and to elevate the serum somatomedin, unattended by growth. In contrast, PRL given to GH-deficient Snell dwarf mice stimulated both bioassayable somatomedin and growth. Perfusion studies have shown that PRL did not affect somatomedin synthesis when hypophysectomized rat livers were used, possibly because of the absence of PRL receptors. Curiously, when normal rat livers were used, PRL stimulated somatomedin activity at 11 AM but not at 3 PM.

Intravenously administered labeled somatomedin localizes primarily in the kidney. The proximal tubule has enzymes that degrade somatomedin, and insulin competes for this pathway. However, nephrectomy does not significantly alter the half-life of somatomedin, as is not the case with insulin. Hepatic metabolism does not seem to be an important mechanism for degradation of somatomedin.

Inhibitors of the biologic action of somatomedins may have a major counterregulatory role, perhaps shunting nutrients from growth to more important functions during critical times. Inhibitors occur in both pathologic and normal states. Inhibitors of sulfate uptake have been found in rats with experimental diabetes mellitus and after hypophysectomy and in humans with malnutrition. In normal rat serum, a factor is present that inhibits somatomedin-stimulated thymidine but not sulfate incorporation into cartilage. Partial characterization has indicated that it has the properties of a pentose and nucleic acid. However, 2 other inhibitors appear to be a steroid and a peptide. Although one inhibitor may be a somatomedin-binding protein, the mechanism of action of others is unknown. The liver is the site of production of at least one inhibitor.

Biologic Actions on Tissues

A. Metabolic Effects: In adipose tissue, somatomedins have the same metabolic actions as insulin but are significantly less potent. All somatomedins stim-

Table 4–10. Effects of hormones on plasma somatomedin levels in humans.

Hormone	Effects and Remarks
GH	Markedly increases somatomedin; is the most potent stimulator.
hPL	May stimulate somatomedin in the fetus.
Thyroxine	Causes weak increase of somatomedin.
Insulin	May increase somatomedin.
PRL	Very weak stimulator. Maintains normal somatomedin levels in hyperprolactinemic children with impaired GH responses.
Adrenal corticosteroids	Increases somatomedin as measured by SM-C radioimmunoassay and competitive binding assay. Decreases somatomedin as measured by some bioassays.
Testosterone	Does not appear to affect somatomedin.
Estrogen	Pharmacologic doses of estrogen decrease somatomedin. Physiologic doses may increase somatomedin.
Progesterone	Increases somatomedin.

ulate glucose transport, oxidation to CO_2, and incorporation into lipid. Somatomedins inhibit lipolysis and epinephrine-stimulated adenylate cyclase activity. In some tissues, basal adenylate cyclase activity is inhibited. The insulinlike actions of somatomedins are initiated by binding to the insulin receptor and not to the specific somatomedin receptor present on adipocytes.

In the rat diaphragm, somatomedins are equipotent with insulin. Both have an immediate stimulatory effect on the transport of amino acids and sugars. This effect does not require protein synthesis and is unaffected by phosphodiesterase inhibitors and thus appears to operate via a different mechanism from that used by GH. However, both somatomedins and GH may be physiologically important for protein synthesis in muscle. In the perfused heart, somatomedin stimulates glucose uptake and lactic acid production.

The actions of somatomedins on chondrocytes have been discussed previously. In fetal calvarial bone cells, somatomedins stimulate the synthesis of DNA, collagen, and collagenase nondigestible protein.

B. Mitogenic Effects: The somatomedins stimulate a wide variety of cultured cells to proliferate in serum-free media. The list includes several types of fibroblasts, myoblasts, smooth muscle cells, GH_3 pituitary cells, chondrocytes, and fetal calvarial cells. Although somatomedins have no direct effect on lymphocytes in serum-free media, they can potentiate concanavalin A–induced DNA synthesis, completely replacing the serum requirement for optimal mitogenic activity for mouse spleen lymphocytes and partially replacing that for human peripheral lymphocytes. Since somatomedin-deficient species do not have an immunologic defect, the measurable somatomedin in GH deficiency is presumably enough to maintain immunologic competence. The immunologic defect previously reported in GH-deficient Snell mice disappears with special attention to animal care.

The concept has been advanced that the growth-promoting effects of somatomedins and insulin are in general mediated through the somatomedin receptors and the metabolic effects through the insulin receptor. However, exceptions are known to exist.

Biologic Effects in Vivo

A. Growth Promotion: The Snell mouse has been successfully used to demonstrate the growth-promoting properties of somatomedins. These mice are genetically deficient in GH, PRL, and TSH. Two groups of investigators have shown that partially pure preparations of somatomedins containing no other hormones stimulate the growth of Snell mice. These exciting results have been confirmed with pure somatomedins in hypophysectomized rats. Earlier attempts to stimulate growth of hypophysectomized rats probably failed because somatomedins have an extremely short half-life when administered without the carrier protein.

Green et al have proposed a dual role for the growth-promoting action of GH. GH can act both directly, by stimulating differentiation of precursor cells; and indirectly, by stimulating somatomedin, which causes proliferation of the differentiated cells. Thus, both GH and somatomedins should be capable of stimulating growth of certain tissues. This theory of Green et al is in harmony with the findings of several other investigators who reported that direct epiphyseal injections of GH stimulate growth.

B. Metabolic Actions: Administration of somatomedin to normal rats stimulates the incorporation of ^{14}C-glucose into adipose tissue and diaphragm. Since insulin does not further increase ^{14}C-glucose incorporation when maximally stimulated by somatomedin, it is apparent that somatomedin and insulin both act on the same transport site. Somatomedins have also been shown to cause thickening of skin and to stimulate sulfate incorporation into bone. In adrenalectomized rats, somatomedin produces more prolonged hypoglycemia than insulin and lowers free fatty acids.

Mechanisms of Action

A. Receptors: Somatomedins are assumed to act like other polypeptide hormones and bind to receptors on the cell surface, thereby triggering a programmed series of intracellular events. Specific receptors have been demonstrated on hPMs, lymphocytes, and human lymphoblastic cells, chondrocytes, adipocytes, fibroblasts, and hepatocytes. Two types of somatomedin receptors have been identified by cross-linking ^{125}I-SM with various tissues and cells. Insulin competes with type I somatomedin receptors that are structurally very similar to insulin receptors; both have a molecular weight over 300,000 and contain a basic subunit of MW 130,000 after the connecting disulfide bridges have been reduced. The second class of somatomedin receptors has a molecular weight of 220,000 but is not composed of subunits and does not bind insulin. Both classes of receptors can be on the same cell, with or without insulin receptors.

B. Intracellular Mediators: No intracellular mediator of the actions of somatomedin has been identified. Calcium should be considered, because calcium can stimulate the uptake of sulfate into cartilage and may be involved with the mechanism of action of other growth factors. The role of cyclic nucleotides is controversial. Initial evidence suggested that somatomedin could lower cAMP levels by inhibiting adenylate cyclase. Subsequent studies questioned this mechanism because the response of basal and stimulated adenylate cyclase to somatomedin varied in different target tissues. Recent investigations have shown that somatomedins may in fact have an opposite effect on intracellular cyclic nucleotide levels. Somatomedins have no direct effect on cAMP-dependent or cAMP-independent protein kinase. Efforts to tie somatomedin actions to cGMP levels have not given convincing results. Since the actions of somatomedin may be immediate, intermediate, or delayed, a single mechanism may not explain these diverse actions.

C. Intracellular Binding Sites: Intracellular binding sites for somatomedins have been found in hepatic membrane fractions and have a different intracellular pattern of distribution from that of insulin receptors. Intracellular incorporation of somatomedins may be a mechanism for down-regulating somatomedin receptors or degrading somatomedin. Since the liver is not a primary target organ for somatomedins, the function of intracellular membranous binding sites probably should be sought in proliferating cells sensitive to somatomedins. Intracellular binding sites could even be recently synthesized receptors in the process of being transported to the plasma membrane. Soluble somatomedin receptors have been identified in the cytosol of the liver, kidney, and placenta. The hepatic soluble receptors may have been shed after synthesis. The renal cytosol receptors appear to be involved in catabolism of somatomedins, and those in the placenta may have a role in regulating fetal growth.

D. Factors Regulating the Cell Cycle: Somatomedins have been shown to be one of 2 types of factors controlling the growth of BALB/c3T3 and other cells. The first is a competence factor that prepares resting cells for DNA synthesis by stimulating their passage into the G_1 phase. However, cells will not exit from the G_1 phase and begin to synthesize DNA unless the second factor, called a progression factor, is present along with epidermal growth factor. Competence factors are platelet-derived growth factor and fibroblast growth factor, and the major progression factors are somatomedins. Recent evidence shows that platelet-derived growth factor up-regulates somatomedin cellular receptors for the progression factor. Thus, without the competence factor, the number of receptors for somatomedin falls off dramatically, and cell division ceases.

Somatomedin Carrier Protein

The somatomedins are unique among the polypeptide hormones in that they are transported in plasma bound to a high-molecular-weight carrier protein (or proteins). The major functions of the carrier protein are to prolong the half-life of somatomedins in plasma from minutes to about 24 hours in humans; to prevent the level of somatomedins from fluctuating, as does that of GH; and to maintain bound somatomedins in an inactive state. The latter is demonstrated by the ability of excess carrier protein to block the biologic effects of somatomedins and the increase in serum somatomedin activity resulting from removal of the carrier protein in most assays. It is possible that the carrier protein has undiscovered independent functions, such as enzymatic activity analogous to that of the peptidases associated with nerve growth factor and epidermal growth factor.

Gel filtration of serum at neutral pH shows 2 major peaks of binding activity at approximately MW 50,000 and MW 150,000 and very little unbound somatomedins. The carrier protein can be separated from its complexed somatomedin by gel filtration at low pH (acid chromatography) and by acid-ethanol extraction. In the normal plasma, there are few unsaturated binding sites, and most of the labeled somatomedins added

appear at MW 50,000, though most of the somatomedin migrates in the MW 150,000 range.

The 150,000-MW species is GH-dependent. In GH deficiency, it is replaced by the 50,000-MW form. The 150,000-MW carrier protein has a subunit structure that consists of an acid-labile unit and an acid-stable subunit of MW 50,000. Isolated hepatocytes produce the low-molecular-weight form. Buffalo rat liver cells that produce BRL-MSA synthesize a carrier protein of approximately MW 60,000 with 2 subunits in the range of MW 31,000. The structural relationship between the low- and high-molecular-weight binding proteins is unknown.

All cells that synthesize somatomedins also synthesize a carrier protein, except for one line of cultured hepatocytes that synthesizes only the binding protein. Genetic evidence has shown that the carrier proteins and somatomedins originate in separate genes. The question of how the synthesis of somatomedin and its carrier protein are coordinated so tightly is unanswered.

Clinical Considerations

A. Somatomedins and Fetal Growth: Somatomedin concentrations in human cord blood have generally correlated well with birth size. However, GH appears to have little or no role in regulating fetal growth, because GH-deficient and anencephalic children have normal birth weights. Nevertheless, somatomedin is easily measured in fetal sera before the 20th week of gestation. The major regulator of fetal somatomedin levels may be placental lactogen or progesterone. The GH-dependent 150,000-MW carrier protein appears only after 32 weeks of gestation. The relative proportion of IGF-II and SM-C in fetal life has not been determined, but the lack of GH dependency suggests that IGF-II may be the fetal somatomedin. This is supported by data showing that fetal rat sera have immunoreactive BRL-MSA (rat IGF-II) levels 20–100 times higher than those in maternal rat sera and elevated rat IGF-II values by the rat placental membrane assay; fetal rat sera also have higher total somatomedin levels by hPM-radioreceptor assay than by SM-C radioimmunoassay. Further evidence of a role for SM-A/IGF-II in fetal growth is the preponderance of type 2 receptors in several fetal tissues and their peaking late in gestation.

In maternal serum during the first part of pregnancy, the SM-C level by radioimmunoassay may fall slightly, but in the last half of pregnancy it increases steadily to almost twice the normal value. At parturition, the increase correlates with the duration of gestation and with maternal levels of placental lactogen. IGF-II levels also increase during the last half of pregnancy. The stimulus for the maternal increase in SM-C and IGF-II is not GH, for both were observed to increase in a pregnant GH-deficient patient. After delivery, SM-C and IGF-II levels fall abruptly.

B. Normal Plasma Somatomedin Levels Throughout Life: In humans, the plasma level of SM-C is lowest at birth and rises progressively throughout childhood. The increase in somatomedin correlates with age and occasionally height but not with weight. Somatomedin levels have been found not to correlate with the growth velocity. The low level of SM-C at the time of greatest growth may be explained by the increased sensitivity of young cartilage to somatomedin.

IGF-II levels are low for the first year of life and then abruptly increase to the adult level. In rats after birth, there is a fall in IGF-II levels, which reach adult values by day 25 and are replaced by SM-C, which then progressively increases.

Girls have been reported to have higher values of SM-C by radioimmunoassay than boys of the same age, and the pubertal spurt of SM-C in girls precedes that in boys by 1–2 years. After puberty, the plasma SM-C level falls to normal adult values. By our hPM-radioreceptor assay and SM-C radioimmunoassay, men were found to have a higher average somatomedin level than women. However, with a different SM-C radioimmunoassay, women were found to have higher levels than men. In women, the SM-C level begins to fall at menopause. In men, a decline also occurs—but approximately 20 years later; sensitivity to GH remains.

CONDITIONS ASSOCIATED WITH SHORT STATURE

GROWTH HORMONE DEFICIENCY

Growth hormone deficiency results in dwarfism. However, the birth weight of GH-deficient children is in the normal range; only later is their condition clinically manifested. The clinical features and treatment of GH deficiency are described in Chapter 5.

Affected children have a low serum somatomedin by bioassay, competitive binding assay, and SM-C and IGF-II radioimmunoassays, but these tests must be interpreted by comparison with standard sera from children of the same age because of the age dependence of somatomedin concentrations (Table 4–11). The SM-C radioimmunoassay is the best diagnostic measurement, but the competitive binding assays also give a better separation of GH-deficient from normal subjects than do bioassays, which can also be affected by other factors. A low value of somatomedins by these assays is consistent with but not diagnostic of GH deficiency, since other conditions can also give low values, eg, malnutrition, marasmus, chronic liver disease, hypothyroidism, and Laron type dwarfism. However, in an otherwise healthy child, a low somatomedin value (especially by SM-C radioimmunoassay) with low or undetectable GH, unresponsive to stimulation, strongly suggests GH deficiency.

GH administration to hypopituitary subjects causes

Table 4–11. Clinical indications for somatomedin determinations.

Condition	Usefulness of Somatomedin Levels
Acromegaly	To establish diagnosis (especially valuable when GH values are in the normal range) and to evaluate therapy.
Excessively tall stature	To differentiate gigantism due to GH excess from cerebral gigantism and normally tall stature.
GH deficiency	Strongly suggests diagnosis in a child with growth failure and no other cause for subnormal somatomedin.
Laron's dwarfism	Elevated GH and low somatomedin levels, unresponsive to GH, required to establish the diagnosis.*
Biologically inactive GH	Low somatomedin, responsive to exogenous GH stimulation, required to make this diagnosis.*
Dwarfism due to resistance to somatomedin	Elevated somatomedin in the presence of normal GH values required to make the diagnosis.*

*After other causes of growth failure have been eliminated.

a detectable elevation of somatomedin as early as 6 hours; peak values are reached between 12 and 24 hours. Daily administration results in a progressive increase in somatomedin that reaches a plateau after 4 days. The values for stimulation of total somatomedins as measured by hPM-radioreceptor assay and by SM-C radioimmunoassay on samples freed of their binding protein correlate with each other. Although somatomedin levels almost always increase after GH therapy and may be dose-dependent, the somatomedin response to GH does not correlate with the resultant growth velocity. Furthermore, an occasional child who responds clinically to GH therapy will not have a rise in SM-C or total somatomedins either acutely or after long-term therapy. In these children, GH also fails to induce the 150,000-MW binding protein. Since most of the somatomedin we measure in serum is actually stored in association with this protein, synthesis and utilization of somatomedin could be normal in these children. Metabolic production rates of somatomedin would answer this question.

LARON TYPE DWARFISM

Laron type dwarfism is a familial form of short stature phenotypically resembling GH deficiency. Somatomedin levels are low, but characteristically the immunoreactive GH is elevated or occasionally normal. The endogenous GH of Laron dwarfs has normal immunoassay and receptor-binding activity, and exogenous GH fails to stimulate not only somatomedin generation but also the other metabolic actions of GH, such as lipolysis. In vitro, GH also fails to stimulate erythroid colony formations. Therefore, Laron dwarfs are considered to have defective GH receptors. Somatomedin therapy may be the only way to restore growth in these children if it can be demonstrated that somatomedins can mediate all the essential actions of GH.

BIOLOGICALLY INACTIVE GROWTH HORMONE SYNDROME

Eight children have been reported with this form of growth retardation. The physical appearance of 2 subjects has been described, and one had the typical features of pituitary dwarfism. Fasting serum GH concentrations and GH responses to provocative stimulation were usually increased. Although the endogenous GH appeared to be normal in several radioimmunoassays, their radioreceptor activity was significantly decreased. In all cases, serum somatomedin levels were subnormal. Exogenous GH stimulated free fatty acid release, somatomedin levels, and growth. It was concluded that the endogenous GH was abnormal in this syndrome. The consensus is that biologically inactive GH is a rare condition in spite of one report to the contrary. In this report, 38% of children with unexplained extreme growth failures, negative physical examinations, and normal GH levels (normal variant short stature) were found to have subnormal SM-C levels. Exogenous GH resulted in an increase in SM-C level and stimulated growth. The major problem with the study was that the baseline growth of these children was much less than that found in children with GH deficiency; this suggested that other factors were involved.

CONGENITAL RESISTANCE TO SOMATOMEDIN

One case of growth retardation due to congenital resistance to somatomedin has been described. Although the child had a normal serum GH level and response to provocative stimuli, his serum somatomedin level was strikingly elevated by bioassay, hPM-radioreceptor assay, and SM-C radioimmunoassay. Exogenous GH had no effect on the somatomedin level and growth. Since the somatomedin was active in the bioassay and radioreceptor assay, it appears that the patient's cells lack the capacity to respond to somatomedin because of a receptor or postreceptor defect.

CHRONIC RENAL DISEASE

Children with chronic renal disease are severely growth-retarded, usually below the third percentile. The cause of short stature in such cases has not been established. GH and insulin levels are elevated. Somatomedin levels measured by bioassay are low, and SM-C by radioimmunoassay is in the low normal range. However, somatomedin values determined by the hPM-radioreceptor assay are elevated into the acromegalic range. The cause of the elevation of somatomedin measured by radioreceptor assay is unknown. The low levels of SM-C by radioimmunoassay suggest that the hPM-radioreceptor assay is detecting another somatomedin, possibly IGF-II. This is substantiated by measurements with the rat placental membrane radioreceptor assay. Although the somatomedin elevation is inversely related to the glomerular filtration rate, it is unlikely to be a reflection of decreased catabolism, for this should not selectively affect one somatomedin. Another explanation could be the presence of an interfering factor; however, various extraction procedures applied to uremic sera have failed to remove an interfering substance. If an abnormal somatomedin exists in chronic renal disease, it is unassociated with growth stimulation or metabolic effects. This could be due to a circulating inhibitor or to down-regulation of the somatomedin receptor analogous to that of the insulin receptor in chronic renal insufficiency. Successful renal transplantation results in a fall of the radioreceptor-active somatomedin to normal. However, growth is still impaired, possibly owing to chronic glucocorticoid administration.

THALASSEMIA MAJOR

Growth retardation is frequently encountered in children with β-thalassemia. GH values and responses are normal, but bioassayable somatomedin levels have been found to be in the range of GH deficiency. Therapy for iron overload with deferoxamine was without effect. In contrast, we have found normal levels of somatomedin by hPM-radioreceptor assay and SM-C radioimmunoassay in a group with β-thalassemia, though all had normal stature. Therapy may have been a factor, since hypertransfusion maintained hemoglobin levels greater than 11 g/dL and deferoxamine therapy was begun early.

MISCELLANEOUS CONDITIONS

Low serum somatomedin concentrations have been found in the presence of elevated GH levels in **anorexia nervosa, marasmus,** and **malnutrition.** With successful therapy, the somatomedin level is normalized, and growth returns in children. There is evidence for a plasma inhibitor in malnutrition.

Hyperadrenocorticism in children usually results in short stature. Somatomedin levels are low by most bioassays, and the success of alternate-day steroid therapy in minimizing growth failure has been correlated with an improved bioassayable serum somatomedin level. However, elevated levels of somatomedin have been found in hyperadrenocorticism by the hPM-radioreceptor assay and the SM-C radioimmunoassay. This suggests that short stature in this condition may be due to a direct steroid effect on cartilage or an inhibitor of the biologic activity of somatomedin.

Serum somatomedin values in **hypothyroidism** are lower than normal, and a comparison of pretreatment values with those measured after thyroid replacement therapy shows a significant difference. **Pygmies** are short because of an isolated defect in SM-C generation. GH and IGF-II levels are normal. GH administration fails to correct the SM-C levels and stimulate growth.

CONDITIONS ASSOCIATED WITH EXCESSIVE GROWTH

ACROMEGALY

The clinical features of acromegaly are discussed in Chapter 4, Part I. Somatomedin values are particularly valuable in the diagnosis and evaluation of therapy for acromegaly. Virtually all patients with acromegaly have elevated values by SM-C radioimmunoassay and competitive binding assays, whereas bioassay measurements are frequently within the normal range. The reason for this discrepancy is not known. Somatomedin levels have the additional advantage of being relatively constant throughout the day, in contrast to the wide fluctuations in the level of GH. Thus, one or two somatomedin measurements in an appropriate clinical setting may substitute for several baseline GH determinations plus provocative and suppression tests.

Rarely, patients with clinical acromegaly have radioimmunoassayable GH levels in the normal range, a finding that may delay therapy. Paradoxic responses to glucose suppression and TRH stimulation can usually be elicited; however, in the cases the author has studied by radioreceptor assay, all have had elevated somatomedin values.

Somatomedins may have their greatest usefulness in evaluating the efficacy of therapy for acromegaly. The successful removal of a GH-producing tumor results in a fall in the serum somatomedin level within 4 days. Persistent elevation of somatomedin is consistent with clinical findings of continued activity, indicating that additional therapy should probably be directed toward normalizing the serum somatomedin. When the serum somatomedin value is used as a criterion for successful therapy, it appears that a basal GH persistently less than 2 ng/mL is required before it can be reasonably concluded that all tumor has been removed or destroyed. Increased morbidity and mortality rates from pulmonary, cardiac, and other diseases in treated acromegalics are probably related to the failure of adequate therapy, since the previous goals were only to reduce the GH levels to less than 5 or 10 ng/mL.

EXCESSIVELY TALL STATURE

GH-producing tumors in childhood, when the epiphyses are actively proliferating, lead to exaggerated linear growth and gigantism. The typical features of acromegaly may not be obvious, but somatomedin levels are elevated. Care should be taken not to confuse the elevated somatomedin levels of gigantism with the normal pubertal increase in somatomedin. Patients with cerebral gigantism have normal somatomedin levels.

BECKWITH-WIEDEMANN SYNDROME

Beckwith-Wiedemann syndrome consists of visceromegaly, macroglossia, omphalocele, hyperinsulinism, and hypoglycemia. An increase in the bioassayable serum somatomedin level has been reported in a child born with this syndrome. The stimulus to increased somatomedin may be hyperinsulinism, since plasma GH is normal. There is no specific treatment other than to supply adequate calories to prevent hypoglycemia. In the reported case, with time, the hyperinsulinism, hypoglycemia, elevated somatomedin, and abnormal growth returned to normal. (See Chapter 5.)

EXCESSIVE GROWTH IN POSTOPERATIVE PATIENTS WITH CRANIOPHARYNGIOMA

An occasional patient with a craniopharyngioma postoperatively has normal or even excessive growth in spite of undetectable GH levels by radioimmunoassay. In these cases, the somatomedin levels have been normal rather than low, and somatomedin may be responsible for the continued growth. What the stimulus is for the normal somatomedin has never been satisfactorily explained. PRL was initially suggested, but subsequent studies disproved this. Insulin is a more likely candidate, since these patients generally have hyperphagia and hyperinsulinism.

CONDITIONS RELATED TO THE METABOLIC ACTION OF SOMATOMEDINS

TUMOR HYPOGLYCEMIA

Hypoglycemia may occasionally be associated with non–insulin-producing tumors of the liver, the adrenal cortex, and retroperitoneum. The pathophysiology of the hypoglycemia is not understood. Insulinlike activity has been isolated from the extracts of 2 tumors, and approximately half of patients have an elevation of serum somatomedin measured either by a rat liver membrane receptor assay or a rat placental membrane receptor assay, which has been reported to be specific for IGF-II. However, the radioimmunoassay for IGF-II, the hPM-radioreceptor assay, and the bioassay for insulinlike activity give normal values, while the radioimmunoassay for SM-C gives a low value. The cause of the spurious radioreceptor assay values is unknown.

DIABETES MELLITUS

Low serum values of bioassayable somatomedin were initially reported in untreated juvenile diabetics and a series of long-term untreated and treated diabetics of presumably mixed origin. Chemically induced diabetes in rats also produces a low serum somatomedin level. A decreased serum somatomedin or a somatomedin inhibitor would appear to explain the poor growth of juvenile diabetics in spite of their hyperresponsiveness to GH. However, modestly elevated bioassayable somatomedin concentrations have recently been found in long-standing insulin-dependent diabetics. We observed by hPM-radioreceptor assay that a group of lean insulin-dependent, well-controlled patients had normal somatomedins. Others have noted normal radioimmunoassayable SM-C that increased after improved control by continuous insulin infusion in juvenile diabetics. It is possible that somatomedins have a dual pathologic role in diabetes mellitus. In juvenile diabetics, low levels could contribute to their retarded growth. However, in older patients, as a result of chronic exposure to excess GH stimulation, the level could eventually rise and contribute to some of the vascular complications of diabetes in view of the ability of somatomedin to bind to endothelial cells and to stimulate collagen synthesis and cell proliferation. Recently, 2 groups have reported increased somatomedin levels in patients with diabetic retinopathy.

RELATION OF SOMATOMEDIN & CANCER

Human chondrosarcomas and fibrosarcomas were discovered to produce a factor with BRL-MSA–like binding activity and, by indirect evidence, to have receptor sites for BRL-MSA. Thus, these tumors may stimulate their own growth by the production of an autocrine hormone and thereby escape some of the body's growth-retarding mechanisms. Human breast cancers in continuous culture have been found to produce a peptide with SM-C–like radioimmunoreactivity and to respond to exogenous SM-C with an increase in growth. This mechanism is probably operating in human breast cancers in vivo, since immunohistochemical data also indicate that human breast carcinomas produce SM-C. Additional evidence of tumor production of somatomedin exists in lower animals. BRL-MSA is produced by a buffalo rat liver tumor cell in continuous culture, and an experimental mouse mammary tumor has been shown to produce somatomedinlike material. Chromosome studies have demonstrated the proximity of ras oncogenes to the somatomedin genes.

REFERENCES

Adams SO et al: Developmental patterns of insulin-like growth factor-I and -II synthesis and regulation in rat fibroblasts. *Nature* 1983;**302**:150.

Ashton IK, Matheson JA: Change in response with age of human articular cartilage to plasma somatomedin activity. *Calcif Tissue Int* 1979;**29**:89.

Atkison PR et al: Release of somatomedin-like activity by cultured WI-38 human fibroblasts. *Endocrinology* 1980;**106**:2006.

Blundell TL et al: Insulin-like growth factor: A model for tertiary structure accounting for immunoreactivity and receptor binding. *Proc Natl Acad Sci USA* 1978;**75**:180.

Clemmons DR, Underwood LE, Van Wyk JJ: Hormonal control of immunoreactive somatomedin production by cultured human fibroblasts. *J Clin Invest* 1981;**67**:10.

Daughaday WH, Mariz IK, Blethen SL: Inhibition of access of bound somatomedin to membrane receptor and immunobinding sites: A comparison of radioreceptor and radioimmunoassay of somatomedin in native and acid-ethanol–extracted serum. *J Clin Endocrinol Metab* 1980;**51**:781.

De Larco JE, Todaro GJ: A human fibrosarcoma cell line producing multiplication stimulating activity (MSA)–related peptides. *Nature* 1978;**272**:356.

D'Ercole AJ, Willson DF, Underwood LE: Changes in the circulating form of serum somatomedin-C during fetal life. *J Clin Endocrinol Metab* 1980;**51**:674.

Dull, TJ et al: Insulin-like growth factor II precursor gene organization in relation to insulin gene family. *Nature* 1984;**310**:777.

Froesch ER et al: Antibody-suppressible and non-suppressible insulin-like activities in serum and their physiologic significance. *J Clin Invest* 1963;**42**:1816.

Furlanetto RW: Nongrowth hormone dependent hormonal regulation of plasma somatomedin levels. Page 197 in: *Insulin-Like Growth Factors/Somatomedins: Basic Chemistry, Biology and Clinical Importance.* Spencer EM (editor). Walter de Gruyter, 1981.

Furlanetto RW et al: Estimation of somatomedin-C levels in normals and patients with pituitary disease by radioimmunoassay. *J Clin Invest* 1977;**60**:648.

Green H, Morikawa M, Nixon T: A dual effector theory of growth hormone action. *Differentiation* 1985;**29**:195.

Hintz RL, Liu F: Demonstration of specific plasma protein binding sites for somatomedin. *J Clin Endocrinol Metab* 1977; **45**:988.

Hintz RL, Liu F: A radioimmunoassay for insulin-like growth factor-II specific for the C-peptide region. *J Clin Endocrinol Metab* 1982;**54**:442.

Holder AT, Spencer EM, Preece MA: Effect of bovine growth hormone and a partially pure preparation of somatomedin on various growth parameters in hypopituitary dwarf mice. *J Clin Invest* 1981;**89**:275.

Howard GA, Spencer EM: Somatomedins A and C directly stimulate bone cell proliferation in vitro. In: *Endocrine Control of Bone and Calcium Metabolism.* Cohn DV et al (editors). Elsevier, 1984.

Isaksson OGP, Jansson JO, Gause IAM: Growth hormone stimulates longitudinal growth directly. *Science* 1982;**216**:1237.

Jansen M et al: Sequence of cDNA encoding human insulin-like growth factor I. *Nature* 1983;**306**:609.

Kasuga M et al: Demonstration of two subtypes of insulin-like growth factor receptors by affinity cross-linking. *J Biol Chem* 1981;**256**:5305.

King GL et al: Direct demonstration of separate receptors for growth and metabolic activities of insulin and multiplication-stimulating activity (an insulinlike growth factor) using antibodies to the insulin receptor. *J Clin Invest* 1980;**66**:130.

Knauer DJ, Smith GL: Inhibition of biological activity of multiplication-stimulating activity by binding to its carrier protein. *Proc Natl Acad Sci USA* 1980;**77**:7252.

Lanes R et al: Dwarfism associated with normal serum growth hormone and increased bioassayable, receptorassayable and immunoassayable somatomedin. *J Clin Endocrinol Metab* 1980;**50**:485.

Laron Z et al: Administration of growth hormone to patients with familial dwarfism with high plasma immunoreactive growth hormone: Measurement of sulfation factor, metabolic and linear growth responses. *J Clin Endocrinol Metab* 1971;**33**:332.

Moses AC et al: Increased levels of multiplication-stimulating activity, an insulin-like growth factor, in fetal rat serum. *Proc Natl Acad Sci USA* 1980;**77**:3649.

Pierson RW, Temin HM: The partial purification from calf serum of a fraction with multiplication-stimulating activity for chicken fibroblasts in cell culture and with non-suppressible insulin-like activity. *J Cell Physiol* 1972;**79**:319.

Rinderknecht E, Humbel RE: Primary structure of human insulin-like growth factor I and its structural homology with proinsulin. *J Biol Chem* 1978;**253**:2769.

Rinderknecht E, Humbel RE: Primary structure of human insulin-like growth factor II. *FEBS Lett* 1978;**89**:283.

Rudman D et al: Children with normal-variant short stature: Treatment with human growth hormone for six months. (2 parts.) *N Engl J Med* 1981;**305**:3, 123.

Salmon WD Jr, Daughaday WH: A hormonally controlled serum factor which stimulates sulfate incorporation by cartilage in vitro. *J Lab Clin Med* 1957;**49**:825.

Schoenle E et al: Insulin-like growth factor I stimulates growth in hypophysectomized rats. *Nature* 1982;**206**:252.

Spencer EM: Lack of response of serum somatomedin to hyperprolactinemia in humans. *J Clin Endocrinol Metab* 1980;**50**:182.

Spencer EM, Mims R, Uthne KO: Somatomedin levels in patients with pituitary microadenomas. In: *Pituitary Microadenomas.* Faglia G, Giovanelli MA, McLeod RM (editors). Academic Press, 1980.

Spencer EM, Ross M, Smith B: The identity of human insulin-like growth factors I and II: Somatomedins C and A and homology with rat IGF I and II. Page 81 in: *Insulin-Like Growth Factors/Somatomedins: Basic Chemistry, Biology and Clinical Importance.* Spencer EM (editor). Walter de Gruyter, 1981.

Spencer EM, Uthne KO: The effect of somatomedin on adenylyl cyclase and guanylyl cyclase activity in various tissues. Page 37 in: *Somatomedins and Growth.* Giordano G, Van Wyk JJ, Minuto F (editors). Academic Press, 1979.

Spencer EM, Uthne K, Arnold W: Growth impairment with elevated somatomedin levels in children with chronic renal insufficiency. *Acta Endocrinol* 1979;**91**:36.

Stiles CD et al: Dual control of cell growth by somatomedins and platelet derived growth factor. *Proc Natl Acad Sci USA* 1979;**76**:1279.

Tricoli JV et al: Location of insulin-like growth factor genes to human chromosomes 11 and 12. *Nature* 1984;**310**:784.

Growth

5

Dennis M. Styne, MD

Assessment of growth in stature is an essential part of the pediatric examination. Growth is an important index of physical and mental health and of the quality of the child's psychosocial environment; chronic problems in any of these areas may be reflected in a decreased growth rate. In this discussion, we will consider influences on normal growth, the normal growth pattern, the measurement of growth, and conditions that lead to disorders of growth.

NORMAL GROWTH

INTRAUTERINE GROWTH

The great changes that take place in the human fetus during intrauterine growth have been summarized by Pierson and Deschamps: From conception to delivery, fetal mass increases 44×10^7 times, compared to a 20-fold increase from birth to adulthood; length increases 3850 times to term, compared to a 3- to 4-fold increase from birth to adulthood. The determinants of normal prenatal growth are poorly understood, though many factors that lead to abnormal prenatal growth have been identified.

Endocrine Factors

Much research remains to be done before the endocrine factors influencing fetal growth will be completely elucidated.

A. Growth Hormone: Although fetal plasma values of growth hormone (GH) are higher than levels reported in most adult acromegalics, GH appears to have little influence on length at birth; infants with GH deficiency have normal birth lengths, and even those with anencephaly (who therefore lack hypothalamic releasing factors) have normal body lengths. Human chorionic somatomammotropin (hCS), a placental hormone similar in structure to GH and prolactin, may not be essential to fetal growth, since patients lacking the hCS gene have achieved normal birth lengths.

B. Thyroid Hormone: The absence of thyroid hormone may have devastating effects on the mental development of a fetus, but hypothyroid newborns are of normal length. In fact, perhaps because of the longer duration of pregnancy in hypothyroid fetuses, the hypothyroid newborn may be longer than average.

C. Insulin: Excessive serum insulin concentrations may be associated with increased length in infants of diabetic mothers and in Beckwith-Wiedemann syndrome, characterized by neonatal hypoglycemia, neonatal gigantism, omphalocele, macroglossia, and hepatomegaly. Inadequate insulin production, found in transient neonatal diabetes mellitus, or insulin resistance, found in the leprechaun syndrome (Donohue syndrome), is associated with short newborn length.

D. Somatomedins (IGF-I and IGF-II): The role of somatomedins in prenatal growth is unclear. IGF-II may play an important role, as suggested by the observation that MSA and IGF-II levels are higher than IGF-I levels in fetal rats and fetal sheep, respectively. (MSA [multiplication-stimulating activity] is chemically similar to IGF-II; see Chapter 4, Part II.) After birth, IGF-II values decrease and IGF-I values increase. There is a correlation of serum IGF-I values with newborn weight in normal infants. Laron's dwarfism, characterized by an inability to generate IGF-I, is associated with low birth length.

Acronyms Used in This Chapter

ACTH	Adrenocorticotropic hormone
cAMP	Cyclic adenosine monophosphate
DNA	Deoxyribonucleic acid
GH	Growth hormone
GnRH	Gonadotropin-releasing hormone
GRH	Growth hormone–releasing hormone
hCG	Human chorionic gonadotropin
hCS	Human chorionic somatomammotropin
hGH	Human growth hormone
IGF	Human insulinlike growth factor (somatomedin)
LH	Luteinizing hormone
MSA	Multiplication-stimulating activity
PTH	Parathyroid hormone
TBG	Thyroid hormone–binding globulin
TRH	Thyrotropin-releasing hormone
TSH	Thyroid-stimulating hormone (thyrotropin)

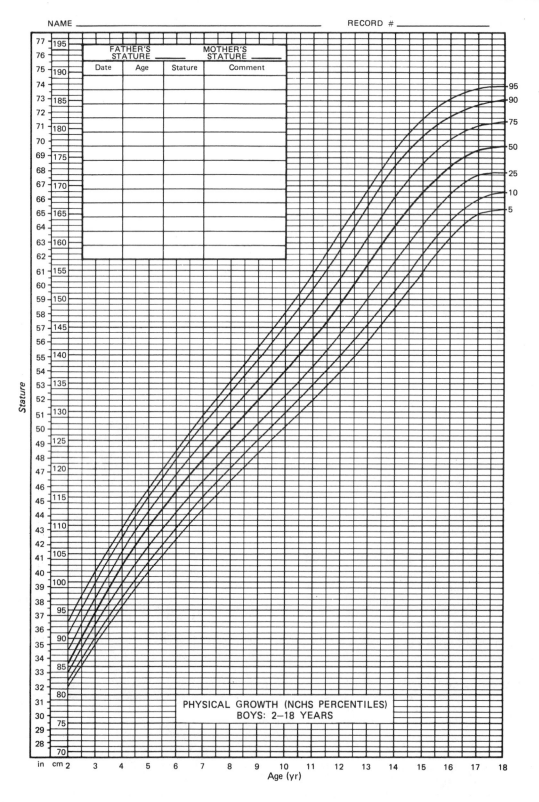

Figure 5–1. Growth chart for boys in the USA. (Redrawn and reprinted with permission of Ross Laboratories, Columbus, OH 43216. © 1980 Ross Laboratories. Sources of data: 1976 study of the National Center for Health Statistics [NCHS; Hyattsville, MD]; Hamill PVV et al: Physical growth: National Center for Health Statistics percentiles. *Am J Clin Nutr* 1979;**32**:607.)

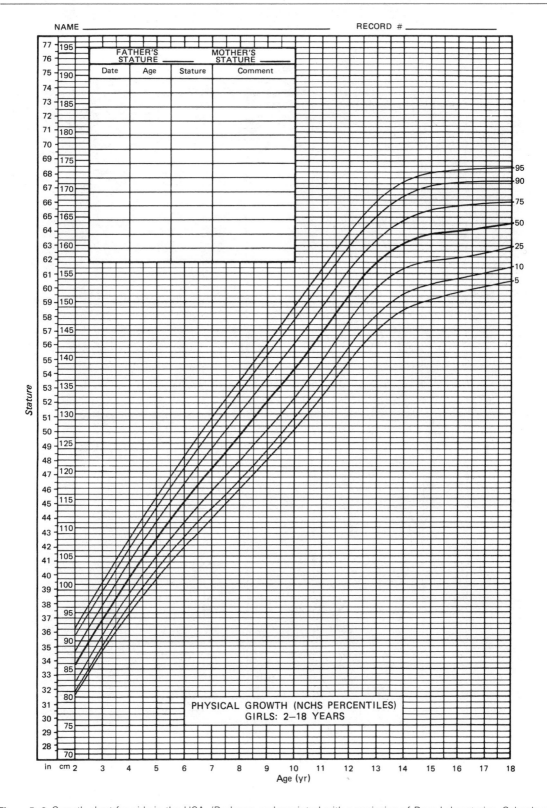

Figure 5–2. Growth chart for girls in the USA. (Redrawn and reprinted with permission of Ross Laboratories, Columbus, OH 43216. © 1980 Ross Laboratories. Sources of data: 1976 study of the National Center for Health Statistics [NCHS; Hyattsville, MD]; Hamill PVV et al: Physical growth: National Center for Health Statistics percentiles. *Am J Clin Nutr* 1979;**32**:607.)

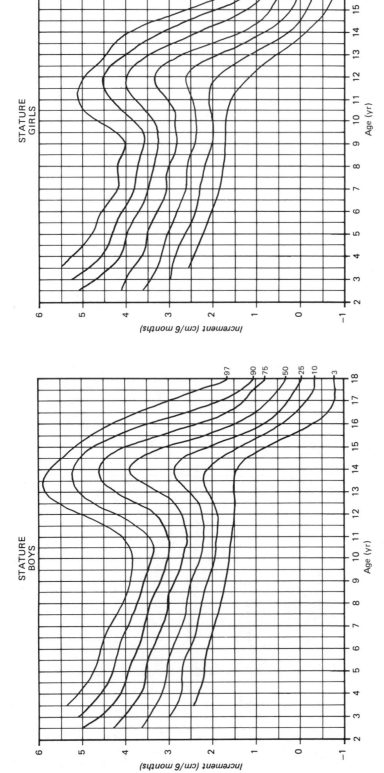

Figures 5–3 and 5–4. Incremental growth charts for boys (Fig 5–3) and girls (Fig 5–4). Height velocity measured over a period of at least 6 months can be compared with the percentiles on the right axis of the charts. (Redrawn and reprinted with permission of Ross Laboratories, Columbus, OH 43216. © 1981 Ross Laboratories. Sources of data: Longitudinal studies of the Fels Research Laboratories (Yellow Springs, OH); Roche AF, Himes JH: Incremental growth charts. *Am J Clin Nutr* 1980;**33**:2041.)

Maternal & Uterine Factors

Maternal factors, often expressed through the uterine environment, exert more influence on birth size than paternal factors. The height of the mother correlates better with fetal size than the height of the father. Worldwide, poor maternal nutrition is the most important condition leading to low birth weight and length; it also predisposes the infant to other serious health hazards after birth. Chronic maternal disease and eclampsia can also lead to poor fetal growth. Maternal alcohol ingestion has been shown to have severe adverse effects on fetal length and mental development and to predispose to other physical abnormalities such as microcephaly, mental retardation, maxillary hypoplasia, and short palpebral fissures. Abuse of other substances, cigarette smoking, and chronic use of some medications (eg, phenytoin) can cause intrauterine growth retardation. Maternal infection—most commonly rubella, toxoplasmosis, and cytomegalovirus—leads to many developmental abnormalities as well as short birth length. In multiple births, the weight of each fetus is usually less than that of the average singleton. Uterine tumors or malformations may decrease fetal growth.

Because infants who are small for gestational age usually do not grow well after birth, any of the factors that cause low birth weight may ultimately have a deleterious effect on postnatal growth and final stature in adulthood. This is in contrast to infants with normal weight for gestational age. Premature infants usually recover to the range of normal height and weight for age by age 2 years. To do this, they must have growth rates that are higher than the average. Thus, a key point in assessing the patient with short stature is determining gestational age at birth and relating it to birth weight and length.

Chromosomal Abnormalities & Malformation Syndromes

Many chromosomal abnormalities that lead to malformation syndromes also cause poor fetal growth. Other malformation syndromes associated with a normal karyotype are characterized by intrauterine growth retardation, but in most cases endocrine abnormalities have not been noted. For further discussion, the reader is referred to other sources listed in the references at the end of this chapter.

POSTNATAL GROWTH

Although we have limited knowledge of the factors affecting prenatal growth, more is known about postnatal growth. Assessment of growth is, of course, easier after birth, and the effects of environmental manipulation and replacement of deficient hormones are easier to document in the child than in the fetus.

Postnatal growth in stature and weight follows a definite pattern in normal children (Figs 5–1 and 5–2). The growth rate is most rapid just after birth and slowest in mid childhood (Figs 5–3 and 5–4). The striking increase in stature known as the pubertal growth spurt then follows, leading to a second peak of growth velocity. The final decrease follows, until fusion of the epiphyses occurs and growth ceases.

Endocrine Factors

A. Growth Hormone and Somatomedins: As discussed in Chapter 4, Part I, somatotropin, or growth hormone (GH), is regulated by hypothalamic somatostatin and growth hormone–releasing hormone (GRH). GH then stimulates somatomedin production, which has a direct influence on the growth of cartilage. In general, serum IGF-I varies with states of GH secretion—decreased in GH deficiency and elevated in acromegaly—but nutrition, chronologic age, and other genetic and metabolic factors can alter this relationship. The replacement of GH in hypopituitary dwarfism leads to striking improvement in growth and elevation of serum IGF-I and has clearly demonstrated the importance of the GH-somatomedin axis in postnatal growth. Plasma somatomedin values are age-dependent. Values are lowest in the neonate, and levels in children are lower than those in adults. Acromegalic levels are reached during puberty, although peak somatomedin values do not closely correlate chronologically with peak height velocity.

B. Thyroid Hormone: Although hypothyroid newborns are not short, they manifest exceedingly poor growth soon after birth if untreated. Acquired hypothyroidism can also lead to a markedly decreased growth rate. Bone age advancement is severely delayed, usually more so than in GH deficiency. The upper to lower segment ratio (Fig 5–7) is also elevated and therefore delayed, owing to poorer limb growth than trunk growth.

C. Sex Steroids: Gonadal steroids exert an important influence on the pubertal growth spurt, while absence of these factors is not important in prepubertal growth. Gonadal and adrenal sex steroids in excess can cause a sharp increase in growth rate as well as the premature appearance and progression of secondary sexual features. If unabated, increased sex steroids will cause advancement of skeletal age, premature epiphyseal fusion, and short adult stature.

D. Glucocorticoids: Cortisone or its analogs in excess can stop growth. The absence of glucocorticoids has little effect on growth if the individual is clinically well in other respects.

Other Factors

A. Genetic Factors: Genetic factors can influence final height. Good correlation is found between mid parental height and the child's height between 3 and 18 years of age; appropriate charts and tables have been developed to display this (Figs 5–5 and 5–6; Tables 5–1 and 5–2).

B. Socioeconomic Factors: Worldwide, the most common cause of short stature is poverty and its effects. Thus, poor nutrition, poor hygiene, and poor health have effects on growth both before and after birth. In people of the same ethnic group and in the

Table 5—1. Parent-specific adjustments (cm) for stature of boys from 3 to 18 years of age.*

Age (yr)	Stature (cm)	Mid Parental Stature (cm)																	
		150	152	154	156	158	160	162	164	166	168	170	172	174	176	178	180	182	184
3	86.0– 87.9	7	6	5	5	4	3	2	1	1	0	−1	−2	−3	−3	−4	−5	−6	−7
	88.0– 97.9	8	7	6	5	4	4	3	2	1	0	−1	−1	−2	−3	−4	−5	−5	−6
	98.0–106.9	8	8	7	6	5	4	4	3	2	1	0	0	−1	−2	−3	−4	−4	−5
4	90.0– 93.9	7	6	5	4	4	3	2	1	0	−1	−1	−2	−3	−4	−5	−5	−6	−7
	94.0–103.9	8	7	6	5	4	3	3	2	1	0	−1	−1	−2	−3	−4	−5	−6	−6
	104.0–112.9	8	8	7	6	5	4	3	3	2	1	0	−1	−1	−2	−3	−4	−5	−6
5	96.0–103.9	8	7	6	5	4	3	2	1	0	0	−1	−2	−3	−4	−5	−6	−7	−8
	104.0–113.9	9	8	7	6	5	4	3	2	1	0	0	−1	−2	−3	−4	−5	−6	−7
	114.0–122.9	9	9	8	7	6	5	4	3	2	1	0	0	−1	−2	−3	−4	−5	−6
6	102.0–111.9	8	7	7	6	5	4	3	2	1	0	−1	−2	−3	−4	−5	−6	−7	−8
	112.0–121.9	9	8	7	7	6	5	4	3	2	1	0	−1	−2	−3	−4	−5	−6	−7
	122.0–130.9	10	9	8	7	6	6	5	4	3	2	1	0	−1	−2	−3	−4	−5	−6
7	108.0–117.9	9	8	7	6	5	4	3	2	1	0	−1	−2	−4	−5	−6	−7	−8	−9
	118.0–127.9	10	9	8	7	6	5	4	3	2	1	0	−1	−2	−4	−5	−6	−7	−8
	128.0–136.9	12	10	9	8	7	6	5	4	3	2	1	0	−1	−2	−4	−5	−6	−7
8	114.0–115.9	10	9	8	6	5	4	3	2	1	−1	−2	−3	−4	−5	−6	−8	−9	−10
	116.0–125.9	11	9	8	7	6	5	4	2	1	0	−1	−2	−3	−5	−6	−7	−8	−9
	126.0–135.9	12	10	9	8	7	6	5	3	2	1	0	−1	−2	−4	−5	−6	−7	−8
	136.0–144.9	13	12	10	9	8	7	6	5	3	2	1	0	−1	−2	−4	−5	−6	−7
9	120.0–121.9	11	9	8	7	6	4	3	2	1	0	−2	−3	−4	−5	−7	−8	−9	−10
	122.0–131.9	11	10	9	8	6	5	4	3	1	0	−1	−2	−3	−5	−6	−7	−8	−10
	132.0–141.9	12	11	10	9	7	6	5	4	2	1	0	−1	−2	−4	−5	−6	−7	−9
	142.0–150.9	13	12	11	10	8	7	6	5	4	2	1	0	−1	−3	−4	−5	−6	−7
10	124.0–127.9	11	10	9	7	6	5	3	2	1	−1	−2	−3	−5	−6	−7	−9	−10	−11
	128.0–137.9	12	11	10	8	7	6	4	3	2	0	−1	−2	−4	−5	−6	−8	−9	−10
	138.0–147.9	13	12	11	9	8	7	5	4	3	1	0	−1	−3	−4	−5	−7	−8	−9
	148.0–158.9	14	13	12	11	9	8	7	5	4	3	1	0	−1	−3	−4	−5	−7	−8
11	128.0–133.9	12	10	9	8	6	5	4	2	1	0	−2	−3	−5	−6	−7	−9	−10	−11
	134.0–143.9	12	11	10	8	7	6	4	3	2	0	−1	−2	−4	−5	−6	−8	−9	−10
	144.0–153.9	14	12	11	10	8	7	5	4	3	1	0	−1	−3	−4	−5	−7	−8	−9
	154.0–162.9	15	13	12	11	9	8	7	5	4	3	1	0	−2	−3	−4	−6	−7	−8
12	132.0–141.9	12	10	9	8	6	5	4	2	1	0	−2	−3	−4	−6	−7	−8	−10	−11
	142.0–151.9	13	11	10	9	7	6	5	3	2	1	−1	−2	−3	−5	−6	−7	−9	−10
	152.0–161.9	13	12	11	9	8	7	5	4	3	1	0	−1	−2	−4	−5	−6	−8	−9
	162.0–170.9	14	13	12	10	9	8	6	5	4	2	1	0	−2	−3	−4	−6	−7	−8
13	136.0–139.9	12	10	9	8	6	5	4	2	1	−1	−2	−3	−5	−6	−7	−9	−10	−12
	140.0–149.9	12	11	10	8	7	6	4	3	1	0	−1	−3	−4	−6	−7	−8	−10	−11
	150.0–159.9	13	12	10	9	8	6	5	4	2	1	−1	−2	−3	−5	−6	−7	−9	−10
	160.0–169.9	14	13	11	10	8	7	6	4	3	2	0	−1	−3	−4	−5	−7	−8	−9
	170.0–178.9	15	13	12	11	9	8	6	5	4	2	1	0	−2	−3	−5	−6	−7	−9
14	142.0–145.9	13	11	10	8	7	5	4	2	1	−1	−2	−4	−5	−7	−8	−10	−11	−13
	146.0–155.9	14	12	11	9	8	6	5	3	1	0	−2	−3	−5	−6	−8	−9	−11	−12
	156.0–165.9	15	13	11	10	8	7	5	4	2	1	−1	−2	−4	−5	−7	−8	−10	−11
	166.0–175.9	15	14	12	11	9	8	6	5	3	2	0	−1	−3	−4	−6	−7	−9	−11
	176.0–184.9	16	15	13	12	10	9	7	6	4	3	1	−1	−2	−4	−5	−7	−8	−10
15	148.0–151.9	14	13	11	9	7	6	4	2	0	−1	−3	−5	−7	−8	−10	−12	−14	−15
	152.0–161.9	15	14	12	10	8	7	5	3	1	0	−2	−4	−6	−7	−9	−11	−13	−14
	162.0–171.9	17	15	13	11	10	8	6	4	3	1	−1	−3	−4	−6	−8	−10	−11	−13
	172.0–181.9	18	16	14	13	11	9	7	6	4	2	0	−1	−3	−5	−7	−8	−10	−12
	182.0–190.9	19	17	16	14	12	10	9	7	5	3	2	0	−2	−4	−5	−7	−9	−11
16	156.0–163.9	17	15	13	11	9	7	5	3	1	−1	−3	−5	−7	−9	−11	−13	−16	−18
	164.0–173.9	19	17	15	13	10	8	6	4	2	0	−2	−4	−6	−8	−10	−12	−14	−16
	174.0–183.9	21	19	17	15	12	10	8	6	4	2	0	−2	−4	−6	−8	−10	−12	−14
	184.0–192.9	23	21	19	17	14	12	10	8	6	4	2	0	−2	−4	−6	−8	−10	−12
17	162.0–165.9	17	15	13	11	9	7	4	2	0	−2	−4	−7	−9	−11	−13	−15	−17	−20
	166.0–175.9	20	17	15	13	11	9	6	4	2	0	−2	−4	−7	−9	−11	−13	−15	−18
	176.0–185.9	22	20	18	16	13	11	9	7	5	3	0	−2	−4	−6	−8	−11	−13	−15
	186.0–194.9	25	23	20	18	16	14	12	9	7	5	3	1	−1	−4	−6	−8	−10	−12
18	160.0–165.9	18	16	13	11	9	6	4	2	0	−3	−5	−7	−10	−12	−14	−17	−19	−21
	166.0–175.9	20	18	16	13	11	9	7	4	2	0	−3	−5	−7	−10	−12	−14	−17	−19
	176.0–185.9	23	21	19	16	14	12	9	7	5	3	0	−2	−4	−7	−9	−11	−14	−16
	186.0–194.9	26	24	22	19	17	15	12	10	8	6	3	1	−1	−4	−6	−8	−11	−13

*See footnote for Table 5—2.

Table 5–2. Parent-specific adjustments (cm) for stature of girls from 3 to 18 years of age.*

Age (yr)	Stature (cm)	Mid Parental Stature (cm)																	
		150	152	154	156	158	160	162	164	166	168	170	172	174	176	178	180	182	184
3	82.0– 83.9	6	5	4	4	3	2	1	1	0	−1	−1	−2	−3	−3	−4	−5	−6	−6
	84.0– 93.9	6	6	5	4	3	3	2	1	1	0	−1	−1	−2	−3	−4	−4	−5	−6
	94.0–102.9	7	7	6	5	4	4	3	2	2	1	0	−1	−1	−2	−3	−3	−4	−5
4	92.0– 93.9	6	6	5	4	3	3	2	1	0	0	−1	−2	−3	−3	−4	−5	−6	−7
	94.0–103.9	7	6	6	5	4	3	2	2	1	0	−1	−1	−2	−3	−4	−4	−5	−6
	104.0–112.9	8	7	7	6	5	4	3	3	2	1	0	0	−1	−2	−3	−3	−4	−5
5	100.0–101.9	8	7	6	5	4	3	2	1	1	0	−1	−2	−3	−4	−5	−5	−6	−7
	102.0–111.9	8	7	6	6	5	4	3	2	1	0	−1	−1	−2	−3	−4	−5	−6	−7
	112.0–120.9	9	8	7	7	6	5	4	3	2	1	1	0	−1	−2	−3	−4	−5	−6
6	106.0–109.9	9	8	7	6	5	4	3	2	1	0	−1	−2	−3	−4	−5	−6	−7	−8
	110.0–119.9	9	9	8	7	6	5	4	3	2	1	0	−1	−2	−3	−4	−5	−6	−7
	120.0–128.9	11	10	9	8	7	6	5	4	3	2	1	0	−1	−2	−3	−4	−5	−6
7	112.0–117.9	9	8	7	6	5	4	3	2	1	0	−1	−2	−3	−4	−5	−6	−7	−8
	118.0–127.9	10	9	8	7	6	5	4	3	2	1	0	−1	−2	−3	−4	−5	−6	−7
	128.0–136.9	11	10	9	8	7	6	5	4	3	2	1	0	−1	−2	−3	−4	−5	−6
8	116.0–123.9	9	8	7	6	5	4	3	2	1	0	−1	−2	−3	−4	−5	−6	−8	−9
	124.0–133.9	10	9	8	7	6	5	4	3	2	1	0	−1	−2	−3	−4	−5	−7	−8
	134.0–142.9	11	10	9	8	7	6	5	4	3	2	1	0	−1	−2	−3	−4	−6	−7
9	122.0–131.9	10	9	8	7	6	5	3	2	1	0	−1	−2	−3	−4	−5	−6	−7	−9
	132.0–141.9	11	10	9	8	7	6	4	3	2	1	0	−1	−2	−3	−4	−5	−7	−8
	142.0–150.9	12	11	10	9	8	6	5	4	3	2	1	0	−1	−2	−3	−5	−6	−7
10	126.0–127.9	10	9	7	6	5	4	3	2	1	0	−1	−2	−3	−5	−6	−7	−8	−9
	128.0–137.9	10	9	8	7	6	5	4	2	1	0	−1	−2	−3	−4	−5	−6	−7	−8
	138.0–147.9	11	10	9	8	6	5	4	3	2	1	0	−1	−2	−3	−4	−5	−7	−8
	148.0–156.9	12	10	9	8	7	6	5	4	3	2	1	0	−1	−3	−4	−5	−6	−7
11	130.0–133.9	10	9	8	6	5	4	3	2	1	0	−1	−2	−3	−4	−6	−7	−8	−9
	134.0–143.9	10	9	8	7	6	5	4	3	1	0	−1	−2	−3	−4	−5	−6	−7	−8
	144.0–153.9	11	10	9	7	6	5	4	3	2	1	0	−1	−2	−3	−5	−6	−7	−8
	154.0–162.9	11	10	9	8	7	6	5	4	3	1	0	−1	−2	−3	−4	−5	−6	−7
12	134.0–139.9	10	9	8	7	6	5	3	2	1	0	−1	−3	−4	−5	−6	−7	−8	−10
	140.0–149.9	11	10	9	7	6	5	4	3	2	0	−1	−2	−3	−4	−6	−7	−8	−9
	150.0–159.9	12	10	9	8	7	6	5	3	2	1	0	−1	−3	−4	−5	−6	−7	−8
	160.0–168.9	12	11	10	9	8	6	5	4	3	2	0	−1	−2	−3	−4	−5	−7	−8
13	140.0–145.9	10	9	8	7	6	4	3	2	1	0	−1	−3	−4	−5	−6	−7	−8	−10
	146.0–155.9	11	10	9	7	6	5	4	3	2	0	−1	−2	−3	−4	−6	−7	−8	−9
	156.0–165.9	12	10	9	8	7	6	5	3	2	1	0	−1	−3	−4	−5	−6	−7	−8
	166.0–174.9	12	11	10	9	8	6	5	4	3	2	1	−1	−2	−3	−4	−5	−7	−8
14	146.0–149.9	10	9	8	6	5	4	3	2	1	0	−1	−3	−4	−5	−6	−7	−8	−9
	150.0–159.9	11	9	8	7	6	5	4	3	1	0	−1	−2	−3	−4	−5	−7	−8	−9
	160.0–169.9	11	10	9	8	7	6	5	3	2	1	0	−1	−2	−3	−5	−6	−7	−8
	170.0–178.9	12	11	10	9	8	6	5	4	3	2	1	0	−2	−3	−4	−5	−6	−7
15	146.0–151.9	10	9	8	7	5	4	3	2	1	−1	−2	−3	−4	−5	−6	−8	−9	−10
	152.0–161.9	11	10	9	7	6	5	4	3	1	0	−1	−2	−3	−4	−6	−7	−8	−9
	162.0–171.9	12	11	10	8	7	6	5	4	2	1	0	−1	−2	−4	−5	−6	−7	−8
	172.0–180.9	13	12	11	9	8	7	6	5	3	2	1	0	−1	−3	−4	−5	−6	−7
16	146.0–151.9	11	10	8	7	6	5	3	2	1	−1	−2	−3	−4	−6	−7	−8	−10	−11
	152.0–161.9	12	10	9	8	7	5	4	3	2	0	−1	−2	−4	−5	−6	−7	−9	−10
	162.0–171.9	13	12	10	9	8	6	5	4	3	1	0	−1	−3	−4	−5	−6	−8	−9
	172.0–180.9	14	13	11	10	9	7	6	5	4	2	1	0	−2	−3	−4	−5	−7	−8
17	148.0–153.9	11	10	9	7	6	5	3	2	1	0	−2	−3	−4	−6	−7	−8	−10	−11
	154.0–163.9	12	11	10	8	7	6	4	3	2	0	−1	−2	−4	−5	−6	−8	−9	−10
	164.0–173.9	13	12	11	9	8	7	5	4	3	1	0	−1	−3	−4	−5	−6	−8	−9
	174.0–182.9	14	13	12	10	9	8	6	5	4	2	1	0	−1	−3	−4	−5	−7	−8
18	148.0–149.9	10	9	8	7	5	4	3	2	1	−1	−2	−3	−4	−6	−7	−8	−9	−10
	150.0–159.9	11	10	8	7	6	5	4	2	1	0	−1	−3	−4	−5	−6	−7	−9	−10
	160.0–169.9	12	11	9	8	7	6	4	3	2	1	0	−2	−3	−4	−5	−6	−8	−9
	170.0–178.9	13	11	10	9	8	7	5	4	3	2	1	−1	−2	−3	−4	−5	−7	−8

*These figures can be used to adjust measured stature to account for parental heights. The average of the mother's and father's heights (mid parental stature) is calculated, and the column closest to the figure is selected. The intersection of a row containing the child's age and height range with the column showing the mid parental height is noted, and the adjustment figure is read from the chart. If the figure has no sign, it is added to the child's height (cm). If there is a negative sign, the number is subtracted from the measured height (cm). The adjusted height is read from the chart in Fig 5–1 (boys) or Fig 5–2 (girls) to determine in what percentile the adjusted height falls. If the child is short but the height percentile adjusted for mid parental height is closer to the 50th percentile, the child probably has inherited a familial tendency toward short stature. If the adjusted height percentile remains low, the child's height is probably inappropriate for the genetic potential of the family, and diagnostic studies may be indicated for an organic cause of short stature. (Reprinted with permission of Ross Laboratories, Columbus, OH 43216. © 1983 Ross Laboratories. Source of data: Himes JH, Roche AF, Thissen D: *Parent-Specific Adjustments for Assessment of Recumbent Length and Stature.* Vol 13 of: *Monographs in Paediatrics.* Karger, 1981.)

Figure 5–5. Adjustment of height based on mid parental stature (Table 5–1). Charts of 3 boys, each 7 years of age. *A* is below the 5th percentile, with a height of 112 cm; taking his mid parental stature of 158 cm into consideration, his adjusted height of 118 cm (arrow) is at the 25th percentile, suggesting that he is short because of familial tendency. *B* is far below the 5th percentile, with a height of 108 cm; his mid parental height of 166 cm causes his adjusted height to rise only 1 cm, suggesting that familial factors may not be the cause of his short stature. The converse is shown by *C*, whose height is 129 cm (95th percentile); mid parental height is 172 cm and adjusted height is equal to measured height, suggesting that the cause of his tall stature is probably not familial.

Figure 5–6. Adjustment of height based on mid parental stature (Table 5–2). Charts of 2 girls, each 7 years old, with height of 112 cm (5th percentile). *A* has a mid parental stature of 168 cm, and her adjusted height is unchanged, suggesting that genetic influences do not explain her short stature. *B* has a mid parental stature of 178 cm, causing her adjusted height (arrow) to fall 5 cm, suggesting that her short stature is more severe than suspected from the original growth chart and that genetic influences are certainly not the cause.

same geographic location, variations in stature are often attributable to these factors. For example, studies have shown that Japanese born and reared in North America were taller than Japanese-born immigrants to North America. Conversely, when socioeconomic factors are equal, the differences in average height between various ethnic groups is probably genetic.

C. Nutrition: The influence of malnutrition accounts for much of the socioeconomic discrepancy in height noted above, but malnutrition may occur in the midst of plenty and must always be suspected in disorders of growth. Chronic disease, which hampers adequate nutrition, often leads to short stature. Severe dieting has been demonstrated to hinder growth at pubertal ages. In infants, feeding problems resulting from inexperience of the parents may account for poor growth. Deliberate starvation of children by parents is an extreme form of child abuse that may be first discovered because of poor growth.

D. Psychologic Factors: Aberrant intrafamilial dynamics, psychologic stress, or psychiatric disease can inhibit growth either by altering endocrine function or by secondary effects on nutrition. The terms psychosocial dwarfism and maternal deprivation denote conditions due to these factors.

E. Chronic Disease: Even apart from the effects of poor nutrition, various chronic systemic diseases can interfere with growth. For example, congestive heart failure and asthma, if uncontrolled, are associated with decreased stature.

Catch-Up Growth

Correction of growth-retarding disorders may be temporarily followed by an abnormally high growth rate as the child approaches normal height for age. This catch-up growth will occur after initiation of therapy for hypothyroidism and GH deficiency, after correction of glucocorticoid excess, and after appropriate treatment of many chronic diseases. Catch-up growth is usually short-lived and is followed by a more average growth rate.

MEASUREMENT OF GROWTH

Accurate measurement of height is an extremely important aspect of the physical examination of children and adolescents. The onset of a chronic disease may often be determined by an inflection point in the growth chart. In other cases, a detailed growth chart will indicate a normal constant growth rate in a child observed to be short for age. If careful growth records are kept, a diagnosis of constitutional delay in growth and adolescence may be made in such a patient; without previous measurements, the child might be subjected to unnecessary diagnostic testing.

Height

The growth charts in most common use indicate the 5th and 95th percentiles as the outer limits of normal. This still leaves 10 out of 100 normal children outside of these boundaries, and it is both unnecessary and impractical to evaluate 10% of the population. It is the duty of the examining physician to accurately determine which short children warrant further evaluation and which ones (and their parents) require only reassurance that the child is healthy. Figs 5–1 and 5–2 furnish data necessary to evaluate height of children at various ages.

Pathologic short stature is usually far below the 5th percentile, but a diagnosis of pathologic short stature should not be based on a single measurement. Serial measurements are required because they allow determination of **growth velocity,** which is a more sensitive index of the growth process than a single determination. A very tall child who develops a postnatal growth problem will not fall below the 5th percentile in height for some time but will fall below the mean in growth velocity soon after the onset of the disorder. As Figs 5–3 and 5–4 indicate, growth velocity varies at different ages, but as a rough guide, a growth rate of less than 4.5 cm per year between age 4 years and the onset of puberty is abnormal. In children under 4 years of age, variations in growth velocity are more difficult to interpret. Normal newborns tend to be clustered in length measurements (partially owing to difficulties in obtaining accurate measurements). In the ensuing months and years, the child's height will enter the channel on the growth chart in which it will continue throughout childhood. Thus, a child whose height is at the mean at birth and falls to the 10th percentile at 1 year of age and to the 5th percentile by 2 years of age may in fact be normal in spite of crossing standard deviation lines in the child's journey to a growth channel at the 5th percentile. Although the growth rate may decrease during these years, it should not be less than the 3rd percentile. A steeper decrease in growth rate may be a sign of disease. It is clear that when a question of abnormal growth arises, previous measurements are always helpful; every physician treating children should record length or height as well as weight at every office visit. Height and height velocity should be determined in relation to the standards for the child's age.

Relation to Mid Parental Height

There is a positive correlation between mid parental height (the average of the heights of both parents) and the stature of a child. This may be taken into account with special charts (Tables 5–1 and 5–2) that indicate the number of centimeters to add or subtract from a child's height to adjust for parental heights when interpreting height for age. An abnormal height is below the 5th percentile for chronologic age when corrected for mid parental height by this chart.

Technique of Measurement

Length and height must be measured accurately. Hasty measurements derived from marks made at an infant's foot and head while the infant is squirming on the examining table are useless. Infants must be measured on a firm horizontal surface with a permanently attached rule, a stationary plate perpendicular to the rule for the head, and a movable perpendicular plate for the feet. One person should hold the head stable while another makes sure the knees are straight and the feet firm against the movable plate. Children over age 2 are measured standing up but cannot be accurately measured on the measuring rod that projects above the common weight scale; the rod is too flexible, and the scale footplate will in fact drop lower when the patient stands on it. Instead, height should be measured with the child standing with heels at the wall, ankles together, and knees and spine straight against a vertical metal rule permanently attached to an upright board or wall. Height is measured at the top of the head by a sliding perpendicular plate (or square wooden block). A Harpenden stadiometer is a mechanical measuring device capable of accurate measurement. Standing height is less than supine length, and it is essential to record the position of measurement each time; shifting from supine height at 2 years to standing height at 2 ½ years can falsely suggest an inadequate growth rate over that 6-month period.

In addition to height or length, other significant measurements include (1) the frontal occipital head circumference; (2) horizontal arm span (between the outspread middle fingertips with the patient standing against a flat backboard); and (3) the upper segment (US) to lower segment (LS) ratio. For the latter, the LS is measured from the top of the symphysis pubica and vertically to the floor with the patient standing straight, and the US is determined by subtracting the LS from the height. (Normal standard US/LS ratios are shown in Fig 5–7.) It is preferable to measure in the metric system, since the smaller gradations make measurements more accurate by eliminating the tendency to round off numbers.

Summary

In summary, we may consider 3 criteria for pathologically short stature: (1) height well below the 5th percentile for chronologic age; (2) growth rate below the 3rd percentile for chronologic age; and (3) height below the 5th percentile for chronologic age when corrected for mid parental height.

SKELETAL (BONE) AGE

Skeletal development is a reflection of physiologic maturation. For example, menarche is better correlated with a skeletal age of 13 years than with a given chronologic age. Skeletal age also affords an indication of remaining growth available to a child and can be used to predict height in adulthood. However, skeletal age cannot serve as a definitive diagnostic factor in any disease; it can assist in diagnosis only when considered along with other aspects.

Bone age is determined by comparing the appearance of epiphyses or shapes of bones on a radio-

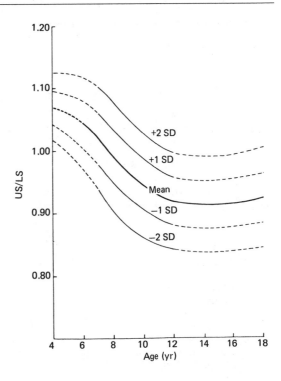

Figure 5–7. Normal upper to lower segment (US/LS) ratios, based on findings in 1015 white children. Values are slightly lower for black children. (Reproduced, with permission, from McKusick V: *Hereditable Disorders of Connective Tissue,* 4th ed. Mosby, 1972.)

graph to an atlas demonstrating normal skeletal maturation for various ages. The Greulich and Pyle atlas of radiographs of the left hand and wrist is most commonly used for comparison with patients' radiographs. The development of various bones, the time of appearance of epiphyses, and the stage of fusion of epiphyses are utilized in the evaluation of skeletal maturation. Any skeletal age more than 2 SD above or below the mean for chronologic age is out of the normal range. Other methods of skeletal age determination such as Tanner and Whitehouse maturity scoring are less widely used in the USA.

For newborn infants, knee and foot radiographs are compared to an appropriate skeletal age atlas; for late pubertal children, just before epiphyseal fusion, the knee atlas will reveal whether any growth remains or whether the epiphyses are fused.

Height prediction may be accomplished by determining skeletal age and height at the time the radiograph was taken and consulting the Bayley-Pinneau tables in the Greulich and Pyle skeletal atlas of the hand. The Roche, Warner, and Theisen (RWT) method of height prediction uses patient weight and mid parental height in addition to the variables noted above. Height prediction by any method becomes more accurate as the child approaches the time of epiphyseal fusion.

DISORDERS OF GROWTH
(Table 5–3)

SHORT STATURE DUE TO NONENDOCRINE CAUSES

1. CONSTITUTIONAL SHORT STATURE

Constitutional short stature is not a disease but rather a variation from normal for the population. It is characterized by moderate short stature (usually not far below the 5th percentile), thin habitus, and retardation of skeletal age. There is frequently a positive family history for similarly affected members and delayed puberty.

All other causes of decreased growth must be ruled out. The patient may be considered physiologically (but not mentally) delayed in development. Characteristic growth patterns include normal birth length and height, with a gradual decrease in percentiles of height for age by 2 years. Onset of puberty is usually delayed for chronologic age but normal for skeletal age. Adult height is in the normal or low normal range (see Fig 16–8).

Table 5–3. Causes of abnormalities of growth.

Short Stature
I. Nonendocrine causes:
  A. Constitutional short stature.
  B. Genetic short stature.
  C. Intrauterine growth retardation.
  D. Syndromes of short stature—
    1. Turner's syndrome and its variants.
    2. Noonan's syndrome (pseudo-Turner's syndrome).
    3. Prader-Willi syndrome.
    4. Laurence-Moon-Biedl syndrome.
    5. Other autosomal abnormalities and dysmorphic syndromes.
  E. Chronic disease—
    1. Cardiac disorders—
      a. Left-to-right shunt.
      b. Congestive heart failure.
    2. Pulmonary disorders—
      a. Cystic fibrosis.
      b. Asthma.
    3. Gastrointestinal disorders—
      a. Malabsorption (eg, celiac disease).
      b. Disorders of swallowing.
    4. Hepatic disorders.
    5. Hematologic disorders—
      a. Sickle cell anemia.
      b. Thalassemia.
    6. Renal disorders—
      a. Renal tubular acidosis.
      b. Chronic uremia.
    7. Immunologic disorders—
      a. Connective tissue disease.
      b. Juvenile rheumatoid arthritis.
      c. Chronic infection.
    8. Central nervous system disorders.
    9. Malnutrition (including that associated with severe dieting or malignant neoplastic disorders and chemotherapy-induced anorexia).
    10. Skeletal dysplasias.

Short Stature (cont'd)
II. Endocrine disorders:
  A. GH deficiency and its variants—
    1. Congenital GH deficiency—
      a. With midline defects.
      b. With other pituitary hormone deficiencies.
      c. Isolated GH deficiency.
      d. Pituitary agenesis.
    2. Acquired GH deficiency—
      a. Hypothalamic-pituitary tumors.
      b. Histiocytosis X.
      c. Central nervous system infections.
      d. Head injuries.
      e. GH deficiency following cranial irradiation.
      f. Central nervous system vascular accidents.
      g. Hydrocephalus.
    3. Variants of GH deficiency—
      a. Laron's dwarfism—syndrome of increased GH and decreased IGF-I.
      b. Biologically inactive GH.
      c. Pygmies.
  B. Psychosocial dwarfism.
  C. Hypothyroidism.
  D. Glucocorticoid excess (Cushing's syndrome)—
    1. Endogenous.
    2. Exogenous.
  E. Pseudohypoparathyroidism.
  F. Disorders of vitamin D metabolism.
  G. Diabetes mellitus with poor control.
  H. Diabetes insipidus, untreated.

Tall Stature
I. Nonendocrine causes:
  A. Constitutional tall stature.
  B. Genetic tall stature.
  C. Syndromes of tall stature—
    1. Cerebral gigantism.
    2. Marfan's syndrome.
    3. Homocystinuria.
    4. Beckwith-Wiedemann syndrome.
    5. XYY syndrome.
    6. Klinefelter's syndrome.
II. Endocrine disorders:
  A. Pituitary gigantism.
  B. Sexual precocity.
  C. Thyrotoxicosis.
  D. Infants of diabetic mothers.

2. GENETIC SHORT STATURE

Short stature may also occur in a familial pattern without retarded bone age or delay in puberty; this is considered "genetic" short stature. Affected children are closer to the mean after correction for mid parental height on the normal population growth charts (Fig 5–5 and 5–6) than they are beforehand. Adult height depends on the mother's and father's heights. Patients with the combination of constitutional short stature and genetic short stature are quite noticeably short due to both factors and are the patients most likely to seek evaluation.

3. INTRAUTERINE GROWTH RETARDATION

The small-for-gestational-age infant will often follow a lifelong pattern of short stature; in comparison, appropriate-for-gestational-age premature infants will usually catch up to the normal range of height and weight by 2 years of age. When compared to appropriate-for-gestational-age infants, intrauterine growth–retarded infants have been noted to have a decrease in cell number at birth; this decrease in number continues throughout childhood. Bone age, age at onset of puberty, and yearly growth rate are normal, and the patients are characteristically thin. Within this grouping are many distinctive genetic or sporadically occurring syndromes. The most common example is Russell-Silver dwarfism, characterized by small size at birth, triangular facies, a variable degree of asymmetry of extremities, and clinodactyly of the fifth finger. Reports of other syndromes in small-for-gestational-age infants can be found in sources listed in the bibliography.

4. SYNDROMES OF SHORT STATURE

Many syndromes have short stature as one of their characteristic features. Some include intrauterine growth retardation and some do not. Common ones are described briefly below.

Laurence-Moon-Biedl syndrome, Prader-Willi syndrome, hypothyroidism, glucocorticoid excess, pseudohypoparathyroidism, and GH deficiency combine obesity with short stature. Moderately obese but otherwise normal children without these conditions tend to have slightly advanced bone age and physiologic maturation with increased stature during childhood and early onset of puberty. Thus, short stature in a chubby child must be considered to have an organic cause until proved otherwise.

Turner's Syndrome & Its Variants

While classic Turner's syndrome of 45,XO gonadal dysgenesis (see Chapter 15) is often correctly diagnosed, it is not always appreciated that any phenotypic female with short stature may have a variant of Turner's syndrome. Thus, every short girl requires a karyotype determination if no other cause for short stature is found (see Chapters 14, 15, and 16).

Noonan's Syndrome (Pseudo-Turner's Syndrome)

This syndrome shares several phenotypic characteristics of Turner's syndrome, but the karyotype is 46,XX in the female or 46,XY in the male, and other features clearly differentiate it from Turner's syndrome; pseudo-Turner's syndrome is an autosomal dominant disorder (see Chapters 13 and 16).

Prader-Willi Syndrome

This condition is characterized by infantile hypotonia, acromicria (small hands and feet), mental retardation, almond-shaped eyes, and extreme obesity. Glucose intolerance and delayed puberty are characteristic. This syndrome is associated with abnormalities of chromosome 15 (see Chapter 16).

Laurence-Moon-Biedl Syndrome

This syndrome of retinitis pigmentosa, polydactyly, and obesity is also associated with poor growth and delayed puberty. It is inherited as an autosomal recessive disorder (see Chapter 16).

Autosomal Karyotypic Disorders & Syndromes

Numerous autosomal karyotypic disorders and syndromes of dysmorphic children with or without mental retardation are characterized by short stature as well. Details of these syndromes can be found in references listed at the end of the chapter.

5. CHRONIC DISEASE

Severe chronic disease of any organ system can cause poor growth in childhood and adolescence. In many cases, there will be adequate physical findings by the time of consultation to permit diagnosis; in some cases, however—most notably celiac disease and regional enteritis—short stature and decreased growth may precede signs of malnutrition or gastrointestinal disease. Patients with chronic disease are usually thin, and poor nutrition may be part of the cause of short stature. Hemoglobin, white blood cell count, erythrocyte sedimentation rate, serum carotene and folate levels, plasma bicarbonate levels, and liver and kidney function should be assessed in short but otherwise apparently normal children before endocrine screening tests are done. Urinalysis should be performed, with attention to specific gravity (to rule out diabetes insipidus) and ability to acidify urine (to evaluate possible renal tubular acidosis). A list of some chronic diseases causing short stature is presented in Table 5–3.

6. MALNUTRITION (OTHER THAN CHRONIC DISEASE)

Malnutrition not due to chronic disease is the most common worldwide cause of short stature. This diagnosis is based on historical and physical findings. The dietary history is of greatest importance. Food faddism or voluntary severe dieting should be considered. There are no simple laboratory tests for diagnosis of malnutrition, although somatomedin levels are low in malnutrition as well as in GH deficiency.

SHORT STATURE DUE TO ENDOCRINE DISORDERS

1. GROWTH HORMONE DEFICIENCY & ITS VARIANTS (Table 5–4)

Current concepts of endocrine regulation of growth propose that GH stimulates growth through intermediary substances, the **somatomedins** (see Chapter 4, Part II). The hypothalamus, through somatostatin and GH-releasing hormone (GRH), controls pituitary gland secretion of GH. GH then stimulates production of somatomedin, which directly increases growth. Earlier theories suggested the liver as the major source of plasma somatomedin that affects cartilage, but recent studies show that a multitude of organs produce somatomedin. In fact, somatomedin may be an autocrine or paracrine factor that influences its own cell of origin or neighboring cells. The plasma somatomedin measured in radioimmunoassays may represent a product that has already exerted its effect and has spilled over into the circulation rather than a product secreted into the circulation to exert its effect on growth at a distance.

Since estimates of the incidence of GH deficiency approach 1:5000–1:10,000 in European populations, the disorder should not be considered rare. Most patients with idiopathic GH deficiency apparently lack GRH but are shown by histologic studies to have adequate pituitary somatotrophs. Patients with pituitary tumors or those rare patients with congenital absence of the pituitary gland lack somatotrophs. Hereditary growth hormone deficiency has been demonstrated in families that lack the gene for the production of growth hormone.

Before 1986, the only clinical method of treatment for GH deficiency was replacement with human GH (hGH) from cadaver donors. In early 1985, three cases of neurologic disease were diagnosed in patients who had received natural hGH 10–15 years before. At least 2 of the 3 cases were diagnosed as having Creutzfeldt-Jakob disease, and the possibility arose that prions contaminating a donor's pituitary gland were transmitted to the GH-deficient patients and caused their death. While no proof of such transmission is available at this writing and despite the fact that newer methods of purifying hGH instituted in 1977 probably would remove such agents, natural growth hormone from all sources has been removed from distribution until the issue can be resolved. Recombinant DNA technology has been applied to increasing production of hGH and will provide a cheaper and more readily available source of the hormone.

GRH has been isolated from pancreatic GH-releasing tumor, sequenced, and synthesized. Hypothalamic GRH has the same structure as GRH from the pancreatic tumors. GRH has potential in the diagnosis of GH deficiency; in experimental studies, GH-deficient patients have demonstrated lower or absent GH secretion after administration of GRH. A few children with idiopathic GH deficiency have been treated with episodic doses of GRH that have restored GH secretion, somatomedin production, and growth. As supplies of synthetic GRH become widely available, this substance may prove to be useful therapy for GH deficiency. Growth disturbances due to diseases of GH release or action are shown in Table 5–4.

Congenital Growth Hormone Deficiency

Congenital GH deficiency is associated with normal birth length but a decrease in growth rate soon after birth. The disorder can be identified by careful measurement in the first year and becomes more obvious by 1–2 years of age. Patients with classic GH deficiency will have short stature, obesity with immature facial appearance, immature high-pitched voice, and some delay in skeletal maturation. Males with GH deficiency may have micropenis, especially if the condition is accompanied by gonadotropin-releasing hormone (GnRH) deficiency (Fig 5–8). GH deficiency in the neonate or child can also lead to symptomatic hypoglycemia and seizures; if ACTH deficiency is also present, the hypoglycemia is usually more severe. The differential diagnosis of neonatal hypoglycemia in a full-term infant who has not sustained birth trauma must include neonatal hypopituitarism. Congenital GH deficiency is also statistically correlated with breech delivery. Intelligence is normal in GH deficiency unless severe hypoglycemia has compromised brain development. When thyrotropin-releasing hormone (TRH) deficiency is also present,

Table 5–4. Postulated disorders of hGH release and action.

Site of Defect	Clinical Condition
Hypothalamus	Idiopathic GH deficiency due to decreased GRH secretion; hypothalamic tumors.
Pituitary gland	Dysplasia, trauma, surgery, or tumor of the pituitary gland.
	Production of an abnormal GH molecule in "biologically inactive GH syndrome."
	Absence of the gene for GH production (type IA GH deficiency).
Sites of somatomedin production	Laron's dwarfism with high GH and low somatomedin concentrations.
	Pygmies with normal GH, low IGF-I, and normal IGF-II concentrations.
Cartilage	Glucocorticoid-induced growth failure.

Figure 5–8. A 12-month-old boy with congenital hypopituitarism. He had hypoglycemic seizures at 12 hours of age. At 1 year, he had another hypoglycemic seizure (plasma glucose, 25 mg/dL) associated with an episode of otitis media, and it was noted that his penis was quite small. He was referred for evaluation because of these findings. At 12 months, length was 66.5 cm (−2 SD) and weight was 8.5 kg (−3 SD). The penis was less than 1.5 cm long, and both testes were descended (each 1 cm in diameter). Plasma GH did not rise above 1 ng/mL after arginine and levodopa testing. (No insulin was given because of the history of hypoglycemia.) LH rose only from 8.6 to 11.7 mIU/mL* after administration of GnRH, 100 μg. Serum thyroxine was low (T$_4$, 6.6 μg/dL; T$_4$ index, 1.5), and after administration of 200 μg of protirelin (TRH), serum TSH rose with a delayed peak characteristic of tertiary hypothyroidism. Plasma ACTH rose only to 53 pg/mL after metyrapone. Thus, he had GH, ACTH, GnRH, and TRH deficiency. He was given 6 doses of 2000 units of chorionic gonadotropin (hCG) intramuscularly over 2 weeks, and plasma testosterone rose to 62 ng/dL. He was then treated with 25 mg of testosterone enanthate every month for 3 months, and his phallus enlarged to 3.5 × 1.2 cm without significant advancement of bone age. With hGH therapy (0.1 unit/kg intramuscularly every other day), he grew at a greater than normal rate for 12 months (catch-up growth), and growth then continued at a normal rate.

*1 ng of LH (preparation LER 960) = 7.8 mIU.

there will be additional signs of hypothyroidism. Less severe forms of partial GH deficiency have been described.

Congenital GH deficiency may occur along with midline anatomic defects. Optic hypoplasia with visual defects ranging from nystagmus to blindness has been described in association with variable hypothalamic deficiency, including diabetes insipidus; absence of the septum pellucidum may also be found on CT scan in about half of patients with this condition. Cleft palate or other forms of dysraphism may be seen with GH deficiency. Children with a single maxillary incisor and GH deficiency have been described. Congenital absence of the pituitary, often found in an autosomal recessive pattern, leads to severe hypopituitarism, including hypoglycemia and hypopituitarism; affected patients have shallow development or absence of the sella turcica.

Hereditary GH deficiency has been described in several kindreds. Recent biochemical techniques have defined the defect in some families. Type IA GH deficiency is inherited in an autosomal recessive pattern; unlike those with classic sporadic GH deficiency, these children are born with somewhat short birth lengths. While they do initially respond to exogenous hGH administration, they soon develop high antibody titers that stop the effect of the therapy. DNA analysis proved that these patients lack the gene for hGH production. Type IB patients have autosomal recessive GH deficiency but no such gene depletion; type II patients have autosomal dominant GH deficiency; and type III patients have X-linked GH deficiency with apparently normal GH genes in both conditions.

Acquired Growth Hormone Deficiency

Onset of GH deficiency in late childhood or adolescence, particularly if accompanied by other pituitary hormone deficiencies, may be due to a hypothalamic-pituitary tumor. The presence of posterior pituitary deficiency in addition to anterior pituitary deficiency makes this even more likely. Conditions that may cause acquired GH deficiency—craniopharyngiomas, germinomas, gliomas, histiocytosis X, etc—are described in Chapter 16. Some patients with constitutional delay in growth and adolescence may have transient GH deficiency before the actual onset of puberty.

Cranial irradiation of the hypothalamic pituitary region for the treatment of head tumors may result in GH deficiency 6–24 months later.

Variants of Growth Hormone Deficiency

Other disorders of GH production or action have been reported that are not manifested in the classic manner of GH deficiency.

Laron's dwarfism is characterized by high plasma GH and low plasma somatomedin concentrations. Growth rate does not increase and somatomedin values do not rise when exogenous hGH is administered. The defect is due to inability to produce somatomedin in response to growth hormone, probably because of impaired receptors for GH. It is inherited as an autosomal recessive disorder.

Patients with radioimmunoassayable but **biologically inactive GH** have low somatomedin values, but treatment with exogenous hGH improves their growth rate and causes a rise in somatomedin levels. The defect may be due to production of an abnormal GH molecule that reacts in radioimmunoassay studies but exerts no biologic activity in the patient. The incidence of this disorder is not known, but it appears to be rare. Several very short, poorly growing children with delayed skeletal maturation, normal GH and somatomedin values, and no signs of organic disease have responded to GH therapy with increased growth rates equal to those of patients with bona fide GH deficiency. These patients may have a variation of constitutional delay in growth or genetic short stature, but a subtle abnormality of GH secretion is possible.

Pygmies have normal plasma GH, low IGF-I, and normal IGF-II concentrations. They do not respond to exogenous GH with improved growth rate or a rise in IGF-I. They have a congenital inability to produce IGF-I, which is of greater importance in stimulating growth than IGF-II.

Diagnosis of Growth Hormone Deficiency

Because basal values of GH are low both in normal children and in GH-deficient patients, the diagnosis of GH deficiency rests upon demonstration of an inadequate rise of serum GH after provocative stimuli. (A rise of < 10 ng/mL is considered inadequate in most laboratories.) Since 10% or more of normal children will not have an adequate rise in GH with one test of GH reserve, several methods of assessing GH

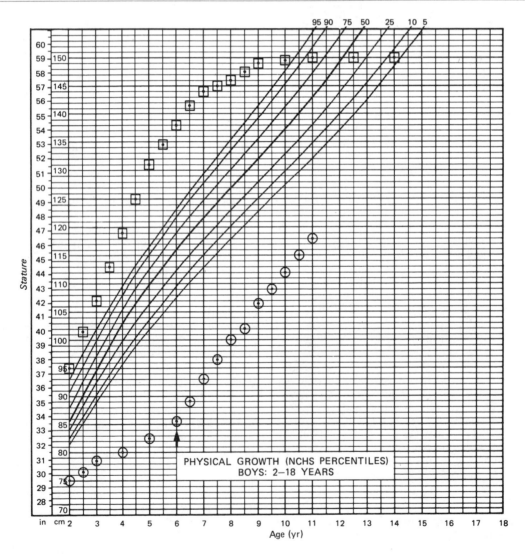

Figure 5–9. Examples of abnormal growth charts. Squares (□) represent the growth pattern of a child (such as patient A in Fig 5–11) with precocious sexual development and early excessive growth leading to premature closure of the epiphyses and cessation of growth. Circles (○) represent growth of a boy (such as patient B in Fig 5–11) with GH deficiency who showed progressively poorer growth until 6 years of age, when he was treated with hGH (arrow), after which catch-up growth occurred.

Figure 5–10. Two examples of abnormal growth plotted on a height velocity chart. *A:* The plot is taken from the data recorded as squares in Fig 5–9, describing a patient with precocious puberty, premature epiphyseal closure, and cessation of growth. *B:* The plot is taken from the data recorded as circles in Fig 5–9, describing a patient with GH deficiency who was treated with hGH (arrow) at age 6. Initial catch-up growth is noted for 2 years, with a lower (but normal) velocity of growth following.

reserve are necessary. Serum GH values should rise during stage III–IV sleep (usually 90 minutes after onset of sleep) and in response to arginine infusion (0.5 g/kg body weight [up to 20 g] over 30 minutes), oral levodopa (125 mg for up to 15 kg body weight, 250 mg for up to 35 kg, or 500 mg for over 35 kg), or clonidine (0.15 mg/m² orally).

GH levels also rise after acute hypoglycemia due to insulin administration; this test carries a risk of seizure if the blood glucose level drops excessively. An insulin tolerance test may be performed if dextrose infusion is available for emergency use, if the patient can be continuously observed by a physician, and if the patient has no history of previous hypoglycemic seizures. The patient must have a normal glucose concentration at the beginning of the test. Regular insulin, 0.075–0.1 unit/kg in saline, may be given as a bolus. In 20–40 minutes, a 50% drop in blood glucose will occur and a rise in serum GH and cortisol should follow. Glucose should be monitored, and an intravenous line must be maintained for emergency dextrose infusion in case the patient becomes unconscious or has a hypoglycemic seizure. If dextrose infusion is necessary, it is imperative that blood glucose not be raised above the normal range, since hyperosmolarity has been reported from overzealous glucose replacement. (See Chapter 4, Part I.)

Patients with **GH neurosecretory dysfunction** have been described who respond to pharmacologic stimuli (levodopa, clonidine, and insulin) but not to physiologic stimuli such as exercise or sleep; these patients may have decreased 24-hour secretion of hGH (or integrated concentrations of hGH) compared to normals, similar to GH-deficient patients. Thus, even pharmacologic testing cannot always determine who has a bona fide need for GH therapy.

Somatomedin values will be low in most GH-deficient subjects, but, as noted above, cases have been reported of short patients with normal somatomedin concentrations who require GH treatment for improvement of growth rate. In addition, starvation will lower somatomedin values in normal children and incorrectly suggest GH deficiency. Likewise, patients with constitutional delay in adolescence will have low IGF-I values for chronologic age but normal values for skeletal age. Thus, somatomedin determinations are not infallible in the diagnosis of GH deficiency. They must be interpreted with regard to nutritional status and skeletal ages.

The above discussion indicates that although phar-

Figure 5–11. Two boys demonstrating extremes of growth. The boy at left in each photograph *(A)* has precocious puberty due to a central nervous system lesion. At 4 4/12 years, he was 125.1 cm tall, which is 5 SD above the mean. (A normal 4-year-old is 101.5 cm tall.) His testes measured 2 × 3.5 cm each, his penis 9.8 × 2.8 cm. He was muscular and had acne and a deep voice. His bone age was 10 years, testosterone 480 ng/dL, and the rise of LH after 100 μg of GnRH was 23.4 mIU/mL, which is pubertal. His brain CT scan revealed a hamartoma of the tuber cinereum. The boy at right *(B)* at 4 2/12 years was 85 cm tall, which is 4.5 SD below the mean. He had the classic physical and historical characteristics of idiopathic GH deficiency, including early growth failure and a cherubic appearance. His plasma GH values did not rise after provocative testing.

macologic tests of GH secretion and plasma soma-tomedin values will usually indicate who has true GH deficiency, the diagnosis will remain in doubt in some cases. This should not lead to the conclusion that all short children should receive GH therapy. Only very short children (height well below the 5th percentile) who grow very slowly (growth velocity below the 3rd percentile for age) with delayed bone ages meticulously studied in research protocols have been shown to benefit from hGH therapy in the absence of proved GH deficiency.

Treatment of Growth Hormone Deficiency

A. Hormonal Replacement: GH-deficient chil-

dren require human growth hormone (hGH) by injection. In the USA, the drug is usually administered in doses of 0.1 unit/kg body weight intramuscularly or subcutaneously 3 times weekly during the period of active growth. Increase in growth rate (Figs 5–9, 5–10, and 5–11) is most marked during the first year of therapy. Older children with bone ages over 10 years do not respond as well and may require larger doses.

There is a species specificity of GH action, and only primate GH can exert growth effects in humans. Until very recently, hGH extracted from cadaver donor pituitary glands has been the only treatment for GH deficiency in humans. Currently, natural hGH is

Figure 5–12. Photograph and growth chart of a 9 1/12-year-old boy with psychosocial dwarfism. He had a long history of poor growth (< 3 cm/yr). The social history revealed that he was given less attention and punished more frequently than his 7 sibs. He ate from garbage cans and begged for food, although he was not completely deprived of food at home. When the photograph was taken (at 9 1/12 years), he was 99 cm tall (–7 SD) and weighed 14.7 kg (–3 SD). His bone age was 5 years, with growth arrest lines visible. Serum thyroxine was 7.8 μg/dL. Peak serum GH varied from nondetectable to 8 ng/mL on different provocative tests between age 6 years and 8 7/12 years. He was placed in a hospital chronic care facility (arrow) for a 6-month period and grew 9 cm, which projects to a yearly growth velocity of 18 cm. On repeat testing, the peak serum GH was 28 ng/mL.

not being distributed until it can be proved that purification techniques eliminate potential contamination with virus or prion particles. Recombinant DNA technology is being utilized to produce larger quantities of hGH, and numerous reports show that this hGH is as effective as natural hGH for stimulating growth in children with hypopituitarism. Since preparations of hGH produced by recombinant DNA techniques are now available, it will be possible to treat many more GH-deficient children with appropriate therapy. It should be noted, however, that results of long-term studies of hGH therapy in non–GH-deficient children are not yet available. Neither the American Academy of Pediatrics nor the drug companies producing hGH have recommended it for any patient without proved classic GH deficiency. Although too often abused in such situations, hGH has no proved effect and no role in athletic training or weight-lifting programs. Glucose intolerance, organomegaly, and skeletal changes such as are found in acromegaly are potential side effects of excessive hGH therapy in non–GH-deficient patients.

B. Supportive Management: Psychologic assessment and counseling are of importance in all types of short stature syndromes, including GH deficiency. Even though academic and social ability is not compromised, the patients' teachers, peers, and even parents may treat them as if they are younger than their chronologic age. Many patients are held back in school because of short stature in spite of normal intelligence. Some patients retain a body image of severe short stature even after normal height has been achieved following treatment. Depression and suicidal behavior can occur in affected adolescents.

2. PSYCHOSOCIAL DWARFISM (Fig 5–12)

Children with psychosocial dwarfism present with poor growth, potbelly, immature appearance, and bizarre eating and drinking habits. Parents may report that the affected child begs for food from neighbors, forages in garbage cans, and drinks from toilet bowls. As a rule this tragic condition occurs in only one of several children in a family. Careful questioning reveals a disordered family situation in which the child is ignored or severely disciplined. Caloric deprivation or physical battering may or may not be a feature of the history.

These children have functional hypopituitarism. Testing will often reveal GH deficiency at first, but after the child is removed from the home, GH function quickly returns to normal. Diagnosis rests upon improvement in behavior or catch-up growth in the hospital or in a foster home. Separation from the family is therapeutic, but the prognosis is guarded. Family psychotherapy may be beneficial.

Growth disorder due to abnormal parent-child interaction in a younger infant is called maternal deprivation. Caloric deprivation due to parental neglect

may be of greater significance in this younger age group.

3. HYPOTHYROIDISM

Thyroid hormone deficiency decreases growth rate and skeletal development and, if onset is at or before birth, leads to mental retardation. Screening programs for the diagnosis of congenital hypothyroidism have been instituted all over the world, and early treatment following diagnosis in the neonatal period will markedly reduce growth failure and mental retardation caused by severe primary hypothyroidism. The more subtle forms of congenital or acquired hypothyroidism in older children (eg, lymphocytic thyroiditis) may lead to growth failure in later life. Characteristics of hypothyroidism are a decreased growth rate and short stature, retarded bone age, and an increased upper to lower segment ratio for chronologic age.

Hypothyroidism cannot be diagnosed solely on the basis of a low plasma total T_4 value; an indication of a low free T_4 value or low free T_4 index is necessary to rule out the relatively frequent cases (one in 10,000) of thyroid hormone–binding globulin (TBG) deficiency, which will artifactually lower total T_4 values into the hypothyroid range. If a test of TBG levels (such as a resin T_3 uptake or plasma TBG concentration) is obtained along with the total T_4, this diagnostic trap can be avoided. Since the majority of cases of hypothyroidism are primary, elevated TSH levels will confirm the diagnosis of bona fide hypothyroidism.

4. CUSHING'S SYNDROME

Excess glucocorticoids (either exogenous or endogenous) will often lead to decreased growth rate before obesity and other signs of Cushing's syndrome develop. The underlying disease may be bilateral adrenal hyperplasia due to abnormal ACTH-cortisol regulation in Cushing's disease, adrenal adenomas, or adrenal carcinoma. The appropriate diagnosis may be missed if urinary cortisol and 17-hydroxycorticosteroid determinations are not interpreted on the basis of the child's body size or if inappropriate doses of dexamethasone are used for testing (appropriate doses are 20 μg/kg/d for the low-dose and 80μg/kg/d for the high-dose suppression test). Furthermore, daily variations in cortisol production necessitate several urinary or plasma cortisol determinations before Cushing's disease can be appropriately diagnosed or ruled out. Exogenous sources of glucocorticoids that cause poor growth may be oral corticosteroids used to treat asthma or even overzealous use of topical corticosteroid ointments or creams. Thus, an accurate history of prior medications is important in diagnosis. Growth failure in Cushing's syndrome may be due to decreased peripheral effect of somatomedin on growing cartilage or decreased GH secretion due to hypothalamic-pituitary effects of elevated glucocorticoid concentrations. Treatment of the underlying disorder (eg, transsphenoidal microadenectomy for Cushing's disease) will restore growth rate to normal (catch-up growth may occur initially) if epiphyseal fusion has not occurred.

5. PSEUDOHYPOPARATHYROIDISM

Pseudohypoparathyroidism is a rare disorder consisting of a characteristic phenotype and chemical signs of hypoparathyroidism, with elevated circulating PTH levels and failure of target tissues to respond to PTH. Children with pseudohypoparathyroidism are short and chubby, with characteristic round faces, short fourth and fifth metacarpal bones, and mental retardation. Serum calcium is low and serum phosphorus is high (as in hypoparathyroidism), but plasma PTH is high. The defect is in the guanylnucleotide-sensitive regulatory protein that couples PTH-occupied receptors to adenylate cyclase. Thus, administration of PTH fails to induce a rise in nephrogenous cAMP or an increase in urinary phosphorus. A rare variant of this disorder (pseudohypoparathyroidism type II) occurs in which administration of PTH produces a rise in nephrogenous cAMP but fails to induce an increase in phosphorus excretion, suggesting a defect distal to the receptor–adenylate cyclase complex. Treatment with high-dose vitamin D and calcium, as well as phosphate-binding agents, will correct the biochemical defects and control hypocalcemic seizures, but it will not improve stature or mentation.

Children with the pseudohypoparathyroid phenotype but with normal circulating levels of calcium, phosphate, and PTH are said to have pseudopseudohypoparathyroidism. They require no calcium or vitamin D therapy. (See Chapter 8.)

6. DISORDERS OF VITAMIN D METABOLISM

Short stature and poor growth are features of rickets in its obvious and more subtle forms. The disease may be vitamin D deficiency due to inadequate oral intake, fat malabsorption, inadequate sunlight exposure, anticonvulsant therapy, or renal or hepatic disease. Classic findings include bowing of the legs, chest deformities (rachitic rosary), and characteristic radiographic findings associated with decreased serum calcium and phosphate levels and elevated serum alkaline phosphatase levels. Vitamin D dependency may be diagnosed when vitamin D is required in doses far higher than necessary to resolve vitamin D deficiency. Short stature may be associated with rickets in renal disorders with hypophosphatemia due to a defect in renal reabsorption of phosphate; examples are Fanconi's syndrome (including cystinosis and other inborn errors of metabolism) and renal tubular acidosis.

When treatment is effective in these disorders (eg, vitamin D for vitamin D deficiency or alkali therapy for appropriate types of renal tubular acidosis), growth rate will improve. (See Chapter 8.)

7. DIABETES MELLITUS

Although well-controlled diabetes mellitus is compatible with normal growth, poorly controlled diabetics often grow slowly. Liver and spleen enlargement in a poorly controlled short diabetic child is indicative of Mauriac's syndrome, which is rarely seen now owing to improved diabetic care. The cause may be poor nutritional status. (See Chapter 19.)

8. DIABETES INSIPIDUS

Polyuria and polydipsia due to inadequate vasopressin (neurogenic diabetes insipidus) or inability of the kidney to respond to vasopressin (nephrogenic diabetes insipidus) will lead to poor caloric intake and decreased growth. With appropriate treatment (see Chapter 6), the growth rate should return to normal. Acquired neurogenic diabetes insipidus may herald a hypothalamic-pituitary tumor, and growth failure may be due to associated GH deficiency.

THE DIAGNOSIS OF SHORT STATURE

As previously stated, an initial decision must be made about whether a child is pathologically short or simply distressed because his or her height is not as close to the 50th percentile as desired by the patient or the parents. Performing unnecessary tests is expensive and may be a source of long-term concern to the parents—a concern that could have been avoided by appropriate reassurance. Alternatively, missing a diagnosis of pathologic poor growth may cause the patient to lose inches of final height.

If a patient's stature, growth rate, or height adjusted for mid parental height is sufficient to warrant evaluation, an orderly approach to diagnosis will eliminate unnecessary laboratory testing. The medical history will provide invaluable information regarding intrauterine course and toxin exposure, birth size and the possibility of birth trauma, mental and physical development, symptoms of systemic diseases (Table 5–3), abnormal diet, and family heights and ages at which pubertal maturation occurred. Evaluation of psychosocial factors affecting the family and the relationship of parents and child can be carried out during the history-taking encounter. Often the diagnosis can be made at this point.

On physical examination, present height and weight should be plotted and compared with any previous data available. If no past heights are available, a history of changes in clothing and shoe sizes or a need to lengthen skirts or pants may reflect prior growth.

Questioning about how the child's stature compares with that of his or her peers and whether the child's height has always been in the same relationship to that of classmates is useful. One of the most important features of the evaluation process is to determine height velocity and compare the child's growth rate with the normal growth rate for age. Adjustment for mid parental height is calculated and nutritional status determined. Arm span, head circumference, and upper to lower segment ratio are measured. Physical stigmas of syndromes or systemic diseases are evaluated. Neurologic examination is essential.

If no specific diagnosis emerges from the physical examination, a set of laboratory evaluations may prove useful. Complete blood count, urinalysis, and serum electrolyte measurements may reveal anemia, abnormalities of hepatic or renal disease (including concentration defects), glucose intolerance, acidosis, calcium disorder, or other electrolyte disturbances. Age-adjusted values must be used, since the normal range of serum alkaline phosphatase and phosphorus values is higher in children than in adults. A sedimentation rate and serum carotene determination may indicate connective tissue disease, Crohn's disease, or malabsorption. Determination of total T_4, TSH, and resin T_3 uptake or free T_4 is appropriate. Skeletal age evaluation will not make a diagnosis; however, if the study shows delayed bone age, the possibility of constitutional delay in growth, hypothyroidism, or GH deficiency must be considered. A somatomedin level, if normal for age, would speak against classic GH deficiency or malnutrition; if low, it must be considered in relation to skeletal age, nutritional status, and general health status. Elevated 24-hour urinary 17-hydroxycorticosteroids (normal, < 4.5 mg/m²) and free cortisol (normal, < 60 μg/m²) signify Cushing's syndrome. If a hypothalamic pituitary disorder is suspected, a skull x-ray or CT scan is indicated. Serum prolactin may be elevated in cases of hypothalamic disorder.

If no diagnosis is apparent after all of the above have been considered and evaluated, more detailed procedures, such as provocative testing for GH deficiency, are indicated. It must be emphasized that a long and expensive evaluation is not indicated until it is likely that psychologic or nutritional factors are not at fault. Likewise, if a healthy-appearing child presents with borderline short stature, normal growth rate, and short familial stature, a period of observation may be more appropriate than laboratory tests.

TALL STATURE DUE TO NONENDOCRINE CAUSES

1. CONSTITUTIONAL TALL STATURE

A person who has been taller than his or her peers and is growing at a velocity within the normal range for bone age, has a moderately advanced bone age, and has no signs of the disorders listed below may be considered to be constitutionally advanced. Predicted final height will usually be in the normal adult range. There may be a history of a close relative who was taller than his or her peers during childhood but who eventually reached normal adult height.

Exogenous obesity in an otherwise healthy child will usually lead to moderate advancement of bone age, slightly increased growth rate, and tall stature in childhood. Puberty will be in the early range of normal, and adult stature will be normal according to genetic influence. As a rule, obesity and short stature should be considered an indication of a potential organic disorder or syndrome.

2. GENETIC TALL STATURE

Children with exceptionally tall parents have a tendency to reach a height above the normal range. The child will be tall for his or her age, will grow at a high normal rate, and the bone age will be close to chronologic age, leading to a tall height prediction.

Occasionally, children will be concerned about being too tall as adults. These worries are more common in girls and will sometimes be of greater concern to the parents than to the patient. It is possible to limit final height by promoting early epiphyseal closure with estrogen in girls or testosterone in boys. Such therapy should not be undertaken without careful consideration of the risks involved, especially those of high-dose estrogen therapy. Such therapy will be ineffective if not started 3–4 years before epiphyseal fusion.

3. SYNDROMES OF TALL STATURE

Cerebral Gigantism

The syndrome of rapid growth in infancy, prominent forehead, high-arched palate, sharp chin, and hypertelorism (Sotos' syndrome) is not associated with GH excess. Mentation is usually impaired. The growth rate decreases to normal in later childhood, but stature remains tall.

Marfan's Syndrome

Arachnodactyly (Marfan's syndrome) is diagnosed by characteristic physical manifestations of tall stature, long thin fingers, hyperextension of joints, lens subluxation, and aortic dilatation. Arm span exceeds height, and the upper to lower segment ratio is quite low owing to long legs.

Homocystinuria

Patients with homocystinuria have phenotypes similar to those with Marfan's syndrome. Additional features of homocystinuria include mental retardation and increased urinary excretion of homocystine.

Beckwith-Wiedemann Syndrome

This syndrome of the large newborn with omphalocele, macroglossia, hypoglycemia with hyperinsulinism due to pancreatic hyperplasia, fetal adrenocortical cytomegaly, and large kidneys with medullary dysplasia is also associated with increased growth in childhood.

XYY Syndrome

Patients with one (47,XYY) or more (48,XYYY) extra Y chromosomes achieve greater than average adult heights. They have normal birth lengths but higher than normal growth rates. Excess GH secretion has not been documented.

Klinefelter's Syndrome

Patients with Klinefelter's syndrome (see Chapter 13) tend toward tall stature, but this is not a constant feature.

TALL STATURE DUE TO ENDOCRINE DISORDERS

1. PITUITARY GIGANTISM

If a GH-secreting pituitary adenoma occurs before epiphyseal fusion, the result will be excessive linear growth rather than just the acral overgrowth characteristic of acromegaly. Height velocity will be abnormally rapid, and other somatic signs that occur in

acromegaly may be found in addition to increased stature (see Chapter 4, Part II). Elevated fasting GH and somatomedin concentrations are diagnostic.

2. SEXUAL PRECOCITY

Early onset of secretion of estrogens or androgens will lead to abnormally increased height velocity. Because bone age is advanced, there will be the paradox of the tall child who, because of early epiphyseal closure, is short as an adult. The conditions include complete and incomplete sexual precocity (including virilizing congenital adrenal hyperplasia) (Figs 5– 9, 5– 10, and 5– 11).

3. THYROTOXICOSIS

Excessive thyroid hormone due to overproduction or overtreatment with thyroxine will lead to increased growth, advanced bone age, and, if occurring in early life, craniosynostosis.

4. INFANTS OF DIABETIC MOTHERS

Glucose intolerance of pregnancy (gestational diabetes) or diabetes mellitus causes large birth size and neonatal hypoglycemia due to pancreatic hyperplasia. A few weeks after birth, postnatal growth and glucose metabolism become normal.

REFERENCES

Normal Growth

Cheek DB, Mellits D, Elliott D: Body water, height, and weight during growth in normal children. *Am J Dis Child* 1966;**112**:312.

Forbes GB: Relation of lean body mass to height in children and adolescents. *Pediatr Res* 1972;**6**:32.

Hamill PVV et al: Physical growth: National Center for Health Statistics percentiles. *Am J Clin Nutr* 1979;**32**:607.

Himes JH, Roche AF, Thissen D: *Parent-Specific Adjustments for Assessment of Recumbent Length and Stature*. Vol 13 of: *Monographs in Paediatrics*. Karger, 1981.

Kaplan SL: Normal and abnormal growth. Pages 83– 104 in: *Pediatrics*, 17th ed. Rudolph A, Hoffman JIE (editors). Appleton-Century-Crofts, 1982.

Marshall WA: *Human Growth and Its Disorders*. Academic Press, 1977.

Roche AF, Himes JH: Incremental growth charts. *Am J Clin Nutr* 1980;**33**:2041.

Smith DW: Growth and its disorders. Vol 15 of: *Major Problems in Clinical Pediatrics*. Schaffer AJ, Markowitz M (editors). Saunders, 1977.

Smith DW et al: Shifting linear growth during infancy: Illustration of genetic factors in growth from fetal life through infancy. *J Pediatr* 1976;**89**:225.

Tanner JM, Whitehouse RH: Clinical longitudinal standards for height, weight, height velocity, weight velocity, and stages of puberty. *Arch Dis Child* 1976;**51**:170.

US Department of Health, Education, and Welfare, Public Health Service: *NCHS Growth Curves for Children: Birth –18 Years, United States*. Publication No. (PHS) 78-1650. Series 11, No. 165, 1977.

Wainer H, Thissen D: Two programs for predicting adult stature of individuals. *Pediatrics* 1976;**58**:369.

Short Stature

Ad Hoc Committee on Growth Hormone Usage, The Lawson Wilkins Pediatric Endocrine Society, and Committee on Drugs: Growth hormone in the treatment of children with short stature. *Pediatrics* 1983;**72**:891.

Aynsley-Green A, Zachmann M, Prader A: Interrelation of the therapeutic effects of growth hormone and testosterone on growth in hypopituitarism. *J Pediatr* 1976;**89**:992.

Bayer L, Robinson SJ: Growth history of children with congenital heart disease. *Radiology* 1973;**108**:655.

Borges JLC et al: Stimulation of growth hormone and somatomedin-C in idiopathic GH-deficient subjects by intermittent, pulsatile administration of synthetic human pancreatic tumor growth hormone–releasing factor–40. *J Clin Endocrinol Metab* 1984;**59**:1.

Clarren SK, Smith DW: The fetal alcohol syndrome. *N Engl J Med* 1978;**298**:1063.

Copeland KC, Underwood LE, Van Wyk JJ: Induction of immunoreactive somatomedin C in human serum by growth hormone: Dose-response relationships and effect on chromatographic profiles. *J Clin Endocrinol Metab* 1980;**50:**690.

Evans WS et al: Intranasal administration of human pancreatic tumor growth hormone–releasing factor–40 stimulates GH release in normal men. *J Clin Endocrinol Metab* 1983;**57:**1081.

Friesen HG: Raben Lecture 1980: A tale of stature. *Endocrine Rev* 1980;**1:**309.

Furlanetto RW, Underwood LE, Van Wyk JJ: Estimation of somatomedin-C levels in normals and patients with pituitary disease by radioimmunoassay. *J Clin Invest* 1977; **60:**648.

Goodman HG, Grumbach MM, Kaplan SL: Growth and growth hormone. 2. Comparison of isolated growth hormone deficiency and multiple pituitary hormone deficiencies in 35 patients with idiopathic hypopituitary dwarfism. *N Engl J Med* 1968;**278:**57.

Groll A et al: Short stature as the primary manifestation of coeliac disease. *Lancet* 1980;**2:**1097.

Harris DA et al: Somatomedin-C in normal puberty and in true precocious puberty before and after treatment with a potent luteinizing hormone–releasing hormone agonist. *J Clin Endocrinol Metab* 1985;**61:**152.

Harrison HE, Harrison HC: *Disorders of Calcium and Phosphate Metabolism in Childhood and Adolescence.* Vol 19 of: *Major Problems in Clinical Pediatrics.* Schaffer AJ, Markowitz M (editors). Saunders, 1979.

Hintz RL et al: Plasma somatomedin and growth hormone values in children with protein-calorie malnutrition. *J Pediatr* 1978;**92:**153.

Horner JM, Thorsson AV, Hintz RL: Growth deceleration patterns in children with constitutional short stature: An aid to diagnosis. *Pediatrics* 1978;**62:**529.

Johnson JD et al: Hypoplasia of the anterior pituitary and neonatal hypoglycemia. *J Pediatr* 1973;**82:**634.

Kaplan SL, Grumbach MM: Pathophysiology of GH deficiency and other disorders of GH metabolism. Pages 45–55 in: *Problems in Pediatric Endocrinology.* La Cauza C, Root AW (editors). Academic Press, 1980.

Kaplan SL et al: Growth and growth hormone. 1. Changes in serum level of growth hormone following hypoglycemia in 134 children with growth retardation. *Pediatr Res* 1968;**2:**43.

Katz HP et al: Growth and growth hormone. 3. Growth hormone release in children with primary hypothyroidism and thyrotoxicosis. *J Clin Endocrinol* 1969;**29:**346.

Kowarski AJ et al: Growth failure with normal serum RIA-GH and low somatomedin activity: Somatomedin restoration and growth acceleration after exogenous GH. *J Clin Endocrinol Metab* 1978;**47:**461.

Laron Z: Syndrome of familial dwarfism and high plasma immunoreactive growth hormone. *Isr J Med Sci* 1974; **10:**1247.

Lovinger RD, Kaplan SL, Grumbach MM: Congenital hypopituitarism associated with neonatal hypoglycemia and microphallus: Four cases secondary to hypothalamic hormone deficiencies. *J Pediatr* 1975;**87(Part 2):**1171.

Meyer-Bahlburg HFL et al: Growth hormone deficiency, brain development, and intelligence. *Am J Dis Child* 1978; **132:**565.

Miller WL, Kaplan SL, Grumbach MM: Child abuse as a cause of post-traumatic hypopituitarism. *N Engl J Med* 1980;**302:**724.

Milner RDG et al: Experience with human growth hormone in Great Britain: The report of the MRC Working Party. *Clin Endocrinol* 1979;**11:**15.

Norman C: Virus scare halts hormone research. *Science* 1985;**228:**1176.

Phillips JA III: Genetic diagnosis: Differentiating growth disorders. *Hosp Pract* (April) 1985;**20:**85.

Pierson M, Deschamps J-P: Growth. In: *Pediatric Endocrinology.* Job J-C, Pierson M (editors). Wiley, 1981.

Pimstone AD, Oberleas D: Zinc: Human nutrition and metabolic effects. *Ann Intern Med* 1970;**73:**631.

Powell GF, Brasel JA, Blizzard RM: Emotional deprivation and growth retardation simulating idiopathic hypopituitarism. *N Engl J Med* 1967;**276:**1271.

Powell GF et al: Emotional deprivation and growth retardation simulating idiopathic hypopituitarism. 2. Endocrinologic evaluation of the syndrome. *N Engl J Med* 1967;**276:**1279.

Prader A, Tanner JM, von Harnack GA: Catch-up growth following illness or starvation. *J Pediatr* 1963;**62:**646.

Pugliese MI et al: Fear of obesity: A cause of short stature and delayed puberty. *N Engl J Med* 1983;**309:**513.

Richards GE et al: Delayed onset of hypopituitarism: Sequelae of therapeutic irradiation of central nervous system, eye, and middle ear tumors. *J Pediatr* 1976;**89:**553.

Rimoin DL: Genetic defects of growth hormone. *Hosp Pract* (Feb) 1971;**6:**113.

Rimoin DL, Horton WA: Short stature. (2 parts.) *J Pediatr* 1978;**92:**523, 697.

Rivarola MA et al: Phenotypic heterogeneity in familial isolated growth hormone deficiency type I-A. *J Clin Endocrinol Metab* 1984;**59:**34.

Roche AF: Growth assessment in abnormal children. *Kidney Int* 1978;**14:**369.

Rogol AD et al: Growth hormone release in response to human pancreatic tumor growth hormone–releasing hormone–40 in children with short stature. *J Clin Endocrinol Metab* 1984;**59:**580.

Rosenfeld RG, Kemp SF, Hintz RL: Constancy of somatomedin response to growth hormone treatment of hypopituitary dwarfism, and lack of correlation with growth rate. *J Clin Endocrinol Metab* 1981;**53:**611.

Rosenfeld RG, Northcraft GB, Hintz RL: A prospective, randomized study of testosterone treatment of constitutional delay of growth and development in male adolescents. *Pediatrics* 1982;**69:**681.

Rosenthal SM et al: Synthetic human pancreas growth hormone–releasing factor (hpGRF[1–44]-NH$_2$) stimulates growth hormone secretion in normal men. *J Clin Endocrinol Metab* 1983;**57:**677.

Safer DJ, Allen RP, Barr E: Growth rebound after termination of stimulant drugs. *J Pediatr* 1975;**86:**113.

Schechter J, Kovacs K, Rimoin D: Isolated growth hormone deficiency: Immunocytochemistry. *J Clin Endocrinol Metab* 1984;**59:**798.

Silver HK, Finkelstein M: Deprivation dwarfism. *J Pediatr* 1967;**7:**317.

Simmons JM et al: Relation of calorie deficiency to growth failure in children on hemodialysis and the growth response to calorie supplementation. *N Engl J Med* 1971;**285:**653.

Sipponen P et al: Familial syndrome with panhypopituitarism, hypoplasia of the hypophysis, and poorly developed sella turcica. *Arch Dis Childhood* 1978;**53:**664.

Sklar CA et al: Hormonal and metabolic abnormalities associated with central nervous system germinoma in children and adolescents and the effect of therapy: Report of 10 patients. *J Clin Endocrinol Metab* 1981;**52:**9.

Smith DW: Recognizable patterns of human malformation. Vol 7 of: *Major Problems in Clinical Pediatrics*. Schaffer AJ (editor). Saunders, 1982.

Spiliotis BE et al: Growth hormone neurosecretory dysfunction. *JAMA* 1984;**251:**2223.

Styne DM, Grumbach MM: Puberty in the male and female: Its physiology and disorders. Pages 313–384 in: *Reproductive Endocrinology*, 2nd ed. Yen SSC, Jaffe RB (editors). Saunders, 1986.

Styne DM et al: Treatment of Cushing's disease in childhood and adolescence by transsphenoidal microadenomectomy. *N Engl J Med* 1984;**310:**889.

Takano K et al: Plasma growth hormone (GH) response to GH-releasing factor in normal children with short stature and patients with pituitary dwarfism. *J Clin Endocrinol Metab* 1984;**58:**236.

Tanner JM, Lejarraga H, Cameron N: The natural history of the Silver-Russell syndrome: A longitudinal study of thirty-nine cases. *Pediatr Res* 1975;**9:**611.

Tanner JM et al: The effect of human growth hormone treatment for 1 to 7 years on the growth of 100 children with growth hormone deficiency, low birth weight, inherited smallness, Turner's syndrome and other complaints. *Arch Dis Child* 1971;**46:**745.

Tanner JM et al: Relative importance of growth hormone and sex steroids for the growth at puberty of trunk length, limb length, and muscle width in growth hormone–deficient children. *J Pediatr* 1976;**89:**1000.

Thomsett MJ et al: Endocrine and neurologic outcome in childhood craniopharyngioma: Review of effect of treatment in 42 patients. *J Pediatr* 1980;**97:**728.

Thorner MO et al: Acceleration of growth in two children treated with human growth hormone–releasing factor. *N Engl J Med* 1985;**312:**2.

Underwood LE, D'Ercole AJ, Van Wyk JJ: Somatomedin-C and the assessment of growth. *Pediatr Clin North Am* 1980;**27:**771.

Van Vliet G et al: Growth hormone can increase growth rate in short normal children: Evaluation of the somatomedin-C generation test in the assessment of children with short stature. *N Engl J Med* 1983;**309:**1016.

Van Wyk JJ, Underwood LE: Growth hormone, somatomedins, and growth failure. *Hosp Pract* (Aug) 1978;**13:**57.

Youlton R, Kaplan SL, Grumbach MM: Growth and growth hormone. 4. Limitations of the growth hormone response to insulin and arginine and of the immunoreactive insulin response to arginine in the assessment of growth hormone deficiency in children. *Pediatrics* 1969;**45:**989.

Zapf J, Walter H, Froesch ER: Radioimmunological determination of insulin-like growth factors I and II in normal subjects and in patients with growth disorders and extrapancreatic tumor hypoglycemia. *J Clin Invest* 1981;**68:**1321.

Tall Stature

Conte FA, Grumbach MM: Epidemiological aspects of estrogen use: Estrogen use in children and adolescents: A survey. *Pediatrics* 1978;**62(Suppl):**1091.

Costin G, Fefferman RA, Kogut MD: Hypothalamic gigantism. *J Pediatr* 1973;**83:**419.

Pierson M, Deschamps J-P: Growth. In: *Pediatric Endocrinology*. Job J-C, Pierson M (editors). Wiley, 1981.

Roche AF: Growth assessment in abnormal children. *Kidney Int* 1978;**14:**369.

Smith DW: Recognizable patterns of human malformation. Vol 7 of: *Major Problems in Clinical Pediatrics*. Schaffer AJ (editor). Saunders, 1982.

Wettenhall HNB, Cahill C, Roche AF: Tall girls: A survey of 15 years of management and treatment. *J Pediatr* 1975;**86:**602.

6

Posterior Pituitary Gland

David J. Ramsay, DM, DPhil

The posterior pituitary gland secretes 2 potent nonapeptides: vasopressin and oxytocin. **Vasopressin** (antidiuretic hormone [ADH]) has important effects on urine flow and thus on water balance. In the presence of vasopressin, the average adult human can produce a urine concentrated to 1200 mosm/kg of water at a flow of approximately 0.5 mL/min. In the absence of vasopressin, as in diabetes insipidus, urine flow may be as high as 15–20 mL/min at a concentration of 30 mosm/kg of water. Vasopressin is also a potent vasoconstrictor agent, and the implications of this action for control of circulation are just beginning to be appreciated.

Oxytocin has important contractile effects on smooth muscle. In particular, it causes contraction of the myoepithelial cells that line the ducts of the mammary gland, thus causing milk ejection, and initiates contractions of the appropriately primed uterus.

ANATOMY & PHYSIOLOGY

The 2 peptides secreted into the bloodstream, arginine vasopressin and oxytocin, each contain 9 amino acids. They are characterized by a ring structure with a disulfide (S–S) linkage (Fig 6–1). In humans, as in most mammals, arginine vasopressin is the peptide associated with urinary concentration. Lysine vasopressin is the form of the peptide in the pig and is much less active in humans, though it has been used therapeutically. Arginine vasopressin has a molecular weight of 1084 and is basic, with an isoelectric point of 10.9.

Acronyms Used in This Chapter

ACTH	Adrenocorticotropic hormone
ADH	Antidiuretic hormone (vasopressin)
cDNA	Complementary deoxyribonucleic acid
CRH	Corticotropin-releasing hormone
DDAVP	Desmopressin acetate; 1-desamino-8-D-arginine vasopressin
mRNA	Messenger ribonucleic acid
SIADH	Syndrome of inappropriate secretion of vasopressin (antidiuretic hormone)

Oxytocin is a less basic peptide with a molecular weight of 1007. In vertebrates, there is a whole family of similar peptides with various amino acid configurations that exert effects on water metabolism and blood pressure. Vasotocin, which is a combination of the structures of vasopressin and oxytocin, has various species-specific effects including water absorption in the kidney and constriction of smooth muscle in the female reproductive tract.

The posterior pituitary gland, or neurohypophysis, develops as a downgrowth from the hypothalamus (Fig 6–2). It consists of fibers and endings of the hypothalamoneurohypophyseal nerve tract and contains many blood vessels, including capillary sinusoids. Humans have approximately 100,000 such nerve fibers in the tracts. The nerve terminals are characterized by a series of repeated swellings along the nerve fiber varying from 1 to 50 μm in thickness.

Synthesis

It is now clear that vasopressin and oxytocin are manufactured in large cell bodies situated mainly in the supraoptic and paraventricular nuclei. The synthesis of the 2 peptides is associated with synthesis of 2 specific binding proteins called **neurophysins**. One molecule of neurophysin I binds one molecule of oxytocin, and one molecule of neurophysin II binds one molecule of vasopressin. Common genetic mechanisms are involved in the synthesis of the peptide and of the neurophysin. For example, the Brattleboro rat, a strain deficient in vasopressin, does not make neurophysin II, although normal quantities of neurophysin I are present. The nucleotide sequences of

Cys — Tyr — Ile — Gln — Asn — Cys — Pro — Leu — Gly — NH₂

Oxytocin

Cys — Tyr — Phe — Gln — Asn — Cys — Pro — Arg — Gly — NH₂

Arginine vasopressin

Figure 6–1. Structures of oxytocin and vasopressin.

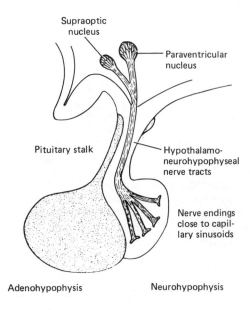

Figure 6–2. The hypothalamoneurohypophyseal system.

bovine arginine vasopressin–neurophysin II and oxytocin–neurophysin I precursors have been determined from cloned cDNA, proving the common precursor hypothesis. The precursors have been termed propressophysin and prooxyphysin.

Secretion & Transport

Neurophysin-peptide combination, often referred to as neurosecretory material, is transported along the axons of the hypothalamoneurohypophyseal nerve tract at a rate of 2–3 mm/h. Complexes are then stored in the nerve terminals in granules. Release of the peptide into the bloodstream occurs following electrical activation of the cell bodies of the nerve tract. For example, intracellular recording techniques have shown groups of neurons that respond to stimuli such as hyperosmolality and certain baroreceptor reflexes. At the nerve terminal, the process of secretion appears to involve the influx of calcium across the membrane. Secretion then proceeds by a process of exocytosis, with release of peptide and associated neurophysin into the bloodstream. The granule membrane is reclaimed by the cell following coating and microvesicle formation.

Extension of Magnocellular System

Oxytocin- and vasopressin-containing neurons project to regions other than the neurohypophysis. The supraoptic nucleus is fairly homogeneous and consists of cell bodies of magnocellular neurons that contain oxytocin or vasopressin and project mainly to the neurohypophysis. This magnocellular projection subserves the neuroendocrine function and accounts for the oxytocin and vasopressin in peripheral blood. In addition to containing some magnocellular neurons,

the paraventricular nucleus contains many smaller (parvocellular) cell bodies. Neurons of the parvocellular type have a widespread distribution and are thought to be involved in integration of central autonomic functions. There are groups of cells that contain oxytocin and vasopressin in other parts of the hypothalamus. Other peptides such as corticotropin-releasing hormone (CRH) and somatostatin have also been localized in parvocellular neurons.

There is an important projection of the vasopressin-containing fibers in the paraventricular nucleus to the zona externa of the median eminence. The release of vasopressin from these terminals allows entry of the peptides into the hypophyseal–portal vascular system and may be connected with the ability of vasopressin to stimulate ACTH secretion. There are caudal projections, mainly of oxytocin-containing neurons, from the paraventricular nucleus to the nucleus of the solitary tract, the dorsal motor nucleus of the vagus, and throughout the substantia gelatinosa and intermediolateral gray matter of the spinal cord. Projections of vasopressin-containing and neurophysin II–containing neurons have been identified in the choroid plexus of lateral ventricles. The oxytocin and vasopressin present in cerebrospinal fluid may originate from nerve endings that do not project to the neurohypophysis.

VASOPRESSIN

Action on the Kidney

Vasopressin has many actions, as set forth in Table 6–1. However, the most important are its actions on the kidney. The major action of vasopressin is to increase the water permeability of the collecting duct epithelium. The luminal membrane of the collecting duct epithelial cell governs the permeability of that epithelium to water. In the absence of vasopressin, permeability of the epithelium to water is very low;

Table 6–1. Actions of vasopressin.

Target Organ	Action
Cortical and outer medullary collecting ducts	↑ Water permeability.
Papillary collecting ducts	↑ Water and urea permeability.
Thick ascending limb of loop of Henle	↑ Salt reabsorption.
Heart	Bradycardia.
Arterioles	Constriction.
Kidney (juxtaglomerular cells)	Suppression of renin release.
Brain	Enhances passive avoidance behavior.
Liver	↑ Glycogenolysis, ↓ fatty acid synthesis.
Adenohypophysis	↑ ACTH release.

and, although the presence of vasopressin markedly increases permeability, vasopressin must first attach to receptors on the peritubular side of the cell in order to exert this action. Vasopressin-sensitive adenylate cyclase is then stimulated, resulting in the generation of cyclic nucleotides within the cell. The sequence of intermediate events is not so clear, but it probably involves activation of the protein kinase system. These intracellular events lead to an increase in the water permeability of the luminal membrane by increasing the number of narrow aqueous channels having radii of about 0.2 nm. Diffusion of water through the membrane is enhanced, and thus the transcellular flow of water is also enhanced. Such changes may involve considerable reorganization of membrane structure—perhaps even microtubule and microfilament formation.

The collecting ducts convey urine from the distal tubule and connecting tubule to the renal pelvis. As the collecting ducts traverse the medulla, the urine passes regions of ever-increasing osmolality up to a maximum in the normal human of 1200 mosm/kg of water at the tip of the papilla. In the presence of vasopressin, collecting duct fluid equilibrates with this hyperosmotic environment, and urine osmolality approaches that of medullary interstitial fluid. Vasopressin also increases the permeability of the papillary collecting duct epithelium to urea. Thus, in the presence of vasopressin, urine flow is low and urine osmolality is approximately 1200 mosm/kg; in its absence, urine flow is high (15–20 mL/min) and urine osmolality approaches 30 mosm/kg.

Other Actions

The physiologic significance of the other actions of vasopressin listed in Table 6–1 is less clear. It has been suggested that the pressor actions of vasopressin are important in the maintenance of blood pressure during hypovolemia. In addition to constriction of vascular smooth muscle, vasopressin modulates baroreceptor reflex activity by increasing the gain, particularly at low arterial pressures.

CONTROL OF WATER BALANCE

Water Requirements

Water balance is controlled by an integrated system that involves precise regulation of water intake via thirst mechanisms and control of water output via vasopressin secretion. Table 6–2 lists the major sources of fluid losses from the human body in temperate environments. Thus, the average individual loses 2.5–3 L of water per day and must take in that amount in order to maintain balance. As long as free access to water is allowed, total body water rarely varies by more than 1–2%. Approximately 1.2 L of the water necessary to maintain balance is taken in food or is provided by oxidative metabolism. The remainder is ingested as water or other fluid beverages.

Table 6–2. Routes of loss of water in an average adult human.

	mL/24 h
Urine	1500
Skin	600
Lungs	400
Feces	100
	2600

Concentration of Urine

The capacity of the kidney to produce a concentrated urine plays an important part in maintenance of water balance. Animals eat a diet that produces osmotically active material which is excreted in urine and thus requires water in which to be excreted. The more concentrated the urine the kidney can produce, the less water is required in order to excrete those solutes. It is not surprising, therefore, that the evolutionary appearance of peptides that can affect water transport coincided with the development of amphibians.

The importance of urinary concentration is demonstrated in Table 6–2. The average human receiving a normal diet excretes 1.5 L of urine per day at an osmolality of approximately 600 mosm/kg of water, ie, twice the concentration of plasma. Without the capacity to concentrate urine, 3 L of water at a concentration of 300 mosm/kg would have to be excreted, and extra amounts of water would have to be provided in the diet. During negative water balance, the urine volume may be reduced to 600 mL/d at a maximum urinary concentration of 1200 mosm/kg. This capacity to concentrate the urine 4 times more than plasma is of extreme importance, since otherwise it would be necessary to provide very large quantities of water in the diet. Animals in arid environments may concentrate urine up to 5 times more than humans and without that capacity would be unable to survive.

Urinary concentration mechanisms can reduce but not completely prevent loss of water in the urine. Even if an individual is maximally concentrating urine, there is still a considerable obligatory fluid loss. This situation is exacerbated in a warm environment, where many liters of fluid may be lost in order to maintain a constant temperature via sweating. The only way in which body fluid can be brought back to normal is by increasing water intake. It is not surprising that there are many similarities between mechanisms involved in the control of thirst and vasopressin secretion.

Control of Thirst & Vasopressin Secretion

Two major mechanisms are involved in the control of thirst and vasopressin secretion: (1) cellular dehydration and (2) extracellular dehydration.

A. Cellular Dehydration: Cellular dehydration occurs when extracellular fluid osmolality is increased by a solute that cannot penetrate cell membranes. As

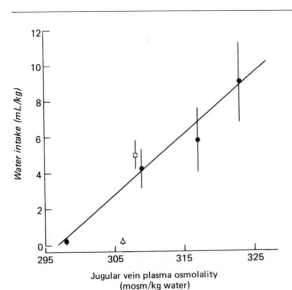

Figure 6–3. Relationship between water intake and jugular vein plasma osmolality. Central osmolality was increased selectively by infusing hypertonic sodium chloride into carotid loops in trained conscious dogs (●). Infusion of hypertonic sucrose was equally effective (□), whereas hypertonic urea (Δ) did not stimulate drinking. (Data from Wood RJ, Rolls BJ, Ramsay DJ: *Am J Physiol* 1977;**323**:88.)

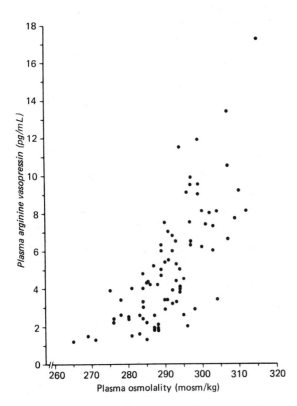

Figure 6–4. Relationship between plasma vasopressin concentration and plasma osmolality in humans during dehydration. (Reproduced, with permission, from Hammer M, Ladefoged J, Olgaard K: *Am J Physiol* 1980;**238**:313.)

the osmolality in intracellular and extracellular fluids is equalized by the passage of water across cell membranes, any increase in extracellular fluid osmolality will cause water to be withdrawn from cells. Verney, in a classic 1947 paper, proposed that osmoreceptor cells were present in the anterior hypothalamus and that when extracellular fluid osmolality increased, all cells—including these hypothesized hypothalamic osmoreceptors—became dehydrated, thus providing the signal for secretion of vasopressin. This theory has now received substantial experimental support. The effect of increasing plasma osmolality in conscious dogs prepared with exteriorized carotid loops on drinking is shown in Fig 6–3. Increasing the osmolality by approximately 10 mosm/kg with a solution of hypertonic sodium chloride or hypertonic sucrose stimulates drinking, whereas solutions of urea and glucose—solutes that penetrate cell membranes and therefore will not cause osmotic withdrawal of water from cells—have no effect on drinking. Fig 6–4 shows the relationship between plasma vasopressin concentration and osmolality in human subjects during dehydration. In this way, increases of only 1% in plasma osmolality cause stimulation of water intake and vasopressin secretion.

Experiments on conscious goats have recently suggested that the central osmoreceptors are sensitive to sodium concentration rather than to osmolality. Furthermore, it is claimed that the receptors are situated in a periventricular site and thus are sensitive to the composition of the cerebrospinal fluid rather than that of the plasma. Although there is some evidence for this hypothesis in ruminants, experiments in rats and dogs have failed to provide evidence for the existence of specific sodium receptors in these species. Moreover, it appears that the osmoreceptors must be situated in an area of the brain where the blood-brain barrier is deficient and thus is influenced by the composition of plasma rather than that of the cerebrospinal fluid. In fact, lesions of the organum vasculosum of the lamina terminalis, one of the circumventricular organs, prevent drinking and vasopressin secretion in response to increased plasma osmolality in the normal physiologic range, although responses to hypovolemia are normal. Although electrical activity of magnocellular neurons in the supraoptic nucleus is sensitive to changes in osmolality, the organum vasculosum of the lamina terminalis is essential for normal osmotic release of vasopressin and stimulation of thirst.

Information on the relationship between plasma vasopressin concentration and plasma osmolality in humans is now available (Fig 6–4). Although there is argument about some points at the lower end of the relationship and about whether the relationship is best represented in a linear or a logarithmic form, the exquisite sensitivity of vasopressin release to changing plasma osmolality is obvious. With plasma vasopressin concentrations of 10–12 pg/mL, the urine is maximally concentrated. Thus, as far as water conservation is concerned, Fig 6–4 represents the physiologic range of variations in plasma vasopressin in humans.

Hematocrit (%)

Figure 6–5. Relationship of plasma vasopressin to isosmotic reductions in blood volume in rats. (Reproduced, with permission, from Dunn FL et al: *J Clin Invest* 1973;**52**:3212.)

B. Extracellular Fluid Dehydration: Both drinking and vasopressin secretion may be stimulated by contraction of the extracellular fluid volume without a change in osmolality. This is referred to as extracellular fluid dehydration. Phenomena such as hemorrhage that reduce extracellular fluid volume result in both drinking and vasopressin secretion. Fig 6–5 demonstrates the relationship between reduction in blood volume and plasma concentrations of vasopressin. Small decreases in volume have minimal effects on vasopressin secretion, but reductions larger than 10% cause a marked stimulation of vasopressin secretion. Indeed, values over 100 pg/mL are not uncommon. These high plasma circulating levels of vasopressin would not appear to have much significance as far as water conservation is concerned, since maximum urinary concentration is reached at much lower plasma levels of vasopressin. However, the high levels of vasopressin secretion following depletion may be important in maintaining blood pressure, acting via the vasoconstrictor function of vasopressin.

C. Interaction of Osmolality and Volume: The pathways involved in hypovolemic stimulation of thirst and vasopressin secretion are still not clear. Two major mechanisms have been proposed, and there is evidence that both are involved. Reductions in blood volume may be sensed by low-pressure receptors in the left and right atria and in the pulmonary circulation. More severe hypovolemia resulting in reduction in blood pressure may be sensed by the arterial baroreceptors. Electrophysiologic evidence shows that information from both low-pressure and high-pressure baroreceptor areas in the circulation is transmitted to

cells in the supraoptic nucleus. In addition to this direct reflex pathway, the renin-angiotensin system may be implicated. It is clear that in all animal species that have been studied, including humans, angiotensin II is an effective dipsogen. In addition, particularly in the presence of a raised plasma osmolality, angiotensin may stimulate vasopressin secretion. Hypovolemia stimulates renin secretion and angiotensin formation reflexly. The relative roles of the direct baroreceptor input and angiotensin mechanisms in the responses to extracellular dehydration have yet to be determined.

The normal day-to-day regulation of water balance therefore involves interaction between osmotic and volume stimuli. In the case of vasopressin secretion, the fall in extracellular fluid volume sensitizes the release of vasopressin to a given osmotic stimulus. Thus, for a given increase in plasma osmolality, the increase in plasma vasopressin concentration will be greater in hypovolemic states compared with normovolemia.

In dehydration, an increase in plasma osmolality results in withdrawal of fluid from cells. Thus, the reduction in total body water is shared equally between intracellular and extracellular fluid compartments. The increase in plasma osmolality and the reduction of extracellular fluid volume act synergistically to stimulate vasopressin release. In salt depletion, however, plasma vasopressin concentrations remain constant or even slightly elevated in spite of a fall in plasma osmolality. Hypovolemia in this situation, as a result of osmotic movements of water from the extracellular into the intracellular fluid space, appears to provide the sensitizing influence.

Thirst mechanisms also involve interactions between extracellular fluid volume and osmolality. During periods of dehydration, increased plasma osmolality provides approximately 70% of the increased thirst drive, and the remaining 30% is due to hypovolemia. In salt depletion, the situation is less clear, but the normal drinking behavior or increased drinking that has been observed in experimental animals has been attributed to the associated hypovolemia.

Satiety

Dehydrated animals have a remarkable capacity to take in the appropriate volume of water in order to repair the deficit. It has been demonstrated that dogs deprived of water for various periods of time drink just the volume of water needed to repair the deficit within 5 minutes. All animals have this capacity, though some species usually take longer to ingest the required amount of fluid. If drinking ceases before complete intestinal absorption of the ingested fluid has occurred, mechanisms other than restoration of volume and composition of extracellular fluid to normal must be involved. These include oropharyngeal and gastric distention factors and perhaps the participation of receptors in the liver. Similar inhibitory influences affect vasopressin secretion. Following voluntary rehydration in dehydrated animals (including humans), plasma vasopressin secretion returns to normal before redilution of the body fluids has been completed.

DIABETES INSIPIDUS

Diabetes insipidus is characterized by the passage of copious amounts of very dilute urine. The disease is due either to failure of the neurohypophysis to secrete adequate quantities of vasopressin (neurogenic diabetes insipidus; also called pituitary, central, or vasopressin-sensitive diabetes insipidus) or failure of the kidney to respond to circulating vasopressin (nephrogenic diabetes insipidus). The loss of large volumes of dilute urine leads to both cellular and extracellular dehydration. Therefore, the disease is associated with polydipsia.

Classification

A. Neurogenic Diabetes Insipidus: The major causes of neurogenic diabetes insipidus are shown in Table 6–3. Operations in the region of the hypothalamus and pituitary gland—eg, removal of chromophobe adenoma—form an important group. Temporary impairment of posterior pituitary function is generally associated with pituitary surgery. Any damage to the hypothalamoneurohypophyseal nerve tracts will result in retrograde degeneration of the fiber tracts that have been interrupted. However, permanent diabetes insipidus will not develop unless over 80% of the pathways have been destroyed.

Idiopathic diabetes insipidus may occur at any age after infancy and affect both sexes. It is characterized by diminution in the number of vasopressin-containing fibers in the nuclei, nerve tracts, and posterior pituitary. Familial diabetes insipidus is a much more rare disorder. The onset occurs in infancy. It is also associated with sparsity of vasopressin-containing fibers. The other causes of diabetes insipidus involve mechanical disturbances to the pituitary or hypothalamus. Supra- or intrasellar tumors may be primary or secondary. A variety of infiltrative, vascular, and infectious causes complete this group. In partial neurogenic diabetes, vasopressin secretion is not completely absent, but plasma arginine vasopressin concentrations are inappropriately low for the plasma osmolality.

B. Nephrogenic Diabetes Insipidus: In this group

Table 6–3. Causes of neurogenic diabetes insipidus.

Hypophysectomy, complete or partial.
Surgery to remove suprasellar tumors.
Idiopathic.
Familial.
Tumors and cysts (intra- and suprasellar).
Histiocytosis.
Granulomas.
Infections.
Interruption of blood supply.

Table 6–4. Causes of nephrogenic diabetes insipidus.

Chronic renal disease: Any renal disease that interferes with collecting duct or medullary function, eg, chronic pyelonephritis.
Hypokalemia.
Protein starvation.
Hypercalcemia.
Sickle cell anemia.
Sjögren's syndrome.
Drugs, eg, lithium, fluoride, methoxyflurane anesthesia, demeclocycline (Declomycin).
Congenital defect.

of diseases (Table 6–4), circulating levels of vasopressin are normal or elevated, but the renal response is suppressed. These can result from a variety of forms of chronic renal disease, particularly those preferentially affecting the medulla and collecting duct system. Thus, if medullary disease (eg, from pyelonephritis) prevents formation of a medullary concentration gradient, urine passing through the collecting duct system cannot become concentrated.

Chronic potassium deficiency leading to hypokalemia is associated with reduction in urinary concentrating capacity. This is partly due to lack of medullary hypertonicity and may be exacerbated by increased medullary production of prostaglandins, thus inhibiting vasopressin action. The neuropathy associated with hypercalcemia generally affects the medullary portions of the kidney first, and this leads to lack of urinary concentration. Drugs such as lithium carbonate and demeclocycline greatly reduce the sensitivity of the renal tubule to vasopressin by virtue of their inhibitory effect on vasopressin-sensitive renal medullary adenylate cyclase. Congenital nephrogenic diabetes insipidus is a rare condition caused by a defect in the response of the renal tubule to vasopressin; it is apt to be associated with insensitivity of medullary adenylate cyclase to vasopressin. It is most common in males with a family history of transmission through apparently normal females, though cases have recently been reported in females.

Psychogenic Polydipsia

In psychogenic polydipsia, or **potomania,** there is a primary increase in drinking, usually in excess of 5 L of water per day, leading to dilution of the extracellular fluid, inhibition of vasopressin secretion, and water diuresis. This type of compulsive water drinking may be associated with a number of psychologic disturbances, and care must be taken to distinguish it from polydipsia due to tumors and other diseases affecting the hypothalamus and interfering with normal drinking pathways.

Differential Diagnosis

It is important to distinguish both types of diabetes insipidus and psychogenic polydipsia from other common causes of polyuria. In general, other forms of polyuria involve osmotic or solute diuresis. For ex-

Table 6–5. Results of diagnostic studies in various types of polyuria.

	Neurogenic Diabetes Insipidus	Nephrogenic Diabetes Insipidus	Psychogenic Polydipsia
Random plasma osmolality	↑	↑	↓
Random urine osmolality	↓	↓	↓
Urine osmolality during mild water deprivation	No change	No change	↑
Urine osmolality during nicotine or hypertonic saline	No change	No change	↑
Urine osmolality following vasopressin intravenously	↑	No change	↑
Plasma vasopressin	Low	Normal or high	Low

ample, in diabetes mellitus, increased excretion of glucose and other solutes requires excretion of increased volumes of water. In osmotic diuresis, the osmolality of the urine tends toward that of plasma. In sharp contrast, the osmolality of the urine in diabetes insipidus and psychogenic polydipsia is very low when compared with that of plasma. Thus, a urine specific gravity less than 1.005 (osmolality < 200 mosm/kg of water) will generally rule out polyuria due to osmotic diuresis. After a careful history has been taken in which special attention is paid to patterns of drinking and urination behavior and the family history, a series of investigations should be instituted to distinguish between the 2 types of diabetes insipidus and psychogenic polydipsia. The physiologic principles are set forth in Table 6–5, and the actual procedures are summarized in Table 6–6.

Table 6–6. Differential diagnosis of diabetes insipidus.

Procedure	Interpretation
Measure plasma and urine osmolality.	A urine osmolality less than that of plasma is consistent with neurogenic or nephrogenic diabetes insipidus; if both urine and plasma are dilute, that is consistent with psychogenic polydipsia.
Dehydration test: If serum osmolality is less than 295 mosm/kg, allow no fluids for 12–18 hours. Measure body weight, urine flow, urine specific gravity, urine and plasma osmolality every 2 hours. Terminate study if body weight falls more than 3%.	A rise in urine osmolality above that of plasma osmolality indicates psychogenic polydipsia. Urine specific gravity less than 1.005 (or 200 mosm/L) indicates either neurogenic or nephrogenic diabetes insipidus.
Measure serum vasopressin at conclusion of dehydration test.	Normal or high vasopressin level usually indicates nephrogenic diabetes insipidus.
Inject 5 units of aqueous vasopressin subcutaneously. Measure urine flow and urine and plasma osmolality.	Rise in urine osmolality above that of plasma osmolality indicates neurogenic diabetes insipidus; failure of urine osmolality to rise indicates nephrogenic diabetes insipidus.

A. Plasma and Urine Osmolality: The first test is to take plasma and urine samples simultaneously for estimation of osmolality. Since in both forms of diabetes insipidus the primary problem is inappropriate water diuresis, the urine will be less concentrated than plasma, whereas the plasma osmolality will be higher than normal. On the other hand, in psychogenic polydipsia, there will be a dilute plasma associated with the production of dilute urine.

B. Water Deprivation: The next step is to examine the effect of water deprivation on urine osmolality under supervision. Supervision is necessary both because the patient with psychogenic polydipsia will go to great lengths to obtain water and because the patient with complete diabetes insipidus may become dangerously dehydrated very rapidly. The patient should be weighed and denied access to water and each voided urine sample measured for specific gravity or osmolality (or both). Whereas the normal individual will soon reduce urine flow to 0.5 mL/min at a concentration greater than that of plasma, the patient with diabetes insipidus will maintain a high urine flow at a specific gravity less than 1.005 (200 mosm/kg of water). A period of 18 hours is usually ample to confirm the diagnosis. The test should be terminated if the body weight falls by more than 3%, since serious consequences of dehydration may ensue. Patients with psychogenic polydipsia will always increase urine osmolality to values greater than those of plasma.

C. Intravenous Hypertonic Saline and Nicotine: Two other tests to stimulate vasopressin secretion are now uncommonly used because they can be hazardous. Intravenous infusion of hypertonic saline should stimulate vasopressin secretion and thus make the diagnosis of psychogenic polydipsia by its effect on urinary concentration. This may be dangerous in patients with heart disease, and the increased solute load may increase urinary concentration. Injection of nicotine should also stimulate vasopressin release in such patients, but the test is associated with untoward effects on the circulation and on central nervous system functions.

D. Vasopressin Test: Once the diagnosis of diabetes insipidus is established, it is necessary to distinguish the vasopressin-insensitive (nephrogenic) disease from the vasopressin-sensitive (neurogenic) form. This is done by injection of aqueous vasopressin (Pitressin). Give 5 units subcutaneously and measure urine osmolality after 1 hour; patients with neurogenic diabetes insipidus will show an increase in urine osmolality to values above that of plasma. It should be remembered that such patients will not show a completely normal response to vasopressin following a single injection. In order to increase the sensitivity of this test, some clinicians prefer to inject vasopressin following the period of mild water deprivation. Under these circumstances, the patient with neurogenic diabetes insipidus will always show urinary concentration.

E. Vasopressin Radioimmunoassays: Sensitive radioimmunoassays for vasopressin are available that allow measurement of plasma vasopressin to be made either from random plasma samples, with infusions of hyperosmotic saline, or during the water deprivation test. Patients with nephrogenic diabetes insipidus secrete normal quantities of vasopressin following water deprivation, allowing a clear distinction to be made from neurogenic forms of diabetes insipidus (Fig 6–6). Patients with partial neurogenic diabetes insipidus show a smaller than normal increase in plasma vasopressin concentration following dehydration or infusion of hypertonic saline.

F. Influence of Endocrine Disease: The diagnosis of neurogenic diabetes insipidus is sometimes difficult to make in the presence of anterior pituitary disease. Low or absent levels of glucocorticoids or thyroid hormone reduce the solute load to the kidney and thus reduce urine flow. Patients with normal plasma levels of vasopressin but hyposecretion of adrenal glucocorticoids will retain a water load. Thus, even if diabetes insipidus is present, coincident thyroid or adrenal insufficiency may mask the polyuria. A history of a prior endocrine disorder should instigate appropriate diagnostic investigation.

Treatment
A. Neurogenic Diabetes Insipidus:
1. Treatment of choice–At present, the drug of choice is desmopressin acetate (DDAVP), a synthetic analog of vasopressin prepared in aqueous solution containing 0.1 mg/mL. It is administered intranasally via a calibrated plastic catheter in doses of 5–20 μg (0.05–0.2 mL) every 12 hours. This agent provides excellent control of polyuria and polydipsia in patients with pituitary diabetes insipidus. It is essential to monitor serum osmolality at regular intervals (initially every 1–2 weeks, later every 3 months) to be certain that the dose is appropriate.

2. Older methods of treatment–Older methods include the following:

Vasopressin in oil (Pitressin Tannate in oil), 5 units intramuscularly, is given every 2–3 days. This material is difficult to suspend, irregularly absorbed, and produces "peaks" and "valleys" in its effect.

Lypressin (Diapid) is a pure synthetic vasopressin administered by intranasal spray. It is effective for only a few hours, so that it must be administered at least every 4–6 hours.

Chlorpropamide (Diabinese) is an orally active hypoglycemic agent that can produce some urinary concentration. It appears to be effective in patients with some capacity to secrete vasopressin by increasing the sensitivity of the renal tubule to vasopressin. The usual dose is 250 mg once or twice daily. Patients receiving chlorpropamide therapy may be subject to severe hypoglycemic episodes, a serious side effect of this form of therapy.

Clofibrate (Atromid-S) may be useful in stimulating vasopressin secretion in some patients with partial deficiencies.

B. Nephrogenic Diabetes Insipidus: The underlying disorder should be treated if possible. It is important to recognize familial disease early, since infants are particularly susceptible to brain damage due to dehydration. Diuretics are helpful, along with dietary salt restriction if necessary. The objective is to maintain the patient in a state of mild sodium depletion and reduce the solute load on the kidney, thus enhancing proximal tubular reabsorption. Reduction in distal tubular flow allows some sodium concentration to take place and minimizes loss of water. Patients with partial sensitivity to vasopressin may be treated with large doses of desmopressin acetate (up to 40 μg/4 h intranasally).

Figure 6–6. Effect of dehydration on plasma vasopressin concentration in normal subjects and patients with polyuria. Note that patients with neurogenic (pituitary) diabetes insipidus cannot increase plasma vasopressin concentration with dehydration, in contrast to patients with psychogenic polydipsia and nephrogenic diabetes insipidus. (Reproduced, with permission, from Robertson GL et al: *J Clin Invest* 1973;52:2346.)

EXCESS VASOPRESSIN SECRETION

A number of diseases are associated with plasma vasopressin concentration that is inappropriately high for that plasma osmolality. Thus, with normal water intake, there is water retention, leading to hyponatremia and hypo-osmolality. The urine is usually more concentrated than plasma. Sodium balance is essentially normal. It is important to rule out renal and endocrine disorders and drug effects that diminish the kidney's capacity to dilute the urine. The syndrome is termed **syndrome of inappropriate secretion of vasopressin (antidiuretic hormone), or SIADH.** The clinical picture can be produced experimentally by giving high doses of vasopressin to a normal subject receiving normal to high fluid intake. Water restriction in patients suspected of having SIADH will result in a return of plasma osmolality and sodium concentration to normal.

Causes of SIADH

The causes of SIADH are outlined in Table 6–7. A number of malignant neoplasms are associated with ectopic production of vasopressin, leading to high plasma vasopressin levels. Bronchogenic carcinomas are particularly apt to be associated with SIADH. Tumors at other sites such as the pancreas and duodenum have also been shown to produce vasopressin. A number of nonmalignant pulmonary diseases such as tuberculosis are associated with high plasma vasopressin concentrations. Tuberculous lung tissue has been shown to contain assayable levels of vasopressin. However, it is not known whether all types of lung disease causing SIADH do so by producing ectopic vasopressin or by stimulation of pituitary vasopressin.

Many different types of central nervous system disorders are associated with increased vasopressin secretion, leading to the clinical picture of SIADH. Temporary causes of SIADH include surgical trauma, anesthesia, pain, and anxiety. A number of drugs implicated in vasopressin release are discussed in the section on diabetes insipidus. Endocrine disorders such as adrenal insufficiency, myxedema, and anterior pituitary insufficiency may be associated with SIADH secondary to hypovolemia and impaired renal excretion of free water. All of these factors—particularly

Table 6–7. Conditions associated with SIADH.

Malignant lung disease, particularly bronchogenic carcinoma.
Nonmalignant lung disease, eg, tuberculosis.
Tumors at other sites (especially lymphoma, sarcoma), eg, duodenum, pancreas, brain, prostate, thymus.
Central nervous system trauma and infections.
Drugs that stimulate vasopressin release, eg, clofibrate, chlorpropamide, and other drugs such as thiazides, carbamazepine, phenothiazines, vincristine, cyclophosphamide.
Endocrine diseases: adrenal insufficiency, myxedema, ataxia, pituitary insufficiency.

in combination with fluid loading—can lead to hyponatremia and hypo-osmolality.

Types of Osmoregulatory Defects

Serial measurements of serum arginine vasopressin in patients with SIADH were used by Robertson et al to describe 4 patterns of osmoregulatory defects in this syndrome. Type A, found in 20% of patients, is characterized by large irregular changes in plasma arginine vasopressin completely unrelated to serum osmolality. This erratic and irregular secretion of arginine vasopressin can be associated with both malignant and nonmalignant disease. Type B is found in about 35% of patients and is associated with excessive secretion of arginine vasopressin but proportionate to osmolality. In these patients, it appears as if the osmotic control of arginine vasopressin secretion is set at a low level or is abnormally sensitive to changes in serum osmolality. Type C, found in 35% of patients, is characterized by a high basal level of arginine vasopressin that rises even higher with a rise in serum osmolality. Type D, found in only 10% of patients, represents a different type of problem. Arginine vasopressin is normally suppressed in hypovolemic states and rises normally with increase in osmolality. Thus, SIADH in these patients may be associated with a change in renal sensitivity to serum arginine vasopressin. Thus far, it has not been possible to correlate the pattern of arginine vasopressin abnormality with the pathology of the syndrome.

Treatment

The treatment of SIADH depends upon the underlying cause. A patient with drug-induced SIADH is treated by withholding the drug. On the other hand, the prognosis of SIADH in a patient with bronchogenic carcinoma is poor. Treatment aims to return plasma osmolality to normal without causing further expansion of the extracellular fluid compartment, as would occur following infusion of hyperosmotic solutions.

A. Fluid Restriction: The simplest form of treatment is fluid restriction, although in the long term the excessive thirst associated with this treatment may be difficult to manage.

B. Diuretics: If plasma osmolality is low and rapid correction is required, diuretics such as furosemide or ethacrynic acid can be employed. These agents prevent a buildup of the concentration gradient in the medulla and thus decrease the effectiveness of vasopressin. Because diuresis is accompanied by significant urinary losses of potassium, calcium, and magnesium, these electrolytes should be returned to the patient by intravenous infusion.

C. Other Methods of Treatment: In an emergency situation with severe hyponatremia, hypertonic saline, ie, 5% saline, administered intravenously at a rate of 3 mL/kg/h, will increase plasma sodium and osmolarity. However, this must be done with great caution, since fluid overload may precipitate heart failure or circulatory collapse. Drugs (mentioned earlier in this chapter) that reduce the effect of vasopressin on the kidney may be useful. Demeclocycline (Declomycin), 1–2 g/d orally, causes a reversible form of diabetes insipidus, countering the effect of SIADH. However, it is nephrotoxic, and renal function (blood urea nitrogen and creatinine) must be monitored carefully. Lithium carbonate has a similar effect, but therapeutic doses are so close to the toxic dose that this drug is rarely useful.

VASOPRESSIN ANTAGONISTS

Improved understanding of structure-activity relationships has made it possible to synthesize agonists and antagonists of neurohypophyseal peptides. Two groups of peptides have been synthesized that antagonize the pressor and antidiuretic actions of arginine vasopressin. The V1 receptors are responsible for the pressor activity of vasopressin and the V2 receptors for the antidiuretic activity. Further refinement of specific antagonists for specific receptors should lead to the development of powerful therapeutic tools.

OXYTOCIN

Oxytocin has a profound effect on uterine smooth muscle. It increases both the frequency and the duration of action potentials during each burst of firing. Thus, administration of oxytocin may initiate contractions in a quiescent uterus or increase the strength and frequency of muscle contractions in an active uterus. The presence of estrogen enhances the action of oxytocin on uterine smooth muscle. Estrogen acts by reducing the membrane potential of smooth muscle cells, thus lowering the threshold of excitation. Toward the end of pregnancy, as estrogen levels become higher, the membrane potential of uterine smooth muscle cells thus becomes less negative, rendering the uterus at full term more sensitive to oxytocin.

There is also an increase in oxytocin receptors in the uterus at this time.

Parturition

Oxytocin is involved in the process of parturition. As the fetus enters the birth canal, the lower segment of the uterus and cervix and then the vagina are dilated. Dilatation of these regions causes reflex release of oxytocin into the bloodstream. Strong uterine contractions are initiated, causing further descent of the fetus, further distention, and further release of oxytocin. However, the precise role of oxytocin in the initiation of labor in humans is still not clear. Patients with diabetes insipidus caused by hypothalamic tumors—and thus a presumed absence of oxytocin secretion—may have normal deliveries, or there may be an increased incidence of forceps deliveries and cesarean sections. The complex neuroendocrine relationships involved in parturition are not yet fully understood.

Lactation

Oxytocin is also involved in lactation. Stimulation of the nipple area gives rise to a neurohumoral reflex involving the secretion of oxytocin. Oxytocin causes contraction of the myoepithelial cells lining the mammary ducts and the ejection of milk contained within them. The milk ejection reflex is essential if the infant is to obtain adequate quantities of milk. The milk ejection reflex may also be conditioned by events related to the infant, such as crying or arrival of the scheduled feeding time. Stress has a potent inhibitory influence on the milk ejection reflex, an event that depends upon central inhibition of oxytocin release in the hypothalamus.

Other Actions

A number of stimuli that also release vasopressin—such as increased plasma osmolality and hypovolemia—cause oxytocin secretion. Since oxytocin is an effective natriuretic agent, particularly at low rates of urine flow, it is possible that it is involved in the regulation of sodium balance. This proposed role for oxytocin remains to be elucidated.

REFERENCES

Bartter FC, Schwartz WB: The syndrome of inappropriate secretion of antidiuretic hormone. *Am J Med* 1967;**42**:790.

Bie P: Osmoreceptors, vasopressin, and control of renal water excretion. *Physiol Rev* 1980;**60**:961.

Cross BA, Leng G (editors): The neurohypophysis: Structure, function and control. *Prog Brain Res* 1983;**60**:1. [Entire issue.]

Krieger DT, Hughes JC: Section III, pp 123–158, in: *Neuroendocrinology*. Sinauer Associates, 1980.

Land H et al: Deduced amino-acid sequence from the bovine oxytocin–neurophysin I precursor cDNA. *Nature* 1983; **302**:342.

Land H et al: Nucleotide sequence of cloned cDNA encoding bovine arginine vasopressin–neurophysin II precursor. *Nature* 1982;**295**:299.

Lauson HD: Metabolism of the neurohypophysial hormones. Section 7 in: *Handbook of Physiology*. Vol 4. American Physiological Society, 1974.

Miller M et al: Recognition of partial defects in antidiuretic hormone secretion. *Ann Intern Med* 1970;**73**:721.

Moses AM, Scheinman SJ, Oppenheim A: Marked hypotonic polyuria resulting from nephrogenic diabetes insipidus with partial sensitivity to vasopressin. *J Clin Endocrinol Metab* 1984;**59**:1044.

Robertson GL, Athar S, Shelton RL: Osmotic control of vasopressin function. In: *Disturbances in Body Fluid Osmolality*. Andreoli TE, Grantham JJ, Rector FC Jr (editors). American Physiological Society, 1977.

Robertson GL, Berl T: Pathophysiology of water metabolism. In: *The Kidney*. Brenner BM, Rector FC Jr (editors). Saunders, 1986.

Robinson AG: DDAVP in the treatment of central diabetes insipidus. *N Engl J Med* 1976;**294:**507.

Russell JT, Brownstein MJ, Gainer H: Biosynthesis of vasopressin, oxytocin, and neurophysins: Isolation and characterization of two common precursors (propressophysin and prooxyphysin). *Endocrinology* 1980;**107:**1880.

Schrier RW, Berl T, Anderson RJ: Osmotic and non-osmotic control of vasopressin release. *Am J Physiol* 1979;**236:**321.

Swanson LW, Sawchenko PE: Hypothalamic integration: Organization of the paraventricular and supraoptic nuclei. *Annu Rev Neurosci* 1983;**6:**269.

Thrasher TN, Keil LC, Ramsay DJ: Lesions of the organum vasculosum of the lamina terminalis (OVLT) attenuate osmotically-induced drinking and vasopressin secretion in the dog. *Endocrinology* 1982;**110:**1837.

Thrasher TN et al: Satiety and inhibition of vasopressin secretion in dehydrated dogs. *Am J Physiol* 1981;**240:**394.

Thrasher TN et al: Thirst and vasopressin release in the dog: An osmoreceptor or sodium receptor mechanism? *Am J Physiol* 1980;**238:**333.

Verney EB: The antidiuretic hormone and the factors which determine its release. *Proc R Soc Lond* 1947;**135:**25.

Weitzman R, Kleeman CR: Water metabolism and the neurohypophysial hormones. In: *Clinical Disorders of Fluid and Electrolyte Metabolism*. Maxwell MH, Kleeman CR (editors). McGraw-Hill, 1980.

Yoshida S, Share L, Yagi K (editors): *Antidiuretic Hormone*. Japan Scientific Societies Press, 1980.

Zerbe RL, Robertson GL: A comparison of plasma vasopressin measurements with a standard indirect test in the differential diagnosis of polyuria. *N Engl J Med* 1981;**305:**1539

Thyroid Gland 7

Francis S. Greenspan, MD, & Basil Rapoport, MB, ChB

PHYSIOLOGY OF THE THYROID GLAND

Thyroid hormones (thyroxine, T_4; triiodothyronine, T_3) (Fig 7–1) play a vital role in fetal development, and throughout life they influence metabolic processes in almost all tissues. The thyroid gland is the only significant source of T_4. While the gland does produce some T_3, which is biologically more active than T_4, most T_3 in humans is produced extrathyroidally from T_4.

The thyroid gland is unique among the endocrine organs in 2 important ways: (1) It maintains a large store of hormone, and (2) it requires iodide for hormone synthesis.

ANATOMY OF THE THYROID

Gross Anatomy

The thyroid consists of a left and right lobe connected (in humans) by an isthmus at the approximate level of the cricoid cartilage (Fig 7–2). The adult thyroid weighs 15–20 g, and assessment of its size

3,5,3',5'-Tetraiodothyronine (thyroxine, T_4)

3,5,3'-Triiodothyronine (T_3)

Figure 7–1. Chemical structures of thyroxine (T_4) and triiodothyronine (T_3).

is important in clinical evaluation of thyroid function. The thyroid is derived from the embryonic thyroglossal duct, which is a midline invagination at the junction of the anterior two-thirds and posterior one-third of the tongue. A remnant of the thyroglossal duct may be observed as a pyramidal thyroid lobe, inserting into the isthmus or into the medial aspect of one of the lobes.

In palpating the thyroid gland, it is important to note the following: (1) The thyroid lobes are largely covered by the sternohyoid and sternothyroid muscles. Enlargement of the thyroid is limited superiorly by the sternothyroid attachment to the thyroid cartilage, but the thyroid gland, when enlarged, can extend superolaterally beneath the sternocleidomastoid. (2) The

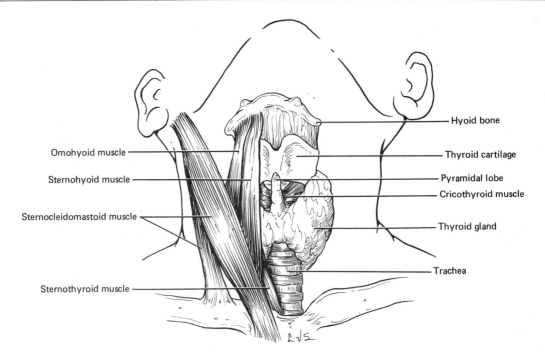

Figure 7–2. Gross anatomy of the human thyroid (anterior view).

thyroid moves upward with the larynx on swallowing. (3) The cricoid cartilage is a landmark for the isthmus. (4) Pyramidal lobe enlargement is a good indication of diffuse rather than local abnormality of the thyroid.

Histology

The basic functional unit of the thyroid is the follicle, a hollow sphere of cells, 15–500 μm in diameter, surrounded by a basement membrane. The wall of the follicle is a single layer of thyroid cells. A few adjacent parafollicular cells (C cells) are larger, clearer on staining, and secrete calcitonin (Fig 7–3A). The follicular cells are cuboidal when quiescent and columnar when active (Figs 7–3B and 7–3C). The

Figure 7–3. *A:* Normal rat thyroid. A single layer of cuboidal epithelial cells surrounds PAS-positive material in the follicular space (colloid). The larger, lighter-staining cells indicated by the arrows (l) are C cells that produce calcitonin. F = follicular cells. *B:* Inactive rat thyroid several weeks after hypophysectomy. The follicular lumens are larger and the follicular cells flatter. *C:* Rat thyroid under intensive TSH stimulation. The animal was fed an iodine-deficient diet and injected with propylthiouracil for several weeks. Little colloid is visible. The follicular cells are tall and columnar. Several mitoses (m) are visible. (Reproduced, with permission, from Halmi NS in: *Histology.* Greep RO, Weiss L [editors]. McGraw-Hill, 1973.)

follicular lumen contains colloid, a viscous gel that is primarily a store of thyroglobulin secreted by the thyroid cells. This store is sufficient for about 100 days of normal thyroid hormone secretion. The follicles are surrounded by a rich capillary network. Blood flow through the thyroid is very high (about 5 mL/g/min) and may be audible with a stethoscope (bruit) when the thyroid is overactive and flow is increased. Networks of sympathetic and parasympathetic nerves also surround the follicles. Their significance is unclear, however, and they do not appear to play a major role in the regulation of thyroid hormone synthesis and secretion.

IODIDE METABOLISM

Adequate ingestion of iodide is a prerequisite for the normal synthesis of thyroid hormones by the thyroid. While the dietary intake of iodide may vary widely, thyroidal secretion of iodine in the form of thyroid hormones is relatively stable. The homeostatic mechanisms at play will be discussed below. The major sources of dietary iodide are water, iodated bread, iodinated salt, and, increasingly, medications, disinfectants, and x-ray contrast material. In addition, kelp, available in health food stores, is being ingested with increasing frequency in the USA.

A typical daily dietary intake of iodide in the USA is now about 500 μg. Iodide is almost completely absorbed in the gastrointestinal tract, where it enters the inorganic iodide pool in the extracellular fluid (Fig 7–4). In the presence of normal renal function, inorganic iodide in the extracellular fluid is rapidly cleared, with a half-life of about 2 hours. Besides dietary iodide, there are 2 other smaller sources contributing to the extracellular fluid iodide pool: (1) iodide released by the deiodination of thyroid hormones in the peripheral tissues (about 60 μg/d) and (2) the release ("leak") of inorganic iodide by the thyroid (about 10–50 μg/d).

The only 2 significant pathways of iodide clearance from the extracellular fluid are the kidneys and the thyroid. Since the thyroid is able to regulate the net amount of iodide it clears from the extracellular fluid (see below), taking up only as much as is needed (about 75 μg/d) for thyroid hormone synthesis, it follows that when the dietary intake of iodide increases, the fractional uptake of extracellular fluid iodide by the thyroid decreases and the proportionate urinary excretion of iodide increases. Conversely, when iodide intake is reduced, the proportionate uptake of extracellular fluid iodide by the thyroid is increased. This is clinically important, because the percentage uptake of radioactive iodide by the thyroid is a useful index of thyroid function (Fig 7–5). In the

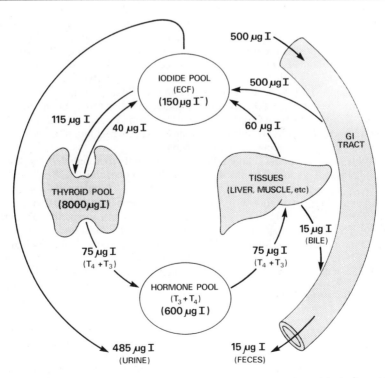

Figure 7–4. Iodine metabolism. The values indicated are representative of those that might be found in a healthy subject ingesting 500 μg of iodine a day. The actual iodine intake varies considerably among different individuals.

Figure 7–5. Typical radioactive iodine uptake (RAIU) curves over 48 hours in patients with normal and abnormal thyroid function. (Reproduced, with permission, from DeGroot LJ, Stanbury JB: *The Thyroid and Its Diseases.* Wiley, 1975.)

USA, particularly since the iodation of bread, the radioactive iodide uptake (RAIU) by the thyroid gland in normal subjects has decreased from about 20–50% of the ingested dose at 24 hours to about 10–25%. RAIU is generally higher in hyperthyroidism and lower in hypothyroidism, although there are exceptions. Measurement of urinary iodide excretion may be useful clinically if it is suspected that the patient has ingested excess iodide.

The largest iodine pool in the body is the slowly turning over thyroid pool (approximately 1% per day; faster in hyperthyroidism). This pool is almost entirely organic iodine in the form of iodinated thyroglobulin stored as colloid within the thyroid follicular lumen.

The thyroid secretes about 75 μg of organic iodine per day in the form of thyroid hormones (chiefly T_4, with a small amount of T_3). Secreted thyroid hormones enter a pool of thyroid hormones, mainly intravascular, bound to thyroid hormone–binding proteins. The iodine content of this hormonal pool is about 600 μg. Cellular uptake of thyroid hormones from this pool is approximately 75 μg of iodine per day in the euthyroid individual. Of this 75 μg of thyroid hormone iodine, about 60 μg reenters the extracellular fluid iodide pool following intracellular enzymatic deiodination of the thyroid hormones. The remainder (15 μg) is conjugated in the liver to the glucuronide and sulfate forms and excreted in the bile and subsequently in the stool. In humans, there is very little enterohepatic recirculation of thyroid hormone.

THYROID HORMONE SYNTHESIS

Thyroglobulin

Thyroglobulin, the precursor of all thyroid hormones, is a very large glycoprotein molecule that is the major protein in the follicular luminal colloid. About 75% of the weight of the entire thyroid gland consists of this protein, though the proportion varies widely depending on the physiologic demands on the gland (Figs 7–3B and 7–3C).

Thyroglobulin is a heterogeneous substance that exists in multiple forms. The most prevalent form and the major precursor for thyroid hormones is a 19S molecule with a molecular weight of 660,000. Ultracentrifugation of thyroglobulin also reveals a small fraction with a sedimentation coefficient of 27S, believed to be a dimer of 19S thyroglobulin. The 19S molecule can in turn dissociate into two 12S components, particularly when the thyroglobulin is poorly iodinated. Studies of the translation of thyroglobulin messenger RNA (mRNA) and the sequencing of this mRNA from a complementary DNA (cDNA) library show that thyroglobulin is synthesized as the 12S subunit.

Human thyroglobulin contains approximately 110 tyrosine residues. It is these residues that are iodinated and ultimately form the thyroid hormones. The relative number of tyrosines in thyroglobulin is not higher than in many other proteins. The propensity of thyroglobulin for iodination is determined instead by its proximity to a very efficient iodination mechanism in the thyroid cell as well as by its tertiary structure, which facilitates iodination. Only a small proportion of the tyrosine residues in thyroglobulin—those that are closest to the surface of the globular molecule—are available for iodination. In geographic areas of iodine sufficiency, a thyroglobulin molecule will contain an average of about 7 molecules of monoiodotyrosine (MIT) and 5 of diiodotyrosine (DIT). In addition, an average of 2 molecules of T_4 will be present, each representing the coupling of 2 molecules of DIT. On average, every third molecule of thyroglobulin will contain one molecule of T_3, formed by the coupling of one DIT with one MIT.

The degree of thyroglobulin iodination varies depending upon the availability of iodide and the efficiency of the iodinating mechanism (see below). Poorly iodinated thyroglobulin contains a relatively high MIT/DIT ratio, which in turn favors increased T_3 synthesis relative to T_4. This is presumably of adaptive significance in that during periods of iodide insufficiency, available iodide is utilized more efficiently by synthesizing a more active hormone. In addition, there is evidence that decreased thyroglobulin iodine content produces a more loosely folded molecule that is more susceptible to proteolysis within the thyroid and will therefore also lead to greater efficiency in the generation of biologically active thyroid hormones.

The mechanism of synthesis of thyroglobulin (Fig 7–6) is the same as that of other glycoproteins. After transcription and processing of thyroglobulin mRNA has taken place, the mRNA is translated by ribosomes in the rough endoplasmic reticulum. The thyroglobulin polypeptide chain is extruded into the lumen of the endoplasmic reticulum. During transport to the Golgi apparatus, thyroglobulin is progressively glycosylated. The molecules are packaged into exocytotic vesicles in the Golgi apparatus. These vesicles fuse with the plasma membrane at the apical border of the follicular cell and release their contents into the follicular lumen. The membrane incorporated into the plasma membrane by this process is believed to recycle by the formation of endocytotic vesicles during the process of hormone secretion (see below).

Figure 7–7. Evidence that iodination of thyroglobulin occurs at or near the apical (follicular) border of the thyroid cell. The figure depicts electron-microscopic autoradiography of part of a rat thyroid cell 30–40 seconds after the administration of sodium ^{125}I to the animal in vivo. The radioactive iodine is represented on a photographic emulsion layer by the silver grains. Few radioactive iodine molecules are localized over the thyroid cell itself, but there are many at the junction of the thyroid cell and the follicular colloid. (× 7000.) (Reproduced, with permission, from Ekholm R: *Endocrinology*. DeGroot LJ et al [editors]. Grune & Stratton, 1979.)

The exact site of thyroglobulin iodination is not established with certainty, but evidence suggests that iodination occurs at the apical (follicular) surface of the thyroid cell. This is based on the autoradiographic localization of radioiodinated thyroglobulin a few seconds after exposure of the thyroid to radioactive iodine (Fig 7–7). In addition, the enzyme necessary for thyroglobulin iodination can be demonstrated at the site by histochemical means.

The process of thyroglobulin biosynthesis and exocytosis into the follicular lumen is believed to be under the dominant control of TSH. Evidence suggests that TSH stimulates both the transcriptional and translational processes, resulting in thyroglobulin synthesis. TSH also rapidly stimulates the exocytosis (extrusion into the follicular lumen) of preformed thyroglobulin.

Thyroglobulin is not the only protein that may be iodinated within the thyroid gland, and other proteins such as albumin may occasionally be iodinated. This, however, occurs to a significant degree only in the abnormal thyroid gland. Because other molecules lack the unique tertiary structure of thyroglobulin necessary for the efficient coupling of iodotyrosines, their iodination does not lead to adequate biologically active thyroid hormone synthesis. Excess iodoalbumin production may be detected by a disproportionately high organic iodine concentration in serum relative to the amount of thyroid hormone present.

Iodide Transport

Iodide is actively transported (''trapped'') from the extracellular fluid into the thyroid follicular cell (Fig 7–8). Once within the cell, inorganic iodide may either be incorporated into protein (''organified'') or diffuse back into the extracellular fluid. At equilib-

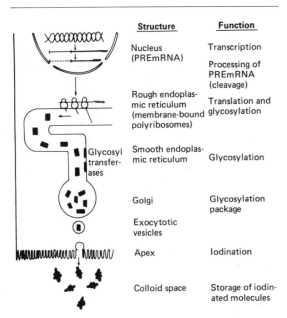

Structure	Function
Nucleus (PREmRNA)	Transcription
	Processing of PREmRNA (cleavage)
Rough endoplasmic reticulum (membrane-bound polyribosomes)	Translation and glycosylation
Smooth endoplasmic reticulum	Glycosylation
Golgi	Glycosylation package
Exocytotic vesicles	
Apex	Iodination
Colloid space	Storage of iodinated molecules

Glycosyl transferases

Figure 7–6. Synthesis of thyroglobulin. See text for details. (Reproduced, with permission, from Dumont J, Vassart G: *Endocrinology*. DeGroot LJ et al [editors]. Grune & Stratton, 1979.)

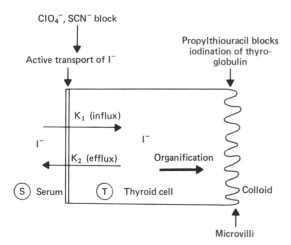

Figure 7–8. The iodide transport mechanism in the thyroid cell. K_1 is the rate constant for iodide being transported from the serum into the thyroid cell and K_2 the diffusion of inorganic iodide from the thyroid cell back into the serum. The iodide transport mechanism involves only inorganic iodide (I^-). SCN^- = thiocyanate; ClO_4^- = perchlorate.

rium, the inorganic iodide concentration ratio between the thyroid cell and the serum (T:S iodide gradient) represents the balance between iodide influx and efflux. It is important to realize that organic iodine, such as iodinated thyroglobulin, does not contribute to this iodide gradient. In the normal thyroid gland, inorganic iodide is organified almost immediately upon entering the cell, so that a high T:S inorganic iodide gradient is not detectable. However, if iodide organification is blocked (see below), a T:S iodide ratio as high as 500:1 has been observed in the mouse thyroid in vitro.

Other structurally related anions such as SCN^-, BF_4^-, NO_3^-, and ClO_4^- competitively inhibit iodide transport. The latter (perchlorate) is used clinically on occasion to evaluate the iodide organification mechanism (Fig 7–9). If the thyroidal iodide organification mechanism is inefficient, inorganic iodide transported into the cell will accumulate. Perchlorate given a few hours after administration of a tracer amount of radioiodide blocks further iodide influx, but passive diffusion of inorganic iodide from the cell back into the extracellular fluid continues. Patients with faulty organification mechanisms have an abnormal "discharge" of radioactivity from the thyroid as it is released back into the extracellular fluid. This is detected by a decrease in radioactivity in the neck. The normal thyroid discharges little of the administered radioiodide with ClO_4^-, because it is readily organified and no longer able to leak out into the serum.

Tissues other than the thyroid also have an active transport mechanism for iodide. These include gastric mucosa, salivary glands, and the choroid plexus. However, unlike the thyroid, these tissues have a

minimal capacity for iodide organification and storage of organic iodine. The active process of I^- concentration against an electrochemical gradient is energy-dependent, requiring oxidative metabolism. Because cardiac glycosides inhibit thyroidal I^- transport, there is much interest in the possible role of Na^+-K^+ ATPase activity in the iodide transport mechanism. Sodium increases I^- influx and inhibits I^- efflux. However, the exact relationship between this enzyme, sodium transport, and the iodide transport mechanism is presently unclear.

Iodide Organification
(Fig 7–10)

Once within the thyroid cell, inorganic iodide is rapidly oxidized by thyroid peroxidase in the presence of H_2O_2 into a reactive intermediate that is then incorporated into the tyrosine residues of acceptor proteins, mainly thyroglobulin. Thyroid peroxidase is a membrane-bound hemoprotein that is relatively unstable and therefore difficult to purify. The exact nature of the reactive oxidized iodide intermediate that binds to acceptor proteins is unknown. Although I_2 (iodine) has been considered, more acceptable alternatives include a sulfenyl iodide or possibly the $I°$ free radical.

The exact mechanism of thyroid H_2O_2 generation is also unknown, but it is probably dependent on

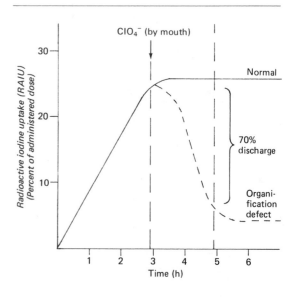

Figure 7–9. Perchlorate discharge of thyroidal inorganic iodine. Two to 3 hours after administration of a tracer dose of radioactive iodide, perchlorate is administered orally, blocking further active transport of iodide into the thyroid cell. In the normal subject (solid line), no significant decrease in radioactivity is detectable over the thyroid gland. In the representative example shown by the dashed line, there is a significant discharge of thyroidal iodide, indicating that iodide organification has been incomplete. ClO_4^- = perchlorate.

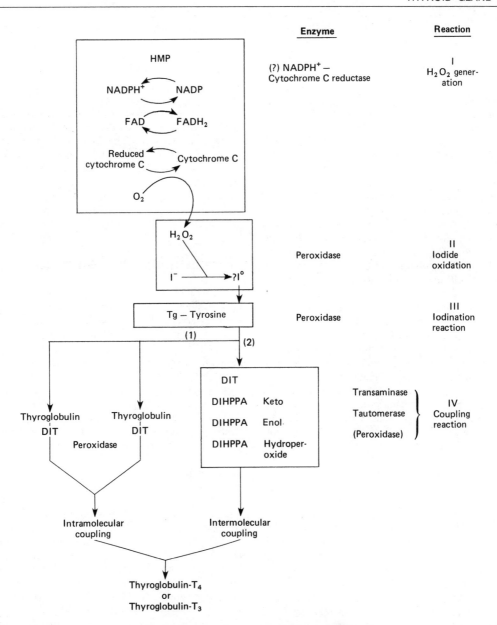

Figure 7–10. Present concepts of thyroglobulin iodination. See text for details. HMP, hexose monophosphate pathway; NADP, nicotinamide adenine dinucleotide phosphate; NADPH$^+$, reduced form of NADP; FAD, flavin adenine dinucleotide; FADH$_2$, reduced form of FAD; I$^-$, iodide; I$^\circ$, iodine free radical; Tg, thyroglobulin; DIT, diiodotyrosine; DIHPPA, diiodo-hydroxyphenylpyruvic acid. (Slightly modified and reproduced, with permission, from Rapoport B, DeGroot LJ: *Semin Nucl Med* 1971;**1**:265.)

reduced pyridine nucleotide oxidation. NADPH–cytochrome C reductase is believed to be involved in thyroidal H$_2$O$_2$ production in that a specific antibody against this enzyme is able to inhibit thyroglobulin iodination in vitro by a thyroid particulate (microsomal) preparation.

As mentioned previously, the site of thyroglobulin iodination is most likely to be apical plasma membrane. This is based on electron-microscopic auto-

radiography of sections of thyroid performed within seconds after the administration of radioactive iodide. That this process occurs at the interface between the thyroid cell and the colloid is consistent with the fact that thyroid peroxidase is membrane-bound and with the direct localization of enzyme activity in apical membrane. Still being investigated, however, are the role of the thyroid peroxidase–like material that is demonstrable histochemically within the interior of the thyroid cell (such as in the Golgi apparatus) and the possible role in iodide organification of multiple pools of intracellular iodide differing in their rates of turnover.

Iodotyrosine Coupling

Iodinated tyrosine residues in thyroglobulin combine to form iodothyronines. Thus, DIT couples with DIT to form thyroxine and MIT with DIT to form triiodothyronine. The exact mechanism by which this coupling reaction occurs is unknown. Two theories currently exist (Fig 7–10): intramolecular coupling and intermolecular coupling. In the former, 2 peptide-linked DIT molecules couple while still part of the thyroglobulin polypeptide chain—a process that may involve generation of free radicals of DIT. In intermolecular coupling, there is evidence that DIT is liberated from thyroglobulin and in turn converted into its pyruvic acid analog diiodohydroxyphenylpyruvic acid (DIHPPA) by tyrosine transaminase. After conversion to its enol form and subsequent oxidation by H_2O_2 and thyroid peroxidase to the DIHPPA hydroperoxide, this intermediate then couples with DIT present within the thyroglobulin molecule to form thyroxine. While this issue remains unsettled, it is clear that thyroid peroxidase plays an important role in the coupling process as well as in initial iodotyrosine formation. Thyroid peroxidase therefore catalyzes all steps in the synthesis of iodothyronines. DIT may itself have a stimulatory effect on iodotyrosine coupling, but the mechanism by which this occurs is poorly understood.

A defect in the coupling mechanism results in diminished T_4 and T_3 formation from DIT and MIT. This may be related to inadequate concentrations of precursor iodotyrosines or to a defect in the enzymes responsible for coupling. As an example of the first possibility, in iodine deficiency, poorly iodinated thyroglobulin contains fewer iodotyrosine molecules overall and more MIT relative to DIT. There may therefore be insufficient DIT residues to permit adequate T_4 formation. As a corollary, there is a proportionate increase in T_3 production relative to T_4. This may represent an adaptive mechanism to environmental iodine deficiency in that T_3 is biologically more potent than T_4. While thyroid peroxidase is important in the coupling mechanism, it is not clearly established whether a deficiency in this enzyme or

some abnormality in its action is responsible for the apparent coupling defect very rarely observed in the human thyroid. The difficulty in determining this is that decreased thyroid peroxidase activity also leads to decreased thyroglobulin iodination, with less MIT and DIT available for coupling.

A number of related drugs are used clinically to treat hyperthyroidism by decreasing thyroid hormone synthesis (Fig 7–11). The thionamide drugs, including methimazole and propylthiouracil, inhibit thyroid peroxidase–catalyzed iodination of thyroglobulin. These drugs may also specifically inhibit the iodotyrosine coupling reaction independently of inhibition of iodotyrosine generation. Propylthiouracil, unlike methimazole, inhibits iodotyrosine coupling in vitro.

THYROID HORMONE SECRETION

Thyroglobulin is stored extracellularly in the follicular lumen. Therefore, as a prerequisite for thyroid hormone secretion into the blood, thyroglobulin must first reenter the thyroid cell and undergo proteolysis. A small quantity of intact thyroglobulin enters the circulation, some by way of the lymphatics.

Autoradiographic studies show that newly iodinated thyroglobulin is stored adjacent to the epithelial border. Continuing synthesis may produce concentric lamellae of colloid with older thyroglobulin in the center. It follows, therefore, that the most recently iodinated thyroglobulin may be the first to be secreted. This has been called the "last come, first served" principle. Not all follicles in the thyroid are of the same size, and their thyroglobulin turnover rates vary considerably. The smaller follicles turn over their contents at a faster rate. Processing of thyroglobulin by the thyroid cell and secretion of the thyroid hormones into the circulation occur in the following sequence (Fig 7–12): (1) Pseudopods from the apical cell surface extend into the colloid in the follicular lumen, and large colloid droplets enter the cytoplasm by endocytosis. Each colloid droplet is enclosed in membrane derived from the apical cell border. Endocytosis of the colloid is dependent on the addition of membrane to the apical surface of the cell that occurs during exocytosis of thyroglobulin—ie, there is membrane recycling. (2) Electron-dense lysosomes migrate apically, meet the incoming colloid droplets, and fuse

Thiouracil   Propylthiouracil   Methimazole

Figure 7–11. Thiocarbamide inhibitors of thyroidal iodide organification.

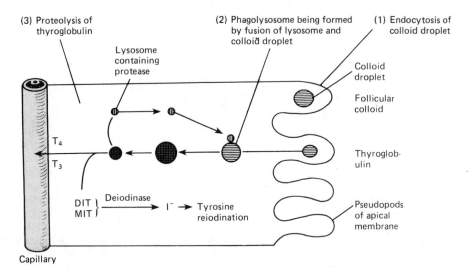

Figure 7–12. Schematic representation of thyroid hormone secretion. See text for details. (Slightly modified and reproduced, with permission, from Rapoport B, DeGroot LJ: *Semin Nucl Med* 1971;1:265.)

with them to produce phagolysosomes. The phagolysosomes continue their migration toward the basal aspect of the cell, during which time they become smaller and more dense as the lysosomal proteases hydrolyze the thyroglobulin. (3) T_4 and, to a much lesser degree, T_3, liberated from thyroglobulin by the proteolytic process, pass from the phagolysosome into the blood by a mechanism that is presently unknown, possibly diffusion. Most of the liberated iodotyrosines (MIT and DIT) are deiodinated by iodotyrosine deiodinase, releasing free iodide. This iodide is partly reutilized for thyroglobulin iodination, but some diffuses out into the circulation (iodide leak).

There is evidence that microtubules and microfilaments play an important role in these steps, presumably by regulating organelle movement. Thus, colchicine and cytochalasin B, which disrupt microtubular and microfilament function, respectively, inhibit thyroid hormone secretion.

Pharmacologic doses of iodide acutely reduce thyroid hormone secretion by an unknown mechanism, possibly by inhibiting thyroid cAMP generation. This slight effect on hormone secretion is clinically insignificant in the normal thyroid. In the hyperfunctioning thyroid, however, iodide has a marked inhibitory effect on hormone secretion that is clinically useful. Continued iodide administration usually inhibits thyroid hormone secretion for only a few weeks. The reason for the escape from this inhibitory effect is not known (and must not be confused with escape from the Wolff-Chaikoff block, discussed below). Lithium acts in a manner similar to iodide, but lithium is rarely used clinically, because it is more toxic.

In addition to the iodotyrosines, which are rapidly deiodinated by NADPH-dependent flavoprotein deiodinase within the thyroid, some T_4 released from

thyroglobulin may also undergo intrathyroidal monodeiodination to T_3. The quantitative significance of this source of T_3 is uncertain. In the normally functioning thyroid gland, however, the secretion of T_3 (whether synthesized de novo or derived from T_4) is relatively small (see below). The deiodination of iodotyrosines and the reutilization of this iodide are very important in the efficient utilization of iodide by the thyroid. This is because perhaps 80% of the iodide in thyroglobulin is in the form of iodotyrosines, which, once secreted into the blood, are rapidly lost in the urine. There is evidence that intrathyroidal iodide released from iodotyrosines exists in a pool separate from iodide entering the thyroid cell directly from the extracellular fluid.

REGULATION OF THYROID FUNCTION

Thyroid hormone synthesis and secretion are regulated by extrathyroidal (thyrotropin) and intrathyroidal (autoregulatory) mechanisms. Although thyrotropin (TSH) is the major modulator of thyroid activity, the importance of autoregulation is receiving increasing recognition.

TSH

TSH is a glycoprotein (MW 28,000; 15% carbohydrate) secreted by specialized cells (thyrotrophs) in the anterior pituitary. TSH consists of 2 polypeptide chains. The alpha chain is nearly identical to the alpha chains of LH, FSH, and chorionic gonadotropin (hCG). TSH specificity is determined by the uniquely different beta chain, which is critical for recognition of the TSH receptor. TSH biologic activity is present only when the 2 chains are combined. The half-life of TSH in plasma is very short (about an hour).

TSH secretion by the pituitary is modulated by thyroid hormone in a negative feedback regulatory mechanism (Fig 7–13). Recent evidence suggests that at the level of the pituitary, it is primarily T_3, produced locally by the monodeiodination of T_4, that inhibits TSH secretion. This is therefore the only site at which the monodeiodination of T_4 to T_3 has been shown to be a prerequisite for the expression of T_4 metabolic activity. In hypothyroidism, there is decreased suppression of TSH secretion, and serum TSH levels are higher than normal. The measurement by radioimmunoassay of high TSH levels in serum is very important clinically in the diagnosis of primary thyroid failure. A direct action of thyroid hormones on the hypothalamus has not been demonstrated.

The "thermostat" setting of the thyroid hormone–TSH feedback loop is modulated by a tripeptide, TSH-releasing hormone (TRH) (Fig 7–14). This factor is present throughout the brain and indeed in

(pyro)Glu-His-Pro-(NH₂)

Figure 7–14. Chemical structure of thyrotropin-releasing hormone (TRH).

other organs, but it is present at highest concentration in the hypothalamus. Hypothalamic production and release of TRH are controlled by poorly understood neural pathways from higher brain centers. TRH reaches the anterior pituitary from the hypothalamus via the hypothalamic-hypophyseal portal system. After binding to specific receptors on the thyrotroph, TRH increases TSH synthesis and secretion. While cAMP can stimulate TSH secretion by the thyrotroph, there is evidence that this agent may not mediate TRH-stimulated TSH release. The present concept is that TRH provides a tonic influence on the negative feedback of thyroid hormone on TSH secretion—ie, TRH is believed to regulate the sensitivity, or the set point, of the thyroid hormone–TSH negative feedback loop. Thyroid hormones, in turn, modulate anterior pituitary responsiveness to TRH by altering the number of TRH receptors on the thyrotrophs. Thus, in animals, administration of thyroid hormones decreases the number of TRH receptors, and in hypothyroidism the number of TRH receptors is increased.

Studies on the role of TRH in the regulation of TSH secretion in humans in vivo have been difficult because physiologically effective concentrations are attained only in the hypothalamic-hypophyseal portal system, and TRH reaching the systemic circulation, where it can be sampled and assayed, is greatly diluted and rapidly cleared with a half-life of a few minutes. In addition, TRH in the systemic circulation is derived from numerous tissues and presumably is represented only to a small degree by the TRH that reaches the systemic circulation after perfusing the pituitary. Because TRH is distributed throughout the central nervous system and because some studies have demonstrated an association between TRH and mood elevation, it is reasonable to speculate that this tripeptide may function as a neurotransmitter in addition to being a tonic regulator of TSH secretion.

Although it is not believed that acute pulses of TRH reach the pituitary and stimulate TSH secretion in vivo, the acute injection of a bolus of synthetic TRH (200–500 μg) rapidly increases TSH secretion (Fig 7–15). This response is of clinical value, particularly in thyrotoxicosis. In this situation, despite TRH stimulation, TSH secretion remains suppressed

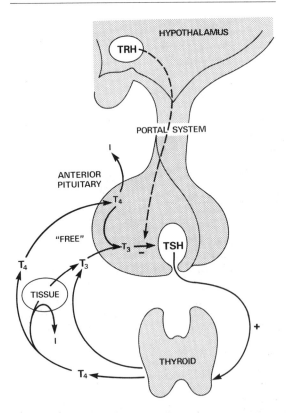

Figure 7–13. The hypothalamic-hypophyseal-thyroid axis. TRH produced in the hypothalamus reaches the thyrotrophs in the anterior pituitary by the hypothalamic-hypophyseal portal system and enhances secretion of TSH by altering the set point of T_3 inhibition of TSH secretion. In the pituitary, it is primarily T_3 that inhibits TSH secretion. T_4 undergoes monodeiodination to T_3 both in the peripheral tissues and in the pituitary itself.

Figure 7–15. Typical serum TSH responses to TRH. The hatched area indicates normal range. (Reproduced, with permission, from Utiger RD: *The Thyroid,* 4th ed. Werner SC, Ingbar SH [editors]. Harper & Row, 1978.)

Figure 7–16. Typical serum TSH responses to TRH in patients with thyroid (primary), pituitary (secondary), and hypothalamic (tertiary) hypothyroidism. The hatched area indicates the normal range. (Reproduced, with permission, from Utiger RD: *The Thyroid,* 4th ed. Werner SC, Ingbar SH [editors]. Harper & Row, 1978.)

by the high (even minimally elevated) thyroid hormone levels (Fig 7–15). However, other influences such as glucocorticoids and starvation may also reduce the TSH response to TRH stimulation. TRH stimulation is also valuable in the diagnosis of the very rare condition known as tertiary (hypothalamic) hypothyroidism, which is distinguished from secondary (pituitary) hypothyroidism by the presence of a TSH response to TRH in the former but not in the latter (Fig 7–16). The TRH test is of little clinical value in primary (thyroidal) hypothyroidism, where the high serum TSH level even before TRH injection is diagnostic and the exaggerated TSH response provides little additional information (Fig 7–16).

Acute injection of TRH also stimulates prolactin release by the pituitary, but it is not clear whether this is physiologically important. In some patients with hypothyroidism, however, serum prolactin levels may be elevated. Dopaminergic stimuli such as levodopa reduce both the prolactin and TSH response to TRH stimulation. In addition, levodopa acutely depresses the elevated TSH levels in primary hypothyroidism. It is unlikely, however, that TRH is the sole releasing factor for both TSH and prolactin, because their secretion may be dissociated under certain circumstances. For example, the nocturnal elevation in prolactin and the acute prolactin response to suckling are not associated with changes in TSH secretion.

Actions of TSH on the Thyroid

TSH has many effects on the thyroid, the net result of which is increased thyroid hormone secretion.

(1) Most TSH actions are produced by binding to specific thyroid plasma membrane receptors with the subsequent stimulation of adenylate cyclase activity and cAMP generation.

(2) TSH affects the iodide transport mechanism in a biphasic manner. There is an initial acute (4-hour) decrease in the iodide thyroid/serum (T:S) ratio. This effect is also produced in vitro by cAMP and reflects an increased rate of I^- efflux. After 4 hours of continued TSH stimulation, the iodide T:S ratio increases as the iodide transport mechanism is enhanced in a process dependent on new protein synthesis.

(3) TSH (and cAMP) stimulate iodide organification (incorporation of iodide into thyroglobulin) primarily by increasing H_2O_2 generation. Exocytosis of thyroglobulin into the follicular lumen is also increased.

(4) Acute TSH stimulation (1–2 minutes) increases pseudopod formation at the apical cell border, followed by endocytosis of colloid, phagolysosome formation, and the subsequent secretion of thyroid hormones (Fig 7–12). As mentioned above, these effects are blocked by colchicine and cytochalasin, which disrupt the cytoskeletal system.

(5) Chronic TSH stimulation increases thyroid

transcriptional and translational activity and ultimately produces hyperplasia and goiter.

(6) Many other effects of TSH on thyroid intermediary metabolism have been described, including increased glucose oxidation (primarily via the pentose phosphate pathway), phospholipid turnover, and increased precursor uptake into thyroid cells. Not all of these effects are produced by cAMP.

Other Thyroid Stimulators

Other stimulators of cAMP generation, particularly epinephrine and prostaglandins, can increase thyroid hormone secretion under experimental conditions. These agents mimic many (not all) of the effects of TSH. In the case of catecholamines, autonomic nerve endings have been demonstrated adjacent to the thyroid follicular cells, and it is conceivable that they may play a role in the regulation of thyroid function. At present, however, their role remains speculative and is most likely a minor one if it exists at all.

Thyroid Autoregulation

The thyroid is able to regulate its uptake of iodide and thyroid hormone synthesis by intrathyroidal mechanisms independent of TSH—ie, these regulatory mechanisms occur even in hypophysectomized animals.

A. Wolff-Chaikoff Block: When increasing amounts of I^- are given to experimental animals, in-

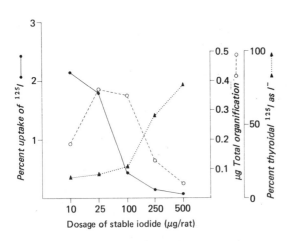

Figure 7–17. The Wolff-Chaikoff block. As increasing doses of iodide are administered to rats, there is an initial increase in iodide organification. At a critical concentration, however, higher doses of iodide given to the animals block iodide organification. The effect of increasing doses of iodide on thyroid hormone synthesis is therefore biphasic. Concomitantly with the increase in the organification block, the intracellular inorganic iodide concentration rises. As the amount of stable iodide injected is increased, there is a decrease in thyroidal uptake of radioactive iodide. (Reproduced, with permission, from DeGroot LJ, Stanbury JB: *The Thyroid and Its Diseases,* 4th ed. Wiley, 1975.)

hibition of iodide organification occurs at a critical level of intrathyroidal inorganic I^- (Fig 7–17). Thyroglobulin iodination and thyroid hormone synthesis subsequently decrease. This is known as the Wolff-Chaikoff block.

The normal thyroid gland escapes from the Wolff-Chaikoff block—and hypothyroidism does not ensue—because of intrathyroidal feedback inhibition of the iodide transport mechanism by an as yet unidentified organic iodine intermediate; ie, there is a reduction in the ability of the thyroid to trap iodide and to maintain a high T:S ratio. Because of diminished active iodide transport, the intrathyroidal inorganic I^- concentration then declines and the "brakes" come off the organification block. A new equilibrium now exists in which thyroid hormone is synthesized at the same rate as before the excess iodide load. The fractional thyroid uptake of iodide from the extracellular fluid is, however, reduced. Conversely, in iodide insufficiency, the iodide transport mechanism becomes more active (independent of TSH) and there is a greater fractional uptake of iodide from the plasma perfusing the thyroid gland. This is reflected in an increased radioactive iodine uptake. In some thyroid diseases (eg, Hashimoto's thyroiditis), escape from the Wolff-Chaikoff block does not occur, and hypothyroidism (iodide myxedema) ensues.

B. Sensitivity to TSH: The thyroid is able to "sense" its organic iodide content and alter its sensitivity to TSH stimulation. For example, when animals receiving a high-iodide diet are injected with TSH, they develop less of a goiter than do iodide-deficient animals injected with the same amount of TSH. An important set point for this, as well as for the iodide transport mechanism, may be at the level of adenylate cyclase. Thus, an organic iodide intermediate also inhibits the cAMP response to TSH stimulation. Very recently, autoregulation by organic iodine of thyroid cellular amino acid and glucose transport has also been recognized. Whether these inhibitors are all the same remains to be determined.

C. Thyroid Hormone Secretion: The Wolff-Chaikoff block must be distinguished from the rapid and transient decrease in thyroid hormone secretion induced by iodide, especially in hyperthyroidism (described above). Although the iodide organification block occurs rapidly, its clinical effects are more delayed because follicular thyroid hormone stores must first be depleted before thyroid hormone secretion declines. On the other hand, in susceptible individuals, a block in hormone secretion can lower serum hormone levels even with full follicular stores of thyroid hormone.

D. Other Examples of Autoregulation: During periods of iodide insufficiency, the ratio of T_3 to T_4 secreted by the thyroid is increased. Since T_3 is more potent than T_4, the thyroid is therefore able to utilize available iodide more efficiently when the supply is limited. Poorly iodinated thyroglobulin is also more susceptible to proteolysis into thyroid hormones than is heavily iodinated thyroglobulin.

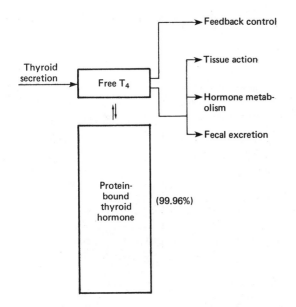

Figure 7–18. Representation of free T_4 (and free T_3) as the biologically active hormone at the level of the pituitary and the peripheral tissues. Most of the thyroid hormones circulating in plasma are protein-bound and have no biologic activity. This pool of bound hormone is in equilibrium with the free hormone pool. (Reproduced, with permission, from DeGroot LJ, Stanbury JB: *The Thyroid and Its Diseases,* 4th ed. Wiley, 1975.)

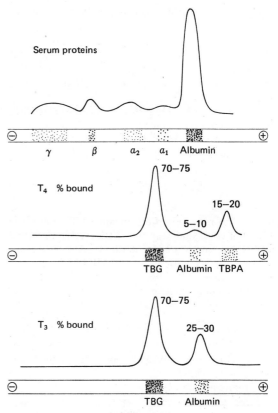

Figure 7–19. Diagrammatic representation of the distribution of radioactive T_4 and T_3 among serum thyroid hormone–binding proteins. *Top:* Paper electrophoretic pattern of serum proteins. *Middle:* Radioactive T_4 was added to serum and was then subjected to paper electrophoresis. The peaks represent the mobility of radioactive T_4 bound to different serum proteins. TBG, thyroid hormone–binding globulin; TBPA, thyroxine–binding prealbumin. *Bottom:* Radioactive T_3 was added to serum and subjected to paper electrophoresis. The peaks indicate the relative distribution of protein-bound radioactive T_3. The figures above each peak indicate the relative hormone distribution among the binding proteins in a normal adult. (Reproduced, with permission, from Rosenfield RL et al: *Pediatric Nuclear Medicine.* James AE Jr, Wagner HN Jr, Cooke RE [editors]. Saunders, 1974.)

THYROID HORMONES IN PLASMA

Plasma Binding Proteins

Thyroid hormones (T_4 and T_3) in plasma are largely bound to protein. Only about 0.04% of the T_4 and 0.4% of the T_3 circulate "free" in the unbound state. The present concept is that only the free hormones enter cells, produce their biologic effects, and are in turn metabolized. Only the free hormone regulates the pituitary feedback mechanism (Fig 7–13). A dynamic equilibrium exists between the plasma and intracellular free hormone pools. Protein-bound thyroid hormones are therefore a very large reservoir that is slowly drawn upon as the free hormone dissociates from the binding proteins and enters the cells (Fig 7–18). Thyroid secretion is precisely regulated to replenish the metabolized thyroid hormones. This maintains a constant level of free hormone. Very little thyroid hormone is lost in the urine, because protein binding minimizes glomerular filtration. Metabolites of T_4 and T_3, on the other hand, are very poorly bound to plasma proteins and are therefore rapidly excreted in the urine.

There are 3 major thyroid hormone–binding proteins in plasma. The hormone-carrying capacity of these proteins can be determined by adding radioactive hormone to serum and subjecting it to electrophoresis (Fig 7–19).

A. Thyroid Hormone–Binding Globulin (TBG): TBG is a monomeric glycoprotein. It is the thyroid hormone–binding protein at lowest concentration in plasma (1–2 mg/dL). Each molecule has a single binding site for T_4 or T_3. Despite its very low concentration, it is the protein with the highest affinity for thyroid hormones ($T_4 > T_3$) and therefore carries most (70%) of the bound thyroid hormones. When fully saturated, it can carry about 20 μg of T_4 per deciliter.

B. Thyroxine-Binding Prealbumin (TBPA): TBPA is present at intermediate concentration in plasma (25 mg/dL). TBPA binds essentially no T_3. Even though its concentration in plasma is 20 times that of TBG, TBPA binds much less T_4 than TBG, because it has a much lower affinity for T_4. Thus, about 20% of T_4 plasma is bound to TBPA—in contrast to approximately 70% of T_4 bound to TBG.

C. Albumin: Albumin has the lowest affinity for T_4 and T_3. However, it binds significant amounts of thyroid hormone (approximately 10% of T_4 and 30% of T_3), because it is present in plasma at very high concentration (about 3500 mg/dL).

D. Kinetics of Thyroid Hormone Interaction With Plasma Binding Proteins: T_4 and T_3 bind reversibly with each binding protein according to the **law of mass action.** For example, in the case of T_4,

$$(T_4) + (TBG) \rightleftharpoons (TBG\text{-}T_4) \qquad \ldots (1)$$

where (T_4) represents free (unbound) T_4, (TBG) is TBG not containing T_4, and $(TBG\text{-}T_4)$ is T_4 bound to TBG (all in molar concentrations). At equilibrium, the rate of association of T_4 and TBG to form TBG-T_4 is the same as the dissociation of TBG-T_4 into its individual components. Thus,

$$kT_4 = \frac{(TBG\text{-}T_4)}{(T_4)(TBG)} \qquad \ldots (2)$$

where kT_4 is the association constant for the interaction of T_4 with TBG.

From equation (2),

$$(T_4) = \frac{(TBG\text{-}T_4)}{kT_4 (TBG)} \qquad \ldots (3)$$

A similar relationship exists for each of the 3 major binding proteins, with their different affinities for T_4 (or T_3), as well as their different absolute concentrations. The free T_4 concentration in serum containing all of these binding proteins is the sum of the values in the numerator (equation 3) for each protein divided by the sum of the respective denominators.

It can therefore be seen from equation (3) that an increase in the concentration of a particular binding protein will initially result in a decrease in the free T_4 concentration (Fig 7–20). In the presence of a normal hypothalamic-pituitary-thyroid axis, there will be a compensatory increase in thyroid hormone secretion until the serum free T_4 level returns to normal. Under these conditions, the normal free T_4 concentration is now associated with an increase in the total (protein-bound) T_4. Daily free T_4 production and clearance rates are the same in both the "initial" and "new" conditions despite the fact that total plasma T_4 concentrations are different.

Because of the high affinity of the binding proteins for thyroid hormones, the concentrations of free T_4 and T_3 in plasma are negligible compared to the concentrations of protein-bound hormones. The former values can therefore be ignored in expressing the total thyroid hormone concentration in plasma. If the thyroid hormone concentration increases to the point of saturation for TBG (approximately 20 μg T_4 per deciliter), as may occur in hyperthyroidism, any further

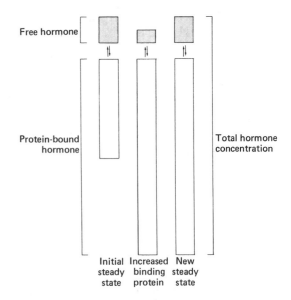

Figure 7–20. The effect of an increase in thyroid hormone–binding protein concentration on the free and protein-bound hormone concentrations. The initial increase in binding protein concentration (as may occur with estrogen administration) increases the amount of bound hormone and transiently decreases the free hormone concentration. There follows a transient increase in thyroid hormone secretion under the stimulus of TSH to replenish the free hormone pool. Another contributing factor is a transient decrease in the metabolic clearance rate of thyroid hormone. A new steady state is attained in which the free hormone secretion, metabolism, and plasma concentration are the same as initially except that the free hormone is now in equilibrium with a larger pool of bound hormone. In subjects receiving thyroid hormone medication, the same daily dose of thyroid hormone is necessary to maintain euthyroidism irrespective of the size of the bound hormone pool.

increase in total serum T_4 concentration is accompanied by a much larger increase in free T_4.

In the converse situation, if the concentration of thyroid hormone–binding protein in plasma is decreased, or if hormonal binding to the proteins is inhibited by, for example, a pharmacologic agent (see below), there is an initial transient increase in the serum free T_4 concentration. This suppresses TSH secretion, and thyroid hormone secretion is consequently reduced. With continued utilization of thyroid hormone by the tissues, the free thyroid hormone level decreases to the normal "euthyroid" level. At equilibrium, the normal free hormone level is now associated with a decreased total (protein-bound) hormone concentration.

The binding of thyroid hormones to plasma binding proteins may vary considerably. Low or high TBG levels are uncommon genetic traits that can produce abnormal levels in total hormone concentrations, with the free (metabolically active) hormone levels re-

Table 7–1. Factors influencing the concentration of protein-bound thyroid hormones in serum.

A. Increased TBG Concentration:
  1. Congenital.
  2. Hyperestrogenic states (pregnancy, estrogen treatment).
  3. Diseases (acute infectious hepatitis, hypothyroidism).
B. Decreased TBG Concentration:
  1. Congenital.
  2. Drugs (androgenic steroids, glucocorticoids).
  3. Major systemic illness (protein malnutrition, nephrotic syndrome, cirrhosis, hyperthyroidism).
C. Drugs Affecting Thyroid Hormone Binding to Normal Concentrations of Binding Protein:
  1. Phenytoin (Dilantin).
  2. Salicylates.
  3. Phenylbutazone.
  4. Mitotane (Lysodren, o,p'-DDD).
  5. Heparin.

maining normal. In addition, a variety of diseases and pharmacologic agents can either decrease the amount of binding protein present in plasma or influence the binding of thyroid hormones to a normal concentration of binding proteins (Table 7–1). Because of the high affinity of TBG for T_4 and T_3, alterations in its concentration have a much greater effect on serum total hormone concentrations than do alterations in TBPA or albumin concentrations.

THYROID HORMONE METABOLISM

T_4 is the major secretory product of the normal thyroid. The major pathway of T_4 metabolism is via the progressive deiodination of the molecule. As shown in Fig 7–21, the initial deiodination of T_4 may occur in the outer ring, producing T_3 ($3,3',5$-T_3); or in the inner ring, producing reverse T_3 (rT_3; $3,3',5'$-T_3). Less than 20% of total T_3 is produced in the thyroid (Fig 7–22). The remaining 80–90% is derived from outer (phenolic) ring monodeiodination of T_4 in the peripheral tissues. T_4 and T_3 in the plasma are metabolized by the peripheral tissues and subsequently excreted. Although the catabolic products of T_4 are generally less biologically active than the parent compound, some metabolites do have biologic activity and, as in the case of T_3, even exceed the biologic potency of T_4 (Table 7–4). It should be noted that data on the bioactivity of compounds other than T_4 and T_3 are based on difficult and inaccurate assays and should be regarded merely as approximations. Almost all (95%) of the reverse T_3 (rT_3) in the plasma is derived from the inner ring monodeiodination of T_4 in the peripheral tissues. Both T_3 and rT_3 are then deiodinated further to the diiodothyronines (T_2) and then to monoiodothyronines. Reverse T_3 and the 3 different T_2 metabolites are essentially biologically inactive and are cleared rapidly from the plasma.

There are 2 separate outer ring deiodinases that convert T_4 to T_3 (and rT_3 to $3,3'$-T_2). The major

Figure 7–21. The deiodinative pathway of thyroxine metabolism. The monodeiodination of T_4 to T_3 represents a "step up" in biologic potency, whereas the monodeiodination of T_4 to reverse T_3 has the opposite effect. Further deiodination of T_3 essentially abolishes hormonal activity.

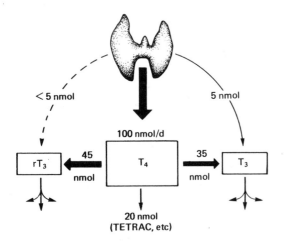

Figure 7–22. Major pathways of thyroxine metabolism in normal adult humans. Rates are expressed in nmol/24 h and are approximations based upon available data. 100 nmol of T_4 is equivalent to approximately 75 μg. rT_3, reverse T_3; TETRAC, tetraiodothyroacetic acid. (Reproduced, with permission, from Cavalieri RR, Rapoport B: Impaired peripheral conversion of thyroxine to triiodothyronine. *Ann Rev Med* 1977;**28**:5765.)

Table 7–3. Representative iodothyronine kinetic values in a euthyroid human.

	T_4	T_3	rT_3
Serum levels			
Total (μg/dL)	8	0.12	0.04
Free (ng/dL)	2.1	0.28	0.24
Body pool (μg)	800	46	40
Distribution volume (L)	10	38	98
Metabolic clearance rate (MCR) (L/d)	1	22	90
Production (disposal) rate (MCR X serum concentration)	80	28	28
Half-life in plasma ($t_{1/2}$) (days)	8	1	0.2

cular volume; ie, T_4 has the smallest distribution volume and the largest pool size. Because of the large plasma pool of T_4 relative to its rate of utilization, the plasma T_4 reservoir turns over relatively slowly. T_3 and, to a greater degree, rT_3 are more loosely bound to plasma proteins and are therefore distributed in a larger volume and cleared more rapidly.

The tissues that concentrate the most thyroid hormone are liver, kidney, and muscle. Brain, spleen, and gonads take up little thyroid hormone. This variation in uptake by different tissues parallels the metabolic effects of T_4 on oxygen consumption in vitro.

It is uncertain how thyroid hormones enter peripheral tissue cells. It was at one time thought that this was a passive diffusion process, but the possibility that there may be specific thyroid hormone receptors on the cell surface and active transport of thyroid hormone into cells is under active investigation. Once within the cell, thyroid hormones either remain free in the cytoplasm or are associated with low-affinity cytosol receptors or high-affinity nuclear and mitochondrial receptors.

In addition to the deiodinative pathways of T_4 metabolism, minor metabolic pathways of uncertain importance include the following:

(1) Oxidative deamination of the iodothyronines into their acetic acid derivatives, eg, tetraiodothyroacetic acid (TETRAC) and triiodothyroacetic acid (TRIAC) (Table 7–4). These compounds retain some biologic activity, but their relative physiologic importance is uncertain.

(2) Phenolic conjugation into glucuronide or sulfate derivatives. The former occurs mainly in the liver and the latter mainly in the kidney. Glucuronide conjugates of T_4 are excreted into the bile and thence in feces. In humans, there is little enterohepatic circulation of thyroid hormone conjugates.

(3) Decarboxylation of thyroxine to thyroxamine.

(4) Cleavage of the ether link between the 2 phenol rings of the iodothyronines.

As mentioned above, 80–90% of T_3 production is from the monodeiodination of T_4 to T_3 (Fig 7–22). This conversion of T_4 to T_3 utilizes approximately 30–40% of the secreted T_4. Virtually all rT_3 (95%) is produced by the monodeiodination of T_4, and this represents another 40% of the T_4 secreted by the thy-

differences between these 2 enzymes (iodothyronine 5'-deiodinase type I and type II) are outlined in Table 7–2.

Because conversion of T_4 to T_3 represents a "step up" in biologic activity whereas conversion of T_4 to rT_3 has the opposite effect (Fig 7–21), the conversion of T_4 to T_3 or rT_3 by inner or outer ring iodothyronine deiodinase is a pivotal regulatory step in determining thyroid hormone biologic activity. It has been proposed that T_4 is a biologically inactive prohormone and that its apparent biologic activity is dependent upon intracellular conversion to T_3. However, other than in the pituitary, all evidence indicates that T_4 itself has intrinsic biologic activity.

The kinetics of T_4, T_3, and rT_3 production, distribution, and clearance are shown in Table 7–3, which indicates typical values that may be seen in a normal human. It can be seen that because of its greater binding affinity to plasma proteins, chiefly TBG, the distribution of T_4 is largely restricted to the intravas-

Table 7–2. Differences between iodothyronine 5'-deiodinase type I and type II.

	Type I	Type II
Tissue (primary localization)	Liver, kidney, muscle	Brain, pituitary, brown adipose tissue
Inhibition by propylthiouracil	Yes	No
Substrate affinity	$rT_3 > T_4$	$T_4 = rT_3$
Enzyme kinetics	Ping-pong	Sequential
Influence of hypothyroidism	Decreased	Increased

Table 7–4. Chemical structures and biologic activity of thyroid hormones.

	Hormone	Common Name	Biologic Activity
	L-3,5,3',5'-Tetraiodothyronine	L-Thyroxine; T₄	100
	L-3,5,3'-Triiodothyronine	T₃	300–800
	L-3,3',5'-Triiodothyronine	Reverse T₃; rT₃	< 1
	DL-3,3'-Diiodothyronine	3,3'-T₂	< 1–3
	DL-3,5-Diiodothyronine	3,5-T₂	7–11
	DL-3',5'-Diiodothyronine	3'5'-T₂	0
	L-3,5,3',5'-Tetraiodothyroacetic acid	TETRAC	? 10–50
	L-3,5,3'-Triiodothyroacetic acid	TRIAC	? 25–35

roid. The remaining 20% of secreted T_4 is excreted in the feces or urine, either in the free form or as conjugates.

A variety of conditions and pharmacologic agents reduce the rate of T_4 monodeiodination to T_3 (Table 7–5). This may lead to decreased serum T_3 concen-trations. The clinical status of a patient is therefore very important in interpreting the significance of a low serum T_3 level. In acute illness or starvation, the low serum T_3 value is usually associated with an elevated serum rT_3 concentration. This reflects pri-marily decreased rT_3 clearance rather than increased

Table 7–5. Conditions or factors associated with decreased conversion of T_4 to T_3.

1. Fetal life.
2. Caloric restriction.
3. Hepatic disease.
4. Major systemic illness.
5. Drugs:
   Propylthiouracil.
   Glucocorticoids.
   Propranolol (mild effect).
   Iodinated x-ray contrast agents (iopanoic acid, ipodate sodium).

Figure 7–23. Basal metabolic rates after injection of equimolar amounts of T_3 and T_4 in a hypothyroid individual. (Reproduced, with permission, from Blackburn C et al: Calorigenic effects of single intravenous doses of L-triiodothyronine and L-thyroxine in myxedematous persons. *J Clin Invest* 1954;33:819.)

rT$_3$ production. While rT$_3$ clearly has little or no agonist activity, there is evidence that it may indeed be a counterhormone in reducing the metabolic activity of more active thyroid hormones.

THYROID HORMONE ACTIONS

Administration of T_4 or T_3—or the pathologic or iatrogenic absence of these hormones—produces general effects on intermediary metabolism and has particular effects on specific organ systems.

Fetal Development

Thyroid hormones are critically important in fetal development, particularly of the neural and skeletal systems. Thus, intrauterine hypothyroidism leads to cretinism (mental retardation and dwarfism). Maternal thyroid hormones do not cross the placenta in sufficient quantity to maintain fetal euthyroidism, and the fetus is therefore dependent upon hormones synthesized by its own thyroid gland (from about 11 weeks' gestation).

Oxygen Consumption & Heat Production

The basal metabolic rate (O$_2$ consumption, at rest, by the whole animal) increases in hyperthyroidism and decreases in hypothyroidism. Severe hyperthyroidism is occasionally associated with fever and severe hypothyroidism with hypothermia. Postnatally, thyroid hormones increase O$_2$ consumption in all tissues except the brain, spleen, and testis. Compared to the effects of TSH on thyroid hormone secretion, most thyroid hormone actions on peripheral tissues are induced relatively slowly over a period of hours or days. For example, T_4 administration to hypothyroid patients does not increase oxygen consumption until 24–48 hours after administration. T_3 acts more rapidly than T_4 but still over a period of hours (Fig 7–23).

Cardiovascular System

Thyroid hormones have marked chronotropic and inotropic effects on the heart. Low cardiac output with bradycardia and slow myocardial contraction and relaxation are characteristic of hypothyroidism. The reverse occurs in hyperthyroidism. The force of contraction in hypothyroidism is normal.

Sympathetic Effects

Many thyroid hormone effects, particularly on the cardiovascular system, are similar to those induced by catecholamines. Hyperthyroid patients are more sensitive to catecholamines. Thyroid hormones increase the number of catecholamine receptors in heart muscle cells. Hepatocyte receptors are unaffected. Thyroid hormones may also amplify catecholamine action at a postreceptor site. Beta-adrenergic inhibition reverses some features of clinical hyperthyroidism, such as eyelid retraction and tachycardia. However, other thyroid hormone actions—eg, effect on O$_2$ consumption—are not prevented by beta-adrenergic blockade. It is clear, therefore, that thyroid hormone action is distinct from catecholamine action. Their exact interrelationship remains to be elucidated.

Pulmonary Effects

Thyroid hormones are necessary for normal hypoxic and hypercapnic drive to the respiratory centers. Hypoventilation with hypoxia and hypercapnia is a consequence of severe hypothyroidism and may require artificial ventilation.

Hematopoiesis

Thyroid hormones increase erythropoiesis, possibly because of increased O$_2$ utilization by tissues leading to increased erythropoietin production. Thyroid hormones also increase 2,3-diphosphoglycerate concentrations in erythrocytes, allowing increased O$_2$

dissociation from hemoglobin and thereby increasing O_2 availability to the tissues. In hypothyroidism, the reverse occurs, and decreased O_2 consumption may lead to "anemia" (which, however, is physiologic).

Endocrine System

Thyroid hormones have a general effect in increasing the metabolism and clearance of various hormones and pharmacologic agents. For example, steroid hormone clearances are increased, leading to compensatory increases in production rates. Thus, administration of thyroid hormones will increase cortisol production and clearance, but the plasma cortisol concentration remains unchanged. Serum prolactin levels are increased in about 40% of patients with primary hypothyroidism. When present, this abnormality is corrected by treatment with thyroid hormone. Insulin requirements in diabetics are frequently increased in hyperthyroidism. The growth hormone response to stimuli such as hypoglycemia is reduced in primary hypothyroidism. Thyroid hormones are necessary for normal LH and FSH secretion. In hypothyroidism, anovulation and menstrual disturbances—particularly menorrhagia—may occur. Decreased renal free water clearance in hypothyroidism may be secondary to enhanced vasopressin activity but is more apt to be related to altered intrarenal hemodynamics. Finally, PTH action may be diminished in hypothyroidism.

Musculoskeletal System

Thyroid hormones have a potent stimulatory effect on bone turnover, increasing both bone formation and resorption. This is associated with increased urinary hydroxyproline excretion. Hypercalcemia is occasionally observed in severe hyperthyroidism. Thyroid hormones increase the rate of muscle relaxation as measured by elicitation of the deep tendon reflexes. This is of clinical value in diagnosing hypothyroidism.

THYROID HORMONE ACTION AT THE MOLECULAR LEVEL

Actions of thyroid hormones have been described at different intracellular sites. There is presently much discussion regarding their relative importance.

RNA Transcription

There is considerable evidence that free T_4 and T_3 enter tissue cells and bind to specific receptors in nuclear acidic proteins associated with chromatin. This is followed by increased RNA transcriptional activity. The physiologic importance of these nuclear binding sites is suggested by their high affinity constant, which is compatible with the prevailing plasma levels of free thyroid hormones. In addition, there is a good correlation between the binding of various analogs of thyroid hormones to nuclear receptors in liver and their metabolic potency. The exact mechanism by which thyroid hormone binding to nuclear protein

receptors leads to increased transcriptional activity is under active investigation.

Protein Translation

T_4 and T_3 increase detectable new protein synthesis in vitro within 5 hours. This is sooner than an effect on transcription can be observed. It is therefore difficult to explain this effect on new mRNA synthesis, and thyroid hormones are therefore believed to alter protein synthesis at a posttranscriptional site as well. Correlation of the induction by thyroid hormones of different enzymes such as mitochondrial malic enzyme and cytosolic α-glycerophosphate dehydrogenase with their respective mRNAs provides further evidence for posttranscriptional effects of thyroid hormones.

Cell Membrane

Thyroid hormones markedly stimulate plasma membrane Na^+-K^+ ATPase activity, which is coupled to Na^+ and K^+ transport across the plasma membrane. This increases ATP utilization. Since a large portion of the O_2 consumption by the entire organism is for maintenance of this transport system, it has been suggested that the effect of thyroid hormone in increasing the basal metabolic rate is related to this effect.

Thyroid hormones have also recently been found to have an acute (within minutes) effect on the plasma membrane of cells such as lymphocytes in that they increase the intracellular transport of glucose and amino acids. The physiologic importance of this phenomenon has not been established.

Mitochondria

Although it was initially thought that thyroid hormones increased oxygen consumption by uncoupling mitochondrial oxidative phosphorylation, leading to inefficient energy utilization, this is now thought to be unlikely. It is possible that ATP synthesis may be increased as a secondary phenomenon—eg, in response to increased ATP utilization in association with increased Na^+ and K^+ transport activity. Nevertheless, mitochondrial receptors of high affinity for thyroid hormones have recently been described, and their importance in mitochondrial function is being investigated.

Effects on Intermediary Metabolism

Thyroid hormones alter the metabolism of carbohydrates, fats, and proteins. It is likely, however, that these effects are not primary but secondary to the mechanisms described above. Cholesterol synthesis and degradation are both increased by thyroid hormones. Since the latter effect predominates, the serum cholesterol level declines in thyroid overactivity and vice versa. Thyroid hormone–induced effects on cholesterol metabolism may be secondary to increased beta-lipoprotein degradation. This may also account for the alteration in serum carotene that parallels the alteration in serum cholesterol. Lipolysis is also increased by thyroid hormones, possibly by enhancing the response to catecholamine stimulation. Glycogenolysis and gluconeogenesis are increased by thyroid hormones, presumably in relation to regeneration of ATP consumed—eg, by increased Na^+-K^+ ATPase activity. Thyroid hormones increase insulin requirements in diabetics. The reasons for this are unclear and may be related to increased insulin degradation or clearance rather than to alterations in carbohydrate metabolism.

THYROID FUNCTION DURING GROWTH & DEVELOPMENT

Fetal Development

Thyroglobulin synthesis begins during the fifth week of intrauterine life, and the iodide transport mechanism becomes active at approximately 12 weeks. During pregnancy, the fetal thyroid is under the control of the fetal hypothalamus and pituitary. Maternal thyroid hormones in their active form can cross the placenta only to a slight extent. A contributing factor to this phenomenon may be that 5' deiodinase is very active in placental tissue. Thus, athyreotic fetuses have detectable but low (hypothyroid) thyroid hormone concentrations.

At maturity, the human fetus has a slightly increased serum TSH and free thyroxine concentration. However, the serum T_3 level is very low—in the range noted in adults during starvation and acute illness. Similarly, the rT_3 concentration is elevated. Immediately after birth, there is a transient increase in TSH secretion, and serum T_3, T_4, and rT_3 levels revert to nearly normal within the first few days and approach normal adult levels during the first year of life.

Thyroid Function in Pregnancy

Serum TBG levels increase approximately 2-fold during pregnancy. A new equilibrium is reached in which the total thyroid hormone concentrations are twice normal but free hormone levels remain normal. Radioactive iodine uptake increases during pregnancy, and the thyroid may increase slightly in size, because of increased renal clearance of iodide and perhaps because of increased iodide utilization by the fetus. The placenta produces a glycoprotein hormone with very weak thyrotropic activity. It is unclear whether this is human chorionic gonadotropin (hCG) itself or another closely related compound that is extracted from the placenta together with hCG. Recent evidence suggests the latter. In normal pregnancy, this substance has little or no effect on thyroid function.

Changes in Thyroid Function With Aging

Although serum T_3 levels are reported to decrease slightly with aging, this observation has been questioned, because elderly persons are more susceptible to a variety of illnesses that may reduce serum T_3 production from T_4 and therefore reduce the average

T_3 level in the group. Irrespective of whether an age-related decrease in T_3 occurs or not, thyroid function in old people appears to be normal as shown by the TSH response to TRH stimulation.

TESTS OF THYROID FUNCTION

Thyroid function tests may be classified as those that (1) measure concentrations of hormones or biologically inactive products secreted by the thyroid gland; (2) directly examine the function of the thyroid gland; (3) test the effects of thyroid hormones on peripheral tissues; (4) evaluate the hypothalamic-pituitary-thyroid axis; and (5) identify and measure pathologic substances in blood not usually present in normal subjects.

MEASUREMENT IN BLOOD OF PRODUCTS SECRETED BY THE THYROID

Measurement of T_4

T_4 is measured by competitive binding assay or by radioimmunoassay. The former test is based on the very high affinity of TBG for T_4. For the latter, an antibody to T_4 (conjugated to a larger protein to be more antigenic) is raised in rabbits. In both instances, the conditions of the assay are such that T_4 is dissociated from endogenous TBG, which therefore does not interfere in the assay. The unknown serum is compared to a series of standards of known T_4 concentration in their ability to competitively inhibit the binding of a tracer amount of radioactive T_4 to TBG or to T_4 antibody.

Under some circumstances, the total T_4 concentration in serum does not accurately reflect metabolic status. As described previously (Table 7–1), thyroid hormone–binding protein concentrations may be altered in a variety of conditions. This leads to altered total T_4 levels but not the metabolically important free T_4 concentrations. Certain drugs—phenytoin and salicylates are the most common offenders—interfere with the binding of T_4 to serum binding proteins. For this reason, it is of clinical value to combine the estimation of the total serum T_4 with an indirect measurement of the free T_4 concentration (see below).

Free T_4 Index & Free T_4

Direct measurement by dialysis of serum free T_4 is a difficult and laborious procedure because of its very low concentration. Although new, ingenious assays for the measurement of free T_4 in serum have been developed, many clinicians still depend on assays that provide an approximation of the absolute free T_4 concentration expressed as a free T_4 index (FT$_4$I). For this purpose, an estimate is made of the binding capacity of the patient's serum for thyroid hormones (Fig 7–24). Radiolabeled T_3 or T_4 (usually T_3) is first added to the serum to be tested and allowed to equilibrate with unlabeled endogenous hormone. An aliquot is then added to either a resin or Sephadex— substances that bind free thyroid hormone with high affinity and therefore compete with serum binding proteins for the free hormone. More T_3 than T_4 is bound to resin because T_3 binds with lower affinity to endogenous binding proteins. The assay using radiolabeled T_3 is therefore more practical than the one using T_4. The resin is then rinsed and counted for radioactivity to determine what percentage of the total radioactivity has been adsorbed. The percentage uptake of total radioactive T_3 by the resin will be greater when there is less binding of the radioactive T_3 to serum binding proteins. Conversely, if serum binding proteins are increased, as in pregnancy, the percentage uptake of radioactive T_3 by the resin will decrease.

Multiplication of the resin or Sephadex uptake value by the total T_4 concentration provides an index of the effective free T_4 concentration independently of changes in hormone binding capacity in serum. It is important to emphasize that this is not a true free T_4 determination but merely an index of this measurement. It has been demonstrated by direct measurement of free T_4 levels by dialysis that there is reasonable proportionality between the true free T_4 level and the free T_4 index, thereby establishing the clinical usefulness of the latter. It may seem confusing that the free T_4 index (FT_4I) is measured with radioactive T_3 (''T_3 resin uptake test''; RT_3U). However, the test is an assessment of the capacity for serum proteins to bind thyroid hormones, and it makes no difference whether T_3 or T_4 is used. T_3 is more useful because it is not as tightly bound to serum proteins as T_4 and because the resin is better able to compete for available free hormone.

In most cases, the combination of the total T_4 and FT_4I is sufficient to establish the thyroid metabolic status of the patient. Under some circumstances, however, even when alterations in thyroid hormone–binding proteins are taken into account by the FT_4I, the value may be misleading and obscure the correct diagnosis. If there is suspicion that the T_4 and FT_4I results are clinically inappropriate, additional tests are necessary. Thus, the FT_4I may be inappropriately low in patients ingesting excessive amounts of T_3 (thy-

Total T_4 (measured separately)	Radioactive T_3 added to serum	Resin Added	% Radioactive T_3 bound to resin	$\times$ Total T_4	= Free T_4 index
(μg/dL)					
10	X X X X X X X Normal TBG	X X + (R) = (R) X X X X	30% ($^3/_{10}$)	10	3.0
15	X X X X X X X X Increased TBG	X X + (R) = (R) X X	20% ($^2/_{10}$)	15	3.0

Figure 7–24. Use of the free T_4 index (FT_4I) to estimate the free T_4 (or free T_3) concentration in serum independently of changes in the thyroid hormone–binding protein concentration. The upper panel represents the TBG concentration in a normal individual and the lower panel that in a subject with an increased TBG concentration. It can be seen that in both situations, the free hormone concentration remains the same; however, the free hormone represents a smaller fraction of the total hormone present in the subject with increased TBG. This leads to a decrease in the amount of radioactive hormone bound by the resin. In both situations, the products of the total T_4 concentration and the fractional uptake of hormone by the resin lead to identical free hormone indices. X = $^{125}T_3$ added to serum. The size of the box is proportional to the content of TBG in serum. X inside box = $^{125}T_3$ bound to TBG. X outside box = $^{125}T_3$ free to bind to resin.

rotoxicosis factitia) or may be normal when hyperthyroidism is associated with relative overproduction of T_3 but not T_4 (T_3 thyrotoxicosis). Phenytoin is a unique drug in that it may lower the FT_4I as well as the total T_4 even though patients remain clinically euthyroid by all other available criteria. The reason for this is unclear. A possible explanation is that intracellular T_4 (or T_3) levels are normal despite depressed serum free T_4 levels.

Occasionally, the FT_4I is inappropriately high. An example of this is the very rare condition of peripheral resistance to thyroid hormones. In addition, during acute illness, euthyroid patients may rarely present with an elevated FT_4I; however, the total T_3 concentration is subnormal. Occasionally, in acute or chronic illness, the resin uptake test for the FT_4I is artificially interfered with by unknown serum factors, and an inappropriately low resin uptake is measured. This results in an artifactually low FT_4I, and the patient may be wrongly diagnosed as being hypothyroid. In these patients, measurement of the true free T_4 by dialysis reveals a normal or even high level. The diagnosis should therefore be reassessed after recovery from the illness. If waiting is not prudent, primary hypothyroidism can be excluded by a serum TSH determination (see below).

The direct measurement of free T_4 (FT_4) by radioimmunoassay is rapidly supplanting the use of the FT_4I. However, many of the commercially available FT_4 tests are susceptible to the same problems (eg, artifacts present in systemic illness) that influence interpretation of the FT_4I.

Measurement of T_3

The T_3 concentration in serum is generally measured by radioimmunoassay (RIA). This should not be confused with the resin T_3 uptake test (RT_3U), which does not measure the serum T_3 level (see above). The competitive binding assay with TBG is more difficult for T_3 than for T_4, because TBG also binds T_4, which is present in serum at a higher concentration than T_3 and which binds with higher affinity to TBG. Measurement of T_3 is of more value in the diagnosis of hyperthyroidism than hypothyroidism, because in hyperthyroidism the increase in T_3 secretion is proportionately greater than the increase in T_4 secretion. This may be manifested occasionally as "T_3 thyrotoxicosis," in which an elevated serum T_3 level is associated with a normal T_4 level. In contrast, in mild hypothyroidism, the serum T_3 level does not fall to the same degree as does the T_4, because TSH stimulation increases the relative secretion of T_3. On the rare occasion when ill patients are found to have a slightly elevated free T_4 index, measurement of the total T_3 level is of great value in excluding hyperthyroidism. In a wide variety of acute and chronic illnesses, the serum total T_3 level is suppressed because of decreased conversion of T_4 to T_3 (Table 7–5).

Free T_3 Index

The total T_3 concentration is influenced by alterations in the concentration of serum binding proteins in the same way as is the serum total T_4 level. Thus, just as the high total T_4 in a patient taking estrogens for contraception is difficult to interpret without determination of the free T_4 index, so must a high total T_3 (RIA) level under these circumstances be interpreted with caution. Use of the free T_3 index is increasing. The test is performed as described above for free T_4 index. The product of the T_3 (RIA) and the RT_3U allows the calculation of a free T_3 index (FT_3I) that is an indicator of the free T_3 level in serum. It is important to mention again that the T_3 resin uptake test (RT_3U), which is merely a test for assessing the capacity for the serum binding proteins to bind thyroid hormones (T_3 or T_4), is not by itself a measure of the T_3 level in serum.

Measurement of Reverse T_3

Reverse T_3 (rT_3) is measured in whole serum by radioimmunoassay. The normal range in adults is approximately 25–75 ng/mL of serum. This is approximately one-third the concentration of the total T_3 concentration. The test is not generally available and is of limited clinical usefulness. Almost all clinical situations can be evaluated without an rT_3 determination on the basis of the serum T_4 and T_3 and their respective free hormone indices. Of potential diagnostic value, however, is the observation that the rT_3 level is elevated in systemic illness when serum T_3 is depressed. In hypothyroidism, on the other hand, both T_3 and rT_3 levels are low.

Measurement of Thyroglobulin

Thyroglobulin is measured in serum by radioimmunoassay. This measurement may be invalidated by the presence in serum of thyroglobulin autoantibodies. The serum thyroglobulin level is normally very low; it is elevated in conditions of thyroid overactivity, in which its secretion is increased along with thyroid hormones. Excess thyroglobulin is also released into the serum when the follicular structure of the thyroid gland is damaged, as in subacute thyroiditis. In these conditions, however, determination of the serum thyroglobulin level is not of diagnostic value. It is of much greater clinical importance in following patients who have had surgery for thyroid cancer. Following total thyroidectomy, thyroglobulin should be undetectable in serum. The de novo appearance of this compound is good evidence that thyroid metastases have developed. In patients with existing thyroid metastases, an increase in the concentration of serum thyroglobulin usually indicates progression of the disease and vice versa.

Measurement of Protein-Bound Iodine (PBI)

Until 2 decades ago, PBI was a major test for measurement of serum thyroid hormone levels. It measures all precipitable iodine-containing proteins. Normally, the iodine content of serum T_4 approximates the PBI. Thus, about 66% of the weight of T_4

is iodine. The normal PBI range is 4–8 μg/dL of serum, about two-thirds of the normal range for the total T_4 concentration. The PBI has been superseded by more specific tests for thyroid hormones, but in rare instances it is still of value. For example, in congenital defects of thyroid hormonogenesis, the PBI may be considerably higher than the serum total T_4 iodine concentration. This indicates the secretion of nonhormonal organic iodine compounds. A similar phenomenon may occur in Hashimoto's thyroiditis. In addition, a variety of organic iodine x-ray contrast materials that may be interfering with thyroid function can be detected by this procedure.

TESTS OF THYROID GLAND FUNCTION

Radioactive Iodine Uptake (RAIU)

The rationale for this test was described in the section on iodide metabolism. Sodium ^{123}I is administered orally, and a gamma scintillation counter is used to measure radioactivity over the area of the thyroid after 24 hours. This interval is chosen because the tracer uptake is at 24 hours near maximum. An earlier measurement is usually done as well, either 4 or 6 hours after radioisotope administration, because the RAIU may occasionally reach a maximum before 24 hours and subsequently decline by 24 hours. Situations in which this decline may be seen include severe thyrotoxicosis with rapid thyroid iodine turnover and early primary thyroid failure (such as in Hashimoto's thyroiditis), where a small remnant of functional thyroid under TSH stimulation is releasing newly synthesized hormone very rapidly without a long period of storage.

Uncommonly, thyrotoxicosis may be associated with a very low or absent thyroid RAIU, which is of diagnostic importance in establishing the condition responsible for the thyrotoxicosis. Examples of low RAIU thyrotoxicosis are (1) subacute thyroiditis, (2) "spontaneously resolving hyperthyroidism," (3) thyrotoxicosis factitia, (4) struma ovarii, (5) excessive iodide intake (jodbasedow effect), and (6) ectopic functional thyroid metastases after total thyroidectomy.

Perchlorate Discharge

The efficiency of the thyroid organification mechanism may be tested by giving $KClO_4$, 0.5 g in solution orally, 2–3 hours after oral administration of radioiodide, and observing its effect on the RAIU (Fig 7–9). Perchlorate inhibits the iodide transport mechanism. In subjects with a normal organification mechanism, ClO_4^- blocks further uptake of radioiodide by the thyroid but does not discharge more than 5% of the accumulated iodide in the next hour. Conversely, if iodide organification is incomplete and inorganic iodide is "backed up" within the thyroid cell, ClO_4^- blocks further I^- transport, but diffusion of I^- out of the cell continues. This is seen as discharge of radio-

active iodide from the thyroid gland, as measured by detectable radioactivity over the gland. A positive test may be observed in (1) congenital iodide organification defects, (2) some cases of Hashimoto's thyroiditis, (3) Graves' disease previously treated with radioactive iodide, and (4) patients who have ingested inhibitors of iodide organification such as methimazole and propylthiouracil. Sensitivity of the test may be enhanced by the administration of 1 mg of stable (nonradioactive) iodide together with the radioactive iodide. This provides additional substrate to stress the organification mechanism. The ClO_4^- discharge test is rarely used, because of its limited diagnostic value given the wide variety of more specific and simpler tests available.

Thyroid Imaging

The size and shape and some features of the internal structure of the thyroid may be assessed by a wide variety of thyroid imaging techniques. Their clinical application will be discussed in greater detail in subsequent sections of this chapter. However, they may be summarized as follows:

A. Radionuclide Scanning: After the administration of radioactive iodide—eg, sodium ^{123}I—an image of the thyroid may be obtained using an appropriate scanning apparatus. With the rectilinear scanner, the scanner moves in a matrix over the patient's neck, and the radioactivity at each point is recorded as a dot on paper or x-ray film (Fig 7–25). The advantage of this scan is that it accurately represents the size of the thyroid and accurately localizes palpable thyroid abnormalities. On the other hand, its resolution is relatively poor, and it takes considerable time for the scan to be completed.

Over recent years, the pinhole collimated gamma camera (scintillation camera) has moved to the fore. The field of the gamma camera is relatively large and encompasses the entire thyroid. This allows a rapid

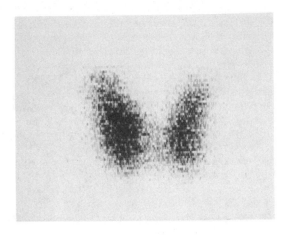

Figure 7–25. Rectilinear thyroid sodium ^{123}I scan performed 6 hours after the ingestion of 100 μCi of sodium ^{123}I. (Courtesy of RR Cavalieri.)

scan of the thyroid without the necessity for moving the camera. The data are usually recorded on Polaroid film (Fig 7–26). Besides speed, the major advantage of this method is increased resolution.

^{99m}Tc pertechnetate is also concentrated by the thyroid and can be used for imaging with high resolution. Unlike radioactive iodine, this isotope is not organified and stored, and the scan is therefore performed very shortly (eg, 20 minutes) after isotope administration. Advantages of this scan in addition to its speed include the fact that it is not interfered with by drugs that block iodide organification. Occasionally, however, thyroid nodules that are "cold" with sodium ^{123}I are not identified with ^{99m}Tc pertechnetate.

B. Fluorescent Scanning: The fluorescent scan provides an image of the distribution of nonradioactive, stable iodine within the thyroid. An approximate quantitation can also be made of the thyroidal iodine store. No radioisotope is administered. An external source of ^{241}Am is directed at the thyroid, resulting in the emission of x-rays by thyroid molecules. By selectively recording emitted 28.5 keV x-rays specific for iodine, an image of the intrathyroidal iodine distribution can be formed. The scan is similar in appearance to the rectilinear radioactive iodine scan (Fig 7–25). The advantage of the fluorescent scan is that it does not require radioactive iodine administration, and the thyroid may be imaged even if the RAIU is zero, such as when the patient is taking exogenous thyroid hormones. Thus, it can be used to determine whether thyroid tissue is absent or when it is present but not trapping radioiodine.

C. Ultrasonography: The application of this technique is similar to that for other organs. Its major use is to differentiate between cystic and solid thyroid lesions that may both appear to be "cold" on radionuclide scanning.

Figure 7–26. Scintiphoto (pinhole collimator) thyroid scan performed 6 hours after the ingestion of 100 μCi of sodium ^{123}I. (Courtesy of RR Cavalieri.)

TESTS OF THE EFFECTS OF THYROID HORMONES ON PERIPHERAL TISSUES

The ultimate test of whether a patient is experiencing the effects of too much or too little thyroid hormone is not a measurement of hormone concentration in the blood or the size and functional activity of the thyroid but the effect of thyroid hormones on the peripheral tissues. Unfortunately, no simple, reproducible, and specific tests are available for this purpose.

Basal Metabolic Rate (BMR)

This test measures a resting subject's oxygen consumption with a spirometer. Oxygen consumption is increased in hyperthyroidism and vice versa. Because of the wide variability of results, attempts were made to standardize the test by correcting for body surface area, age, and sex and by making sure patients were truly at rest. The test is expensive, time-consuming, subject to a variety of influencing factors, and not very sensitive and is rarely used today.

Photomotogram

This simple apparatus can be used to measure the speed of relaxation of the Achilles tendon reflex. The patient kneels on a chair with the foot positioned in such a way as to interrupt a photoelectric light beam. The Achilles tendon is tapped with a hammer, which initiates a timer, and when the foot returns to its original position the timer is stopped and indicates the length of time taken for return of the foot to the original position. The approximate half-relaxation time is 230–350 ms. This test is of limited value in hypothyroidism, in which the relaxation time is typically prolonged. Although relaxation time is faster in hyperthyroidism, there is a large overlap with the normal range and the test is therefore of little clinical value. The test is influenced by a wide variety of other neuromuscular conditions as well as by pharmacologic agents, and in the author's opinion it is of limited diagnostic value.

Q–Kd Interval

Measurement of the Q–Kd interval provides an assessment of the effect of thyroid hormones on the rate of myocardial contraction. The test measures time elapsed between initiation of the QRS complex on the ECG and the arrival of the pulse wave in the brachial artery as measured by the Korotkoff sound. The Q–Kd interval is typically decreased in hyperthyroidism and increased in hypothyroidism. The limitations of the test are similar to those described for the photomotogram, and it too is rarely used.

Biochemical Changes

Thyroid hormones influence the concentration of a vast array of tissue and blood compounds as well as the activity of many different enzymes. Unfortunately, however, none of these changes are specific enough, sensitive enough, or convenient enough to measure to make them of clinical importance. Perhaps the most useful is the serum cholesterol, which is elevated in hypothyroidism and decreased in hyperthyroidism. Serum creatine phosphokinase (CPK) and lactate dehydrogenase (LDH) may also be increased in hypothyroidism.

EVALUATION OF THE HYPOTHALAMIC-PITUITARY-THYROID AXIS

Measurement of Serum TSH

Factors that influence TSH secretion have been described above. TSH is measured in blood by radioimmunoassay. This test is the most sensitive, convenient, and specific test for the diagnosis of primary hypothyroidism (Fig 7–27). A TSH test that has recently become available is sufficiently sensitive to measure TSH levels in the serum of euthyroid patients and therefore may distinguish between euthyroidism and hyperthyroidism. This ultrasensitive TSH test may therefore supplant the TRH test (see below) in the diagnosis of mild hyperthyroidism. However, the validity for this use still requires confirmation. There is increasing evidence that the measurement of TSH by radioimmunoassay does not always correlate precisely with the degree of TSH bioactivity. Clinically, however, this is not important, and there is generally an excellent correlation between TSH immunoactivity and biologic activity.

Thyrotropin-Releasing Hormone (TRH) Test

In a sense, the TRH test may be regarded as a test of the metabolic effects of thyroid hormones on the peripheral tissues—in this case, specifically the thyrotrophs. In hyperthyroidism, the TSH response to TRH is dampened or abolished, and in primary hypothyroidism the maximum response is enhanced (Figs 7– 15 and 7– 16). The TSH response to TRH is slightly greater in females than in males. A normal response is a 2- to 5-fold increase over basal serum TSH 15– 30 minutes after intravenous injection of 500 μg of TRH.

TRH is usually administered intravenously (400 or 500 μg as a single bolus), but it may also be given orally, intramuscularly, or by continuous intravenous infusion. When TRH is given intravenously as a bolus injection, the serum TSH level increases rapidly, reaching a maximum 15– 30 minutes after injection, and then declines more slowly over a period of a few hours (Figs 7– 15 and 7– 16). The greatest value of this test is in the diagnosis of mild hyperthyroidism, for which it is the most sensitive test. As an indication of its sensitivity, the administration of exogenous thyroid hormones to normal subjects—at a dose insufficient to raise serum hormone levels above the normal range—suppresses the TSH response to TRH stimulations. The test is of less value in primary hypothyroidism (thyroidal failure), in which the high, unstimulated TSH value is in itself sufficient evidence for the diagnosis. While the TSH response to TRH is augmented in hypothyroidism, this increase is generally proportionate to the elevation in the basal TSH concentration and therefore provides little additional information.

The TRH test is the only test available to distinguish between secondary (pituitary) and tertiary (hypothalamic) hypothyroidism (Fig 7– 16). In the former, there is a decreased or absent TSH response to TRH stimulation. In the latter, despite a low serum TSH in association with low serum T_4 and T_3 levels, there is an adequate—but sometimes delayed—TSH response to TRH injection.

TSH Stimulation Test

This test measures the responsiveness of the thyroid to exogenous TSH. Originally used to test the degree of thyroid reserve in primary hypothyroidism, it has been superseded by direct measurement of the

Figure 7–27. Diagnostic value of serum TSH concentration (determined by radioimmunoassay) in primary hypothyroidism. Patients with secondary hypothyroidism and hyperthyroidism have undetectable serum TSH concentrations. The dark areas indicate undetectable levels. Note that TSH levels may be undetectable in normal subjects also. (Reproduced, with permission, from Hershman JM, Pittman JA Jr: Control of thyroid secretion in man. *N Engl J Med* 1971;**285**:997.)

endogenous TSH level in serum. The test is time-consuming, expensive, and potentially dangerous. Bovine TSH (10 units) is administered intramuscularly daily for 3 days. The thyroid RAIU is measured before and after TSH administration. It is important to skin test patients before administration of bovine TSH, because serious allergic responses have occurred.

Thyroid Suppression With T₃

In Graves' disease, thyroid function is autonomous and no longer under the control of the hypothalamic-pituitary axis. Because thyroid overactivity is produced by a factor other than TSH, suppression of endogenous TSH by administration of T_3 will not reduce the thyroid RAIU. The standard T_3 suppression test involves the initial measurement of the thyroid RAIU followed by the administration for 5–7 days of 100 μg of T_3 per day in divided doses. After this period, the RAIU is measured again. T_3 suppression should reduce the RAIU in normal subjects by at least 50%. Although the T_3 suppression test and the TRH test are both useful in the evaluation of selected thyrotoxicosis patients, there are important differences between them. The TSH response to TRH is blunted when the pituitary senses excess thyroid hormone, irrespective of the condition producing the thyrotoxicosis. In contrast, the T_3 suppression test is not used to diagnose thyrotoxicosis but rather thyroid autonomy. Nonsuppressibility of the RAIU is not sufficient for the diagnosis of thyrotoxicosis. For example, after radioactive iodine treatment for Graves' disease, the patient may be euthyroid but still have a T_3-nonsuppressible thyroid.

MEASUREMENT OF PATHOLOGIC THYROID AUTOANTIBODIES

Thyroglobulin Autoantibodies & Thyroid Microsomal Autoantibodies

These antibodies are present in the serum of patients with autoimmune thyroid disease and to a lesser degree in some other thyroid conditions. The clinical value of their measurement will be discussed in subsequent sections of this chapter. The most commonly used method for measuring these antibodies is by a hemagglutination technique. Thyroglobulin or thyroid microsomal proteins are absorbed onto tannic acid–treated sheep red blood cells. Antibodies against these antigens agglutinate the cells, and dilution of the patient's serum allows determination of antibody titer. Thyroglobulin autoantibodies and thyroid microsomal autoantibodies may also be measured by more sensitive immunoradiometric assays, of which there are numerous variations.

Thyroid-Stimulating Immunoglobulins (TSI)

Many different tests have been used for the measurement of TSI. Most have been too impractical or insensitive for general clinical use.

A. Long-Acting Thyroid Stimulator (LATS): This was the initial assay for the measurement of TSI. The assay measures the ability of patients' sera to release radioiodine from the thyroid glands of mice prelabeled with radioiodine. The difficulties with this assay are that it is time-consuming, expensive, and of limited sensitivity and specificity. The false-negative rate is approximately 50%. Many other factors also influence the bioassay animals, leading to difficulty in interpreting the results.

B. LATS Protector: This is an adaptation of the LATS assay. Advantage is taken of the species-specificity of TSI. Thus, human thyroid tissue absorbs LATS activity from LATS-positive serum. Serum or IgG from a patient with active Graves' disease prevents adsorption of LATS to the thyroid tissue and therefore "protects" it. Different human sera can therefore be assessed in terms of their efficacy in protecting a standard LATS serum of known activity from adsorption to thyroid tissue. The LATS is measured by the mouse bioassay method described above. The disadvantage of the LATS protector assay is that it is even more laborious than the LATS assay. However, false-negative results in Graves' disease are reduced, and the test would be of clinical value if it were easier to perform.

C. Thyroid cAMP Assays: Serum—or IgG—from a patient with Graves' disease is tested for its ability to stimulate cAMP generation in human thyroid tissue—either slices or plasma membranes. Initial studies have indicated a 10–30% false-negative rate. A major disadvantage of the slice assay is the need for fresh human thyroid tissue. Variations on the assay include quantitation of colloid droplets in thyroid follicular cells and measurement of thyroid hormones secreted by the tissue slices. None of these assays are practical enough for extensive clinical use. Recently, the cAMP response in human thyroid cells cultured in monolayers has been adapted for the bioassay of TSI. The sensitivity and practicality of this new assay now permit the routine determination of TSI.

D. TSH Binding Inhibition (TBI): This assay utilizes the binding of radiolabeled bovine TSH to human thyroid plasma membrane preparations. This binding is inhibited to varying degrees by sera or IgG from patients with active Graves' disease. It is important to realize that the TBI assay is not truly a TSI assay in that it does not measure biologic activity. Another name for the test is TSH displacement assay (TDA). While this assay is convenient and has a relatively low false-negative rate, it is plagued by false-positive results. Thus, a wide variety of nonspecific interfering substances, such as thyroglobulin, inhibit TSH binding. There is also a low correlation between the results obtained in the TBI assay and in the thyroid slice cAMP assay using the same test sera.

DISORDERS OF THE THYROID GLAND

Patients with thyroid disease will usually complain of (1) thyroid enlargement, or goiter; (2) symptoms of thyroid deficiency, or hypothyroidism; (3) symptoms of thyroid hormone excess, or hyperthyroidism; or (4) complications of a specific form of hyperthyroidism, Graves' disease, which may present with striking prominence of the eyes (exophthalmos) or, rarely, thickening of the skin over the lower legs (thyroid dermopathy).

The **history** should include evaluation of symptoms related to the above complaints, discussed in more detail below. Exposure to ionizing radiation in childhood has been associated with an increased incidence of thyroid disease, including cancer. Iodide ingestion in the form of kelp or iodide-containing cough preparations may induce goiter, hypothyroidism, or hyperthyroidism. Lithium carbonate, used in the treatment of manic-depressive psychiatric disorder, can also induce hypothyroidism and goiter. Residence in an area of low dietary iodide is associated with iodine-deficiency goiter, or "endemic goiter." Although dietary iodide is generally adequate in developed countries, there are still areas low in natural iodine (ie, undeveloped countries in Africa, Asia, South America, and inland mountainous areas). Finally, the family history should be explored with particular reference to goiter, hyperthyroidism, or hypothyroidism, as well as immunologic disorders such as diabetes, rheumatoid disease, pernicious anemia, or myasthenia gravis, which may be associated with an increased incidence of thyroid disease. Multiple endocrine neoplasia type IIa (Sipple's syndrome) with medullary carcinoma of the thyroid gland is an autosomal dominant condition.

Physical examination of the thyroid gland is illustrated in Fig 7–28. The thyroid is firmly attached

Figure 7–28. Examination of the thyroid gland. *A:* Observe the neck, especially as the patient swallows. *B:* Examine from the front, rotating the gland slightly with one thumb while palpating the other lobe with the other thumb. *C:* Examine from behind, using 3 fingers and the same technique. *D:* The size of each lobe or of thyroid nodules can be measured by first drawing an outline on the skin.

to the anterior trachea midway between the sternal notch and the thyroid cartilage; it is often easy to see and to palpate. The patient should have a glass of water for comfortable swallowing. There are 3 maneuvers: (1) With a good light coming from behind the examiner, have the patient swallow a sip of water. Observe the gland as it moves up and down. Enlargement and nodularity can often be noted. (2) Palpate the gland anteriorly. Gently press down with one thumb on one side of the gland to rotate the other lobe forward, and palpate as the patient swallows. (3) Palpate the gland from behind the patient with the middle 3 fingers on each lobe while the patient swallows. An outline of the gland can be traced on the skin of the neck and measured (Fig 7–28D). Nodules can be measured in a similar way. Thus, changes in the size of the gland or in nodules can be followed.

Each lobe of the normal thyroid gland measures about 2 cm in vertical dimension and about 1 cm in horizontal dimension above the isthmus. An enlarged thyroid gland has been called **goiter** (derived from French; ultimately from Latin *guttur* "throat"). Generalized enlargement is termed **diffuse goiter;** irregular or lumpy enlargement is called **nodular goiter.**

HYPOTHYROIDISM

Hypothyroidism is a clinical syndrome resulting from a deficiency of thyroid hormones, which in turn results in a generalized slowing down of metabolic processes. Hypothyroidism in infants and children results in marked slowing of growth and development, with serious permanent consequences including mental retardation. Hypothyroidism with onset in adulthood causes a generalized slowing down of the organism, with the deposition of glycosaminoglycans in intracellular spaces, particularly in skin and muscle, producing the clinical picture of **myxedema.** The symptoms of hypothyroidism in adults are largely reversible with therapy.

Etiology
(Table 7–6)

Hypothyroidism may be classified in a number of ways. It may be primary (thyroid failure), secondary (to pituitary TSH deficit), or tertiary (due to hypothalamic deficiency of TRH); or there may be an abnormality of the thyroxine (T_4) receptor in the cell, inducing peripheral resistance to the action of thyroid hormones. Hypothyroidism can also be classified as goitrous or nongoitrous, but this is probably unsatisfactory since Hashimoto's thyroiditis may produce hypothyroidism with or without goiter. The incidence of various causes of hypothyroidism will vary depending on geographic and environmental factors such as dietary iodide and goitrogen intake, the genetic characteristics of the population, and the age distribution of the population (pediatric or adult). The causes of hypothyroidism, listed in the approximate order of

Table 7–6. Etiology of hypothyroidism.

Primary:
1. Hashimoto's thyroiditis:
   a. With goiter.
   b. "Idiopathic" thyroid atrophy, presumably end-stage autoimmune thyroid disease, following either Hashimoto's thyroiditis or Graves' disease.
2. Radioactive iodine therapy for Graves' disease.
3. Subtotal thyroidectomy for Graves' disease or nodular goiter.
4. Excessive iodide intake (kelp, radiocontrast dyes).
5. Subacute thyroiditis.
6. Rare causes in the USA:
   a. Iodide deficiency.
   b. Other goitrogens such as lithium; antithyroid drug therapy.
   c. Inborn errors of thyroid hormone synthesis.

Secondary: Hypopituitarism due to pituitary adenoma, pituitary ablative therapy, or pituitary destruction.

Tertiary: Hypothalamic dysfunction (rare).

Peripheral resistance to the action of thyroid hormone.

their frequency in an adult population in the USA, are presented in Table 7–6.

Hashimoto's thyroiditis is probably the most common cause of hypothyroidism. In younger patients, it is more likely to be associated with goiter; in older patients, the gland may be totally destroyed by the immunologic process, and the only trace of the disease will be a persistently positive test for thyroid microsomal autoantibodies. Similarly, the end stage of Graves' disease may be hypothyroidism. This is accelerated by destructive therapy such as administration of radioactive iodine or subtotal thyroidectomy. Thyroid glands involved in autoimmune disease are particularly susceptible to excessive iodide intake (eg, ingestion of kelp tablets or iodide-containing cough preparations) or administration of iodide-containing radiographic contrast media. In these situations, the large amounts of iodide block thyroid hormone synthesis, producing hypothyroidism with goiter. Although the process may be temporarily reversed by withdrawal of iodide, the underlying disease will often progress, and permanent hypothyroidism will usually supervene. Hypothyroidism may occur during the late phase of subacute thyroiditis; this is usually transient, but it is permanent in about 10% of patients. Iodide deficiency is rarely a cause of hypothyroidism in the USA but may be more common in underdeveloped countries. Certain drugs can block hormone synthesis and produce hypothyroidism with goiter; at present, the most common pharmacologic cause of hypothyroidism (other than iodide) is lithium carbonate, used for the treatment of manic-depressive states. The antithyroid drugs propylthiouracil and methimazole in continuous dosage will do the same. Inborn errors of thyroid hormone synthesis will result in severe hypothyroidism if the block in hormone synthesis is complete or will result in mild hypothyroidism if the block is partial.

Pituitary and hypothalamic deficiencies as causes for hypothyroidism are quite rare and are usually associated with other symptoms and signs. Peripheral resistance to thyroid hormones is extremely rare, occurs in families, and is characterized by high serum concentrations of T_4 and T_3, goiter, and features of hypothyroidism rather than hyperthyroidism.

Pathogenesis

Thyroid hormone deficiency affects every tissue in the body, so that the symptoms are multiple. Pathologically, the most characteristic finding is the accumulation of glycosaminoglycans—mostly hyaluronic acid—in interstitial tissues. Accumulation of this hydrophilic substance accounts for the interstitial edema that is particularly evident in the skin, heart muscle, and striated muscle. The accumulation is due not to excessive synthesis but to decreased destruction of glycosaminoglycans.

Clinical Presentations

A. Newborn Infants (Cretinism): The term cretinism was originally applied in endemic goiter areas to infants with mental retardation, short stature, a characteristic puffy appearance of the face and hands, and (frequently) deaf mutism and pyramidal tract signs (Fig 7-29). In the USA, neonatal screening programs have revealed that approximately one out of 4000 neonates will have a low T_4 and elevated TSH, indicative of primary neonatal hypothyroidism. This may be due to failure of the thyroid to descend during embryonic development from its origin at the base of the tongue to its usual site in the lower anterior neck, which results in an ''ectopic thyroid'' gland that functions poorly. Another cause of neonatal hypothyroidism is placental transfer of thyroid antibodies in a mother with Hashimoto's thyroiditis, which results in blocking of TSH action or antibody-related immune destruction of the fetal thyroid. Rare causes of neonatal hypothyroidism include administration during pregnancy of iodides, antithyroid drugs, or radioactive iodine for thyrotoxicosis.

The symptoms of hypothyroidism in newborns include respiratory difficulty, cyanosis, jaundice, poor feeding, hoarse cry, umbilical hernia, and marked retardation of bone maturation. The proximal tibial epiphysis and distal femoral epiphysis are present in almost all full-term infants with a body weight of over 2500 g. Absence of these epiphyses strongly suggests hypothyroidism. Because early treatment is essential to prevent permanent mental retardation, neonatal screening programs have been introduced to measure serum T_4 or TSH: A serum T_4 under 6 μg/dL or a serum TSH over 30 μU/mL is indicative of neonatal hypothyroidism. The diagnosis can then be confirmed by radiologic evidence of retarded bone age.

B. Children: Hypothyroidism in children is characterized by retarded growth and evidence of mental retardation. In the adolescent, precocious puberty may

Figure 7-29. A 9-month-old infant with hypothyroidism (cretinism). Note the puffy face, protuberant abdomen, umbilical hernia, and muscle weakness (infant cannot sit up unassisted).

Figure 7-30. Hypothyroidism in adult (myxedema). Note puffy face, puffy eyes, frowsy hair, and dull and apathetic appearance.

occur, and there may be enlargement of the sella turcica in addition to short stature. This is not due to pituitary tumor but probably to pituitary hypertrophy associated with excessive TSH production.

C. Adults: In adults, the common features of hypothyroidism include easy fatigability, coldness, weight gain, constipation, menstrual irregularities, and muscle cramps. Physical findings include a cool, dry skin, puffy face and hands, hoarse, husky voice, and slow reflexes (Fig 7–30). Reduced conversion of carotene to vitamin A and increased blood levels of carotene may give the skin a yellowish color.

Cardiovascular signs include bradycardia and cardiac enlargement; the enlargement may be due in part to interstitial edema and left ventricular dilatation but is often due to pericardial effusion (Fig 7–31). The ECG reveals low voltage of QRS complexes and P and T waves, with improvement on therapy (Fig 7–32). The degree of pericardial effusion can easily be determined by echocardiography. Cardiac output is reduced, although congestive heart failure and pulmonary edema are rarely noted. Although there is controversy about whether myxedema induces coronary artery disease, there is evidence that coronary

Figure 7–31. *Top:* Chest x-ray studies of patient with hypothyroid cardiomyopathy. *Left:* Before therapy, showing pronounced cardiomegaly. *Right:* Six months after institution of thyroxine therapy, the heart size has returned to normal. (Reproduced, with permission, from Reza MJ, Abbasi AS: Congestive cardiomyopathy in hypothyroidism. *West J Med* 1975;**123**:228.) *Bottom:* ECG of a 29-year-old woman with hypothyroidism *(A)* before and *(B)* after 2 months of therapy with levothyroxine sodium (Synthroid). CW, chest wall; RVW, right ventricular wall; RVC, right ventricular cavity; IVS, interventricular septum; LVC, left ventricular cavity; PWLV, posterior wall left ventricle. Note disappearance of pericardial effusion following levothyroxine therapy. (Reproduced, with permission, from Sokolow M, McIlroy MB: *Clinical Cardiology*, 4th ed. Lange, 1986.)

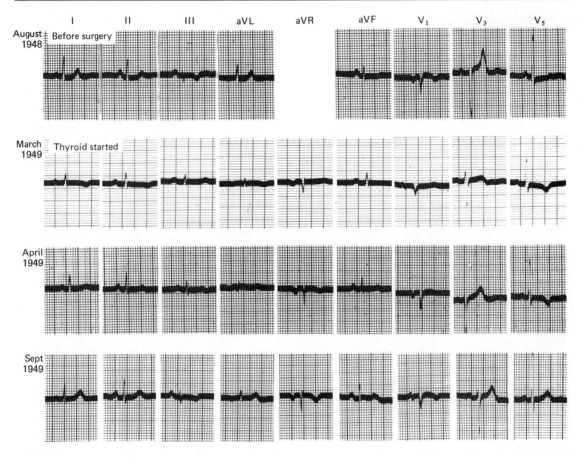

Figure 7–32. Hypothyroidism in a 47-year-old woman following thyroidectomy for hyperthyroidism in September 1948. BMR −51 in March 1949. Note progressive improvement in T waves after thyroid replacement was started in March 1949. (Reproduced, with permission, from Sokolow M, McIlroy MB: *Clinical Cardiology,* 4th ed. Lange, 1986.)

artery disease is more common in patients with hypothyroidism, particularly in older patients. For this reason, it is important to start levothyroxine replacement therapy in myxedematous patients over age 50 with very small doses, increasing the dose slowly over a period of several months.

Pulmonary function in adult hypothyroidism is characterized by shallow, slow respirations and impaired ventilatory responses to hypercapnia or hypoxia. This feature is important in the development of myxedema coma.

Intestinal peristalsis is markedly slowed, resulting in chronic constipation and occasionally severe fecal impaction.

Renal function is impaired, with decreased glomerular filtration rate and impaired ability to excrete a water load. This predisposes the myxedematous patient to water intoxication if excessive free water is administered.

There are at least 4 mechanisms that may contribute to **anemia** in patients with hypothyroidism: (1) impaired hemoglobin synthesis as a result of thyroxine deficiency; (2) iron deficiency from increased iron loss with menorrhagia, as well as impaired intestinal absorption of iron; (3) folate deficiency from impaired intestinal absorption of folic acid; and (4) pernicious anemia, with vitamin B_{12}-deficient megaloblastic anemia. The pernicious anemia is often part of a spectrum of autoimmune diseases: myxedema due to chronic thyroiditis, with thyroid autoantibodies present; pernicious anemia with parietal cell autoantibodies present; diabetes mellitus with islet cell autoantibodies present; adrenal insufficiency with adrenal autoantibodies present; etc.

Many patients complain of symptoms referable to the **neuromuscular system,** eg, severe muscle cramps, paresthesias, and muscle weakness.

Central nervous system symptoms may include chronic fatigue, lethargy, and inability to concentrate.

Hypothyroidism produces impaired peripheral metabolism of estrogens, with altered FSH and LH secretion, resulting in anovulatory cycles and infertility. This may also be associated with severe menorrhagia.

Patients with myxedema are usually quite placid but can be severely depressed or even extremely agitated (''myxedema madness'').

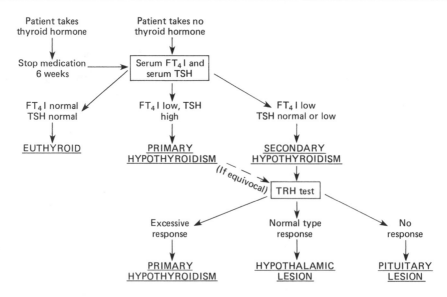

Figure 7–33. Diagnosis of hypothyroidism. Either free thyroxine (FT$_4$) or free thyroxine index (FT$_4$I) may be used with TSH for evaluation.

Diagnosis

The laboratory diagnosis of hypothyroidism is not difficult (Fig 7–33). A low serum T$_4$, low resin T$_3$ uptake, low free thyroxine, and elevated serum TSH are characteristic of primary hypothyroidism. Serum T$_3$ levels are variable and may be within the normal range. A positive test for thyroid autoantibodies suggests underlying Hashimoto's thyroiditis. In patients with pituitary myxedema, the FT$_4$I or FT$_4$ will be low but serum TSH will not be elevated. To differentiate pituitary from hypothalamic disease, the TRH test is most helpful (Fig 7–16). An elevated basal TSH level with excessive response indicates primary hypothyroidism. Absence of TSH response to TRH indicates pituitary deficiency. A partial or "normal" response indicates that pituitary function is intact but that a defect exists in hypothalamic secretion of TRH. Since pituitary or hypothalamic hypothyroidism is rare, TRH tests are usually unnecessary in the diagnosis of hypothyroidism.

The patient may be taking thyroid medication (levothyroxine or desiccated thyroid tablets) when first seen. A positive test for thyroid autoantibodies would suggest underlying Hashimoto's thyroiditis, in which case the medication should be continued. If antibodies are absent, the medication should be withdrawn for 6 weeks and determinations made for FT$_4$I or FT$_4$ and for TSH. The 6-week period of withdrawal is necessary because of the long half-life of thyroxine (8 days) and to allow the pituitary gland to recover after a long period of suppression. The pattern of recovery of thyroid function after withdrawal of T$_4$ is noted in Fig 7–34. In hypothyroid individuals, TSH becomes markedly elevated at 5–6 weeks and T$_4$ remains sub-normal, whereas both are normal after 6 weeks in euthyroid controls.

In patients with hypothyroidism, a delay in muscle contraction and relaxation is usually evident on physical examination, particularly in the biceps reflex. The speed of contraction and partial relaxation of the Achilles tendon reflex can be measured by the "photomotogram." The response in hypothyroidism (300–600 ms) overlaps the normal response (230–350 ms), so that the test is not useful for the diagnosis of hypothyroidism. However, the test is quite useful to follow patients under therapy. Improvement in reflex contraction and relaxation time will coincide with the clinical response to appropriate therapy.

The clinical picture of fully developed myxedema is usually quite clear, but the symptoms and signs of mild hypothyroidism may be very subtle. Patients with hypothyroidism will at times present with unusual features—neurasthenia with symptoms of muscle cramps, paresthesias, and weakness; anemia; disturbances in reproductive function, including infertility, delayed puberty, or menorrhagia; idiopathic edema or pleuropericardial effusions; retarded growth; obstipation; chronic rhinitis or hoarseness due to edema of nasal mucosa on vocal cords; and severe depression progressing to emotional instability or even frank paranoid psychosis. In such cases, the diagnostic studies outlined above will confirm or rule out hypothyroidism as a contributing factor.

Complications

A. Myxedema Coma: Myxedema coma is the end stage of untreated hypothyroidism. It is characterized by progressive weakness, stupor, hypothermia, hy-

Figure 7–34. Changes in T_4, T_3, TSH, and TRH response following abrupt withdrawal of suppressive thyroxine therapy. Note that in euthyroid individuals the T_4 may not return to normal until 6 weeks after withdrawal of therapy and that serum TSH is never elevated. In hypothyroid patients, TSH may be elevated as early as 2 weeks after withdrawal of therapy, and TRH response is exaggerated. LLN = lower limit of normal; ULN = upper limit of normal. (Reproduced, with permission, from Wood LC: Controversial questions in thyroid disease. Workshop in the Thyroid, American Thyroid Association, Nov 1979, as adapted from Vagenakis AG et al: Recovery of pituitary thyrotropic function after withdrawal of prolonged thyroid suppression therapy. *N Engl J Med* 1975;293:681.)

poventilation, hypoglycemia, hyponatremia, water intoxication, shock, and death. Although rare now, in the future it may occur more frequently in association with the increasing use of radioiodine for the treatment of Graves' disease, with resulting permanent hypothyroidism. Since it occurs most frequently in older

patients with underlying pulmonary and vascular disease, the mortality rate is extremely high.

The patient (or a family member if the patient is comatose) may recall previous thyroid disease, radioiodine therapy, or thyroidectomy. The medical history is of gradual onset of lethargy progressing to stupor or coma. Examination shows bradycardia and marked hypothermia, with body temperature as low as 24 °C (75 °F). The patient is usually an obese elderly woman with yellowish skin, a hoarse voice, a large tongue, thin hair, puffy eyes, ileus, and slow reflexes. There may be signs of other illnesses such as pneumonia, myocardial infarction, cerebral thrombosis, or gastrointestinal bleeding.

Laboratory clues to the diagnosis of myxedema coma include lactescent serum, high serum carotene, elevated serum cholesterol, and increased cerebrospinal fluid protein. Pleural, pericardial, or abdominal effusions with high protein content may be present. Serum tests will reveal a low T_4(RIA), low RT_3U, and usually a markedly elevated TSH. Thyroidal radioactive iodine uptake is low, and thyroid autoantibodies are usually strongly positive, indicating underlying thyroiditis. The ECG shows sinus bradycardia and low voltage. If laboratory studies are not readily available, which is frequently the case, the diagnosis must be made clinically.

The pathophysiology of myxedema coma involves 3 major aspects: (1) CO_2 retention and hypoxia, (2) fluid and electrolyte imbalance, and (3) hypothermia. CO_2 retention has long been recognized as an integral part of myxedema coma and had been attributed to such factors as obesity, heart failure, ileus, immobilization, pneumonia, pleural or peritoneal effusions, central nervous system depression, and weak chest muscles. More recently, Zwillich et al have demonstrated that the ventilatory responses to hypoxia are markedly depressed in patients with myxedema, as are the ventilatory responses to hypercapnia. These authors suggest that the failure of the myxedema patient to respond to hypoxia or hypercapnia may be associated with hypothermia. Thyroid hormone therapy in patients with myxedema markedly improves the ventilatory response to hypoxia. Because of the impaired ventilatory drive, assisted respiration is almost always necessary in patients with myxedema coma. The major fluid and electrolyte disturbance is water intoxication, which presents as hyponatremia and is managed by water restriction. Hypothermia is frequently not recognized, because the ordinary clinical thermometer only goes down to about 34 °C (94 °F); a laboratory type thermometer that registers a broader scale must be used to obtain accurate body temperature readings. The low body temperature may be due to diminished thyroxine stimulation of the sodium-potassium transport mechanism and decreased ATPase activity. Active rewarming of the body is contraindicated, because it may induce vasodilatation and vascular collapse. A rise in body temperature is a useful indication of therapeutic effectiveness of thyroxine.

Other disorders that may precipitate myxedema coma include heart failure, pulmonary edema, pleural or peritoneal effusions, ileus, and anemia. Adrenal insufficiency occurs occasionally in association with myxedema coma, but it is relatively rare and usually associated with either pituitary myxedema or concurrent autoimmune adrenal insufficiency (Schmidt's syndrome). Drug intoxication is quite common, and myxedema coma that develops in the hospital may be precipitated by administration of sedatives or narcotics. Seizures, bleeding episodes, hypocalcemia, or hypercalcemia may be present.

It is important to differentiate pituitary myxedema from primary myxedema. In pituitary myxedema, adrenal insufficiency may be present, and adrenal replacement is essential. Clinical clues to the presence of pituitary myxedema include a history of amenorrhea or impotence and physical evidence of scanty pubic or axillary hair. Laboratory findings will usually reveal normal serum cholesterol and normal or low pituitary TSH levels. On skull x-ray, the sella turcica may be enlarged. The treatment of myxedema coma is discussed below.

B. Myxedema With Heart Disease: Hypothyroidism has a direct effect upon the myocardium, causing interstitial edema, nonspecific myofibrillary swelling, and pericardial effusion, manifested by bradycardia and diminished cardiac output. These complications are usually completely reversible with appropriate therapy.

C. Myxedema With Coronary Artery Disease: Since myxedema frequently occurs in older persons, it is often associated with underlying coronary artery disease. In this situation, the low levels of circulating thyroid hormone actually protect the heart against increased demands that would result in increasing angina pectoris or myocardial infarction. Correction of the myxedema must be done very cautiously in order not to provoke arrhythmia, angina, or acute myocardial infarction. In some patients, it is necessary to perform coronary bypass surgery to improve coronary circulation before full replacement therapy can be instituted.

Treatment of Hypothyroidism

Hypothyroidism is treated with levothyroxine, which is available in pure form and is stable and inexpensive (Table 7–7). Levothyroxine is converted

in the body in part to T_3, so that both hormones become available even though only one is administered. Desiccated thyroid is unsatisfactory because of its variable hormone content, and triiodothyronine (as liothyronine) is unsatisfactory because of its rapid absorption and rapid disappearance from the bloodstream. The half-life of levothyroxine is about 8 days, so it need be given only once daily. Although only 40–60% of the preparation is absorbed, blood levels are easily monitored by following the free thyroxine index and serum TSH levels. Replacement doses of levothyroxine in adults range from 0.05 to 0.3 mg/d, with a mean of 0.18 mg/d. In infants under 1 year of age, the dose of levothyroxine is about 6 μg/kg/d; in older children (2–12 years), the dose is about 3–4 μg/kg/d; and in adults, the dose is about 2.2 μg/kg/d, or about 1 μg/lb/d.

Treatment of Myxedema With Heart Disease

In long-standing hypothyroidism or in older patients, particularly those with cardiovascular disease, it is imperative to start treatment slowly. Levothyroxine is given in a dosage of 0.025 mg/d for 2 weeks, increasing by 0.025 mg every 2 weeks until a daily dose of 0.1 or 0.15 mg is reached. It usually takes about 2 months for a patient to come into equilibrium on full dosage. In these patients, the heart is very sensitive to the level of circulating thyroxine, and if angina pectoris or cardiac arrhythmia develops, it is essential to reduce the dose of thyroxine immediately. In younger patients, or patients with mild disease, full replacement may be started immediately.

Treatment of Myxedema Coma

Myxedema coma is an acute medical emergency and should be treated in the intensive care unit. Blood gases must be monitored regularly, and the patient usually requires intubation and mechanical ventilation. Associated illnesses such as infections must be treated by appropriate therapy. Intravenous fluids should be administered with caution, and excessive free water intake must be avoided.

Because patients with myxedema coma absorb all drugs poorly, it is imperative to give levothyroxine intravenously. Holvey et al pointed out that these patients have marked depletion of serum thyroxine and a large number of empty binding sites on thyrox-

Table 7–7. Equivalence and cost of preparations available for the treatment of hypothyroidism.

	Average Daily Adult Dose (mg/d)	Approximate Daily Cost*	Comment
Levothyroxine (T_4)	0.15	$ 0.03	Best preparation.
Liothyronine sodium (T_3)	0.05	0.04	Difficult to monitor. Multiple doses required.
Desiccated thyroid	90	0.015	Variable potency.
Thyroglobulin	90	0.025	Difficult to monitor.
Liotrix (T_4/T_3 mixture)	(a) T_4 0.075, T_3 0.019 (b) T_4 0.09, T_3 0.023	0.05	Two different formulas.

*Data from *Guide to Prescription Drug Costs,* HCFA Publication 02104, Department of Health and Human Services, April, 1980.

ine-binding globulin and therefore should receive an initial loading dose of thyroxine intravenously, followed by a small daily intravenous dose. An initial dose of 300– 400 μg of levothyroxine is administered intravenously, followed by 50 μg of levothyroxine intravenously daily. This preparation is commercially available. Intravenous triiodothyronine (liothyronine) is not commercially available, and fresh, sterile solutions of liothyronine in alkaline buffer must be prepared daily. The clinical guides to improvement are a rise in body temperature and the return of normal cerebral function. Hydrocortisone hemisuccinate, 100 mg intravenously followed by 50 mg intravenously every 6 hours, is indicated if the patient has associated adrenal or pituitary insufficiency—and indeed has been recommended for all patients with myxedema coma. If the adrenal or pituitary status is not known, it is probably desirable to support the patient with intravenous hydrocortisone, but adrenal function is probably adequate in most patients with myxedema coma.

When giving levothyroxine intravenously in large doses, there is an inherent risk of precipitating angina, heart failure, or arrhythmias in older patients with underlying coronary artery disease. Thus, this type of therapy is not recommended for ambulatory patients with myxedema; it is better to start slowly and build up the dose as noted above.

Course & Prognosis

The course of untreated myxedema is one of slow deterioration leading eventually to myxedema coma and death. The results of treatment are very gratifying. Because of the long half-life (8 days) of thyroxine, it takes time to establish equilibrium on a fixed dose. Therefore, it is important to monitor the free thyroxine index and TSH levels every 4– 6 weeks until a normal balance is reached. Thereafter, the patient must be maintained on replacement therapy for life, with free thyroxine index and TSH monitoring about once a year.

The mortality rate of myxedema coma was about 80% at one time. The prognosis has been vastly improved by recognition of the importance of mechanically assisted respiration and the use of intravenous levothyroxine. At present, the outcome probably depends upon how well the underlying disease problems can be managed.

HYPERTHYROIDISM & THYROTOXICOSIS

Thyrotoxicosis is the clinical syndrome that results when tissues are exposed to high levels of circulating thyroid hormone. In most instances, thyrotoxicosis is due to hyperactivity of the thyroid gland, or hyperthyroidism. Occasionally, thyrotoxicosis may be due to other causes such as excessive ingestion of thyroid hormone or excessive secretion of thyroid hormone from ectopic sites. The various forms of thyrotoxicosis

Table 7–8. Conditions associated with thyrotoxicosis.

1. Diffuse toxic goiter (Graves' disease).
2. Toxic adenoma (Plummer's disease).
3. Toxic multinodular goiter (Marine-Lenhart syndrome).
4. Subacute thyroiditis.
5. Hyperthyroid phase of Hashimoto's thyroiditis.
6. Thyrotoxicosis factitia.
7. Rare forms of thyrotoxicosis: ovarian struma, metastatic thyroid carcinoma (follicular), hydatidiform mole, TSH-secreting pituitary tumor.

are listed in Table 7– 8. These syndromes will be discussed individually below.

1. DIFFUSE TOXIC GOITER (Graves' Disease)

Graves' disease is the most common form of thyrotoxicosis and may occur at any age, more commonly in females than in males. The syndrome consists of one or more of the following features: (1) thyrotoxicosis, (2) goiter, (3) ophthalmopathy (exophthalmos), and (4) dermopathy (pretibial myxedema).

Etiology

The cause of Graves' disease is not known. There is a strong familial predisposition in that about 15% of patients with Graves' disease have a close relative with the same disorder, and about 50% of relatives of patients with Graves' disease have circulating thyroid autoantibodies. Females are involved about 5 times more commonly than males. The disease may occur at any age, with a peak incidence in the 20- to 40-year age group. Human leukocyte antigen (HLA) typing has indicated an increased frequency of HLA-B8 and DR3 in Occidental and HLA-Bw35 in Oriental patients with Graves' disease and in their relatives, indicating a genetic factor in the pathogenesis of the disease.

Pathogenesis

The present concept of the pathogenesis of Graves' disease is that it is an autoimmune disease in which T lymphocytes become sensitized to antigens within the thyroid gland and stimulate B lymphocytes to synthesize antibodies to these antigens (Fig 7– 35). One such antibody may be directed against the TSH receptor site in the thyroid cell membrane and has the capacity to stimulate the thyroid cell to increased growth and function. This antibody has been called thyroid-stimulating immunoglobulin (TSI). Initially it was measured by bioassay in mice and was called long-acting thyroid stimulator (LATS). However, LATS could be detected in this heterologous assay in only about 50% of patients. When human thyroid tissue was used for detection of this antibody (either by increase in colloid droplet formation or increase in cAMP production), TSI could be detected in over

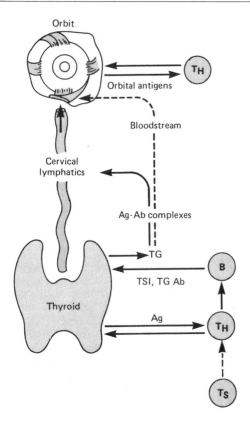

Figure 7–35. One theory of the pathogenesis of Graves' disease. There is a defect in suppressor T lymphocytes (T$_S$) that allows helper T lymphocytes (T$_H$) to stimulate B lymphocytes (B) to synthesize thyroid autoantibodies. The thyroid-stimulating immunoglobulin (TSI) is the driving force for thyrotoxicosis. Thyroglobulin autoantibodies (TG Ab) may combine with thyroglobulin (TG), forming immune complexes (Ag-Ab complexes) that can reach the orbit via the superior cervical lymphatic channels or by way of the bloodstream. These immune complexes can bind to orbital muscle and set up an inflammatory reaction in the muscle, causing the ophthalmopathy. T lymphocytes may then become sensitized to orbital antigens, maintaining prolonged ophthalmopathy. It is not yet clear what "triggers" the immunologic cascade.

90% of patients with Graves' disease. The presence of this circulating antibody was positively correlated with active disease and with relapse of the disease. It is not clear what "triggers" the acute episode. Volpé has suggested that there is a defect in immunoregulation with failure of "suppressor" T lymphocyte function, allowing "helper" T lymphocytes to stimulate B lymphocytes to produce immunoglobulins directed against the thyroid gland, some of which would have the capacity to stimulate the thyroid gland as TSI. Kriss et al have proposed that the ophthalmopathy of Graves' disease is due to deposition in orbital muscles of immune complexes such as thyroglobulin-antithyroglobulin complexes, initiating an immune complex inflammatory reaction. An alternative theory for

the pathogenesis of ophthalmopathy is that it is due to lymphocyte-mediated autoimmune disease involving orbital muscle. Both theories may be correct. The pathogenesis of the thyroid dermopathy (pretibial myxedema) and the rare subperiosteal inflammation has not yet been clarified.

Many of the symptoms of thyrotoxicosis suggest a possible synergism between epinephrine and thyroxine. Thus, findings include tachycardia, tremor, sweating, lid lag, and stare. Yet circulating levels of epinephrine are normal. This situation has been clarified by the discovery of an increased number of epinephrine binding sites in heart muscle in animals treated with thyroxine, suggesting that the increased epinephrine sensitivity of patients with thyrotoxicosis may be due to these increased epinephrine receptors.

Clinical Findings

A. Symptoms and Signs: In younger individuals, common manifestations include palpitations, nervousness, easy fatigability, hyperkinesia, diarrhea, excessive sweating, and preference for cold. Thyroid enlargement, thyrotoxic eye signs (see below), and mild tachycardia commonly occur. In addition, in children there is rapid growth with accelerated bone maturation. In older patients, cardiovascular and myopathic manifestations often predominate. Loss of muscle mass may be so severe that the patient cannot rise from a chair without assistance. In patients over the age of 60, the most common presenting complaints are palpitation, dyspnea on exertion, tremor, nervousness, and weight loss.

The eye signs of Graves' disease have been classified by the American Thyroid Association as noted in Table 7–9. Note that this classification utilizes the mnemonic "NO SPECS." Class 1 involves spasm of the upper lids associated with active thyrotoxicosis and usually resolves spontaneously when the thyrotoxicosis is adequately controlled. Classes 2 through 6 represent true infiltrative disease involving orbital

Table 7–9. Classification of eye changes in Graves' disease.*

Class	Definition
0	No signs or symptoms.
1	Only signs, no symptoms. (Signs limited to upper lid retraction, stare, lid lag.)
2	Soft tissue involvement (symptoms and signs).
3	Proptosis (measured with Hertel exophthalmometer).†
4	Extraocular muscle involvement.
5	Corneal involvement.
6	Sight loss (optic nerve involvement).

*Reproduced, with permission, from Werner SC: Classification of the eye changes of Graves' disease. *J Clin Endocrinol Metab* 1969;**29**:782 and 1977;**44**:203.
†Upper limits of normal according to race: Oriental, 18 mm; white, 20 mm; black, 22 mm. Increase in proptosis of 3–4 mm is mild involvement; 5–7 mm, moderate involvement; and over 8 mm, severe involvement. Other classes can be similarly graded as mild, moderate, or severe.

Figure 7–36. Patient with mild ophthalmopathy of Graves' disease. *Left:* Before radioactive iodine therapy. Note white sclera visible above and below the iris as well as mild periorbital edema. *Classification* (see Table 7–9): class 1, mild; class 2, mild; class 3, mild. *Right:* After radioactive iodine therapy. Marked improvement is noted.

Figure 7–37. Severe ophthalmopathy of Graves' disease. Note marked periorbital edema, injection of corneal blood vessels, and proptosis. There was also striking limitation of upward and lateral eye movements and reduced visual acuity. *Classification* (see Table 7–9): class 1, severe; class 2, severe; class 3, severe; class 4, severe; class 5, none; class 6, mild.

Figure 7–38. *A:* Hertel exophthalmometer. *B:* Proper use of the exophthalmometer. The edges of the instrument are placed on the lateral orbital ridges, and the distance from the orbital bone to the anterior cornea is read on the scale contained within the prisms.

muscles and orbital tissues (Figs 7–36 and 7–37). Class 2 represents soft tissue involvement with periorbital edema, congestion or redness of the conjunctiva, and swelling of the conjunctiva (chemosis). Class 3 represents proptosis as measured by the Hertel exophthalmometer. This instrument is illustrated in Fig 7–38A. It consists of 2 prisms with a scale, mounted on a bar. The prisms are placed on the lateral orbital ridges, and the distance from the orbital ridge to the anterior cornea is measured on the scale (Fig 7–38B). The upper limits of normal according to race are listed in the footnote to Table 7–9. Class 4 represents muscle involvement. The muscle most commonly involved in the infiltrative process is the inferior rectus, with involvement impairing upward gaze. The muscle second most commonly involved is the medial rectus, with involvement impairing lateral gaze. Class 5 represents corneal involvement (keratitis), and class 6 represents loss of vision from optic nerve involvement. Infiltrative ophthalmopathy is due to infiltration of the extraocular muscles with lymphocytes and edema fluid in an acute inflammatory reaction. This produces muscle enlargement with proptosis, periorbital edema, chemosis, and congestion of the conjunctiva (Fig 7–37). In addition, the impaired muscle movement results in diplopia. Ocular muscle enlargement has been demonstrated beautifully in orbital CT scans (Fig 7–39). When muscle swelling occurs posteriorly, toward the apex of the orbital cone, the optic nerve is compressed, and it is when this happens that loss of vision is likely to occur.

Thyroid dermopathy consists of thickening of the skin, particularly over the lower tibia, due to accumulation of glycosaminoglycans. It is relatively rare, occurring in about 2–3% of patients with Graves' disease (Fig 7–40). It is usually associated with ophthalmopathy. The skin is markedly thickened and cannot be picked up between the fingers. Sometimes dermopathy involves the entire lower leg and may

Figure 7–40. Dermopathy of Graves' disease. Marked thickening of the skin is noted, usually over the pretibial area. Thickening will occasionally extend downward over the ankle and the dorsal aspect of the foot but almost never above the knee.

extend onto the feet. Bony involvement (osteopathy), with subperiosteal bone formation and swelling, is particularly evident in the metacarpal bones (Fig 7–41). This too is a relatively rare finding. A more common finding in Graves' disease is separation of the nail from its bed, or onycholysis (Fig 7–42).

B. Laboratory Findings: T_3 is secreted in excess quantity early in the development of Graves' disease and in recurrences of Graves' disease. Thus, high levels of T_3 by radioimmunoassay and an elevated thyroid radioactive iodine uptake are the characteristic laboratory findings in Graves' disease. In addition, resin T_3 uptake and serum T_4 levels will also be elevated and TSH will be suppressed. Thyroid autoantibodies are usually present, particularly thyroid-stimulating immunoglobulin.

In patients with equivocal findings, it may be necessary to resort to special studies. The thyroid gland is normally suppressed when exogenous thyroid hormone is administered. In Graves' disease, the gland is driven by thyroid-stimulating immunoglobulin and is therefore nonsuppressible. Failure of radioiodine uptake to decrease or serum T_4 to fall after administration of triiodothyronine (liothyronine) in doses of 75–100 μg/d for 7–21 days is an indication that the gland is functioning autonomously and is strongly

Figure 7–39. Orbital CT scan in a patient with severe ophthalmopathy and visual failure. Note the marked enlargement of extraocular muscles posteriorly, with compression of the optic nerve at the apex of the orbital cone.

Figure 7–41. X-ray of hand of patient with thyroid osteopathy. Note marked periosteal thickening of the proximal phalanges.

Figure 7–42. Onycholysis (separation of the nail from its bed) in Graves' disease usually resolves spontaneously as the patient improves.

suggestive of Graves' disease. In addition, failure of TSH to rise following administration of TRH intravenously suggests that circulating levels of thyroid hormone are excessive and have suppressed the pituitary gland. The suppression test is useful in younger patients who have symptoms and signs of ophthalmopathy but whose findings in other thyroid function tests are normal. The TRH test is very useful in older patients who present with cardiac symptoms and no striking elevation of circulating thyroid hormone levels. The suppression test is contraindicated in these older patients, because of the hazard of cardiac complications. Echography and CT scans of the orbit have revealed muscle enlargement in most patients with Graves' disease even when there is no clinical evidence of ophthalmopathy. In patients with clinical evidence of ophthalmopathy, orbital muscle enlargement is frequently striking (Fig 7–37).

Differential Diagnosis

Graves' disease occasionally presents in an unusual or atypical fashion, in which case the diagnosis may not be obvious. Marked muscle atrophy may suggest severe myopathy that must be differentiated from primary neurologic disorder. Older patients with Graves' disease may present with symptoms of heart involvement, especially refractory atrial fibrillation or heart failure. This is characterized by high-output heart failure or chronic atrial fibrillation relatively insensitive to digoxin. Finally, patients with Graves' disease may present with infertility and amenorrhea as the primary symptoms. In all of these instances, the diagnosis of Graves' disease can usually be made with the above clinical and laboratory studies.

In the recently recognized syndrome called "familial dysalbuminemic hyperthyroxinemia," there is present in serum an abnormal albumin that preferentially binds T_4 but not T_3. This results in elevation of serum T_4 and FT_4I, but free T_4, T_3, and TSH are normal. It is important to differentiate this euthyroid state from hyperthyroidism. In addition to the lack of clinical features of hyperthyroidism, a normal serum T_3 and TSH level and a normal TRH response will rule out Graves' disease or toxic nodular goiter.

Complications

Thyrotoxic crisis ("thyroid storm") is the acute exacerbation of all of the symptoms of thyrotoxicosis, often presenting as a syndrome of such severity as to be life-threatening. Occasionally, thyroid storm may be mild and present simply as an unexplained febrile reaction after thyroid surgery in a patient who has been inadequately prepared. More commonly, it occurs in a more severe form, after surgery, radioactive iodine therapy, or parturition in a patient with thyrotoxicosis who has been inadequately controlled, or during a severe, stressful illness or disorder such as uncontrolled diabetes, trauma, acute infection, severe drug reaction, or myocardial infarction. The clinical manifestations of thyroid storm are marked hypermetabolism and excessive adrenergic response. Fever ranges from 38 to 41 °C (from 100 to 106 °F) and is associated with flushing and sweating. There is marked tachycardia, often with atrial fibrillation and high pulse pressure and occasionally with heart failure. Central nervous system symptoms include marked agitation, restlessness, delirium, and coma. Gastrointestinal symptoms will include nausea, vomiting, diarrhea, and jaundice. A fatal outcome will be associated with heart failure and shock.

At one time it was thought that "dumping" of stored thyroxine and triiodothyronine was responsible for thyroid storm. Careful studies have revealed that the serum levels of T_4 and T_3 in patients with thyroid storm are not higher than in thyrotoxic patients without this condition. There is no evidence that thyroid storm is due to excessive production of triiodothyronine. There is evidence that in thyrotoxicosis there are increased numbers of binding sites for catecholamines, so that heart and nervous tissues have increased sensitivity to circulating catecholamines. In addition, there is decreased binding to TBG, with elevation of free T_3 and T_4. The present theory is that in this setting, with increased binding sites available for catecholamines, an acute illness, infection, or surgical stress triggers an outpouring of catecholamines which, in association with high levels of free T_4 and T_3, precipitate the acute problem.

The most striking clinical diagnostic feature of thyrotoxic crisis is hyperpyrexia out of proportion to other findings. Laboratory findings include elevated serum T_4, FT_4I, and T_3 by radioimmunoassay.

Treatment

Although autoimmune mechanisms are responsible for the syndrome of Graves' disease, management has been largely directed toward controlling the hyperthyroidism. Three good methods are available: (1) antithyroid drug therapy, (2) surgery, and (3) radioactive iodine therapy.

A. Antithyroid Drug Therapy: In general, antithyroid drug therapy is most useful in young patients with small glands and mild disease. The drugs (propylthiouracil or methimazole) are given until the disease undergoes spontaneous remission. This occurs in 20–40% of patients treated for 6 months to 15 years. Although this is the only therapy that leaves an intact thyroid gland, it does require a long period of observation, and the incidence of relapse is high, perhaps 60–80% even in selected patients. Antithyroid drug therapy is generally started with large divided doses; when the patient becomes clinically euthyroid, maintenance therapy may be achieved with a lower single morning dose. A common regimen consists of giving propylthiouracil, 100–150 mg every 6 hours initially, and then in 4–8 weeks reducing the dose to 50–200 mg once or twice daily. Propylthiouracil has one advantage over methimazole in that it partially inhibits the conversion of T_4 to T_3, so that it is effective in bringing down the levels of activated thyroid hormone more quickly. On the other hand, methimazole has a longer duration of action and is more useful if a single daily dose is desirable. The laboratory tests of most value in monitoring the course of therapy are serum T_3 (by RIA) and free thyroxine.

1. Duration of therapy–The optimal duration of therapy of antithyroid drugs is quite variable. Sustained remissions can be predicted in patients with the following characteristics: (1) The thyroid gland returns to normal size. (2) The patient can be controlled on a relatively small dose of antithyroid drugs. (3) TSI is no longer detectable in the serum. (4) The thyroid gland becomes normally suppressible following the administration of liothyronine.

2. Reaction to drugs–Reactions to antithyroid drugs most commonly involve either a rash (about 5% of patients) or agranulocytosis (about 0.5% of patients). The rash may frequently be managed by simple addition of antihistamines and is not necessarily an indication for discontinuing the medication unless it is severe and generalized. Agranulocytosis is an indication for immediate cessation of antithyroid drug therapy, institution of appropriate antibiotic therapy, and shifting to an alternative type of therapy. Agranulocytosis is usually heralded by sore throat and fever. Thus, all patients receiving antithyroid drugs are instructed that if sore throat or fever develops, they should immediately stop taking the drug and see a physician, who should obtain a white count and differential count. Cholestatic jaundice, hepatocellular toxicity, and acute arthralgia are rare side effects but require cessation of drug therapy when they do occur.

B. Surgical Treatment: Subtotal thyroidectomy is the treatment of choice for patients with very large glands or multinodular goiters.

The patient is prepared with antithyroid drugs until euthyroid (about 6 weeks). In addition, starting 2 weeks before the day of operation, the patient is given saturated solution of potassium iodide, 5 drops twice daily. This regimen has been shown empirically to diminish the vascularity of the gland and to simplify surgery.

There is disagreement about how much thyroid tissue should be removed. Total thyroidectomy is usually not necessary unless the patient has severe progressive ophthalmopathy (see below). On the other hand, if too much thyroid tissue is left behind, the disease will relapse. Most surgeons leave 2–3 g of thyroid tissue on either side of the neck. Although some patients do not require thyroid supplementation following thyroidectomy for Graves' disease, some patients do.

Hypoparathyroidism and recurrent laryngeal nerve injury occur as complications of surgery in about 1% of cases.

C. Radioactive Iodine Therapy: Therapy with sodium ^{131}I is the preferred treatment for most patients over age 21. In many patients without underlying heart disease, radioactive iodine may be given immediately in a dosage of 80–120 μCi/g of thyroid weight estimated on the basis of physical examination and sodium ^{123}I rectilinear scan. The dosage is corrected for iodine uptake according to the following formula:

$$80-120 \ \mu Ci/g \ \times \ \begin{array}{c} \text{Estimated} \\ \text{weight of} \\ \text{gland in} \\ \text{grams} \end{array} \ \times \ \frac{100}{\begin{array}{c} \text{24-Hour radio-} \\ \text{active iodine} \\ \text{uptake (\%)} \end{array}} \ = \ \text{Dose in } \mu Ci$$

In patients with underlying heart disease, severe thyrotoxicosis, or large glands (> 100 g), it is often desirable to achieve a euthyroid state before radioactive iodine is started. These patients are treated with antithyroid drugs (as above) until they are euthyroid; medication is then stopped for 5–7 days; radioactive iodine uptake is then determined and a scan is done; and a dose of 120–150 $\mu Ci/g$ of estimated thyroid weight is calculated on the basis of this uptake. A slightly larger dose is necessary in patients previously treated with antithyroid drugs. Following the administration of radioactive iodine, the gland will shrink and the patient will usually become euthyroid over a period of 6–12 weeks.

The major complication of radioactive therapy is hypothyroidism, which ultimately develops in 80% or more of patients who are adequately treated. However, this complication may indeed be the best assurance that the patient will not have a recurrence of hyperthyroidism. Serum free thyroxine index and TSH levels should be followed, and if they show the development of hypothyroidism, prompt replacement therapy with levothyroxine, 0.1–0.2 mg daily, is instituted.

It is of interest that hypothyroidism may occur after any type of therapy for Graves' disease and may occasionally be the outcome of ''burned-out'' Graves' disease. Accordingly, all patients with Graves' disease require lifetime follow-up to be certain that they remain in a euthyroid state.

D. Other Medical Measures: During the acute phase of thyrotoxicosis, beta-adrenergic blocking agents are extremely helpful. Propranolol, 10–40 mg every 6 hours, will control tachycardia, hypertension, and atrial fibrillation. This drug is gradually withdrawn as serum thyroxine levels return to normal. Adequate nutrition, including multivitamin supplements, is essential. Barbiturates accelerate T_4 metabolism, and phenobarbital may be helpful both for its sedative effect and to lower T_4 levels.

Treatment of Complications

A. Thyrotoxic Crisis: Thyrotoxic crisis (thyroid storm) requires vigorous management. Propranolol, 1–2 mg slowly intravenously or 40–80 mg every 6 hours orally, is extremely helpful in controlling the severe cardiovascular symptoms. In the presence of severe heart failure or asthma, one can use reserpine, 1 mg intramuscularly every 6 hours, or guanethidine, 1–2 mg/kg in divided doses orally daily. Hormone release is retarded by the administration of sodium iodide, 1 g intravenously over a 24-hour period, or saturated solution of potassium iodide, 10 drops twice

daily. Hormone synthesis is blocked by the administration of propylthiouracil, 250 mg every 6 hours. The conversion of T_4 to T_3 is partially blocked by the combination of propranolol and propylthiouracil and the administration of hydrocortisone hemisuccinate, 50 mg intravenously every 6 hours. Supportive therapy includes a cooling blanket and acetaminophen to help control fever. Aspirin is probably contraindicated, because of its tendency to bind to TBG and displace thyroxine, rendering more thyroxine available in the free state. Fluids, electrolytes, and nutrition are important. For sedation, phenobarbital is probably best because it accelerates the peripheral metabolism and inactivation of thyroxine and triiodothyronine, ultimately bringing these levels down. Oxygen, diuretics, and digitalis are indicated for heart failure. Finally, it is essential to treat the underlying disease process that may have precipitated the acute exacerbation. Thus, antibiotics, anti-allergy drugs, and postoperative care are indicated for management of these problems. As an extreme measure (rarely needed) to control thyrotoxic crisis, plasmapheresis or peritoneal dialysis may be used to remove high levels of circulating thyronines.

B. Ophthalmopathy: Management of ophthalmopathy due to Graves' disease involves treatment of thyroid disease. In the opinion of one of the authors (FSG), total surgical excision of the thyroid gland or total ablation of the thyroid gland with radioactive iodine is indicated. Although there is controversy over the need for total ablation, removal or destruction of the thyroid gland certainly prevents exacerbations and relapses that may worsen residual ophthalmopathy. Keeping the patient's head elevated will diminish periorbital edema. For the severe acute inflammatory reaction, a short course of corticosteroid therapy is frequently effective, eg, prednisone, 100 mg daily orally in divided doses for 7–14 days, then every other day for 6–12 weeks. If corticosteroid therapy is not effective, external x-ray therapy to the retro-orbital area may be helpful. The dose is usually 2000 rads in 10 fractions given over a period of 2 weeks. The lens and anterior chamber structures must be shielded.

In very severe cases with threat to vision, orbital decompression can be used. One type of orbital decompression involves the transantral approach through the maxillary sinus, removing the floor and the lateral walls of the orbit. This has been extremely effective, and exophthalmos can be reduced by 5–7 mm in each eye by this technique. After the acute process has subsided, the patient is frequently left with double vision or lid abnormalities due to muscle fibrosis and contracture. These can be corrected by cosmetic lid surgery or eye muscle surgery.

Thyrotoxicosis & Pregnancy

Thyrotoxicosis during pregnancy presents a special problem. Radioactive iodine is contraindicated, because it crosses the placenta freely and may injure the fetal thyroid. Two good alternatives are available. If the disease is detected during the first trimester, the patient can be prepared with propylthiouracil, and subtotal thyroidectomy can be performed safely during the mid trimester. It is essential to provide thyroid supplementation during the balance of the pregnancy. Alternatively, the patient can be treated with antithyroid drugs throughout the pregnancy, postponing the decision regarding long-term management until after delivery. The dosage of antithyroid drugs must be kept to the minimum necessary to control symptoms, because these drugs cross the placenta and may affect the function of the fetal thyroid gland. If the disease can be controlled by initial doses of propylthiouracil of 300 mg or less and maintenance doses of 50– 150 mg/d, the likelihood of fetal hypothyroidism is extremely small. The free thyroxine index should be maintained in the upper range of normal by downward adjustment of propylthiouracil dosage. Supplemental thyroxine is not necessary. Breast feeding is not contraindicated, because propylthiouracil is not concentrated in the milk.

Graves' disease may occur in the newborn infant. There seem to be 2 neonatal forms of the disease. In both types, the mother has a current or recent history of Graves' disease. In the first type, the child is born small, with weak muscles, tachycardia, fever, and frequently respiratory distress or neonatal jaundice. Examination reveals an enlarged thyroid gland and occasionally reveals prominent, puffy eyes. The heart rate is rapid, temperature is elevated, and heart failure may ensue. Laboratory studies reveal an elevated FT_4I, a markedly elevated T_3, and usually a low TSH—in contrast to normal infants who have elevated TSH at birth. Bone age may be accelerated. TSI is often found in the serum of both the infant and the mother. The pathogenesis of this syndrome is thought to involve transplacental transfer of TSI from mother to fetus, with subsequent development of thyrotoxicosis. The disease is self-limited and subsides over a period of 4– 12 weeks, coinciding with the fall in the child's TSI. Therapy includes propylthiouracil in a dose of 5– 10 mg/kg/d (in divided doses at 8-hour intervals); strong iodine (Lugol's) solution, 1 drop (8 mg potassium iodide) every 8 hours; and propranolol, 2 mg/kg/d in divided doses. In addition, adequate nutrition, antibiotics for infection if present, sedatives if necessary, and supportive therapy are indicated. If the child is very toxic, corticosteroid therapy (prednisone, 2 mg/kg/d) will partially block conversion of T_4 to T_3 and may be helpful in the acute phase. The above medications are gradually reduced as the child improves and can usually be discontinued by 6– 12 weeks.

A second form of neonatal Graves' disease occurs in children from families with a high incidence of Graves' disease. Symptoms develop more slowly and may not be noted until the child is 3– 6 months old. This syndrome is thought to be a true genetic inheritance of defective lymphocyte immunoregulation. It is much more serious in terms of severity, with a 20% mortality rate and evidence of persistent brain dysfunction even after successful treatment. The hyper-thyroidism may persist for months or years and requires prolonged therapy.

Course & Prognosis

In general, the course of Graves' disease is one of remissions and exacerbations over a protracted period of time unless the gland is destroyed by surgery or radioactive iodine. Although some patients may remain euthyroid for long periods after treatment, many eventually develop hypothyroidism. Lifetime follow-up is therefore indicated for all patients with Graves' disease.

2. OTHER FORMS OF THYROTOXICOSIS

Toxic Adenoma (Plummer's Disease)

Thyrotoxicosis may develop because of a single adenoma, usually a follicular adenoma, hypersecreting T_3 and T_4. These lesions start out as a "hot nodule" on the thyroid scan, slowly increase in size, and gradually suppress the other lobe of the thyroid gland (Fig 7– 43).

The typical patient is an older individual (usually over 40) who has noted recent growth of a long-standing thyroid nodule. Symptoms of weight loss, weakness, shortness of breath, palpitation, tachycardia, and heat intolerance are noted. Eye signs are almost never present. Physical examination reveals a definite nodule on one side, with very little thyroid tissue on the other side. Laboratory studies usually reveal marked elevation in serum T_3 levels, with only borderline elevation of thyroxine levels. The scan reveals that the nodule is "hot." Toxic adenomas are

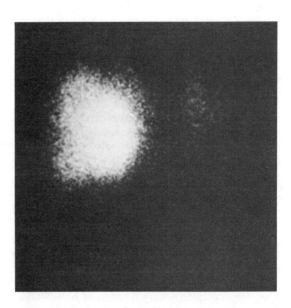

Figure 7–43. Toxic nodule of the right lobe of the thyroid gland as it appears on ^{99m}Tc pertechnetate scan. Note that the left lobe of the gland has been almost completely suppressed. (Courtesy of JM Lowenstein.)

almost always follicular adenomas and almost never malignant. They are easily managed by administration of antithyroid drugs such as propylthiouracil, 100 mg every 6 hours, or methimazole, 10 mg every 6 hours, followed by unilateral lobectomy; or with radioactive iodine. Sodium ^{131}I in doses of 20–30 mCi is usually required to destroy the benign neoplasm. Radioactive iodine is preferable for smaller toxic nodules, but larger ones are best managed by operation.

Toxic Multinodular Goiter
(Marine-Lenhart Syndrome)

This disorder occurs in older patients with long-standing multinodular goiter. Ophthalmopathy is extremely rare. Clinically, the patient presents with tachycardia, heart failure, or arrhythmia and sometimes weight loss, nervousness, tremors, and sweating. Laboratory studies reveal a striking elevation in serum T_3 levels, with less striking elevation in serum T_4 levels. Radioiodine scan reveals multiple functioning nodules in the gland, although occasionally one may see an irregular, patchy distribution of radioactive iodine (Fig 7–44).

Hyperthyroidism in patients with multinodular goiters can often be precipitated by the administration of iodides (jodbasedow effect, or iodide-induced hyperthyroidism). It was at first thought that jodbasedow effect occurred only in iodine-deficient geographic areas and that administration of iodides supplied the "building blocks" for hypersecretion of T_4 and T_3. However, Vagenakis et al have reported that 4 out of 8 patients with nontoxic goiters who lived in a high-iodine area (Boston) and who received 5 drops of saturated solution of potassium iodide daily developed hyperthyroidism. Thus, large doses of iodide can in-

duce hyperthyroidism in any patient with a nontoxic goiter regardless of the geographic locality.

The management of this problem is somewhat difficult. Ideally, subtotal thyroidectomy would be the treatment of choice, but these patients are often poor operative risks. Alternatively, one can give relatively large doses of radioactive iodine, but the multinodular goiter will not be destroyed, and repeated doses of radioactive iodine may be necessary. Antithyroid drugs are effective only on a temporary basis to bring the patient to a euthyroid state. They should be used prior to surgery or radioactive iodine therapy in order to diminish the stress of these procedures. Propranolol may be helpful to control the cardiac problems.

Subacute Thyroiditis

This entity will be discussed in a separate section, but it should be mentioned here that thyroiditis may present as an acute release of T_4 and T_3 with symptoms of thyrotoxicosis. The typical patient is a young person with a history of malaise and complaints of neck pain, tachycardia, weight loss, and sweating. The thyroid gland is large and slightly tender. Laboratory findings reveal elevated free thyroxine index and serum T_3 but a very low radioactive iodine uptake, often less than 1%. The erythrocyte sedimentation rate is usually markedly elevated. This disease will usually subside spontaneously, although the patient may require propranolol to control cardiovascular symptoms and aspirin for local pain and discomfort.

Hashimoto's Thyroiditis

Hashimoto's thyroiditis can also go through an acute phase with increased T_3 and T_4 release, producing transient hyperthyroidism. This too is associated with high T_3 and T_4 levels and very low radioactive iodine uptake. It is important to differentiate Hashimoto's thyroiditis from true Graves' disease, since the former will resolve spontaneously and does not require surgery, antithyroid drug therapy, or radioactive iodine. In most cases, propranolol is the only therapy required.

Thyrotoxicosis Factitia

This is a psychoneurotic disturbance in which excessive amounts of thyroxine or thyroid hormone are ingested, usually for purposes of weight control. The individual is often someone connected with medicine to whom thyroid medication is easily available. Features of thyrotoxicosis, including weight loss, nervousness, palpitation, tachycardia, and tremor, may be present, but no goiter or eye signs. Characteristically, the serum T_4 and T_3 levels are elevated and radioactive iodine uptake nil. Management requires careful discussion of the hazards of long-term thyroxine therapy, particularly cardiovascular damage and muscle wasting. Formal psychotherapy may be necessary.

Figure 7–44. Toxic multinodular goiter as it appears on ^{99m}Tc pertechnetate scan. Note multiple functioning thyroid nodules. (Courtesy of JM Lowenstein.)

Rare Forms of Thyrotoxicosis

A. Struma Ovarii: In this syndrome, teratoma of

the ovary contains thyroid tissue, and the thyroid tissue becomes hyperactive. Mild features of thyrotoxicosis result, such as weight loss and tachycardia, but there is no evidence of goiter or eye signs. Free thyroxine index and serum T_3 are usually mildly elevated, and the radioiodine uptake in the neck will be nil. Body scan reveals uptake of radioiodine in the pelvis. The disease is curable with removal of the teratoma.

B. Thyroid Carcinoma: Carcinoma of the thyroid, particularly follicular carcinoma, may concentrate radioactive iodine, but only rarely does it retain the ability to convert this iodide into active hormone. There have been a few instances of metastatic thyroid cancer presenting with hyperthyroidism. The clinical picture consists of weakness, weight loss, and palpitation, without goiter or ophthalmopathy. Body scan reveals areas of uptake usually distant from the thyroid, eg, bone or lung. Treatment with large doses of radioactive iodine may destroy the metastatic deposits.

C. Hydatidiform Mole: Hydatidiform mole produces chorionic gonadotropin, which has intrinsic TSH-like activity. This may induce thyroid hyperplasia, increased iodine turnover, and mild elevation of serum T_4 and T_3 levels. It is rarely associated with overt thyrotoxicosis and is totally curable by removal of the mole.

D. Syndrome of Inappropriate TSH Secretion: A group of patients have recently been reported with elevated serum immunoreactive TSH in association with elevated serum free thyroxine values. This has been called the "syndrome of inappropriate TSH secretion." Two types of problems are found: (1) TSH-secreting pituitary adenoma and (2) nonneoplastic pituitary hypersecretion of TSH.

Patients with TSH-secreting pituitary adenomas usually present with mild thyrotoxicosis and goiter, usually with amenorrhea. There are no eye signs of Graves' disease. Study reveals elevated total and free serum T_4 and T_3. There is no response to TRH, and the increased radioactive iodine uptake is not suppressible with exogenous thyroid hormone. On the other hand, serum TSH, usually undetectable in Graves' disease, is elevated. Visual field examination may reveal temporal defects, and CT scanning of the sella reveals a pituitary tumor. Management usually involves control of the thyrotoxicosis with antithyroid drugs and removal of the pituitary tumor via transsphenoidal hypophysectomy. If the tumor cannot be completely removed, it may be necessary to treat residual tumor with radiation therapy and to control thyrotoxicosis with radioactive iodine.

Nonneoplastic pituitary hypersecretion of TSH is essentially a form of pituitary (and occasionally peripheral) resistance to T_3 and T_4. Thus, increasing levels of T_3 and T_4 fail to suppress pituitary TSH secretion, and TSH pours out. Patients with only pituitary resistance to T_3 and T_4 present with goiter and hyperthyroidism, elevated free T_4, elevated TSH, normal response to TRH, and a normal response to T_3 suppression. These patients act as if the pituitary set point for T_3 suppression is at a higher than normal

level. Patients with both pituitary and peripheral resistance to thyroid hormones will present with goiter, elevated T_3 and T_4, and elevated TSH, but they are euthyroid or mildly hypothyroid. This syndrome is familial and has been called **Refetoff's syndrome.**

Management of these syndromes is difficult. If the patient is hypothyroid or euthyroid, T_3 therapy may be effective in maintaining a euthyroid state and reducing TSH. In the hyperthyroid patient, bromocriptine may lower TSH and control thyrotoxic symptoms.

NONTOXIC GOITER

Etiology

Nontoxic goiter usually represents enlargement of the thyroid gland from TSH stimulation, which in turn results from inadequate thyroid hormone synthesis. Table 7–10 lists some of the causes of nontoxic goiter. Iodine deficiency was the most common cause of nontoxic goiter or "endemic goiter"; with the widespread use of iodized salt and the introduction of iodides into fertilizers, animal feeds, and food preservatives, iodide deficiency in developed countries is relatively rare. The only remaining areas of endemic goiter are in inland, undeveloped regions such as the Himalayas, the Andes, Central Africa, and New Guinea. It does not exist in the USA. Estimated optimal iodine requirements for adults are in the range of 150–300 $\mu g/d$. In endemic goiter areas, the daily urinary excretion of iodine falls below 50 $\mu g/d$; in areas where iodine is extremely scarce, excretion falls below 20 $\mu g/d$. The mechanism for goiter formation is thought to be low iodine intake, impaired hormone formation, increased TSH secretion, and hyperplasia of thyroid cells.

Dietary goitrogens are a rare cause of goiter, and of these the most common is iodide itself. Large doses of iodides used (for example) in the treatment of chronic pulmonary disease may in susceptible individuals produce goiter and hypothyroidism. Withdrawal of iodide reverses the process. Other goitrogens include lithium carbonate, used for the treatment of manic-depressive psychosis, and some vegetable foodstuffs such as thioglucosides, found in cabbage, and goitrin, found in certain roots and seeds. Cyanogenic glycosides found in cassava can release thiocyanates that may cause goiter, particularly in the presence of iodide defi-

Table 7–10. Etiology of nontoxic goiter.

1. Iodine deficiency.
2. Goitrogen in the diet.
3. Hashimoto's thyroiditis.
4. Subacute thyroiditis.
5. Inadequate hormone synthesis due to inherited defect in thyroidal enzymes necessary for T_4 and T_3 biosynthesis.
6. Inherited deficiency in T_4 receptor in cell membrane (rare).
7. Neoplasm, benign or malignant.

ciency. The role of these vegetable goitrogens in the production of goiter is not clearly established.

Thyroid enlargement may occur in adolescents, particularly at the time of menarche, or as a result of pregnancy or ingestion of oral contraceptive drugs. It was at first thought that these goiters were due to increased thyroxine-binding globulin and increased demands upon the thyroid to maintain a larger extra-thyroidal hormone pool. However, many of these patients have underlying chronic lymphocytic thyroiditis (Hashimoto's thyroiditis), which is the real cause of the goiter. Hashimoto's thyroiditis is a common illness, particularly in women. Hormone synthesis is impaired, and thyroid enlargement develops. In subacute thyroiditis, thyroid enlargement occurs in association with acute inflammatory changes, presumably due to viral infection (see below).

Nontoxic goiter may occur as a result of synthesis resulting from genetic deficiencies in enzymes necessary for hormone biosynthesis (thyroid dyshormonogenesis). These effects may be complete, resulting in a syndrome of cretinism with goiter; or partial, resulting in nontoxic goiter with mild hypothyroidism. At least 5 separate biosynthetic abnormalities have been reported: (1) impaired transport of iodine; (2) deficient peroxidase with impaired oxidation of iodide to iodine and failure to incorporate iodine into thyroglobulin; (3) impaired coupling of iodinated tyrosines to triiodothyronine or tetraiodothyronine; (4) absence or deficiency of iodotyrosine deiodinase, so that iodine is not conserved within the gland; and (5) excessive production of metabolically inactive iodoprotein by the thyroid gland. In addition, it has been demonstrated that impaired formation of thyroglobulin, or synthesis of abnormal thyroglobulin, may result in inadequate hormone production. In all of these syndromes, impaired production of thyroid hormones presumably results in TSH release and goiter formation.

Finally, thyroid enlargement can be due to a benign lesion, such as adenoma, or to a malignant one such as carcinoma.

Pathogenesis

It has been demonstrated quite clearly that the pathogenetic mechanism of nontoxic goiter due to dyshormonogenesis involves first diffuse hyperplasia, followed by focal hyperplasia with necrosis and hemorrhage, and finally the development of new areas of focal hyperplasia. Thus, a diffuse nontoxic goiter progresses over a period of time to a multinodular nontoxic goiter.

Clinical Findings

A. Symptoms and Signs: Patients with nontoxic goiter usually present with thyroid enlargement, which may be diffuse or multinodular. The gland may be relatively firm but is often extremely soft. Over a period of time, the gland becomes larger and larger, so that in long-standing multinodular goiter, huge goiters may develop and extend inferiorly to present as substernal goiter. The patient may complain of pressure symptoms in the neck, particularly on moving the head upward or downward, and of difficulty in swallowing. Vocal cord paresis is rare. There may be symptoms of mild hypothyroidism, but most of these patients are euthyroid. Thyroid enlargement represents compensated hypothyroidism.

B. Laboratory Findings: Laboratory studies will reveal a low or normal free thyroxine index and, usually, normal levels of TSH. It is assumed that at the time the studies are made the patient has come into equilibrium or balance, so that TSH levels are not elevated. In patients with dyshormonogenesis due to abnormal iodoprotein synthesis, PBI may be elevated out of proportion to serum T_4, because of secretion of nonhormonal organic iodide compounds.

C. Scan Studies: Isotope scanning usually reveals a patchy uptake, frequently with focal areas of uptake corresponding to ''hot'' nodules. Radioactive uptake usually is suppressible on administration of thyroid hormones such as liothyronine. Echography may reveal cystic changes in one or more of the nodules, representing previous hemorrhage and necrosis.

Differential Diagnosis

The major problem of differential diagnosis is to rule out cancer. This will be discussed in more detail in the section on thyroid carcinoma.

Treatment

With the exception of those due to neoplasm, the management of nontoxic goiter consists simply of giving thyroid hormones until TSH is completely sup-

Figure 7–45. Multinodular goiter at the time of surgery. The asymmetric enlargement and the nodularity are apparent, as is the rightward deviation of the trachea resulting from marked enlargement of the lobe.

pressed. Levothyroxine in doses of 0.15–0.2 mg daily will suppress pituitary TSH and result in slow regression of the goiter as well as correction of hypothyroidism. Long-standing goiters may have areas of necrosis, hemorrhage, and scarring that will not regress on thyroxine therapy. However, the lesions will not grow while the patient is taking thyroxine.

The gross appearance of a multinodular goiter at the time of surgery is presented in Fig 7–45. Note that the left lobe of the gland extends from the middle of the thyroid cartilage to just above the clavicle. The pressure of this enlargement has caused deviation of the trachea to the right. The surface of the gland is irregular, with many large and small nodules. Although these multinodular goiters are rarely malignant, the size of the mass with resulting pressure symptoms may require subtotal thyroidectomy.

Course & Prognosis

Patients with nontoxic goiter must usually take levothyroxine for life. They should avoid iodides, which may induce either hyperthyroidism or, in the absence of thyroxine therapy, hypothyroidism. Occasionally, single adenomas or several adenomas will become hyperplastic and produce toxic nodular goiter (discussed above). Nontoxic goiter is often familial, and other members of the family should be examined and observed for the possible development of goiter.

Surgery is not necessary for nontoxic goiter unless obstructive symptoms develop or marked substernal extension occurs. Substernal goiter does not respond to levothyroxine therapy and must be removed surgically.

THYROIDITIS

1. SUBACUTE THYROIDITIS

Subacute thyroiditis (De Quervain's thyroiditis, granulomatous thyroiditis) is an acute inflammatory disorder of the thyroid gland most likely due to viral infection. A number of viruses, including mumps virus, coxsackievirus, and adenoviruses, have been implicated, either by finding the virus in biopsy specimens taken from the gland or by demonstration of rising titers of viral antibodies in the blood during the course of the infection. Pathologic examination reveals moderate thyroid enlargement and a mild inflammatory reaction involving the capsule. Histologic features include destruction of thyroid parenchyma and the presence of many large phagocytic cells, including giant cells.

Clinical Findings

A. Symptoms and Signs: Subacute thyroiditis usually presents with fever, malaise, and soreness in the neck, which may extend up to the angle of the jaw or toward the ear lobes on one or both sides of the neck. Initially, the patient may have symptoms of

Figure 7–46. Changes in serum T_4 and radioactive iodine uptake in patients with subacute thyroiditis. In the initial phase, serum T_4 is elevated and the patient may have symptoms of thyrotoxicosis, but radioactive iodine uptake is markedly suppressed. The illness may pass through phases of euthyroidism and hypothyroidism before remission. (Data adapted, with permission, from Woolf PD, Daly R: Thyrotoxicosis with painless thyroiditis. *Am J Med* 1976; 60:73.)

hyperthyroidism with palpitations, agitation, and sweats. There is no ophthalmopathy. On physical examination, the gland is exquisitely tender, so that the patient will object to pressure upon it. There are no signs of local redness or heat suggestive of abscess formation. Clinical signs of toxicity, including tachycardia, tremor, and hyperreflexia, may be present.

B. Laboratory Findings: Laboratory studies will vary with the course of the disease. Initially, T_3 by RIA, T_4 by RIA, and resin T_3 uptake are usually elevated, whereas serum TSH and thyroid radioactive iodine uptake are extremely low. The erythrocyte sedimentation rate is markedly elevated, sometimes as high as 100 mm/h by the Westergren scale. Thyroid autoantibodies are usually not detectable in serum. As the disease progresses, T_4 and T_3 will drop, TSH will rise, and symptoms of hypothyroidism are noted. Later, radioactive iodine uptake will rise, reflecting recovery of the gland from the acute insult (Fig 7–46).

Differential Diagnosis

Subacute thyroiditis can be differentiated from other viral illnesses by the involvement of the thyroid gland. It is differentiated from Graves' disease by the presence of low thyroid radioiodine uptake at a time when T_3 and T_4 levels are elevated.

Treatment

In most cases, only symptomatic treatment is necessary, eg, aspirin, 0.6 g 4 times daily. If pain, fever, and malaise are disabling, a short course of corticosteroids such as prednisone, 20 mg 3 times daily for

7–10 days, may be necessary to reduce the inflammation. Therapy with thyroid hormones, either levothyronine, 25 μg 3 times daily, or levothyroxine, 0.2 mg once daily, may be necessary during the hypothyroid phase of the illness in order to prevent reexacerbation of the disease induced by the rising TSH levels. In most patients, complete recovery occurs, but in about 10% of cases permanent hypothyroidism ensues and long-term thyroxine therapy is necessary.

Course & Prognosis

Subacute thyroiditis usually resolves spontaneously over weeks or months. Occasionally, the disease may begin to resolve and then suddenly get worse, sometimes involving first one lobe of the thyroid gland and then the other. Exacerbations come at a time when the T_4 levels have fallen, TSH has risen, and the gland is starting to recover function. Rarely, the course may extend over several years, with repeated bouts of inflammatory disease.

2. CHRONIC (HASHIMOTO'S) THYROIDITIS

Chronic thyroiditis (Hashimoto's thyroiditis, lymphocytic thyroiditis) is probably the most common cause of hypothyroidism and goiter in the USA. It is certainly the major cause of goiter in children and in young adults and is probably the major cause of "idiopathic myxedema," which represents an end stage of Hashimoto's thyroiditis with total atrophy of the gland. **Riedel's struma** is probably a variant of Hashimoto's thyroiditis with extensive fibrosis extending outside the gland and involving overlying muscle and surrounding tissues. Riedel's struma presents as a stony hard mass that must be differentiated from thyroid cancer.

Etiology & Pathogenesis

Hashimoto's thyroiditis is thought to be an autoimmune disease in which there is a defect in "suppressor" T cells, and "helper" T cells stimulate B lymphocytes to produce autoantibodies to thyroidal antigens, including microsomal and thyroglobulin autoantibodies. During the early phases of Hashimoto's thyroiditis, thyroglobulin autoantibodies are markedly elevated, and microsomal autoantibodies are not so high. Later, thyroglobulin autoantibodies may disappear, but the microsomal autoantibodies will be present for many years. Pathologically, there is massive infiltration of lymphocytes into the thyroid gland, with total destruction of normal thyroidal architecture. There may be actual formation of lymphoid follicles and germinal centers. The follicular epithelial cells are frequently enlarged and contain a basophilic cytoplasm (Hurthle cells). Destruction of the gland results in a fall in serum T_3 and T_4 levels and a rise in TSH: Initially, TSH may maintain adequate hormonal synthesis by the development of thyroid enlargement or goiter, but in many cases the gland fails, and hypothyroidism with or without goiter ensues.

Hashimoto's thyroiditis is part of a spectrum of thyroid diseases that includes Graves' disease at one end and idiopathic myxedema at the other (Fig 7–47). It is familial and may be associated with other autoimmune diseases such as pernicious anemia, adrenocortical insufficiency, idiopathic hypoparathyroidism, myasthenia gravis, and vitiligo. **Schmidt's syndrome** consists of Hashimoto's thyroiditis, idiopathic adrenal insufficiency, hypoparathyroidism, diabetes mellitus, ovarian insufficiency (rarely), and candidal infections. Schmidt's syndrome represents destruction of multiple endocrine glands on an autoimmune basis.

Clinical Findings

A. Symptoms and Signs: Hashimoto's thyroiditis usually presents with goiter in a patient who is euthyroid or has mild hypothyroidism. The sex distribution is about 4 females to one male. The process is painless, and the patient may be unaware of the goiter unless it becomes very large.

B. Laboratory Findings: There are multiple defects in iodine metabolism. Peroxidase activity is decreased, so that organification of iodine is impaired. This can be demonstrated by a positive perchlorate discharge test. In addition, iodination of metabolically inactive protein material occurs, so that there will be a disproportionately high serum PBI compared to serum T_4. Radioiodine uptake may be high, normal, or low. Circulating thyroid hormone levels are usually normal or low, and if low, TSH will be elevated.

The most striking laboratory finding is the high titer of autoantibodies to thyroidal antigens in the serum. Thyroglobulin and microsomal autoantibody

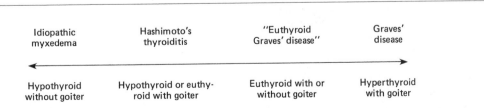

Figure 7–47. Spectrum of autoimmune disease of the thyroid gland. The clinical manifestations of autoimmune disease of the thyroid gland range from idiopathic myxedema, through nontoxic goiter, to diffuse toxic goiter, or Graves' disease. At times one can see progression of autoimmune disease from one form to another in the same patient.

tests are strongly positive in most patients with Hashimoto's thyroiditis.

An additional diagnostic test that has recently become available is the fine needle aspiration biopsy. With this technique, biopsy samples will reveal a heavy infiltration of lymphocytes as well as the presence of Hurthle cells on the smear.

Differential Diagnosis

Hashimoto's thyroiditis must be differentiated from other causes of nontoxic goiter. This is best done by antibody studies and if necessary by fine needle aspiration biopsy.

Complications & Sequelae

The major complication of Hashimoto's thyroiditis is progressive hypothyroidism. Rarely, a patient with Hashimoto's thyroiditis may develop lymphoma of the thyroid gland, but whether the 2 conditions are causally related is not clear. Thyroid lymphoma is characterized by rapid growth of the gland despite continued thyroid hormone therapy; the diagnosis of lymphoma must be made by surgical biopsy.

There is no evidence that adenocarcinoma of the thyroid gland occurs more frequently in patients with Hashimoto's thyroiditis, but the 2 diseases—chronic thyroiditis and carcinoma—can coexist in the same gland. Cancer must be suspected when a solitary nodule or thyroid mass grows or fails to regress while the patient is receiving maximal tolerated doses of thyroxine. Fine needle aspiration biopsy may be helpful in differential diagnosis.

Treatment

Treatment consists of giving levothyroxine, 0.15–0.3 mg daily. These doses are slightly higher than physiologic replacement in an effort to suppress TSH and allow regression of the goiter. Surgery is rarely indicated.

Course & Prognosis

Without treatment, Hashimoto's thyroiditis may progress from goiter and hypothyroidism to myxedema. The myxedema is totally corrected by adequate thyroxine therapy. Because Hashimoto's thyroiditis may be a part of a syndrome of multiple autoimmune diseases, the patient should be followed for other illnesses such as pernicious anemia, adrenal insufficiency, hypothyroidism, or diabetes mellitus.

Hashimoto's thyroiditis may go through periods of activity when large amounts of T_4 and T_3 are released or "dumped," resulting in symptoms of thyrotoxicosis. This syndrome, which has been called **spontaneously resolving hyperthyroidism,** is characterized by low radioiodine uptake. However, it can be differentiated from subacute thyroiditis in that the gland is not tender, the erythrocyte sedimentation rate is not elevated, autoantibodies to thyroidal antigens are strongly positive, and fine needle aspiration biopsy reveals lymphocytes and Hurthle cells. Therapy is symptomatic, usually requiring only propranolol, until

symptoms subside; T_4 supplementation may then be necessary.

Since Hashimoto's thyroiditis is part of a spectrum of autoimmune thyroid disease that includes Graves' disease, patients with Hashimoto's thyroiditis may develop true Graves' disease, occasionally with severe ophthalmopathy or dermopathy. The chronic thyroiditis may blunt the severity of the thyrotoxicosis, so that the patient may present with eye or skin complications of Graves' disease without marked thyrotoxicosis, a syndrome often called euthyroid Graves' disease. The thyroid gland will invariably be nonsuppressible, and this, plus the presence of thyroid autoantibodies, will help to make the diagnosis. The ophthalmopathy and dermopathy are treated as if thyrotoxic Graves' disease were present.

3. OTHER FORMS OF THYROIDITIS

The thyroid gland may be subject to acute abscess formation in patients with septicemia or acute bacterial endocarditis. Abscesses cause symptoms of pyogenic infection, with local pain and tenderness, swelling, and warmth and redness of the overlying skin. Needle aspiration may be helpful to confirm the diagnosis and identify the organism. Treatment includes antibiotic therapy and occasionally incision and drainage. A thyroglossal duct cyst may become infected and present as acute suppurative thyroiditis. This too will respond to antibiotic therapy and occasionally incision and drainage.

Ionizing radiation can induce both acute and chronic thyroiditis. Thyroiditis may occur acutely in patients treated with large doses of radioiodine and may be associated with release of thyroid hormones and an acute thyrotoxic crisis. Such an occurrence is extremely rare, however; the author has seen only 2 cases in several thousand patients treated for Graves' disease with radioactive iodine.

External radiation was used many years ago for the treatment of benign conditions such as severe acne and chronic tonsillitis or adenoiditis. This treatment was frequently associated with the development of focal thyroiditis and at times with goiter and hypothyroidism. If cancer can be ruled out by physical examination and other studies, these patients should be treated with long-term thyroxine therapy as described above in the discussion of Hashimoto's thyroiditis.

EFFECTS OF ACUTE & CHRONIC ILLNESS ON THYROID FUNCTION

The effects of thyroid hormone are controlled by a number of factors, including the following: (1) T_3 and T_4 feedback on TSH secretion; (2) autoregulation of hormone synthesis, depending on iodide availability; (3) peripheral metabolism of T_4, with activation by conversion to T_3 or inactivation by conversion to rT_3; and (4) the binding equilibrium between serum thyroid-binding proteins and tissue receptors. Acute and chronic illnesses have striking effects on these systems, particularly the peripheral metabolism of T_4 to T_3.

The peripheral metabolism of T_4 is diagrammed in Fig 7–21. Activation of the inner ring deiodinase accelerates conversion of T_4 to rT_3 and conversion of T_3 to 3,3′-T_2, markedly lowering the circulating level of T_3. This occurs physiologically in the fetus and pathologically in circumstances of carbohydrate restriction, as in malnutrition, starvation, anorexia nervosa, and diabetes mellitus (Table 7–5). Among the drugs that tend to lower the circulating levels of T_3, corticosteroids and iodinated dyes are the most effective and propylthiouracil and propranolol are relatively weak. Finally, acute illness such as myocardial infarction, febrile illness, trauma, burns, and surgery, as well as chronic illness—especially chronic liver disease, chronic renal disease, and cancer in advanced stages—also inhibit conversion of T_4 to T_3. These conditions result in what has been called the low T_3 syndrome.

Low T_3 syndrome is characterized by normal or slightly elevated T_4, low T_3, increased rT_3, and a normal TSH. Typical findings are presented in Fig 7–48 (adapted from Chopra et al, 1979). Data from normal, "sick," and hypothyroid individuals are compared. The "sick" patients have relatively normal serum T_4, compared with true hypothyroid patients, who have a very low T_4. T_3 is low in both "sick" and hypothyroid patients, but rT_3 is elevated in the "sick" group in comparison with both the normal and the hypothyroid groups. TSH is markedly elevated in the hypothyroid patients and normal in the "sick" patients. Further evidence that the "sick" patients are not hypothyroid can be obtained by the TRH test, which is normal in "sick" patients and hyperresponsive in hypothyroid patients (Fig 7–16).

There are 2 important areas of differential diagnosis in this syndrome: (1) Hypothyroidism must be ruled out, since failure to treat hypothyroidism in the presence of other illness could be catastrophic. The normal T_4, elevated rT_3, and normal TSH will rule out hypothyroidism. (2) Occasionally, T_4 may be slightly elevated, perhaps to compensate for the low T_3. In this case, patients may be confused with hyperthyroid patients but can be differentiated by the low T_3 and a normal TRH test.

A group of patients have been reported with a **low T_3, low T_4 syndrome.** Generally, they are much sicker and are usually in the intensive care unit. Indeed, the presence of both low T_3 and low T_4 has been associated with high mortality rates and poor outcomes. This syndrome is characterized by low T_4, low T_3, high rT_3, normal TSH, and usually an impaired response to TRH. Typical findings are presented in Fig 7–49. Note that T_4 and T_3 are low, but reverse T_3 is markedly elevated, and TSH is normal, in contrast to findings in hypothyroid patients. It is not clear why patients with this syndrome are not hypothyroid. A possible explanation has been suggested by Chopra et al (1979), who noted that although the T_4 level was low, a greater percentage of T_4 was dialyzable, and the actual level of free T_4 was increased. This was not detected by the free thyroxine index; it was only detected by dialysis measurements. Chopra et al postulate an inhibitor of T_4-binding to thyroid-binding proteins to account for these findings.

Clinical Implications of Low T_3 Syndrome

The clinical implications of these observations are important. The presence of low T_3 in milder diseases and low T_4 and low T_3 in very severe diseases suggests that these findings are related to the severity of the disease process. It is essential to rule out hyperthyroidism in low T_3 syndrome with elevated T_4 and to rule out hypothyroidism in both syndromes. Measurements

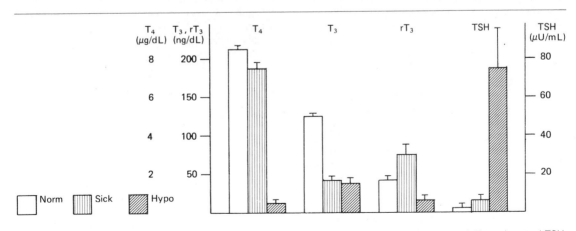

Figure 7–48. Low T_3 syndrome. Note that euthyroid sick patients have normal T_4, low T_3, elevated rT_3, and normal TSH, compared to normal and hypothyroid patients. (Reproduced, with permission, from Chopra IJ et al: Misleading low free thyroxine index and usefulness of reverse triiodothyronine measurements in nonthyroidal illness. *Ann Intern Med* 1979;**90**:905.)

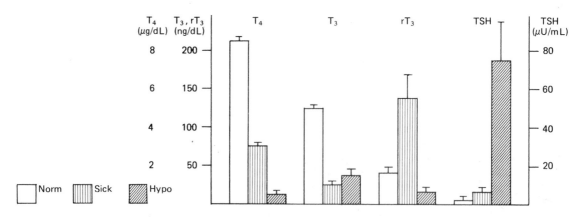

Figure 7–49. Low T_3, low T_4 syndrome. Note that very sick patients have low T_4, low T_3, elevated rT_3, and normal TSH, compared with normal and hypothyroid patients. (Reproduced, with permission, from Chopra IJ et al: Misleading low free thyroxine index and usefulness of reverse triiodothyronine measurements in nonthyroidal illness. *Ann Intern Med* 1979;**90**:905.)

of TSH and TRH response may be necessary. Finally, the FT_4I may not adequately reflect the level of free T_4 in severely ill patients, and direct determination of free T_4 may be necessary to clarify the thyroid status.

Management of Low T_3 Syndromes

Patients with these syndromes should not be treated with thyroid hormones to restore normal blood levels, since there is no evidence that treatment with T_3 or T_4 will be helpful and there are many reasons why such treatment might be hazardous. It is thought that these aberrations of thyroid hormone metabolism are an adaptive mechanism that may in some way protect the organism from excessive metabolic activity in the presence of serious illness. Certainly, one should correct any caloric or carbohydrate deprivation and treat the underlying illness, which will usually be accompanied by a return of thyroid hormone metabolism to normal.

THYROID NODULES & THYROID CANCER

In 95% of cases, thyroid cancer presents as a nodule or lump in the thyroid. In occasional instances, enlarged cervical lymph nodes will be the first sign of the disease. The latter is particularly apt to be the case in children, although on careful examination a small primary focus in the form of a thyroid nodule can usually be felt. Rarely, distant metastasis in lung or bone is the first sign of thyroid cancer.

Thyroid nodules are extremely common, particularly among women. The prevalence of thyroid nodules in the USA has been estimated to be about 4% of the adult population. In young children, the incidence is less than 1%; in persons aged 11–18 years,

about 1.5%; and in persons over age 60, about 5%.

In contrast to thyroid nodules, thyroid cancer is a rare condition—0.004% per year according to the Third National Cancer Survey. Thus, most thyroid nodules are benign, and a method must be utilized for identifying those that are likely to be malignant.

Etiology of Benign Thyroid Nodules

Benign conditions that can produce nodularity in the thyroid gland are listed in Table 7–11. They include focal areas of chronic thyroiditis, a dominant portion of a multinodular goiter, or a cyst involving either thyroid tissue, parathyroid tissue, or thyroglossal duct remnants. Other benign conditions include agenesis of one lobe of the thyroid, with hypertrophy of the other lobe presenting as a mass in the neck. It is usually the left lobe of the thyroid that fails to develop, and the hypertrophy occurs in the right lobe. Scarring in the gland following surgery—or regrowth of the gland after surgery or radioiodine therapy—can present with nodularity. Finally, benign neoplasms in the thyroid include follicular adenomas

Table 7–11. Etiology of benign thyroid nodules.

1. Focal thyroiditis.
2. Dominant portion of multinodular goiter.
3. Thyroid, parathyroid, or thyroglossal cysts.
4. Agenesis of a thyroid lobe.
5. Postsurgical remnant hyperplasia or scarring.
6. Postradioiodine remnant hyperplasia.
7. Benign adenomas:
   a. Follicular:
      Colloid or macrofollicular.
      Fetal.
      Embryonal.
      Hurthle cell.
   b. Rare: Teratoma, lipoma, hemangioma.

Table 7–12. Risk factors useful in distinguishing benign from malignant thyroid lesions.

	More Likely Benign	More Likely Malignant
History	Family history of benign goiter. Residence in endemic goiter area.	Family history of medullary cancer of thyroid. Previous therapeutic irradiation of head or neck. Recent growth of nodule. Hoarseness, dysphagia, or obstruction.
Physical characteristics	Older woman. Soft nodule. Multinodular goiter.	Child, young adult, male. Solitary, firm nodule clearly different from rest of gland ("dominant nodule"). Vocal cord paralysis, firm lymph nodes, distant metastases.
Serum factors	High titer of thyroid autoantibodies.	Elevated serum calcitonin. Elevated serum thyroglobulin (?).
Scanning techniques ^{123}I or $^{99m}TcO_4$	"Hot nodule."	"Cold nodule."
Echo scan	Cyst (pure).	Solid or semicystic.
Biopsy (needle)	Benign appearance on cytologic examination.	Malignant or suggestion of malignancy.
Levothyroxine therapy (0.2 mg/d or more for 3 months or longer)	Regression.	No regression.

such as colloid or macrofollicular adenomas, fetal adenomas, embryonal adenomas, and Hurthle cell or oxyphil adenomas. Rare types of benign lesions include teratomas, lipomas, and hemangiomas. With the exception of thyroid hyperplasia of the right lobe of the gland in the presence of agenesis of the left lobe—and some follicular adenomas—all of the above lesions present as "cold" nodules on isotope scanning.

Differentiation of Benign & Malignant Lesions of the Thyroid Gland

Risk factors that predispose to benign or malignant disease are set forth in Table 7–12 and discussed below.

A. History: A family history of goiter suggests benign disease, as does residence in an area of endemic goiter. On the other hand, a family history of medullary carcinoma, a history of recent growth, or a history of hoarseness, dysphagia, or obstruction strongly suggests cancer.

Probably the most important historical feature is exposure to ionizing radiation. The incidence of thyroid lesions after irradiation is summarized in Table 7–13. As little as 6.5 rads to the thyroid gland received during the radiation treatment of tinea capitis has been reported to cause cancer in 0.11% of exposed children; the incidence of thyroid cancer in sibling controls was 0.02%. Radiation therapy to the thymus was used many years ago for the treatment of respiratory problems or poor growth in infants. The thyroid received dosages of 100–400 rads, and the incidence of thyroid cancer attributed to this source ranged from 0.5 to 5%. X-ray therapy to the neck and chest given to children or adolescents for acne, tonsillitis, adenoiditis, otitis media, or skin lesions with thyroid doses ranging from 200 to 1500 rads produced nodular goiter with an incidence of around 27% and thyroid cancer with an incidence of 5–7%. These tumors developed 10–40 years after radiation was administered, with a peak incidence at 20–30 years. Radiation fallout with a thyroid dose of 700–1400 rads has

Table 7–13. Thyroid lesions after irradiation.

		Incidence (%)		
Areas Treated	Estimated Dose to Thyroid (rads)	Nodular Goiter	Cancer	Source
Scalp	6.5	. . .	0.11	Modan et al (1974)
Thymus				
Total group	119	1.8	0.8	Hemplemann et al (1975)
Subgroup	399	7.6	5.0	
Neck, chest	807	27.2	5.7	Favus et al (1975)
	180–1500	26.2	6.8	Refetoff et al (1975)
Radiation fallout	<50	. . .	0.4	Parker et al (1974)
	>50	. . .	6.7	Sampson et al (1969)
	175 (γ) and 700–1400 (β)	39.6	5.7	Conard et al (1970)
^{131}I therapy	±10,000	0.17	0.08	Dobyns et al (1974)

produced nodular goiter in approximately 40% of patients exposed and thyroid cancer in about 6%. On the other hand, radioiodine therapy, which exposes the thyroid to a dosage of around 10,000 rads, was rarely associated with the development of thyroid cancer, presumably because the thyroid gland is largely destroyed by these doses of radioiodine so that—although the incidence of postradiation hypothyroidism is high—the incidence of thyroid cancer is extremely low.

Ninety percent of patients with radiation-induced thyroid cancer develop papillary carcinoma; the remainder develop follicular carcinoma. Medullary carcinoma and anaplastic carcinomas have been rare following radiation exposure. Data from several large series suggest that the incidence of cancer in a patient who presents with a solitary cold nodule of the thyroid gland and a history of therapeutic radiation of the head, neck, or chest is around 50%.

B. Physical Characteristics: Physical characteristics associated with a low risk for thyroid cancer include older age, female sex, soft thyroid nodules, and the presence of a multinodular goiter. Individuals at higher risk for thyroid cancer include children, young adults, and males. A solitary firm or dominant nodule that is clearly different from the rest of the gland increases the risk of malignancy. Vocal cord paralysis, enlarged lymph nodes, and suspected metastases are strongly suggestive of malignancy.

C. Serum Factors: A high titer of thyroid autoantibodies in serum is associated with a low risk of thyroid cancer and suggests chronic thyroiditis as the cause of thyroid enlargement. On the other hand, an elevated serum calcitonin, particularly in patients with a family history of medullary carcinoma, strongly suggests the presence of thyroid cancer. Elevated serum thyroglobulin titers may be associated with metastatic follicular or papillary thyroid carcinoma but are usu-

ally not helpful in determining the nature of the thyroid nodule.

D. Scanning Techniques: Scanning procedures can be used to identify "hot" or "cold" nodules, ie, those that take up more or less radioactive iodine than surrounding tissue. Hot nodules are almost never malignant, whereas cold ones may be. Scintillation camera photographs with ^{99m}Tc pertechnetate give the best resolution (Fig 7–50). Echo scans can distinguish cystic and solid lesions. A pure cyst is almost never malignant. Lesions that have internal echoes or are solid on echo scan may be benign or malignant. CT scanning or magnetic resonance imaging (MRI) may be helpful in defining substernal extension or deep thyroid nodules in the neck.

E. Needle Biopsy: The major advance in management of the thyroid nodule in recent years has been the fine needle aspiration biopsy. Large needle aspiration biopsies of the thyroid for diagnostic purposes were in use from about 1930, but Soderstrom in 1952 introduced the technique of fine needle aspiration biopsy. Since then, fine needle biopsy has been widely used in Sweden, Europe, and Japan, and, more recently, in the USA. With this technique, a 23- or 25-bore needle is used, and the diagnosis relies on cytologic rather than histologic examination. It is nontraumatic, simple, easily repeated, and very acceptable to the patient.

Fine needle aspiration biopsy clearly separates thyroid nodules into 3 groups:

1. Malignant thyroid nodules–The technique is almost 100% diagnostic.

2. Follicular neoplasms–About 15% of these lesions are malignant, and about 85% are benign. Some follicular neoplasms may be hot; most of them are cold.

3. Benign thyroid nodules–The rate of false-negative results with fine needle aspiration biopsy is

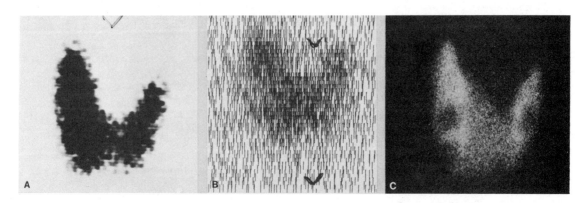

Figure 7–50. Demonstration of resolution obtained utilizing different scanning techniques: *A:* ^{123}I scintiscan with rectilinear scanner. *B:* Fluorescent scan with rectilinear scanner. *C:* ^{99m}Tc pertechnetate scan with the pinhole collimated gamma camera. Note the presence of 2 "cold" nodules, one in each lobe of the thyroid, easily detected in *C* but not clearly delineated in the other 2 scans. The lesion in the right lobe was palpable, about 1 cm in diameter, and was shown to be follicular carcinoma on needle biopsy. The lesion in the left lobe was either a metastatic tumor or a second primary follicular carcinoma. (Courtesy of MD Okerlund.)

about 4%. Results are accurate in about 96% of cases, as demonstrated by subsequent surgery or long-term follow-up of patients with lesions originally reported to be benign.

F. Suppressive Therapy: Finally, benign lesions may regress after thyroxine therapy, whereas malignant ones are very unlikely to regress. Therefore, marked regression of the nodule following administration of levothyroxine, 0.2 mg orally daily for 3 months or more, is suggestive of a benign lesion.

G. Decision Matrix Analysis of Benign and Malignant Lesions: A decision matrix for the management of a thyroid nodule is outlined in Fig 7–51. A patient with a thyroid nodule should have a fine needle aspiration biopsy as the initial screening test for a thyroid mass. If a diagnosis of malignancy is made, the patient is referred directly to the surgeon. If the cytologic report shows that the nodule is benign, the patient is given thyroxine, and if the lesion regresses, the patient is maintained on thyroxine indefinitely. If there is no regression, the lesion is biopsied, or if it grows or changes in consistency, it may be excised. In patients who are reported to have follicular neoplasms, scanning is employed. If the scan reveals the

nodule to be hot, the patient is simply observed, at times with thyroxine therapy. If the lesion is cold and there is an increased chance of malignancy (large lesion, firm nodule, young patient), the patient might be referred directly to the surgeon. If the risk is low (small lesion, soft nodule, older patient), the patient is given thyroxine. If there is no regression with thyroxine in the latter case, the lesion should probably be excised.

There are 2 groups that represent special problems: patients with thyroid cysts and patients who have received radiation therapy. Although thyroid cysts are almost always benign, occasionally one can find cancer in the wall of the cyst. For this reason, recurrent cysts should be studied with ultrasonography, and if there is evidence of a septated lesion or growth in the wall of the lesion, the lesion should be surgically removed. In patients who have received radiation therapy, there may be multiple lesions, some benign and some malignant. Therefore, in the presence of a cold nodule in a patient who has had radiation exposure, surgery is recommended directly.

If this protocol is followed, there will be a marked reduction in surgery for benign thyroid nodules, and

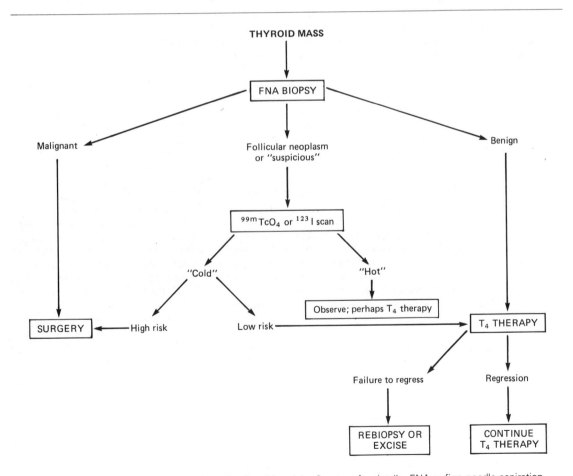

Figure 7–51. Decision matrix for workup of a thyroid nodule. See text for details. FNA = fine needle aspiration.

the incidence of malignancy at the time of surgery will be about 40%. The cost savings is enormous, since unnecessary surgery is eliminated and the cost of thyroid nodule "workup" is cut in half. In addition, there is no delay in making the diagnosis and referring the patient with thyroid cancer for appropriate therapy.

THYROID CANCER

Pathology

The types and approximate frequency of malignant thyroid tumors are listed in Table 7–14.

A. Papillary Carcinoma: Papillary carcinoma of the thyroid gland usually presents as a firm, solitary, "cold," "solid" nodule clearly different from the rest of the gland. In multinodular goiter, the cancer will be a "dominant nodule"—larger, firmer, and (again) clearly different from the rest of the gland. About 10% of papillary carcinomas, especially in children, present with enlarged cervical nodes, but careful examination will usually reveal a "cold" nodule in the thyroid. Rarely, there will be hemorrhage, necrosis, and cyst formation in the malignant nodule, but on echo scan there will be clearly defined internal echoes that serve to differentiate the semicystic malignant lesion from the nonmalignant "pure cyst." Finally, papillary carcinoma may be found incidentally as a microscopic focus of cancer in the middle of a gland removed for other reasons such as Graves' disease.

Microscopically, the tumor consists of single layers of thyroid cells arranged in vascular stalks, with papillary projections extending into microscopic cyst-like spaces. The nuclei of the cells are large and pale and frequently contain clear, glassy intranuclear inclusion bodies. About 40% of papillary carcinomas form laminated calcified spheres, often at the tip of a papillary projection, called "psammoma bodies." These are usually diagnostic of papillary carcinoma. These cancers usually extend by intraglandular metastasis and by local lymph node invasion. They grow very slowly and remain confined to the thyroid gland and local lymph nodes for many years. In older patients, they may become more aggressive and invade locally into muscles and trachea. In later stages, they can spread to the lung. Death is usually due to local disease, with invasion of deep sectors in the neck;

less commonly, death may be due to extensive pulmonary metastases. In some older patients, a slowly growing papillary carcinoma will begin to grow rapidly and convert to undifferentiated or anaplastic carcinoma. This "late anaplastic shift" is another cause of death from papillary carcinoma. Many papillary carcinomas secrete thyroglobulin, which can be used as a marker for recurrence or metastasis of the cancer.

B. Follicular Carcinoma: Follicular carcinoma is characterized by the maintenance of small follicles, although colloid formation is poor. Indeed, follicular carcinoma may be indistinguishable from follicular adenoma except by capsular invasion or vascular invasion. The tumor is slightly more aggressive than papillary carcinoma and can spread either by local invasion of lymph nodes or by blood vessel invasion with distant metastases to bone or lung. Microscopically, the cells are cuboidal, with large nuclei arranged around follicles that frequently contain colloid. These tumors often retain the ability to concentrate radioactive iodine, to form thyroglobulin, and, rarely, to synthesize T_3 and T_4. Thus, the rare "functioning thyroid cancer" is almost always a follicular carcinoma. This characteristic makes these tumors more likely to respond to radioactive iodine therapy. In untreated patients, death is due to local extension or to distant bloodstream metastasis with extensive involvement of bone, lungs, and viscera.

A variant of follicular carcinoma is the "Hurthle cell" carcinoma, characterized by large individual cells with pink-staining cytoplasm filled with mitochondria. They behave like follicular cancer. Mixed papillary and follicular carcinomas behave more like papillary carcinoma. Most follicular carcinomas secrete thyroglobulin, and this feature can be used to follow the course of disease.

C. Medullary Carcinoma: Medullary cancer is a disease of the C cells (parafollicular cells) derived from the ultimobranchial body and capable of secreting calcitonin, histaminase, prostaglandins, serotonin, and other peptides. Microscopically, the tumor consists of sheets of cells separated by a pink-staining substance that has characteristics of amyloid. This material stains with Congo red. Amyloid consists of chains of calcitonin laid down in a fibrillary pattern—in contrast to other forms of amyloid, which may have immunoglobulin light chains or other proteins deposited in a fibrillary pattern.

Medullary carcinoma is somewhat more aggressive than papillary or follicular carcinoma but not as aggressive as undifferentiated thyroid cancer. It extends locally into lymph nodes and into surrounding muscle and trachea. It may invade lymphatics and blood vessels and metastasize to lungs and viscera. Calcitonin secreted by the tumor is a marker for medullary carcinoma and can be used both to discover the tumor and as an index of cure or recurrence. About two-thirds of medullary carcinomas are familial, and about one-third are isolated instances of the cancer. The familial tumors may be associated with multiple endocrine neoplasia type IIa (Sipple's syndrome),

Table 7–14. Approximate frequency of malignant thyroid tumors.

Papillary carcinoma (including mixed papillary and follicular)	60%
Follicular carcinoma	20%
Medullary carcinoma	5%
Undifferentiated carcinomas	14%
Miscellaneous (including lymphoma, fibrosarcoma, squamous cell carcinoma, malignant hemangioendothelioma, teratomas, and metastatic carcinomas)	1%

characterized by medullary carcinoma, pheochromocytomas, and parathyroid adenomas; or they may be associated with type IIb, characterized by medullary carcinoma, pheochromocytomas, and multiple neuromas of the tongue, lips, and bowel (see Chapter 25). At times, only the medullary carcinoma is familial, and no other endocrine glands are involved. The important thing is that if medullary carcinoma is diagnosed, all family members should be screened for possible medullary carcinoma. The best screening test is serum calcitonin after pentagastrin stimulation.

D. Undifferentiated (Anaplastic) Carcinoma:
Undifferentiated thyroid gland tumors include small cell, giant cell, and spindle cell carcinomas. They usually occur in older patients with a long history of goiter in whom the gland suddenly—over weeks or months—begins to enlarge and produce pressure symptoms, dysphagia, or vocal cord paralysis. Death from massive local extension usually occurs within 6–36 months. These tumors are very resistant to therapy.

E. Miscellaneous Types:

1. Lymphoma–The only type of rapidly growing thyroid cancer that is responsive to therapy is the lymphoma, which may develop as a part of a generalized lymphoma or may be primary in the thyroid gland. Thyroid lymphoma occasionally develops in a patient with long-standing Hashimoto's thyroiditis and may be difficult to distinguish from chronic thyroiditis. It is characterized by lymphocyte invasion of thyroid follicles and blood vessel walls, which helps to differentiate thyroid lymphoma from chronic thyroiditis. If there is no systemic involvement, the tumor may respond dramatically to radiation therapy.

2. Metastatic thyroid cancer–Many systemic cancers metastasize to the thyroid gland, including

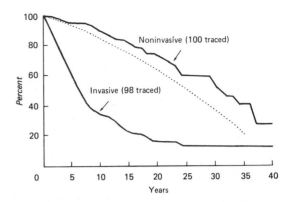

Figure 7–53. Follicular carcinoma. Survivorship curves (6 operative deaths excluded) for patients with slight or equivocal capsular invasion and those with moderate or marked invasion (including recurrent and inoperable tumors). Dotted line is curve for normal persons of comparable age and sex. (Reproduced, with permission, from Woolner LB et al: Long term survival rates. In: *Thyroid Cancer.* Vol 12. Hedinger CE [editor]. UICC Monograph Series. Springer-Verlag, 1969.)

cancers of the breast and kidney, bronchogenic carcinoma, and malignant melanoma. The primary site of involvement is usually obvious. Occasionally, the diagnosis is made by needle biopsy or open biopsy of a rapidly enlarging cold thyroid nodule. The prognosis is that of the primary tumor.

Natural History of Thyroid Cancer

Papillary carcinoma of the thyroid (the most common type) may exist as a microscopic focus in the gland. The incidence of microscopic foci of thyroid cancer at autopsy has varied from 4% in several series in the USA to as high as 25% in persons of Japanese descent living in the Hawaiian Islands. The lesion does not shorten life and is probably of no clinical significance. Woolner et al have shown that in patients with "occult" or microscopic papillary carcinoma— or small intrathyroidal papillary carcinoma—the survival rate is about the same as that of individuals without thyroid cancer. On the other hand, if there is evidence of extrathyroidal extension of the cancer, life expectancy is markedly affected (Fig 7–52). Similarly, in persons with small, noninvasive follicular carcinoma, the survival rate does not differ from that of control groups; whereas in the case of follicular carcinoma that has invaded blood vessels or in which there is evidence of extrathyroidal extension, survival is poor (Fig 7–53). Medullary carcinoma shows a similar pattern, with good survival for intrathyroidal small lesions and impaired survival for patients with extrathyroidal extension (Fig 7–54). Patients with anaplastic carcinomas have a very poor prognosis; almost all are dead within 3 years (Fig 7–55).

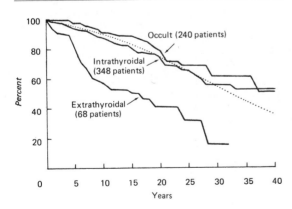

Figure 7–52. Papillary carcinoma. Survivorship curves for occult, intrathyroidal, and extrathyroidal lesions. Dotted line is curve for normal persons of comparable age and sex. (Reproduced, with permission, from Woolner LB et al: Long term survival rates. In: *Thyroid Cancer.* Vol 12. Hedinger CE [editor]. UICC Monograph Series. Springer-Verlag, 1969.)

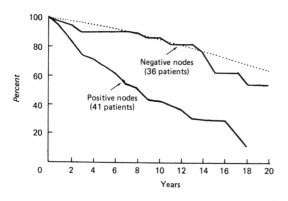

Figure 7–54. Medullary carcinoma. Survivorship curves for patients with metastatic involvement of cervical lymph nodes at time of initial surgery and those without such involvement. Dotted line is curve for normal persons of comparable age and sex. (Reproduced, with permission, from Woolner LB et al: Long term survival rates. In: *Thyroid Cancer.* Vol 12. Hedinger CE [editor]. UICC Monograph Series. Springer-Verlag, 1969.)

Figure 7–55. Anaplastic carcinoma. Survivorship curve, plotted in months. (Reproduced, with permission, from Woolner LB et al: Long term survival rates. In: *Thyroid Cancer.* Vol 12. Hedinger CE [editor]. UICC Monograph Series. Springer-Verlag, 1969.)

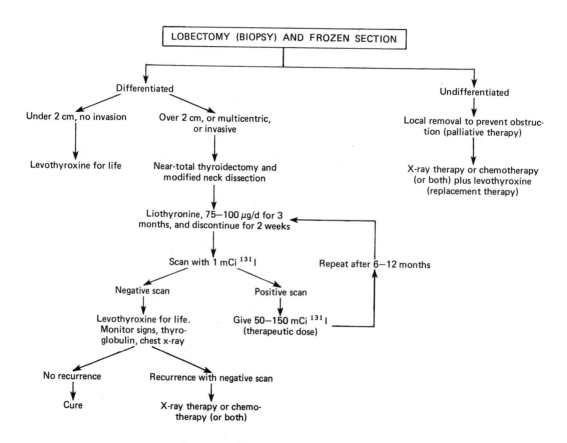

Figure 7–56. Management of thyroid cancer.

Factors Related to Survival of Patients With Thyroid Cancer

Mazzaferri et al have reviewed factors related to survival of patients with thyroid cancer, including the type of malignancy and the size of the lesion. Papillary, follicular, or medullary carcinomas over 2 cm in diameter have a worse prognosis than small, well-circumscribed lesions. Invasion of the thyroid capsule with local extension into surrounding muscle and fascia is associated with a poor prognosis. On the other hand, lymph node involvement, particularly in young persons, may not represent a worsening of the prognosis. However, lymph node involvement in patients over 40 years of age implies a worse prognosis. Blood vessel invasion is an adverse prognostic feature. Several studies have shown that papillary carcinoma and follicular carcinoma are more virulent in patients under 7 or over 40 years of age.

Management of Thyroid Cancer (Fig 7–56)

A. Papillary and Follicular Carcinoma: Lobectomy is satisfactory for small (< 2 cm) papillary and follicular thyroid carcinomas, but near-total thyroidectomy is required for larger lesions or for cancers with evidence of extrathyroidal extension. Modified neck dissection is indicated if there is evidence of lymph node metastases. Prophylactic neck dissections are not recommended.

Radioiodine scan and therapy are indicated for patients with large papillary or follicular carcinomas (> 2 cm) or with evidence of intra- or extrathyroidal extension. Postoperatively, the patient receives liothyronine (Cytomel), 75– 100 μg daily in divided doses for about 3 months; the medication is then stopped for 2 weeks, and the patient is scanned with 1 mCi of ^{131}I. Liothyronine is used for replacement therapy because it is cleared from the blood rapidly; after 2 weeks off therapy, TSH levels are sufficiently high to obtain good scanning studies. If there is evidence of residual radioactive iodine uptake in the neck or elsewhere, radioactive iodine (^{131}I) is effective treatment. The scan is repeated at intervals of 6– 12 months until no further uptake is observed; the patient is then maintained on full replacement therapy with levothyroxine, 0.2– 0.3 mg daily, to suppress serum TSH to undetectable levels.

Follow-up at intervals of 6– 12 months should include careful examination of the neck for recurrent masses. If a lump is noted, needle biopsy examination is indicated to confirm or rule out cancer. Serum thyroglobulin will usually be undetectable after total thyroidectomy and levothyroxine therapy. A rise in serum thyroglobulin suggests recurrence of thyroid cancer. Chest x-ray every 2– 3 years may reveal pulmonary metastases, although a rising serum thyroglobulin concentration is a more sensitive indicator. If the patient does develop a mass in the neck, a rise in serum thyroglobulin, or a mass on chest x-ray, ^{131}I scan should be repeated following the technique outlined above. If the lesions concentrate ^{131}I, this may be useful in treatment; if they do not concentrate ^{131}I, local excision or local x-ray therapy may be useful. For recurrences that cannot be managed by these modalities, chemotherapy should be considered.

B. Medullary Carcinoma: Patients with medullary carcinoma should be followed in a similar way, except that the marker for recurrent medullary cancer is serum calcitonin. Histaminase and other peptides are also secreted by these tumors, but assays for these substances are not generally available. If a patient has a persistently elevated serum calcitonin concentration after total thyroidectomy and regional node dissection, selective venous catheterization and sampling for serum calcitonin may reveal the location of the metastases. If this fails to localize the lesion (as is often the case), the patient must be followed until the metastatic lesion shows itself as a palpable mass or a shadow on the chest x-ray or CT scan. Rarely, metastatic medullary carcinoma can be treated with ^{131}I; usually, however, local excision and levothyroxine therapy are best. Chemotherapy for medullary carcinoma has not been effective.

C. Anaplastic Carcinoma: Anaplastic carcinoma of the thyroid has a very poor prognosis. Treatment consists of isthmusectomy (to confirm the diagnosis and to prevent tracheal compression) and palliative x-ray therapy. Thyroid lymphomas are quite responsive to x-ray therapy; giant cell, squamous cell, spindle cell, and anaplastic carcinomas are unresponsive. Chemotherapy is not very effective for anaplastic carcinomas. Doxorubicin (Adriamycin), 75 mg/m^2 as a single injection or divided into 3 consecutive daily injections repeated at 3-week intervals, has been useful in some patients with disseminated thyroid cancer unresponsive to surgery, TSH suppression, or radiation therapy. This drug is quite toxic; side effects include cardiotoxicity, myelosuppression, alopecia, and gastrointestinal symptoms.

D. X-Ray Therapy: Local x-ray therapy has been useful in the treatment of solitary metastatic lesions, particularly follicular or papillary tumors, that do not concentrate radioactive iodine. It is particularly effective in isolated nonfunctional bone metastases.

Prognosis

The prognosis is very poor for undifferentiated thyroid cancer (Fig 7– 55) but much better for the more differentiated types. Cady et al point out that age and sex of the patient at the time of diagnosis are the most important variables affecting prognosis in differentiated thyroid cancer. They define a "high-risk" group of men over 40 and women over 50 with a recurrence rate of 33% and a death rate of 27%. In contrast, they found that in a "low-risk" group of men under 40 and women under 50, the recurrence rate was 11% and the death rate 4%. These data suggest that although every effort should be made to provide appropriate therapy for all patients with thyroid cancer—surgery, radioiodine, and thyroxine— older patients will not do as well as younger ones despite best efforts.

REFERENCES

Thyroid Physiology & Tests

Bernal J, Refetoff S: The action of thyroid hormone. *Clin Endocrinol (Oxf)* 1977;**6**:227.

Bilezikan JP, Loeb JN: The influence of hyperthyroidism and hypothyroidism on α- and β-adrenergic receptor systems and adrenergic responsiveness. *Endocr Rev* 1983;**4**:378.

Braverman LE, Ingbar SH: Changes in thyroidal function during adaptation to large dose of iodide. *J Clin Invest* 1963;**42**:1216.

DeGroot LJ: Kinetic analysis of iodine metabolism. *J Clin Endocrinol Metab* 1966;**26**:149.

DeGroot LJ, Niepomniszcze H: Biosynthesis of thyroid hormone: Basic and clinical aspects. *Metabolism* 1977; **26**:665.

Dumont JE: The action of thyrotropin on thyroid metabolism. *Vitam Horm* 1971;**29**:287.

Edelman IS: Thyroid thermogenesis. *N Engl J Med* 1974; **290**:1303.

Field JB: Thyroid-stimulating hormone and cyclic adenosine 3′,5′-monophosphate in the regulation of thyroid gland function. *Metabolism* 1975;**24**:381.

Hershman JM: Clinical application of thyrotropin-releasing hormone. *N Engl J Med* 1974;**290**:886.

Ingbar SH: Autoregulation of the thyroid: Response to iodide excess and depletion. *Mayo Clin Proc* 1972;**47**:814.

Kidd A et al: Progress in endocrinology and metabolism: Immunologic aspects of Graves' and Hashimoto's diseases. *Metabolism* 1980;**29**:80.

Larsen PR: Thyroid-pituitary interaction: Feedback regulation of thyrotropin secretion by thyroid hormones. *N Engl J Med* 1982;**306**:23.

Mayberry WE et al: Radioimmunoassay for human thyrotrophin: Clinical value in patients with normal and abnormal thyroid function. *Ann Intern Med* 1971;**74**:471.

Oppenheimer JH: Thyroid hormone action at the nuclear level. *Ann Intern Med* 1985;**102**:374.

Pierce JG: Eli Lilly lecture. The subunits of pituitary thyrotropin: Their relationship to other glycoprotein hormones. *Endocrinology* 1971;**89**:1331.

Pittman JA et al: Hypothalamic hypothyroidism. *N Engl J Med* 1971;**285**:844.

Roti E et al: The placental transport, synthesis and metabolism of hormones and drugs which affect thyroid function. *Endocr Rev* 1983;**4**:131.

Wolff J: Iodide goiter and the pharmacologic effects of excess iodide. *Am J Med* 1969;**47**:101.

Wolff J, Chaikoff IL: Plasma inorganic iodide as a homeostatic regulator of thyroid function. *J Biol Chem* 1948; **174**:555.

Hypothyroidism

Blum M: Myxedema coma. *Am J Med Sci* 1972;**264**:432.

Catz B, Russell S: Myxedema, shock and coma. *Arch Intern Med* 1961;**108**:407.

Crowley WF Jr et al: Noninvasive evaluation of cardiac function in hypothyroidism: Response to gradual thyroxine replacement. *N Engl J Med* 1977;**296**:1.

Fisher DA et al: Results of screening one million North American infants. *J Pediatr* 1979;**94**:700.

Holvey DN et al: Treatment of myxedema coma with intravenous thyroxine. *Arch Intern Med* 1964;**113**:89.

Maeda M et al: Changes in serum triiodothyronine, thyroxine and thyrotropin during treatment with thyroxine in severe

primary hypothyroidism. *J Clin Endocrinol Metab* 1976; **43**:10.

Rees-Jones RW, Rolla AR, Larsen PR: Hormonal content of thyroid replacement preparations. *JAMA* 1980;**243**:459.

Santos AD et al: Echocardiographic characterization of the reversible cardiomyopathy of hypothyroidism. *Am J Med* 1980;**68**:675.

Stock JM, Surks MI, Oppenheimer JH: Replacement dosage of L-thyroxine in hypothyroidism: A reevaluation. *N Engl J Med* 1974;**290**:529.

Vagenakis AG et al: Recovery of pituitary thyrotropic function after withdrawal of prolonged thyroid-suppression therapy. *N Engl J Med* 1975;**293**:681.

van der Gaag RD, Drexhage HA, Dussault JH: Role of maternal immunoglobulins blocking TSH-induced thyroid growth in sporadic forms of congenital hypothyroidism. *Lancet* 1985;**1**:246.

Zwillich CW et al: Ventilatory control in myxedema and hypothyroidism. *N Engl J Med* 1975;**292**:662.

Hyperthyroidism

Bierwaltes WH: The treatment of hyperthyroidism with iodine-131. *Semin Nucl Med* 1978;**8**:95.

Bradley EL III, DiGirolamo M, Tarcan Y: Modified subtotal thyroidectomy in the management of Graves' disease. *Surgery* 1980;**87**:623.

Braverman LE: Thyrotoxicosis: Therapeutic considerations. *Clin Endocrinol Metab* 1978;**7**:221.

Burman JD, Baker JR Jr: Immune mechanisms in Graves' disease. *Endocr Rev* 1985;**6**:183.

Burrow GN: Hyperthyroidism during pregnancy. *N Engl J Med* 1978;**298**:150.

Davis PJ, Davis FB: Hyperthyroidism in patients over the age of 60 years. *Medicine* 1974;**53**:161.

Dobyns BM: Prevention and management of hyperthyroid storm. *World J Surg* 1978;**2**:293.

Fisher DA: Pathogenesis and therapy of neonatal Graves' disease. *Am J Dis Child* 1976;**130**:133.

Gardner DF, Utiger RD: The natural history of hyperthyroidism due to Graves' disease in remission: Sequential studies of pituitary thyroid regulation and various serum parameters. *J Clin Endocrinol Metab* 1979;**49**:417.

Gorman CA: The presentation and management of endocrine ophthalmopathy. *Clin Endocrinol Metab* 1978;**7**:67.

Gorman CA, Robertson JS: Radiation dose in the selection of ^{131}I or surgical treatment for toxic thyroid adenoma. *Ann Intern Med* 1978;**89**:85.

Jacobson DH, Gorman CA: Endocrine ophthalmopathy: Current ideas concerning etiology, pathogenesis and treatment. *Endocr Rev* 1984;**5**:200.

Kriss JP, Konishi J, Herman M: Studies on the pathogenesis of Graves' ophthalmopathy (with some related observations regarding therapy). *Recent Prog Horm Res* 1975; **31**:533.

MacGregor AM et al: Prediction of relapse in hyperthyroid Graves' disease. *Lancet* 1980;**1**:1101.

Rapoport B et al: Clinical experience with a human thyroid cell bioassay for thyroid-stimulating immunoglobulin. *J Clin Endocrinol Metab* 1984;**58**:332.

Ruiz M et al: Familial dysalbuminemic hyperthyroxinemia, a syndrome that can be confused with thyrotoxicosis. *N Engl J Med* 1982;**306**:635.

Solomon DH, Kleeman KE: Concepts of pathogenesis of Graves' disease. *Adv Intern Med* 1976;**22**:273.

Toft AD (editor): Hyperthyroidism. *Clin Endocrinol Metab* 1985;**14**:299. [Entire issue.]

Tolis G et al: Pituitary hyperthyroidism: Case report and review of the literature. *Am J Med* 1978;**64**:177.

Vanderlaan WP: Antithyroid drugs in practice. *Mayo Clin Proc* 1972;**41**:962.

Volpé R: The pathogenesis of Graves' disease: An overview. *Clin Endocrinol Metab* 1978;**7**:3.

Syndrome of Inappropriate TSH Secretion

Bernal J, Refetoff S, DeGroot LJ: Abnormalities of triiodothyronine binding to lymphocyte and fibroblast nuclei from a patient with peripheral tissue resistance to thyroid hormone action. *J Clin Endocrinol Metab* 1978;**47**:1266.

Refetoff S, Dewind LT, DeGroot LJ: Familial syndrome combining deaf-mutism, stippled epiphyses, goiter and abnormally high PBI: Possible target organ refractoriness to thyroid hormone. *J Clin Endocrinol Metab* 1967;**27**:279.

Weintraub BD et al: Inappropriate secretion of thyroid-stimulating hormone. *Ann Intern Med* 1981;**95**:339.

Nontoxic Goiter

Stanbury JB: Familial goiter. Page 206 in: *The Metabolic Basis of Inherited Disease*, 4th ed. Stanbury JB, Wyngaarden JB, Frederickson DS (editors). McGraw-Hill, 1978.

Stanbury JB, Metzel BS (editors): *Endemic Goiter and Endemic Cretinism.* Wiley, 1980.

Thilly CH et al: Fetal hypothyroidism and maternal thyroid status in severe endemic goiter. *J Clin Endocrinol Metab* 1978;**47**:354.

Thyroiditis

Amino N et al: Measurement of circulating thyroid microsomal antibodies by the tanned red cell hemagglutination technique: Its usefulness in the diagnosis of autoimmune disease. *Clin Endocrinol* 1976;**5**:115.

Khangure MS et al: A long term follow-up of patients with autoimmune thyroid disease. *Clin Endocrinol* 1977;**6**:41.

Larsen PR: Serum triiodothyronine, thyroxine and thyrotropin during hyperthyroid, hypothyroid and recovery phases of subacute non-suppurative thyroiditis. *Metabolism* 1974;**23**:467.

Mori T, Kriss JP: Measurement by competitive binding radioassay of serum antimicrosomal and antithyroglobulin antibodies in Graves' disease and other thyroid disorders. *J Clin Endocrinol Metab* 1971;**33**:688.

Nikolai TF et al: Lymphocytic thyroiditis with spontaneously resolving hyperthyroidism (silent thyroiditis). *Arch Intern Med* 1980;**140**:478.

Papapetrou PD et al: Long-term treatment of Hashimoto's thyroiditis with thyroxine. *Lancet* 1972;**2**:1045.

Volpé R, Row VV, Ezrin C: Circulating viral and thyroid antibodies in subacute thyroiditis. *J Clin Endocrinol* 1967;**12**:1275.

Weetman AP, McGregor AM: Autoimmune thyroid disease: Developments in our understanding. *Endocr Rev* 1984;**5**:309.

Yoshida H et al: Association of serum antithyroid antibodies with lymphocytic infiltration of the thyroid gland: Studies of 70 autopsied cases. *J Clin Endocrinol Metab* 1978;**46**:859.

Effects of Chronic Illness on Thyroid Function

Cavalieri RR, Rapoport B: Impaired peripheral conversion of thyroxine to triiodothyronine. *Annu Rev Med* 1977;**28**:57.

Chopra IJ et al: Misleadingly low free thyroxine index and usefulness of reverse triiodothyronine measurement in nonthyroidal illness. *Ann Intern Med* 1979;**90**:905.

Gardner DF et al: Effect of triiodothyronine replacement on the metabolic and pituitary responses to starvation. *N Engl J Med* 1979;**300**:579.

Gavin LA, Rosenthal M, Cavalieri RR: The diagnosis dilemma of isolated hyperthyroxinemia in acute illness. *JAMA* 1979;**242**:251.

Schimmel M, Utiger RD: Thyroidal and peripheral production of thyroid hormone: Review of recent findings and their clinical implications. *Ann Intern Med* 1977;**87**:760.

Thyroid Nodules & Thyroid Cancer

Beierwaltes WH: The treatment of thyroid carcinoma with radioactive iodine. *Semin Nucl Med* 1978;**8**:79.

Blum M, Rothschild M: Improved nonoperative diagnosis of the solitary "cold" thyroid nodule: Surgical selection based on risk factors and three months of suppression. *JAMA* 1980;**243**:242.

Clark OH: Thyroid nodules and thyroid cancer: Surgical aspects. *West J Med* 1980;**133**:1.

DeGroot LJ et al (editors): *Radiation-Associated Thyroid Carcinoma.* Grune & Stratton, 1977.

Greenspan FS: Radiation exposure and thyroid cancer. *JAMA* 1977;**237**:2089.

Greenspan FS: Thyroid nodules and thyroid cancer. *West J Med* 1974;**121**:359.

Harwood J, Clark OH, Dunphy JE: Significance of lymph node metastases in differentiated thyroid cancer. *Am J Surg* 1978;**136**:107.

Lowhagen T et al: Aspiration Biopsy Cytology (ABC) in tumors of the thyroid gland suspected to be malignant. *Surg Clin North Am* 1979;**59**:3.

Mazzaferri EL et al: Papillary thyroid carcinoma: The impact of therapy in 576 patients. *Medicine* 1977;**56**:171.

Miller JM, Hamburger JI, Kim S: Diagnosis of thyroid nodules: Use of fine-needle aspiration and needle biopsy. *JAMA* 1979;**241**:481.

Parker LN et al: Thyroid carcinoma after exposure to atomic radiation: A continuing survey of a fixed population, Hiroshima and Nagasaki, 1958–1971. *Ann Intern Med* 1974;**80**:600.

Sampson RJ et al: Thyroid carcinoma in Hiroshima and Nagasaki. 1. Prevalence of thyroid carcinoma at autopsy. *JAMA* 1979;**209**:65.

Sarkar SK et al: Subsequent fertility and birth histories of children and adolescents treated with ^{131}I for thyroid cancer. *J Nucl Med* 1976;**17**:460.

Sokal JE: The problem of malignancy in nodular goiter recapitulation and a challenge. *JAMA* 1959;**170**:405.

Vander JB, Gaston A, Dauber TR: The significance of nontoxic thyroid nodules. *Ann Intern Med* 1968;**69**:537.

Woolner LB et al: Thyroid carcinoma: General considerations and follow-up data on 1181 cases. In: *Thyroid Neoplasia*. Young S, Inman DR (editors). Academic Press, 1968.

8

The Calciotropic Hormones & Metabolic Bone Disease

Claude D. Arnaud, MD, & Felix O. Kolb, MD

EXTRACELLULAR & BONE MINERAL HOMEOSTASIS

A highly integrated and complex endocrine system maintains calcium, phosphate, and magnesium homeostasis in all vertebrates. It involves an interplay between the actions of 2 polypeptide hormones, parathyroid hormone (PTH) and calcitonin (CT), and a sterol hormone, 1,25-dihydroxycholecalciferol, or $1,25(OH)_2D_3$.* Biosynthesis and secretion of the polypeptide hormones are regulated by a negative feedback mechanism that involves the activity of ionic calcium in the extracellular fluid (Fig 8–1). The biosynthesis of $1,25(OH)_2D_3$ from the major circulating metabolite of vitamin D, 25-hydroxycholecalciferol ($25OHD_3$), takes place in the kidney and is regulated by PTH and CT, as well as by the extracellular fluid concentrations of calcium and phosphate. Other hormones, such as insulin, cortisol, growth hormone (GH), thyroxine, epinephrine, estrogen, testosterone, somatomedin, and inorganic phosphate, together with some compounds not yet identified and certain physical phenomena, undoubtedly have roles in modifying and regulating organ responses to PTH, CT, and $1,25(OH)_2D_3$.

PTH, CT, and $1,25(OH)_2D_3$ regulate the flow of minerals into and out of the extracellular fluid compartment through their actions on intestine, kidney, and bone (Table 8–1; Fig 8–2). The target cells of these organs function as a cellular barrier between the extracellular fluid compartment and the intestinal lumen, the renal tubular lumen, and the bone fluid compartment (adjacent to mobilizable bone mineral) (Fig 8–3). These target cells are highly specialized for solute transport against a concentration gradient and thus are often described as being polarized.

*The nomenclature of the calciotropic hormones and vitamin D metabolites discussed in this chapter is generally in agreement with the recommendations of the Endocrine Society and conforms to the editorial practices of the *Journal of Clinical Endocrinology and Metabolism*. Note especially the following: vitamin D_3 = cholecalciferol; vitamin D_2 = ergocalciferol; 25-hydroxycholecalciferol = $25OHD_3$; 25-hydroxyergocalciferol = $25OHD_2$; 1,25-dihydroxycholecalciferol (often written 1α,25-dihydroxy . . . in other texts) = $1,25(OH)_2D_3$; 24,25-dihydroxycholecalciferol = $24,25(OH)_2D_3$. A few others of lesser importance are mentioned briefly in the section entitled Vitamin D.

Acronyms Used in This Chapter

ACTH	Adrenocorticotropic hormone
ATP	Adenosine triphosphate
cAMP	Cyclic adenosine monophosphate
CT	Calcitonin
GFR	Glomerular filtration rate
GH	Growth hormone
Gpp(NH)p	5'-Guanyl-imidodiphosphate
HAM	Hypoparathyroidism-Addison's disease-mucocutaneous candidiasis (syndrome)
iCT	Immunoreactive calcitonin
iPTH	Immunoreactive parathyroid hormone
MEDAC	Multiple endocrine deficiency-auto-immune–candidiasis (syndrome)
MEN	Multiple endocrine neoplasia
OAF	Osteoclast-activating factor
PRL	Prolactin
PTH	Parathyroid hormone
RNA	Ribonucleic acid

Role of Parathyroid Hormone
Target Tissues

Under normal circumstances, PTH prevents serum calcium from falling below physiologic concentrations by stimulating calcium movement from intestinal and renal tubular lumina and from the bone fluid compartment into the blood. Whereas its effects on bone and kidney are direct, PTH acts indirectly on the intestine, through the mediation of vitamin D. The hormone stimulates (directly and through its hypophosphatemic effects) the conversion of $25OHD_3$ to $1,25(OH)_2D_3$ in the kidney via a $25OHD_3$ 1α-hydroxylase in the mitochondria of the renal tubule. The $1,25(OH)_2D_3$ thus formed stimulates intestinal calcium absorption. PTH also prevents serum phosphate levels from rising above normal physiologic concentrations by increasing renal tubular excretion of phosphate. This regulatory action is important because phosphate, like calcium, is also released into the blood by PTH-induced bone resorption. This function can be particularly appreciated in patients with end-stage renal failure associated with severe hyperparathyroidism. These patients develop hyperphosphatemia because large quantities of phosphate are released from bone, and the kidney can no longer excrete them.

Figure 8–1. Plasma immunoreactive PTH (iPTH) and CT (iCT) as a function of plasma total calcium in pigs given EDTA to decrease plasma calcium or given calcium infusions to increase plasma calcium. Note that as serum calcium increases, serum iPTH falls and serum iCT rises; as serum calcium decreases, the reverse occurs. ($r = -0.942$ for iPTH and 0.964 for iCT; p for both is $< .001$.) (Reproduced, with permission, from Arnaud CD et al, in: *Calcitonin: Proceedings of the Second International Symposium.* Taylor S [editor]. Heinemann, 1969.)

Role of Calcitonin

Calcitonin prevents abnormal increases in both serum calcium and serum phosphate. It decreases the translocation of calcium from the renal tubule and bone fluid compartment into the blood and thus can be considered as a counterregulator of PTH. The ef-fects of CT on vitamin D metabolism and on the intestinal absorption of calcium are uncertain.

Integrated Actions of PTH, CT, & 1,25(OH)₂D₃

It is likely that PTH and CT regulate the entry of

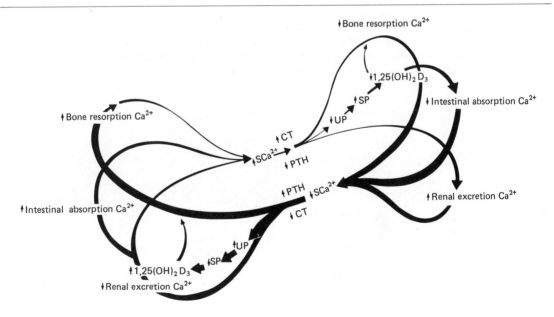

Figure 8–2. Regulation of calcium homeostasis. Three overlapping control loops interlock and relate to one another through the level of blood concentrations of ionic calcium, PTH, and CT. Each loop involves a calciotropic hormone target organ (bone, intestine, kidney). The limbs on the left depict physiologic events that increase the blood concentration of calcium (SCa²⁺), and the limbs on the right, events that decrease this concentration. UP = urine phosphorus, SP = serum phosphorus. See text for detailed descriptions. (Modified and reproduced, with permission, from Arnaud CD: *Fed Proc* 1978;**37**:2558.)

Table 8–1. Actions of major calcium-regulating hormones.

	Bone	Kidney	Intestine
Parathyroid hormone (PTH)	Increases resorption of calcium and phosphate.	Increases reabsorption of calcium; decreases reabsorption of phosphate; increases conversion of $25OHD_3$ to $1,25(OH)_2D_3$; decreases reabsorption of bicarbonate.	No direct effects.
Calcitonin (CT)	Decreases resorption of calcium and phosphate.	Decreases reabsorption of calcium and phosphate. Questionable effect on vitamin D metabolism.	No direct effects.
Vitamin D	Maintains Ca^{2+} transport system.	Decreases reabsorption of calcium.	Increases absorption of calcium and phosphate.

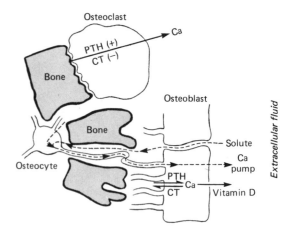

Figure 8–4. Relationships among calciotropic hormones, bone cells, and calcium transport. Bone crystal is represented by the shaded areas. The osteoclast, with an active "ruffled border," is shown resorbing bone—a process stimulated by PTH (+) and inhibited by CT (–). The "osteoblasts" (perhaps better called "surface osteocytes") are not forming bone but are actively extruding calcium from the bone fluid (between cells and crystals) under the influence of hormones. Processes connecting deep osteocytes are shown participating in transport of calcium (dotted arrows).

calcium into polarized cells of the surface membrane of bone and the renal tubular lumen. $1,25(OH)_2D_3$ acts primarily to maintain the cellular calcium transport system in the intestine, which causes the active extrusion of calcium against a concentration gradient from the interior of the cell (ionized calcium concentration = 10^{-7} to 10^{-6} mol/L), across the antiluminal membrane, and into the extracellular fluid (ionized calcium concentration = 10^{-3} mol/L) (Fig 8–4). Thus, the calciotropic hormones, especially PTH and $1,25(OH)_2D_3$, are interdependent. The renal production of $1,25(OH)_2D_3$ depends upon the prevailing concentration of PTH in the blood, and the ability of PTH to increase plasma calcium depends upon a calcium transport system maintained by $1,25(OH)_2D_3$.

Interrelationship of Calcium & the Calciotropic Hormones

The relationships among the several components involved in maintaining mineral homeostasis are il-

Figure 8–3. Cellular barrier separating the extracellular fluid compartment from the intestinal and renal tubular lumina and from the bone fluid compartment. PTH, CT, and $1,25(OH)_2D_3$ act on these cells (directly or indirectly) to regulate the flow of calcium into and out of the extracellular fluid (ECF) compartments. (See Fig 8–2.) (Reproduced, with permission, from Rasmussen H et al: *Fed Proc* 1970;**29**:1190.)

lustrated in Fig 8–2. Each of the 3 overlapping feedback loops involves one of the target organs of the calciotropic hormones and the 4 controlling elements, ie, plasma calcium, PTH, CT, and $1,25(OH)_2D_3$. The left limbs of the loops depict physiologic events that increase plasma calcium, and the right limbs, events that decrease plasma calcium. Under physiologic conditions, there are small fluctuations in plasma calcium. Decreases in plasma calcium increase PTH se-

cretion and decrease CT secretion. These changes in hormone secretion lead to increased bone resorption, decreased renal excretion of calcium, and increased intestinal calcium absorption via PTH stimulation of $1,25(OH)_2D_3$ production (left side of Fig 8–2). As a consequence of these events, plasma calcium rises slightly above its physiologic concentrations, inhibiting PTH secretion and stimulating CT secretion. These changes in plasma hormone concentrations de-

Figure 8–5. Proposed intracellular pathway of the biosynthesis of PTH. The initial product of synthesis on the ribosomes, preproPTH, is converted into proPTH by removal of (1) the NH_2-terminal methionyl residues (methionyl aminopeptidase) and (2) the NH_2-terminal sequence (−29 through −7) of 23 amino acids (by "clipase") during synthesis and within seconds afterward, respectively. The conversion of preproPTH to proPTH probably occurs during transport of the polypeptide into the cisterna of the rough endoplasmic reticulum. By 20 minutes after synthesis, proPTH reaches the Golgi region and is converted into PTH by (3) removal of the NH_2-terminal hexapeptide. PTH is either stored in secretory granules or released into the cell cytoplasm, where it remains until it is released into the circulation in response to a fall in the blood concentration of calcium. The intact PTH, PTH(1–84), undergoes at least 2 cleavages while in the secretory granule (and possibly in the cytoplasm) (4) and (5). These cleavages generate amino-, mid-, and carboxy-region fragments. The mid- and carboxy-region fragments are secreted into the circulation along with PTH(1–84), whereas the amino-region fragments are further degraded by the cell. The PTH(1–84) released into the circulation undergoes metabolic degradation in the liver and kidney (6), and this adds to the pool of circulating fragments. The time required for these events to occur is shown. (Modified and reproduced, with permission, from Habener JF et al: *Recent Prog Horm Res* 1977;**33**:287.)

crease bone resorption, increase renal excretion of calcium, and decrease intestinal absorption of calcium (right side of Fig 8–2), causing plasma calcium to fall below the physiologic level. This sequence of events probably occurs within milliseconds, so that plasma calcium is maintained at physiologic levels within minimal oscillation. The "butterfly" scheme in Fig 8–2 not only demonstrates the relationships among elements that control mineral homeostasis under physiologic conditions but also suggests how potential pathogenetic mechanisms and adaptive responses elicited by disease or treatment would operate in this system.

PARATHYROID HORMONE

Structure & Biosynthesis

PTH is an 84-amino-acid, linear polypeptide with a molecular weight of 9500. Its biosynthesis and intracellular processing are complex (Fig 8–5). The original gene product of the parathyroid cell is a 115-amino-acid precursor called preproparathyroid hormone (preproPTH). The hydrophobic 23-amino-acid "pre" sequence acts to bind the polyribosome-precursor complex to the endoplasmic reticulum, providing access to the cisternal space and, presumably, to the enzyme ("clipase") that removes the "pre"

HUMAN– ◯   BOVINE– ◯   PORCINE– ◿

Figure 8–6. Parathyroid hormone. The figure shows the structure of human PTH and indicates at which positions the amino acid residues differ for bovine and porcine PTH. (From Keutmann HT et al: *Biochemistry* 1978;**17**:5723.)

sequence, leaving the 90-amino-acid proPTH structure. The proPTH is converted to PTH in the Golgi apparatus by proteolytic removal ("tryptic clipase") of the remaining 6-amino-terminal amino acid sequence. Here, the 84-amino-acid polypeptide is readied for secretion either in a secretory granule or in its free form. There is no evidence that either of the PTH precursor molecules or the "pre" or "pro" peptide sequences normally find their way into the circulation. In contrast to the rapid regulation of PTH *secretion,* PTH *biosynthesis* is only slowly influenced by changes in concentration of extracellular ionic calcium.

Intracellular stores of PTH may be regulated by a degradative pathway that is stimulated by high and inhibited by low extracellular calcium. This degradative pathway is currently of considerable interest. Not only may it provide an important mechanism for regulating PTH economy, but the fragments of the hormone produced during intracellular degradation and secreted from the cell may also provide a major source of the multiple immunoreactive forms of PTH known to circulate in the blood (see below).

The amino acid sequences of bovine, porcine, and human PTH have been determined (Fig 8–6). The differences among them prevent complete immunologic cross-reactivity. This probably accounts for the difficulties in developing radioimmunoassays for the measurement of human PTH using antisera directed against the more readily available bovine or porcine peptides. All of the structural information required for full biologic activity of native 84-amino-acid PTH lies in the 34 amino acids at the amino terminus. The active fragments of the bovine and human hormones, multiple fragments of the mid and carboxyl regions of the bovine and human hormones, and recently the full sequence of human parathyroid hormone have been synthesized and are available for investigational use. Studies of the mid- and carboxy-region fragments have shown them to be biologically inert.

Control of Secretion

PTH is rapidly released from the parathyroid gland in response to decreases in the plasma ionic calcium. It acts on kidney and bone and indirectly on intestine to restore the concentration of this cation to just above the normal set point (Fig 8–1), which in turn inhibits secretion of the hormone. This negative feedback cycle is depicted in Fig 8–2. The concentration of extracellular ionic calcium is the major regulator of PTH secretion. Other factors influence secretion only indirectly. For example, plasma phosphate alters the degree to which calcium is complexed, and arterial blood pH alters the degree to which it binds to albumin (normally about 50% of the total). The effects of extracellular magnesium concentrations on secretion are qualitatively similar to but physiologically less important than those induced by ionic calcium. Paradoxically, severe, prolonged hypomagnesemia markedly inhibits secretion of PTH and may be associated with hypocalcemia (see section on hypoparathyroidism). Known direct PTH secretagogues of questionable physiologic importance include beta-adrenergic agonists, prostaglandins, and histamine. These agents, as well as decreased ionic calcium, stimulate the production of cyclic 3',5'-adenosine monophosphate (cAMP) in parathyroid cells in vitro, and it is presumed that this compound mediates their actions on hormone secretion.

Metabolism & Circulating Forms

Circulating PTH is heterogeneous, consisting of the intact 84-amino-acid polypeptide and multiple fragments of the hormone (Fig 8–7). These fragments are derived from the mid and carboxyl regions of the hormone molecule and thus are likely to be biologically inert. There is no evidence that biologically active fragments are secreted by the parathyroid gland or that they are present in the circulation. The relative quantities of intact PTH and its fragments in serum are not known precisely at present, but there are more circulating fragments than intact hormone. This difference is due primarily to the longer survival time of the fragments in the circulation (see Fig 8–7 legend). The fragments are derived both by release from the parathyroid gland and from the degradative metabolism of intact 84-amino-acid PTH (liver and kidney); the quantitative importance of these sources is uncertain.

Biologically active PTH normally circulates in the blood at extremely low concentrations (< 50 pg/mL).

It is likely that there are individual, constitutionally dependent "set point" values for plasma ionic calcium above which glandular secretion rates are decreased and below which they are increased. However, the steady-state levels of PTH and the size of the glands are probably determined primarily by the degree to which the parathyroid glands must adapt to individual, chronic, environmentally induced changes in the plasma level of ionic calcium (eg, dietary calcium and phosphate). In normal humans (Fig 8–8), as in lower animals (Fig 8–1), there is an inverse relationship between the fasting levels of serum calcium and serum immunoreactive PTH.

Actions

The major function of PTH is to correct hypocalcemia. As Fig 8–2 shows, it performs this function by (1) conservation of calcium by the kidney, (2) release of calcium from bone, (3) enhanced absorption of calcium from the gut (indirectly via vitamin D), and (4) reduction in plasma phosphate.

A. Effects of PTH on Kidney: PTH acts on the kidney (1) to increase renal tubular reabsorption of calcium and magnesium and (2) to increase phosphate and bicarbonate excretion by inhibiting their proximal tubular resorption. These latter effects have several important indirect effects on the homeostasis of extracellular calcium. Hormone-induced bicarbonaturia tends to produce acidosis, which decreases the ability

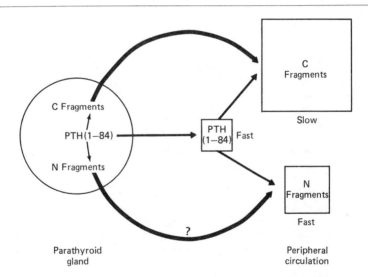

Figure 8–7. Metabolic alterations in PTH(1–84) that result in its immunoheterogeneity in gland extracts and biologic fluids. This scheme is based on study of abnormal parathyroid tissue and hyperparathyroid serum. Data on normal glands and serum are not available. An uncertain proportion of intraglandular PTH(1–84) is proteolytically cleaved into amino-region fragments (N fragments) and carboxy-region fragments (C fragments). All of these PTH molecular species are released into the circulation (approximately 80% PTH[1–84] and 20% fragments). Once in the circulation, PTH(1–84) undergoes proteolytic cleavage in liver and kidney, generating N and C fragments that are added to the circulating pool of hormone fragments. The rate of disappearance of C fragments from the circulation is slow ($t_{1/2}$ 20–40 minutes), whereas that of PTH(1–84) and of N fragments is fast ($t_{1/2}$ < 10 minutes). These differences in metabolic turnover probably account for the large pool of C fragments and small pools of PTH(1–84) and N fragments in the blood under steady-state conditions (see text). (Reproduced, with permission, from DiBella FP et al: Page 338 in: *Excerpta Medica Int Cong Ser* No. 421, 1977.)

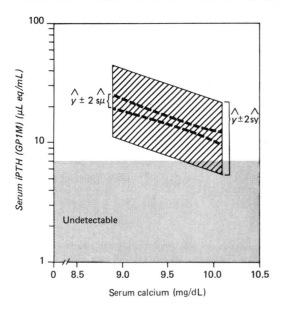

Figure 8–8. Serum immunoreactive PTH (iPTH) (log scale) as a function of total serum calcium in 150 normal human subjects ($r = -0.424$; $p < .001$). $y \pm 2\ s\mu$ = mean ± 2 SEM; $y \pm 2$ sy = mean ± 2 SD. GP1M is the antiserum (mid region) used in the radioimmunoassay. (Reproduced, with permission, from Purnell D et al: *Am J Med* 1974; 56:801.)

of circulating albumin to bind calcium, thus increasing ionic calcium by physicochemical means. Hormone-induced phosphaturia ensures that the increased release of phosphate from bone, which occurs obligately during hormone-induced calcium mobilization from bone, does not produce hyperphosphatemia. Increased serum phosphate would tend to complex calcium and thereby counteract the physiologic effect of PTH to increase plasma ionic calcium.

The most important indirect effect of the phosphaturic action of the hormone is illustrated in the intestinal feedback loop in Fig 8–2. PTH, either directly or indirectly by its hypophosphatemic action, stimulates renal tubular $25OHD_3$ 1α-hydroxylase to convert the major circulating metabolite of cholecalciferol, $25OHD_3$, to its major biologically active metabolite, $1,25(OH)_2D_3$. This latter compound acts directly on intestinal mucosal cells to increase calcium absorption and on bone to increase resorption.

In the process of stimulating adenylate cyclase in renal tubular cells (see below), PTH increases urinary excretion of cAMP. Presumably, cAMP is released into the tubular fluid following its intracellular synthesis. Urinary cAMP is increased by administration of other hormones, including epinephrine and glucagon, but its renal production and excretion are almost entirely due to PTH. It can therefore be used as an indirect measure of PTH secretion or action, as noted below.

B. Effects of PTH on Bone: PTH increases the

net release of calcium and phosphate from bone into extracellular fluid (Fig 8–4). This is a direct result of the hormone's effect on the differentiation or activities of bone cells (osteogenic precursors, osteoblasts, osteoclasts, and osteocytes). These events appear to depend upon a permissive effect of $1,25(OH)_2D_3$, but the precise cellular mechanism of this important hormonal relationship is poorly understood. The physiology and pathophysiology of mineral metabolism demonstrate a wide range of interactions between PTH (tropic) and vitamin D (permissive), and these interactions will be noted below in the sections on hypoparathyroidism, hyperparathyroidism, and metabolic bone disease.

Mechanisms of Action

PTH binds to specific plasma membrane receptors of target cells. These occupied receptors interact with a guanyl nucleotide–regulated membrane-bound protein that in turn activates membrane-bound adenylate cyclase to convert ATP to cAMP (Fig 8–9). cAMP, by virtue of its ability to initiate a cascade of enzyme-activated intracellular phosphorylations, is considered

Figure 8–9. Mechanism of PTH action on membrane-bound adenylate cyclase. PTH(1–34) is the biologically active PTH agonist ⁸Nle-¹⁸Nle-²³Tyr-bPTH(1–34)amide, and PTH(3–34) is the biologically inactive PTH antagonist ⁸Nle-¹⁸Nle-³⁴Tyr-bPTH(3–34)amide. Both of these are capable of binding to the PTH receptor (R). However, only PTH(1–34) is capable of converting the receptor to a high-affinity state, so that guanyl nucleotide regulatory protein (N) can be stimulated to bind guanosine triphosphate (GTP). The binding of GTP to N converts R to a low-affinity state, inducing dissociation of PTH(1–34) *and* the formation of an N-adenylate cyclase (AC) complex, leading to the activation of this enzyme and the increased production of intracellular cAMP. In contrast, the binding of PTH(3–34) to R does not change the affinity of R; consequently, R cannot interact with N or induce activation of adenylate cyclase.

to be one of possibly several intracellular "second messengers" responsible for mediating the final expression of the action of the hormone. The details of these enzyme activations and the manner in which they relate to discrete effects of the hormone are unknown. Other potential second messengers of PTH (eg, calcium itself) that might act in concert with or modulate the actions of cAMP are currently being investigated.

Information concerning the structural requirements for the action of PTH at the site of its receptor is rapidly becoming available. The region of the molecule essential for receptor binding is the amino acid sequence 25–30, and for receptor activation, the 1–7 sequence. Recently, 2 analogs of bovine PTH that are truncated at the amino terminus have been developed. One of these is ^{8}Nle-^{18}Nle-^{34}Tyr-bPTH(3–34)amide, or bPTH(3–34)amide. This analog has both agonist and antagonist properties in vitro. It binds to PTH receptors in the kidney to the same degree as bPTH(1–34) but is much less potent in converting the receptor to the high-affinity state necessary to activate adenylate cyclase (Fig 8–9). Although bPTH(3–34)amide acts as an antagonist in vitro, it fails to antagonize concomitantly administered PTH in vivo. The other analog, ^{34}Tyr-bPTH(7–34)amide, has antagonist but no agonist properties in vitro. Preliminary studies indicate that it antagonizes PTH in vivo but that large doses are required, possibly owing to the fact that its ability to bind to PTH receptors is weak. In spite of this, the development of this analog represents an important advance in the effort to design a PTH antagonist that can rapidly reverse hypercalcemia in patients with severe hyperparathyroidism.

Assay in Biologic Fluids

The major tool for measuring PTH in biologic fluids is radioimmunoassay. Values for serum iPTH vary from laboratory to laboratory, however, because of the differences in the source (bovine or human) and purity of the PTH preparations used as standards and in the specificity of the antisera. Therefore, interpretation of serum iPTH values requires knowledge of the normal range for each assay system. Until recently, most radioimmunoassays of human PTH have used ^{125}I-labeled bovine PTH as the radioligand and cross-reacting antisera directed against porcine or bovine PTH. Use of synthetic human PTH or its fragments, which have recently become commercially available, may help to minimize some of the inconsistencies in the future. However, variations in the specificities of antisera used in different assays will continue to result in different iPTH values for the same serum sample. Such differences reflect true differences in the concentrations of the various forms of circulating PTH.

At present, all available antisera that have a sufficiently high affinity for PTH to be useful in radioimmunoassays are multivalent and contain antibodies directed at multiple regions of the PTH molecule. Antisera directed against the mid or carboxyl region of the PTH molecule recognize inactive mid- or carboxy-region fragments and intact biologically active PTH, while antisera directed against the amino region recognize amino-region fragments and intact PTH. Because the quantities of mid- and carboxy-region fragments in the circulation are greater than those of amino-region fragments or intact PTH, values for serum iPTH are higher when measured with mid- and carboxy-region assays than with amino-region assays.

Mid- and carboxy-region assays have provided surprisingly good diagnostic tools in the evaluation of patients suspected of having parathyroid disease, even though the resulting values for serum iPTH primarily reflect circulating biologically inactive hormone (ie, mid- and carboxy-region fragments). This is fortunate because the concentrations of intact PTH in the circulation are so low that, with rare exception, they are beyond the sensitivity limits of all the amino-region assays yet developed.

Ideally, radioimmunoassays for PTH should do the following: (1) be able to measure serum iPTH in over 95% of normal subjects; (2) demonstrate an inverse relationship between serum iPTH and total serum calcium over the normal range of serum calcium (Fig 8–8); (3) show consistently low or undetectable serum iPTH values in all patients with hypoparathyroidism as well as in all patients with hypercalcemia of nonparathyroid origin, other than cancer; and (4) demonstrate iPTH values greater than the upper limits of normal in 90% of patients with surgically proved primary hyperparathyroidism.

Until recently, bioassays for PTH lacked sufficient sensitivity for the study of circulating PTH. This obstacle has now been overcome by 2 novel approaches. One is a cytochemical bioassay that is based on the PTH-specific stimulation of glucose 6-phosphate dehydrogenase in guinea pig renal slices. This assay is extremely sensitive, measuring femtogram amounts of PTH. Its disadvantage is its technical complexity. The other assay, which is more convenient, uses a nonhydrolyzable analog of guanosine triphosphate— ie, 5′-guanyl-imidodiphosphate, or Gpp(NH)p—to greatly augment the sensitivity of adenylate cyclase to PTH in canine kidneys in vitro. In the presence of Gpp(NH)p, as little as 10 pg/mL of intact PTH elicits significant stimulation. However, even with this sensitivity, the measurement of PTH in normal serum requires the immunoextraction of 3 mL of serum. This assay is accurate, precise, and simple and can be performed rapidly.

Radioligand-binding studies have been used to probe the PTH receptor, but no clinically useful radioreceptor assay for PTH has been developed.

CALCITONIN

Structure & Biosynthesis

Calcitonin (CT), a 32-amino-acid polypeptide with a molecular weight of 3700 and a disulfide bridge between residues 1 and 7 (Fig 8–10), is biosynthesized and secreted by the ultimobranchial (parafollic-

Figure 8–10. Amino acid sequence of CTs. Note the similarity between human and rat CT and the substantial differences in amino acid sequence from the porcine, bovine, and ovine CTs. Salmon and eel CTs are actually more similar to human CT than are hormones from ungulates. In the 7 amino acids in the N-terminal ring, the only substitution is serine for glycine. (Modified and reproduced, with permission, from Hirsch PF: *J Exp Zool* 1971;**178**:139.)

ular, "C") cells. Recent work has shown that human CT is cleaved from a high-molecular-weight precursor and that this precursor also contains a second discrete peptide, katacalcin. Katacalcin circulates in normal subjects in roughly equimolar relationship to CT and, like CT, is secreted in excess in medullary carcinoma of the thyroid. It is not known whether katacalcin has an important role in humans.

The ultimobranchial cells develop from neural crest tissue during embryonic life. They form a discrete organ in submammalian vertebrates called the ultimobranchial gland. In the mammal, the anlage of the cells merges with the embryonic thyroid gland, ultimately becoming dispersed in the central region of each lobe (of the thyroid gland), adjacent to the follicular cells.

The amino acid sequences of CT from many species (porcine, bovine, human, rat, salmon, eel) have been determined (Fig 8–10). They are different enough so that immunologic cross-reactivity between them is incomplete. In fact, radioimmunoassay of human CT was not possible until synthetic human CT became available so that specific antibodies directed against it could be used. The entire CT molecule is required for full biologic activity, as is the intact 1–7 disulfide bridge. Salmon CT has an amino acid sequence markedly different from those of mammalian CTs and is about 30 times more potent. Synthetic salmon CT is commercially available and can be used for treatment of metabolic bone disease (see Paget's Disease, below).

Control of Secretion

CT is rapidly released by the "C" cells in response to small increases in plasma ionic calcium. It acts on kidney and bone to restore the level of this cation to just below a normal set point, which in turn inhibits secretion of the hormone (Fig 8–2). CT thus is a physiologic antagonist of PTH. The hormones act in concert to maintain the normal concentration of ionic calcium in extracellular fluid (Fig 8–2).

There is a positive correlation between plasma calcium and plasma immunoreactive CT (iCT) in normal subjects when plasma calcium is increased above the normal range (by oral calcium ingestion) (Fig 8–11). Induced hypercalcemia causes an increase in plasma iCT in about 40–60% of normal women and 70–80% of normal men. Although pentagastrin injection also increases plasma iCT, it is unlikely that gastrin is a physiologic CT secretagogue. Other CT secretagogues of unknown physiologic significance include glucagon, beta-adrenergic agonists, and alcohol.

Metabolism & Circulating Forms

CT exists in several molecular forms both in ultimobranchial tissue and in plasma. In contrast to PTH, however, the major circulating species are not

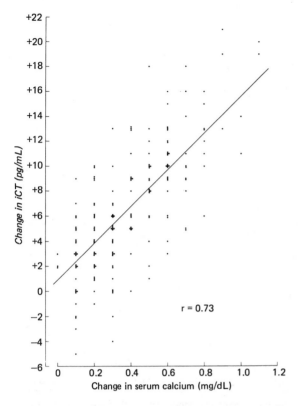

Figure 8–11. Changes in iCT plotted against corresponding changes in serum calcium after calcium ingestion. The data represent the responses of 10 subjects to each of 3 different oral calcium doses. (Reproduced, with permission, from Austin LA et al: *J Clin Invest* 1979;**64**:1721.)

hormone fragments but consist of as many as 4 or 5 immunoreactive forms with molecular weights larger than 32-amino-acid CT. It is likely that some of these forms are polymers of CT with interchain disulfide molecular linkages. The different antisera used in radioimmunoassays recognize these forms differently, and therefore the normal range for plasma CT must be established for each assay. The plasma concentrations of monomeric iCT are extremely low (< 50 pg/mL).

Actions

The importance of CT in the calcium homeostasis of adult humans is not established. An excess or deficiency of PTH or vitamin D produces dramatic clinical disorders. In contrast, an excess or deficiency of CT, as occurs in medullary thyroid carcinoma or postthyroidectomy, respectively, produces few discernible and no serious abnormalities of mineral metabolism. The basal plasma levels of CT and its responsiveness to induced hypercalcemia or pentagastrin injection are lower in women than in men and decrease with age. In adult humans, CT may function primarily to restrain the bone resorptive effects of PTH. If this is the case, the long-term combination of a progressive decrease

in CT secretion and reserve—and an increase in PTH secretion with aging—may contribute to the osteoporosis of menopause and aging (see Osteoporosis, below).

When bone turnover rates are high, CT administration rapidly produces hypocalcemia and hypophosphatemia. These effects are largely due to decreased bone resorption secondary to inhibition of activities of bone-resorbing cells (osteoclasts). CT also increases urinary calcium and phosphate, but its action on the kidney is transient and variable. Current evidence does not support a direct effect of CT on the intestinal absorption of calcium. However, several recent reports suggest that the hormone may have a negative influence on the renal production of $1,25(OH)_2D_3$. Such an effect would be consistent with the concept of CT as a physiologic antagonist of PTH.

Mechanisms of Action

CT receptors have been demonstrated in the plasma membranes of target cells (kidney). The hormone stimulates adenylate cyclase in bone and kidney in some species (human and rat), but whether cAMP is a major intracellular mediator of CT action has not been established.

Assay in Biologic Fluids

The major tool for measuring CT in biologic fluids has been radioimmunoassay. Antibodies against human CT generally cross-react with rat CT, but antibodies against porcine or bovine CT cross-react poorly with human and rat CT. Although iCT in human plasma is heterogeneous, synthetic human CT is generally used as an assay standard. As with PTH, most antisera to human CT are multivalent, and assays using them measure the different circulating forms of CT differently. Thus, as noted above, the normal ranges for plasma iCT vary from laboratory to laboratory.

The single most important factor determining the clinical utility of a CT radioimmunoassay is its sensitivity. This is because many patients with CT-secreting medullary cancers of the thyroid gland have normal basal levels of plasma iCT and can be identified only with provocative tests (ie, calcium infusion, pentagastrin injection; see below). An assay that cannot measure basal levels of iCT cannot demonstrate an abnormal increase in plasma iCT.

Since the introduction of the original rat hypocalcemic assay for CT, there has been little progress in the development of bioassays for this hormone. Although CT receptors have been demonstrated, radioreceptor assays are too insensitive for the measurement of CT in biologic fluids.

VITAMIN D

Physiology, Metabolism, & Action

It is now firmly established that vitamin D and its metabolites are sterol hormones and that their metab-

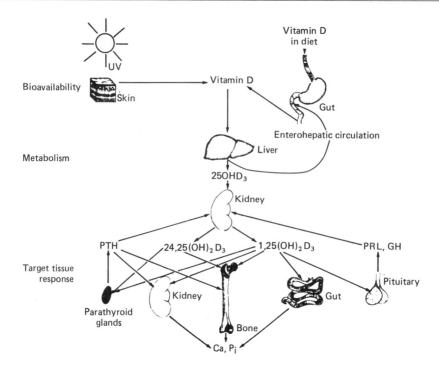

Figure 8–12. The vitamin D endocrine system. **Bioavailability:** Vitamin D is made available to the body by photogenesis in the skin and by absorption from the intestine. Part of the intestinal absorption involves endogenous vitamin D products secreted in bile (enterohepatic circulation). **Metabolism:** Vitamin D must be hydroxylated first in the liver to $25OHD_3$ and then in the kidney to $1,25(OH)_2D_3$ and $24,25(OH)_2D_3$. Other metabolites and other tissues capable of metabolizing the vitamin D metabolites are known. **Target tissue response:** The 3 principal target tissues are kidney, bone, and intestine, but the parathyroid glands and the anterior pituitary may also be target tissues. Their hormone products (PTH, PRL, and GH) help regulate vitamin D metabolism in the kidney, and PTH, at least, also has independent effects on the regulation of calcium and phosphate homeostasis in bone and kidney. (Reproduced, with permission, from Bikle DD: *Advances in Internal Medicine,* 1982. Year Book, 1982.)

olism and mechanism of action have much in common with those of the other steroid hormones (Fig 8–12). Vitamin D_3 (cholecalciferol) is primarily synthesized in the skin by ultraviolet irradiation of 7-dehydrocholesterol. Vitamin D_2 (ergocalciferol), which is used to fortify dairy products, is produced by ultraviolet irradiation of the plant sterol ergosterol.

A. Activation of Vitamin D: The parent compound, vitamin D, essentially lacks biologic activity and requires metabolic transformation to attain potency.

1. 25-Hydroxylation–The first step in this activation (Fig 8–12) involves 25-hydroxylation by microsomal enzymes—a process that occurs chiefly in the liver. This conversion does not appear to be tightly regulated, and the circulating concentration of 25-hydroxycholecalciferol $(25OHD_3)$,* estimated to be about 30 ng/mL in normal individuals, is primarily a function of the bioavailability of vitamin D. Therefore, it is subject to both seasonal and regional variation, owing to differences in both diet and sunlight

*See the footnote at the beginning of this chapter for a comment on the nomenclature of vitamin D metabolites.

exposure. $25OHD_3$ is the most abundant circulating form of the hormone, and it is transported in serum bound to a specific globulin (vitamin D–binding protein), as are the other vitamin D metabolites.

2. 1α-Hydroxylation–The next step in the bioactivation of vitamin D, 1α-hydroxylation of $25OHD_3$, occurs in the mitochondria of the renal tubules. This hydroxylation is tightly regulated and constitutes the rate-limiting step in the production of the active metabolite, $1,25(OH)_2D_3$.* Production of $1,25(OH)_2D_3$ is controlled by a number of regulators in accordance with the body's mineral requirements. Hypophosphatemia and hypocalcemia appear to be the primary stimuli for activating renal 1α-hydroxylase. The stimulus created by low calcium levels is probably mediated by PTH, which stimulates 1α-hydroxylase activity either directly or by its hypophosphatemic effects (Figs 8–2 and 8–12). Evidence that CT inhibits the activity of 1α-hydroxylase is less strong. In addition, $1,25(OH)_2D_3$ may regulate its own synthesis directly or by suppressing the parathyroid glands, where receptors for this metabolite have been reported.

B. Concentrations of Vitamin D Metabolites: In

normal individuals, $1,25(OH)_2D_3$ is estimated to circulate at concentrations as low as 30 pg/mL. This metabolite is more rapidly cleared from plasma than its more abundant precursor, $25OHD_3$, and is about 100 times more potent in stimulating intestinal calcium absorption. It is thus generally considered to be the major biologic effector of the vitamin D endocrine system. However, the fact that $25OHD_3$ circulates in concentrations 1000 times greater than $1,25(OH)_2D_3$ suggests that $25OHD_3$ may have intrinsic biologic importance as well.

C. Other Hydroxylation Pathways: Hydroxylation of $25OHD_3$ to $24,25(OH)_2D_3$ occurs mainly in the kidney and represents an alternative metabolic fate for $25OHD_3$. The regulation of this pathway generally appears to be reciprocal to that leading to $1,25(OH)_2D_3$: for example, PTH stimulates production of $1,25(OH)_2D_3$ but suppresses that of $24,25(OH)_2D_3$. At present, the physiologic importance of $24,25(OH)_2D_3$ is unclear. It may be involved in normal bone formation, but it is more likely that 24-hydroxylation represents the initial step in the metabolic elimination of $25OHD_3$. Additional vitamin D metabolites have been identified, including $25,26(OH)_2D_3$, $1,24,25(OH)_3D_3$, $1,25,26(OH)_3D_3$, and $25OH-26,23$-lactone. Excretion of vitamin D metabolites occurs primarily in the bile, and evidence has been presented for enterohepatic circulation of both $25OHD_3$ and $1,25(OH)_2D_3$.

Role of Vitamin D

It is generally accepted that the principal physiologic role of vitamin D is to increase plasma levels of calcium and phosphate and thus maintain conditions favorable for bone mineralization. The most extensively studied physiologic action of $1,25(OH)_2D_3$, however, is its role in facilitating the absorption of calcium and phosphate by the intestine, and much of our knowledge concerning the molecular mechanism of action of vitamin D has been derived from studies of the intestinal cell. Intestinal cytosolic receptors for $1,25(OH)_2D_3$ have been demonstrated; they function to translocate the hormone into the cell nucleus, where the association of the hormone-receptor complex with chromatin influences transcription and promotes the production of at least one new protein, calcium-binding protein, which is presumed to facilitate transcellular calcium transport. According to this view, vitamin D acts as a classic steroid hormone; however it has also been suggested that the hormone may have cellular actions independent of de novo protein synthesis.

$1,25(OH)_2D_3$ receptors have also been demonstrated in bone, parathyroid glands, pancreas, pituitary, placenta, and other tissues. It is possible, therefore, that vitamin D acts directly on these tissues. Vitamin D may also have a role, as yet poorly defined, in muscle function. The recent identification of several additional target organs for $1,25(OH)_2D_3$, such as the hematolymphopoietic tissue, suggests a role far beyond its known importance in mineral metabolism.

Some lymphomas and granulomatous disorders such as sarcoidosis may show ectopic production of $1,25(OH)_2D_3$ from its precursors, which may explain the hypercalcemia observed in these disorders. $1,25(OH)_2D_3$ may also have a regulatory role in connection with bone marrow stem cells and their progeny, including cells of T lymphocyte lineage.

Assay in Biologic Fluids

Two general approaches using radiolabeled vitamin D derivatives have been developed for measurement of the various vitamin D sterols in vitro: competitive protein-binding analysis and radioimmunoassay. The sensitive technique of competitive protein-binding analysis takes advantage of naturally occurring specific proteins that have high affinity for the vitamin D metabolites and are present either in serum (vitamin D–binding protein) or in intestinal target cells (cytosolic receptors). Both of these techniques involve competition in vitro between a radioligand and the vitamin D sterol of interest for available sites on the binding protein. Antisera for use in radioimmunoassays are developed against immunogenic derivatives of the vitamin D sterol molecule.

Existing competitive protein-binding assays and radioimmunoassays are not inherently specific for a single circulating vitamin D metabolite, because other closely related vitamin D metabolites compete to some extent for available binding sites on the binding protein or antibody. Furthermore, other components of blood, including plasma proteins and lipids, may cause nonspecific interference. To increase the specificity and sensitivity of the assays, it is necessary to first extract the vitamin D sterols from plasma using a suitable lipophilic solvent and then isolate the particular metabolite of interest chromatographically (using Sephadex LH-20 followed by high-pressure liquid chromatography). Simplified, rapid fractionation techniques that have been introduced recently should make the measurement of $25OHD_3$ and $1,25(OH)_2D_3$ more convenient.

A sensitive bioassay for $1,25(OH)_2D_3$ has been developed using the hormone's ability to mobilize calcium in embryonic bone organ cultures in vitro as an index of activity. This assay is comparable in sensitivity to competitive protein-binding assays and radioimmunoassays, but the procedure is tedious and requires experience to perform.

DISORDERS OF PARATHYROID FUNCTION

HYPOPARATHYROIDISM

Deficient secretion of PTH is characterized clinically by symptoms of neuromuscular hyperactivity and biochemically by hypocalcemia, hyperphosphatemia, and diminished to absent circulating iPTH.

Etiology

There are 3 major categories of PTH-deficient hypoparathyroidism: surgical, idiopathic, and functional.

Surgical hypoparathyroidism is the most common type. It may occur after any surgical procedure in which the anterior neck is explored, including thyroidectomy, removal of abnormal parathyroid glands, and excision of malignant neck lesions. Parathyroid glands need not actually be removed for hypoparathyroidism to ensue; in such cases, it is presumed that the blood supply to the parathyroid glands has been interrupted. Surgical hypoparathyroidism is relatively unusual (0.5–1%) when experienced surgeons perform neck explorations and when such procedures are quick and easy; however, the incidence increases alarmingly with surgical inexperience or with prolonged, extensive procedures requiring frequent blood vessel ligation.

Idiopathic hypoparathyroidism is a broad category of disorders undoubtedly with more than one cause. It can be divided into 2 subcategories depending on the age at onset: that occurring at an early age and that occurring late in life. Aside from congenital absence of the glands (as in DiGeorge's syndrome), the syndromes occurring at an early age are of genetic origin, usually with an autosomal recessive mode of transmission. This type of hypoparathyroidism is termed "multiple endocrine deficiency–autoimmune–candidiasis (MEDAC) syndrome" or "juvenile familial endocrinopathy" or "hypoparathyroidism–Addison's disease–mucocutaneous candidiasis (HAM) syndrome" (see Chapter 25). Circulating autoantibodies specific for parathyroid and adrenal tissue are frequently present but correlate poorly with clinical manifestations. Candidiasis is usually the first problem to appear (early childhood) and is resistant to both local antifungal measures and treatment of endocrine deficiencies. Hypoparathyroidism generally occurs about 4 years after the onset of candidiasis, at a mean age of 9 years, and Addison's disease about 5 years later, at a mean age of 14 years. Pernicious anemia (with autoantibodies to parietal cells and intrinsic factor), ovarian failure, and autoimmune thyroiditis with hypothyroidism also occur in this category of patients. Sporadic cases of MEDAC syndrome have been reported; in most of these cases, patients are seen at a later age, and some have hypoparathyroidism only.

The late-onset form of idiopathic hypoparathyroidism occurs sporadically without circulating glandular autoantibodies. Except for rare instances of hemochromatotic and metastatic involvement, the cause of parathyroid gland destruction in these cases is unknown.

Functional hypoparathyroidism occurs in patients who have undergone long periods of hypomagnesemia. Such patients include those with selective defects in gastrointestinal magnesium absorption, generalized gastrointestinal malabsorption, or alcoholism. Since magnesium is required for PTH release from the glands, serum iPTH is characteristically low or undetectable. Hypocalcemia is also present. Treatment with magnesium salts is followed within minutes by an increase in serum iPTH and, ultimately, by restoration of eucalcemia. Magnesium is probably also required for the peripheral action of PTH, and hypocalcemia in patients with functional hypoparathyroidism may be partly due to failure of the hormone to act normally on its target tissues.

Less well understood is the neonatal hypoparathyroidism in infants of mothers with primary hyperparathyroidism. It is thought that in utero exposure to maternal hypercalcemia results in prolonged suppression of fetal parathyroid glands and failure of the parathyroid glands to respond to hypocalcemic stimuli after birth.

Pathology

Although it has not been documented, it is likely that small remnants of viable parathyroid tissue are present in many patients with surgical hypoparathyroidism. Patients with MEDAC syndrome may have lymphocytic infiltration and fibrosis of glands. In the few patients with late-onset idiopathic hypoparathyroidism who have been examined, fatty infiltration, fibrosis, and atrophy have been found.

Long-standing cases of hypoparathyroidism have characteristic soft tissue calcifications in the lens and basal ganglia of the brain. All types of bone cells are diminished, and both formation and resorption surfaces in bone are decreased.

Pathologic Physiology

The pathophysiologic and biochemical consequences of parathyroid gland removal can be appreciated by referring to the "butterfly" diagram (Fig 8–2). In this disease, the right limbs of the 3 feedback loops predominate, with (1) decreased bone resorption; (2) decreased renal phosphate excretion, increased serum phosphate, decreased $1,25(OH)_2D_3$, and decreased intestinal absorption of calcium; and (3) increased renal excretion of calcium for the prevailing serum concentration of calcium. There is hypocalcemia and usually hyperphosphatemia, if dietary phosphate intake has been normal. Urinary calcium is usually low unless eucalcemia has been restored with treatment. In the latter case, urinary calcium is generally higher than it was before the development of hypoparathyroidism, and it occasionally reaches hypercalciuric levels. Nephrogenous cAMP is decreased (Fig 8–19), but it increases promptly following administration of PTH.

Hypocalcemia and alkalosis (due to decreased bicarbonate excretion; see above), if sufficiently severe, cause increased neuromuscular excitability with consequent tetany and, rarely, convulsions. Chronic hypocalcemia per se may also cause (1) basal ganglia calcification and occasional extrapyramidal neurologic syndromes; (2) papilledema and increased intracranial pressure; (3) psychiatric disorders; (4) skin, hair, and fingernail abnormalities; (5) candidal infections; (6) inhibition of normal dental development; (7) lenticular cataracts; (8) intestinal malabsorption; (9) prolongation of the QT and ST intervals of the ECG; (10) in rare cases, 2:1 heart block and, even more rarely, heart failure requiring digitalis and diuretics; and finally (11) increased serum concentrations of creatine phosphokinase and lactic dehydrogenase.

Classification

Parfitt has divided clinical hypoparathyroidism into 5 categories based primarily on the concentration of serum calcium. Grades 1 and 2 represent patients with no hypocalcemia and inconstant spontaneous hypocalcemia, respectively; grades 3, 4, and 5 represent patients whose serum calcium is below 8.5, 7.5, and 6.5 mg/dL, respectively. The clinical manifestations of hypoparathyroidism depend upon the severity and chronicity of the hypocalcemia.

Clinical Features

A. Neuromuscular Manifestations: In general, the rate of decrease in serum calcium appears to be the major determinant for development of neuromuscular complications (see below) of hypocalcemia. Thus, complications are most likely to occur within 1–2 days after parathyroidectomy, when serum calcium decreases acutely, and at serum calcium values that may be considerably higher (eg, 8 mg/dL) than might be found in patients who have had severe hypocalcemia (eg, 6 mg/dL) for long periods. Immediately after neck surgery in the region of the parathyroid glands, and for several days afterward, it is important to observe patients carefully for the development of the clinical signs (see below) heralding tetany rather than to rely on the absolute level of serum calcium.

Nerves exposed to low concentrations of calcium show decreased thresholds of excitation, repetitive responses to a single stimulus, reduced accommodation, and, in extreme cases, continuous activity. Such abnormal neural function occurs spontaneously in both sensory and motor fibers in hypocalcemic states and gives rise to neuromuscular manifestations.

1. Paresthesias–Numbness and tingling may occur around the mouth, in the tips of the fingers, and sometimes in the feet.

2. Tetany–An attack of tetany usually begins with prodromal paresthesias and is followed by spasms of the muscles of the extremities and face. The hands (Fig 8–13), forearms, and, less commonly, the feet become contorted in a characteristic way. First, the thumb is strongly adducted, followed by flexion of the metacarpophalangeal joints, extension of the interphalangeal joints (fingers together), and flexion of the wrist and elbow joints. This somewhat grotesque spastic condition, although quite painful when full-blown, is more alarming than dangerous.

3. Hyperventilation–Because of the alarm re-

sulting from tetany, patients may hyperventilate and secrete increased amounts of epinephrine. Hyperventilation causes hypocapnia and alkalosis, which in turn worsen hypocalcemia by causing increased binding of ionic calcium to plasma proteins. Prolonged hyperventilation in normal subjects can lower serum ionic calcium and produce tetany, but great care should be exercised in attributing such findings to hyperventilation alone.

4. Adrenergic symptoms–Increased epinephrine secretion produces further anxiety, tachycardia, sweating, and peripheral and circumoral pallor.

5. Convulsions–Patients with hypoparathyroidism may have convulsions. Convulsions are much more common in young people with the disease and are of 2 types: one is a more generalized form of tetany followed by prolonged tonic spasms; the other is a typical epileptiform seizure (grand mal, jacksonian, focal, or petit mal). The latter type is associated with electroencephalographic findings typical of epilepsy. Because restoration of eucalcemia results in a decrease in the number of seizures without improvement in the electroencephalographic findings associated with seizures, it is thought that hypocalcemia lowers the excitation threshold of preexisting epilepsy. The characteristic electroencephalographic changes associated with hypocalcemia disappear after restoration of eucalcemia. Laryngeal spasm with obstruction may occur during tetany and may precipitate seizures because of hypoxia. The relatively unusual finding of papilledema and increased intracranial pressure resulting from hypocalcemia in association with convulsions mimics the clinical picture of brain tumor.

6. Signs of latent tetany–Latent tetany can be detected by several relatively specific physical signs. **Chvostek's sign** is elicited by tapping the facial nerve just anterior to the ear lobe, just below the zygomatic arch, or between the zygomatic arch and the corner of the mouth. The response ranges from twitching of the lip at the corner of the mouth to twitching of all

Figure 8–13. Position of hand in hypocalcemic tetany (Trousseau's sign). (Reproduced, with permission, from Ganong WF: *Review of Medical Physiology,* 12th ed. Lange, 1985.)

of the facial muscles on the stimulated side. Simple twitching at the corner of the mouth occurs in 25% of normal subjects, but more extensive muscle contraction (ala nasi and orbital muscles) is a reliable sign of latent tetany.

Trousseau's sign (Fig 8–13) should be sought with a sphygmomanometer cuff. The cuff is inflated to above systolic blood pressure for at least 2 minutes while the hand is observed carefully. A positive response consists of the development of typical carpal spasm (Fig 8–13), with relaxation occurring 5–10 seconds after the cuff is deflated. An apparent spasm that disappears instantly may not be significant. Trousseau's sign is the most reliable sign of latent tetany, and serial tests for it should be performed and the results recorded in the immediate postoperative period after anterior neck surgery.

7. Extrapyramidal signs–Extrapyramidal neurologic syndromes, including classic parkinsonism, occur in patients with chronic hypoparathyroidism. Such manifestations are presumed to be related in some way to the basal ganglion calcification that is present in most patients. Many untreated patients without extrapyramidal syndromes are unduly sensitive to the dystonic side effects of phenothiazine drugs, suggesting that basal ganglion calcification may have more general pathologic importance than was once believed. Successful treatment of hypocalcemia may improve the neurologic disorder and is sometimes associated with decreases in basal ganglion calcification on x-ray.

B. Other Clinical Manifestations:

1. Posterior lenticular cataract–This is the most common sequela of hypoparathyroidism. Cataracts must be present and growing for 5–10 years before visual impairment occurs. Fully mature cataracts in hypoparathyroidism are confluent and produce total opacity of the lens. Such cataracts are different from senile cataracts, which are frequently confined to one segment of the lens. Successful treatment of hypocalcemia generally halts the progression of cataracts, and in rare cases the opacities may diminish in size.

2. Cardiac manifestations–Prolongation of the QT interval in the ECG (corrected for rate) is associated with hypocalcemia. Resistance to digitalis, hypotension, and refractory congestive heart failure with cardiomegaly may occur; these are reversed by normalization of the serum calcium.

3. Dental manifestations–Abnormalities in enamel formation, delayed or absent dental eruption, and defective dental root formation with short or blunted roots indicate that hypocalcemia was present during childhood.

4. Malabsorption syndrome–Intestinal malabsorption with steatorrhea is uncommon in hypoparathyroidism but may be present in patients with long-standing untreated disease. It is presumed to be due to decreased serum calcium because it is reversed by successful treatment of hypocalcemia but not by a gluten-free diet. Management is difficult because treatment of hypoparathyroidism largely depends on the ability to increase calcium transport across a normal gastrointestinal tract with drugs.

Diagnosis

A. Serum Calcium: Detection of hypoparathyroidism depends upon being alert to its possible presence in certain clinical situations. Accurate annual measurements of serum calcium are indicated (1) in patients who have had anterior neck surgery or (2) in those suspected of having MEDAC syndrome. Cutaneous candidiasis, cataracts, incidentally discovered basal ganglion calcifications, convulsions, numbness and tightening of the fingers, facial muscle spasm (spontaneous or self-induced), delayed dentition, and developmental retardation are all indications for prompt serum calcium measurement.

B. Serum Phosphorus: In the absence of renal failure, the diagnosis of hypoparathyroidism is virtually certain if hypocalcemia and hyperphosphatemia are found. Some patients, however, may be relatively phosphate-depleted because of dietary restriction, malabsorption, or the ingestion of aluminum hydroxide gels. In patients who have undergone parathyroidectomy for primary hyperparathyroidism, osseous avidity for minerals may be so great as to actually produce hypophosphatemia. In the first instance, the exclusion of nonparathyroid disorders as the cause of hypocalcemia becomes important. In the second, the question arises whether hypocalcemia is due to true hypoparathyroidism or to "bone hunger" alone.

C. Serum iPTH: In both circumstances, measurement of serum iPTH is crucial for the correct diagnosis. Increased values in a range appropriate to the degree of hypocalcemia would essentially exclude the presence of hypoparathyroidism and suggest end-organ resistance to PTH (pseudohypoparathyroidism, vitamin D deficiency, vitamin D dependency) or secondary hyperparathyroidism due to such disorders as dietary deficiency of calcium, intestinal malabsorption of calcium, or excessive intake of drugs containing absorbable phosphate (eg, neutral phosphate in the treatment of X-linked hypophosphatemic rickets).

An undetectable serum iPTH confirms the diagnosis of hypoparathyroidism if the assay technique used is sensitive enough to measure serum iPTH in the large majority of normal subjects. Serum iPTH may be detectable in some patients with hypoparathyroidism if the assay employed is very sensitive. Presumably, these patients have grade 1 parathyroid insufficiency. However, it is important to recognize that such low values may be due to nonspecific effects of serum per se in radioimmunoassays that do not adequately control for this factor.

Patients with functional hypoparathyroidism due to hypomagnesemia also have low to undetectable levels of serum iPTH. Identification of these individuals depends upon the measurement of serum magnesium and the demonstration that treatment with magnesium salts restores eucalcemia and increases serum iPTH.

Treatment

A. Therapeutic Difficulties: Theoretically, the most appropriate therapy for hypoparathyroidism would be physiologic replacement of PTH. There are practical limitations to this approach, including the need to administer the hormone parenterally and the current high cost of suitable commercial human PTH preparations. Such treatment might become feasible in the future for patients poorly controlled by conventional regimens.

Because of the absence of PTH and the consequent hyperphosphatemia, $25OHD_3$ 1α-hydroxylase, the renal enzyme that converts $25OHD_3$ to $1,25(OH)_2D_3$, is relatively inactive in patients with hypoparathyroidism. Thus, little if any circulating $25OHD_3$ is converted to $1,25(OH)_2D_3$, and there are low to undetectable serum levels of this metabolite. In fact, hypoparathyroid patients are for this reason resistant to pharmacologic doses of vitamin D.

Although lowering of serum phosphate levels with diets low in phosphate (ie, restricting dairy products and meat) and oral aluminum hydroxide gels (to bind intestinal phosphate) might be expected to increase the conversion of $25OHD_3$ to $1,25(OH)_2D_3$, such treatment has received little attention. Rather, treatment with pharmacologic doses of ergocalciferol or its more potent analog dihydrotachysterol, in combination with oral calcium, has been the mainstay of treatment. Severe hypercalcemia is often a complication of this treatment if serum calcium is not monitored frequently. Serum calcium should be measured weekly at the initiation of treatment with vitamin D, then monthly during dosage adjustment, and at least every 3 months during long-term follow-up. A single episode of vitamin D intoxication can irreversibly impair renal function. Furthermore, toxicity can persist for weeks to months because of the effective tissue storage of vitamin D and its circulating metabolite $25OHD_3$. Treatment of vitamin D intoxication is similar to that described for severe hypercalcemia (discussed below). Hydration and furosemide are most important, and in some patients corticosteroids (60 mg prednisone or 300 mg cortisone daily in 4 divided doses), which appear to antagonize vitamin D action, are necessary.

B. Emergency Measures for Tetany: Tetany due to hypoparathyroidism requires emergency treatment with intravenous calcium. The aim is to prevent laryngeal stridor and convulsions. After a patent airway is assured, 10–20 mL of a 10% solution of calcium gluconate (90 mg elemental calcium per 10 mL) should be given slowly (not more than 10 mL/min) until symptoms are relieved or until serum calcium rises above 7 mg/dL. Hypercalcemia is to be avoided; maintaining calcium at levels between 7.5 and 9 mg/dL is adequate. Caution should be exercised in patients taking digitalis, because calcium potentiates the action of this drug on the heart; electrocardiographic monitoring is thus necessary during intravenous calcium therapy for these patients. Therapy with vitamin D should be initiated as soon as possible (see below).

It may be necessary to maintain serum calcium at levels that prevent tetany for several days before vitamin D becomes effective. This is accomplished with the combined administration of oral and intermittent intravenous calcium. Oral calcium is begun as soon as possible, starting with 200 mg of elemental calcium (as calcium carbonate, 40% calcium) every 2 hours and gradually increasing to 500 mg every 2 hours if necessary. If serum calcium falls below 7.5 mg/dL after 6 hours of the combined regimen, a continuous calcium infusion should be started. Five hundred milliliters of 5% glucose and water containing 10 mL of 10% calcium gluconate is given over 6 hours initially, with the quantity of calcium increased in increments of 5 mL every 6 hours until satisfactory control is achieved. Anticonvulsive agents (phenytoin, phenobarbital, etc) may be helpful in management of patients with convulsions resistant to calcium therapy and should be given as soon as such resistance is suspected. Phenothiazine drugs should be avoided because they may induce severe dyskinesia.

C. Severe Hypocalcemia: In patients with hyperparathyroidism and bone disease who have undergone successful excision of one or more hyperfunctioning parathyroid glands, hypocalcemia may be profound and resistant to treatment ("hungry bone" syndrome). As much as 10 g of elemental calcium administered intravenously by infusion over 24 hours may be required to increase serum calcium above 7.5 mg/dL. Such patients are notoriously resistant to vitamin D, but responses are regularly achieved with $1,25(OH)_2D_3$ (calcitriol [Rocaltrol]) in doses ranging from 0.5 to 2 μg daily or with parathyroid extract (300–1000 units intramuscularly or intravenously). The manufacture of parathyroid extract has been discontinued, but synthetic human PTH(1–34) should become available soon.

D. Severe Hypoparathyroidism: Most patients with grades 4 and 5 hypoparathyroidism require some form of long-term vitamin D treatment (Table 8–2). Success is usually achieved with the regimen suggested by Parfitt: dihydrotachysterol (Hytakerol), 4 mg/d as a single dose for 2 days, then 2 mg/d for 2 days, then 1 mg/d, adjusting this dose as required by serum calcium measurements (1 mg is equivalent to about 120,000 USP units or 3 mg of vitamin D_2). Ideally, serum calcium should be maintained between 8.5 and 9 mg/dL. This leaves a margin for an increase in serum calcium to levels that are not dangerous. The major advantage of dihydrotachysterol is its relatively rapid onset of action and short half-life. With regard to the latter, hypercalcemia due to inadvertent overdoses of dihydrotachysterol is relieved within 1–3 weeks after the drug is discontinued, whereas toxicity from vitamin D_2 persists for 6–18 weeks. Dihydrotachysterol offers another advantage in that parathyroid function can be tested relatively soon after withdrawal of the drug. Hypocalcemia within 2 weeks of withdrawal strongly suggests the persistence of hypoparathyroidism. The disadvantage of dihydrotachysterol is that it is more expensive than ergocalciferol.

Table 8–2. Vitamin D preparations used in the treatment of hypoparathyroidism.

	Potency*	How Supplied	Daily Dose (Range)	Time Required for Toxic Effects to Subside
Ergocalciferol (ergosterol, vitamin D_2)	40,000 USP units/mg.	Capsules of 25,000 and 50,000 units; solution, 500,000 units/mL.	25,000–200,000 units.	6–18 weeks.
Dihydrotachysterol (Hytakerol)	120,000 USP units/mg.	Tablets of 0.125, 0.2, and 0.4 mg.	0.2–1 mg.	1–3 weeks.
Calcifediol (Calderol)	. . .	Capsules of 20 and 50 μg.	20–200 μg.	3–6 weeks.
Calcitriol (Rocaltrol)	. . .	Capsules of 0.25 and 0.5 μg.	0.25–5 μg.	½–2 weeks.

*Number of units of vitamin D provided by 1 mg of the preparation.

1. Ergocalciferol (vitamin D_2)–The most commonly available FDA-approved vitamin D preparation is ergocalciferol, or vitamin D_2 (Table 8–2). In initiating treatment with this drug, it is important to prevent hypercalcemia. This can be accomplished consistently by giving small doses in the beginning (0.6 mg/d, or 25,000 units/d) and increasing them gradually after steady-state levels of serum calcium are achieved at each dosage level. However, restoration of eucalcemia in this way sometimes requires an inordinately long time, and it is recommended that high doses (1.25–2.5 mg/d, or 50,000–100,000 units/d) be given early, tapering to 0.6–1.25 mg/d as serum calcium concentrations approach 9 mg/dL. Most patients can be managed successfully with 1.25–2.5 mg/d. The occasional patient who requires more than 3.75 mg/d (150,000 units/d) is a candidate for the shorter-acting analogs or metabolites of vitamin D.

Little information is available concerning the long-term management of hypoparathyroidism with the cholecalciferol metabolites calcifediol (Calderol) and calcitriol (Rocaltrol). Both appear to be effective and pharmacologically superior to ergocalciferol with respect to rapidity of onset and termination of action, but—except in patients who are particularly difficult to manage—neither seems to offer major advantages over dihydrotachysterol, and both are even more expensive than dihydrotachysterol. The initiation and termination of action appear to be faster for calcitriol than for dihydrotachysterol. Calcitriol has been approved by the FDA for the treatment of hypoparathyroidism.

2. Calcium–Since the major action of vitamin D preparations is to increase intestinal calcium absorption, dietary calcium must be adequate during treatment of hypoparathyroidism. This can be achieved with a total (dietary and supplemental) intake of 1 g or more daily in patients under age 40 and 2 g in patients over age 40. Supplements can be provided by administering calcium as the gluconate, lactate, chloride, or carbonate salt. There are disadvantages for each. Calcium gluconate and lactate tablets contain relatively small quantities of elemental calcium, so that large numbers of tablets must be given. Calcium chloride tablets contain large quantities of calcium but tend to produce gastric irritation. Calcium carbonate tablets (the preferred preparation) also contain large

quantities of calcium but tend to produce alkalosis, which may aggravate hypocalcemia.

E. Moderate Hypoparathyroidism: Patients with grade 3 hypoparathyroidism may require only calcium supplementation (1–5 g daily) and moderate degrees of phosphate restriction (combined with aluminum hydroxide gels) to maintain serum calcium in the desired range of 8.5–9 mg/dL. This avoids the risk of vitamin D intoxication and should be tried in appropriate circumstances.

Complications

Aside from hypercalcemia, hypercalciuria may be a complication of successful treatment. Hypercalciuria develops because PTH is no longer maintaining normal renal tubular reabsorption of calcium (Fig 8–2). Accurate measurement of 24-hour urine calcium is therefore necessary to avert possible renal stone formation as serum calcium approaches normal levels during calcium and vitamin D treatment. Thiazide diuretics, which increase renal tubular reabsorption of calcium, may be useful in such cases and may have the added advantage of partially restoring eucalcemia. In fact, such treatment has been used successfully without vitamin D in the management of mild hypoparathyroidism.

Prognosis

Long-term restoration of serum calcium to normal or nearly normal ranges usually results in improvement in most manifestations of surgical and idiopathic hypoparathyroidism, including the skin disorders and associated candidiasis. Unfortunately, the latter appears to persist in MEDAC syndrome, and resolution usually can be achieved only with iodoquinol or with systemic amphotericin B (alone or combined with transfer factor) therapy. The increasing use of parathyroid autotransplantation in surgery for disorders requiring extensive removal of thyroid or parathyroid tissue may lower the incidence of permanent hypoparathyroidism.

PSEUDOHYPOPARATHYROIDISM & PSEUDOPSEUDOHYPO-PARATHYROIDISM

Pseudohypoparathyroidism is a rare familial disorder characterized by target tissue resistance to PTH, hypocalcemia, increased parathyroid gland function, and a variety of congenital defects in the growth and development of the skeleton, including short stature and short metacarpal and metatarsal bones. Patients with pseudopseudohypoparathyroidism have the developmental defects without the biochemical abnormalities of pseudohypoparathyroidism. There are also patients with pseudohypoparathyroidism who have target tissue resistance to the hormone but no developmental abnormalities, and others with developmental abnormalities who experience spontaneous cure of biochemical abnormalities. There are even patients who have developmental abnormalities and clinical hypoparathyroidism in the face of typical osteitis fibrosa cystica. This syndrome is known as pseudohypohyperparathyroidism.

Etiology

Clearly, the complex abnormalities mentioned in the foregoing paragraph cannot be ascribed to a single underlying biochemical defect. Although abnormal target tissue responses to PTH may be the basic disorder, it is likely that defects in any one of a number of limiting steps, from receptor binding of the hormone to final expression of the cellular actions of PTH, could be involved.

At present, the only proved biochemical defect of this type is one in which the guanyl nucleotide-sensitive regulatory protein that couples PTH-occupied receptors to adenylate cyclase is decreased by half in the red blood cells of some patients with pseudohypoparathyroidism (Fig 8-9). In such patients, this defect appears to produce resistance to several other hormones that apparently exert their actions by stimulating the production of increased cellular cAMP (vasopressin, glucagon). Other possible mechanisms, as yet largely untested, include secretion of a biologically inert form of PTH, circulating inhibitors of PTH action, an intrinsic abnormality of PTH receptors, autoantibodies to the PTH receptor, a defect in adenylate cyclase, a specific and defined disturbance in the process by which PTH alters the distribution of ions across membranes, and abnormalities of cellular protein kinases or other hormone-dependent enzymes.

Patients with pseudohypoparathyroidism generally fail to respond normally to the administration of large doses of PTH with an increase in urinary phosphate excretion and in nephrogenous cAMP (type I). A few patients have normal cAMP responses but diminished phosphate responses (type II), whereas others (rarely) may have the reverse. Studies describing these apparently paradoxic findings imply that cAMP may not be involved in all of the biologic actions of PTH. However, these results could also be explained in other ways, including (1) the possibility that urinary excretion of cAMP does not accurately reflect all of the cAMP-related cellular events critical to PTH action and (2) the likelihood that only small changes in intracellular cAMP are required for PTH action.

Serum levels of $1,25(OH)_2D_3$ have been reported to be low in pseudohypoparathyroidism, and defective conversion of $25OHD_3$ to $1,25(OH)_2D_3$ has therefore been suggested as the mechanism involved in abnormal mineral homeostasis in these patients. This argument is supported by reports of success in restoring serum calcium and urinary phosphate excretion to normal levels with administration of $1,25(OH)_2D_3$, but again, other explanations are probably more valid. There is recent evidence that generation of increased renal tubular cAMP is involved in stimulation of 1α-hydroxylation of $25OHD_3$. If such is the case, one could postulate that normal tissue responsiveness to PTH is necessary for production of $1,25(OH)_2D_3$, and its absence in pseudohypoparathyroidism would account for the low levels of serum $1,25(OH)_2D_3$ in this disease. Furthermore, administration of $1,25(OH)_2D_3$ might be expected to increase the responsiveness of bone to PTH in patients with deficient production of $1,25(OH)_2D_3$ simply because the hypercalcemic action of PTH depends on the presence of biologically active metabolites of vitamin D. Finally, the phosphaturia induced in pseudohypoparathyroidism by $1,25(OH)_2D_3$ administration could be due to the restoration of eucalcemia; it is well known that phosphaturia occurs when serum calcium is restored toward normal in patients with surgical hypoparathyroidism.

Genetic Basis of Pseudohypoparathyroidism

Although pseudohypoparathyroidism is inherited, its mode of transmission is unclear. The 2:1 female:male ratio of occurrence suggests an X-linked dominant mechanism; however, it is difficult to explain how the developmental defects of pseudohypoparathyroidism can be inherited in the absence of abnormalities in the adenylate cyclase system. Furthermore, 4 cases of male-to-male transmission of the developmental defects have been recorded.

Incidence

Pseudohypoparathyroidism and pseudopseudohypoparathyroidism are rare. Most cases are concentrated in a few centers in the USA.

Pathologic Physiology

Qualitatively, the biochemical findings in patients with pseudohypoparathyroidism are identical to those observed in patients with surgical or idiopathic hypoparathyroidism, except that serum iPTH is increased appropriately for the degree of hypocalcemia. The pathophysiology of the disease is best understood by reference to Fig 8-2. PTH action is blocked in all 3 of the left limbs of the target tissue feedback loops. The results (in the right limbs) are (1) decreased bone resorption, caused by decreased bone cell responsiveness to PTH; (2) increased serum phosphate,

Figure 8–14. Hands of a patient with pseudohypoparathyroidism. *A:* Note the short fourth finger. *B:* Note the "absent" fourth knuckle. *C:* Film shows the short fourth metacarpal. (Reproduced, with permission, from Potts JT: Page 1359 in: *The Metabolic Basis of Inherited Disease,* 4th ed. Stanbury JB, Wyngaarden JB, Fredrickson DS [editors]. McGraw-Hill, 1978.)

caused by decreased renal tubular responsiveness to the phosphaturic effects of PTH and decreased production of $1,25(OH)_2D_3$ with decreased intestinal calcium absorption; and (3) increased renal excretion of calcium for the degree of hypocalcemia, which is caused again by decreased renal tubular responsiveness to the hypocalciuric effects of PTH. The consequent hypocalcemia stimulates PTH secretion. There is no good explanation for the hypocalcemia in patients with pseudohypohyperparathyroidism who (paradoxically) have osteitis fibrosa cystica and elevated levels of alkaline phosphatase (see below).

In patients with pseudohypoparathyroidism who are hypocalcemic, the parathyroid glands are hyperplastic. Aside from the unique developmental abnormalities noted below, the findings are the same as those of surgical hypoparathyroidism.

Clinical Features

Most of the symptoms and signs of pseudohypoparathyroidism are the same as those of surgical hypoparathyroidism and idiopathic hypoparathyroidism and are due almost entirely to hypocalcemia. However, there are certain unique developmental features. Many patients are mentally retarded, short and stocky, and obese with rounded faces. Many have one or more short metacarpal or metatarsal bones, which is manifested by formation of a dimple over the head of the involved metacarpals on making a fist. The fingers (especially the fourth) may be short (Fig 8–14). The calvarium is thickened in one-third of patients, and there may be delayed dentition, defective enamel, and absence of teeth. There may also be exostoses, ectopic ossification, coxa vara or coxa valga, bowing of the radius, tibia, and fibula, and hypothyroidism.

Diagnosis

The diagnosis of pseudohypoparathyroidism is likely when the developmental abnormalities described above are present. When serum calcium and phosphorus are normal in such a patient, the diagnosis of pseudopseudohypoparathyroidism is almost certain, although some of the same abnormalities may be present (occasionally) in patients with Turner's, Gardner's, or basal cell nevus syndrome. If hypocalcemia and hyperphosphatemia are present, the diagnosis of pseudohypoparathyroidism is likely. Increased serum iPTH and markedly diminished phosphaturic and nephrogenous cAMP responses to PTH distinguish pseudohypoparathyroidism from surgical, idiopathic, or functional hypoparathyroidism in patients with equivocal signs or absence of developmental abnormalities. If the serum phosphorus is normal or low in a hypocalcemic patient, secondary hyperparathyroidism due to vitamin D or dietary calcium deficiency or to intestinal malabsorption of calcium must be excluded. Measurement of serum $25OHD_3$ should be helpful in the first instance, and dietary history or analysis in the second. The third (intestinal malabsorption) may present difficulties because hypocalcemia per se may produce malabsorption, and unless magnesium deficiency is present, patients with primary intestinal malabsorption usually have increased levels of serum iPTH. Therapeutic tests are needed in this situation. When successful treatment of malabsorption with a gluten-free diet restores eucalcemia, the diagnosis is probably gluten-sensitive enteropathy. If correction of hypocalcemia with a regimen used in the treatment of hypoparathyroidism cures the malabsorption syndrome, pseudohypoparathyroidism is a likely diagnosis.

Treatment

The treatment of pseudohypoparathyroidism is identical to that for hypoparathyroidism. No therapy is usually necessary for pseudopseudohypoparathyroidism.

PRIMARY HYPERPARATHYROIDISM

Primary hyperparathyroidism represents an overlapping group of syndromes that are caused by excessive, relatively uncontrolled secretion of PTH by one or more hyperfunctioning parathyroid glands. Hypercalcemia, the biochemical hallmark of the disorder, fails to inhibit gland activity in the normal manner. Most patients today are relatively asymptomatic and are detected by routine measurements of serum calcium. Symptoms, when present, can be remarkably varied and vague. The classic presentation of nephrolithiasis, osteitis fibrosa cystica, and soft tissue calcification is rare today.

Etiology

The cause of primary hyperparathyroidism is unknown. A genetic factor may be involved, since several families have been described in which the disease is inherited as an autosomal dominant trait. Investigations of the incidence of thyroid carcinoma in patients who have had neck x-rays have shown a greater than expected number of cases of primary hyperparathyroidism, implicating this factor as one possible underlying cause. However, it is difficult to interpret such studies because there is little information about the general incidence and natural history of primary hyperparathyroidism.

Calcium infusions in hyperparathyroid patients with mild hypercalcemia incompletely suppress serum iPTH. This strongly suggests that increased hormone secretion in these patients is due, at least in part, to a set point error in the level of ionic calcium at which abnormal tissue is suppressed. This defect has recently been directly confirmed in vitro. Isolated parathyroid cells from hyperfunctioning glands require higher concentrations of calcium in the medium to decrease PTH secretion than do cells obtained from normal glands.

Incidence

Routine automated measurement of serum calcium has vastly increased detection of primary hyperparathyroidism. In one recent, well-controlled study, the annual rate of disease detection was 3.5 times greater after the introduction of routine screening of serum calcium than it was before. The incidence of primary hyperparathyroidism increases dramatically in both men and women after age 50; it is 2–4 times more common in women. In a careful epidemiologic study, the age-adjusted incidence was estimated to be 42 per 100,000. However, studies of selected patient populations (with most patients over 40 years of age) have revealed as many as 1/1000 to 1/200 patients with the disease.

Pathology

A. Parathyroid Glands: Histologically, abnormal parathyroid glands from patients with primary hyperparathyroidism have been characterized as being hyperplastic, adenomatous, or malignant. Unfortunately, controlled studies of histologic interpretations by pathologists have shown that it is difficult or impossible to distinguish between adenomas and hyperplasia. Furthermore, abnormal but nonmalignant parathyroid tissue may, in rare cases, have many of the histologic features of malignant tissue. Thus, to classify parathyroid lesions, it is generally necessary to rely on gross pathologic features observed during surgery. The surgeon determines the number, size, and gross appearance of abnormal glands present. The pathologist then determines whether biopsy specimens are parathyroid tissue. Single-gland involvement (‘‘adenoma’’) occurs in about 80% of patients with hyperparathyroidism and multiple-gland involvement (‘‘hyperplasia’’) in about 20%. The diagnosis of true carcinoma of the gland is based on a combination of gross appearance of the lesion, histologic features, and, ultimately, the biologic behavior of the abnormal tissue. Less than 2% of hyperfunctioning glands are malignant. Familial primary hyperparathyroidism and the hyperparathyroidism associated with multiple endocrine neoplasia almost always involve multiple glands. Abnormal parathyroid glands usually weigh 0.2–2 g (27–75 mg is normal) and have a characteristic yellow-red color and ‘‘bulging’’ appearance in situ. Occasionally, very large glands (> 10 g) are observed. The severity of the clinical manifestations—especially the degree of hypercalcemia—is generally proportionate to the quantity of hyperfunctioning tissue. The predominant cell type in most abnormal glands is the chief cell; it can be arrayed in sheets or cords or may appear in follicles. So-called water-clear cells and oxyphilic cells may be admixed, and in rare cases one of these may predominate. There is no question that the chief cell synthesizes and secretes PTH. The functions of the water-clear and oxyphilic cells are unknown.

B. Bone: In virtually all patients with primary hyperparathyroidism, histomorphometric analysis of bone biopsies of the iliac crest shows the effects of excess PTH on bone. These effects include increased bone resorption surfaces, increased numbers of osteoclasts, osteocytic osteolysis, and, in moderate to severe cases, marrow fibrosis. Only far-advanced disease is associated with classic bone cysts and fractures. These patients have a mineralization defect characterized by large quantities of unmineralized collagen and disorganized (woven rather than lamellar) bone.

C. Kidney: About 20–30% of patients have nephrolithiasis, which is frequently complicated by pyelonephritis. Gross nephrocalcinosis or calcification of the renal papillae is unusual, but microscopic examination of kidneys with special calcium stains has sometimes revealed peritubular and tubular calcifications at autopsy. The incidence of such soft tissue calcification in patients with mild to moderate disease is unknown. However, it may be relatively frequent, since chondrocalcinosis and calcific tendinitis can be demonstrated on x-rays in 7.5–18% of cases.

D. Other Organs: Calcification of other organs such as stomach, lung, and heart has been observed in patients with hyperparathyroid crisis (serum calcium > 15 mg/dL).

E. Muscle: Myopathy is relatively common in primary hyperparathyroidism, and muscle biopsy may show neuropathic atrophy of both type I and type II muscle fibers. These histologic changes parallel clinical, neurologic, and neuromuscular dysfunction.

Pathologic Physiology

As might be expected, the constant, incompletely controlled release of PTH from hyperfunctioning parathyroid tissue causes exaggerated physiologic responses in target organs.

A. Hypercalcemia: Because the excess hormone stimulates the transport of calcium into the blood from the intestinal and renal tubular lumina as well as from bone (Fig 8–2), the intestine and kidney are unable to correct the hypercalcemia. Thus, patients with primary hyperparathyroidism, in contrast to those with other (nonparathyroid) hypercalcemic diseases, lack the first lines of defense against hypercalcemia, increased renal and intestinal loss of calcium. Early in the course of the disease, when serum calcium values are less than 11.5 mg/dL (normal range, 8.9–10.1 mg/dL), urinary calcium can be relatively low for the degree of hypercalcemia. It is only when serum calcium values are greater than 12 mg/dL, when the renal tubular mechanism for resorbing calcium is overwhelmed, or when there is an unrelated decrease in the renal tubular capacity to resorb calcium that the kidney's adaptive mechanism for correcting hypercalcemia becomes operative and hypercalcemia develops. Unfortunately, this chronic adaptation (hypercalciuria), along with other changes in urine composition that occur in primary hyperparathyroidism (eg, increased pH due to bicarbonaturia), contributes to the urolithiasis and urinary tract infections that are so common in these patients.

Many patients with primary hyperparathyroidism have decreased renal tubular reabsorption of phosphate, hyperphosphaturia, and hypophosphatemia. In normal people or in patients with a diminished capacity to convert $25OHD_3$ to $1,25(OH)_2D_3$, the renal tubular effects of PTH aid mineral homeostasis by stimulating $1,25(OH)_2D_3$ production and by clearing from the blood phosphate that was removed from bone during resorption of calcium. However, in patients with primary hyperparathyroidism, hypercalcemia is aggravated by the increased production of $1,25(OH)_2D_3$ and by a decrease in the amount of serum phosphate available to form complexes with serum ionic calcium.

B. Calcium in Soft Tissues: Other mechanisms for correcting hypercalcemia are required as the disease progresses. These generally result in a "trade-off" between a decrease in serum calcium and the development of organ disease. One such mechanism is the deposition of calcium in soft tissues that occurs because the normal solubility product of $Ca^{2+} \times PO_4^{3-}$ in serum (approximately 40) is exceeded. This may cause joint pain due to calcific tendinitis and chondrocalcinosis, or it may compromise renal function (secondary to nephrocalcinosis).

C. Vitamin D Deficiency: Another adaptive mechanism is the development of vitamin D deficiency, which may render patients with even severe hyperparathyroidism eucalcemic or nearly so. In this instance, a patient with only marginal stores of vitamin D may develop vitamin D deficiency because of the long-term increase in the conversion of $25OHD_3$ to $1,25(OH)_2D_3$ that is caused by the increased circulating levels of PTH. Such patients may have severe osteomalacia.

D. Increased Degradation of PTH: A final adaptive mechanism may be a hypercalcemia-reduced increase in the degradation of biologically active forms of PTH peripherally (eg, in the liver and possibly the kidney) and in parathyroid tissue itself. Evidence in support of such effects of ionic calcium is available in both animals and humans. Thus, it is possible that plasma calcium per se may not only regulate PTH secretion but may also be important in determining the relative quantities of biologically active PTH and inactive hormone fragments in the circulation. The one adaptive mechanism that might be expected to play an important role in correcting the hypercalcemia of primary hyperparathyroidism is increased secretion of CT. However evidence indicates that this does not occur in most patients; and in some patients (particularly women), CT reserve actually appears to be diminished.

E. Hyperchloremic Acidosis: Patients with primary hyperparathyroidism generally have mild to moderate hyperchloremic acidosis. This is due chiefly to excess PTH, which decreases the urinary concentration of hydrogen ion and increases urinary bicarbonate excretion. These effects also tend to aggravate existing hypercalcemia, first by impairing the ability of blood albumin to bind ionic calcium and secondly by increasing the dissolution of bone mineral.

F. Increased Urinary cAMP: Urinary cAMP is increased in as many as 80% of patients with primary hyperparathyroidism. This presumably reflects an increase in PTH-stimulated renal cell adenylate cyclase activity. Interestingly, some studies indicate that the phosphaturic and cAMP responses to exogenously administered PTH are blunted in patients with primary hyperparathyroidism, suggesting a state of refractoriness or "desensitization" of one or more of the cellular components responsible for these effects. This "desensitization" and the increase in urinary cAMP excretion have been used as diagnostic tests for the presence of hyperparathyroidism (see below).

G. Osteitis Fibrosa Cystica: Patients with radiologic evidence of osteitis fibrosa cystica frequently have increased serum concentrations of the bone isoenzyme of alkaline phosphatase. This bone enzyme is produced by osteoblasts and probably is one of several enzymes involved in osseous mineralization. These patients also excrete greater than normal quantities of hydroxyproline in their urine. This amino acid is unique to collagen, the major structural protein in bone. Such combined increases in serum alkaline phosphatase and urinary excretion of hydroxyproline have been interpreted as gross reflections of increased bone turnover in primary hyperparathyroidism.

Clinical Features

A. Symptoms: Patients with primary hyperparathyroidism are usually asymptomatic or have nonspecific symptoms such as weakness and easy fatigability. When symptoms do occur, they can generally be attributed to one of 2 causes: (1) hypercalcemia with associated hypercalciuria or (2) osteitis fibrosa cystica.

1. Hypercalcemia and associated hypercalciuria—The symptoms attributable to hypercalcemia involve a number of systems: (1) central nervous system: impaired mentation, loss of memory for recent events, emotional lability, depression, anosmia, somnolence, and even coma; (2) neuromuscular: weakness (especially of the proximal musculature); (3) rheumatologic: joint pain due to associated gout, intra-articular deposition of calcium pyrophosphate crystals (pseudogout), calcific tendinitis, and chondrocalcinosis; (4) dermatologic: pruritus, probably due to metastatic calcification in the skin; (5) gastrointestinal: anorexia, nausea, vomiting, dyspepsia, and constipation; and (6) renal: polyuria, nocturia, renal colic due to lithiasis, nephrocalcinosis that sometimes leads to renal failure, and associated symptoms of uremia. All of these abnormalities are related to the degree of elevation of ionic calcium in extracellular fluid, but the correlation is a crude one. One patient may be severely incapacitated at a level of serum calcium that produces only moderate symptoms in another.

Severe pancreatitis and intractable peptic ulcer have been observed in individual patients with primary hyperparathyroidism and are thought to be due to hypercalcemia. However, the evidence that these disorders occur with increased frequency in primary hyperparathyroidism is weak. Hypertension occurs with increased frequency, even in patients with mild hyperparathyroidism, but its cause is unknown.

2. Osteitis fibrosa cystica—Symptomatic bone disease (osteitis fibrosa cystica) is now unusual. Patients may complain of diffuse bone pain or, very rarely, may have a pathologic fracture through a bone cyst.

B. Signs: Most patients show no signs of the disorder. Such signs as are present are usually confined to the neuromuscular system or to organ systems in which soft tissue calcification is present. Neurologic abnormalities are nonspecific and include impaired mentation, mental depression, psychosis, hypoactive deep tendon reflexes, joint hyperextensibility, sensory loss for perception of pain and vibration, proximal muscle weakness (particularly the thighs), abnormal tongue movements (resembling fasciculations), lingual atrophy, ataxic gait, and abnormally strong (hard) fingernails.

1. Soft tissue calcification—Soft tissue calcification can result in arthritis (chondrocalcinosis or calcific tendinitis), conjunctivitis (conjunctival calcium phosphate crystals), and "band keratopathy," which is characterized by deposition in the cornea of opaque calcium phosphate in vertical lines parallel to and within the ocular limbus, usually laterally (3 o'clock and 9 o'clock). "Band keratopathy" can best be seen by slit lamp examination. It is rare in hyperparathyroidism unless serum phosphate is also elevated (eg, after the onset of renal failure).

2. Enlarged glands—It is seldom possible to palpate enlarged parathyroid glands. A nodule felt in the neck of a patient with primary hyperparathyroidism is much more likely to be in the thyroid than in the parathyroid gland.

3. Bone tenderness and deformities—Rarely, patients may exhibit bone tenderness on examination. Bone deformities, fractures through an osteoclastic cyst, the presence of an epulis (brown tumor of the jaw), and "pseudoclubbing" due to collapsed terminal phalanges have been described even more rarely.

C. X-Ray Findings: The most specific and frequent radiographic sign of osteitis fibrosa cystica is subperiosteal bone resorption. This is best demonstrated in magnified fine-grain industrial x-rays of the fingers (especially the index finger). An example from a patient with severe primary hyperparathyroidism is shown in Fig 8–15A. Note the radial surface of the distal phalanx, where the cortex is almost completely resorbed, leaving only fine wisps of cortical bone. Other radiographic manifestations of the disease range from generalized osteopenia to bone cysts ("brown tumors") and erosion of distal phalangeal tufts or the distal ends of clavicles. Severe osteitis fibrosa cystica involving the skull is shown in Fig 8–15B.

Soft tissue calcifications (eg, calcific tendinitis, chondrocalcinosis, nephrocalcinosis, pulmonary calcifications) may be incidental findings on routine films. The latter 2 can be well demonstrated with scanning techniques using radioactively labeled diphosphonate compounds.

Nephrocalcinosis is rarely seen on x-ray, but nephrolithiasis is common. The stones are usually radiopaque (ie, calcium oxalate and calcium phosphate

Figure 8–15. *A:* Magnified x-ray of index finger on fine-grain industrial film showing classic subperiosteal resorption in a patient with severe primary hyperparathyroidism. Note the left (radial) surface of the distal phalanx, where the cortex is almost completely resorbed, leaving only fine wisps of cortical bone. *B:* Skull x-ray from a patient with severe secondary hyperparathyroidism due to prolonged end-stage renal disease. Extensive areas of demineralization alternate with areas of increased bone density, resulting in an exaggerated picture of the "salt and pepper" skull x-ray, which used to be a classic finding in primary hyperparathyroidism. This is rarely seen now and cannot be visualized easily in x-ray reproductions. Although it is difficult to appreciate at this magnification, the dental lamina dura is absent, another classic x-ray finding in severe hyperparathyroidism. (Both films courtesy of H Genant.)

stones) and can be seen on plain films. Nephrotomograms are helpful in identifying, localizing, and measuring them. This latter procedure is important in determining the "activity" of the stone disease. An increase in stone diameter with time can be taken as evidence of "active" stone disease and is probably an indication for treatment of hyperparathyroidism. Primary hyperparathyroidism may also be associated, although less commonly, with uric acid stones (not radiopaque). Thus, x-ray examination of the urinary tract with contrast material is also important.

Differential Diagnosis

In general, the major problem in the differential diagnosis of primary hyperparathyroidism is distinguishing it from other conditions associated with hypercalcemia (Table 8–3). Thiazide diuretic therapy and nonhematologic malignant diseases are the most common ones. Less common but equally important are (1) hematologic malignant diseases involving bone (myeloma, lymphoma, leukemia); (2) granulomatous diseases (sarcoidosis, tuberculosis, berylliosis); (3) endocrine disorders, including thyrotoxicosis and acute adrenal insufficiency; (4) familial hypocalciuric hypercalcemia (benign familial hypercalcemia); (5) in-

toxication with calcium, vitamin D, vitamin A, or lithium; (6) extensive skeletal immobilization (eg, in a spica body cast) in normal young people and prolonged bed rest in patients with osteolytic or metabolic bone disease; and (7) idiopathic hypercalcemia of infancy. More than one cause of hypercalcemia may coexist in the same patient (eg, hyperparathyroidism and sarcoidosis).

Table 8–3. Differential diagnosis of hypercalcemia.

Due to increased serum PTH
  Primary and "tertiary" hyperparathyroidism
  Some nonhematologic malignant diseases
Not due to increased serum PTH
  Drug-induced hypercalcemia (thiazides, furosemide, vitamin D, calcium, vitamin A, lithium)
  Granulomatous diseases (sarcoidosis, tuberculosis, berylliosis)
  Genetic diseases (familial hypocalciuric hypercalcemia)
  Immobilization
  "Idiopathic" hypercalcemia
  Some nonhematologic malignant diseases
  Malignant hematologic diseases
  Nonparathyroid endocrine diseases (Addison's disease, hyper- and hypothyroidism)

A. Pathogenesis of Hypercalcemia: Hypercalcemic disorders can be divided into those due to excess PTH and those due to other factors. Only primary hyperparathyroidism and a large subgroup of nonhematologic malignant diseases fall into the first category. The remainder fall into the second category and are characterized by suppression of PTH secretion.

B. Nonparathyroid Hypercalcemia: The underlying causes of hypercalcemia in the conditions in the second category are varied and, for the most part, uncertain. They will not be discussed here except to show how they can be excluded from the differential diagnosis of primary hyperparathyroidism. The most important ones are the hypercalcemia of cancer and familial hypocalciuric hypercalcemia.

1. Hypercalcemia of cancer–It is unlikely that a bony metastasis produces chronic hypercalcemia simply by physical displacement of bone. Rather, malignant tumors probably produce the same osteolytic humoral factors after metastasis to bone as they do before. These factors include PTH-like substances, prostaglandins, and osteoclast-activating factor (OAF). It is presumed that any one or a combination of these humors might be secreted systemically by parent tumors or released by bony metastases in sufficient quantities to stimulate local osteolysis and produce hypercalcemia. There is little question that OAF is involved in the production of hypercalcemia in patients with hematologic cancers, especially multiple myeloma. Until recently, it was thought that hypercalcemia in patients with nonhematologic cancers was, in large part, due to ectopic secretion of prostaglandins, but studies with inhibitors of prostaglandin synthesis have shown that plasma calcium rarely falls after their administration. This finding suggests that prostaglandins are relatively unimportant in the production of hypercalcemia in cancer.

Fuller Albright in 1948 postulated that PTH was responsible for solid-tumor hypercalcemia in some patients. In the absence of renal failure, many of these patients have the same degree of hypophosphatemia as patients with moderate to severe primary hyperparathyroidism. Normal (80%) to increased (20%) values for serum iPTH have been reported by some laboratories in as many as 70–80% of hypercalcemic patients with nonhematologic cancers. Serum values for iPTH using the same radioimmunoassay in patients with primary hyperparathyroidism and equal degrees of hypercalcemia are much higher than in patients with the hypercalcemia of cancer. These results suggest that the presence of iPTH in the sera of patients with cancer-associated hypercalcemia is either an incidental finding not etiologically related to the hypercalcemia or that it is quantitatively misrepresented by assays used to detect it and that, in fact, sufficient quantities of a biologically active PTH-like compound with low PTH immunoreactivity circulate in the plasma of these patients and account for the hypercalcemia. Studies concerning the heterogeneity of circulating bioactive and immunoreactive PTH in patients with the syndrome of ectopic hyperparathyroidism (cancer-associated hypercalcemia) favor the latter alternative. Moreover, a recent study shows that nephrogenous cAMP excretion in many patients with cancer-associated hypercalcemia is the same as or greater than that in patients with primary hyperparathyroidism. However, in this study, cancer patients had not only greater hypercalciuria but also much lower values for serum $1,25(OH)_2D_3$ than did patients with primary hyperparathyroidism. These findings suggest that the range of biologic actions of the PTH-like substance in patients with ectopic disease may be different from that of native PTH. Alternatively, another, non-PTH humor coincidentally released by solid tumors associated with hypercalcemia may decrease $1,25(OH)_2D_3$ production.

Current studies directed at discovering hypercalcemic substances produced by malignant tissue have used either extracts of tumors or conditioned media from cultures of tumors associated with hypercalcemia. Compounds that either bind and activate the PTH receptor or stimulate bone resorption and bind to the epidermal growth factor receptor have been identified. Whether these compounds are pathogenetically important in cancer-associated hypercalcemia needs to be determined.

2. Familial hypocalciuric hypercalcemia (familial benign hypercalcemia)–This syndrome is probably the second most important disorder in the differential diagnosis of primary hyperparathyroidism. It is inherited as an autosomal dominant trait and is characterized usually by asymptomatic or mild hypercalcemia, hypocalciuria, mild hypermagnesemia (variably present), and normal to low levels of serum iPTH. Parathyroid exploration in a number of patients has shown either normal parathyroid glands or equivocal "hyperplasia," and subtotal parathyroidectomy has consistently failed to restore eucalcemia. Recent studies have shown that the nephrogenous cAMP responses to exogenous and endogenous PTH are greater in patients with familial hypocalciuric hypercalcemia than in normal subjects or in patients with primary hyperparathyroidism. These observations suggest that the hypercalcemia in this familial syndrome may be partly due to renal hypersensitivity to the hypocalciuric effects of PTH. However, the persistence of increased renal tubular reabsorption of calcium after parathyroidectomy and the notable absence of the characteristic sequelae of primary hyperparathyroidism (eg, renal stones and osteitis fibrosa cystica) indicate that tissue hypersensitivity to PTH is probably not the sole cause of the disorder.

Severe parathyroid hyperplasia may occur in infants born of parents with this syndrome. Thus, measurement of serum calcium is indicated in all such infants. Hypercalcemia associated with findings compatible with hyperparathyroidism (increased serum iPTH) should be treated promptly by subtotal parathyroidectomy.

Diagnosis

The presence of hypercalcemia is established when

at least 3 measurements of total serum calcium are greater than normal. Venous blood should be drawn in the morning under fasting conditions with minimal venous stasis. The normal range for the total serum calcium is 8.9–10.1 mg/dL. Laboratories reporting a wider normal range (eg, 9–11 mg/dL) may have based it on measurements of serum calcium in subjects not documented as normal or may have a significant problem with calcium contamination. The latter is frequently due to use of a conventional chalkboard (chalk contains calcium) in the laboratory or to use of contaminated test tubes when drawing blood. Such sources of error must be eliminated, since large numbers of patients with mild hypercalcemia (eg, 10.1–11 mg/dL) will go undetected if the normal range for serum calcium is too wide. In the case of laboratory contamination, wide swings in serum calcium in individual subjects will be observed, leading to diagnostic confusion and to waste of patient and laboratory resources in the further investigation of artifactual hypercalcemia.

Freshly drawn blood specimens adjusted for pH must be used for measurements of serum ionic calcium. Special electrodes are required. In practice, since most calcium is bound to serum albumin, a rough estimate of true calcium can be made by adding or subtracting 0.8 mg/dL for each g/dL of albumin that is above or below normal. Special formulas and nomograms are also available. The QT interval in the ECG is shortened (adjusted for heart rate) when serum ionic calcium is significantly elevated.

A. Review of History of Present Illness: Hypercalcemia generally reflects serious underlying disease that may not have been suspected during the initial evaluation. Because of this, the patient with hypercalcemia should first have a repeat history and physical examination with specific objectives in mind. These include detailed evaluations of duration of illness, drug intake, the possible presence of non–mineral-related endocrine disease, a history of nephrolithiasis with documentation (old x-rays), symptoms of cancer, a family history of endocrine and mineral disorders, and the possible presence of palpable lymph nodes or masses, skin pigmentation or lesions (metastases), and thyromegaly, hepatomegaly, or splenomegaly.

1. Nephrolithiasis and body weight–Illness of long duration associated with nephrolithiasis and maintenance of normal weight favors a diagnosis of primary hyperparathyroidism; illness of short duration associated with weight loss without nephrolithiasis favors a nonparathyroid cause of hypercalcemia, particularly cancer.

2. Thiazide drugs–A history of thiazide intake might explain an increase in serum calcium to 11 mg/dL, but higher values usually indicate that this drug has merely increased the hypercalcemia of another condition (eg, mild primary hyperparathyroidism).

3. Vitamin D intake–This may not have been elicited in the initial history. Vitamin D can cause severe hypercalcemia in adults when taken in doses exceeding 50,000 units/d. Furthermore, patients with any disorder that causes hypercalcemia may be abnormally sensitive to vitamin D. Thus, intake of less than 50,000 units/d may aggravate existing hypercalcemia in sarcoidosis and primary hyperparathyroidism; what may appear initially to be a severe form of the primary disorder may prove ultimately to be relatively mild when vitamin D intake is curtailed.

4. Calcium intake–Excess calcium intake (> 5 g/d) in the form of calcium carbonate antacids can cause severe hypercalcemia in susceptible individuals, especially when coupled with additional intake of alkali (bicarbonate) (‘‘milk alkali syndrome’’). This condition is rare in its pure form. Most patients actually have underlying primary hyperparathyroidism and are taking calcium carbonate and alkali for associated gastric hyperacidity.

5. Family history–The family history may contain important clues to the correct diagnosis and treatment of a hypercalcemic patient. It is essential to inquire about the presence of hypercalcemia, nephrolithiasis, neck exploration, metabolic bone disease, intractable peptic ulcer disease, and endocrine tumors in family members, since primary hyperparathyroidism occurs as part of several familial multiple endocrine neoplasia (MEN) syndromes (see Chapter 25). There are few distinctive laboratory findings in the syndrome of familial hypocalciuric hypercalcemia, and a definitive diagnosis can be made only by documenting hypercalcemia in the patient's immediate relatives. A history of unsuccessful parathyroid surgery in more than one hypercalcemic relative is unfortunately characteristic of this condition. It is helpful if the surgeon is given information regarding possible multiple endocrine neoplasia or familial hyperparathyroidism before neck exploration is undertaken. Multiple parathyroid gland enlargement (‘‘hyperplasia’’) is almost certain to be present in both of these conditions, and subtotal parathyroidectomy (removal of 3½ glands) rather than single-gland removal would be indicated. Finally, mothers of infants with severe neonatal tetany should be suspected of having primary hyperparathyroidism.

B. Radioimmunoassay of Parathyroid Hormone: There has been a revolutionary change in the laboratory investigation of hypercalcemia in recent years owing to the development of sensitive and specific radioimmunoassays for serum PTH. Whereas patients were once extensively evaluated for nonparathyroid disorders that could cause hypercalcemia, the trend now is to use serum iPTH and calcium measurements to assign patients either to a group likely to benefit from surgical resection of parathyroid lesions or to one that requires further diagnostic evaluation for the cause of hypercalcemia (Fig 8–16).

1. iPTH in primary hyperparathyroidism–The results of a study using sensitive radioimmunoassay technique for measuring serum PTH that is specific for the mid (43–68) region of the molecule in the diagnosis of primary hyperparathyroidism are illustrated in Fig 8–17. Ninety percent of patients with surgically proved disease had serum iPTH values that

Figure 8–16. Use of PTH radioimmunoassay in the diagnosis and management of patients with hypercalcemia.

Figure 8–17. Serum iPTH values as a function of serum calcium concentration in 450 patients with surgically proved primary hyperparathyroidism. The area enclosed by the solid lines represents the normal range ±2 SD for serum iPTH and serum calcium. Note that there is a 10% overlap of serum iPTH with the normal range and that over 95% of normal sera and all hyperparathyroid sera have measurable iPTH. Formal discriminate analysis of serum iPTH and serum calcium distinguishes all hyperparathyroid patients from normal subjects. GP1M specifies the antiserum used in the assay. (Reproduced, with permission, from Arnaud CD et al: Page 19 in: *Excerpta Medica Int Cong Ser* No. 346, 1975.)

exceeded the upper limit of normal, and 10% had values that were in the upper range of normal but inappropriately high for the total calcium concentration in the same serum sample. Not shown are serum iPTH values in patients with nonparathyroid hypercalcemia (eg, sarcoidosis, vitamin D intoxication). These are low or undetectable except in ectopic hyperparathyroidism due to nonparathyroid cancer (see below) or in patients with coexisting primary hyperparathyroidism. Thus, it is possible, by measuring calcium and iPTH in a single morning fasting serum sample, to correctly categorize 80–90% of hypercalcemic patients who may benefit from resection of hyperfunctioning parathyroid glands and a similar percentage of patients who have nonparathyroid hypercalcemia and require further study. The practical advantages of using serum iPTH as the principal laboratory probe to "triage" hypercalcemic patients are obvious. In most patients with primary hyperparathyroidism, a correct diagnosis can be made in an outpatient setting, eliminating the costs and inconveniences of hospitalization and the repeated indirect tests required to make a less definitive diagnosis by exclusion.

2. iPTH in hypercalcemia of cancer–Values of serum iPTH measured with a carboxy-region assay are much lower for a given serum calcium in hyperparathyroidism due to nonparathyroid cancer (ectopic) than in primary hyperparathyroidism (Fig 8–18). This interesting phenomenon is apparently due in part to the finding that patients with ectopic hyperparathyroidism have lower quantities of mid- and carboxy-region fragments but essentially equivalent quantities of intact PTH in comparison with patients with primary hyperparathyroidism. Irrespective of the pathophysiologic mechanisms involved, the relationships shown in Fig 8–18 help to indicate how a physician should manage hypercalcemic and hypophosphatemic patients suspected but not proved to have cancer (eg, those with weight loss, anemia, and high erythrocyte sedimentation rates). If serum calcium values are over 12.5 mg/dL and serum iPTH is within the normal range or only slightly increased, more intensive efforts should be made to identify a neoplastic lesion and to follow the patient with medical treatment. If the situation is not clarified after 6–12 months, the patient should be reevaluated for the presence of primary hyperparathyroidism (Fig 8–16).

C. Serum and Urine Biochemistry: Several serum and urine measurements may be helpful in assigning hypercalcemic patients to parathyroid or nonparathyroid categories. Hyperphosphatemia in the absence of severe renal failure favors a nonparathyroid cause. Hypophosphatemia, when dietary phosphate is adequate and when oral phosphate-binding agents are not being ingested, favors primary hyperparathyroidism but is frequently present in ectopic hyperparathyroidism. Increased serum chloride favors primary hyperparathyroidism. Increased serum alkaline phosphatase is more common in patients with cancer than in those with primary hyperparathyroidism and, in the absence of radiographic evidence of osseous hyperparathyroidism, should suggest the possibility of ectopic hyperparathyroidism. Globulin abnormalities in serum protein electrophoresis point toward multiple myeloma or sarcoidosis, but increases in gamma globulin that disappear after parathyroidectomy have been observed in primary hyperparathyroidism. Although increases in the erythrocyte sedimentation rate and anemia have been recorded in primary hyperparathyroidism, these findings suggest a nonparathyroid cause of hypercalcemia, particularly cancer.

Measurement of urine calcium in hypercalcemic patients is generally useful only when it is low. This finding may be the only clue to familial hypocalciuric hypercalcemia. Because of the therapeutic importance of making this diagnosis (ie, avoiding neck exploration), measurement of 24-hour urine calcium is recommended in the routine evaluation of any hypercalcemic patient before exploration is performed.

D. Nephrogenous cAMP: About 40–50% of the cAMP excreted in the urine is derived from renal tubular cells. Its production and cellular release into the urine are almost entirely under the control of PTH. This component of urinary cAMP can be accurately estimated and is termed nephrogenous cAMP. Since

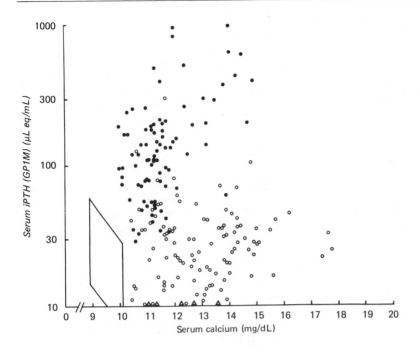

Figure 8–18. Relationship between serum iPTH (as measured by a mid-region assay) and serum calcium in patients with primary hyperparathyroidism (black dots) and hypercalcemic patients with cancer (open dots). Note that for a given serum calcium value, serum iPTH is lower in patients with cancer. In 5 of 105 patients with cancer, serum iPTH was undetectable (open triangles). Area enclosed with solid lines indicates normal range ±2 SD for serum iPTH and serum calcium. GP1M is the antiserum used in the assay. (Reproduced, with permission, from Benson RC Jr et al: *Am J Med* 1974;**56**:823.)

it is above normal in about 80% of patients with primary hyperparathyroidism (Fig 8–19) and in a large proportion of patients with ectopic hyperparathyroidism, it is not helpful in distinguishing between these 2 common disorders. However, because low levels of nephrogenous cAMP are present in patients who have nonparathyroid hypercalcemia but not cancer,

the test may be useful in patients with equivocal increases in serum iPTH. In such patients, a low level of nephrogenous cAMP would suggest that the serum iPTH value was artifactual and would argue against primary hyperparathyroidism, whereas a normal or increased level would confirm the validity of the serum iPTH value and favor this condition.

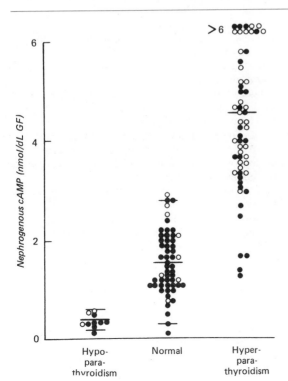

Figure 8–19. Nephrogenous cAMP, expressed as a function of glomerular filtration rate, in control subjects and patients with primary hyperparathyroidism. The open circles represent the subjects and patients with renal impairment (mean creatinine clearance < 80 mL/min). Closed circles represent subjects with normal renal function. The longer horizontal bars represent the mean values; shorter bars show ±2 SD. GF = glomerular filtrate. (Reproduced, with permission, from Broadus AE et al: *J Clin Invest* 1977;**60**:771.)

E. Other Diagnostic Tests: The glucocorticoid suppression test may be used in unusual situations when the results of all of the tests discussed above are equivocal. It is based on the observation that the hypercalcemia of conditions such as vitamin D intoxication, sarcoidosis, lymphoproliferative syndromes, and myeloma generally responds to the administration of 50–100 mg of cortisone or 40–60 mg of prednisone given daily in divided doses for 10 days, as shown by a decrease in serum calcium. This response is unusual in primary or ectopic hyperparathyroidism. However, results should be interpreted cautiously, since the mechanisms involved in steroid-induced suppression of hypercalcemia are poorly understood, and variables other than steroids (eg, hydration) may influence the level of serum calcium during the test. A positive test result (ie, a significant decrease in serum calcium) is a contraindication to neck exploration and signals the need for investigation for a nonparathyroid cause of hypercalcemia. A negative test result would be consistent with a diagnosis of primary or ectopic hyperparathyroidism.

Other diagnostic tests used less frequently include measurements of phosphate clearance (increased in primary hyperparathyroidism) and of urinary cAMP after PTH administration (usually decreased in primary hyperparathyroidism, most likely because of a "desensitization" mechanism).

F. Radiographs: It is essential to obtain high-quality x-rays of the hands on fine-grain industrial film in all patients whose hypercalcemia is a diagnostic problem. Although the finding of definitive subperiosteal bone resorption is relatively unusual (occurring in about 8–10% of patients with primary hyperparathyroidism), it is diagnostic of hyperparathyroidism and probably represents the most reliable and readily available evidence that neck exploration is needed in patients with severe, life-threatening hypercalcemia.

G. Preoperative Localization of Abnormal Parathyroid Tissue: Abnormal parathyroid tissue that is causing primary hyperparathyroidism will be discovered and excised in over 90% of initial neck explorations performed by a competent parathyroid surgeon. Thus, there is no need for invasive procedures to localize glandular tissue prior to first surgery except under very unusual circumstances (see below).

Generally, localization procedures are reserved for patients whose first neck exploration was not successful or who suffer recurrent disease. These procedures can be divided into noninvasive and invasive. Noninvasive procedures include esophagography, ultrasonography, computed tomography, and scanning with ^{201}Tl plus ^{99m}Tc. Invasive procedures include arteriography, differential venous catheterization with measurement of iPTH in the serum samples obtained, and needle aspiration of a mass localized by ultrasonography.

1. Esophagography–Esophagography may occasionally identify a relatively large parathyroid gland deep in the tracheoesophageal groove that was inadvertently missed on first exploration because of its aberrant shape. However, the procedure is usually unrewarding.

2. Ultrasonography, computed tomography, and scanning with ^{201}Tl plus ^{99m}Tc–Ultrasound technology has improved so rapidly that it is now possible to identify parathyroid lesions in the neck as small as 1 cm in diameter. Further technologic development in this area is expected, and routine ultrasound evaluation prior to initial neck exploration may become accepted practice. Because lesions can be identified in real time with this procedure, it has been possible to obtain needle aspiration biopsies of them. With use of routine and immunohistologic procedures and either immunoassays or bioassays of extracts of aspirated tissue, lesions located by ultrasonography can be identified as parathyroid in origin, thus giving the surgeon a histologic diagnosis preoperatively.

Whereas ultrasonography is generally not useful in identifying mediastinal lesions, computed tomography should be employed routinely with ultrasonography and esophagography in the patient harboring one or more missed or recurrent parathyroid lesions.

^{201}Tl is avidly concentrated by parathyroid tissue; when it is used in combination with ^{99m}Tc scans of the neck to identify thyroid tissue, parathyroid lesions can be effectively localized. This procedure is relatively new, and the incidence of false-positive and false-negative results obtained with it are unknown. Both false-positive and false-negative results have been obtained using ultrasonography and computed tomography, and at their present stage of development, it is prudent to use more than one of these procedures in patients with recurrent hyperparathyroidism and in patients whose first neck explorations were unsuccessful.

These procedures may help in the diagnosis of a severely hypercalcemic patient who has not undergone previous neck exploration. In such a case, identification of a mass lesion in a location consistent with normal or aberrant parathyroid tissue strongly suggests the presence of primary hyperparathyroidism and argues for early neck exploration, even before serum iPTH has been measured.

3. Thyroid arteriography–Of the invasive procedures, thyroid arteriography is most useful to the surgeon when a lesion is identified. However, as with the noninvasive procedures, the results are specific only in the sense that the location of an identified lesion is consistent with that of a normal or aberrant parathyroid gland. Neurologic complications such as transient occipital blindness and hemiplegia have been recorded; therefore, the procedure should be avoided in patients at risk for neurovascular disease. Use of small quantities of contrast medium by a radiologist with long experience in the technique minimizes the risk of complications.

4. Selective venous catheterization–Ideally, differential catheterization of the neck and mediastinal veins for the purpose of obtaining serum for iPTH analysis should be performed after veins have been identified by arteriography. The procedure is simple if a lesion has been identified by arteriography. If arteriography has not identified a lesion, all of the accessible small veins of the neck and mediastinum should be entered and sampled. It is often difficult to obtain blood from small veins because the lumina are obstructed by the catheter tip. The blood in the larger veins may be easier to aspirate, but the blood flow is so great that "step-up" increases in serum iPTH can be obliterated even if the catheter tip is near a small vein draining a parathyroid tumor. It is important to use a bioassay for PTH or one of the radioimmunoassays that recognize only intact PTH (ie, assays specific for intact PTH or amino-region fragments) in measurements of iPTH in sera obtained during venous catheterization. "Step-up" differences in iPTH concentrations between peripheral sera ànd sera from veins draining parathyroid lesions are greater when such assays are used, owing to the relatively low concentrations of intact PTH in the peripheral circulation. By contrast, mid- or carboxy-region assays measure the high concentrations of mid- or carboxy-region fragments in the peripheral circulation and provide smaller "step-up" increases. Venous catheterization studies must be interpreted with caution; because of the distortion in venous anatomy produced by individual variation, previous surgery, and venous anastomoses, the best result that can be obtained is usually lateralization of a parathyroid lesion. In general, less than a 2-fold "step-up" should be ignored unless all other values for iPTH are almost identical. It is important to recognize that significant increases in iPTH have been recorded in sera draining normal parathyroid glands. This finding argues against the use of differential venous sampling in the initial diagnosis of hyperparathyroidism.

Natural History of Hyperparathyroidism

The natural history of primary hyperparathyroidism is not well understood. This is because most patients in whom the diagnosis is made undergo neck exploration and removal of the abnormal glands and are cured.

A large proportion of patients have "biochemical" hyperparathyroidism—ie, only a slightly increased serum calcium (10.1–11 mg/dL) and no clinical manifestations of the disease. A study of 150 such patients at the Mayo Clinic showed that a minority (10–30%) will develop a more severe form of the disease within 5 years, but no clinical or biochemical measurement was predictive of such progression.

It is presumed that patients with mild to moderately severe primary hyperparathyroidism started with the "biochemical" form of the disease. However, some of these patients attain a degree of disease stability; some have been observed for as long as 10–15 years without apparent progression. Except for a few who progress to severe disease, the remaining patients in this group probably have slow progression with gradual development of osteopenia and deterioration of renal function. Patients with severe primary hyperparathyroidism (serum calcium > 15 mg/dL) will almost certainly die of the complications sooner or later unless the disease is diagnosed and appropriately treated.

Resection of benign parathyroid lesions is usually curative. Recurrences are rare in patients with single-gland disease but relatively common in multiple-gland disease. It is unclear whether successful surgical treatment restores impaired renal function. Stone formation generally ceases unless factors other than primary hyperparathyroidism are operative. There have been anecdotal reports of relief of severe psychiatric symptoms after removal of abnormal parathyroid glands. All but the more severe forms of osteitis fibrosa cystica improve within months and resolve completely within a year after parathyroidectomy. Recent studies suggest that surgical treatment of hyperparathyroidism in patients with postmenopausal or senile osteoporosis results in improvement of osteopenia. This is important because as many as 8–10% of patients with age-related osteopenia have increased circulating levels of iPTH and may suffer from some form of curable hyperparathyroidism.

Treatment of Hypercalcemia
A. Medical Treatment:
1. Chronic moderate hypercalcemia (serum calcium 12–15 mg/dL)–Medical management of diseases causing nonparathyroid hypercalcemia generally results in prompt resolution of this biochemical abnormality. Far-advanced malignant disorders (solid or hematologic tumors) are exceptions, and long-term chronic treatment of cancer-related hypercalcemia in such cases is a therapeutic challenge. There is no satisfactory protocol for managing this problem, and it is a fertile area for pharmacologic research.

a. Glucocorticoids–Glucocorticoids appear to be the major resource for treatment of hypercalcemia associated with hematologic malignant neoplasms. They should be given in relatively high doses (eg, prednisone, 60–120 mg/d given orally in divided doses) and for relatively long periods (1 month) before the treatment is considered a failure.

b. Mithramycin–Mithramycin (Mithracin), a toxic antibiotic that inhibits bone resorption, may be useful in the treatment of hypercalcemia due to both hematologic and solid malignant neoplasms. The usual dosage is 25 μg/kg by intravenous push. When hypercalcemia recurs, this same dose may be given again, provided platelet counts have not been dangerously suppressed and renal function has not become impaired. Lower doses (10–15 μg/kg) have been used successfully with fewer side effects.

c. Phosphate–Oral phosphate may be used as an antihypercalcemic agent in patients who have not been taking glucocorticoids. (The combination of oral phosphate and glucocorticoids occasionally induces nephrolithiasis, although the cause is unknown.) Either neutral phosphate or potassium phosphate may be given in doses as high as 2–4 g/d orally in divided doses. Initial doses should be relatively low (1–2 g of elemental phosphorus as phosphate per day orally in divided doses every 6 hours), because of gastrointestinal side effects; these disappear with time. Serum calcium, phosphate, and creatinine should be measured regularly to determine if phosphate treatment is effective and to detect the possible development of hyperphosphatemia or renal function impairment. Compliance can be assessed by measurement of 24-hour urine phosphorus. In general, decreases in serum calcium during phosphate therapy do not occur unless serum phosphate concentrations increase. Increases in serum phosphorus above 5 mg/dL should be avoided because of the danger of inducing extraskeletal calcifications. Phosphate therapy can be used as a temporary measure during diagnostic studies. Phosphate therapy may cause hypokalemia, requiring administration of potassium supplements.

d. Calcitonin–Although it would seem rational to use CT, normal doses (100 units/d) have been disappointing. There are recent reports of good results with high doses of CT (400– 1000 units every 12 hours) or with CT plus glucocorticoids (CT, 100 units twice daily, and prednisone, 60 mg daily).

e. Estrogen–Because estrogens decrease bone resorption and serum calcium in postmenopausal osteoporosis, estrogens have been used successfully to lower serum calcium in primary hyperparathyroidism. In the absence of contraindications (eg, personal or family history of uterine or breast cancer), maintenance doses (eg, 0.625– 1.25 mg conjugated estrogens [Premarin, etc]) should be given to all postmenopausal patients with primary hyperparathyroidism under medical management.

f. Other agents–Based on the presence of both adrenergic and histamine receptors on parathyroid cells, alpha- and beta-adrenergic blockers and cimetidine have been tried in primary hyperparathyroidism, with variable results.

2. Acute severe hypercalcemia (serum calcium > 15 mg/dL)–The medical therapy of acute severe hypercalcemia is quite different from that of chronic moderate hypercalcemia. Treatment should be started as soon as severe hypercalcemia has been detected, because the condition is life-threatening.

a. Hospitalization–If possible, the patient should remain ambulatory, since immobilization may increase serum calcium in some patients. Serum calcium, magnesium, sodium, and potassium must be monitored every 2– 4 hours. In patients with heart disease who are in danger of developing heart failure from volume overload, central venous pressure should be monitored so that appropriate measures can be taken if the pressure increases.

b. Calcium restriction–Dietary calcium should be restricted immediately, and all drugs that might cause hypercalcemia (thiazides, vitamin D, etc) should be discontinued.

c. Reduction of digitalis–If the patient is taking digitalis, it may be wise to reduce the dose because the hypercalcemic patient may be more sensitive to the toxic effects of this drug. Ideally, the patient should be admitted to an intensive care unit for electrocardiographic monitoring while antihypercalcemic measures are being instituted. Beta-adrenergic blocking agents are useful in protecting the heart against the adverse effects of severe hypercalcemia, especially serious arrhythmias.

d. Hydration and diuretics–The mainstay of therapy is a regimen of hydration with saline solutions plus diuresis with furosemide or ethacrynic acid. The objective is to increase the urinary excretion of calcium rapidly, thus decreasing the exchangeable calcium pool and the serum calcium concentration. Saline is given to increase sodium excretion, since sodium clearance and calcium clearance parallel one another during water or osmotic diuresis. Furosemide inhibits the tubular reabsorption of calcium and aids in maintaining diuresis. Approximately 4– 6 L of isotonic saline should be given intravenously daily, along with 20– 100 mg of furosemide every 1– 2 hours (intravenously or orally) or 10– 40 mg of ethacrynic acid every 1– 2 hours (intravenously or orally). Such a regimen should increase urinary calcium to 500– 1000 mg/d and lower serum calcium by 2– 6 mg/dL after 24 hours.

e. Potassium and magnesium depletion and dehydration–These complications of therapy must be anticipated and appropriate replacement therapy instituted early.

f. Maintenance regimen–After serum calcium has decreased to a reasonably safe level (< 13 mg/dL), a chronic regimen may be instituted. This should consist of furosemide (40– 160 mg/d orally) or ethacrynic acid (50– 200 mg/d orally), sodium chloride tablets (400– 600 meq/d orally), and at least 3 L of fluid per day. Serum calcium, magnesium, and potassium should be monitored daily at first and then weekly when serum calcium has stabilized. Magnesium and potassium should be replaced as necessary.

g. Other drugs–Two other drugs are used in patients with hypercalcemia associated with cancer.

(1) Indomethacin–Although responses are infrequent, indomethacin (25 mg every 6 hours orally) may be tried. The rationale is that the hypercalcemia may be due to increased bone resorption caused by excessive prostaglandin released by the cancer.

(2) Mithramycin–Mithramycin is given in 2– 4 doses of 10– 15 μg/kg intravenously on alternate days early in the course of treatment of acute hypercalcemia. It is probably unwise to give mithramycin if primary hyperparathyroidism is suspected, because the patient is likely to require surgery and mithramycin can cause marked thrombocytopenia. Patients receiving mithramycin should be followed carefully with platelet counts, serum creatinine, and liver function tests because of its possible toxicity to the liver, kidney, and marrow.

B. Surgery for Removal of Abnormal Parathyroid Tissue: Surgical treatment should be considered in all patients with an established diagnosis of primary hyperparathyroidism. It is not clear that the biochemical form of the disease necessarily progresses to the stage at which clinically significant sequelae

Table 8–4. Categories of treatment for patients
with primary hyperparathyroidism.

Criteria	Preferred Treatment
1. One or more of the following: Serum calcium > 11 mg/dL. Osteitis fibrosa cystica. Progressive osteopenia. Metabolically active nephro- lithiasis. Decreased renal function. Intractable peptic ulcer. Pancreatitis. Serious psychiatric disease. Severe hypertension.	Surgical removal of parathy- roid lesion.
2. Unsuccessful surgery, or recur- rence with manifestations noted in category 1.	Surgical removal of parathy- roid lesion; preoperative localization may be indi- cated.
3. Serum calcium < 11 mg/dL. Abnormal serum iPTH. Absence of manifestations noted in category 1.	Surgical removal of parathy- roid lesion or medical man- agement (see text).
4. Surgery contraindicated.	Medical management for hy- percalcemia and prevention of nephrolithiasis (see text).

develop. However, most of these patients have his-tologic evidence of hyperparathyroidism on bone bi-opsy. Age is not a contraindication to neck explora-tion. Indeed, it is better to perform elective parathy-roidectomy and manage hypercalcemia in that way than to deal with it later as a complication of another serious illness (eg, myocardial infarction).

1. Indications for surgery–In the long-term fol-low-up of biochemical hyperparathyroidism com-mented upon earlier, a group of arbitrary criteria were developed as indications for neck exploration (Table 8–4): (1) serum calcium higher than 11 mg/d; (2) radiographic evidence of metabolic bone disease; (3) active nephrolithiasis; (4) demonstration of de-creased renal function; and (5) development of one or more "complications" of hyperparathyroidism such as serious psychiatric disease, peptic ulcer that is re-sistant to treatment, pancreatitis, and severe hyper-tension. In any patient in whom long-term medical management of the disease is planned, certain studies should be obtained routinely (Fig 8–16). *At a mini-mum,* these should include a yearly history and phys-ical examination, serum calcium, creatinine clear-ance, and bone mineral content of the spine; x-rays of the hand on fine-grain industrial film to detect subperiosteal bone resorption; and a plain film of the abdomen to detect renal calcifications. If inactive nephrolithiasis has been found on initial examination, nephrotomograms should be done to determine if new stones have formed or existing ones have enlarged. By definition, either of the latter would indicate re-currence of active stone disease, which would in turn be an indication for surgery.

2. Parathyroid surgeon–The most critical con-

sideration in the surgical management of primary hy-perparathyroidism is selection of a surgeon with ex-tensive experience in parathyroid surgery and the abil-ity to distinguish between an enlarged or abnormal parathyroid gland or lesion and a normal gland.

3. Surgical procedures–Two different proce-dures are currently used. The most widely accepted procedure consists of identifying all 4 parathyroid glands (using biopsy if necessary) followed by re-moval of a single enlarged parathyroid gland or of 3½ glands if multiple glands are involved (Table 8– 5). If abnormal parathyroid tissue cannot be identified, hemithyroidectomy should be performed, preferably on the side of a "missing" gland, because an intra-thyroidal lesion may be present. All remaining para-thyroid glands or remnants are marked with nonab-sorbable sutures to facilitate future identification of parathyroid tissue if repeat surgery for recurrent hy-perparathyroidism is necessary.

The less commonly used procedure consists of exploring one side of the neck first and removing any single enlarged parathyroid gland. If the second gland on the same side is normal, the other side is not explored. If the second gland is abnormal, it is re-moved and the other side of the neck is explored and all parathyroid tissue removed except for one-half of a gland. This second approach leaves the unoperated side without scar tissue and makes it easier to explore at some future time for recurrent hyperparathyroidism. However, it fails to establish whether multiple glands are involved, since enlarged glands may be present on the unoperated side.

No matter which approach is taken, it is important to make accurate records of the number and location of glands identified and removed (preferably by de-tailed diagram). This information is essential in find-ing the missed glands if hypercalcemia persists or recurs.

4. Parathyroid autotransplantation–Autotrans-plantation of a portion of an enlarged parathyroid gland to the muscles of the forearm can be beneficial in special circumstances, such as when the last known parathyroid gland is removed because of recurrent primary hyperparathyroidism. Without transplanta-tion, patients of this type may become hypoparathy-roid. The functioning of such transplants can be easily assessed by measuring serum PTH in venous blood from both forearms. A "step-up" in the concentration

Table 8–5. Extent of parathyroidectomy.

Number of Glands Involved	Procedure
All 4	Removal of 3 glands and all but 35–50 mg of the fourth gland; suture tagging of remnant.
Two or 3	Removal of all but half of a normal gland; suture tagging of remaining half.
One	Removal of involved gland; identification of remain- ing glands (often by biopsy); suture tagging of re- maining glands.

of serum iPTH in the transplanted forearm in comparison with the nontransplanted one is indicative of a functioning graft. If such patients develop hypercalcemia, portions of the transplanted gland can be removed easily.

5. Ectopic location–About 20% of abnormal parathyroid glands are in the mediastinum. However, 95% of these are in the superior part of the cavity, attached to the thymus or mediastinal fat pad. These abnormal glands are readily identified and removed during routine neck exploration by lifting the contents of the superior mediastinum into the neck incision. The remaining 5% are located elsewhere in the mediastinum and can only be made accessible for excision by splitting the sternum. Before the advent of localization procedures (see above), the success rate in removing abnormal parathyroid tissue from the mediastinum was only 50%. The decision to perform mediastinal exploration largely depends on the accuracy and completeness of the information obtained during initial neck exploration. If the exploration was inadequate or the records incomplete, repeat neck exploration is probably indicated. A recent study in which patients of this type were explored again showed an 80% success rate in finding missed abnormal parathyroid glands in the neck or superior mediastinum attached to the thymus. In rare cases, a fifth or sixth parathyroid gland may be present and abnormal.

C. Postoperative Care:

1. Hypocalcemia–If surgery is successful, serum calcium concentrations decrease to the normal range or lower within 24–48 hours. It is possible to determine if all abnormal parathyroid tissue has been removed by measuring decreased cAMP in a "spot" urine collection within 2 hours after parathyroidectomy. Patients with significant bony demineralization may develop severe hypocalcemia postoperatively. This is presumably due to the avidity of demineralized bone for extracellular fluid calcium ("hungry bone syndrome"). It can be distinguished from the development of hypoparathyroidism by the absence of hyperphosphatemia and the presence of increased serum iPTH. Treatment may be difficult and requires large quantities of intravenous calcium given continuously by infusion plus calcium carbonate given orally in doses of 1–10 g/d, depending upon the serum calcium response. Ergocalciferol (vitamin D_2) (usually 50,000–100,000 units daily) is of uncertain value. In the authors' experience, $1,25(OH)_2D_3$ (calcitriol, Rocaltrol) in relatively large doses (1–2 μg/d) has been useful.

2. Hypoparathyroidism–Most patients who develop hypocalcemia and mild hyperphosphatemia have temporary hypoparathyroidism, as evidenced by low normal serum levels of iPTH. A few of these patients will develop permanent hypoparathyroidism that requires treatment.

3. Other complications–Worsening of renal function (temporary or permanent), metabolic acidosis, hypomagnesemia, pancreatitis, and gout or pseudogout are other complications that may occur in the postoperative period. The problem of deterioration of renal function should be anticipated in patients who have abnormal renal function before the operation, and prophylactic infusions of mannitol should be given early in the postoperative period to initiate and maintain osmotic diuresis. Likewise, exacerbations of gout or pseudogout should be anticipated in patients with intra-articular calcifications or a history of arthritic attacks.

4. Follow-up–Follow-up is recommended for about 10 years. This is especially important for patients with multiple-gland disease, because of the likelihood of recurrence. Another concern is the rare but real possibility that an excised lesion (in spite of histologic evidence of benignity) may have been malignant. In such cases, early detection of hypercalcemia may permit definitive surgical treatment before the development of local or distant metastases.

SECONDARY HYPERPARATHYROIDISM OF CHRONIC RENAL FAILURE

An increase in PTH secretion that is adaptive and unrelated to intrinsic disease of the parathyroid glands is called secondary hyperparathyroidism. The disorder is associated with prolonged stimulation of the parathyroid glands by chronic decreases in the concentration of ionic calcium in the blood. Several conditions cause chronic hypocalcemia and secondary hyperparathyroidism (Table 8–6). However, except in extreme cases, chronic renal failure is the only one in which secondary hyperparathyroidism produces clinically significant manifestations. Thus, this section will emphasize hyperparathyroidism associated with chronic renal failure.

Interest in the hyperparathyroidism of chronic renal failure and its associated bone disease, **renal osteodystrophy,** is a fairly recent development. Before the advent of hemodialysis, the sequelae of progressive nephron destruction were not studied seriously, because the life expectancy of patients with chronic renal failure was so short. Since these patients are now maintained with dialysis and renal transplantation, the problems of chronic management must be identified and solved.

Table 8–6. Major causes of chronic hypocalcemia other than parathyroprival hypoparathyroidism.

Dietary deficiency of vitamin D or calcium.
Decreased intestinal absorption of vitamin D or calcium due to primary small bowel disease, short bowel syndrome, and postgastrectomy syndrome.
Drugs that cause rickets or osteomalacia such as phenytoin, phenobarbital, cholestyramine, and laxatives.
States of tissue resistance to vitamin D.
Excessive intake of inorganic phosphate compounds.
Pseudohypoparathyroidism.
Severe hypomagnesemia.
Chronic renal failure.

Pathogenesis of Secondary Hyperparathyroidism in Chronic Renal Failure

Serum iPTH progressively increases in patients with chronic renal failure as glomerular filtration rate (GFR) decreases below 40 mL/min (Fig 8– 20). This relationship might have been predicted on the basis of older studies that showed increases in serum phosphorus concentrations at this same level of GFR (40 mL/min). However, it was not until the investigations of Bricker et al that the role of decreased renal filtration of phosphate and subsequent hyperphosphatemia in the genesis of renal hyperparathyroidism was appreciated. According to their hypothesis, each decrement in GFR is accompanied by a transient increase in serum phosphorus, which in turn leads to a transient decrease in serum calcium and a compensatory increase in secretion of PTH. Restoration of serum calcium and serum phosphorus toward normal occurs as a result of the effects of increased serum PTH on mobilization of bone mineral and renal tubular reabsorption of phosphate, respectively. As the cycle is repeated, secondary hyperparathyroidism progressively worsens and parathyroid hyperplasia develops.

The evidence in support of the hypothesis of Bricker et al is impressive. First, a reduction in phosphate intake in proportion to the reduction in GFR prevents renal hyperparathyroidism in dogs that have had progressive renal failure for as long as 1 year. Second, there is a consistent positive correlation between serum concentrations of phosphate and iPTH in patients with chronic renal failure (Fig 8– 21). Third, reductions in the serum concentrations· of phosphate by dietary restriction and administration of aluminum hydroxide gels in patients with chronic renal failure are associated with increases in serum calcium and decreases in serum iPTH.

The hyperphosphatemia of chronic renal failure may also have a negative influence on the production of $1,25(OH)_2D_3$, even before the destruction of nephrons is so complete that the renal $25OHD_3$-converting enzymes are eliminated. As illustrated in Fig 8– 2, such an effect would result in a decrease in the intestinal absorption of calcium—a well-established finding in patients with chronic renal failure. This decrease would contribute further to hypocalcemia and secondary hyperparathyroidism. It is well known that serum concentrations of $1,25(OH)_2D_3$ are low in patients with end-stage renal disease, but there have been no systematic studies of the relation between serum concentrations of this vitamin D metabolite and the degree of chronic renal failure.

The osseous manifestations of progressive increases in PTH secretion and decreases in $1,25(OH)_2D_3$ production by the kidney are evident in patients with chronic renal failure. They include classic osteitis fibrosa cystica similar to that seen in primary hyper-

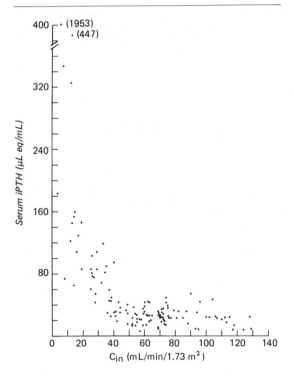

Figure 8 –20. Serum iPTH as a function of the renal clearance of inulin in normal subjects and patients with varying degrees of renal failure. The assay used GP1M as the antiserum. (Reproduced with permission, from Arnaud CD et al: Page 349 in: *Urinary Calculi: Recent Advances in Aetiology, Stone Structure, and Treatment.* International Symposium on Renal Stone Research, 1973.)

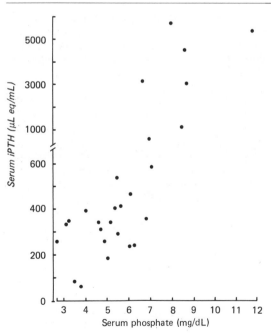

Figure 8 –21. Relationship between serum iPTH and serum phosphate in patients with renal failure. (Reproduced, with permission, from Bordier PJ et al: *Kidney Int* 1975;7[Suppl 2]:102.)

parathyroidism (Fig 8– 15A and 8– 15B) and osteo-malacia (Fig 8– 30). In addition, osteosclerosis and osteoporosis are often present at the same time. The causes of these 2 disorders are unknown and are probably multiple. It is thought that the osteosclerosis is related to the hyperphosphatemia, and the osteoporosis to diminished sex hormone function and the metabolic acidosis of uremia. Finally, it is well established that the bones of patients with chronic renal failure are resistant to the calcemic actions of PTH. Although there may be several underlying reasons for such resistance, it is commonly thought that the major factors are the decreased serum concentration of $1,25(OH)_2D_3$ and the dependency of PTH on normal vitamin D metabolism for its action on bone.

The pathogenesis of renal hyperparathyroidism during the progressive destruction of nephrons is illustrated in Fig 8– 22. The processes schematically described result in the classic biochemical and physiologic abnormalities of mineral and bone metabolism observed in patients with chronic renal failure, including hypocalcemia, hyperphosphatemia, decreased intestinal absorption of calcium and negative calcium balance, marked increases in circulating PTH, and the different bone diseases noted above.

Natural History

A. Chronic Renal Failure: The natural history of disorders of mineral and bone metabolism that are associated with chronic renal failure is not well under-stood. A group of untreated patients with chronic renal failure of varying severity and duration who were not undergoing hemodialysis has been studied in order to provide such information. In spite of the limitations imposed on interpretation of results from a cross-sectional study, it was possible to roughly categorize the development of mineral abnormalities as a function of time and severity (Fig 8– 23). The first detectable abnormality appears to be an increase in serum iPTH. This occurs when GFR falls below 40 mL/min and before there are detectable changes in serum phosphate or calcium. This is not unexpected, if increased PTH secretion represents the major mechanism by which the organism adapts to renal phosphate retention. The important question is whether this adaptive mechanism, which appears to be so successful in maintaining extracellular calcium and phosphate homeostasis under physiologic conditions, is in the best interest of the patient with renal failure or whether externally applied therapeutic measures designed to achieve the same purpose might serve such a patient better in the long run.

In the study noted above, all of the patients who had mild to moderate degrees of chronic renal failure (serum creatinine ≤ 3 mg/dL) had histomorphometric evidence of excess circulating PTH in bone biopsies, and many had subperiosteal bone resorption on hand radiographs (stage I), in spite of normal serum levels of calcium and phosphorus. Thus, it appears that maintenance of normal levels of serum calcium and phosphorus in patients with early renal failure by adaptive increases in PTH secretion occurred as a result of an important trade-off—loss of osseous integrity.

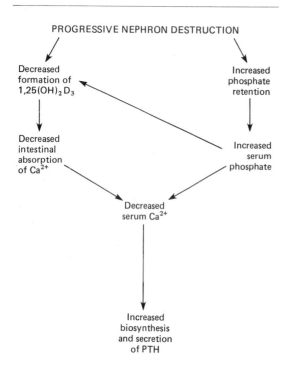

Figure 8 –22. Pathogenesis of parathyroid hyperplasia during progressive destruction of nephrons. (Reproduced, with permission, from Arnaud CD et al: *Kidney Int* 1973;**4**:89.)

Figure 8 –23. Stages of biochemical and osseous abnormalities in renal osteodystrophy as a function of time and nephron loss. (Reproduced, with permission, from Bordier PJ et al: *Kidney Int* 1975;**7**[Suppl 2]:102.)

Figure 8–24. Relationship between serum iPTH and serum calcium. *Top:* Stage III and stage IV patients with high iPTH values. *Bottom:* Stage I and stage II patients with relatively low iPTH values. (Reproduced, with permission, from Bordier PJ et al: *Kidney Int* 1975;**7**[Suppl 2]:102.)

Stage II was marked by the development of hypocalcemia, hyperphosphatemia, and further increases in serum iPTH. A transition to this stage probably reflects the development of severe vitamin D deficiency caused by the hyperphosphatemia and the loss of $1,25(OH)_2D_3$ hydroxylase that occurs with progressive destruction of the kidney. Deficiency of $1,25(OH)_2D_3$ results in superimposition of osteomalacia on osteitis fibrosa cystica, which, having developed during stage I, now becomes worse. It is probably the degree and duration of the hypocalcemia of stage II that determine whether patients enter stages III and IV. These stages are characterized by worsening hyperparathyroidism, restoration of the serum calcium first to normal and then to hypercalcemic levels, and development of severe hyperphosphatemia. In fact, it is likely that some time during the transition from stage II to stage III, hyperparathyroidism becomes self-perpetuating and relatively autonomous (referred to by some as "tertiary" hyperparathyroidism). Phosphorus, as well as calcium, is released from bone during the process of PTH-induced bone resorption, and the initial perturbation causing hyperparathyroidism—hyperphosphatemia—is aggravated by the adaptive process originally developed to control it. In this manner, the negative feedback system that operates between bone and parathyroid glands when a normal kidney is present may be transformed into a biologically unstable "positive feedback" system when phosphorus cannot be excreted by a functioning kidney. Evidence of a defect in the ability of hypercalcemia to suppress PTH secretion in stage III and stage IV patients is illustrated in Fig 8–24. Whereas the expected negative correlation between serum iPTH and serum calcium is evident in stage I and stage II patients (lower panel), a positive correlation between these 2 variables exists in stage III and stage IV patients. The determinants of the transformation from stage II to stage III are poorly understood, but they probably include dietary levels of calcium, phosphate, and vitamin D and the rapidity with which the patient loses nephrons. During stages III and IV, osteitis fibrosa cystica and osteomalacia become even more prominent, and, because the product of the serum concentrations of calcium and phosphate increases to levels that favor precipitation, soft tissue calcification ensues.

B. "Aluminum" Osteodystrophy: A newly recognized syndrome of osteodystrophy that does not conform to the bone disease characterizing the 4 stages shown in Fig 8–23 has been described in patients with chronic renal failure. This syndrome is present in relatively few patients (5–10%) with renal osteodystrophy. Its cause is unknown, although accumulation of aluminum in bone (especially at the calcification front) due to the aluminum contained in dialysis baths or phosphate-binding agents has been recently implicated. Patients with this disorder have bone pain and multiple fractures and tend to develop hypercalcemia. Thus, superficially at least, they resemble patients with stage III or stage IV disease. However, instead of severe degrees of osteitis fibrosa cystica and hyperparathyroidism, these patients have a bone disease characterized by low-turnover osteomalacia and osteoporosis with only small or moderate increases in serum iPTH. Patients who have been subjected to parathyroidectomy have responded poorly or not at all. This is in striking contrast to patients with true stage IV renal hyperparathyroidism and osteodystrophy, who almost always respond favorably as long as they are carefully managed to prevent recrudescence of hyperparathyroidism after subtotal parathyroidectomy. The effectiveness of deferoxamine, a drug that chelates aluminum, is currently being assessed in the treatment of "aluminum" osteodystrophy.

Clinical Features

The clinical manifestations of renal hyperparathyroidism and osteodystrophy are related to hypocalcemia in stage II patients and to soft tissue calcifications, osteodystrophy, and pruritus in stage III and stage IV patients. Although not common, symptoms of neuromuscular irritability and tetany similar to those in hypoparathyroidism may occur. Osteodystrophy causes bone pain due to either osteitis fibrosa or multiple fractures (frequently of the ribs). Soft tissue calcification of the joints (usually the shoulder) may be evident in rare cases as hard irregular masses over the joints. Pruritus is most debilitating when it occurs, and its cause is poorly understood. However, it routinely abates after successful medical or surgical management of hyperparathyroidism. Radiographs of the skeleton commonly show the ravages of osteitis fibrosa cystica (Fig 8–15A and 8–15B), osteomalacia (Fig 8–30), and osteosclerosis. This latter condition is classically observed as the "rugger jersey sign" (referring to the striped shirts worn by British rugby teams) and is caused by increased density of the upper and lower margins of vertebral bodies, separated by central horizontal zones of decreased density. Soft tissue calcifications often seen on x-ray in the later stages are most prominent in large vessels and joints but have been observed in extreme cases in lung, stomach, and heart. It is thought that soft tissue calcification of small blood vessels is responsible for the rare development of necrotic skin lesions on legs, abdomen, and fingertips.

Treatment

Little effort has been made to interrupt the adaptive cycle described in the section on pathogenesis and to prevent the development of the pathologic "positive feedback" between bone and parathyroid glands during the course of renal failure. This is probably because patients are generally asymptomatic and reluctant to take medicines early in the course of renal failure. In addition, no long-term prospective studies have been reported showing that appropriate therapy instituted early and directed at preventing the development of positive phosphorus balance, negative calcium balance, and hyperparathyroidism will significantly decrease the incidence or severity of mineral and bone complications that occur in the late stages of renal failure, during hemodialysis, or after kidney transplantation. However, investigations during the past 10 years have shown that restoration of serum calcium and phosphorus levels toward normal by the use of oral phosphate-binding gels and calcium concentrations of 6–7 mg/dL in the dialysate for patients undergoing hemodialysis decreases serum levels of iPTH (Fig 8–25) and causes improvement in established renal osteodystrophy (Fig 8–26). It is therefore likely that the component of renal osteodystrophy that is due to hyperparathyroidism could be prevented if steps were taken *early* in the course of chronic renal failure to avoid adaptive increases in PTH secretion. Since the stimulus to PTH secretion is hypocalcemia induced by hyperphosphatemia and decreased intestinal absorption of calcium, it is logical to assume that a combination of ingestion of a low-phosphate diet, administration of phosphate-binding gels, and treatment with relatively large doses of absorbable calcium and physiologic doses of $1,25(OH)_2D_3$ (calcitriol)

Figure 8–25. Serial values of plasma iPTH, calcium, and phosphate during treatment of a patient with low and then high calcium levels in the dialysate. Plasma phosphate was reduced to 6 mg/dL by oral administration of aluminum hydroxide gel, after which dialysate calcium concentrations were progressively increased to 8 mg/dL. (Reproduced, with permission, from Goldsmith RS et al: *Am J Med* 1971;**50**:692.)

might be successful in restoring extracellular calcium and phosphorus homeostasis and preventing secondary hyperparathyroidism.

A. Management of Stage I Renal Osteodystrophy: The major difficulty in this stage is determining when to begin treatment in individual patients, because serum calcium and phosphorus concentrations are usually within the normal range early in the course of chronic renal failure. In spite of this, serum iPTH is increased during the first stage (Fig 8–23). Unfortunately, this change may be difficult to detect with some radioimmunoassays. Assays specific for the mid or carboxyl region of the PTH molecule show that serum iPTH is increased uniformly in patients with chronic renal failure. Although an increased level of serum iPTH may reflect diminished clearance of carboxy-terminal fragments by diseased kidneys, mid- and carboxy-region assays show that institution of the therapy noted below results in a progressive decline in serum iPTH toward the normal range. This result suggests that there is either a decrease in PTH secretion or improved clearance of carboxy-terminal fragments by the kidney. The latter possibility is a remote one, and it is likely that the observed decreases in serum iPTH reflect success in directly interrupting the development of adaptive hyperparathyroidism.

Figure 8–26. X-rays of index finger of a patient before *(left)* and after *(right)* plasma phosphate was reduced to normal with aluminum hydroxide gel and 6 months of dialysis against a bath of 8 mg/dL calcium. (Reproduced, with permission, from Vosik WM et al: *Mayo Clin Proc* 1972;**47**:110.)

1. Dietary restriction of phosphorus–It appears that the single most important marker for stage I renal osteodystrophy—and the major indication for considering a patient with chronic renal failure for treatment with dietary restriction of phosphate, calcium supplementation, and vitamin D therapy—is an abnormally high serum iPTH value as measured by a mid- or carboxy-region assay. Although dietary restriction of phosphate may be sufficient for some patients, others may require the addition of phosphate-binding antacids in order to reduce serum iPTH.

2. Removal of phosphate–There are many aluminum-containing phosphate-binding antacids on the market. Alu-Capsules, high-potency liquid Basaljel, and aluminum hydroxide–containing cookies (commercially prepared or baked at home) appear to be the most effective and the best tolerated because of their almost complete absence of aluminum taste. The patient should be offered a variety of preparations and dosage forms and should be allowed to choose an acceptable combination. Dosage must be adjusted for each patient, and prolonged hypophosphatemia should be avoided. The initial dose should be between 0.25 and 0.5 g/d; the dose should be increased if serum

phosphate and serum iPTH fail to decrease. For maximal effect on dietary phosphate absorption, antacids should always be taken with meals.

3. Calcium supplementation–Because low-phosphate diets are also low in calcium, it is necessary to provide supplementation with some form of absorbable calcium. Calcium carbonate is preferred because it is cheap and well tolerated and combats renal acidosis. Calcium supplementation is necessary even when the patient is on a normal diet, because enteral absorption of calcium is usually decreased in chronic renal failure. Serum calcium should be monitored because a few patients develop hypercalcemia. However, doses as high as 5 g/d may be tolerated well.

4. Vitamin D therapy–It is reasonable to maintain patients with early renal failure on relatively small doses (1000–2000 units/d) of ergocalciferol (vitamin D_2), providing no more than 10 times the daily requirement. Experience with $1,25(OH)_2D_3$ (calcitriol) in patients with stage I disease has not yet been reported.

B. Management of Stage II Renal Osteodystrophy: Most patients with end-stage renal failure present with the mineral and osseous abnormalities found in stage II disease. The hallmarks of this stage are hypocalcemia, hyperphosphatemia, and increases in serum iPTH greater than those in stage I. Generally, serum iPTH measured by a mid- or carboxy-region assay is 10–20 times normal values.

Since stages III and IV tend to be much less reversible by medical means than stage I or stage II, it is important to manage the patient with stage II disease aggressively. In treating such a patient, one must recognize that the hypocalcemia seen in stage II probably reflects a fortuitous protective adaptation of the organism to severe hyperparathyroidism. In other words, the permissive influence of vitamin D on the bone-resorbing action of PTH has been largely removed by the final destruction of the kidneys, and the devastating effects of enormously high concentrations of circulating PTH have been naturally averted. Thus, it is probably important to delay the introduction of vitamin D or one of its biologically active metabolites or analogs until the hyperparathyroidism has been partially brought under control. This can be done in almost all dialyzed patients by restoring serum calcium and phosphorus to normal levels by the simple manipulation of dietary and dialysate calcium and dietary phosphate described above. Serum phosphate should be reduced to less than 5 mg/dL before attempts to increase serum calcium are made; this prevents increases in the calcium × phosphate product greater than 70 and the tendency to soft tissue calcifications. The regimen is most easily initiated in the hospital and should take no longer than 1 week. After serum iPTH begins to decrease, some form of vitamin D therapy may be introduced. The most effective form of vitamin D therapy has not yet been determined. A combination of metabolites may be necessary to restore both intestinal calcium absorption and bone formation processes to normal. Currently, dihydrotachysterol (0.125 mg twice weekly to 1 mg daily) is used extensively and is probably the drug of choice. Equivalent doses of ergocalciferol or any of the available vitamin D metabolites (Table 8–2) may also be used.

C. Management of Patients on Dialysis: Stage I and II Renal Osteodystrophy: When stage I and II patients who are treated as described in the previous section reach the end stage of renal failure and it becomes necessary for them to begin a hemodialysis program, they will have only minor hyperparathyroidism and renal osteodystrophy. These patients should present few problems in continuing prophylaxis. Since a PTH-induced increase in release of phosphate from bone into the circulation has been at least partly averted, dietary phosphate need not be severely restricted, and the dose of phosphate-binding agent needed to maintain serum phosphorus in the normal range should be tolerated by the average patient. Although these patients may require only supplements of vitamin D_2 (ergocalciferol) to avoid development of osteomalacia, one or more active vitamin D metabolites is occasionally necessary.

Dialysis patients with stage II renal osteodystrophy should respond to the treatment outlined for patients in stage II who are not on hemodialysis. The important consideration in patients on hemodialysis is to avoid aggravating negative calcium balance, which occurs when dialysate calcium concentrations are below 5.7 mg/dL. In fact, it is possible and probably desirable to use hemodialysis as a means of producing positive calcium balance by employing calcium concentrations of 6.5–8 mg/dL. However, this should not be attempted until serum phosphate concentrations are below 5 mg/dL, because extraosseous mineralization may be induced when the serum calcium × phosphate product is 70 or more. This therapeutic regimen is illustrated in Fig 8–25, where the reduction of plasma phosphate to 3 mg/dL combined with the gradual introduction of dialysate calcium concentrations of 8 mg/dL resulted in an increase in plasma calcium from 8 to 10 mg/dL and a concomitant and permanent decrease in plasma iPTH from values up to 20 times normal to values just above the upper limits of normal within a period of 2.5 months. Once abnormal mineral metabolism is brought under control, dialysate calcium concentrations should be reduced to about 6.5 mg/dL.

D. Management of Stage III and IV Renal Osteodystrophy: Stage III disease can be identified by the presence of hyperphosphatemia and eucalcemia with serum iPTH values (as measured by mid- or carboxy-region assay) from 50 to 100 times normal levels; in stage IV disease, there is hypercalcemia with elevations of serum iPTH to 200–1000 times normal levels. Whether patients with stage III or IV disease should be treated with the regimen illustrated in Fig 8–25 is controversial. It is clear that with heroic effort, it can be successfully applied to these patients. Fig 8–26 shows improvement in bone disease in one such patient. Ordinarily, patients with stage III or IV renal osteodystrophy should probably be treated initially

with subtotal parathyroidectomy in order to decrease the size of the parathyroid gland mass, followed by the regimen described for patients with stage II renal osteodystrophy. This rather radical approach is justified because mineral complications and persistence of hyperparathyroidism after renal transplantation are less severe in patients whose hyperparathyroidism and osteodystrophy were well controlled before transplantation. It generally takes much longer to bring stage III and stage IV patients under control, and success is less common than in patients with stage II disease. Therefore, considering the unpredictable availability of donor kidneys for transplantation and the probable desirability of having hyperparathyroidism and renal osteodystrophy under control prior to transplantation, it is important to decide as soon as possible whether patients have stage III or stage IV renal osteodystrophy. When in doubt, the clinician should institute an intensive regimen of medical treatment, and if marked improvement in hyperparathyroidism and osteodystrophy is not observed within 3–6 months, subtotal parathyroidectomy should be considered.

E. Renal Transplantation: Depending upon the stage of renal hyperparathyroidism and osteodystrophy, successful renal transplantation may reverse the entire course of these complications. Patients who receive transplants during stage I or II achieve normal levels of serum iPTH, calcium, and phosphorus within months. Patients who receive transplants during stage III or IV may never achieve normal levels of serum iPTH and often suffer from hypercalcemia and hypophosphatemia for years, even when the transplanted kidney is functioning normally. Ultimately, some patients in this latter group require subtotal parathyroidectomy, but the indications for the procedure in such patients are poorly defined.

Prognosis & Future Prospects

It is becoming clear that the outcome of the mineral and osseous complications of end-stage renal failure depends upon early recognition and treatment of these complications, particularly before hemodialysis is started. At present, it is uncertain whether such an approach will succeed in the long-term management of patients, because some elements of the prophylactic regimen described in this section may be unavailable or unacceptable to the patient. The most important of these is an oral phosphate-binding preparation that will be enthusiastically accepted by patients. Another is a reliable, inexpensive PTH radioimmunoassay, specific for the mid or carboxyl region of the molecule, for patient follow-up. Finally, the underlying cause of the newly described syndrome of low-turnover osteomalacia in patients with end-stage renal failure must be determined (see above). It is possible that this syndrome is related to the widespread use of phosphate-binding agents that contain aluminum; if so, its incidence will increase. This might mean that an entirely new approach to the treatment of renal osteodystrophy would have to be developed.

DISORDERS OF CALCITONIN (CT) SECRETION

No clinical disorder has been reported to date in which hypocalcitoninemia plays a definitive role. However, there are a number of conditions in which hypercalcitoninemia is found—most notably medullary carcinoma of the thyroid gland (see also Chapter 7).

MEDULLARY CARCINOMA OF THE THYROID GLAND

Medullary carcinoma is a malignant tumor of the parafollicular cells of the thyroid gland. It occurs sporadically but may also be inherited as an autosomal dominant trait as part of the type II multiple endocrine neoplasia (MEN) syndrome. (See Chapters 7 and 25.) This syndrome includes medullary carcinoma of the thyroid gland and pheochromocytoma. There are 2 variants of the syndrome: type IIa and type IIb. Patients with MEN type IIa have a normal appearance but a high incidence of hyperparathyroidism, most frequently due to enlargement of multiple parathyroid glands. Patients with MEN type IIb have a striking appearance due to labial and mucosal ganglioneuromas, a marfanoid habitus, and other somatic abnormalities. Hyperparathyroidism is unusual in this variant.

Incidence

Medullary carcinoma constitutes 3.5–10% of all thyroid cancers. The sex incidence is almost equal (male:female ratio of 1.3:1 in sporadic cases and 1:1 in familial cases). In general, familial cases present at a younger age than do sporadic ones.

Pathology

Medullary carcinoma appears as a solid, often hard mass confined to but not encapsulated in the thyroid gland. It is often unilateral in sporadic cases and bilateral in familial cases. The lesion is composed of sheets of cells with granular cytoplasms and usually contains irregular masses of amyloid and fibrous tissue. Most patients who present with a thyroid mass already have metastases to cervical lymph nodes. Some masses spread to the upper mediastinum. Metastases beyond the mediastinum, usually delayed until late in the natural history of the disease, most commonly occur in lungs, liver, bones, and adrenal glands.

Pathophysiology

Medullary carcinomas secrete large quantities of CT and respond to provocative stimuli such as intravenous pentagastrin or hypercalcemia induced by intravenous calcium. Although CT produces hypocalcemia and hypophosphatemia in experimental animals, these biochemical findings are unusual in patients with medullary carcinoma in spite of extremely high levels of immunoreactive calcitonin (iCT). This paradox is probably due to a combination of factors, including homologous desensitization of tissues that normally respond to the actions of CT.

Medullary carcinomas may secrete many other bioactive substances in addition to CT, each with the potential of causing symptoms. These include biogenic amines, ACTH and corticotropin-releasing hormone, prostaglandins, nerve growth factor, and possibly a PRL-releasing hormone. Diarrhea is present in about 20% of patients. This symptom relents after surgical excision of the tumor and is therefore thought to be humorally mediated. Cushing's syndrome is present in about 5% of cases, secondary to secretion of excessive ACTH.

Clinical Features

Most patients with sporadic medullary carcinoma present with an asymptomatic thyroid mass. Patients with MEN type IIb may complain of neuromas and their marfanoid appearance. Hypercalcemia may be detected in the course of routine blood screening in patients with MEN type IIa with primary hyperparathyroidism. Most importantly, hypertension in patients with MEN type IIa or IIb may reflect the presence of pheochromocytoma, which may be more life-threatening than medullary carcinoma.

Paraneoplastic syndromes (eg, Cushing's syndrome) as well as intractable diarrhea and flushing should alert the physician to the possible existence of medullary carcinoma. A family history of more than one case of thyroid cancer should certainly raise a suspicion of MEN type IIa in a patient with bizarre symptoms.

Other neural manifestations of MEN type IIb include medullated nerves in the cornea on slit lamp examination of the eye and ganglioneuromas of the gastrointestinal tract. The latter may cause gastrointestinal obstruction as well as megacolon.

Medullary cancers occasionally calcify. Thus, the discovery of a calcified thyroidal mass does not indicate that it is benign; rather, this is probably an indication for measurement of serum iCT (see below).

Diagnosis

The cornerstone of the laboratory investigation of patients suspected of having medullary carcinoma is radioimmunoassay of plasma CT. Although not absolutely specific for the tumor (see below), increased serum levels of iCT in patients with a thyroid mass, a family history of medullary carcinoma, or pheochromocytoma virtually establish the diagnosis. Other conditions in which increased levels of serum iCT have been reported include (1) ectopic secretion by almost any malignant tumor (especially small cell carcinoma of the lung), (2) chronic renal failure, (3) gastrointestinal disorders such as endocrine tumors of the pancreas and pernicious anemia, (4) subacute Hashimoto's thyroiditis, and (5) pregnancy.

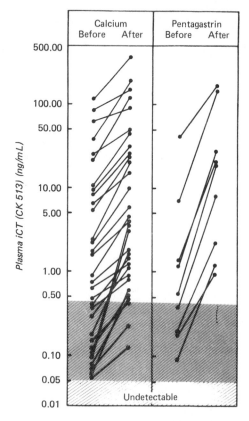

Figure 8–27. Maximal plasma iCT concentrations measured with antiserum CK 513 in patients with histologically proved medullary thyroid carcinoma or C cell hyperplasia before and after administration of calcium (left panel) or pentagastrin (right panel). The upper limit of stimulated plasma iCT concentrations in normal persons (shaded areas) is 0.42 ng/mL. (Reproduced, with permission, from Sizemore GW et al: *Surg Clin North Am* 1977;**57**:633.)

The diagnostic accuracy of CT radioimmunoassay is greatly enhanced when combined with provocative tests. As many as 30% of members of a family with MEN type IIa or IIb who harbor small medullary carcinomas will have normal basal levels of plasma iCT. Their neoplastic disease can only be detected by provocative tests with intravenous administration of pentagastrin, 0.5 mg over 5– 10 seconds, or calcium chloride, 150 mg over 10 minutes (Fig 8– 27). Plasma iCT increases abnormally in most cases within 2– 5 minutes. The CT radioimmunoassay used should be sensitive enough to measure plasma iCT in the normal range. Otherwise, the assay is unlikely to detect relatively small increases above the stimulated normal range, thus making the test impossible to interpret.

To rule out familial medullary carcinoma, iCT should be measured during a provocative test in all available first-degree relatives of patients with medullary carcinoma, regardless of the family history. In a few affected patients with minimal parafollicular cell disease, false-negative results may be obtained

with any of the tests mentioned. Provocative tests should therefore be performed annually in first-degree relatives who have had negative tests. About half of the members of a given family in which one member has MEN type IIa or IIb eventually develop medullary cancer. Early detection will permit definitive surgical treatment.

Treatment

In patients with medullary carcinoma, pheochromocytoma must be excluded or treated first. Medullary carcinoma is then treated by total thyroidectomy. Total thyroidectomy is especially important in patients with MEN type IIa or IIb, because medullary carcinoma is almost always bilateral and polycentric. Lymph nodes in the midline compartment should be removed and those in both internal jugular chains sampled. If jugular lymph nodes are involved, modified neck dissection should be performed. Postoperatively, all patients should be studied with provocative tests to determine if residual tumor is present. They should also be given thyroid hormone replacement. The overall prevalence of residual or metastatic medullary cancer after such surgery is about 35%. Most of these patients are older and have had regional metastases at the time of surgery. Long-term follow-up with provocative tests every year is advised for all patients. Although it is usually difficult to determine the location of metastases that are responsible for a positive test, local recurrences can be suspected and dealt with surgically. There is no known effective chemotherapeutic, radiopharmaceutical, or radiation treatment of medullary carcinoma.

Prognosis

Patients with sporadic medullary carcinoma have the least favorable prognosis because metastases are usually present at the time of diagnosis; only 46% of these patients survive for 10 years. Patients with MEN type IIa appear to fare better, with few deaths reported. Conversely, in a Mayo Clinic series of 107 patients with MEN type IIb, 67% have had residual disease after surgery and 18% died of medullary cancer. The reasons for the apparent difference in prognosis between MEN type IIa and MEN type IIb are unknown.

HYPERCALCIURIA

Hypercalciuria is usually detected in the course of evaluation of a patient with renal stone disease. It is variably defined as excretion of more than 300 mg of calcium per 24 hours in men and 250 mg per 24 hours in women. Urinary calcium excretion depends on many factors, but the most important is dietary intake of calcium. It is the *concentration* of calcium in the urine that determines whether calcium will interact with anionic constituents (particularly oxalate) of the urine to form stones. Thus, prevention of calcium-containing stones requires reduction in urinary concentrations of calcium and oxalate. It has recently been shown that increased excretion of uric acid in the urine is not only responsible for the formation of uric acid stones but may also be important in the formation of calcium oxalate stones. This means that the clinician should pay careful attention to uric acid excretion in patients with calcium oxalate stones and should attempt to reduce it if it is elevated.

The present section will concentrate on evaluation of the metabolic causes of hypercalciuria and calcium-containing stones, with the exception of infection, medullary sponge kidney, and renal tubular acidosis. The reader should consult the references at the end of this chapter for excellent reviews on cystine, uric acid, and magnesium ammonium phosphate stones.

Epidemiologic Considerations

Hypercalciuria appears to be common in the general population, but there is little accurate information about its incidence. The true incidence of stone disease is also unknown, although it is likely that 1–3% of people in most industrialized countries have had or will have a renal stone. Geography, race, and occupation probably have some influence on the incidence of stone disease, but the underlying factors are poorly understood. The frequency of calcium phosphate stones is equal in men and women. They occur in patients with sterile alkaline urines—ie, in cases of renal tubular acidosis, protracted use of carbonic anhydrase inhibitors, or primary hyperparathyroidism. Calcium oxalate stones occur more frequently in men (3–8:1) and in patients with idiopathic hypercalciuria.

Biochemical Characteristics of Calcium Stones

The most common anionic constituent of calcium-containing stones is oxalate. Calcium phosphate is also often present (mixed stones). Urinary saturation with calcium phosphate or calcium oxalate correlates roughly with the stone content of either anion. Hypercalciuria is observed in patients who make either mixed or unmixed stones, regardless of whether urinary calcium excretion is expressed as concentration, quantity per unit of time, or as the ratio of calcium to creatinine. Oxalate excretion is increased in patients who form calcium oxalate stones, and urinary pH is increased in those who form mixed stones.

Pathogenesis of Hypercalciuria

The reader is again referred to the "butterfly" diagram (Fig 8–2) while studying the pathogenetic concepts discussed below.

A. Hypercalcemia: In the presence of a normal rate of renal glomerular filtration, hypercalcemia due to any cause (see section on primary hyperparathyroidism), if sufficiently severe, results in hypercalciuria. One exception is benign familial hypercalcemia (familial hypocalciuric hypercalcemia), in which hypocalciuria is the biochemical hallmark of the disease.

Another is mild hyperparathyroidism, in which urinary calcium may be normal in spite of hypercalcemia because of the hypocalciuric effects of excess PTH. However, even in such cases of hyperparathyroidism, calcium stones are common and may be due to the presence of other risk factors, such as hyperoxaluria, hyperuricosuria, and increased urine pH. For the most part, renal stone disease occurs primarily in patients who have had chronic hypercalcemia. In fact, this historical information is sometimes important in making the differential diagnosis of hypercalcemia (Table 8–3). Hypercalcemia in patients with documented stone disease is much more likely to be due to primary hyperparathyroidism than to cancer.

B. Diet: High dietary intake of protein causes both increased intestinal absorption and increased urinary excretion of calcium. These effects are poorly understood, but evidence indicates that dietary protein has a greater influence than dietary calcium on urinary calcium when calcium intake is in the range of 800–1400 mg/d. Urolithiasis has been reported in patients who have inordinately high protein intakes.

Increased dietary carbohydrate increases urinary calcium excretion at least in part because it increases the glomerular filtration rate. The calciuric response to a carbohydrate load is greater in stone-formers and their relatives than in normal subjects, but there is no difference between these groups in fractional urinary calcium excretion.

Lactose ingestion also increases urinary excretion of calcium, but lactose appears to act primarily by facilitating intestinal absorption of calcium. Lactose is known to be highly lithogenic in animals, and milk restriction may be important in the management of some patients with calcium stones (see below).

Urinary calcium increases in parallel with dietary intake of elemental calcium. It is presumed that much of the absorbed calcium is transferred from intestine to blood by a passive transport process, because with a high calcium intake, the hormonal mechanisms that regulate active calcium transport across the intestine adapt to decrease active transport (Fig 8–2). Therefore, decreasing the dietary intake of calcium in patients with hypercalciuric stone disease would seem to be appropriate. However, the situation is not so simple. Although calcium restriction reduces urinary calcium excretion, it also increases intestinal absorption and renal excretion of oxalate and, in the long term, results in secondary hyperparathyroidism. Increased calcium intake, on the other hand, decreases intestinal absorption and renal excretion of oxalate by inducing calcium oxalate precipitation in the gut while increasing urinary calcium. Therefore, either of these dietary manipulations could aggravate calcium stone disease in hypercalciuric patients, and the authors cannot recommend them. Instead, a nutritionally adequate intake of calcium (600–800 mg/d) should be maintained in most patients and pharmacologic agents used (see treatment section below) to lower urinary calcium excretion.

C. Intestinal Hyperabsorption of Calcium: Most

patients with hypercalciuria that is unrelated to chronic states of hypercalcemia, drugs, or diet absorb too much calcium. Many of these patients have decreased serum levels of iPTH and decreased nephrogenous cAMP, presumably reflecting decreased PTH secretion caused by small increases in serum calcium within the normal range. In general, serum phosphorus is below the normal mean; and in one-third of patients, serum levels of $1,25(OH)_2D_3$ are increased. Clearly, in these latter patients, the normal adaptive decrease in $1,25(OH)_2D_3$ production in response to hyperabsorption of calcium and decreased levels of serum PTH fails to occur. It has been suggested that hypophosphatemia due to a renal phosphate leak is responsible (see intestinal loop of Fig 8–2). In this pathogenetic scheme, the renal phosphate leak is postulated to be the primary defect, and hyperabsorption of calcium and hypercalciuria are secondary to the effects of increased serum levels of $1,25(OH)_2D_3$.

The cause of intestinal hyperabsorption of calcium in the remaining two-thirds of patients with hypercalciuria, whose serum concentrations of $1,25(OH)_2D_3$ are normal or low, is unknown. It is possible that endocrine abnormalities not yet identified may be present. On the other hand, these patients may represent a group whose hyperabsorption of calcium is due to an intrinsic defect in the intestine, in which greater than normal quantities of calcium are transported from intestinal lumen to blood.

D. "Renal Leak" of Calcium: It is generally agreed that few patients with hypercalciuria have a true "renal calcium leak." It is possible, however, that some patients with intestinal hyperabsorption of calcium also have a renal tubule defect that permits excessive urinary excretion of calcium. Patients whose hypercalciuria is due solely to a renal leak of calcium have serum concentrations of calcium in the lower range of normal; this results in small increases in serum levels of PTH, which increase bone resorption and the production of $1,25(OH)_2D_3$. The resulting increase in serum levels of $1,25(OH)_2D_3$ causes intestinal hyperabsorption of calcium and produces pathophysiologic changes that superficially resemble hypercalciuria due to "primary" intestinal hyperabsorption of calcium. Thus, only the increased levels of serum iPTH and increased nephrogenous cAMP distinguish patients with hypercalciuria due to renal calcium leak from those with hypercalciuria due to intestinal hyperabsorption of calcium. A sensitive radioimmunoassay of PTH (preferably of the mid or carboxyl region) that can measure serum iPTH in the normal range is required for these diagnostic criteria to be applied systematically. Severe, long-standing hypercalciuria may result in increased bone turnover and osteopenia.

Diagnosis

A. Measurement of Urine Calcium: The diagnosis of hypercalciuria is made by measuring the calcium excreted in the urine over a 24-hour period while the patient is ingesting a diet containing normal amounts of calcium (about 800–1000 mg/d). Values greater than 250 mg/24 h in women and 300 mg/24 h in men indicate the presence of hypercalciuria. Patients who present with renal stone disease should undergo a full evaluation, including measurement of the 24-hour urinary excretion of calcium, phosphate, creatinine, oxalate, and uric acid. If a renal stone is not available, patients should strain their urine. A biochemical and crystallographic analysis of the stone should be made so that the patient can be instructed in decreasing the urinary concentrations of the stone's constituents. Particular attention should be paid to excluding other metabolic disorders such as primary hyperparathyroidism, which may be primary or contributing factors. When nephrolithiasis is present, it is important to obtain baseline radiographic studies of the kidneys (intravenous urogram and nephrotomograms) to identify the number and size (diameter) of stones present. Similar follow-up studies will give an indication of the activity of the stone disease. (Growth of a stone or appearance of a new stone indicates that stone disease is active.) If a patient is in the inactive phase of nephrolithiasis, specific drug therapy is probably not indicated. If the patient is passing gravel, stone disease is active, and intensive therapy is indicated.

B. History: In seeking the underlying cause of hypercalciuria, a careful history, including diet and drug intake, is important. A history of an extremely high intake of protein, dairy products, or carbohydrates may account for hypercalciuria. Excessive self-medication with calcium-containing antacids, low-phosphate diets, or phosphate-binding antacids can also produce hypercalciuria. The mechanism involved in the latter 2 phenomena is poorly understood. Hypercalciuric patients who are vegetarians may be especially prone to the development of nephrolithiasis, because their diet may be high in oxalate-containing foods or inadequate in phosphate content.

C. Serum iPTH: Although a number of provocative tests of the calciuric and nephrogenous cAMP responses to ingested calcium have been described for distinguishing between intestinal hyperabsorption of calcium and renal leak of calcium, measurement of serum iPTH is the most helpful test available. As noted in the section on pathogenesis, increased serum iPTH in the presence of low normal serum calcium reflects the presence of a renal leak of calcium, whereas normal or decreased serum iPTH in conjunction with high normal serum calcium generally reflects hyperabsorption of calcium. Further study of patients with increased serum iPTH levels may be necessary to distinguish them from patients with primary hyperparathyroidism associated with a renal leak of calcium. For some reason, this latter syndrome occurs most frequently in women, and although unusual, it should be suspected whenever a woman presents with hypercalciuria, because removal of the parathyroid lesion is curative. In most cases, primary hyperparathyroidism can be excluded in patients with increased serum iPTH by determining if serum iPTH decreases during thiazide administration. As will be discussed in the treatment section, thiazide diuretics increase the tubular reabsorption of calcium and thereby increase serum calcium. If serum iPTH decreases with thiazide administration, hyperparathyroidism is probable and occurs secondary to a renal leak of calcium. If serum iPTH fails to decrease with thiazides, the patient probably has associated primary hyperparathyroidism.

Treatment

A. Hypercalciuria Without Nephrolithiasis: Specific drug therapy (see below) should probably be avoided in patients with hypercalciuria without nephrolithiasis. Excessive intake of protein, carbohydrates, dairy products, antacids, and low-phosphate diets should be discontinued or curtailed. Patients should be instructed to avoid foods high in oxalate and to consume at least 2500–3000 mL of water per day.

B. Hypercalciuria With Nephrolithiasis: Surgical treatment of obstructive uropathy caused by nephrolithiasis is always indicated. Medical management is indicated for prevention of calcium stone disease.

1. Hypercalciuria–All of the therapeutic measures mentioned above should be used, except that water intake should be greater (4000 mL/d). The patient should be instructed to drink one or 2 glasses of water in the middle of the night because the concentration of urinary solutes is greatest then. If stones contain oxalate, the patient should be instructed in the preparation and planning of a low-oxalate diet. Some foods to be avoided are listed in Table 8–7.

2. Active nephrolithiasis–If nephrolithiasis is active (see above), one or more of 4 therapeutic agents should be used: (1) thiazide diuretics, (2) orthophosphate, (3) the xanthine oxidase inhibitor allopurinol, and (4) magnesium oxide and pyridoxine. Thiazide diuretics and orthophosphate have been reported to reduce the rate of stone recurrence. Thiazide diuretics decrease hypercalciuria by increasing the tubular reabsorption of calcium. Medication should be given at 12-hour intervals—eg, 50 mg of hydrochlorothiazide, twice daily. The only significant complications of thiazide therapy are potassium depletion and annoying polyuria; potassium supplements of 20–40 meq/d should be administered to most patients. Oral supplements of orthophosphate decrease urinary calcium by an unknown mechanism. One to 1.5 g of elemental phosphorus should be administered in 3 divided doses daily as neutral phosphate compounds (eg, K-Phos Neutral, 4–6 tablets/d). Few side effects other than

Table 8–7. High-oxalate foods.

Vegetables	Fruits	Miscellaneous
Asparagus	Concord grapes	Almonds
Beans	Cranberries	Cashews
Beets and beet greens	Currants	Cocoa
Brussels sprouts	Oranges	Tea
Potatoes	Pineapple	
Rhubarb	Plums	
Spinach	Strawberries	

occasional diarrhea have been reported with this therapy, and long-term studies have shown no significant changes in serum iPTH. Orthophosphate therapy is indicated only for patients with sterile urines, because it accelerates stone growth in individuals with ammonium phosphate stones caused by urea-splitting organisms. Magnesium oxide (200 mg/d) plus large doses of pyridoxine (100–150 mg/d) may be of value in the treatment of idiopathic calcium oxalate stones, but systematic studies of the efficacy of this regimen have been meager.

3. Uric acid excretion–Finally, it is clear that many patients with calcium oxalate stones excrete abnormally large quantities of uric acid. Treatment of these patients with allopurinol (100–200 mg twice daily) reduces the urinary excretion of uric acid and the rate of stone formation when combined with thiazide diuretics. The mechanism of this action of allopurinol is unknown.

METABOLIC BONE DISEASE

Functions of Bone

Bone has 3 major functions: (1) It provides rigid support to extremities and body cavities containing vital organs. In disease situations in which bone is weak or defective, erect posture may be impossible, and vital organ function may be compromised. (An example is the cardiopulmonary dysfunction that occurs in patients with severe kyphosis due to vertebral collapse.) (2) Aside from rigid support, bones are crucial to locomotion in that they provide efficient levers and sites of attachment for muscles. With bony deformity, these levers become defective, and severe abnormalities of gait develop. (3) Finally, as has been discussed in previous sections of this chapter, bone provides a large reservoir of ions, such as calcium, phosphorus, magnesium, and sodium, that are critical for life and can be mobilized when the external environment fails to provide them.

Structure of Bone

As a living tissue, bone is unique in that it is not only rigid and resists forces that would ordinarily break brittle materials but is also light enough to be moved by coordinated muscle contractions. These characteristics are functions of the strategic locations of 2 major types of bone (Fig 8–28). Cortical bone, composed of densely packed, mineralized collagen laid down in layers, provides rigidity and is the major component of tubular bones. Trabecular (cancellous) bone is spongy in appearance, provides strength and elasticity, and constitutes the major portion of the axial skeleton. Disorders in which cortical bone is defective or scanty lead to fractures of the long bones, whereas disorders in which trabecular bone is defective or scanty lead to vertebral fractures. Fractures of long bones may also occur because normal trabecular bone reinforcement is lacking.

Two-thirds of the weight of bone is due to mineral; the remainder is due to water and collagen. Minor organic components such as proteoglycans, lipids, noncollagenous proteins, and acidic proteins containing γ-carboxyglutamic acid are probably important, but their functions are poorly understood.

A. Bone Mineral: The mineral of bone is present in 2 forms. The major form consists of hydroxyapatite in crystals of varying maturity. The remainder is amorphous calcium phosphate, which lacks a coherent x-ray diffraction pattern, has a lower calcium-to-phosphate ratio than pure hydroxyapatite, occurs in regions of active bone formation, and is present in larger quantities in young bone.

B. Formation and Resorption of Bone: Bone is resorbed and formed continuously throughout life, and these important processes are dependent upon 3 major types of bone cells, each with different functions.

1. Osteoblasts–Osteoblasts form new bone on surfaces of bone previously resorbed by osteoclasts. The osteoblasts are thought to be derived from a population of dividing cells on bone surfaces that arise from mesenchymal cells in bone connective tissue. Osteoblasts are actively involved in the synthesis of matrix components of bone (primarily collagen) and probably facilitate the movement of mineral ions between extracellular fluids and bone surfaces (Figs 8–3 and 8–4). The physiologic importance of such ion transport by osteoblasts—if it occurs at all—is controversial, but there is widespread agreement that osteoblast-mediated transport of calcium and phosphate is involved in the mineralization of collagen, which in turn is crucial to the formation of bone. In the process of bone formation, osteoblasts gradually become encased in the bone matrix they have produced.

2. Osteocytes–Once osteoblasts are trapped in the mineralized matrix, their functional and morphologic characteristics are changed and they are then called osteocytes. Protein synthetic activity decreases markedly, and the cells develop multiple processes that reach out through lacunae in bone tissue to "communicate" with processes of other osteocytes within a unit of bone (osteon) and also with the cell processes of surface osteoblasts (Fig 8–4). The physiologic importance of osteocytes is controversial, but they are believed to act as a cellular syncytium that permits translocation of mineral in and out of regions of bone removed from surfaces.

3. Osteoclasts–The osteoclast is a multinucleated giant cell that is responsible for bone resorption (Fig 8–4). It is probably derived from circulating mononucleated macrophages, which differentiate into the mature osteoclasts by fusion in the bone environment. These cells contain all of the enzymatic components that, when secreted into their environs, are capable of solubilizing matrix and releasing calcium and phosphate. Once released, mineral is transported through the osteoclast into the extracellular fluid and ultimately into blood. Opinion has varied over the years concerning the relative importance of osteoclastic resorption of bone and the translocation of mineral from the surface of bone into the extracellular space by surface osteoblasts in extracellular mineral homeostasis.

C. Structural Features of Bone: Microscopically, there are 2 types of bone structure: woven and lamellar. Both may be found in either cortical or trabecular bone. However, whereas woven bone is a normal constituent of embryonic bone, it usually reflects the presence of disease in adult bone.

Lamellar bone is stronger than woven bone and is formed more slowly. It progressively replaces woven bone as the skeleton develops after birth. Whereas woven bone is characterized by nonparallelism of collagen fibers, with many osteocytes per unit area of matrix and mineral that is poorly incorporated into collagen fibrils, lamellar bone has a parallel arrangement of collagen fibers, few osteocytes per unit area of matrix, and a mineral phase that is within the collagen fibrils. Cortical lamellar bone is present in concentric layers surrounding vascular channels that comprise the haversian systems of cortical bone (osteons) (Fig 8–28). By contrast, the lamellar bone of trabeculae is present in layers and is laid down in long sheaves and sheets.

Dynamics of Bone

The term "modeling" as applied to bone denotes processes involved in formation of the macroscopic skeleton. Thus, modeling ceases at maturity (age 18–20). The term "remodeling" denotes those processes occurring at bone surfaces before and after adult development which are required to maintain the structural integrity of bone. Abnormalities of remodeling are responsible for metabolic bone diseases, and these will be discussed in this section. These abnormalities involve alterations in the balance between bone formation and bone resorption that lead to diminished structural integrity of bone and ultimately compromise its functions.

Normally, in spite of continuous bone remodeling, there is no net gain or loss of skeletal mass after longitudinal growth has ceased. This has led to the view that bone resorption and formation are closely "coupled" and that this coupling is the result of the coordinated activity of "packets" of interacting osteoblasts and osteoclasts. These "packets" have been termed "basic multicellular units." The temporal activity of such a unit is characterized by osteoclastic resorption of a defined quantity of bone (on the surface in trabecular bone and by actual excavation in cortical bone), followed by repair of the defect by osteoblasts. Such repair occurs as a result of laying down of collagen (osteoid) and its subsequent mineralization.

By use of sequential, timed labeling of bone with orally administered tetracycline (which binds to recently mineralized collagen) and quantitative histomorphometric analysis of transiliac bone biopsies from

Cortical (compact) bone

Figure 8–28. Diagram of some of the main features of the microstructure of mature bone seen in both transverse section *(top)* and longitudinal section. Areas of cortical (compact) and trabecular (cancellous) bone are included. The central area in the transverse section simulates a microradiograph, with the variations in density reflecting variations in mineralization. Note the general construction of the osteons, the distribution of the osteocyte lacunae, the haversian canals, resorption spaces, and the different views of the structural basis of bone lamellation. See text for description. (Reproduced, with permission, from page 217 in: *Gray's Anatomy.* 35th ed. Warwick R, Williams PL [editor]. Longman, 1973.)

normal adult humans, it has been possible to time the activities of a basic multicellular unit. Such estimates indicate that osteoclastic resorption proceeds for about 1 month in a normal 30-year-old adult, and osteo-blastic repair takes about 3 months.

The term "sigma" denotes the total duration of activity of a typical basic multicellular unit (ie, 4 months). This concept of "sigma" has added a new

dimension to conventional views about the pathogen-esis of metabolic bone disease. Thus, not only might alterations in the relative numbers and activities of osteoblasts and osteoclasts be important in production of an imbalance of bone formation and bone resorp-tion, but abnormalities in the relative durations of activities of these 2 cell types could underly such an imbalance.

Analysis of Bone Biopsy

Presently, quantitative histomorphometric analysis of transiliac bone biopsies has achieved almost the status of a fine art. The procedure is employed in centers established to evaluate metabolic bone disease from both diagnostic and therapeutic points of view. The procedure is most useful (1) in establishing a diagnosis of osteomalacia (see below) and (2) in determining if, in a given patient, diminished bone density is associated with quantitatively significant changes in "sigma" and its bone formation and bone resorption components.

OSTEOMALACIA

Osteomalacia is failure of the organic matrix (osteoid) of bone to mineralize normally. Rickets, which will be only briefly discussed in this chapter, is failure of normal mineralization and maturation of the growth plate at the epiphysis in children.

Etiology & Incidence

A number of factors are critical for normal bone mineralization. An absence or defect of any of them may lead to osteomalacia. The most frequent underlying biochemical causes of mineralization defects—individually or in combination—are a decrease in the product of the concentrations of calcium and phosphate in the extracellular fluid such that the supply of minerals to bone-forming surfaces is inadequate; abnormal functioning of bone-forming cells; abnormal or defective collagen production; and a decrease in the pH below 7.6 at sites of mineralization.

Table 8–8 lists the major disorders that can lead to osteomalacia, including those due to vitamin D deficiency, phosphate deficiency, systemic acidosis, drug toxicity, and primary defects of bone. Because of the vague symptomatology of osteomalacia (see below), the disease is often not suspected and is probably much more common than is usually thought.

A. Vitamin D Deficiency: Whereas it was formerly thought that vitamin D deficiency due to inadequate sunlight exposure rarely caused osteomalacia, certain social and environmental developments have almost certainly led to an increased incidence of this problem. This is particularly true in the case of the elderly, who are frequently institutionalized or stay indoors at home and fail to receive either adequate sunlight exposure or dietary supplements of vitamin D.

Although the facts are difficult to document, industrialization without adequate smog control will almost certainly result in an increased incidence of osteomalacia and rickets by filtering out the ultraviolet wavelengths of light from the atmosphere. This can be prevented by systematic supplementation with vitamin D.

With the increase in world population, extreme northern and southern latitudes could become more populated. People living there would be susceptible

Table 8–8. Etiology of osteomalacia.

Vitamin D deficiency
  Inadequate sunlight exposure without dietary supplementation.
    House- or institution-bound people.
    Atmospheric smog.
    Long-term residence in far northern and far southern latitudes.
    Excessive covering of body with clothing.
  Gastrointestinal disease that interrupts the normal enterohepatic recycling of vitamin D and its metabolites, resulting in their fecal loss.
    Chronic steatorrhea (pancreatic).
    Malabsorption (gluten-sensitive enteropathy).
    Surgical resection of large parts of intestine.
    Formation of biliary fistulas.
  Impaired synthesis of $1,25(OH)_2 D_3$ by the kidney.
    Nephron loss, as occurs in chronic kidney disease (see section on renal hyperparathyroidism).
    Functional impairment of $1,25(OH)_2 D_3$ hydroxylase (eg, in hypoparathyroidism).
    Congenital absence of $1,25(OH)_2 D_3$ hydroxylase (vitamin D–dependency rickets type I).
    Suppression of $1,25(OH)_2 D_3$ production by endogenously produced substances (cancer).
  Target cell resistance to $1,25(OH)_2 D_3$—eg, absent or diminished number of $1,25(OH)_2 D_3$ receptors, as in vitamin D–dependency rickets type II.

Phosphate deficiency
  Dietary.
    Low intake of phosphate.
    Excessive ingestion of aluminum hydroxide.
  Impaired renal tubular reabsorption of phosphate.
    X-linked hypophosphatemia.
    Adult-onset hypophosphatemia.
    Other acquired and hereditary renal tubular disorders associated with renal phosphate loss (Fanconi's syndrome, Wilson's disease).
    Tumor-associated hypophosphatemia.

Systemic acidosis
  Chronic renal failure.
  Distal renal tubular acidosis.
  Ureterosigmoidoscopy.
  Chronic acetazolamide and ammonium chloride administration.

Drug-induced osteomalacia
  Excessive diphosphonate administration.
  Excessive fluoride administration.
  Anticonvulsant administration.

Toxin-induced osteomalacia
  Aluminum.
  Lead.
  Cadmium.

Primary mineralization defects
  Hypophosphatasia.
  Osteopetrosis.
  Fibrogenesis imperfecta ossium.

to osteomalacia and rickets because of the diminished amount of ultraviolet irradiation.

In people who habitually cover their bodies with excessive clothing, the migration from areas of intense ultraviolet exposure to areas of marginal ultraviolet exposure can lead to the development of osteomalacia and rickets. This phenomenon has been reported in Great Britain in immigrants from India, Pakistan, and other Commonwealth countries since the 1950s.

1. Malabsorption–One of the most common causes of osteomalacia due to vitamin D deficiency is gastrointestinal disease associated with malabsorption of vitamin D and calcium. This is particularly true of disorders in which the enterohepatic circulation of vitamin D is interrupted. The biologically active metabolites of vitamin D that are normally secreted into the bile are either diverted (biliary fistula) or not reabsorbed (chronic steatorrhea, gluten-sensitive enteropathy, surgical resection of large parts of the distal jejunum and ileum). In these situations, not only is exogenous vitamin D poorly absorbed, but the body's stores of vitamin D and its metabolites that originate from skin biosynthesis are also depleted by biliary or fecal loss.

2. Impaired renal synthesis–As noted in previous sections, impaired synthesis of $1,25(OH)_2D_3$ by the kidney can lead to osteomalacia. This can occur in chronic kidney disease, in which there is extensive nephron loss, or when other conditions are unfavorable for the synthesis of $1,25(OH)_2D_3$, such as in hypoparathyroidism when serum phosphate is increased (Fig 8–2).

3. Genetic defects–Two recessively inherited vitamin D deficiency states associated with rickets and osteomalacia are characterized by resistance to treatment with large doses of vitamin D. In one, vitamin D–dependency rickets type I, serum concentrations of $1,25(OH)_2D_3$ are very low. This disease is thought to be due to a defect in $1,25(OH)_2D_3$ hydroxylase in the kidney. In the other, vitamin D–dependency rickets type II, serum concentrations of $1,25(OH)_2D_3$ are high. This disease is thought to be due to target cell resistance to the action of $1,25(OH)_2D_3$. Patients have been described recently whose cultured skin fibroblasts are deficient in receptors for $1,25(OH)_2D_3$.

4. Oncogenic disease–Osteomalacic syndromes have been associated with certain tumors. Although proof is not yet available, it is thought that the underlying cause of the bone disease is a humoral substance secreted by the tumor that suppresses the synthesis of $1,25(OH)_2D_3$.

B. Lowering of Phosphorus: Any sustained lowering of serum phosphorus will ultimately result in rickets and osteomalacia. Phosphate deficiency can occur as a result of failure of intestinal absorption of phosphate (dietary lack or sequestering of phosphate in the intestine by binding of the mineral to aluminum hydroxide in antacids) or excessive renal excretion of phosphate. Vegetarians who do not include dairy products in their diets are particularly susceptible to phosphate deficiency, as are elderly or debilitated individuals who are fed a diet low in phosphate. Although it is likely that only excessive use of phosphate-binding antacids will result in a deficiency in phosphate severe enough to produce osteomalacia, the potential for this disorder is great

because these drugs are widely available.

The classic example of rickets and osteomalacia due to renal phosphate wasting is the heritable disease X-linked hypophosphatemia, in which a renal phosphate transport defect is manifest. Similar renal phosphate wasting and osteomalacia occur in many patients with Fanconi's syndrome and in patients with adult-onset hypophosphatemia.

Severe phosphate wasting is occasionally associated with benign or malignant lesions, such as sclerosing hemangiomas, angiosarcomas, hemangiopericytomas, and nonossifying fibromas. Some of these involve bone and others soft tissues. Surgical removal of these lesions almost always restores serum phosphate and urinary phosphate excretion to normal and heals the osteomalacia, suggesting that the tumors secrete a humoral substance that either promotes phosphaturia or interferes with vitamin D metabolism.

Aside from chronic renal failure, the disorders listed in Table 8–8 that cause systemic acidosis and osteomalacia are uncommon. The evidence that they produce osteomalacia on the basis of systemic acidosis per se is based only on therapeutic responses achieved when blood pH is restored to normal with bicarbonate therapy. Thus, it is possible that the acidosis acts indirectly, by inducing other systemic abnormalities that then produce osteomalacia.

The mechanisms involved in the development of osteomalacia due to drugs and the primary mineralization defects listed in Table 8–8 are largely unknown.

Pathology

There is little (if anything) unusual about the gross characteristics of the bones of patients with osteomalacia, except perhaps that they are easier to biopsy because they are soft. Histomorphometrically, however, there are major deviations from normal, primarily related to the thickness and surface coverage of unmineralized osteoid and the degree of mineralization of osteoid. Characteristically, the average thickness of osteoid exceeds 20 μm (normal, 15 $\pm$ 2.3 μm), and over 20% of the bone surface is covered by osteoid (normal, 2.1 $\pm$ 1%). The "calcification front" at the junction of mineralized bone and osteoid, which is normally marked intensely by tetracycline labels incorporated into bone prior to biopsy, is barely visible. These changes in the quantity of osteoid are due not to increased synthesis of collagen by bone-forming cells but rather to a failure in collagen mineralization. The rate of collagen synthesis may actually be decreased. Because the rate of mineralization is slowed, "sigma" (see above) is prolonged.

Pseudofractures, which are characteristic of osteomalacia, are defects in cortical bone that are bordered by osteoid-encased lamellar bone, with interspersed areas of variably mineralized woven bone.

Depending upon the stage of development of osteomalacia or rickets, bone resorption surfaces may be increased or decreased. After secondary hyperparathyroidism due to hypocalcemia has been established, increased osteoclastic resorption may be observed. Late in the course of development of the disease, when osteoid covers the greater portion of mineralized surfaces, little exposed mineral is available for osteoclastic attack, and bone resorption surfaces are decreased.

Pathophysiology

A. Vitamin D Deficiency: The most useful information about the pathogenesis of osteomalacia and rickets has been provided by studies of the natural history of these diseases. It has not been possible, because of ethical considerations, to conduct longitudinal investigations of the parameters of calcium metabolism in patients with rickets and osteomalacia. However, measurements of these parameters have been reported in individual patients suffering from rickets or osteomalacia of varying degrees of severity. Fig 8–29, which provides an idealized scheme of the results of these studies, depicts 3 stages of development of vitamin D–deficiency rickets or osteomalacia. These stages are characterized by unique changes in the serum concentrations of calcium, phosphate, iPTH, and 25OHD$_3$ and the severity of radiographically assessed bone lesions.

B. Stages of Osteomalacia: In the first stage of rickets or osteomalacia, there is mild hypocalcemia, appropriately increased serum iPTH, normal or slightly decreased serum phosphate, and decreased serum 25OHD$_3$, which is approximately half the

PROGRESSIVE DEPLETION OF 25OHD$_3$

Figure 8–29. Serum biochemical changes and severity of bone disease in the 3 stages of rickets or osteomalacia. See text for description. (Reproduced, with permission, from Arnaud SB et al: *Vitamin D and Problems in Uremic Bone Disease.* Walter de Gruyter, 1975.)

mean value for age-matched normal controls.

In the second stage, serum 25OHD$_3$ decreases slightly or not at all. The serum calcium concentration is restored to normal, but paradoxically, there is only a small decrease in serum iPTH. Hypophosphatemia and bone lesions worsen.

In the third stage, when florid rickets or osteomalacia becomes manifest, serum 25OHD$_3$ decreases to almost undetectable levels. Hypocalcemia again is apparent and is more severe than in stage I; the degree of hypophosphatemia is the same as for stage II; and serum iPTH increases further and is again appropriate for the degree of hypocalcemia.

The underlying defect leading to these biochemical and osseous changes is the decrease in production of 1,25(OH)$_2$D$_3$, which is due to the diminished availability of the major circulating metabolite of vitamin D, 25OHD$_3$. As Fig 8–2 shows, decreased 1,25(OH)$_2$D$_3$ results in decreased intestinal calcium absorption, decreased bone resorption, hypocalcemia, increased PTH secretion, and hypophosphatemia (stage I). The resulting decreased calcium × phosphate product in serum is insufficient for the normal mineralization of bone, and the osteomalacic process is initiated. The increased PTH secretion and hypophosphatemia represent compensatory phenomena designed to correct the hypocalcemia, but they occur at the expense of osseous demineralization caused by hyperparathyroidism. As stage I shifts to stage II, the severity of the hyperparathyroidism restores serum calcium toward normal. This restoration probably depends upon increased production of 1,25(OH)$_2$D$_3$ from residual stores of 25OHD$_3$; this increased production is the result of the stimulation of renal 1α-hydroxylase by increased serum levels of PTH. The mechanism whereby increased PTH secretion is maintained in spite of normocalcemia in this stage is poorly understood. A negative feedback relationship between vitamin D metabolites and PTH secretion may exist, wherein normal levels of vitamin D metabolites are required for physiologic concentrations of serum calcium to suppress parathyroid gland activity. During the transition from stage II to stage III, vitamin D stores are depleted, and in spite of the hyperparathyroidism and hypophosphatemia, 1,25(OH)$_2$D$_3$ production stops because 25OHD$_3$, the substrate, is lacking. In stage III, hypocalcemia develops again and is worse than in stage I because of an even greater decrease in intestinal absorption of calcium. PTH secretion increases further in response to hypocalcemia; however, because vitamin D is required for PTH to resorb bone, this compensatory mechanism fails and hypocalcemia persists. In this stage, hypocalcemia and hypophosphatemia become so severe that the serum calcium × phosphate product is too low for normal bone formation, and florid osteomalacia or rickets becomes evident.

C. Phosphate Deficiency: The pathogenesis of the rickets or osteomalacia associated with phosphate deficiency is poorly understood but is presumed to be related to a decrease in the serum calcium × phosphate product below the level required for normal bone formation. Dietary phosphate deficiency is known to be associated with increases in serum concentrations of $1,25(OH)_2D_3$ and calcium and in urinary excretion of calcium. Serum concentrations of iPTH are appropriately decreased, and the PTH-induced demineralization of bone seen in vitamin D deficiency is not observed. Thus, as long as phosphate deficiency is not complicated by deficiencies in vitamin D or calcium, the biochemical changes seen in vitamin D deficiency, rickets, or osteomalacia do not occur.

D. Acidosis: The pathogenesis of the rickets and osteomalacia associated with acidosis is also poorly understood. Possible underlying causes include inhibition of mineralization due to a decrease in pH below 7.6 at calcification sites, acidosis-induced hypophosphatemia, and acidosis-induced resistance to the actions of vitamin D. In addition, the hypercalciuria often observed in acidosis may cause hyperparathyroidism, and the combined effects on bone of the excess PTH and negative calcium balance may be important in the ultimate bone disease associated with acidosis.

Clinical Features

A. Symptoms and Signs: The clinical manifestations of osteomalacia in adults often go unrecognized. This is especially true in patients with osteomalacia due to a vitamin D deficiency caused by disorders of the gastrointestinal tract, because the symptoms of the primary disorder are so prominent. Thus, diffuse skeletal pain and muscular weakness without a specific pattern may be overlooked, and the diagnosis of bone disease may not be suspected until roentgenograms reveal osteomalacia as an incidental finding.

There are few if any characteristic clinical signs of osteomalacia, except for deformities caused by

fractures in the ribs, vertebrae, and long bones. Such extensive disease is rare. Classically, patients with osteomalacia have a characteristic waddling gait that is due both to proximal muscular weakness and to pain and discomfort during movement of limbs. Some patients have severe muscular hypotonia and paradoxically brisk deep tendon reflexes. This latter finding is probably due to associated hypocalcemia. In contrast to hypoparathyroidism, osteomalacia is rarely associated with hypocalcemic tetanic manifestations. This difference is probably due to the presence of hyperphosphatemia and lower levels of serum ionized calcium in patients with hypoparathyroidism.

B. Laboratory Findings: The serum biochemistry of osteomalacia and rickets is described above. The values of serum calcium, phosphate, iPTH, and $25OHD_3$ clearly depend upon the stage of the disease at the time the patient is seen (Fig 8– 29). Generally, low levels of $25OHD_3$ indicate that osteomalacia is severe, but this is not always true. Increased serum alkaline phosphatase is characteristic. The cause of this abnormality is not well understood; it is probably related to increased but ineffective activity of osteoblasts.

C. X-Ray Findings: The radiologic features of osteomalacia also depend upon the stage of the disease and may be dramatic. There is usually some decrease in bone density. Cortices may be thinned, and roentgenograms of the vertebrae may reveal both loss of trabeculae and blurring of trabecular markings. In stage I and early stage II osteomalacia, radiologic changes may be indistinguishable from those seen in osteoporosis. The most characteristic finding in osteomalacia—and one that is almost pathognomonic—is the radiolucent band termed a **pseudofracture,** a defect in bone that is perpendicular to the bone surface (Fig 8– 30A and B). These bands, which may be present at multiple sites, are usually symmetric and

Figure 8–30. *A:* X-rays of the radius and ulna of a patient with severe osteomalacia, showing healing of a pseudofracture (arrows) during 7 months of treatment with ergocalciferol. *B:* X-ray of the pelvis, showing pseudofractures (Looser's zones, or Milkman's fractures) in a woman with severe osteomalacia. (Courtesy of G Gordan.)

bilateral; the characteristic locations include the inner aspects of the femur, the pubic rami, the outer edges of the scapulas, the upper fibula, and the metatarsals. Pseudofractures almost always occur where major arteries cross bones. It is thought that trauma due to arterial pulsation or other factors is responsible for their location and symmetry. Pseudofractures are also termed Looser's zones or Milkman's fractures, after the individuals who first described them.

Paradoxically, patients with untreated osteomalacia due to specific defects in renal tubular phosphate transport may show increased rather than decreased osseous density and even bony spurs on x-rays. However, such hyperostotic bone is abnormal. It fractures easily and consists of thickened cortices and trabeculae invested in large quantities of thickened osteoid. The cause of this hyperostosis is unknown.

Differential Diagnosis

Osteomalacia and rickets are usually suspected on the basis of the history or the presence of other disorders that frequently cause osteomalacia and rickets. Patients with muscular weakness and skeletal pain should be screened. Children with histories of irritability, poor growth and development, and convulsions should also be investigated. Patients who are taking drugs that have been associated with the development of osteomalacia (Table 8–8) are at risk for this disease and should be evaluated annually for hypocalcemia, hypophosphatemia, and hypocalciuria. Decreased urinary calcium is one of the earliest biochemical signs of osteomalacia and is probably due to increased PTH secretion secondary to mild hypocalcemia. Patients with chronic intestinal disease, particularly those with gluten-sensitive enteropathy or pancreatic insufficiency, should also be considered to have osteomalacia unless this is disproved. Nutritional deprivation and chronic deprivation of sunlight exposure also increase the risk of osteomalacia. Patients with a family history of short stature should be investigated for one of the inherited forms of osteomalacia.

Screening tests for the presence of osteomalacia should include measurements of total serum calcium; serum phosphate, magnesium, iPTH (using a mid- or carboxy-region assay), 25OHD$_3$, and alkaline phosphatase; and urinary calcium. The presence of hypocalcemia, hyperphosphatemia, increased iPTH, hyper- or hypophosphatasia, or hypocalciuria should prompt further investigations, including x-rays of the skeleton and a radionuclide bone scan (pseudofractures show increased uptake on bone scan). If these latter procedures do not reveal pseudofractures, a transiliac bone biopsy with double tetracycline labeling should be performed. Patients with full-blown osteomalacia due to vitamin D deficiency will have all of the above biochemical findings as well as pseudofractures, and the bone biopsies only offer confirmation. Measurement of 72-hour excretion of fat in the stool is recommended to exclude intestinal malabsorption as a factor in the development of osteo-

malacia, because this disease is often unaccompanied by overt symptoms. Serum levels of 25OHD$_3$ are generally low but may be normal in patients whose diets contain vitamin D at the time of investigation. After restoration of serum 25OHD$_3$ concentrations to normal levels, there is a long time lag before the restoration of other important minerals to normal and the healing of bone lesions. Serum concentrations of 1,25(OH)$_2$D$_3$ should be measured in children whose rickets or osteomalacia appears to be resistant to therapeutic doses of vitamin D. Low values will be found in patients with vitamin D–dependency rickets type I and extremely high values in patients with vitamin D–dependency rickets type II.

More often than not, osteomalacia due to mild degrees of vitamin D deficiency is manifested only by small increases in serum iPTH and hypocalciuria. In such cases, only bone biopsy will establish the diagnosis.

A. Hypophosphatemia: Most patients with osteomalacia due to untreated phosphate deficiency (Table 8–8) have normal serum concentrations of calcium, 25OHD$_3$, and iPTH. This distinguishes them from individuals with vitamin D deficiency. However, excessive treatment of these patients with inorganic phosphate frequently produces mild hypocalcemia and increased serum levels of iPTH. Aside from the occasional presence on x-rays of increased bone density in patients with X-linked hypophosphatemic rickets and variable evidence of osteitis fibrosa cystica in patients with vitamin D deficiency, there appears to be no difference between osteomalacic lesions due to vitamin D deficiency and those due to phosphate deficiency.

B. Inherited Osteomalacia: All patients suspected of having an inherited form of osteomalacia should be studied for the presence of renal tubular acidosis using ammonium chloride loading and measurement of urine pH. This is important because successful therapy of renal tubular acidosis depends upon treatment with alkali. Such treatment is not part of the regimen recommended for osteomalacia caused by vitamin D or phosphate deficiencies.

C. Hypoparathyroidism: The differentiation of hypoparathyroidism from osteomalacia is generally not difficult. Patients with hypoparathyroidism usually have hyperphosphatemia (rather than hypophosphatemia) and a history of thyroidectomy. In rare instances, hypoparathyroidism is associated with steatorrhea; in these cases, both hypophosphatemia and osteomalacia may be present, and measurement of serum iPTH may be the key in making the correct diagnosis. Serum concentrations of iPTH are low or undetectable in hypoparathyroidism, but they are generally increased in patients with osteomalacia, unless severe hypomagnesemia is also present.

D. Hypophosphatasia: The finding of a serum alkaline phosphatase at the lower limits of normal should prompt measurement of plasma levels and urinary excretion of phosphorylethanolamine, which are markedly elevated in patients with hypophosphatasia.

E. Tumor: The clinician should search for subcutaneous and bone tumors in all patients with osteomalacia, since such tumors may be the underlying cause of the osteomalacia and their removal may cure the disease.

Treatment

A. Vitamin D: Patients with rickets or osteomalacia due to simple dietary deficiency of vitamin D or lack of exposure to sunlight respond well to small daily supplements of ergocalciferol and calcium or regular periods of exposure to ultraviolet light (artificial or natural). Administration of oral doses of ergocalciferol (0.05 mg [2000 IU] daily) for several months will heal the bone disease and restore serum calcium, phosphate, alkaline phosphatase, and iPTH to normal in most cases. This dose is insufficient to influence the course of rickets or osteomalacia due to any other cause. Although $1,25(OH)_2D_3$ (calcitriol) has been successful in the treatment of simple rickets and osteomalacia due to inadequate sunlight exposure, dihydrotachysterol has not.

Vitamin D treatment usually results in an increase in serum phosphorus within several days, but serum calcium may not increase for a week or more. In fact, in some patients with severe rickets or osteomalacia, serum calcium may actually decrease for a short period, and in children the development of tetany and convulsions has been described. Phosphate supplements are contraindicated during the early stages of treatment with vitamin D because they may aggravate hypocalcemia.

B. Calcium: Decreases in serum calcium have been ascribed to rapid movement of calcium from the extracellular fluids into bone as a result of its vitamin D–induced mineralization. For this reason—and to provide adequate calcium for bone mineralization—it is important to administer calcium (2 g of elemental calcium daily for children and 1 g for adults) along with vitamin D. Serum alkaline phosphatase and iPTH decrease slowly over a period of several weeks, but improvement in radiographic abnormalities may not be apparent for several months. The previously absent mineralization front in osteoid that underlies osteoblasts appears rapidly. This occurs even before important changes in the serum concentrations of calcium and phosphate and has been interpreted as evidence that vitamin D affects bone mineralization directly.

C. Malabsorption Therapy: Patients with rickets or osteomalacia due to intestinal malabsorption may not respond to treatment with vitamin D compounds, because the vitamin is poorly absorbed. Those patients with gluten-sensitive enteropathy respond to ingestion of a gluten-free diet if sunlight exposure is adequate or small doses of oral vitamin D are given. Patients with other forms of malabsorption (Table 8–8) may require up to 5 mg (200,000 IU) per day of oral ergocalciferol, and some may require 40,000–80,000 IU of ergocalciferol (calciferol) given intravenously or intramuscularly. Unfortunately, preparations of vitamin D suitable for parenteral use are not generally available. Oral calcifediol and calcitriol in larger-than-usual doses may also be effective.

D. Long-Term Therapy: Patients with impaired synthesis of $1,25(OH)_2D_3$ or target cell resistance to $1,25(OH)_2D_3$ should be treated with calcitriol (Rocaltrol), although they may respond to large doses of either ergocalciferol or calcifediol. The treatment of patients with renal osteodystrophy or hypoparathyroidism has already been discussed. Patients with vitamin D–dependency rickets types I and II have been treated traditionally with large doses of ergocalciferol. Regimens must be individually tailored and careful lifelong follow-up maintained. Initial doses should be 25 μg (1000 IU) of ergocalciferol per kilogram of body weight per day. After approximately 2 months of treatment, the response to this dose is evaluated with x-rays of bony lesions and measurements of serum calcium, phosphate, iPTH, and alkaline phosphatase. If no improvement is observed, the dose of vitamin D is increased by 25%; if signs of healing are observed, the dose is increased by only 15%. Similar evaluations should be made every 2 months, with appropriate increases in vitamin D dose until a satisfactory maintenance dose has been determined. The requirement for ergocalciferol varies among patients but is usually in the range of 40–50 μg/kg/d. Serum calcium should be measured every 3–4 months for life. The development of hypercalcemia can be avoided by maintaining serum concentrations of calcium in the low normal range. Vitamin D therapy should be discontinued at the earliest sign of hypercalcemia. If detected early, serum calcium returns to the normal range within a week; if it remains normal for 2 weeks, vitamin D therapy can be reinstituted at a dose 15% lower than that which caused the hypercalcemia. Successful therapy is marked by "catch-up" skeletal growth, followed by normal growth.

Liquid forms of vitamin D should be used in patients with vitamin D–dependency rickets, because precise doses can be metered out to the patient with a small, well-calibrated syringe. Table 8–9 lists available liquid preparations of vitamin D_2.

Calcifediol (100–900 μg/d) has been used successfully in the treatment of vitamin D–dependency rickets, but it is expensive and offers little advantage over ergocalciferol except that hypercalcemia resolves sooner after calcifediol is discontinued. Calcitriol, on the other hand, should provide an important advantage because of its rapid onset and termination of action. Long-term experience in the treatment of patients with vitamin D–dependency rickets with calcitriol has not yet accrued. The doses of dihydrotachysterol required

Table 8–9. High-potency ergocalciferol (vitamin D_2) preparations in liquid form.

Ergocalciferol oral solution, 8000 IU vitamin D_2 per milliliter. Calciferol, 500,000 IU vitamin D_2 per milliliter (should be diluted to 100,000 IU/mL [1:5] with edible vegetable oil before dispensing).

for successful treatment of these patients are large, and this drug offers no special advantage over vitamin D.

E. Hypophosphatemic Rickets: The treatment of X-linked hypophosphatemic rickets is extremely challenging and requires persistence and excellent relationships with family members, so that patients will be compliant in their ingestion of phosphate. Lifelong treatment with orthophosphate supplements by mouth in doses ranging from 1 to 5 g of elemental phosphorus per day in divided doses every 5–6 hours will heal the rickets and osteomalacia of this disease. Phosphate supplements (Table 8–10) may be distasteful and can cause diarrhea initially, but with persistence, serum concentrations of phosphorus are restored toward normal (4 mg/dL), and side effects generally disappear. The only major complication of phosphate therapy is the development of secondary hyperparathyroidism. The reason for this complication is poorly understood, since normal children who maintain similar levels of serum phosphate do not develop secondary hyperparathyroidism. Secondary hyperparathyroidism can be prevented only by coincident treatment with a vitamin D preparation that prevents decreases in ionized calcium that are ordinarily caused by phosphate therapy. Although ergocalciferol in doses of 0.1–1.25 mg (4000–50,000 IU) daily was used previously, it has recently been determined that calcitriol is equally effective or even more effective. Calcitriol is recommended in the treatment of patients with X-linked hypophosphatemia because hypercalcemia resolves rapidly after its discontinuation and because it may have specific antirachitic effects.

In following patients with X-linked hypophosphatemia who are under treatment with phosphate supplements and vitamin D, procedures similar to those described in the treatment of vitamin D dependency should be used. Serum calcium, phosphate, and iPTH should be measured at intervals of 3–4 months. If hypercalcemia supervenes, vitamin D should be discontinued and then reinstituted at a lower dose when eucalcemia is restored. If serum iPTH increases much above the upper limit of the normal range, orthophosphate should be withheld temporarily; in some cases, however, it may be necessary to increase the dose of vitamin D. Renal function should be monitored carefully by measuring serum creatinine serially. Twenty-four-hour urinary phosphorus can be monitored to assess patient compliance with the phosphate regimen. Values in excess of 1000–2000 mg/d suggest compliance, but it must be remembered that patients and parents may be interested in pleasing the physician, and patients may take phosphate supplements immediately prior to 24-hour collection of urine but not chronically as prescribed.

F. Renal Tubular Acidosis: Rickets and osteomalacia due to distal renal tubular acidosis are expeditiously treated by correcting the acidosis with sodium bicarbonate, potassium bicarbonate, or both. Adults require 5–10 g/d and children 1–5 g/d. Response to therapy should be monitored by measurements of blood pH, with values maintained at nearly physiologic levels. Rickets may heal slowly, and the response may be accelerated by the addition of vitamin D (in relatively high doses) to the treatment regimen. Therapy should be monitored by measuring serum calcium, and the dose of vitamin D should be regulated accordingly. Once rickets has healed, vitamin D therapy is rarely required, but it is probable that lifelong treatment with alkali will be necessary.

G. Rickets Due to Tumor: The response of tumor-associated rickets and osteomalacia to surgical removal of the offending tumor is dramatic. Serum phosphate increases within 1–2 days, and bone lesions heal within 6 months to 1 year.

H. Hypophosphatasia: In treatment of bone lesions associated with hypophosphatasia, use of conventional drugs (eg, vitamin D and calcium) has been unsatisfactory. Recently, increases in alkaline phosphatase and some degree of healing have been observed with doses of fluoride ion in the range of 40 mg/d. Spontaneous remissions have been reported.

OSTEOPOROSIS

Osteoporosis is a generalized disorder of bone characterized by a decrease in the quantity of bone but no change in its quality. The decrease in quantity results in increased bone fragility and fractures following minimal or no trauma.

Table 8–10. Phosphate supplements for oral administration in hypophosphatemia.

Acidic phosphate (Joulie's solution)		
Dibasic sodium phosphate	102	Dissolve the phosphate salt in about 750 mL of warm water to which the
($Na_2HPO_4 \cdot 7H_2O$) (reagent grade)		phosphoric acid has been added. Make the solution up to 1L with distilled
Phosphoric acid NF (85%)	58.8	water. Store at room temperature. The concentration of phosphorus in this
Distilled water, qs ad	1000	solution is 2.76 g/dL; the pH is 4.3.
Neutral phosphate solution		
$NaH_2PO_4 \cdot H_2O$ (reagent grade)	18.2	Mix the phosphate salts and dispense in dry form as packets. Dissolve the
$Na_2HPO_4 \cdot 7H_2O$ (reagent grade)	145	packet of salts in distilled water by gently warming. Store in refrigerator at
Distilled water, qs ad	1000	$4°C$. Shake well if precipitate forms. Each batch lasts several days. The concentration of phosphorus in this solution is 2.08 g/dL; the pH is neutral.
Neutra-Phos-K, K-Phos Neutral; others		
Inorganic phosphorus, 250 mg		Dissolve capsules in water and take orally. Take tablets orally with water.
per capsule or tablet		

Table 8–11. Classification of osteoporosis according to frequency of occurrence.

Frequent	Infrequent
Postmenopausal	Juvenile
Senile	Young adult
Hypogonadism (oophorectomy)	Osteogenesis imperfecta
Corticosteroid-induced	Chromosomal abnormalities
Immobilization	Migratory
Neoplasms (eg, myeloma)	Disappearing bones
	Cushing's syndrome
	Hyperthyroidism
	Iron storage disease

Etiology & Incidence

Osteoporosis occurs most frequently in post-menopausal women and the aged. It has been estimated that at least 20% of women have suffered one or more fractures (vertebral, wrist, or proximal femur) by age 65 and as many as 40% have fractures thereafter. This enormous increase in fracture rate in comparison to the rate in premenopausal women is directly related to the progressive decrease in bone mass that occurs with aging in women. Osteoporosis is a major source of morbidity in this population. Decreases in bone mass in men are delayed until after age 60, when fracture rates progressively increase. As many as 5–20% of older patients hospitalized with hip fracture die of cardiopulmonary problems, thus making hip fracture due to osteoporosis one of the more frequent indirect causes of death in North America. As many as 50% of the patients who survive become dependent on nursing home care.

The major types of osteoporosis are listed in Table 8–11 according to frequency of occurrence. The specific cause of the most common form of osteoporosis—that associated with menopause and aging—is unknown, but the major risk and complicating factors are listed in Table 8–12.

A. Estrogen and Calcium Deficiency: There is little question that loss of sex hormone function is of major importance in bone loss associated with aging. Well-controlled trials in several centers have shown that treatment of perimenopausal or oophorectomized women with physiologic doses of estrogen prevents bone loss, in contrast to control subjects given low doses of estrogen or placebo. It has also been established that older persons not only ingest less calcium-containing foods than young men and women but also generally require considerably more calcium in their diets (1400 mg of elemental calcium daily versus 800 mg daily, respectively) to maintain total body calcium balance. Thus, it appears likely that sex hormone deficiency at menopause and calcium deficiency are the major etiologic factors in the osteoporosis of aging.

Although many elderly persons lose bone, not all develop fractures. The absolute quantity of bone present at the time sex hormone and calcium deficiencies develop ultimately determines whether fractures will occur. Hence, if the rate of bone loss is similar among individuals, the critical point of bone "weakness"

permitting fracture with minimal trauma will be reached more rapidly in individuals beginning with small amounts of bone than in those beginning with large amounts.

B. Other Factors: Less important risk factors in the development of osteoporosis include alcohol abuse, smoking, immobilization, and lack of exercise. The means by which these factors accelerate bone loss are poorly understood, but they are controllable and should be considered in the treatment of osteoporosis due to any cause. Complicating factors include the conditions that may be associated with vitamin D deficiency, excessive circulating concentrations of PTH, thyroid hormone, or corticosteroids, and a variety of drugs. Particularly important among the latter are corticosteroids, thyroid hormone, and anticonvulsants, which are all commonly used for disorders unrelated to osteoporosis. The true extent and frequency with which osteoporosis is associated with chemotherapy in the treatment of cancer or with heparin therapy are unknown.

C. Juvenile Osteoporosis: Juvenile osteoporosis is rare, and its cause is unknown. It occurs in late childhood and adolescence and is self-limited, lasting about 5 years. Young adult osteoporosis is also rare. It occurs at a later age (20–40), but in contrast to juvenile osteoporosis, it may progress rapidly to an

Table 8–12. Risk factors and complicating factors in osteoporosis.

Genetic factors
  Nonblack race
  Northern European stock
  Small bone mass
  Defects in collagen synthesis or structure
Nutritional deficiency
  Calcium and phosphate
  Vitamin D (sunlight deprivation without dietary
    supplementation)
  Vitamin C
  Protein
Hypogonadism
Drugs
  Alcohol
  Corticosteroids
  Thyroid hormone
  Anticonvulsants
  Cancer chemotherapy
  Heparin
  Caffeine
Smoking
Gastrointestinal disease
  Gastric or intestinal resection
  Malabsorption
  Pancreatic insufficiency
  Hepatic disease
Renal disease
Hyperparathyroidism
Hyperthyroidism
Immobilization and lack of exercise
Excessive exercise (eg, jogging), leading to
    weight loss, amenorrhea, or both

almost total collapse of the axial skeleton and death from respiratory failure. Its cause is also unknown.

D. Osteogenesis Imperfecta: Osteogenesis imperfecta is a relatively common heritable disorder of bone that is probably caused by defects in collagen synthesis or structure. The most severely affected individuals suffer multiple fractures early in life that ultimately produce severe deformity and growth retardation. Other manifestations include bluish-gray scleras (an inconstant finding), ligamentous laxity, and hearing loss in adults. It has been suggested that some patients who develop osteoporosis in later life may have mild forms of osteogenesis imperfecta.

E. Chromosomal Abnormalities: Although sex hormone deficiency may be responsible in part for the osteoporosis observed in patients with chromosomal abnormalities (eg, Turner's XO and Klinefelter's XXY syndromes), other unknown factors are probably also involved.

F. Immobilization: The osteoporosis of immobilization can be localized (associated with casts for fractures or with painful limbs), generalized (associated with prolonged bed rest or space travel), or neurologic (associated with paraplegia or quadriplegia). The causes are unknown, but absence of stress and muscle pull on bone is an underlying factor in all of these disorders.

G. Vitamin C Deficiency and Hemochromatosis: Osteoporosis may be associated with severe vitamin C deficiency and hemochromatosis. Vitamin C is a cofactor in the enzymatic hydroxylation of proline and lysine in collagen. Because of this, a deficiency in vitamin C is thought to produce abnormalities in collagen biosynthesis and maturation that interfere with bone formation. A similar mechanism may be involved in the osteoporosis of hemochromatosis; the abnormal accumulation of iron may promote oxidation of vitamin C, resulting in its depletion. Hemochromatosis of the testes, which causes hypogonadism and sex hormone deficiency, is almost certainly an important contributing factor in the production of osteoporosis of this disorder.

H. Migratory Osteoporosis and Sudeck's Atrophy: There are 2 rare forms of local osteoporosis that appear to be unrelated to immobilization. The first is transitory or regional migratory osteoporosis. It is characterized by painful loss of bone, usually in the upper femoral shafts, which almost always reverses without treatment. The second is the syndrome of "disappearing bones," in which one or more parts of limb bones disappear radiologically and are replaced by fibrous tissue. This disorder probably represents an extreme form of Sudeck's atrophy of bone which occurs after trauma or fracture. It is variably reversible, and no specific treatment is available. The underlying causes of these conditions are unknown.

Anatomic & Chemical Pathology

Osteoporosis can often be detected during transiliac bone biopsy. The biopsy needle saws through the outer table of bone with little difficulty, and ex-

treme care is needed to avoid crushing the specimen. Examination of such a specimen shows that the mass of bone per unit volume of bone tissue is reduced, but its mineral content per unit mass is normal. In contrast, the bone in osteomalacia has a reduced mineral content per unit mass.

Tetracycline labeling of bone in vivo has shown that bone formation decreases with age and bone resorption remains constant. Microradiographic studies show increases in bone resorption surfaces, probably resulting from the failure of bone formation processes to repair previously resorbed bone. Since it has not yet been possible to investigate the dynamic properties of human bone cells, it is still unknown whether bone cell function in osteoporosis is abnormal.

Pathogenesis

A. Postmenopausal and Senile Osteoporosis: The pathogenesis of postmenopausal and senile osteoporosis is poorly understood, but important observations during the past decade have led to a hypothesis with therapeutic implications. Although evidence is incomplete, it is likely that sex hormones protect bone against the destructive effects of PTH. Thus, the incidence of osteoporosis in postmenopausal women with hypoparathyroidism is decreased, and estrogen treatment in patients with hyperparathyroidism reduces blood calcium levels toward normal. Most importantly, estrogen treatment in patients with postmenopausal osteoporosis causes decreased bone resorption surfaces (as observed in transiliac bone biopsies), small decreases in serum levels of calcium, and appropriate increases in serum levels of iPTH. By inference, therefore, the loss of sex hormone function at the menopause may permit normal levels of circulating PTH to act on bone unopposed, resulting in relatively greater bone resorption in comparison with formation. Negative bone balance ensues, and the resulting increase in the release of calcium from bone causes small increases in the serum levels of calcium, which in turn decreases serum levels of iPTH. The consequences of chronic decreases in PTH secretion are manifest and can be predicted from Fig 8–2. Serum concentrations of phosphate increase because of a decrease in PTH-induced phosphate excretion. The combination of decreased PTH secretion and increased serum phosphate results in diminished $1,25(OH)_2D_3$ production and decreased intestinal calcium absorption. Likewise, urinary calcium excretion is increased as a result of a decrease in PTH-induced renal tubular reabsorption of calcium. These adaptive mechanisms are normally quite effective in preventing increases in serum calcium due to environmental perturbations (eg, increased intestinal absorption of calcium). They can only be considered maladaptive when increases in serum calcium are induced by a primary defect in bone that causes a relative increase in resorption over formation (eg, postmenopausal osteoporosis). Thus, if the sequence of events described above is correct, the decrease in intestinal absorption of calcium and increase in renal excretion of calcium observed in postmenopausal osteoporosis represent epiphenomena of negative bone balance that can only aggravate the primary bone lesions by producing a negative balance in total body calcium.

Serum iPTH has been shown to increase with age in apparently normal subjects. Although this could be due to an intrinsic change in the secretory activity of the parathyroid glands, it is likely that a combination of a dietary deficiency in calcium in the aged, diminished intestinal calcium absorption, and possibly decreased renal function is responsible. Significant increases in serum iPTH above the normal mean value are generally not observed under the age of 60, and they could themselves be responsible for the osteoporosis observed in old people. More intriguing, however, is the possibility that the adverse effects of sex hormone deficiency and secondary hyperparathyroidism due to calcium deficiency merge as age progresses and are responsible for the ultimate clinical picture of advanced osteoporosis in the very old. A working classification of the osteoporosis of aging, based on these 2 pathogenetic schemes, has been proposed: type I denotes osteoporosis due to sex hormone deficiency, and type II denotes that due to secondary hyperparathyroidism.

It has recently been suggested that decreased secretion of calcitonin in women may be an additional etiologic factor.

B. Glucocorticoid-Induced Osteoporosis: Glucocorticoid-induced osteoporosis occurs in patients with Cushing's disease and in other patients treated with glucocorticoids. Diminished bone mass can be observed within months following initiation of high-dose steroid therapy and can result in the rapid compromise of skeletal integrity. Corticosteroids have many effects on extracellular mineral and bone metabolism. They almost certainly interfere with normal production of bone collagen by osteoblasts, and there is evidence in cultured bone cells in vitro that they increase cellular sensitivity to PTH. Corticosteroids also inhibit intestinal absorption of calcium. The mechanism of this action is poorly understood, but it may involve interference with the normal metabolism of vitamin D to its biologically active metabolite $1,25(OH)_2D_3$, as well as direct toxic effects on the intestinal cell. Negative calcium balance due to decreased intestinal absorption of calcium is almost always manifest, and the resulting mild hypocalcemia causes appropriate increases in serum concentrations of iPTH. The secondary hyperparathyroidism and possibly the increased sensitivity of bone to PTH are reflected histomorphometrically in an increase in bone resorption surfaces. Thus, the combined effects of diminished bone formation and increased bone resorption result in severe negative bone balance and a rapid decrease in bone mass.

C. Hyperthyroidism: There are dramatic histomorphometric changes in the bones of patients with hyperthyroidism. These are characterized by increased osteoclastic resorption and increased osteoblastic bone formation. Osteoid seams are frequently increased in width owing to accelerated matrix production, and marrow fibrosis may be present. These changes are almost certainly due to the direct effects of thyroid hormones on bone cells and are reflected by increased urinary excretion of hydroxyproline and hydroxylysine and increased serum concentrations of alkaline phosphatase. Alterations in extracellular mineral homeostasis are not always obvious, probably because the increases in bone formation and bone resorption are equivalent. Nevertheless, mild hypercalcemia is occasionally observed and is associated with adaptive decreases in serum iPTH, increases in serum phosphate due to decreased phosphate excretion, marked hypercalciuria, and decreases in intestinal absorption of calcium.

The bone loss that occurs in hyperthyroidism rarely achieves clinical significance in the young but may sufficiently aggravate the bone loss in postmenopausal women or old men to precipitate fractures.

Quantitative Measurement of Bone Mass

There are 3 approaches to quantitative assessment of bone mass. The first uses careful x-rays of the hands and measurements of the periosteal and endosteal diameters of a metacarpal bone (the second, third, or fourth). The thickness of the cortical bone is determined by subtracting the internal diameter from the external diameter. Measurements are best made with a precision caliper. The precision of this measurement is about ± 2%.

The second approach uses photon beam absorptiometry, introduced by Cameron and Sorenson. The single-beam method measures the attenuation by bone (usually the radius) of gamma ray emission from isotopes (^{125}I or ^{247}Am). Commercial instruments are now available, and with careful application the precision of measurements is also about ± 2%. The disadvantage of this technique is that accessible limb bones have little trabecular bone, and measurements thus reflect chiefly cortical bone. Since most osteoporosis of clinical significance involves principally trabecular bone, there is a large overlap in values for normal subjects and patients with proved osteoporosis.

The recently developed dual-photon absorptiometry method can measure mass in almost any bone in the body. Thus, the bones most frequently fractured in patients with osteoporosis (vertebrae and femoral neck) can be assessed directly. The overlap in bone mass values between normal subjects and patients with proved osteoporosis is considerably less than that observed using the single-beam technique.

Another promising technique, introduced by Genant and Cann, uses computer-assisted tomography to obtain direct measurements of bone mass in any part of a given vertebra. Variability of this technique using the most advanced instruments is less than ± 2%.

It appears that dual-photon absorptiometry and computer-assisted tomography are similar in their ability to differentiate bone mass in normal subjects from that in patients with proved osteoporosis, but they have never been directly compared in this regard. Both techniques should ultimately provide the clinician with accurate measurements of changes in bone mass during observation or treatment. They should also help in assessing the value of various new treatments for osteoporosis.

Clinical Features

A. Symptoms and Signs: Patients with uncomplicated osteoporosis without bone fractures are usually asymptomatic. The first manifestation of reduced bone mass is usually a wrist fracture or a vertebral crush fracture caused by a small amount of force. A fresh vertebral fracture produces severe localized pain in the back that frequently radiates anteriorly into the chest, sometimes resembling the pain of a cardiopulmonary catastrophe. Torso movement aggravates the pain and recumbency relieves it, with improvement occurring within 1–2 months. Subsequent vertebral fractures may occur and may contribute to chronic back pain, but more often the intensity of pain is poorly related to the degree of spinal deformity seen on x-rays. During the acute phase of fracture, spot tenderness occurs over the back, but neurologic signs are rare.

1. Dorsal kyphosis and loss of height–The single most prominent finding in patients with well-established osteoporosis is dorsal kyphosis (so-called dowager's hump) and loss of height. Accurate measurements of height and arm span are most important in assessing the development and progress of osteoporosis in patients who have undergone oophorectomy or orchiectomy or in patients undergoing routine evaluation after the age of 45 years. Normally, total erect height equals arm span but becomes progressively less than arm span with vertebral collapse.

All of the classic signs of hip fracture are present in patients with osteoporosis who are afflicted with this problem, but because most patients are aged, the incidence of fatal complications is increased.

Figure 8–31. *A:* Magnified x-rays of thoracic vertebrae from a woman with osteoporosis. Note the relative prominence of vertical trabeculae and the absence of horizontal trabeculae. *B:* Lateral x-ray of the lumbar spine of a woman with postmenopausal osteoporosis. Note the increased density of the superior and inferior cortical margins of vertebrae, the marked demineralization of vertebral bodies, and the central compression of articular surfaces of vertebral bodies by intervertebral disks. (Courtesy of G Gordan.)

2. Signs of other disorders–Patients with osteoporosis due to causes other than sex hormone deficiency and aging may have symptoms and signs related to the underlying disorder (eg, Cushing's syndrome due to excessive corticosteroids).

B. Laboratory Findings: Serum calcium, phosphate, alkaline phosphatase, and iPTH are within normal ranges in patients with osteoporosis due to sex hormone deficiency and aging. In the acute phase of development, urinary calcium and hydroxyproline may be slightly increased, but these indices have no diagnostic value. Significant abnormalities in serum calcium, phosphate, alkaline phosphatase, iPTH, and serum proteins should be regarded with suspicion, and one or more of the complicating factors listed in Table 8–12 should be sought.

C. X-Ray Findings: X-rays of the skeleton do not show a decrease in osseous density until at least 30% of bone mass has been lost. Although such a decrease in density may be observed in all bones, the most valuable x-rays for diagnostic purposes are those of the lateral lumbar and thoracic spine. One should look for loss of horizontal trabeculae and prominent end plates of the vertebral bodies (Fig 8–31A). Intervertebral disks are more prominent than is normal, and mechanical failure of vertebrae is manifested by wedging and protrusion of the disk into the body of the vertebra (Fig 8–31B). The latter finding has been termed "codfish spine" because this species has biconcave vertebral bodies.

X-rays of the upper part of the femur that are taken so as to accentuate trabecular patterns may be most helpful in assessing the clinical importance of reduced bone mass (Singh index) (Fig 8–32). Disappearance of the superior trabecular pattern that traverses the greater trochanter (arrow in grade 3 sketch) probably indicates that the osteoporosis is severe enough to increase the risk of hip fracture.

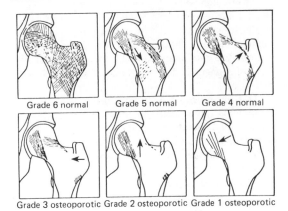

Grade 6 normal   Grade 5 normal   Grade 4 normal

Grade 3 osteoporotic   Grade 2 osteoporotic   Grade 1 osteoporotic

Figure 8–32. The effects of increasingly severe osteoporosis on the pattern of trabecular bone in the upper end of the femur. Arrows show progressive radiologic disappearance of trabecular groups. (Reproduced, with permission, from Singh M et al: *Ann Intern Med* 1972;**77**:63.)

Differential Diagnosis

Without radiographic evidence of vertebral fractures or a history of fracture of other bones with minimal trauma, the detection of significant decreases in bone mass may be difficult. Even with the use of the most sophisticated techniques (see previous section), single values for bone mass may be within the normal range for age after 20% of the skeleton has been lost. Serial measurements showing progressive loss of bone are necessary in order to estimate the original bone mass that might have been present in an individual patient before osseous destruction. The physician should also be aware of conditions and risk factors that may lead to loss of bone mass (Table 8–12). Therapeutic or prophylactic measures should be instituted as rapidly as possible and systematic measurements made at regular intervals to determine the progress of the disease or the effect of treatment.

There are many disorders that mimic or complicate postmenopausal or senile osteoporosis. The routine history and physical examination are very useful in discovering them. The history will reveal drug treatment, gastric or intestinal resections, oophorectomy, sunlight deprivation, and immobilization. Physical examination may reveal the presence of Cushing's syndrome or hyperthyroidism as well as the presence of hepatomegaly or splenomegaly. Liver enlargement suggests liver disease and, in men, the possibility of hemochromatosis. Small, soft testicles should raise suspicions about hypogonadism due to a variety of causes, including Klinefelter's syndrome (see Chapter 13). Short stature in a woman may be a sign of Turner's syndrome (see Chapter 15).

Multiple myeloma and diffuse metastasis of malignant tumors to the vertebrae are commonly misdiagnosed as postmenopausal or senile osteoporosis. These conditions should be suspected when the history indicates that the patient may have cancer. In the absence of historical clues, unusually rapid progression of osseous destruction often indicates the presence of cancer. In such cases, bone marrow examination or direct biopsy of lesions may be most helpful.

Total serum calcium, phosphate, magnesium, alkaline phosphatase, albumin and globulin, iPTH, cortisol, and thyroxine should be measured in all patients with osteoporosis. In patients with postmenopausal or senile osteoporosis, the values for all of these indices should be within the normal range. Abnormalities indicate the presence of disorders that mimic or complicate postmenopausal or senile osteoporosis, and a specific diagnosis should be established as soon as possible. Serum $1,25(OH)_2D_3$ should be measured in patients suspected of sunlight deprivation or malabsorption, and in men, measurement of serum testosterone is indicated to exclude hypogonadism.

Treatment

The treatment of osteoporosis depends on establishing its underlying cause to the extent possible. Patients with endocrine abnormalities can usually be treated by either hormone replacement (hypogonadism) or removal of hyperfunctioning endocrine tissue. In most instances, drugs that induce osteoporosis can be discontinued or replaced by other drugs, or the dosage can be reduced. In the case of corticosteroid therapy, measures designed to help prevent osteoporosis should be considered. Alternate-day corticosteroid therapy in conjunction with oral calcium supplements (1–2 g of elemental calcium daily) to decrease PTH secretion may be helpful in this regard.

Once it has been established that a patient is at risk or has postmenopausal osteoporosis, the risk factors listed in Table 8–12 should be eliminated whenever possible. Small women of northern European ancestry whose Singh index (Fig 8–32) for the upper femoral trabecular pattern is grade 3 or below should be warned that hip fracture is likely to occur with minimal trauma. These patients should eliminate hazards that might cause them to fall (eg, waxed floors and throw rugs).

At first evaluation, baseline measurement of bone mass should be obtained using one or more of the following techniques: determination of the mean cortical thickness of the metacarpals, photon absorptiometry of the radius, and either dual-photon absorptiometry or computed tomography to determine the density of one lumbar vertebra (see above).

A. Calcium: After 24-hour urinary calcium is measured (to rule out idiopathic hypercalciuria), oral calcium supplements of 1–2 g of elemental calcium daily are begun. Such therapy increases intestinal absorption of calcium, decreases serum levels of iPTH, and decreases resorption surfaces. If undue hypercalciuria is noted, thiazides are indicated.

B. Estrogens: It has been shown that estrogen prevents bone loss in oophorectomized and perimenopausal women, and a recent study indicates that calcium and estrogen together markedly decrease the fracture rate in osteoporotic women. However, noncyclic estrogen therapy is controversial because some reports indicate that such treatment may increase the incidence of uterine cancer. The conservative approach would be to maintain calcium supplements for a year, at which time bone mass should be measured again and estrogen treatment started if values are significantly below previously obtained baseline values. The more aggressive approach would be to administer cyclic ethinyl estradiol (0.02 mg/d) or conjugated estrogen (0.625 mg/d) for 3 of every 4 weeks. Then progesterone (1–10 mg) should be given during the last week that estrogen is administered. In patients with a uterus, menstrual bleeding may be expected during the week off estrogen and progesterone. However, it should be recognized that the possible adverse effects of long-term progesterone therapy have not been fully evaluated. Absolute contraindications to estrogen therapy include a personal or family history of breast or genital cancer. It is possible that anabolic steroid preparations (eg, stanozolol) may offer an alternative form of therapy to these women.

C. Fluoride: Fluoride ion is the only form of treatment available that has been demonstrated to increase bone mass. Radiographic evidence shows that spinal density increases in patients with osteoporosis who have been given sodium fluoride (50 mg/d), oral calcium (1 g/d), and vitamin D (50,000 IU every 3–5 days). In another study, the combination of fluoride, calcium, and estrogen appeared to decrease fracture rates to a greater extent than did the combination of estrogen and calcium; vitamin D alone had no influence on fracture rates. It is important to recognize that numerous side effects occur with fluoride therapy, including joint swelling and gastrointestinal intolerance. Most importantly, fluoride is at present an investigational drug not approved by the FDA for treatment of osteoporosis.

D. Androgens for Men: Men with osteoporosis should be treated in a manner similar to that described for women, except that androgens should be given instead of estrogens. Unfortunately, androgens may aggravate prostatic hyperplasia. Combined androgen and estrogen therapy (eg, Deladumone) may be of value in this regard.

E. Phosphate: Although phosphate supplements might be expected to increase bone formation, they are associated with development of secondary hyperparathyroidism and apparent worsening of bone disease in patients with osteoporosis. The effect of combining phosphate with other drugs of proved efficacy has yet to be studied extensively.

F. Calcitonin: Calcitonin (Calcimar) was expected to provide the ideal therapy for osteoporosis because of its supposed inhibitory action on bone resorption. However, calcitonin increases serum iPTH and does little to inhibit bone resorption unless calcium supplements are used to prevent hyperparathyroidism. Calcitonin has recently been approved by the FDA for the treatment of osteoporosis in doses of 100 IU/d. It must be given parenterally and is expensive but may be an alternative to estrogen therapy when this drug is contraindicated or not tolerated.

G. Parathyroid Hormone: In an effort to increase bone formation, synthetic human PTH(1–34) has been given to osteoporotic patients in low doses. Early results suggest that such treatment produces positive calcium balance and increases trabecular bone formation. The combination of PTH treatment with other drugs designed to decrease bone resorption has not been tried.

H. Diphosphonate Compounds: Diphosphonate compounds have been shown to decrease bone resorption and therefore might be expected to have a beneficial effect in patients with osteoporosis. Using the only compound currently available in the USA (etidronate disodium), one study has demonstrated a reduction in both bone formation and bone resorption in osteoporotic patients. Although this drug is known to produce osteomalacia when given in high doses, other diphosphonate compounds do not. It is therefore possible that these latter agents may prove to be of use in the treatment of osteoporosis.

I. Life-Style: It is important to encourage osteoporotic patients to make adequate sunlight exposure, dietary intake of calcium, and physical exercise a part of their lives. Such measures usually decrease chronic back pain and promote a sense of well-being. Adequate back supports are most important.

PAGET'S DISEASE
(Osteitis Deformans)

Although Paget's disease of bone is a disorder of bone remodeling, it cannot be classified strictly as a metabolic bone disease, because the abnormalities are focal. The disease is characterized by histologic and gross osseous deformities due to local uncontrolled bone resorption, which is caused by excessive numbers of osteoclasts and osteoblasts and ultimately leads to formation of structurally fragile osseous tissue. Any bone of the body may be involved, but the most frequent sites are the femur, tibia, skull, lumbosacral spine, and pelvis. The disease is usually asymptomatic, and except for a similar bone disease in young children called hereditary bone dysplasia with hyperphosphatasia, or "juvenile Paget's disease," patients generally come to medical attention only after age 40.

Paget's disease occurs in a fairly distinct geographic distribution. About 4% of people over 40 years of age in Germany and England have the disease, whereas it is considerably less common in North America and relatively rare in Scandinavia, Africa, and the Near and Far East. It is likely that fewer than 2% of patients with radiographic evidence of Paget's disease are symptomatic. The disease may occur in families and has been reported in identical twins.

Coexistence of primary hyperparathyroidism and Paget's disease has been noted, but this observation must be interpreted cautiously in light of the fact that both disorders are common, and when one is detected, the usual laboratory investigations will almost certainly reveal the other, if present.

Etiology

Recently, the old idea that Paget's disease may be due to some chronic inflammatory process has been revived. Nuclear inclusions resembling virus particles have been observed in the osteoclasts of patients with Paget's disease, suggesting that its underlying cause may be a slow virus.

Pathology

The gross pathologic features of Paget's disease in its full-blown state consist of diffuse bony deformities, including marked enlargement of the skull, expansion and compression of the vertebrae, platybasia with compression of the cerebellum and spinal cord, anterior and lateral bowing of the extremities, and protrusion of the femoral head into the acetabulum as a result of pelvic involvement. Histologically, all bone cell types are increased in number and apparently in activity. Lamellar bone in the cortex and trabeculae is progressively replaced by woven bone, so that its gross architecture becomes chaotic. As lesions progress, woven bone is replaced by randomly laid lamellar bone; sections thus present a characteristic mosaic structure when observed under polarized light. Osteoid volume is increased but the calcification front is normal, indicating that new bone formation is occurring at a rapid rate. Osteoclasts show great variation in size and may contain up to 100 nuclei. Osteoblasts may be very large, with irregularly shaped nuclei. Osteocytic osteolysis is a prominent finding. Areas of bone that have undergone a full "pagetic cycle" retain architectural abnormalities, but cell numbers and activity are normal.

Pathogenesis

Although bone mineral turnover may be many times greater than normal in Paget's disease, calcium balance is generally maintained because the rates of bone resorption and formation are similar. Only when Paget's disease is complicated by disorders causing further increases in bone resorption (eg, prolonged immobilization or primary hyperparathyroidism) will abnormalities of extracellular mineral metabolism become evident. The hypercalcemia of immobilization may be extremely severe and lead to suppression of PTH secretion, hypercalciuria, decreased intestinal absorption of calcium, and negative calcium balance. If primary hyperparathyroidism is present, hypercalcemia may be more severe than might be predicted by the levels of serum iPTH.

Characteristically, serum alkaline phosphatase levels are markedly increased. These increased levels are probably due to the increased numbers of osteoblasts present in pagetic bone, since serum alkaline phosphatase activity appears to correlate well with histomorphometric values for active bone formation surface. Serum acid phosphatase activity may also be increased in some patients, and this increase is thought to be due to increased numbers of osteoclasts present in lesions.

Urinary excretion of hydroxyproline is increased in most patients, owing to increased rates of synthesis and destruction in bone collagen.

Clinical Features

A. Symptoms and Signs: Relatively few patients with radiologically proved Paget's disease have significant symptoms. The diagnosis is often made as an incidental finding on x-rays taken for other reasons. The chief symptom is bone pain over lesions. Joint symptoms produced by Paget's disease may be difficult to distinguish from those of arthritis. Deafness in patients with Paget's disease of the skull is usually related to bony abnormalities of the internal and external auditory apparatus rather than compression of the eighth nerve by temporal bone enlargement. Vertebral crush fractures occur frequently. In rare cases, there are severe neurologic complications resulting from spinal cord compression and dislocation of cervical vertebrae.

Fractures of long bones may occur. Incomplete ("fissure") fractures, frequently painful, are usually present on the convex surfaces of lower limb bones and may progress to complete fracture with minimal or no trauma. Fractures usually heal rapidly. Redness with increased skin temperature over pagetic bone is a common finding; rarely, bruits may be heard. Increased cardiac output is common in patients with extensive disease. These vascular manifestations are probably due to increased blood flow in involved areas both in bone and in overlying skin. High-output congestive heart failure may occur in patients with underlying heart disease.

The risk of osteogenic sarcoma is greater in patients with Paget's disease than in the population at large. Its major sites are the humerus and skull.

B. Laboratory Findings: Serum calcium, phosphate, magnesium, and iPTH are usually normal. Abnormalities should be taken as evidence of a superimposed condition, such as immobilization or primary hyperparathyroidism. Serum alkaline phosphatase levels are markedly increased, and acid phosphatase levels may also be increased. Urinary hydroxyproline is usually increased except in patients with minimal disease.

C. X-Ray Findings: There is a vast spectrum of characteristic radiologic abnormalities, ranging from pure osteolytic lesions to areas that show both osteolysis and sclerosis. Subperiosteal bone resorption has not been noted in Paget's disease; when present, it suggests primary hyperparathyroidism. The classic bony abnormality seen in the extremities is a large, uniform resorption front that appears as a V-shaped wedge on x-ray (Fig 8–33). As the front advances along the shaft, sclerotic bone is laid down behind it, resulting in anterior or lateral bowing. Thick bony trabeculae are common and may fill in the medullary cavity of bones. The skull is often grossly enlarged, and the mixture of sclerotic and lytic areas gives rise to the classic "cotton wool" appearance on x-ray. Initially, the skull may show a purely osteolytic lesion (osteoporosis circumscripta). Thickening of long bones and vertebrae occurs frequently, and crush factors cause varying degrees of kyphosis.

The development of radionuclide bone scans using ^{99m}Tc-labeled diphosphonate or pyrophosphate and ^{67}gallium citrate has aided greatly in documenting the extent of the disease and revealing lesions that may not be apparent radiologically (Fig 8–34).

Differential Diagnosis

The diagnosis of Paget's disease is relatively straightforward. It is based on the presence of typical bone lesions on x-ray or radionuclide bone scans; normal levels of serum calcium, phosphate, and iPTH; increased serum levels of alkaline phosphatase; and increased excretion of total hydroxyproline in the urine. The only major disorder that mimics Paget's disease is cancer that has metastasized to bone. Osteoblastic metastases such as those from the prostate may be indistinguishable from Paget's lesions on x-ray or radionuclide scanning, and alkaline phosphatase may be increased. The only distinguishing feature may be

Figure 8–33. X-rays of the right femur in a patient with juvenile Paget's disease before *(left)* and after *(right)* 10 months of treatment with calcitonin. Note the advancing V-shaped resorption front (arrow). A striking improvement in the appearance of diseased bone is seen after treatment. (Reproduced, with permission, from Doyle P et al: *Br J Radiol* 1974;**47**:9.)

a marked elevation in the serum level of acid phosphatase in prostatic cancer; this enzyme is only occasionally increased in Paget's disease. In most instances in which metastatic cancer is suspected, confirmation by biopsy either of the primary lesion or of bone metastases is necessary. In contrast, osteolytic lesions such as those that occur in multiple myeloma do not produce markedly abnormal bone scans. Serum alkaline phosphatase may be increased in patients who have metastatic osteolytic lesions due to liver metastases, and fractionation of serum alkaline phosphatase will show that the bulk of the enzyme is not derived from bone. Ultimately, lesions must be biopsied to determine whether bone metastases are present. The development of a sarcoma in association with a pagetic bone lesion is suggested by the appearance of a lytic area within dense bone, a marked increase in pain over the lesion, and an unexplained increase in serum alkaline phosphatase levels.

Treatment

The consensus at present is that only patients with symptoms should be treated. However, the underlying

Figure 8–34. Bone scan of patient with severe Paget's disease of the skull, ribs, spine, pelvis, right femur, and acetabulum. Note localization of bone-seeking isotope (^{99m}Tc-labeled diphosphonate) in these areas.

calcitonin or diphosphonate treatment in an individual patient is almost arbitrary. The advantage of calcitonin is that radiologic evidence of healing has been observed in some patients after treatment. The advantage of diphosphonates is that they can be administered orally. Osteogenic sarcoma developing in pagetic lesions is virtually unresponsive to any form of therapy.

The treatment of juvenile Paget's disease is similar to the treatment of adult Paget's disease, although calcitonin appears to be the drug of choice.

A. Calcitonin: In North America, only synthetic salmon calcitonin (Calcimar) is presently available, but synthetic human calcitonin should be available soon. Porcine calcitonin, extracted from pig thyroid glands, was used in the initial pharmacologic studies of treatment of Paget's disease; its availability is limited, and there is no reason to prefer it over salmon or human calcitonin.

The rationale for the use of calcitonin is that it decreases bone resorption. When administered to patients with Paget's disease in doses of about 100 units/d subcutaneously or intramuscularly, it markedly decreases the number of active osteoclasts. Urinary hydroxyproline decreases within 24 hours after the initial injection, but serum alkaline phosphatase does not begin to fall until approximately 2 weeks after treatment is started. Brief but significant hypocalcemia and hypophosphatemia occur shortly after administration, and appropriate increases in serum iPTH in response to the hypocalcemia have been observed. Serum calcium, phosphate, and iPTH return to normal within 4–6 hours and remain so until calcitonin is administered again. Negative calcium balance improves, with decreases in urinary and fecal calcium excretion. Radiologic improvement may not occur for months or years; the criteria for healing are decreased bone volume, increased density of cortices with restoration of a normal corticomedullary junction, and restoration of normal trabecular bone. Histomorphometry of bone biopsy specimens is difficult to evaluate because of the dynamics of untreated pagetic lesions. It has been shown, however, that along with a decrease in osteoclast numbers, there is a decrease in the surface of bone covered by osteoblasts, as well as replacement of woven bone by lamellar bone.

Although it is difficult to evaluate pain objectively, there is apparent relief of pain and bone tenderness within weeks following initiation of therapy. Objective signs of response include a decrease in redness and heat of the skin over involved bones and decreases in cardiac output. Neurologic signs (when present) may improve, but hearing rarely improves. Withdrawal of calcitonin treatment usually results in the return of symptoms and progression of bone lesions.

On the basis of decreases in alkaline phosphatase and urinary excretion of hydroxyproline, it appears that most patients given calcitonin have good long-term responses. However, some patients respond only briefly, with the indices returning to previously high levels in months. Others experience prolonged re-

cause of symptoms is sometimes difficult to determine because the pain of degenerative arthritis often mimics that of Paget's disease. When doubt exists, a therapeutic trial of nonsteroidal anti-inflammatory agents should be given before therapy for Paget's disease is initiated. In patients who fail to respond to these agents, one of several courses can be followed; each has its advantages and disadvantages. Before any treatment is started, patients with mild disease and without deformity should be reassured that most patients with the disease do not develop the disfiguring deformities they may have read or heard about.

During the last 10 years, calcitonin, diphosphonates, and mithramycin have become available for treatment. They all suppress the number and activity of the abnormal bone cells, but they act by different mechanisms. As will be noted below, mithramycin is a toxic drug of last resort. Presently, the choice of missions followed by late recrudescence of the disease. There is no rational explanation for these relapses except in a very few patients who develop high titers of calcitonin antibodies when a nonhuman species of calcitonin is used. In such cases, human calcitonin usually produces a remission.

The ideal dose and schedule for treatment of Paget's disease with calcitonin have not been determined. It is conventional to give 100 Medical Research Council (MRC) units subcutaneously per day, although therapeutic effects have been observed at half this dose. Patients generally administer the drug themselves with a tuberculin syringe after instruction about rotation of injection sites. In patients with Paget's disease who also have hypercalcemia due to immobilization, higher doses (200–400 MRC units) should be given intravenously by slow infusion over 24 hours. A dramatic decrease in serum calcium usually occurs.

Some patients develop side effects that necessitate discontinuation of treatment. These include flushing, fatigue, nausea, diarrhea, vomiting, pain at the injection site, rash, and a sense of being disconnected from reality. In most cases, these symptoms can be minimized by administering calcitonin at bedtime or lowering the dosage.

Low titers of antibodies to salmon calcitonin develop in about half of patients, but only 10% develop antibody titers high enough to cause relapse. In such cases, human calcitonin should be used (if available), since it has not been shown to produce antibodies.

B. Diphosphonate: The diphosphonates are analogs of pyrophosphate, with a P–C–P rather than a P–O–P structure, and are resistant to enzymatic and chemical hydrolysis. They are adsorbed onto the surface of bone mineral and thus inhibit both bone resorption and formation. Evidence indicates that they also are taken up by bone cells and may interfere with bone cell activity.

Currently, only etidronate disodium (Didronel) is available in North America. In doses of 5 mg/kg/d orally, etidronate disodium causes a dramatic decrease in serum alkaline phosphatase and total urinary hydroxyproline excretion, as well as symptomatic im-

provement in most patients with Paget's disease. Unfortunately, the intestinal absorption of this drug is inconstant, so that it must be given after an overnight fast or 2–3 hours after a meal. Most of the drug accumulates in bone and is not metabolized. It is excreted unchanged in the urine. If it is well absorbed, doses higher than 5 mg/kg/d may cause osteomalacia.

Etidronate is given in courses of about 3–6 months and is reinstituted when serum alkaline phosphatase and total hydroxyproline levels increase after remission. Remissions vary in duration but have lasted as long as 2 years or more. Pagetic lesions have been shown to regress histologically in bone biopsies, but radiographic evidence of healing has rarely been reported.

Etidronate causes few side effects. Diarrhea occurs occasionally but can often be prevented by administering the agent with foods low in calcium content; this decreases absorption to a variable degree, but patients still achieve therapeutic effects. Serum concentrations of phosphate increase within a week after starting treatment, especially with doses larger than 5 mg/kg, but serum concentrations of calcium remain normal, and there is no change in serum iPTH. The effect on serum phosphate is probably related to the drug's effect on renal tubular handling of phosphate.

In patients with very severe disease or in those who fail to respond to either drug, larger doses (eg, 10–15 mg/kg/d of etidronate) or alternating or combination therapy with etidronate and calcitonin may produce a biochemical response.

C. Mithramycin: As noted in the discussion of the treatment of hypercalcemia, mithramycin (Mithracin) is a cytotoxic antibiotic that inhibits RNA synthesis. It decreases serum alkaline phosphatase levels and urinary hydroxyproline excretion in patients with Paget's disease. It is given intravenously in doses of about 10–15 μg/kg at weekly intervals until biochemical remission occurs or toxic effects appear. Toxicity may be severe and includes liver dysfunction, renal failure, and suppression of platelet production. For this reason, it should be used only under the most desperate circumstances (eg, spinal cord compression).

REFERENCES

EXTRACELLULAR & BONE MINERAL HOMEOSTASIS

Albright F, Reifenstein EC Jr: *The Parathyroid Glands and Metabolic Bone Disease.* Williams & Wilkins, 1948.

Arnaud CD: Calcium homeostasis: Regulatory elements and their integration. *Fed Proc* 1978;**37**:2557.

Aurbach GD (editor): Vol 7: Parathyroid Gland. Section 7: *Endocrinology.* In: *Handbook of Physiology.* Greep RO, Astwood EB (editors). Williams & Wilkins, 1976.

Aurbach GD et al: Parathyroid hormone, calcitonin and the calciferols. Page 922 in: *Textbook of Endocrinology,* 6th ed. Williams RH (editor). Saunders, 1981.

Avioli LV, Raisz LG: Bone metabolism and disease. Page 1709 in: *Metabolic Control and Disease.* Bondy PK, Rosenberg LE (editors). Saunders, 1980.

Bringhurst FR, Potts JT: Calcium and phosphate distribution, turnover and metabolic actions. Page 551 in: *Endocrinology.* Vol 2. DeGroot LJ et al (editors). Grune & Stratton, 1979.

Neer RM: Calcium and inorganic phosphate homeostasis. Page 669 in: *Endocrinology.* Vol 2. DeGroot LJ et al (editors). Grune & Stratton, 1979.

Raisz LG: Bone metabolism and calcium regulation. Page 32 in: *Metabolic Bone Disease.* Vol 1. Avioli LV, Krane SM (editors). Academic Press, 1977.

Rasmussen H, Bordier P: *The Physiology and Cellular Basis of Metabolic Bone Disease.* Williams & Wilkins, 1974.

PARATHYROID HORMONE

Structure & Biosynthesis

Cohn DV, Elting JJ: Synthesis and secretion of parathormone and secretory protein I by the parathyroid gland. Page 1 in: *Bone and Mineral Research Annual 2*. Peck WA (editor). Elsevier, 1984.

Habener JF et al: Parathyroid hormone: Biochemical aspects of biosynthesis, secretion, action, and metabolism. *Physiol Rev* 1984;**64**:985.

Kemper B et al: Structure and function of bovine parathyroid hormone messenger RNA. Page 19 in: *Proceedings of the Seventh International Conference on Calcium Regulating Hormones*. Cohn DV, Talmage RV, Mathews JL (editors). Excerpta Medica, 1981.

Keutmann H: Chemistry of parathyroid hormone. Page 593 in: *Endocrinology*. Vol 2. DeGroot LJ et al (editors). Grune & Stratton, 1979.

Kronenberg HM et al: Studies of parathyroid hormone biosynthesis using recombinant DNA technology. Page 5 in: *Proceedings of the Seventh International Conference on Calcium Regulating Hormones*. Cohn DV, Talmage RV, Mathews JL (editors). Excerpta Medica, 1981.

Control of Secretion

Anast CS et al: Evidence for parathyroid failure in magnesium deficiency. *Science* 1972;**177**:606.

Brown EM et al: Set-point for calcium: Its role in normal and abnormal parathyroid secretion. Page 35 in: *Proceedings of the Seventh International Conference on Calcium Regulating Hormones*. Cohn DV, Talmage RV, Mathews JL (editors). Excerpta Medica, 1981.

Cohn DV, Elting JJ: Synthesis and secretion of parathormone and secretory protein I by the parathyroid gland. Page 1 in: *Bone and Mineral Research Annual 2*. Peck WA (editor). Elsevier, 1984.

Cohn DV et al: Secretion of parathormone from two independently controlled intracellular pools. Page 28 in: *Proceedings of the Seventh International Conference on Calcium Regulating Hormones*. Cohn DV, Talmage RV, Mathews JL (editors). Excerpta Medica, 1981.

Fischer JA et al: The acute parathyroid hormone response to changes in ionized calcium during phosphate infusions. *Eur J Clin Invest* 1973;**3**:151.

Fischer JA et al: Acute parathyroid hormone response to epinephrine in vivo. *J Clin Invest* 1973;**52**:2434.

Fischer JA et al: Regulation of parathyroid hormone secretion in vitro and in vivo. *Calcif Tissue Int* 1982;**34**:313.

Heath H III: Biogenic amines and the secretion of parathyroid hormone and calcitonin. *Endocr Rev* 1980;**1**:319.

Mayer GP: Parathyroid hormone secretion. Page 607 in: *Endocrinology*. Vol 2. DeGroot LJ et al (editors). Grune & Stratton, 1979.

Oldham SB et al: Dynamics of parathyroid hormone secretion in vitro. *Am J Med* 1971;**50**:650.

Metabolism & Circulating Forms

Berson SA, Yalow RS: Immunochemical heterogeneity of parathyroid hormone in plasma. *J Clin Endocrinol Metab* 1968;**28**:1037.

DiBella FP et al: Hyperfunctioning parathyroid glands: Major source of immunoheterogeneity. Proceedings of the Sixth Parathyroid Conference. *Excerpta Medica* 1978;**421**:337.

Fischer JA et al: Calcium-regulated parathyroid hormone peptidase. *Proc Natl Acad Sci USA* 1972;**69**:2341.

Flueck JA et al: Immunoheterogeneity of parathyroid hormone in venous effluent serum from hyperfunctioning parathyroid glands. *J Clin Invest* 1977;**60**:1367.

Hruska KA et al: Metabolism of immunoreactive parathyroid hormone in the dog: Role of the kidney and the effect of chronic renal disease. *J Clin Invest* 1975;**56**:39.

Martin KV et al: The peripheral metabolism of parathyroid hormone. *N Engl J Med* 1979;**301**:1092.

Martin KV et al: Selective uptake of intact parathyroid hormone by the liver: Differences between hepatic and renal uptake. *J Clin Invest* 1976;**58**:781.

Mayer GP et al: Effects of plasma calcium concentrations on the relative proportion of hormone and carboxyl-terminal fragments in parathyroid venous blood. *Endocrinology* 1979;**104**:1778.

Segre GV: Heterogeneity and metabolism of parathyroid hormone. Page 613 in: *Endocrinology*. Vol 2. DeGroot LJ et al (editors). Grune & Stratton, 1979.

Segre GV et al: Parathyroid hormone in human plasma: Immunochemical characterization and biological implications. *J Clin Invest* 1972;**51**:3163.

Silverman R, Yalow RS: Heterogeneity of parathyroid hormone. *J Clin Invest* 1973;**52**:1958.

Actions

Albright F, Reifenstein EC Jr: *The Parathyroid Glands and Metabolic Bone Disease*. Williams & Wilkins, 1948.

Bijvoet OLM: Kidney function in calcium and phosphate metabolism. Page 118 in: *Metabolic Bone Disease*. Vol 1. Avioli LV, Krane SM (editors). Academic Press, 1977.

Dennis VW et al: Renal handling of phosphate and calcium. *Annu Rev Physiol* 1979;**41**:257.

Klahr S, Hruska KA: Effects of parathyroid hormone on the renal reabsorption of phosphorus and divalent cations. Page 65 in: *Bone and Mineral Research Annual 2*. Peck WA (editor). Elsevier, 1984.

Knox FG et al: Phosphate transport along the nephron. *Am J Physiol* 1977;**233**:261.

Parsons JA: Parathyroid physiology and the skeleton. Page 159 in: *Biochemistry and Physiology of Bone*. Vol 4. Bourne GH (editor). Academic Press, 1976.

Raisz LG: Bone metabolism and calcium regulation. Page 32 in: *Metabolic Bone Disease*. Vol 1. Avioli LV, Krane SM (editors). Academic Press, 1977.

Shelling DH: *The Parathyroids in Health and Disease*. Mosby, 1935.

Mechanisms of Action

Arnaud CD et al: Further studies on the interrelationship between parathyroid hormone and vitamin D. *J Clin Invest* 1966;**45**:1955.

Aurbach GD, Chase LR: Cyclic 3′,5′-adenylic acid in bone and the mechanism of action of parathyroid hormone. *Fed Proc* 1970;**29**:1179.

Draper MW: The structure of parathyroid hormone: Its effects on biological action. *Mineral Electrolyte Metab* 1982;**8**:159.

Draper MW et al: Photoaffinity labeling of the canine renal receptor for parathyroid hormone. *J Biol Chem* 1982;**257**:3714.

Dziak R, Stern PH: Calcium transport in isolated bone cells. 3. Effects of parathyroid hormone and cyclic 3′,5′-AMP. *Endocrinology* 1975;**97**:1281.

Forte L, Nichols GA, Anast CS: Renal adenylate cyclase and the interrelationship between parathyroid hormone and vitamin D in the regulation of urinary phosphate and adenosine cyclic 3′,5′monophosphate excretion. *J Clin Invest* 1976;**57**:559.

Goltzman D: Biochemical mode of action of parathyroid hormone. Page 631 in: *Endocrinology*. Vol 2. DeGroot LJ et al (editors). Grune & Stratton, 1979.

Klahr S, Hruska KA: Effects of parathyroid hormone on the renal reabsorption of phosphorus and divalent cations. Page 65 in: *Bone and Mineral Research Annual 2*. Peck WA (editor). Elsevier, 1984.

Nissenson RA: Functional properties of parathyroid hormone receptors. *Mineral Electrolyte Metab* 1982;**8**:151.

Nissenson RA et al: Parathyroid hormone receptors in kidney and bone: Relation to adenylate cyclase activation. Page 44 in: *Proceedings of the Seventh International Conference on Calcium Regulating Hormones*. Cohn DV, Talmage RV, Mathews JL (editors). Excerpta Medica, 1981.

Rasmussen H, Pechet M, Fast D: Effect of dibutyryl cyclic adenosine 3',5'-monophosphate, theophylline and other nucleotides upon calcium and phosphate metabolism. *J Clin Invest* 1968;**47**:1843.

Rasmussen H et al: The relationship between vitamin D and parathyroid hormone. *J Clin Invest* 1963;**42**:1940.

Teitelbaum AP et al: Coupling of the canine renal parathyroid hormone receptor to adenylate cyclase: Modulation by guanyl nucleotides and N-ethylmaleimide. *Endocrinology* 1982;**111**:1524.

Assay in Biologic Fluids

Arnaud C, Tsao HS, Littledike ET: Radioimmunoassay of human parathyroid hormone in serum. *J Clin Invest* 1971;**50**:21.

Arnaud CD et al: Influence of immunoheterogeneity of circulating parathyroid hormone on results of radioimmunoassays of serum in man. *Am J Med* 1974;**56**:785.

Berson SA et al: Immunoassay of bovine and human parathyroid hormone. *Proc Natl Acad Sci USA* 1963; **49**:613.

Bikle DD (editor): *Assay of Calcium-Regulating Hormones*. Springer-Verlag, 1983.

Fischer JA, Binswanger U, Dietrich FM: Human parathyroid hormone: Immunological characterization of antibodies against a glandular extract and the synthetic amino-terminal fragments 1–12 and 1–34 and their use in the determination of immunoreactive hormone in human sera. *J Clin Invest* 1974;**54**:1382.

Frame B, Potts JT (editors): Clinical application of parathyroid hormone assays. Page 3 of: *Clinical Disorders of Bone and Mineral Metabolism*. Section I. International Congress Series 617. Excerpta Medica, 1983.

Goltzman D et al: Cytochemical bioassay of parathyroid hormone: Characteristics of the assay and analysis of circulating hormonal forms. *J Clin Invest* 1980;**65**:1309.

Nissenson RA et al: Endogenous biologically active human parathyroid hormone: Measurement by guanyl nucleotide-amplified renal adenylate cyclase assay. *J Clin Endocrinol Metab* 1981;**52**:840.

CALCITONIN

Austin LA, Heath HH III: Calcitonin: Physiology and pathophysiology. *N Engl J Med* 1981;**304**:269.

Austin LA et al: Regulation of calcitonin secretion in normal man by changes of serum calcium within the physiologic range. *J Clin Invest* 1979;**64**:1721.

Bikle DD (editor): *Assay of Calcium-Regulating Hormones*. Springer-Verlag, 1983.

Heath HH III, Sizemore GW: Plasma calcitonin in normal man: Differences between men and women. *J Clin Invest* 1977;**60**:1135.

Owyang C et al: Comparison of the effects of pentagastrin injection and meal-stimulated gastrin on plasma calcitonin in normal man. *Am J Dig Dis* 1978;**23**:1084.

Pont A: Secretion and metabolism of calcitonin in man. Page 641 in: *Endocrinology*. Vol 2. DeGroot LJ et al (editors). Grune & Stratton, 1979.

Potts JT, Aurbach GD: Chemistry of the calcitonins. Page 423 of Vol 7: Parathyroid Gland. Section 7: *Endocrinology*. In: *Handbook of Physiology*. Greep RO, Astwood EB (editors). Williams & Wilkins, 1976.

Talmage RV, Cooper CW: Physiology and mode of action of calcitonin. Page 647 in: *Endocrinology*. Vol 2. DeGroot LJ et al (editors). Grune & Stratton, 1979.

Talmage RV et al: The physiological significance of calcitonin. Page 74 in: *Bone and Mineral Research Annual 1*. Peck WA (editor). Excerpta Medica, 1983.

VITAMIN D

Bikle DD (editor): *Assay of Calcium-Regulating Hormones*. Springer-Verlag, 1983.

Bikle DD: The vitamin D endocrine system. Page 45 in: *Advances in Internal Medicine*. Stollerman GH (editor). Year Book, 1982.

Cohn DV et al (editors): Mechanism of action of vitamin D. Page 229 in: *Endocrine Control of Bone and Calcium Metabolism*. Section VII. International Congress Series 619. Excerpta Medica, 1984.

DeLuca HF: Metabolism and mechanism of action of vitamin D. Page 7 in: *Bone and Mineral Research Annual 1*. Peck WA (editor). Elsevier, 1983.

DeLuca HF, Holick MF: Vitamin D: Biosynthesis, metabolism and mode of action. Page 653 in: *Endocrinology*. Vol 2. DeGroot LJ et al (editors). Grune & Stratton, 1979.

Eisman JE et al: 1,25-Dihydroxyvitamin D in biological fluids: A simplified and sensitive assay. *Science* 1976;**193**:1021.

Frame B, Potts JT (editors): Vitamin D in clinical medicine. Page 65 of: *Clinical Disorders of Bone and Mineral Metabolism*. Section III. International Congress Series 617. Excerpta Medica, 1983.

Manolagas SC, Deftos LJ: The vitamin D endocrine system and the hematolymphopoietic tissue. (Editorial.) *Ann Intern Med* 1984;**100**:144.

Normal AW et al (editors): *Vitamin D: Chemical, Biochemical and Clinical Endocrinology of Calcium Metabolism. Proceedings of the Fifth Workshop on Vitamin D*. Walter de Gruyter, 1982.

DISORDERS OF PARATHYROID FUNCTION

Hypoparathyroidism

Avioli LV: The therapeutic approach to hypoparathyroidism. *Am J Med* 1974;**57**:34.

Kooh SW et al: Treatment of hypoparathyroidism and pseudohypoparathyroidism with metabolites of vitamin D: Evidence for impaired conversion of 25-hydroxyvitamin D to 1,25 dihydroxyvitamin D. *N Engl J Med* 1975;**293**:840.

Lewis T: Trousseau's phenomenon in tetany. *Clin Sci* 1942;**4**:361.

Medalle R, Waterhouse C: A magnesium-deficient patient presenting with hypocalcemia and hyperphosphatemia. *Ann Intern Med* 1972;**79**:76.

Neer RM et al: Effect of 1α-hydroxyvitamin D_3 and 1,25-dihydroxyvitamin D_3 on calcium and phosphorus metabolism in hypoparathyroidism. *Metabolism* 1975;**24**:1403.

Nusynowitz ML, Frame B, Kolb FO: The spectrum of the hypoparathyroid states. *Medicine* 1976;**55**:105.

Palmer RF, Searles HH, Boldrey EB: Papilledema and hypoparathyroidism simulating brain tumor. *J Neurosurg* 1959;**16**:378.

Parfitt AM: The incidence of hypoparathyroid tetany after thyroid operations: Relationship to age, extent of resection and surgical experience. *Med J Aust* 1971;**1**:1103.

Parfitt AM: The spectrum of hypoparathyroidism. *J Clin Endocrinol Metab* 1972;**34**:152.

Parfitt AM: Surgical, idiopathic and other varieties of parathyroid hormone–deficient hypoparathyroidism. Page 755 in: *Endocrinology*. Vol 2. DeGroot LJ et al (editors). Grune & Stratton, 1979.

Porter RH et al: Treatment of hypoparathyroid patients with chlorthalidone. *N Engl J Med* 1978;**298**:577.

Rude RK, Oldham SB, Singer FR: Functional hypoparathyroidism and parathyroid hormone end-organ resistance in human magnesium deficiency. *Clin Endocrinol* 1976; **5**:209.

Rude RK et al: PTH secretion in magnesium deficiency. *J Clin Endocrinol Metab* 1978;**47**:800.

Russell R: Hypoparathyroidism and malabsorption. *Br Med J* 1967;**3**:781.

Spinner MW et al: Familial distribution of organ-specific antibodies in the blood of patients with Addison's disease and hypoparathyroidism and their relatives. *Clin Exp Immunol* 1969;**5**:461.

Suh SM et al: Pathogenesis of hypocalcemia in primary hypomagnesemia: Normal end-organ responsiveness to parathyroid hormine, impaired parathyroid gland function. *J Clin Invest* 1973;**52**:153.

Pseudohypoparathyroidism
& Pseudopseudohypoparathyroidism

Albright F et al: Pseudohypoparathyroidism: An example of the "Seabright-bantam syndrome." *Endocrinology* 1942;**20**:922.

Chase LR, Melson GL, Aurbach GD: Pseudohypoparathyroidism: Defective excretion of 3′,5′-AMP in response to parathyroid hormone. *J Clin Invest* 1969;**48**:1822.

Costello JM, Dent CE: Hypo-hyperparathyroidism. *Arch Dis Child* 1963;**38**:397.

Drezner M, Neelon FA, Lebavitz HE: Pseudohypoparathyroidism type II: A possible defect in the reception of the cyclic AMP signal. *N Engl J Med* 1973;**289**:1056.

Frame B, Potts JT (editors): Pseudohypoparathyroidism (PHP) and related disorders. Page 449 in: *Clinical Disorders of Bone and Mineral Metabolism*. Section XVII. International Congress Series 617. Excerpta Medica, 1983.

Kolb FO, Steinbach HL: Pseudohypoparathyroidism with secondary hyperparathyroidism and osteitis fibrosa. *J Clin Endocrinol Metab* 1962;**22**:59.

Kooh SW et al: Treatment of hypoparathyroidism and pseudohypoparathyroidism with metabolites of vitamin D to 1,25-dihydroxyvitamin D. *N Engl J Med* 1975;**293**:840.

Potts JT Jr: Pseudohypoparathyroidism. Page 769 in: *Endocrinology*. Vol 2. DeGroot LJ et al (editors). Grune & Stratton, 1979.

Sinha TK, Bell NH: 1,25-Dihydroxyvitamin D_3 and pseudohypoparathyroidism. *N Engl J Med* 1976;**294**:612.

Van Dop C, Bourne HR: Pseudohypoparathyroidism. *Annu Rev Med* 1983;**34**:259.

Primary Hyperparathyroidism

Benson RC et al: Immunoreactive forms of circulating parathyroid hormone in primary and ectopic hyperparathyroidism. *J Clin Invest* 1974;**54**:175.

Benson RC et al: Radioimmunoassay of parathyroid hormone in hypercalcemic patients with malignant disease. *Am J Med* 1974;**56**:821.

Broadus AE, Stewart AF: Humoral mechanisms of hypercalcemia. Page 311 in: *Bone and Mineral Research Annual 2*. Peck WA (editor). Elsevier, 1984.

Broadus AE et al: A detailed evaluation of oral phosphate therapy in selected patients with primary hyperparathyroidism. *J Clin Endocrinol Metab* 1983;**56**:953.

Broadus AE et al: Nephrogenous cyclic adenosine monophosphate as a parathyroid function test. *J Clin Invest* 1977;**60**:771.

Christenssen T et al: Prevalence of hypercalcemia in health screening in Stockholm. *Acta Med Scand* 1976;**200**:131.

Clark OH, Way LW, Hunt TK: Recurrent hyperparathyroidism. *Ann Surg* 1976;**184**:391.

Dauphine RT, Riggs BL, Scholz DA: Back pain and vertebral crush fractures: An unemphasized mode of presentation for primary hyperparathyroidism. *Ann Intern Med* 1975;**83**:365.

Doppman JL: Parathyroid localization: Arteriography and venous sampling. *Radiol Clin North Am* 1976;**14**:163.

Doppman JL et al: Computed tomography for parathyroid localization. *J Comput Assist Tomogr* 1977;**1**:30.

Foley TP Jr et al: Familial benign hypercalcemia. *J Pediatr* 1972;**81**:1060.

Frame B, Potts JT (editors): Management of hypercalcemic hyperparathyroidism. Page 149 in: *Clinical Disorders of Bone and Mineral Metabolism*. Section VI. International Congress Series 617. Excerpta Medica, 1983.

Frame B, Potts JT (editors): Pathogenesis of hyperparathyroidism. Page 129 in: *Clinical Disorders of Bone and Mineral Metabolism*. Section V. International Congress Series 617. Excerpta Medica, 1983.

Gallagher JC, Wilkinson R: The effect of ethinylestradiol on calcium and phosphorus metabolism of post-menopausal women with primary hyperparathyroidism. *Clin Sci Mol Med* 1973;**34**:785.

Gaz RD, Wang CA: Management of asymptomatic hyperparathyroidism. *Am J Surg* 1984;**147**:498.

Genant HK et al: Primary hyperparathyroidism: A comprehensive study of clinical, biochemical and radiographic manifestations. *Radiology* 1973;**109**:513.

Goldsmith RE et al: Familial hyperparathyroidism: Description of a large kindred with physiological observations and a review of the literature. *Ann Intern Med* 1976;**94**:36.

Habener JF, Potts JT Jr: Clinical features of primary hyperparathyroidism. Page 693 in: *Endocrinology*. Vol 2. DeGroot LJ et al (editors). Grune & Stratton, 1979.

Heath H III, Hodgson SF, Kennedy MA: Primary hyperparathyroidism: Incidence, morbidity, and potential economic impact in a community. *N Engl J Med* 1980;**302**:189.

Heath H III, Purnell DC: Asymptomatic hypercalcemia and primary hyperparathyroidism. Page 189 in: *Calcium Disorders*. Heath DA, Marx SJ (editors). Butterworth, 1982.

Heath H III, Purnell DC: Urinary cyclic 3′,5′-adenosine monophosphate responses to exogenous and endogenous parathyroid hormone in familial benign hypercalcemia and primary hyperparathyroidism. *J Lab Clin Med* 1980;**96**:974.

Lambert PW, Heath H III, Sizemore GW: Pre- and postoperative studies of plasma calcitonin in primary hyperparathyroidism. *J Clin Invest* 1979;**63**:602.

Marcus R et al: Conjugated estrogen in the treatment of postmenopausal women with hyperparathyroidism. *Ann Intern Med* 1984;**100**:633.

Marx SJ et al: Adenosine 3',5'-monophosphate response to parathyroid hormone: Familial hypocalciuric hypercalcemia versus typical primary hyperparathyroidism. *J Clin Endocrinol Metab* 1980;**50**:546.

Neer RM, Potts JT Jr: Medical management of hypercalcemia and hyperparathyroidism. Page 725 in: *Endocrinology.* Vol 2. DeGroot LJ et al (editors). Grune & Stratton, 1979.

Okerlund MD et al: A new method with high sensitivity and specificity for localization of abnormal parathyroid glands. *Ann Surg* 1984;**200**:381.

Prinz RA et al: Radiation associated hyperparathyroidism: A new syndrome? *Surgery* 1977;**82**:296.

Purnell DC et al: Primary hyperparathyroidism: A prospective clinical study. *Am J Med* 1971;**50**:670.

Purnell DC et al: Treatment of primary hyperparathyroidism. *Am J Med* 1974;**56**:800.

Rude RK et al: Urinary and nephrogenous adenosine 3',5'-monophosphate in the hypercalcemia of malignancy. *J Clin Endocrinol Metab* 1981;**52**:765.

Scheible W, Deutsch AL, Leopold GR: Parathyroid adenoma: Accuracy of preoperative localization by high-resolution real-time sonography. *JCU* 1981;**9**:325.

Scholz DA, Purnell DC: Asymptomatic primary hyperparathyroidism: Ten-year prospective study. *Mayo Clin Proc* 1981;**56**:473.

Seyberth HW et al: Prostaglandins as mediators of hypercalcemia associated with certain types of cancer. *N Engl J Med* 1975;**293**:1278.

Stark DD et al: Parathyroid imaging: Comparison of high-resolution CT and high-resolution sonography. *AJR* 1983;**141**:633.

Stewart AF et al: Biochemical evaluation of patients with cancer-associated hypercalcemia: Evidence for humoral and nonhumoral groups. *N Engl J Med* 1980;**30**:1377.

Suki WN et al: Acute treatment of hypercalcemia with furosemide. *N Engl J Med* 1970;**283**:836.

Tomlinson S et al: Reversible resistance to the renal action of parathyroid hormone in man. *Clin Sci Mol Med* 1976;**51**:59.

Wang CA: Surgery of the parathyroid glands. *Adv Surg* 1971;**5**:109.

Wells SA Jr et al: Parathyroid autotransplantation in primary parathyroid hyperplasia. *N Engl J Med* 1976;**29**:57.

Secondary Hyperparathyroidism of Chronic Renal Failure

Alfrey AC: Aluminum intoxication. (Editorial.) *N Engl J Med* 1984;**310**:1113.

Arnaud CD: Hyperparathyroidism and renal failure. *Kidney Int* 1973;**4**:80.

Arnaud CD, Goldsmith RS: Successful medical management of osteitis fibrosa due to tertiary hyperparathyroidism. *Mayo Clin Proc* 1972;**47**:110.

Bordier PJ, Marie PJ, Arnaud CD: Evolution of renal osteodystrophy: Correlation of bone histomorphometry and serum mineral and immunoreactive parathyroid hormone values before and after treatment with calcium carbonate or 25-hydroxycholecalciferol. *Kidney Int [Suppl]* 1975;**No. 2**:102.

Bricker NS: On the pathogenesis of the uremic state: An exposition of the "trade-off" hypothesis. *N Engl J Med* 1972;**286**:1093.

Brickman AS et al: Clinical effects of 1,25-dihydroxyvitamin D₃ in uremic patients with overt osteodystrophy. *Contrib Nephrol* 1980;**18**:29.

Coburn J et al: Pathophysiology and treatment of uremic bone disease. (Editorial.) *Calcif Tissue Int* 1983;**35**:712.

Coburn JW et al: A skeletal mineralizing defect in dialysis patients: A syndrome resembling osteomalacia but unrelated to vitamin D. *Contrib Nephrol* 1980;**18**:172.

David DS (editor): *Calcium Metabolism in Renal Failure and Nephrolithiasis.* Wiley, 1981.

Fournier AE et al: Etiology of hyperparathyroidism and bone disease during hemodialysis. 2. Factors affecting serum immunoreactive parathyroid hormone. *J Clin Invest* 1971;**50**:599.

Frame B, Potts JT (editors): Renal osteodystrophy. Page 249 in: *Clinical Disorders of Bone and Mineral Metabolism.* Section X. International Congress Series 617. Excerpta Medica, 1983.

Goldsmith RS et al: Control of secondary hyperparathyroidism during long-term hemodialysis. *Am J Med* 1971;**50**:692.

Johnson WJ et al: Prevention and reversal of progressive secondary hyperparathyroidism in patients maintained by hemodialysis. *Am J Med* 1974;**56**:827.

Massry SG et al: Skeletal resistance to parathyroid hormone in renal failure. *Ann Intern Med* 1973;**78**:357.

Ott SM et al: The prevalence of bone aluminum deposition in renal osteodystrophy and its relation to the response to calcitriol therapy. *N Engl J Med* 1982;**30**:709.

Parker TF et al: Jejunal absorption and secretion of calcium in patients with chronic renal disease on hemodialysis. *J Clin Invest* 1974;**54**:358.

Portale AA et al: Effect of dietary phosphorus on circulating concentrations of 1,25-dihydroxyvitamin D and immunoreactive parathyroid hormone in children with moderate renal insufficiency. *J Clin Invest* 1984;**73**:1580.

Slatopolsky E et al: On the pathogenesis of hyperparathyroidism in chronic experimental and renal insufficiency in the dog. *J Clin Invest* 1971;**50**:492.

Slatopolsky E et al: On the prevention of secondary hyperparathyroidism in experimental chronic renal disease using "proportional reduction" of dietary phosphorus intake. *Kidney Int* 1972;**2**:147.

Stanbury SW, Lumb GA: Parathyroid function in chronic renal failure: A statistical survey of the plasma and biochemistry in azotaemic renal osteodystrophy. *Q J Med* 1966;**35**:1.

DISORDERS OF CALCITONIN SECRETION

Austin LA, Heath H III: Calcitonin, physiology and pathophysiology. *N Engl J Med* 1981;**304**:269.

Chong GC et al: Medullary carcinoma of the thyroid gland. *Cancer* 1975;**35**:695.

Graze K et al: Natural history of familial medullary thyroid carcinoma: Effect of a program for early diagnosis. *N Engl J Med* 1978;**299**:980.

Saad MF et al: The prognostic value of calcitonin immunostaining in medullary carcinoma of the thyroid. *J Clin Endocrinol Metab* 1984;**59**:850.

Schwartz KE et al: Calcitonin in nonthyroidal cancer. *J Clin Endocrinol Metab* 1979;**49**:438.

Silva OL et al: Calcitonin as a marker for bronchogenic cancer. *Cancer* 1979;**44**:680.

Sizemore GW et al: Epidemiology of medullary carcinoma of the thyroid gland: A 5 year experience (1971– 1976). *Surg Clin North Am* 1977;**57**:633.

Williams ED: Medullary carcinoma of the thyroid. Page 777 in: *Endocrinology.* Vol 2. DeGroot LJ et al (editors). Grune & Stratton, 1979.

HYPERCALCIURIA

Chadwick KS et al: Mechanism for hyperoxaluria in patients with ileal dysfunction. *N Engl J Med* 1973;**289**:172.

Coe FL: Treated and untreated recurrent calcium nephrolithiasis in patients with idiopathic hypercalciuria, hyperuricosuria, or no metabolic disorder. *Ann Intern Med* 1977;**87**:404.

Coe FL, Bushinski DA: Pathophysiology of hypercalciuria. *Am J Physiol* 1984;**247**:1.

Coe FL (editor): *Hypercalciuric States: Pathogenesis, Consequences and Treatment*. Grune & Stratton, 1984.

Danielson BG et al: Treatment of idiopathic calcium stone disease. (Editorial.) *Calcif Tissue Int* 1983;**35**:715.

Finlayson B: Calcium stones: Some physical and clinical aspects. Page 337 in: *Calcium Metabolism in Renal Failure and Nephrolithiasis*. David DS (editor). Wiley, 1977.

Frame B, Potts JT (editors): Idiopathic hypercalciuria. Page 401 in: *Clinical Disorders of Bone and Mineral Metabolism*. Section XV. International Congress Series 617. Excerpta Medica, 1983.

Kolb FO: Non-operative management of renal calculi. *J Genitourin Med* (March) 1979;**1**:29.

Pak CY: Ambulatory evaluation of nephrolithiasis. *Am J Med* 1980;**69**:19.

Pak CY (editor): Symposium on urolithiasis. *Kidney Int* 1978;**13**:341.

Pak CY et al: Mechanism for calcium urolithiasis among patients with hyperuricosuria: Supersaturation of urine with respect to monosodium urate. *J Clin Invest* 1977;**59**:426.

Seldin DW, Wilson JD: Renal tubular acidosis. Page 1548 in: *The Metabolic Basis of Inherited Disease*, 4th ed. Stanbury JB et al (editors). McGraw-Hill, 1972.

Shen FH, Baylink DJ: Increased serum 1,25-dihydroxyvitamin D in idiopathic hypercalciuria. *J Lab Clin Med* 1977;**90**:955.

Smith LH et al: Management of cystinuria and cystine-stone disease. *J Urol* 1959;**81**:61.

Smith LH et al: Orthophosphate therapy in calcium renal lithiasis. Page 188 in: *Urinary Calculi*. Delatt LC et al (editors). Karger, 1973.

Thomas WC Jr: *Renal Calculi: A Guide to Management*. Thomas, 1976.

Yendt ER et al: Effects of thiazides in idiopathic hypercalciuria. *Am J Med Sci* 1966;**251**:449.

Yendt ER et al: The use of thiazides in the prevention of renal calculi. *Can Med Assoc J* 1970;**102**:614.

METABOLIC BONE DISEASE

General

Bordier PJ, Tun-Chot S: Quantitative histology of metabolic bone disease. *Clin Endocrinol Metab* 1972;**1**:197.

Byers PD: The diagnostic value of bone biopsies. Page 183 in: *Metabolic Bone Disease*. Vol 1. Avioli LV, Krane SM (editors). Academic Press, 1977.

Frame B, Potts JT (editors): Assessment of trabecular bone status. Page 27 in: *Clinical Disorders of Bone and Mineral Metabolism*. Section II. International Congress Series 617. Excerpta Medica, 1983.

Frost HM: Tetracycline based analysis of bone remodeling. *Calcif Tissue Res* 1969;**3**:211.

Genant HK: Osteoporosis. 1. Advanced radiologic assessment using quantitative computed tomography. *West J Med* 1983;**139**:75.

Health and Public Policy Committee, American College of Physicians: Radiologic methods to evaluate bone mineral content. *Ann Intern Med* 1984;**100**:908.

Jowsey J: *The Bone Biopsy*. Plenum, 1977.

Mazess RB: The noninvasive measurement of skeletal mass. Page 223 in: *Bone and Mineral Research Annual 1*. Peck WA (editor). Excerpta Medica, 1983.

Meunier PJ: Histomorphometry of the skeleton. Page 191 in: *Bone and Mineral Research Annual 1*. Peck WA (editor). Excerpta Medica, 1983.

Meunier PJ, Bersot C: Endocrine influences on bone cells and bone remodeling evaluated by clinical histomorphometry. Page 445 in: *Endocrinology of Calcium Metabolism*. Parson JA (editor). Raven Press, 1982.

Parfitt AM: The cellular basis of bone turnover and bone loss. *Clin Orthop* 1977;**127**:236.

Rasmussen HR, Bordier PJ: *The Physiological and Cellular Basis of Metabolic Bone Disease*. Williams & Wilkins, 1974.

Teitelbaum SL, Bates M: Relationships of static and kinetic hisomorphometric features of bone. *Clin Orthop* 1980; **156**:238.

Osteomalacia

Arnaud CD et al: Serum parathyroid hormone levels in acquired vitamin D deficiency of infancy. *Pediatrics* 1972; **49**:837.

Arnaud CD et al: Serum parathyroid hormone in X-linked hypophosphatemia. *Science* 1971;**173**:845.

Arnaud CD et al: Vitamin D dependency: An inherited postnatal syndrome with secondary hyperparathyroidism. *Pediatrics* 1970;**46**:871.

Arnaud SB et al: 25-Hydroxyvitamin D and the pathogenesis of vitamin D deficiency. Page 229 in: *Pediatric Diseases Related to Calcium*. DeLuca HF, Anast C (editors). Elsevier/North Holland, 1980.

Arnaud SB et al: 25-Hydroxyvitamin D_3: Evidence of an enterohepatic circulation in man. *Proc Soc Exp Biol Med* 1975;**149**:570.

Arnaud SB et al: The interrelationships between vitamin D and parathyroid hormone in disorders of mineral metabolism in man. Page 397 in: *Vitamin D and Problems in Uremic Bone Disease*. Walter de Gruyter, 1975.

Arnaud SB et al: Serum 25-hydroxyvitamin D (25OHD) and the pathogenesis of osteomalacia in patients with nontropical sprue. *Gastroenterology* 1977;**72**:1025.

Balsan S et al: 1,25-Dihydroxyvitamin D_3 and 1α-hydroxyvitamin D_3 in children: Biologic and therapeutic effects in nutritional rickets and different types of vitamin D resistance. *Pediatr Res* 1975;**9**:586.

Bartter FC: Hypophosphatasia. Page 1295 in: *The Metabolic Basis of Inherited Disease*, 3rd ed. Stanbury JB et al (editors). McGraw-Hill, 1972.

Brooks MH et al: Vitamin D dependent rickets type II: Resistance of target organs to 1,25-dihydroxyvitamin D. *N Engl J Med* 1978;**298**:996.

Clow C et al: Management of hereditary metabolic disease: The role of allied health personnel. *N Engl J Med* 1971; **284**:1292.

Dent CE, Smith R: Nutritional osteomalacia. *Q J Med* 1969;**38**:195.

Dent CE, Stamp TCB: Hypophosphatemic osteomalacia presenting in adults. *Q J Med* 1971;**158**:303.

Dent CE, Winter CE: Osteomalacia due to phosphate depletion from excessive aluminum hydroxide ingestion. *Br Med J* 1974;**1**:551.

Drezner MK, Feinglos MN: Osteomalacia due to 1-alpha-25-dihydroxycholecalciferol deficiency: Association with a giant cell tumor of bone. *J Clin Invest* 1977;**60**:1045.

Dunnigan MG et al: Acquired disorders of vitamin D metabolism. Page 125 in: *Calcium Disorders*. Heath DA, Marx SJ (editors). Butterworth, 1982.

Frame B, Parfitt AM: Osteomalacia: Current concepts. *Ann Intern Med* 1978;**89:**966.

Fraser D: Hypophosphatasia. *Am J Med* 1957;**22:**730.

Fraser D et al: Hyperparathyroidism as the cause of hyperaminoaciduria and phosphaturia in human vitamin D deficiency. *Pediatr Res* 1967;**1:**425.

Fraser D et al: Pathogenesis of hereditary vitamin D-dependent rickets: An inborn error of vitamin D metabolism involving defective conversion of 25-hydroxyvitamin D to 1α,25-dihydroxyvitamin D. *N Engl J Med* 1973;**289:**817.

Glorieux FH et al: Use of phosphate and vitamin D to prevent dwarfism and rickets in X-linked hypophosphatemia. *N Engl J Med* 1972;**287:**481.

Goldring SR, Krane SM: Disorders of calcification: Osteomalacia and rickets. Page 853 in: *Endocrinology*. Vol 2. DeGroot LJ et al (editors). Grune & Stratton, 1979.

Haddad JG Jr: Serum 25-hydroxycalciferol levels and bone mass in children on anticonvulsant therapy. *N Engl J Med* 1975;**292:**550.

Maclaren NK, Lifshitz F: Vitamin D-dependency rickets in institutionalized, mentally retarded children on long-term anti-convulsant therapy. 2. The response to 25-hydroxycholecalciferol and vitamin D. *Pediatr Res* 1973;**7:**914.

Morgan DB et al: The osteomalacia syndrome after stomach operations. *Q J Med* 1970;**39:**395.

Morris RC et al: Renal acidosis. *Kidney Int* 1972;**1:**332.

Nassim JR et al: The effects of vitamin D and gluten-free diet in idiopathic steatorrhea. *Q J Med* 1958;**28:**141.

Ryan EA, Reiss E: Oncogenic osteomalacia. *Am J Med* 1984;**77:**501.

Salassa RM, Jowsey J, Arnaud CD: Hypophosphatemic osteomalacia associated with "nonendocrine" tumors. *N Engl J Med* 1970;**283:**65.

Scriver CR et al: Hereditary rickets. Page 1 in: *Calcium Disorders*. Heath DA, Marx SJ (editors). Butterworth, 1982.

Stamp TCB, Round JM: Seasonal changes in human plasma levels of 25-hydroxyvitamin D. *Nature* 1974;**247:**563.

Steinbach HL, Noetzli M: Roentgen appearance of the skeleton in osteomalacia and rickets. *Am J Roentgenol Radium Ther Nucl Med* 1964;**91:**955.

Osteoporosis

Adinoff AD, Hollisten JR: Steroid-induced fractures and bone loss in patients with asthma. *N Engl J Med* 1983;**309:**265.

Aitben JM: The prevention of osteoporosis. Page 47 in: *Calcium Disorders*. Heath DA, Marx SJ (editors). Butterworth, 1982.

Arnaud CD et al: On the role of parathyroid hormone in the osteoporosis of aging. Page 215 in: *Osteoporosis: Recent Advances in Pathogenesis and Treatment*. DeLuca HF et al (editors). University Park Press, 1981.

Avioli LV: Osteoporosis. Page 280 in: *Bone and Mineral Research Annual 1*. Peck WA (editor). Excerpta Medica, 1983.

Avioli LV (editor): *The Osteoporotic Syndrome: Detection, Prevention and Treatment*. Grune & Stratton, 1983.

Baylink DJ: Glucocorticoid-induced osteoporosis. (Editorial.) *N Engl J Med* 1983;**309:**306.

Cann CE et al: Decreased spinal mineral content in amenorrheic women. *JAMA* 1984;**251:**626.

Daniell HW: Osteoporosis of the slender smoker. *Arch Intern Med* 1976;**136:**298.

DeLuca HF et al: Vitamin D and its possible role in etiology and treatment of osteoporosis. Page 203 in: *Osteoporosis: Recent Advances in Pathogenesis and Treatment*. DeLuca HF et al (editors). University Park Press, 1981.

Frame B, Potts JT (editors): Osteoporosis: Pathogenesis, prevention and treatment. Page 317 in: *Clinical Disorders of Bone and Mineral Metabolism*. Section XIII. International Congress Series 617. Excerpta Medica, 1983.

Frost HM: Mechanical microdamage, bone remodelling and osteoporosis: A review. Page 231 in: *Osteoporosis: Recent Advances in Pathogenesis and Treatment*. DeLuca HF et al (editors). University Park Press, 1981.

Gallagher JC, Riggs BL: Current concepts in nutrition: Nutrition and bone disease. *N Engl J Med* 1978;**298:**193.

Gallagher JC et al: Effect of estrogen on calcium absorption and serum vitamin D metabolites in postmenopausal osteoporosis. *J Clin Endocrinol Metab* 1980;**51:**1359.

Gallagher JC et al: Epidemiology of fractures of the proximal femur in Rochester, Minnesota. *Clin Orthop* 1980;**150:**163.

Gallagher JC et al: Examination of prevalence rates of possible risk factors in a population with a fracture of the proximal femur. *Clin Orthop* 1980;**153:**158.

Gallagher JC et al: Intestinal calcium absorption and serum vitamin D metabolites in normal subjects and osteoporotic patients: Effect of age and dietary calcium. *J Clin Invest* 1979;**64:**729.

Genant HK et al: Osteoporosis. 2. Prevention of bone loss and fractures in women and risks of menopausal estrogen therapy. *West J Med* 1983;**139:**204.

Gordan GS, Picchi J, Roof BS: Antifracture efficacy of long-term estrogens for osteoporosis. *Trans Assoc Am Physicians* 1973;**86:**326.

Gruber HE et al: Long-term calcitonin therapy in postmenopausal osteoporosis. *Metabolism* 1984;**33:**295.

Hahn TJ: Corticosteroid-induced osteopenia. *Arch Intern Med* 1978;**138:**882.

Heaney RP: Unified concept of the pathogenesis of osteoporosis: Updated. Page 369 in: *Osteoporosis: Recent Advances in Pathogenesis and Treatment*. DeLuca HF et al (editors). University Park Press, 1981.

Heaney RP, Recker RR: Osteoporosis-related nutritional influences on bone: Calcium. Page 253 in: *Osteoporosis: Recent Advances in Pathogenesis and Treatment*. DeLuca HF et al (editors). University Park Press, 1981.

Heath H III: Athletic women, amenorrhea, and skeletal integrity. (Editorial.) *Ann Intern Med* 1985;**102:**258.

Horsman A et al: The effect of estrogen dose on postmenopausal bone loss. *N Engl J Med* 1983;**309:**1405.

Ireland P, Fordtran JS: Effect of dietary calcium and age on jejunal calcium absorption in humans studied by intestinal perfusion. *J Clin Invest* 1973;**52:**2672.

Jee WS, Clark I: Glucocorticoid-induced osteoporosis. Page 331 in: *Osteoporosis: Recent Advances in Pathogenesis and Treatment*. DeLuca HF et al (editors). University Park Press, 1981.

Jowsey J et al: Calcium and salmon calcitonin in treatment of osteoporosis. *J Clin Endocrinol Metab* 1978;**47:**633.

Lane JM et al: Osteoporosis: Current diagnosis and treatment. *Geriatrics* 1984;**39:**40.

Lindsay R et al: Long-term prevention of postmenopausal osteoporosis by estrogen. *Lancet* 1976;**2:**1038.

Marcus R et al: Menstrual function and bone mass in elite women distance runners: Endocrine and metabolic features. *Ann Intern Med* 1985;**102:**158.

Owen RA et al: The national cost of acute care of hip fractures associated with osteoporosis. *Clin Orthop* 1980;**150:**172.

Peck WA: Corticosteroids and bone. *Calcif Tissue Int* 1984;**36**:4.

Riggs BL: Treatment of osteoporosis with sodium fluoride: An appraisal. Page 366 in: *Bone and Mineral Research Annual 2*. Peck WA (editor). Elsevier, 1984.

Riggs BL, Melton LJ: Evidence for two distinct syndromes of involutional osteoporosis. (Editorial.) *Am J Med* 1983;**75**:899.

Riggs BL et al: Differential changes in bone mineral density of the appendicular skeleton with aging: Relationship to spinal osteoporosis. *J Clin Invest* 1981;**67**:328.

Riggs BL et al: Effect of the fluoride/calcium regimen on vertebral fracture occurrence in postmenopausal osteoporosis. *N Engl J Med* 1982;**306**:446.

Riggs BL et al: Effect of oral therapy with calcium and vitamin D in primary osteoporosis. *J Clin Endocrinol Metab* 1976;**42**:1139.

Riggs BL et al: Short- and long-term effects of estrogen and synthetic anabolic hormones in post-menopausal osteoporosis. *J Clin Invest* 1972;**51**:1659.

Riggs BL et al: A syndrome of osteoporosis, increased parathyroid hormone and inappropriately low 1,25-dihydroxyvitamin D. *Mayo Clin Proc* 1978;**53**:701.

Rigotti NA et al: Osteoporosis in women with anorexia nervosa. *N Engl J Med* 1984;**311**:1601.

Seeman E et al: Risk factors for spinal osteoporosis in men. *Am J Med* 1983;**75**:977.

Seeman E et al: The treatment of postmenopausal and senile osteoporosis. Page 69 in: *Calcium Disorders*. Heath DA, Marx SJ (editors). Butterworth, 1982.

Singh M et al: Femoral trabecular pattern index for evaluation of spinal osteoporosis. *Ann Intern Med* 1972;**77**:63.

Smith DM et al: The loss of bone mineral with aging and its relationship to risk of fracture. *J Clin Invest* 1975;**56**:311.

Tsai K-S et al: Impaired vitamin D metabolism with aging in women: Possible role in pathogenesis of senile osteoporosis. *J Clin Invest* 1984;**73**:1668.

Paget's Disease

Altman RD, Singer F (editors): Proceedings of the KROC Foundation Conference on Paget's Disease of Bone. *Arthritis Rheum* 1980;**23(10-Suppl)**:1073.

Cawley MI: Complications of Paget's disease of bone. *Gerontology* 1983;**29**:276.

Fleish H: Biphosphonates: Mechanisms of action and clinical applications. Page 319 in: *Bone and Mineral Research Annual 1*. Peck WA (editor). Excerpta Medica, 1983.

Frame B, Potts JT (editors): Paget's disease. Page 377 in: *Clinical Disorders of Bone and Mineral Metabolism*. Section XIV. International Congress Series 617. Excerpta Medica, 1983.

Huvos AG et al: Osteogenic sarcoma associated with Paget's disease of bone: A clinicopathologic study of 65 patients. *Cancer* 1983;**52**:1489.

Kanis JA, Russell RGG (editors): Symposium: Diphosphonates and Paget's disease of bone. *Metab Bone Dis Relat Res* 1981;**3**:219.

Krane SM: Etidronate disodium in the treatment of Paget's disease of bone. *Ann Intern Med* 1982;**96**:619.

Perry HM III et al: Alternate calcitonin and etidronate disodium therapy for Paget's bone disease. *Arch Intern Med* 1984;**144**:929.

Singer FR: *Paget's Disease of Bone*. Plenum Press, 1977.

Singer FR, Mills BG: Evidence for a viral etiology of Paget's disease of bone. *Clin Orthop* 1983;**178**:245.

Singer FR, Mills BG: Paget's disease of bone: Etiology and therapeutic aspects. Page 394 in: *Bone and Mineral Research Annual 2*. Peck WA (editor). Elsevier, 1984.

Siris ES, Jacobs TP, Canfield RE: Paget's disease of bone. *Bull NY Acad Med* 1980;**56**:285.

Strewler GJ: Paget's disease of bone. *West J Med* 1984;**140**:763.

Wallach S: Treatment of Paget's disease. *Adv Intern Med* 1982;**27**:1.

9 Glucocorticoids & Adrenal Androgens

J. Blake Tyrrell, MD, & Peter H. Forsham, MD

The adrenal cortex produces several steroid hormones of which the most important are cortisol, aldosterone, and the adrenal androgens. Disorders of the adrenal glands lead to classic endocrinopathies such as Cushing's syndrome, Addison's disease, hyperaldosteronism, and the syndromes of congenital adrenal hyperplasia. This chapter describes the physiology and disorders of the glucocorticoids and the adrenal androgens. Disorders of aldosterone secretion are discussed in Chapter 10 and congenital defects in adrenal hormone biosynthesis in Chapters 10 and 15.

Advances in diagnostic procedures have simplified the evaluation of adrenocortical disorders; in particular, the assay of plasma glucocorticoids, androgens, and ACTH has allowed more rapid and precise diagnosis. In addition, advances in surgical and medical treatment have improved the outlook for patients with these disorders.

EMBRYOLOGY & ANATOMY

Embryology

The adrenal cortex is of mesodermal origin and is identifiable as a separate organ in the 2-month-old fetus. At 2 months' gestation, the cortex is composed of a **fetal zone** and a **definitive zone** similar to the adult adrenal cortex. The adrenal cortex then increases rapidly in size; at mid gestation, it is considerably larger than the kidney and much larger than the adult gland in relation to total body mass. The fetal zone makes up the bulk of the weight of the adrenal cortex at this time.

The fetal adrenal is under the control of ACTH by mid pregnancy, but the fetal zone is deficient in the activity of 3β-hydroxysteroid dehydrogenase (see section on biosynthesis of cortisol and adrenal androgens, below) and thus produces mainly dehydroepiandrosterone (DHEA) and DHEA sulfate, which serve as precursors of maternal-placental estrogen production after conversion in the liver to 16α-hydroxylated derivatives. The definitive zone synthesizes a number of steroids and is the major site of fetal cortisol synthesis.

Anatomy

The anatomic relationship of the fetal and defin-

Acronyms Used in This Chapter

ACTH	Adrenocorticotropic hormone
ADH	Antidiuretic hormone (vasopressin)
cAMP	Cyclic adenosine monophosphate
CBG	Corticosteroid-binding globulin
CRH	Corticotropin-releasing hormone
DHEA	Dehydroepiandrosterone
DNA	Deoxyribonucleic acid
DOC	Deoxycorticosterone
GH	Growth hormone
GnRH	Gonadotropin-releasing hormone
HLA	Human leukocyte antigen
LH	Luteinizing hormone
LPH	Lipotropin
mRNA	Messenger ribonucleic acid
PMN	Polymorphonuclear neutrophil
PRL	Prolactin
PTH	Parathyroid hormone
REM	Rapid eye movement
RNA	Ribonucleic acid
SHBG	Sex hormone–binding globulin
TRH	Thyrotropin-releasing hormone
TSH	Thyroid-stimulating hormone (thyrotropin)

itive zones is maintained until birth, at which time the fetal zone gradually disappears, with a consequent decrease in adrenocortical weight in the 3 months following delivery. During the next 3 years, the adult adrenal cortex develops from cells of the outer layer of the cortex and differentiates into the 3 adult zones: glomerulosa, fasciculata, and reticularis.

The adult adrenal glands, with a combined weight of 8–10 g, lie in the retroperitoneum above or medial to the upper poles of the kidneys (Fig 9–1). A fibrous capsule surrounds the gland; the yellowish outer cortex comprises 90% of the adrenal weight, the inner medulla about 10%.

The adrenal cortex is richly vascularized and receives its main arterial supply from branches of the inferior phrenic artery, the renal arteries, and the aorta. These small arteries form an arterial plexus beneath the capsule and then enter a sinusoidal system that penetrates the cortex and medulla, draining into a single central vein in each gland. The right adrenal vein drains directly into the posterior aspect of the

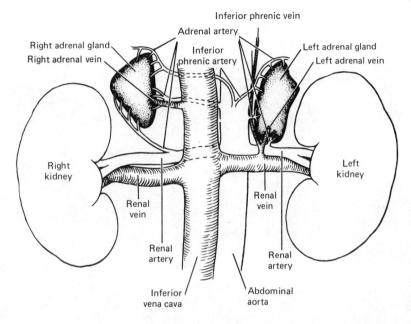

Figure 9–1. Location and blood supply of the adrenal glands (schematic). (Reproduced, with permission, from Baxter JD, Tyrrell JB: The adrenal cortex. In: *Endocrinology and Metabolism.* Felig P et al [editors]. McGraw-Hill, 1981.)

vena cava; the left adrenal vein enters the left renal vein.

Microscopic Anatomy

Histologically, the adult cortex is composed of 3 zones: an outer zona glomerulosa, a zona fasciculata, and an inner zona reticularis (Fig 9–2). However, the inner 2 zones appear to function as a unit (see below). The **zona glomerulosa,** which produces aldosterone, is deficient in 17α-hydroxylase activity and thus cannot produce cortisol or androgens (see below and Chapter 10). The zona glomerulosa lacks a well-defined structure, and the small lipid-poor cells are scattered beneath the adrenal capsule. The **zona fasciculata** is the thickest layer of the adrenal cortex and produces cortisol and androgens. The cells of the zona fasciculata are larger and contain more lipid and thus are termed "clear cells." These cells extend in columns from the narrow zona reticularis to either the zona glomerulosa or to the capsule. The inner **zona reticularis** surrounds the medulla and also produces cortisol and androgens. The "compact" cells of this narrow zone lack significant lipid content but do contain lipofuscin granules. The zonae fasciculata and reticularis are regulated by ACTH; excess or deficiency of this hormone alters their structure and function. Thus, both zones atrophy when ACTH is deficient; when ACTH is present in excess, hyperplasia and hypertrophy of these zones occur. In addition, chronic stimulation with ACTH leads to a gradual depletion of the lipid from the clear cells of the zona fasciculata at the junction of the 2 zones; these cells thus attain the characteristic appearance of the com-

pact reticularis cells. With chronic excessive stimulation, the compact reticularis cells extend outward and may reach the outer capsule. It is postulated that the zona fasciculata cells can respond acutely to ACTH stimulation with increased cortisol production, whereas the reticularis cells maintain basal glucocorticoid secretion and that induced by prolonged ACTH stimulation.

BIOSYNTHESIS OF CORTISOL & ADRENAL ANDROGENS

Steroidogenesis

The major hormones secreted by the adrenal cortex are cortisol, the androgens, and aldosterone. The carbon atoms in the steroid molecule are numbered as shown in Fig 9–3, and the major biosynthetic pathways and hormonal intermediates are illustrated in Figs 9–4 and 9–5.

A. Zones and Steroidogenesis: Because of enzymatic differences between the zona glomerulosa and the inner 2 zones, the adrenal cortex functions as 2 separate units, with differing regulation and secretory products. Thus, the zona glomerulosa, which produces aldosterone, lacks 17α-hydroxylase activity and cannot synthesize 17α-hydroxypregnenolone and 17α-hydroxyprogesterone, which are the precursors of cortisol and the adrenal androgens. The synthesis of aldosterone by this zone is primarily regulated by the renin-angiotensin system and by potassium, as discussed in Chapter 10.

The zona fasciculata and zona reticularis (Fig 9–4)

Figure 9–2. Photomicrographs of the adrenal cortex (H&E stain). *A:* A low-power general view. I, the glomerulosa; II, the fasciculata; III, the reticularis. × 80. *B:* The capsule and the zona glomerulosa. × 330. *C:* The zona fasciculata. × 330. *D:* The zona reticularis. × 330. (Reproduced, with permission, from Junqueira LC, Carneiro J: *Basic Histology*, 5th ed. Lange, 1986.)

CH₃
21
20 C=O
18
CH₃ 17
11 12 13 16
19 C D
CH₃ 9 14 15
1
2 10 8
A B
3 5 7
O 4 6

C21 steroid (progesterone)

O

HO

C19 steroid (dehydroepiandrosterone)

Figure 9–3. Structure of adrenocortical steroids. The letters in the formula for progesterone identify the A, B, C, and D rings; the numbers show the positions in the basic C21 steroid structure. The angular methyl groups (positions 18 and 19) are usually indicated simply by straight lines, as in the lower formula. Dehydroepiandrosterone is a "17-ketosteroid" formed by cleavage of the side chain of the C21 steroid 17-hydroxypregnenolone and its replacement by an O atom. (Reproduced, with permission, from Ganong WF: *Review of Medical Physiology,* 12th ed. Lange, 1985.)

Figure 9–4. Steroid biosynthesis in the zona fasciculata and zona reticularis of the adrenal cortex. The major secretory products are underlined. The enzymes for the reactions are numbered on the left and at the top of the chart, with the steps catalyzed shown by the shaded bars. ① = Cholesterol 20,22-hydroxylase:20,22-desmolase complex; ② = 3β-hydroxysteroid dehydrogenase:Δ⁵-oxosteroid isomerase complex; ③ = 21-hydroxylase; ④ = 11β-hydroxylase; ⑤ = 17α-hydroxylase; ⑥ = 17,20-desmolase; ⑦ = sulfokinase. (Modified and reproduced, with permission, from Ganong WF: *Review of Medical Physiology*, 12th ed. Lange, 1985.)

Cholesterol

Pregnenolone

Progesterone

11-Deoxycorticosterone

Corticosterone

18-Hydroxycorticosterone

Aldosterone

Figure 9–5. Steroid biosynthesis in the zona glomerulosa. The steps from cholesterol to corticosterone are the same as in the zona fasciculata and zona reticularis. However, the zona glomerulosa contains the enzymes for converting corticosterone to aldosterone, whereas it lacks 17α-hydroxylase activity. (Modified and reproduced, with permission, from Ganong WF: *Review of Medical Physiology,* 12th ed. Lange, 1985.)

produce cortisol, androgens, and small amounts of estrogens. These zones, primarily regulated by ACTH, do not contain the enzymatic system necessary to dehydrogenate 18-hydroxycorticosterone and thus do not synthesize aldosterone. (See Chapter 10.)

B. Cholesterol Uptake and Synthesis: Synthesis of cortisol and the androgens by the zonae fasciculata and reticularis begins with cholesterol, as does the synthesis of all steroid hormones. Plasma lipoproteins are the major source of adrenal cholesterol, though synthesis within the gland from acetate also occurs. A small pool of free cholesterol within the adrenal is available for rapid synthesis of steroids when the adrenal is stimulated. When stimulation occurs, there is also increased hydrolysis of stored cholesteryl esters to free cholesterol, increased uptake from plasma lipoproteins, and increased cholesterol synthesis within the gland.

C. Cholesterol Metabolism: The conversion of cholesterol to pregnenolone is the rate-limiting step

in adrenal steroidogenesis and the major site of ACTH action on the adrenal. This step occurs in the mitochondria, is mediated by the side-chain cleavage enzyme complex (cholesterol 20,22-hydroxylase:20,22-desmolase), and involves 2 hydroxylations and then the side-chain cleavage of cholesterol. Pregnenolone is then transported outside the mitochondria before further steroid synthesis occurs.

D. Synthesis of Cortisol: Cortisol synthesis proceeds by the 17α-hydroxylation of pregnenolone within the smooth endoplasmic reticulum to form 17α-hydroxypregnenolone. This steroid is then converted to 17α-hydroxyprogesterone after conversion of its 5,6 double bond to a 4,5 double bond by the 3β-hydroxysteroid dehydrogenase:Δ⁵-oxosteroid isomerase enzyme complex, which is also located within the smooth endoplasmic reticulum. An alternative but apparently less important pathway in the zonae fasciculata and reticularis is from pregnenolone → progesterone → 17α-hydroxyprogesterone (Fig 9–4).

The next step, which is again microsomal, involves the 21-hydroxylation of 17α-hydroxyprogesterone to form 11-deoxycortisol; this compound is further hydroxylated within mitochondria by 11β-hydroxylase to form cortisol. The zonae fasciculata and reticularis also produce 11-deoxycorticosterone (DOC), 18-hydroxydeoxycorticosterone, corticosterone, and 18-hydroxycorticosterone. However, as noted above, the absence of mitochondrial 18-hydroxysteroid dehydrogenase prevents production of aldosterone by these zones of the adrenal cortex (Fig 9–5).

E. Synthesis of Androgens: The production of adrenal androgens from pregnenolone and progesterone requires prior 17α-hydroxylation and thus does not occur in the zona glomerulosa. The major quantitative production of androgens is by conversion of 17α-hydroxypregnenolone to the 19-carbon compounds (C19 steroids) DHEA and its sulfate conjugate DHEA sulfate. Thus, 17α-hydroxypregnenolone undergoes removal of its 2-carbon side chain at the C17 position by microsomal 17,20-desmolase, yielding DHEA with a keto group at C17. DHEA is then converted to DHEA sulfate by a reversible adrenal sulfokinase. The other major adrenal androgen, androstenedione, is produced from 17α-hydroxyprogesterone by 17,20-desmolase and to a lesser extent from DHEA. Androstenedione can be converted to testosterone, though adrenal secretion of this hormone is minimal. The adrenal androgens, DHEA, DHEA sulfate, and androstenedione, have minimal intrinsic androgenic activity, and they contribute to androgenicity by their peripheral conversion to the more potent androgens testosterone and dihydrotestosterone. Although DHEA and DHEA sulfate are secreted in greater quantities, androstenedione is qualitatively more important, since it is more readily converted peripherally to testosterone.

Regulation of Secretion

A. Secretion of CRH and ACTH: ACTH is the trophic hormone of the zonae fasciculata and reticu-

Figure 9–6. Mechanism of action of ACTH on cortisol-secreting cells of the adrenal cortex. AC = adenylate cyclase; R = receptor. (Reproduced, with permission, from Ganong WF: *Review of Medical Physiology,* 12th ed. Lange, 1985.)

laris and the major regulator of cortisol and androgen production by the adrenal cortex. ACTH in turn is regulated by the hypothalamus and central nervous system via neurotransmitters and corticotropin-releasing hormone (CRH). The neuroendocrine control of CRH and ACTH secretion is discussed in Chapters 3 and 4 and involves 3 mechanisms to be discussed below.

B. ACTH Effects on the Adrenal Cortex: The delivery of ACTH to the adrenal cortex leads to the rapid synthesis and secretion of steroids; plasma levels of these hormones rise within minutes after ACTH administration. ACTH increases RNA, DNA, and protein synthesis. Chronic stimulation leads to adrenocortical hyperplasia and hypertrophy; conversely, ACTH deficiency results in decreased steroidogenesis and is accompanied by adrenocortical atrophy, decreased gland weight, and decreased protein and nucleic acid content.

C. ACTH and Steroidogenesis: ACTH binds to high-affinity plasma membrane receptors of adrenocortical cells, thereby activating adenylate cyclase and increasing cAMP, which in turn activates intracellular phosphoprotein kinases (Fig 9– 6). This process stimulates the rate-limiting step of cholesterol to Δ^5-pregnenolone conversion and initiates steroidogenesis. The exact mechanisms of ACTH stimulation of the side-chain cleavage enzyme are unknown, as is their relative importance; however, ACTH has a number of effects, including increased free cholesterol formation as a consequence of increased cholesterol esterase activity and decreased cholesteryl ester synthetase; increased lipoprotein uptake by the adrenal cortex; increased content of certain phospholipids, which may increase cholesterol side-chain cleavage; and increased binding of cholesterol to the cytochrome P-450 cholesterol cleavage enzyme in mitochondria.

D. Neuroendocrine Control: Cortisol secretion is closely regulated by ACTH, and plasma cortisol levels

parallel those of ACTH (Fig 9– 7). There are 3 mechanisms of neuroendocrine control: (1) episodic secretion and the circadian rhythm of ACTH, (2) stress responsiveness of the hypothalamic-pituitary adrenal axis, and (3) feedback inhibition by cortisol of ACTH secretion.

1. Circadian rhythm–Circadian rhythm is superimposed on episodic secretion; it is the result of central nervous system events that regulate both the number and magnitude of CRH and ACTH secretory episodes. Cortisol secretion is low in the late evening and continues to decline in the first several hours of sleep, at which time plasma cortisol levels may be undetect-

Figure 9–7. Fluctuations in plasma ACTH and glucocorticoids (11-OHCS) throughout the day. Note the greater ACTH and glucocorticoid rises in the morning before awakening. (Reproduced, with permission, from Krieger DT et al: *J Clin Endocrinol Metab* 1971;**32**:266.)

able. During the third and fifth hours of sleep, there is an increase in secretion; but the major secretory episodes begin in the sixth to eighth hours of sleep (Fig 9–7) and then begin to decline as wakefulness occurs. About half of the total daily cortisol output is secreted during this period. Cortisol secretion then gradually declines during the day, with fewer secretory episodes of decreased magnitude; however, there is increased cortisol secretion in response to eating and exercise.

Although this general pattern is consistent, there is considerable intra- and interindividual variability, and the circadian rhythm may be altered by changes in sleep pattern, light-dark exposure, and feeding times. The rhythm is also changed by (1) physical stresses such as major illness, surgery or trauma, or starvation; (2) psychologic stress, including severe anxiety, endogenous depression, and the manic phase of manic-depressive psychosis; (3) central nervous system and pituitary disorders; (4) Cushing's syndrome; (5) liver disease and other conditions that affect cortisol metabolism; (6) chronic renal failure; and (7) alcoholism. Cyproheptadine inhibits the circadian rhythm, possibly by its antiserotoninergic effects, whereas other drugs usually have no effect.

2. Stress responsiveness–Plasma ACTH and cortisol secretion are also characteristically responsive to physical stress. Thus, plasma ACTH and cortisol are secreted within minutes following the onset of stresses such as surgery and hypoglycemia (Fig 9–8), and these responses abolish circadian periodicity if the stress is prolonged. Stress responses originate in the central nervous system and increase hypothalamic CRH and thus pituitary ACTH secretion. Stress responsiveness of plasma ACTH and cortisol is abolished by prior high-dose glucocorticoid administration

Figure 9–9. Feedback inhibition of plasma ACTH levels during intravenous cortisol infusion at a rate of 50 mg/h in patients with Addison's disease. ACTH values are expressed as percentages of mean basal levels. (Reproduced, with permission, from Fehm HL et al: *J Clin Invest* 1979; **63**:247.)

Figure 9–8. Plasma cortisol responses to major surgery (continuous line) and minor surgery (broken line) in normal subjects. Mean values and standard errors for 20 patients are shown in each case. (Reproduced, with permission, from Plumpton FS, Besser GM, Cole PV: *Anaesthesia* 1969; **24**:3.)

and in spontaneous Cushing's syndrome; conversely, the responsiveness of ACTH secretion is enhanced following adrenalectomy.

3. Feedback inhibition–The third major regulator of ACTH and cortisol secretion is that of feedback inhibition by glucocorticoids of CRH, ACTH, and cortisol secretion. Glucocorticoid feedback inhibition occurs at both the pituitary and hypothalamus and involves 2 distinct mechanisms—fast and delayed feedback inhibition (Fig 9–9).

Fast feedback inhibition of ACTH secretion is rate-dependent; ie, it depends on the rate of increase of the glucocorticoid but not the dose administered. This phase is rapid, and basal and stimulated ACTH secretion both diminish within minutes after the plasma glucocorticoid level increases. This fast feedback phase is transient and lasts less than 10 minutes, suggesting that this effect is not mediated via cytosolic glucocorticoid receptors but rather via actions on the cell membrane.

Delayed feedback inhibition after the initial rate-dependent effects of glucocorticoids further suppresses CRH and ACTH secretion by mechanisms that are both time- and dose-dependent. Thus, with continued glucocorticoid administration, ACTH levels continue to decrease and become unresponsive to stimulation. The ultimate effect of prolonged glucocorticoid administration is suppression of CRH and ACTH release and atrophy of the zonae fasciculata and reticularis as a consequence of ACTH deficiency. The suppressed hypothalamic-pituitary-adrenal axis fails to respond to stress and stimulation. Delayed feedback appears to act via the classic glucocorticoid receptor (see below), thus reducing synthesis of the messenger RNA for pro-opiomelanocortin, the precursor of ACTH.

E. ACTH Effects on Regulation of Androgen Production: Adrenal androgen production in adults is also regulated by ACTH; both DHEA and androstenedione exhibit circadian periodicity in concert with ACTH and cortisol. In addition, plasma concentrations of DHEA and androstenedione increase rapidly with ACTH administration and are suppressed by glucocorticoid administration, confirming the role of endogenous ACTH in their secretion. DHEA sulfate, because of its prolonged metabolic clearance rate, does not exhibit a diurnal rhythm. Thus, adrenal androgen secretion is regulated by ACTH, and, in general, the secretion of these hormones parallels that of cortisol. The existence of a separate anterior pituitary hormone that regulates adrenal androgen secretion has been postulated but not yet proved.

CIRCULATION OF CORTISOL & ADRENAL ANDROGENS

Cortisol and the adrenal androgens circulate bound to plasma proteins. The plasma half-life of cortisol (70– 90 minutes) is determined by the extent of plasma binding and by the rate of metabolic inactivation.

Plasma Binding Proteins

Cortisol and adrenal androgens are secreted in an unbound state; however, these hormones bind to plasma proteins upon entering the circulation. Cortisol binds mainly to corticosteroid-binding globulin (CBG, transcortin) and to a lesser extent to albumin, whereas the androgens bind chiefly to albumin. The precise physiologic role of plasma protein binding is unclear, since bound steroids are biologically inactive and the active fraction is that which circulates unbound. Furthermore, CBG is not required for cortisol transport to target tissues or for full biologic activity of the steroid. The plasma proteins may provide a pool of circulating cortisol by delaying metabolic clearance, thus preventing more marked fluctuations of plasma free cortisol levels during episodic secretion by the gland.

Free & Bound Cortisol

In basal conditions, about 10% of the circulating cortisol is free, about 75% is bound to CBG, and the remainder is bound to albumin. The plasma free cortisol level is approximately 1 μg/dL, and it is this biologically active cortisol which is regulated by ACTH.

A. Corticosteroid-Binding Globulin (CBG): CBG has a molecular weight of about 50,000, is produced by the liver, and binds cortisol with high affinity. The CBG in plasma has a cortisol-binding capacity of about 25 μg/dL. When total plasma cortisol concen-

trations rise above this level, the free concentration rapidly increases and exceeds its usual fraction of 10% of the total cortisol. Other endogenous steroids do not appreciably affect cortisol binding to CBG under usual circumstances; an exception is in late pregnancy, when progesterone may occupy about 25% of the binding sites on CBG. Synthetic steroids do not bind significantly to CBG—with the exception of prednisolone, which has a high affinity. CBG levels are increased in high-estrogen states (pregnancy; estrogen or oral contraceptive use), hyperthyroidism, diabetes, certain hematologic disorders, and on a genetic basis. CBG concentrations are decreased in familial CBG deficiency, hypothyroidism, and protein deficiency states such as severe liver disease or nephrotic syndrome.

B. Albumin: Albumin has a much greater capacity for cortisol binding but a lower affinity. It normally binds about 15% of the circulating cortisol, and this proportion increases when the total cortisol concentration exceeds the CBG binding capacity. Synthetic glucocorticoids are extensively bound to albumin; eg, 77% of dexamethasone in plasma is bound to albumin.

C. Androgen Binding: Androstenedione, DHEA, and DHEA sulfate circulate weakly bound to albumin. However, testosterone is bound extensively to a specific globulin, sex hormone–binding globulin (SHBG). (See Chapters 13 and 14.)

METABOLISM OF CORTISOL & ADRENAL ANDROGENS

The metabolism of the steroids renders them inactive and increases their water solubility, as does their subsequent conjugation with glucuronide or sulfate groups. These inactive conjugated metabolites are more readily excreted by the kidney. The liver is the major site of steroid catabolism and conjugation, and 90% of these metabolized steroids are excreted by the kidney.

Conversion & Excretion of Cortisol

Cortisol is modified extensively before excretion in urine; less than 1% of secreted cortisol appears in the urine unchanged.

A. Hepatic Conversion: Hepatic metabolism of cortisol involves a number of metabolic conversions of which the most important (quantitatively) is the irreversible inactivation of the steroid by Δ^4-reductases, which reduce the 4,5 double bond of the A ring. Dihydrocortisol, the product of this reaction, is then converted to tetrahydrocortisol by a 3-hydroxysteroid dehydrogenase. Cortisol is also converted extensively to biologically inactive cortisone, which is then metabolized by the enzymes described above to yield tetrahydrocortisone. Tetrahydrocortisol and tetrahydrocortisone can be further altered to form the cortoic acids. These conversions result in the excretion of approximately equal amounts of cortisol and cortisone metabolites. Cortisol and cortisone are also metabolized to the cortols and cortolones and to a lesser extent by other pathways. Cortisol is also converted to 6β-hydroxycortisol, which is water-soluble and excreted unchanged in the urine.

B. Hepatic Conjugation: Over 95% of cortisol and cortisone metabolites are conjugated by the liver and then reenter the circulation to be excreted in the urine. Conjugation is mainly with glucuronic acid at the 3α-hydroxyl position and to a lesser extent as the sulfate at the 21-hydroxyl group.

C. Variations in Clearance and Metabolism: The metabolism of cortisol is altered by a number of circumstances. It is decreased in infants and in the elderly. It is impaired in chronic liver disease, leading to decreased renal excretion of cortisol metabolites; however, the plasma cortisol level remains normal. Hypothyroidism decreases both metabolism and excretion; conversely, hyperthyroidism accelerates these processes. Cortisol clearance may be reduced in starvation and anorexia nervosa and is also decreased in pregnancy because of the elevated CBG levels. The metabolism of cortisol to 6β-hydroxycortisol is increased in the neonate, in pregnancy, with estrogen therapy, and in patients with liver disease or severe chronic illness. Cortisol metabolism by this pathway is also increased by drugs that induce hepatic microsomal enzymes, including barbiturates, phenytoin, mitotane (o,p'-DDD), aminoglutethimide, and rifampin. These alterations generally are of minor physiologic importance, since secretion, plasma levels, and cortisol half-life are normal. However, they result in decreased excretion of the urinary metabolites of cortisol measured as 17-hydroxycorticosteroids. These conditions and drugs have a greater influence on the metabolism of synthetic glucocorticoids and may result in inadequate plasma levels of the administered glucocorticoid because of rapid clearance and metabolism.

Conversion & Excretion of Adrenal Androgens

Adrenal androgen metabolism results either in degradation and inactivation or the peripheral conversion of these weak androgens to their more potent derivatives testosterone and dihydrotestosterone. DHEA is readily converted within the adrenal to DHEA sulfate, the adrenal androgen secreted in greatest amount. DHEA secreted by the gland is also converted to DHEA sulfate by the liver and kidney, or it may be converted to Δ^4-androstenedione. DHEA sulfate may be excreted without further metabolism; however, both it and DHEA are also metabolized to 7α- and 16α-hydroxylated derivatives and by 17β-reduction to Δ^5-androstenediol and its sulfate. Androstenedione is converted either to testosterone or by reduction of its 4,5 double bond to etiocholanolone or androsterone, which may be further converted by 17β-reduction to etiocholanediol and androstanediol, respectively. Testosterone is converted to dihydrotestosterone in androgen-sensitive tissues by 5α-reduction, and it in turn is mainly metabolized by 3α-reduction to androstanediol. The metabolites of these androgens are conjugated either as glucuronides or sulfates and excreted in the urine. (See Figs 13–2 and 14–5.)

BIOLOGIC EFFECTS

GLUCOCORTICOIDS

Although glucocorticoids were originally so called because of their influence on glucose metabolism, they are currently defined as steroids that exert their effects by binding to specific cytosolic receptors which mediate the actions of these hormones. These glucocorticoid receptors are present in virtually all tissues, and glucocorticoid-receptor interaction is responsible for most of the known effects of these steroids. Alterations in the structure of the glucocorticoids have led to the development of synthetic compounds with greater glucocorticoid activity. The increased activity of these compounds is due to increased affinity for the glucocorticoid receptors and delayed plasma clearance, which increases tissue exposure. In addition, many of these synthetic glucocorticoids have negligible mineralocorticoid effects and thus do not result in sodium retention, hypertension, and hypokalemia. This section describes the molecular mechanisms of glucocorticoid action and the effects on individual metabolic functions and tissues.

Molecular Mechanisms

A. Glucocorticoid Receptors: Glucocorticoid action is initiated by entry of the steroid into the cell and binding to the cytosolic glucocorticoid receptor proteins (Fig 9–10). After binding, activated hormone-receptor complexes enter the nucleus and interact with nuclear chromatin acceptor sites. These events cause the expression of specific genes and the transcription of specific mRNAs. The resulting proteins affect the glucocorticoid response, which may be inhibitory or stimulatory depending on the specific tissue affected. Although glucocorticoid receptors are similar in many tissues, the proteins synthesized vary widely and are the result of expression of specific genes in different cell types. The mechanisms of this specific regulation are unknown.

B. Other Mechanisms: Although interaction of glucocorticoids with cytosolic receptors and their subsequent stimulation of gene expression are responsible for most glucocorticoid effects, other effects may occur through different mechanisms. The most significant example is that of glucocorticoid-induced fast feedback inhibition of ACTH secretion (see above). This effect occurs within minutes of glucocorticoid administration, and its rapidity suggests that it is not due to RNA and protein synthesis but rather to glucocorticoid-induced changes in secretory function or cell membranes.

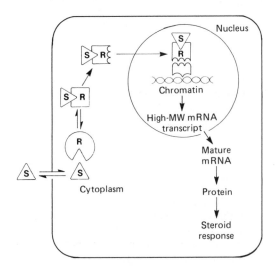

Figure 9–10. Steps in steroid hormone action. Activation of the intracellular receptors by steroid hormones is followed by nuclear binding of the complex and stimulation of mRNA synthesis. R = receptor; S = steroid hormone. (Reproduced, with permission, from Catt KJ, Dufau ML: Hormone action: Control of target-cell function by peptide, thyroid, and steroid hormones. In: *Endocrinology and Metabolism.* Felig P et al [editors]. McGraw-Hill, 1981.)

Glucocorticoid Agonists & Antagonists

The study of glucocorticoid receptors has led to the definition of glucocorticoid agonists and antagonists. These studies have also identified a number of steroids with mixed effects termed partial agonist, partial antagonist, or partial agonist–partial antagonist.

A. Agonists: In humans, cortisol, synthetic glucocorticoids (eg, prednisolone, dexamethasone), corticosterone, and aldosterone are glucocorticoid agonists. The synthetic glucocorticoids have substantially higher affinity for the glucocorticoid receptor, and these have greater glucocorticoid activity than cortisol when present in equimolar concentrations. Corticosterone and aldosterone have substantial affinity for the glucocorticoid receptor; however, their plasma concentrations are normally much lower than that of cortisol, and thus these steroids do not have significant physiologic glucocorticoid effects.

B. Antagonists: Glucocorticoid antagonists bind to the glucocorticoid receptors but do not elicit the nuclear events required to cause a glucocorticoid response. These steroids compete with agonist steroids such as cortisol for the receptors and thus inhibit agonist responses. Other steroids have partial agonist activity when present alone; ie, they elicit a partial glucocorticoid response. However, in sufficient concentration, they compete with agonist steroids for the receptors and thus competitively inhibit agonist responses; ie, these partial agonists may function as partial antagonists in the presence of more active glu-

cocorticoids. Steroids such as progesterone, 11-deoxycortisol, DOC, testosterone, and 17β-estradiol have antagonist or partial agonist–partial antagonist effects; however, the physiologic role of these hormones in glucocorticoid action is probably negligible, because they circulate in low concentrations.

Intermediary Metabolism

Glucocorticoids in general inhibit DNA synthesis. In addition, in most tissues they inhibit RNA and protein synthesis and accelerate protein catabolism. These actions provide substrate for intermediary metabolism; however, accelerated catabolism also accounts for the deleterious effects of glucocorticoids on muscle, bone, connective tissue, and lymphatic tissue. In contrast, RNA and protein synthesis in liver is stimulated.

A. Hepatic Glucose Metabolism: Glucocorticoids increase hepatic gluconeogenesis by stimulating the gluconeogenetic enzymes phosphoenolpyruvate carboxykinase and glucose 6-phosphatase. They also have a permissive effect in that they increase hepatic responsiveness to the gluconeogenetic hormones (glucagon, catecholamines), and they also increase the release of substrates from peripheral tissues, particularly muscle. This latter effect may be enhanced by the glucocorticoid-induced reduction in peripheral amino acid uptake and protein synthesis. Glucocorticoids also increase glycerol and free fatty acid release by lipolysis and increase muscle lactate release. These steroids also enhance hepatic glycogen synthesis and storage by stimulating glycogen synthetase activity and to a lesser extent by inhibiting glycogen breakdown. These effects are insulin-dependent. (See Fig 19–9.)

B. Peripheral Glucose Metabolism: Glucocorticoids also alter carbohydrate metabolism by inhibiting peripheral glucose uptake in muscle and adipose tissue. This effect and the others described above may result in increased insulin secretion in states of chronic glucocorticoid excess.

C. Effects on Adipose Tissue: In adipose tissue, the predominant effect is increased lipolysis with release of glycerol and free fatty acids. This is partially due to direct stimulation of lipolysis by glucocorticoids, but it is also contributed to by decreased glucose uptake and enhancement by glucocorticoids of the effects of lipolytic hormones. Although glucocorticoids are lipolytic, increased fat deposition is a classic manifestation of glucocorticoid excess. This paradox may be explained by the increased appetite caused by high levels of these steroids and by the lipogenic effects of the hyperinsulinemia that occurs in this state. The reason for abnormal fat deposition in states of cortisol excess is unknown. In these instances, fat is classically deposited centrally in the face, cervical area, trunk, and abdomen; the extremities are usually spared.

D. Summary: The effects of the glucocorticoids on intermediary metabolism can be summarized as follows: (1) Effects are minimal in the fed state. However, during fasting, glucocorticoids contribute to the maintenance of plasma glucose levels by increasing gluconeogenesis, glycogen deposition, and the peripheral release of substrate. (2) Hepatic glucose production is enhanced, as is hepatic RNA and protein synthesis. (3) The effects on muscle are catabolic, ie, decreased glucose uptake and metabolism, decreased protein synthesis, and increased release of amino acids. (4) In adipose tissue, lipolysis is stimulated. (5) In glucocorticoid deficiency, hypoglycemia may result, whereas in states of glucocorticoid excess there may be hyperglycemia, hyperinsulinemia, muscle wasting, and weight gain with abnormal fat distribution.

Effects on Other Tissues & Functions

A. Connective Tissue: Glucocorticoids in excess inhibit fibroblasts, lead to loss of collagen and connective tissue, and thus result in thinning of the skin, easy bruising, stria formation, and poor wound healing.

B. Bone: The physiologic role of glucocorticoids in bone metabolism and calcium homeostasis is unknown; however, in excess, they have major deleterious effects. Glucocorticoids directly inhibit bone formation by decreasing cell proliferation and the synthesis of RNA, protein, collagen, and hyaluronate. Glucocorticoids also directly stimulate bone-resorbing cells, leading to osteolysis and increased urinary hydroxyproline excretion. In addition, they potentiate the actions of PTH and 1,25-dihydroxycholecalciferol $(1,25[OH]_2D_3)$ on bone, and this may further contribute to net bone resorption.

C. Calcium Metabolism: Glucocorticoids also have other major effects on mineral homeostasis. They markedly reduce intestinal calcium absorption, which tends to lower serum calcium. This results in a secondary increase in PTH secretion, which maintains serum calcium within the normal range by stimulating bone resorption. In addition, glucocorticoids may directly stimulate PTH release. The mechanism of decreased intestinal calcium absorption is unknown, though recent studies have shown that it is not due to decreased synthesis or decreased serum levels of the active vitamin D metabolites; in fact, $1,25(OH)_2D_3$ levels are normal or even increased in the presence of glucocorticoid excess. Increased $1,25(OH)_2D_3$ synthesis in this setting may result from decreased serum phosphorus levels (see below), increased PTH levels, and direct stimulation by glucocorticoids of renal 1α-hydroxylase. Glucocorticoids also increase urinary calcium excretion, and hypercalciuria is a consistent feature of cortisol excess. They also reduce the tubular reabsorption of phosphate, leading to phosphaturia and decreased serum phosphorus concentrations.

Thus, glucocorticoids in excess result in negative calcium balance, with decreased absorption and increased urinary excretion. Serum calcium levels are maintained, but at the expense of net bone resorption. Decreased bone formation and increased resorption ultimately result in the disabling osteopenia that is often a major complication of spontaneous and iatrogenic glucocorticoid excess (see Chapter 8).

D. Growth and Development: Glucocorticoids accelerate the development of a number of systems and organs in fetal and differentiating tissues, although the mechanisms are unclear. As discussed above, glucocorticoids are generally inhibitory, and these stimulatory effects may be due to glucocorticoid interactions with other growth factors. Examples of these development-promoting effects are increased surfactant production in the fetal lung and the accelerated development of hepatic and gastrointestinal enzyme systems.

Glucocorticoids in excess inhibit growth in children, and this adverse effect is a major complication of therapy. This may be a direct effect on bone cells, although decreased growth hormone (GH) secretion and somatomedin generation also contribute (see Chapter 5).

E. Blood Cells and Immunologic Function:

1. Erythrocytes–Glucocorticoids have little effect on erythropoiesis and hemoglobin concentration. Although mild polycythemia and anemia may be seen in Cushing's syndrome and Addison's disease, respectively, these alterations are more likely to be secondary to altered androgen metabolism.

2. Leukocytes–Glucocorticoids influence both leukocyte movement and function. Thus, glucocorticoid administration increases the number of intravascular polymorphonuclear leukocytes by increasing PMN release from bone marrow, by increasing the circulating half-life of PMNs, and by decreasing PMN movement out of the vascular compartment. Glucocorticoid administration reduces the number of circulating lymphocytes, monocytes, and eosinophils, mainly by increasing their movement out of the circulation. The converse—ie, neutropenia, lymphocytosis, monocytosis, and eosinophilia—is seen in adrenal insufficiency. Glucocorticoids also decrease the migration of inflammatory cells (PMNs, monocytes, and lymphocytes) to sites of injury, and this is probably a major mechanism of the anti-inflammatory actions and increased susceptibility to infection that occur following chronic administration. Glucocorticoids also decrease lymphocyte production and the mediator and effector functions of these cells.

3. Immunologic effects–Glucocorticoids influence multiple aspects of immunologic and inflammatory responsiveness, including the mobilization and function of leukocytes, as discussed above. They also impair release of effector substances, antigen processing, antibody production and clearance, and other specific bone marrow–derived and thymus-derived lymphocyte functions.

F. Cardiovascular Function: Glucocorticoids may increase cardiac output, and they also increase peripheral vascular tone, possibly by augmenting the effects of other vasoconstrictors, eg, the catecholamines. Thus, refractory shock may occur when the glucocorticoid-deficient individual is subjected to stress. Glucocorticoids in excess may cause hypertension independently of their mineralocorticoid effects; however, the incidence and the precise cause of this problem are unclear.

G. Renal Function: These steroids affect water and electrolyte balance by actions mediated either by mineralocorticoid receptors (sodium and water retention, hypokalemia, and hypertension) or via glucocorticoid receptors (increased glomerular filtration rate due to increased cardiac output or due to a direct renal effect). Thus, corticosteroids such as betamethasone or dexamethasone that have little mineralocorticoid activity increase sodium and water excretion. Glucocorticoid-deficient subjects therefore have decreased glomerular filtration rates and are unable to excrete a water load. This may be contributed to by increased ADH secretion, which may occur in glucocorticoid deficiency.

H. Central Nervous System Function: Glucocorticoids readily enter the brain, and although their physiologic role in central nervous system function is unknown, their excess or deficiency may profoundly alter behavior and cognitive function.

1. Excessive glucocorticoids–In excess, the glucocorticoids initially cause euphoria; however, with prolonged exposure, a variety of psychologic abnormalities occur, including irritability, emotional lability, and depression. Hyperkinetic or manic behavior is less common; overt psychoses occur in a small number of patients. Many patients also note impairment in cognitive functions, most commonly memory and concentration. Other central effects include increased appetite, decreased libido, and insomnia, with decreased REM sleep and increased stage II sleep.

2. Decreased glucocorticoids–Patients with Addison's disease are apathetic and depressed and tend to be irritable, negativistic, and reclusive. They have decreased appetite but increased sensitivity of taste and smell mechanisms.

I. Effects on Other Hormones:

1. Thyroid function–Glucocorticoids in excess affect thyroid function. Although basal TSH levels are usually normal, TSH responsiveness to thyrotropin-releasing hormone (TRH) is frequently subnormal. Serum total thyroxine (T_4) concentrations are usually low normal; however, thyroxine-binding globulin is decreased, and free T_4 levels are normal. Total and free T_3 (triiodothyronine) concentrations may be low, since glucocorticoid excess decreases the conversion of T_4 to T_3 and increases conversion to reverse T_3. Despite these alterations, manifestations of hypothyroidism are not apparent.

2. Gonadal function–Glucocorticoids also affect gonadotropin and gonadal function. In males, they inhibit gonadotropin secretion, as evidenced by decreased responsiveness to administered gonadotropin-releasing hormone (GnRH) and subnormal plasma testosterone concentrations. In females, glucocorticoids also suppress LH responsiveness to GnRH, resulting in suppression of estrogens and progestins with inhibition of ovulation and amenorrhea.

J. Miscellaneous Effects:

1. Peptic ulcer–The role of steroid excess in the production or reactivation of peptic ulcer disease is controversial. Ulcers in spontaneous Cushing's syndrome and with modest exposure to glucocorticoid therapy are unusual, although current data suggest that steroid-treated patients with established ulcers and those on high-dose therapy may be at increased risk.

2. Ophthalmologic effects–Intraocular pressure varies with the level of circulating glucocorticoids and parallels the circadian variation of plasma cortisol levels. In addition, glucocorticoids in excess increase intraocular pressure in patients with open-angle glaucoma. Glucocorticoid therapy may also cause cataract formation.

ADRENAL ANDROGENS

The direct biologic activity of the adrenal androgens (androstenedione, DHEA, and DHEA sulfate) is minimal, and they function primarily as precursors for peripheral conversion to the active androgenic hormones testosterone and dihydrotestosterone. Thus, DHEA sulfate secreted by the adrenal undergoes limited conversion to DHEA; this peripherally converted DHEA and that secreted by the adrenal cortex can be further converted in peripheral tissues to androstenedione, the immediate precursor of the active androgens.

The actions of testosterone and dihydrotestosterone are described in Chapter 13. This section will deal only with the adrenal contribution to androgenicity.

Effects in Males

In males with normal gonadal function, the conversion of adrenal androstenedione to testosterone accounts for less than 5% of the production rate of this hormone, and thus the physiologic effect is negligible. In adult males, excessive adrenal androgen secretion has no clinical consequences; however, in boys, it causes premature penile enlargement and early development of secondary sexual characteristics.

Effects in Females

In females, ovarian androgen production is low; thus, the adrenal substantially contributes to total androgen production by the peripheral conversion of androstenedione. In the follicular phase of the menstrual cycle, adrenal precursors account for two-thirds of testosterone production and one-half of dihydrotestosterone production. During midcycle, the ovarian contribution increases, and the adrenal precursors account for only 40% of testosterone production.

In females, abnormal adrenal function as seen in Cushing's syndrome, adrenal carcinoma, and congenital adrenal hyperplasia results in excessive secretion of adrenal androgens, and their peripheral conversion results in androgen excess, manifested by acne, hirsutism, and virilization.

LABORATORY EVALUATION

Cortisol and the adrenal androgens are measured by specific plasma assays that have simplified the evaluation of adrenal dysfunction. Certain urinary assays, particularly measurement of 24-hour urine free cortisol, can also be useful. In addition, plasma concentrations of ACTH can be determined. The plasma steroid methods commonly used measure the total hormone concentration and are therefore influenced by alterations in plasma binding proteins. Furthermore, since ACTH and the plasma concentrations of the adrenal hormones fluctuate markedly (Fig 9–7), single plasma measurements are frequently unreliable. Thus, plasma levels must be interpreted cautiously, and more specific diagnostic information is usually obtained by performing appropriate stimulation and suppression tests.

Plasma ACTH

A. Methods of Measurement: Plasma ACTH measurements by radioimmunoassay are extremely useful in the diagnosis of pituitary-adrenal dysfunction; however, they are less commonly available than assays for other polypeptide hormones (see Chapter 4). In general, antisera that react with the biologically active 1–24 sequence of human ACTH are preferable, since they do not detect biologically inactive fragments. The normal range of plasma ACTH is 20–100 pg/mL in the morning, and the sensitivity of these assays is 5–20 pg/mL. ACTH is unstable, and specimens must be handled carefully. They should be collected in heparinized plastic syringes and tubes on ice, centrifuged immediately after collection, and then frozen until assayed.

B. Interpretation: Plasma ACTH levels are most useful in differentiating pituitary causes from adrenal causes of adrenal dysfunction: (1) In **adrenal insufficiency** due to primary adrenal disease, plasma ACTH levels are elevated, usually over 250 pg/mL. Conversely, in pituitary ACTH deficiency and secondary hypoadrenalism, plasma ACTH levels are less than 50 pg/mL. (2) In **Cushing's syndrome** due to primary glucocorticoid-secreting adrenal tumors, plasma ACTH is suppressed, and a level less than 20 pg/mL is diagnostic. In patients with Cushing's disease (pituitary ACTH hypersecretion), plasma ACTH levels are normal or only modestly elevated (40–200 pg/mL). Plasma ACTH levels in the ectopic ACTH syndrome range from 100 to several thousand picograms per milliliter. They are usually markedly elevated; however, overlap occurs with levels seen in Cushing's disease. (3) Plasma ACTH levels are also markedly elevated in patients with the common forms of **congenital adrenal hyperplasia** and are useful in the diagnosis and management of these disorders (see Chapters 10 and 15).

Plasma β-Lipotropin & β-Endorphin

β-Lipotropin (β-LPH) is secreted in equimolar amounts with ACTH and is measured by radioimmunoassay. Because of its greater stability and ease of measurement, it has some advantage over the measurement of ACTH. Alterations in β-LPH levels in disease states parallel those of ACTH as described above. Most assays of β-LPH also measure β-endorphin, and thus separation of these hormones is required for precise measurement of β-endorphin. This can be accomplished by chromatography; however, the clinical utility of β-endorphin measurements has not been established.

Plasma Cortisol

A. Methods of Measurement: Plasma cortisol methods of measurement in current use include radioimmunoassay, competitive protein-binding assay, fluorimetric assay, and high-performance liquid chromatography. These methods measure total cortisol (both bound and free) in plasma. Methods that measure plasma free cortisol—ie, that not bound to CBG—are not yet clinically available.

1. Radioimmunoassays–Radioimmunoassays of plasma cortisol depend on inhibition of binding of radiolabeled cortisol to an antibody by the cortisol present in a plasma sample. Current assays are very sensitive, so that small plasma volumes can be used. In addition, cross-reactivity of current antisera with other endogenous steroids is minimal, and radioimmunoassay thus gives a reliable measurement of total plasma cortisol levels. Commonly used drugs and medications do not interfere with this assay.

2. Competitive protein-binding assay–This test is similar in principle to radioimmunoassay except that CBG is utilized to bind cortisol instead of an antibody. Although other endogenous steroids bind CBG with high affinity, their plasma concentrations are usually much lower than that of cortisol, and they therefore do not cause significant interference. The synthetic glucocorticoids prednisolone and 6α-methylprednisolone bind to CBG in appreciable amounts and may interfere with the assay, although other hormones and medications do not.

3. Fluorimetric assay–This test measures the fluorescence of steroids with 11-hydroxyl groups and thus measures plasma 11-hydroxycorticosteroids. Cortisol is the major hormone measured, but the method also detects corticosterone and 21-deoxycortisol. The latter 2 steroids are usually present in low concentrations and thus do not cause significant interference. Synthetic glucocorticoids do not cross-react in this assay. Since plasma has nonspecific background fluorescence, this method overestimates the plasma cortisol concentration by 2–3 μg/dL. Background fluorescence may be increased in the plasma of uremic or jaundiced patients, and spironolactone, quinacrine, quinidine, fusidic acid, niacin, and heparin preparations containing benzyl alcohol interfere with the assay.

4. High-performance liquid chromatography–This test also provides a specific method of cortisol determination. Other endogenous steroids are excluded by chromatography, but it is possible that prednisone and prednisolone might interfere. Drug interference does not occur.

B. Interpretation: The diagnostic utility of single plasma cortisol concentrations is limited by the episodic nature of cortisol secretion and its appropriate elevations during stress. As explained below, more information is obtained by dynamic testing of the hypothalamic-pituitary-adrenal axis.

1. Normal values–Normal plasma cortisol levels vary with the method used. With radioimmunoassay and the competitive protein-binding radioassay, levels at 8 AM range from 3 to 20 μg/dL and average 10–12 μg/dL. Values obtained later in the day are lower and at 4 PM are approximately half of morning values. At 10 PM to 2 AM, the plasma cortisol concentrations by these methods are usually under 3 μg/dL. With the fluorimetric assay, values at 7–8 AM are 5–25 μg/dL, with a mean of 20 μg/dL.

2. Levels during stress–Cortisol secretion increases in patients who are acutely ill, during surgery, and following trauma; thus, plasma concentrations may be elevated.

3. High-estrogen states–The total plasma cortisol concentration is also elevated with increased CBG binding capacity, which occurs most commonly when circulating estrogen levels are high, eg, during pregnancy and when exogenous estrogens or oral contraceptives are being used. In these situations, plasma cortisol may reach levels 2–3 times normal.

4. Other conditions–CBG levels may be increased or decreased in other situations, as discussed above in the sections on circulation and metabolism. Total plasma cortisol concentrations may also be increased in severe anxiety, endogenous depression, starvation, anorexia nervosa, alcoholism, and chronic renal failure.

Urinary Corticosteroids

A. Free Cortisol:

1. Methods of measurement–The assay of unbound cortisol excreted in the urine is an excellent method for the diagnosis of Cushing's syndrome. Normally, less than 1% of the secreted cortisol is excreted unchanged in the urine. However, in states of excess secretion, the binding capacity of CBG is exceeded, and plasma free cortisol therefore increases, as does its urinary excretion. Urine free cortisol is measured in a 24-hour urine collection by radioimmunoassay or competitive protein-binding assay after extraction of the cortisol.

2. Normal values–The normal range of these assays is nil to 110 μg/24 h, and elevated levels are found in over 90% of patients with spontaneous Cushing's syndrome.

3. Diagnostic utility–This method is particularly useful in differentiating simple obesity from Cushing's syndrome, since levels are not elevated in obesity, as are the urinary 17-hydroxycorticosteroids (see below). The levels may be elevated in the same conditions that increase plasma cortisol (see above), including a slight elevation during pregnancy. This test is not useful in adrenal insufficiency, because of the lack of sensitivity of the method at low levels and because low cortisol excretion is often found in normal persons.

B. 17-Hydroxycorticosteroids and 17-Ketogenic Steroids: These urinary steroids are less frequently measured at present, because of the greater utility of plasma cortisol and urine free cortisol measurements. Urinary 17-ketosteroid measurements are discussed in the following section on androgens.

1. 17-Hydroxycorticosteroids–

a. Methods of assay–Urine 17-hydroxycorticosteroids are assayed by the colorimetric Porter-Silber reaction, which detects cortisol and cortisone metabolites.

b. Normal values–Normal values are 3–10 mg/24 h, or 2–6.5 mg/g of urine creatinine.

c. Altered excretion–Total excretion is increased in obesity; however, these values are normal when corrected for creatinine excretion. 17-Hydroxycorticosteroids are increased in hyperthyroidism and decreased in hypothyroidism, starvation, liver disease, renal failure, and pregnancy. Drugs that induce hepatic microsomal enzymes increase cortisol conversion to 6β-hydroxycortisol, which is not measured by the 17-hydroxycorticosteroid method, and therefore reduce 17-hydroxycorticosteroid excretion (see section on metabolism).

d. Drug interference–Direct drug interference with the colorimetric reaction occurs with spironolactone, chlordiazepoxide, hydroxyzine, meprobamate, phenothiazines, and quinine.

2. 17-Ketogenic steroids–The 17-ketogenic steroids include not only the metabolites of cortisol but also those of a number of other steroids, eg, pregnanetriol. The procedure for measurement first converts these steroids to 17-ketosteroids, and they are then measured colorimetrically by the Zimmermann reaction. Normal values are 6–20 mg/24 h. This is less specific for cortisol metabolites than measurement of 17-hydroxycorticosteroids and is less reliable in the diagnosis of Cushing's syndrome. Values are increased by penicillin G and decreased by glucose, meprobamate, and radiographic contrast agents.

C. Cortisol Secretion Rate: There are several research techniques available to measure the cortisol secretion rate, which normally is 8–25 mg/d. The rate is decreased in adrenal insufficiency and increased in Cushing's syndrome, obesity, hyperthyroidism, and pregnancy. Expression of the secretion rate in terms of creatinine excretion allows differentiation of Cushing's syndrome from exogenous obesity. Thus, in normals and in obese subjects, cortisol secretion is less than 20 mg/24 h/g of urinary creatinine, whereas in patients with Cushing's syndrome values greater than 26 mg/24 h/g of creatinine are obtained. Although useful, these methods are not generally available.

Dexamethasone Suppression Tests

A. Low-Dose Tests: These procedures are used to establish the presence of Cushing's syndrome regardless of its cause. Dexamethasone, a potent glucocorticoid, normally suppresses pituitary ACTH release with a resulting fall in plasma and urine corticosteroids, thus assessing feedback inhibition of the hypothalamic-pituitary-adrenal axis. In Cushing's syndrome, this mechanism is abnormal, and steroid secretion fails to be suppressed in the normal way. Dexamethasone in the doses used does not interfere with the measurement of plasma and urinary corticosteroids.

1. Overnight 1-mg dexamethasone suppression test–This is a suitable screening test for Cushing's syndrome. Dexamethasone, 1 mg orally, is given as a single dose at 11 PM, and the following morning a plasma sample is obtained for cortisol determination. Cushing's syndrome is excluded if the plasma cortisol level is less than 5 μg/dL. If the level is greater than 10 μg/dL—in the absence of conditions causing false-positive responses—Cushing's syndrome is the probable cause, and the diagnosis should be confirmed with other procedures.

Over 98% of patients with Cushing's syndrome have abnormal responses. Although false-negative results are rare, they may occur in patients in whom dexamethasone metabolism is abnormally slow, since plasma levels of dexamethasone in these patients are higher than normally achieved and result in apparently normal suppression of cortisol. Simultaneous measurement of plasma dexamethasone and cortisol levels will identify these patients; however, dexamethasone measurements are available only on a research basis.

False-positive results occur in 15% of patients with obesity and in 25% of hospitalized and chronically ill patients. Acute illness, depression, anxiety, alcoholism, high-estrogen states, and uremia may also cause false-positive results. Patients taking phenytoin, barbiturates, and other inducers of hepatic microsomal enzymes may have accelerated metabolism of dexamethasone and thus fail to achieve adequate plasma levels to suppress ACTH.

2. Two-day low-dose test–This test is performed by administering dexamethasone, 0.5 mg every 6 hours for 2 days. Twenty-four-hour urine collections are obtained before and on the second day of dexamethasone administration. The test provides the same information as the overnight 1-mg test but is more time-consuming and requires urine collections. However, it is very useful when the results of other tests are equivocal. In response to this procedure, patients *without* Cushing's syndrome suppress urine 17-hydroxycorticosteroids to less than 4 mg/24 h or to less than 1 mg/g of urinary creatinine on the second day of dexamethasone administration. The response of urine free cortisol is less well standardized; however, a reduction in excretion to less than 25 μg/24 h appears to exclude Cushing's syndrome. Although the plasma cortisol response has been less extensively studied, a morning cortisol level of less than 5 μg/dL (obtained 6 hours after the last dose of dexamethasone has been given) is considered a normal response.

About 95% of patients with Cushing's syndrome

have abnormal responses. False-positive results occur rarely in patients with obesity and in high-estrogen states. However, false-positive results do occur with acute and chronic illness, depression, alcoholism, and phenytoin therapy.

B. High-Dose Tests: High-dose dexamethasone tests differentiate Cushing's disease (pituitary ACTH hypersecretion) from the ectopic ACTH syndrome and adrenal tumors, since the hypothalamic-pituitary axis in Cushing's disease is suppressible with supraphysiologic doses of glucocorticoids, whereas cortisol secretion is autonomous in patients with adrenal tumors or ectopic ACTH syndrome and is therefore nonsuppressible. Exceptions to these responses are discussed in the section on diagnosis of Cushing's syndrome.

1. Overnight high-dose dexamethasone suppression test–This test is faster and simpler to perform than the standard 2-day test described below. After a baseline morning cortisol specimen is obtained, a single dose of dexamethasone, 8 mg orally, is administered at 11 PM, and plasma cortisol is measured at 8 AM the following morning. In Cushing's disease, plasma cortisol levels are reduced to less than 50% of baseline values in 95% of patients, whereas steroid secretion in patients with ectopic ACTH syndrome or cortisol-producing adrenal tumors is not suppressed to this extent and is usually unchanged. This single-dose test is more reliable than the 2-day high-dose test and can be regarded as the procedure of choice.

2. Two-day high-dose test–This test is performed by administering dexamethasone, 2 mg orally every 6 hours for 2 days. Twenty-four-hour urine samples are collected before and on the second day of dexamethasone administration. Patients with Cushing's disease have a reduction in urine 17-hydroxycorticosteroid excretion to less than 50% of baseline values, whereas those with adrenal tumors or the ectopic ACTH syndrome usually have little or no reduction in urinary 17-hydroxycorticosteroids. Urine free cortisol or plasma cortisol appears to give equally adequate responses, and the same criteria apply; the response of urine 17-ketogenic steroids appears to be less reliable. Regardless of the parameter measured, 15–30% of patients with Cushing's disease fail to achieve 50% suppression of corticosteroid levels, thus limiting the reliability of the procedure.

Pituitary-Adrenal Reserve

Determinations of pituitary-adrenal reserve are used to evaluate the patient's adrenal and pituitary resources and to assess the ability of the hypothalamic-pituitary-adrenal axis to respond to stress. ACTH administration directly stimulates adrenal secretion; metyrapone inhibits cortisol synthesis, thereby stimulating pituitary ACTH secretion; and insulin-induced hypoglycemia stimulates ACTH release by increasing CRH secretion. More recently, CRH has been utilized to directly stimulate pituitary corticotrophs to release ACTH and β-LPH. The relative utility of these procedures is discussed below in the section on adrenocortical insufficiency and also in Chapter 4.

A. ACTH Stimulation Testing:

1. Procedure and normal values–The rapid ACTH stimulation test measures the acute adrenal response to ACTH and is used to diagnose both primary and secondary adrenal insufficiency. A synthetic human α^{1-24}-ACTH called tetracosactrin or cosyntropin (Cortrosyn) is used. It has full biologic potency and a lower incidence of allergic reactions than occurred with animal ACTH derivatives. Fasting is not required, and the test may be performed at any time of the day. A baseline cortisol sample is obtained; cosyntropin is administered in a dose of 0.25 mg intramuscularly or intravenously; and additional samples for plasma cortisol are obtained at 30 or 60 minutes following the injection. With the fluorimetric cortisol assay, the response is normal if the basal plasma cortisol level is greater than 5 μg/dL, with an increment greater than 7 μg/dL and a peak level greater than 18 μg/dL at 30 minutes. When cortisol is measured by immunoassay, competitive protein-binding assay, or liquid chromatography, the normal response is a peak cortisol level greater than 15–18 μg/dL, with an increment greater than 5 μg/dL.

2. Subnormal responses–If the cortisol response to the rapid ACTH stimulation test is inadequate, adrenal insufficiency is present. In primary adrenal insufficiency, destruction of cortical cells reduces cortisol secretion and increases pituitary ACTH secretion. Therefore, the adrenal is already maximally stimulated, and there is no further increase in cortisol secretion when exogenous ACTH is given; ie, there is decreased adrenal reserve. In secondary adrenal insufficiency due to ACTH deficiency, there is atrophy of the zonae fasciculata and reticularis, and the adrenal thus is unresponsive to acute stimulation with exogenous ACTH. In either primary or secondary types, a subnormal response to the rapid ACTH stimulation test accurately predicts deficient responsiveness of the axis to insulin hypoglycemia, metyrapone, and surgical stress.

3. Normal responses–A normal response to the rapid ACTH stimulation test excludes both primary adrenal insufficiency (by directly assessing adrenal reserve) and overt secondary adrenal insufficiency with adrenal atrophy. However, a normal response does not rule out partial ACTH deficiency (decreased pituitary reserve) in patients whose basal ACTH secretion is sufficient to prevent adrenocortical atrophy. These patients may be unable to further increase ACTH secretion and thus may have subnormal pituitary ACTH responsiveness to stress or hypoglycemia. In such patients, further testing with metyrapone or hypoglycemia may be indicated. For further discussion, see the section on diagnosis of adrenocortical insufficiency.

4. Aldosterone secretion–The rapid ACTH stimulation test also increases aldosterone secretion and has been used to differentiate primary from secondary adrenocortical insufficiency. In the primary form with destruction of the cortex, both cortisol and aldosterone are unresponsive to exogenous ACTH. However, in secondary adrenal insufficiency, the zona glomerulosa, which is controlled by the renin-angiotensin system, is usually normal. Therefore, the aldosterone response to exogenous ACTH is normal. The normal increment in plasma aldosterone is more than 4 ng/dL.

5. Three-day tests–Three-day ACTH stimulation tests are rarely used at present, since the rapid ACTH test and measurements of plasma ACTH are usually sufficient to diagnose and establish the cause of adrenocortical insufficiency.

B. Metyrapone Testing: Metyrapone testing is used to diagnose adrenal insufficiency and to assess pituitary-adrenal reserve. The test procedures are detailed in Chapter 4. Metyrapone blocks cortisol synthesis by inhibiting the 11β-hydroxylase enzyme that converts 11-deoxycortisol to cortisol. This stimulates ACTH secretion, which in turn increases the secretion and plasma levels of 11-deoxycortisol. Urinary 17-hydroxycorticosteroid levels also increase because of increased excretion of the metabolites of 11-deoxycortisol that are measured by this method. The overnight metyrapone test is most commonly used and is best suited to patients with suspected pituitary ACTH deficiency; patients with suspected primary adrenal failure are usually evaluated with the rapid ACTH stimulation test as described above and discussed in the section on diagnosis of adrenocortical insufficiency. The normal response to the overnight metyrapone test is a plasma 11-deoxycortisol level greater than 7 μg/dL and indicates both normal ACTH secretion and adrenal function. A subnormal response establishes adrenocortical insufficiency but does not differentiate primary and secondary forms. A normal response to metyrapone accurately predicts normal stress responsiveness of the hypothalamic-pituitary axis and correlates well with responsiveness to insulin-induced hypoglycemia.

C. Insulin-Induced Hypoglycemia Testing: The details of this procedure are described in Chapter 4. Hypoglycemia induces a central nervous system stress response, increases CRH release, and in this way increases ACTH and cortisol secretion. It therefore measures the integrity of the axis and its ability to respond to stress. With fluorimetric cortisol determination, the normal plasma cortisol response is an increment greater than 8 μg/dL and a peak level greater than 18–20 μg/dL. When the competitive protein-binding method is used, cortisol increases by more than 5 μg/dL. The plasma ACTH response to hypoglycemia is not well standardized. A normal plasma cortisol response to hypoglycemia excludes adrenal insufficiency and decreased pituitary reserve. Thus, patients with normal responses do not require cortisol therapy during illness or surgery.

D. CRH Testing: The procedure for CRH testing is described in Chapter 4. Current experience with CRH testing is limited, although it has been established that ACTH responses are exaggerated in patients with primary adrenal failure and absent in patients with hypopituitarism. Delayed responses may occur in patients with hypothalamic disorders. Whether this procedure will have major clinical utility and supplant any of the procedures described above remains to be determined.

Androgens

Androgen excess is usually evaluated by the measurement of basal levels of these hormones, since suppression and stimulation tests are not as useful as in disorders affecting the glucocorticoids.

A. Plasma Levels: Assays are currently available for total plasma levels of DHEA, DHEA sulfate, androstenedione, testosterone, and dihydrotestosterone; these tests are of greater diagnostic utility than the traditional measurement of urinary androgen metabolites measured as urinary 17-ketosteroids.

Because it is present in greater quantities, DHEA sulfate can be measured directly in unextracted plasma. However, because of their similar structures and lower plasma concentrations, the other androgens require extraction and purification steps prior to assay. This is accomplished by solvent extraction followed by chromatography, and the purified steroids are then measured by radioimmunoassay or competitive protein-binding radioassay. These methods allow measurement of multiple steroids in small volumes of plasma.

B. Free Testosterone: Plasma free testosterone (ie, testosterone not bound to SHBG) can be measured and is a more direct measure of circulating biologically active testosterone than the total plasma level. These methods require separation of the bound and free hormone prior to assay and are technically difficult. The plasma free testosterone concentration in normal women averages 5 pg/mL, representing approximately 1% of the total testosterone concentration. In hirsute women, average levels are 16 pg/mL, with a wide range.

C. SHBG Binding Capacity: The binding capacity of SHBG can be measured, although these methods are not in general use. SHBG binding capacity is higher in women; it is increased in pregnancy, in women receiving exogenous estrogens, in hepatic cirrhosis, and in hyperthyroidism and is decreased in hirsute women with increased androgens and in patients with acromegaly.

D. Urinary 17-Ketosteroids: Measurement of urinary androgen metabolites (eg, the 17-ketosteroids) is much less useful in the evaluation of androgen excess than the plasma methods described above. The biologically active androgens testosterone and dihydrotestosterone account for less than 1% of total urinary 17-ketosteroids; the major steroids measured are the metabolites of DHEA and DHEA sulfate. The ketosteroids are separated by solvent extraction and measured colorimetrically by the Zimmermann reaction. Normal values are 5–15 mg/24 h in women and 7–17 mg/24 h in men. A number of drugs interfere with this method. Thus, penicillin, spironolactone, chlorpromazine, ethinamate, meprobamate, and nalidixic acid falsely elevate the values, whereas chlor-

diazepoxide, propoxyphene, progestins, reserpine, and etryptamine acetate reduce them.

DISORDERS OF ADRENOCORTICAL INSUFFICIENCY

Deficient adrenal production of glucocorticoids or mineralocorticoids results in adrenocortical insufficiency, which is either the consequence of destruction or dysfunction of the cortex (primary adrenocortical insufficiency, Addison's disease) or secondary to deficient pituitary ACTH secretion (secondary adrenocortical insufficiency). Secondary adrenocortical insufficiency due to glucocorticoid therapy is the most common cause.

PRIMARY ADRENOCORTICAL INSUFFICIENCY (Addison's Disease)

Etiology & Pathology

Addison's disease is idiopathic (autoimmune adrenal atrophy, autoimmune adrenalitis, lymphocytic adrenalitis) in about 80% of cases and is associated with disordered organ-specific immunity and a high incidence of other immunologic and autoimmune endocrine disorders (see Chapter 25). About 20% of cases occur as complications of tuberculosis. Other rare causes are listed in Table 9–1. The disorder itself is rare, with a reported prevalence of 39 per million population in the United Kingdom and 60 per million in Denmark. It is more common in females, with a female:male ratio of 2.6:1. Tuberculous adrenal de-

Table 9–1. Causes of primary adrenocortical insufficiency.*

Major causes
    Autoimmune (about 80%)
    Tuberculosis (about 20%)
Rare causes
    Adrenal hemorrhage and infarction
    Fungal infections
    Metastatic and lymphomatous replacement
    Amyloidosis
    Sarcoidosis
    Hemochromatosis
    Radiation therapy
    Surgical adrenalectomy
    Enzyme inhibitors (metyrapone, aminoglutethimide, trilostane)
    Cytotoxic agents (mitotane; o,p'-DDD)
    Congenital (enzyme defects, hypoplasia, familial glucocorticoid deficiency)

*Modified and reproduced, with permission, from Baxter JD, Tyrrell JB, in: *Endocrinology and Metabolism.* Felig P et al (editors). McGraw-Hill, 1981.

struction is most common in males, giving an overall female:male ratio of 1.25:1. Addison's disease is usually diagnosed in the third to fifth decades; mean ages of 34 and 38 years have been reported for the idiopathic and tuberculous types, respectively.

A. Idiopathic Adrenocortical Insufficiency: Lymphocytic infiltration of the adrenal cortex is the characteristic histologic feature. The adrenals are small and atrophic, and the capsule is thickened. The adrenal medulla is preserved, though cortical cells are largely absent, show degenerative changes, and are surrounded by a fibrous stroma and lymphocytic infiltrates.

Idiopathic Addison's disease is frequently accompanied by gonadal failure, hyperthyroidism, hypothyroidism, Hashimoto's thyroiditis, diabetes mellitus, vitiligo, hypoparathyroidism, and pernicious anemia (Table 9–2). One or more of these disorders is present in 40–53% of patients with idiopathic Addison's disease, and there is an even higher incidence of circulating autoantibodies to affected glands and tissues.

1. Schmidt's syndrome–The association of Addison's disease with these conditions has been termed Schmidt's syndrome, autoimmune endocrine failure, and polyglandular failure syndrome. Genetic and HLA associations are discussed in Chapter 25. These disorders are not present in Addison's disease due to specific causes.

2. Ovarian failure–This occurs in approximately 25% of female patients and usually presents as secondary amenorrhea. Patients with both ovarian and adrenal failure also have a very high incidence of hypoparathyroidism and thyroid disease. Hypoparathyroidism is most frequent in those with primary amenorrhea.

3. Testicular failure–Testicular failure is uncommon and occurs in fewer than 5% of males with idiopathic Addison's disease.

4. Thyroid disorders–Clinical thyroid disorders occur in 16% of patients. The incidence of subclinical thyroiditis is even higher; about 80% of patients with idiopathic Addison's disease have lymphocytic infiltration of the thyroid, and there is a high incidence of elevated TSH levels. Hyperthyroidism occurs in 7% of patients, of whom the majority are female;

Table 9–2. Frequency of other autoimmune disorders in patients with idiopathic adrenocortical insufficiency.*

	Percent
Primary ovarian failure	23
Thyroid disorders	16
Insulin-dependent diabetes mellitus	12
Vitiligo	9
Hypoparathyroidism	6
Pernicious anemia	4

*Modified and reproduced, with permission, from Baxter JD, Tyrrell JB, in: *Endocrinology and Metabolism.* Felig P et al (editors). McGraw-Hill, 1981.

Table 9–3. Incidence of circulating autoantibodies in idiopathic adrenocortical insufficiency.*

	Percent
Adrenal	64
Thyroid	
Cytoplasm	45
Thyroglobulin	22
Stomach	
Parietal cells	30
Intrinsic factor	9
Parathyroid	26
Gonad	17
Islet cell	8

*Reproduced, with permission, from Baxter JD, Tyrrell JB, in: *Endocrinology and Metabolism.* Felig P et al (editors). McGraw-Hill, 1981.

clinical hypothyroidism or Hashimoto's thyroiditis with goiter occurs in 9% of patients.

5. Diabetes mellitus–This is present in about 12% of patients with idiopathic Addison's disease and is typically type I (insulin-dependent). The mean age at diagnosis of the 2 disorders is approximately 30 years. Sex distribution is equal, and islet cell autoantibodies are common in these patients.

6. Hypoparathyroidism–Hypoparathyroidism occurs in 6% of patients with idiopathic Addison's disease. These 2 disorders occur at younger ages than the other disorders listed above, with a mean age at diagnosis of 12 years. There is also an increased incidence of early ovarian failure, usually presenting as primary amenorrhea, in patients with idiopathic Addison's disease and hypoparathyroidism.

7. Other disorders–These include vitiligo in 9% and pernicious anemia in about 4% of patients. Subclinical atrophic gastritis, hypochlorhydria, and achlorhydria also occur.

8. Circulating autoantibodies–The incidence of autoantibodies to adrenal and other tissue antigens is increased in patients with idiopathic Addison's disease (Table 9–3) but not in patients with adrenal failure due to other causes. Circulating adrenal autoantibodies are present in over 60% of patients with idiopathic Addison's disease. Thyroid autoantibodies occur in 45% of patients with idiopathic Addison's disease and are present more frequently (2:1) in female patients. Gastric parietal cell and intrinsic factor autoantibodies are present in 30% and 9%, respectively; parathyroid autoantibodies in 26%; autoantibodies to steroid-producing cells in 17%; and islet cell autoantibodies in 8% of patients with idiopathic Addison's disease.

B. Adrenocortical Insufficiency Due to Invasive and Hemorrhagic Disorders: Invasive or hemorrhagic disorders causing adrenocortical failure result in total or near-total destruction of both glands. With septicemia or hemorrhage, the adrenal is rapidly destroyed, whereas gradual destruction usually occurs in conditions such as tuberculosis.

1. Adrenal tuberculosis and other destructive

causes–Adrenal tuberculosis is due to hematogenous infection of the cortex and usually occurs as a complication of systemic tuberculous infection (lung, gastrointestinal tract, or kidney). The adrenal glands are replaced by caseous necrosis; both cortical and medullary tissue is destroyed. Calcification of the adrenals is frequent and is radiologically demonstrable in about 50% of cases.

Other destructive causes also result in loss of both cortical and medullary tissue. Histologic examination reveals scarring, inflammatory changes, or replacement of adrenal tissue with tumor or infiltrates. Adrenal calcification occurs less commonly than with tuberculosis.

2. Bilateral adrenal hemorrhage–Hemorrhage may cause acute adrenal insufficiency. In children, fulminant meningococcemia and *Pseudomonas* septicemia are the most common causes. In adults (mostly > age 50), anticoagulant therapy given for other major illnesses is responsible for one-third of cases. Other causes in adults include septicemia, coagulation disorders, adrenal vein thrombosis, adrenal metastases, trauma, abdominal surgery, and obstetric gestational and postpartum complications.

The adrenal glands are often massively enlarged; there is replacement of the medulla and inner cortex by hemorrhage and ischemic necrosis of the outer cortex, so that only a few subcapsular cortical cells survive. Venous thrombosis frequently accompanies the hemorrhage. In surviving patients, the hematomas may calcify.

C. Familial Glucocorticoid Deficiency: Familial glucocorticoid deficiency is a rare disorder in which there is hereditary adrenocortical unresponsiveness to ACTH. This leads to adrenal insufficiency with subnormal glucocorticoid and adrenal androgen secretion and elevated plasma ACTH levels.

In this disorder, cortisol secretion is unresponsive to both endogenous and exogenous ACTH stimulation. However, aldosterone secretion responds to both posture change and sodium deprivation, except in a few subjects who have partial aldosterone deficiency. Presentation is usually in childhood and may be accompanied by achalasia. Histologically, there is preservation of the zona glomerulosa, with degenerative changes in the zonae fasciculata and reticularis. These features and the absence of lymphocytic infiltration of the adrenal cortex differentiate this condition from idiopathic adrenocortical insufficiency.

Pathophysiology

Loss of more than 90% of both adrenal cortices results in the clinical manifestations of adrenocortical insufficiency. Gradual destruction such as occurs in the idiopathic and invasive forms of the disease leads to chronic adrenocortical insufficiency. However, more rapid destruction occurs in many cases; about 25% of patients are in crisis or impending crisis at the time of diagnosis. With gradual adrenocortical destruction, the initial phase is that of decreased adrenal reserve; ie, basal steroid secretion is normal, but secretion does not increase in response to stress. Thus, acute adrenal crisis can be precipitated by the stresses of surgery, trauma, or infection, which require increased corticosteroid secretion. With further loss of cortical tissue, even basal secretion of mineralocorticoids and glucocorticoids becomes deficient, leading to the manifestations of chronic adrenocortical insufficiency. Destruction of the adrenals by hemorrhage results in sudden loss of both glucocorticoid and mineralocorticoid secretion, accompanied by acute adrenal crisis.

With decreasing cortisol secretion, plasma levels of ACTH and β-lipotropin (β-LPH) are increased because of decreased negative-feedback inhibition of their secretion. In chronic states, the elevated ACTH levels cause hyperpigmentation; this is usually absent when adrenal destruction is rapid.

Clinical Features

A. Symptoms and Signs: Cortisol deficiency causes weakness, fatigue, anorexia, nausea and vomiting, hypotension, and hypoglycemia. Mineralocorticoid deficiency produces renal sodium wasting and potassium retention and can lead to severe dehydration, hypotension, hyponatremia, hyperkalemia, and acidosis.

1. Chronic primary adrenocortical insufficiency–The chief symptoms (Table 9–4) are hyperpigmentation, weakness and fatigue, weight loss, anorexia, and gastrointestinal disturbances.

Hyperpigmentation is the classic physical finding, and its presence in association with the above manifestations should suggest primary adrenocortical insufficiency. Generalized hyperpigmentation of the skin and mucous membranes is the earliest manifestation of Addison's disease. It is increased in sun-exposed areas and accentuated over pressure areas such as the knuckles, toes, elbows, and knees. It is accompanied by increased numbers of black or dark-brown freckles. The classic hyperpigmentation of the buccal mucosa and gums is preceded by generalized hyperpigmentation of the skin; adrenal insufficiency should also be suspected when there is increased pigmentation of the palmar creases, nail beds, nipples, areolae, and perivaginal and perianal mucosa. Scars that have formed after the onset of ACTH excess become hyperpigmented, whereas older ones do not. Although

Table 9–4. Clinical features of primary adrenocortical insufficiency.[*]

	Percent
Weakness, fatigue, anorexia, weight loss	100
Hyperpigmentation	92
Hypotension	88
Gastrointestinal disturbances	56
Salt craving	19
Postural symptoms	12

[*]Reproduced, with permission, from Baxter JD, Tyrrell JB, in: *Endocrinology and Metabolism.* Felig P et al (editors). McGraw-Hill, 1981.

pigmentation of the buccal mucosa, palmar creases, vulva, and anus is a normal phenomenon in dark-skinned races, patients frequently describe increase in pigmentation of these sites. Pigmentation of the tongue is an abnormal finding in all races.

General weakness, fatigue and malaise, anorexia, and weight loss are invariable features of the disorder. Weight loss may reach 15 kg with progressive adrenal failure. Gastrointestinal disturbances, especially nausea and vomiting, occur in most patients; diarrhea is less frequent. An increase in gastrointestinal symptoms during an acute adrenal crisis may confuse the diagnosis by suggesting a primary intra-abdominal process.

Hypotension is present in about 90% of patients and causes orthostatic symptoms and occasionally syncope. In more severe chronic cases and in acute crises, recumbent hypotension or shock is almost invariably present. Vitiligo occurs in 4–17% of patients with idiopathic Addison's disease but is rare in Addison's disease due to other causes. Salt craving occurs in about 20% of patients.

Severe hypoglycemia may occur in children. This finding is unusual in adults but may be provoked by fasting, fever, infection, or nausea and vomiting, especially in acute adrenal crisis.

Amenorrhea is common in Addison's disease. It may be due to weight loss and chronic illness or to primary ovarian failure. Loss of axillary and pubic hair may occur in women as a result of decreased secretion of adrenal androgens.

2. Acute adrenal crisis–Acute adrenal crisis represents a state of acute adrenocortical insufficiency and occurs in patients with Addison's disease who are exposed to the stress of infection, trauma, surgery, or dehydration due to salt deprivation, vomiting, or diarrhea.

The symptoms are listed in Table 9–5. Anorexia and nausea and vomiting increase and worsen the volume depletion and dehydration. Hypovolemic shock may occur, and adrenal insufficiency should be considered in any patient with unexplained vascular collapse. Abdominal pain may occur and mimics an acute abdominal emergency. Weakness, apathy, and confusion are usual. Fever is usual and may be due to infection or to hypoadrenalism per se. Hyperpigmentation is present unless the onset of adrenal insufficiency is rapid and should suggest the diagnosis.

Additional findings that suggest the diagnosis are hyponatremia, hyperkalemia, lymphocytosis, eosinophilia, and hypoglycemia.

Table 9–5. Clinical features of acute adrenal crisis.

Hypotension and shock
Fever
Dehydration, volume depletion
Nausea, vomiting, anorexia
Weakness, apathy, depressed mentation
Hypoglycemia

Table 9–6. Clinical features of adrenal hemorrhage.*

	Percent
General features	
Hypotension and shock	74
Fever	59
Nausea and vomiting	46
Confusion, disorientation	41
Tachycardia	28
Cyanosis or lividity	28
Local features	
Abdominal, flank, or back pain	77
Abdominal or flank tenderness	38
Abdominal distention	28
Abdominal rigidity	20
Chest pain	13
Rebound tenderness	5

*Reproduced, with permission, from Baxter JD, Tyrrell JB, in: *Endocrinology and Metabolism.* Felig P et al (editors). McGraw-Hill, 1981.

Shock and coma may rapidly lead to death in untreated patients.

3. Acute adrenal hemorrhage–(See Table 9–6.) Bilateral adrenal hemorrhage and acute adrenal destruction in an already compromised patient with major medical illness follow a progressively deteriorating course. The usual manifestations are abdominal, flank, or back pain and abdominal tenderness. Abdominal distention, rigidity, and rebound tenderness are less frequent. Hypotension, shock, fever, nausea and vomiting, confusion, and disorientation are common; tachycardia and cyanosis are less frequent.

With progression, severe hypotension, volume depletion, dehydration, hyperpyrexia, cyanosis, coma, and death ensue.

The diagnosis of acute adrenal hemorrhage should be considered in the deteriorating patient with unexplained abdominal or flank pain, vascular collapse, hyperpyrexia, or hypoglycemia.

B. Laboratory, X-Ray, and Electrocardiographic Findings:

1. Gradual adrenal destruction–Hyponatremia and hyperkalemia are classic manifestations of the mineralocorticoid deficiency of primary adrenal insufficiency and should suggest the diagnosis. Hematologic manifestations include normocytic, normochromic anemia, neutropenia, eosinophilia, and a relative lymphocytosis. Azotemia with increased concentrations of blood urea nitrogen and serum creatinine is due to volume depletion and dehydration. Mild acidosis is frequently present. Hypercalcemia of mild to moderate degree occurs in about 6% of patients.

Abdominal radiographs reveal adrenal calcification in half of patients with tuberculous Addison's disease and in some patients with other invasive or hemorrhagic causes of adrenal insufficiency.

Electrocardiographic features are low voltage, a vertical QRS axis, and nonspecific ST–T wave abnormalities secondary to abnormal electrolytes.

2. Acute adrenal hemorrhage–Hyponatremia and

hyperkalemia occur in only a small number of cases, but azotemia is a usual finding. Increased circulating eosinophils may suggest the diagnosis.

SECONDARY ADRENOCORTICAL INSUFFICIENCY

Etiology

Secondary adrenocortical insufficiency due to ACTH deficiency is most commonly a result of exogenous glucocorticoid therapy. Pituitary or hypothalamic tumors are the most common causes of naturally occurring pituitary ACTH hyposecretion. These and other less common causes are reviewed in Chapter 4.

Pathophysiology

ACTH deficiency is the primary event and leads to decreased cortisol and adrenal androgen secretion. Aldosterone secretion remains normal except in a few cases. In the early stages, basal ACTH and cortisol levels may be normal; however, ACTH reserve is impaired, and ACTH and cortisol responses to stress are therefore subnormal. With further loss of basal ACTH secretion, there is atrophy of the zonae fasciculata and reticularis of the adrenal cortex; and, therefore, basal cortisol secretion is decreased. At this stage, the entire pituitary adrenal axis is impaired; ie, there is not only decreased ACTH responsiveness to stress but also decreased adrenal responsiveness to acute stimulation with exogenous ACTH.

The manifestations of glucocorticoid deficiency are similar to those described for primary adrenocortical insufficiency. However, since aldosterone secretion by the zona glomerulosa is usually preserved, the manifestations of mineralocorticoid deficiency are absent.

Clinical Features

A. Symptoms and Signs: Secondary adrenal insufficiency is usually chronic, and the manifestations may be nonspecific. However, acute crisis can occur in undiagnosed patients or in corticosteroid-treated patients who do not receive increased steroid dosage during periods of stress.

The clinical features of secondary adrenal insufficiency differ from those of primary adrenocortical insufficiency in that pituitary secretion of ACTH and β-LPH is deficient and hyperpigmentation is therefore not present. In addition, mineralocorticoid secretion is usually normal. Thus, the clinical features of ACTH and glucocorticoid deficiency are nonspecific.

Volume depletion, dehydration, and electrolyte abnormalities are usually absent. Hypotension is usually not present except in acute presentations. Hyponatremia may occur as a result of water retention and inability to excrete a water load but is not accompanied by hyperkalemia. Prominent features are weakness, lethargy, easy fatigability, anorexia, nausea, and occasionally vomiting. Arthralgias and myalgias also occur. Hypoglycemia is occasionally the

presenting feature. Acute decompensation with severe hypotension or shock unresponsive to vasopressors may occur.

B. Associated Features: Patients with secondary adrenal insufficiency commonly have additional features that suggest the diagnosis. A history of glucocorticoid therapy or, if this is not available, the presence of cushingoid features suggests prior glucocorticoid use. Hypothalamic or pituitary tumors leading to ACTH deficiency usually cause loss of other pituitary hormones (hypogonadism and hypothyroidism). Hypersecretion of GH or prolactin (PRL) from a pituitary adenoma may be present.

C. Laboratory Findings: Findings on routine laboratory examination consist of normochromic, normocytic anemia, neutropenia, lymphocytosis, and eosinophilia. Serum sodium, potassium, creatinine, and bicarbonate and blood urea nitrogen are usually normal; plasma glucose may be low, though severe hypoglycemia is unusual.

DIAGNOSIS OF ADRENOCORTICAL INSUFFICIENCY

Although the diagnosis of adrenal insufficiency should be confirmed by assessment of the pituitary adrenal axis, therapy should not be delayed nor should the patient be subjected to procedures that may increase volume loss and dehydration and further contribute to hypotension. If the patient is acutely ill, therapy should be instituted and the diagnosis established when the patient is stable.

Diagnostic Tests

Since basal levels of adrenocortical steroids in either urine or plasma may be normal in partial adrenal insufficiency, tests of adrenocortical reserve are necessary to establish the diagnosis (Fig 9–11). These tests are described in the section on laboratory evaluation and in Chapter 4.

Rapid ACTH Stimulation Test

The rapid ACTH stimulation test assesses adrenal reserve and is the initial procedure in the assessment of possible adrenal insufficiency, either primary or secondary.

Subnormal responses to exogenous ACTH administration are an indication of decreased adrenal reserve and establish the diagnosis of adrenocortical insufficiency. Further diagnostic procedures are not required, since subnormal responses to the rapid ACTH stimulation test indicate lack of responsiveness to metyrapone, insulin-induced hypoglycemia, or stress. However, this test does not permit differentiation of primary and secondary causes. This is best accomplished by measurement of basal plasma ACTH levels, as discussed below.

A normal response to the rapid ACTH stimulation test excludes primary adrenal failure, since a normal cortisol response indicates normal cortical function.

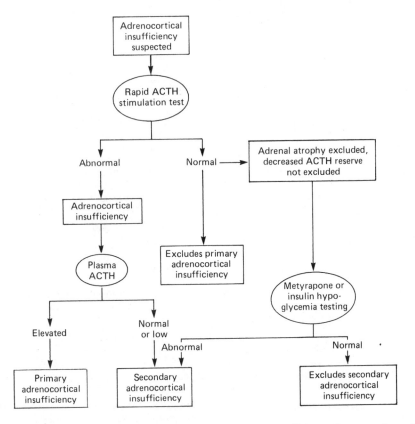

Figure 9–11. Evaluation of suspected primary or secondary adrenocortical insufficiency. Boxes enclose clinical decisions, and circles enclose diagnostic tests. (Redrawn and reproduced, with permission, from Baxter JD, Tyrrell JB: The adrenal cortex. In: *Endocrinology and Metabolism.* Felig P et al [editors]. McGraw-Hill, 1981.)

However, normal responsiveness does not exclude partial secondary adrenocortical insufficiency in those few patients with decreased pituitary reserve and decreased stress responsiveness of the hypothalamic-pituitary-adrenal axis who maintain sufficient basal ACTH secretion to prevent adrenocortical atrophy. If this situation is suspected clinically, pituitary ACTH responsiveness may be tested directly with metyrapone or insulin-induced hypoglycemia. (See section on laboratory evaluation and below.)

Plasma ACTH Levels

If adrenal insufficiency is present, plasma ACTH levels are used to differentiate primary and secondary forms. In patients with primary adrenal insufficiency, plasma ACTH levels are over 250 pg/mL and usually range from 400 to 2000 pg/mL. With pituitary ACTH deficiency, plasma ACTH levels range from 0 to 50 pg/mL and are usually less than 20 pg/mL (Fig 9–12).

Partial ACTH Deficiency

When partial ACTH deficiency and decreased pituitary reserve are suspected despite normal respon-

siveness to the rapid ACTH stimulation test, the following procedures may be used for more direct assessment of hypothalamic-pituitary function:

A. Methods of Testing: The overnight **metyrapone test** is used in patients with suspected hypothalamic or pituitary disorders when hypoglycemia is contraindicated and in those with prior glucocorticoid therapy. **Insulin-induced hypoglycemia** is used in patients with suspected hypothalamic or pituitary tumors, since both ACTH and GH responsiveness can be assessed (see Chapter 4).

B. Interpretation: A normal response to either metyrapone or hypoglycemia excludes secondary adrenocortical insufficiency. (See section on laboratory evaluation.) Subnormal responses, in the presence of a normal response to ACTH administration, establish the diagnosis of secondary adrenal insufficiency.

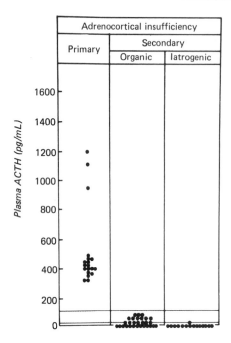

Figure 9–12. Basal plasma ACTH levels in primary and secondary adrenocortical insufficiency. (Reproduced, with permission, from Irvine WJ, Toft AD, Feek CM: Addison's disease. In: *The Adrenal Gland.* James VHT [editor]. Raven Press, 1979.)

TREATMENT OF ADRENOCORTICAL INSUFFICIENCY

Acute Addisonian Crisis (Table 9–7)

Treatment for acute addisonian crisis should be instituted as soon as the diagnosis is suspected. Therapy includes administration of glucocorticoids; correction of dehydration, hypovolemia, and electrolyte abnormalities; general supportive measures; and treatment of coexisting or precipitating disorders.

A. Cortisol (Hydrocortisone): Parenteral cortisol in soluble form (hydrocortisone hemisuccinate or phosphate) is the glucocorticoid preparation most commonly used. This agent has sufficient sodium-retaining potency so that additional mineralocorticoid therapy is not required in patients with primary adrenocortical insufficiency who have deficient secretion of both aldosterone and cortisol.

Cortisol in doses of 100 mg intravenously is given every 6 hours for the first 24 hours. The response to therapy is usually rapid, with improvement occurring within 12 hours or less. If improvement occurs and the patient is stable, 50 mg every 6 hours is given on the second day, and in most patients the dosage may then be gradually reduced to approximately 10 mg 3 times daily by the fourth or fifth day. (See section on maintenance therapy, below.)

1. In severely ill patients, especially in those with

Table 9–7. Treatment of acute adrenal crises.

Glucocorticoid replacement

(1) Administer cortisol (as hydrocortisone phosphate or hemi-succinate), 100 mg intravenously every 6 hours for 24 hours.

(2) When the patient is stable, reduce the dosage to 50 mg every 6 hours.

(3) Taper to maintenance therapy by day 4 or 5 and add mineralocorticoid therapy as required.

(4) Maintain or increase the dose to 200–400 mg/d if complications persist or occur.

General and supportive measures

(1) Correct volume depletion, dehydration, and hypoglycemia with intravenous saline and glucose.

(2) Evaluate and correct infection and other precipitating factors.

additional major complications (eg, sepsis), higher cortisol doses (100 mg intravenously every 6– 8 hours) are maintained until the patient is stable.

2. In primary Addison's disease, mineralocorticoid replacement, in the form of fludrocortisone (see below), is added when the total cortisol dosage has been reduced to 50– 60 mg/d.

3. In secondary adrenocortical insufficiency with acute crisis, the primary requirement is glucocorticoid replacement and is satisfactorily supplied by the administration of cortisol, as outlined above. If the possibility of excessive fluid and sodium retention in such patients is of concern, equivalent parenteral doses of synthetic steroids such as prednisolone or dexamethasone may be substituted.

4. Intramuscular cortisone acetate is contraindicated in acute adrenal failure for the following reasons: (1) absorption is slow; (2) it requires conversion to cortisol in the liver; (3) adequate plasma levels of cortisol are not obtained; and (4) there is inadequate suppression of plasma ACTH levels, indicating insufficient glucocorticoid activity.

B. Intravenous Fluids: Intravenous glucose and saline are administered to correct volume depletion, hypotension, and hypoglycemia. Volume deficits may be severe in Addison's disease, and hypotension and shock may not respond to vasopressors unless glucocorticoids are administered. Hyperkalemia and acidosis are usually corrected with cortisol and volume replacement; however, an occasional patient may require specific therapy for these abnormalities.

Maintenance Therapy (Table 9–8)

Patients with Addison's disease require lifelong therapy, usually with both glucocorticoids and mineralocorticoids. Cortisol (hydrocortisone) is the glucocorticoid preparation most often used. The total dosage is usually 25– 30 mg/d orally, given as 15– 20 mg in the morning on arising and 10 mg at 4– 5 PM. Other glucocorticoids such as oral cortisone acetate (37.5 mg/d), which is rapidly absorbed and converted to cortisol, or equivalent doses of synthetic steroids

Table 9–8. Regimen for maintenance therapy of primary adrenocortical insufficiency.*

(1) Cortisol, 15–20 mg in AM and 10 mg at 4–5 PM.
(2) Fludrocortisone, 0.05–0.1 mg orally in AM.
(3) Clinical follow-up: Maintenance of normal weight, blood pressure, and electrolytes with regression of clinical features.
(4) Patient education plus identification card or bracelet.
(5) Increased cortisol dosage during "stress."

*Reproduced, with permission, from Baxter JD, Tyrrell JB, in: *Endocrinology and Metabolism.* Felig P et al (editors). McGraw-Hill, 1981.

(eg, prednisone or prednisolone) may also be used.

Cortisol in twice-daily doses gives satisfactory responses in most patients; however, some patients may require only a single morning dose, and others may require 3 doses per day to maintain well-being and normal energy levels. Insomnia as a side effect of glucocorticoid administration can usually be prevented by administering the last daily dose at 4–5 PM.

Fludrocortisone (9α-fluorocortisol; Florinef) is used for mineralocorticoid therapy; the usual doses are 0.05–0.1 mg/d orally in the morning. Because of the long half-life of this agent, divided doses are not required. About 10–20% of addisonian patients can be managed with cortisol and adequate dietary sodium intake alone and do not require fludrocortisone.

Secondary adrenocortical insufficiency is treated with the cortisol dosages described above for the primary form. Fludrocortisone is rarely required.

Response to Therapy; Clinical Assessment

There are no currently available biochemical procedures for assessing the response to treatment of adrenocortical insufficiency. Measurement of plasma cortisol and ACTH levels is of no particular value, because of the wide variability in plasma levels in relationship to the timing of the cortisol dose and the time of plasma sampling. Measurement of urine free cortisol levels has been suggested, but a significant advantage has not yet been substantiated.

The adequacy of glucocorticoid and mineralocorticoid replacement is currently best evaluated by the clinical response to therapy. Thus, in appropriately treated patients, there is improvement or resolution of the features of glucocorticoid and mineralocorticoid deficiency, and most patients lead normal lives without significant disability.

A. Cortisol Therapy: Adequate treatment results in the disappearance of weakness, malaise, and fatigue. Anorexia and other gastrointestinal symptoms resolve, and weight returns to normal. The hyperpigmentation invariably improves but may not entirely disappear. Inadequate cortisol administration leads to persistence of these symptoms of adrenal insufficiency, and excessive pigmentation will remain. Greater than physiologic doses of glucocorticoids result in weight gain and may cause cushingoid features.

B. Mineralocorticoid Therapy: This should be monitored by frequent measurement of blood pressure and of serum electrolytes. With adequate treatment, the blood pressure is normal without orthostatic change, and serum sodium and potassium remain within the normal range. Hypertension and hypokalemia result if the fludrocortisone dose is excessive; conversely, undertreatment may lead to fatigue and malaise, orthostatic symptoms, and subnormal supine or upright blood pressure, with hyperkalemia and hyponatremia.

Prevention of Adrenal Crisis

The development of acute adrenal insufficiency in previously diagnosed and treated patients is almost entirely preventable in cooperative individuals. The 2 essential elements are patient education and increased glucocorticoid dosages during illness.

The patient should be informed about the necessity for lifelong therapy, the possible consequences of acute illness, and the necessity for increased therapy and medical assistance during acute illness. An identification card or bracelet should be carried or worn at all times.

The cortisol dose should be increased by the patient to 60–80 mg/d with the development of minor illnesses; the usual maintenance dosage may be resumed in 24–48 hours if improvement occurs. Increased mineralocorticoid therapy is not required.

If symptoms persist or become worse, the patient should continue increased cortisol doses and call the physician.

Vomiting may result in inability to ingest or absorb oral cortisol, and diarrhea in addisonian patients may precipitate a crisis because of rapid fluid and electrolyte losses. Patients must understand that if these symptoms occur, they should seek immediate medical assistance so that parenteral glucocorticoid therapy can be given.

Steroid Coverage for Surgery (Table 9–9)

Patients with primary or secondary adrenocortical

Table 9–9. Steroid coverage for surgery.*

(1) Correct electrolytes, blood pressure, and hydration if necessary.
(2) Give hydrocortisone phosphate or hemisuccinate, 100 mg intramuscularly, on call to operating room.
(3) Give hydrocortisone phosphate or hemisuccinate, 50 mg intramuscularly or intravenously, in the recovery room and every 6 hours for the first 24 hours.
(4) If progress is satisfactory, reduce dosage to 25 mg every 6 hours for 24 hours and then taper to maintenance dosage over 3–5 days. Resume previous fludrocortisone dose when the patient is taking oral medications.
(5) Maintain or increase cortisol dosage to 200–400 mg/d if fever, hypotension, or other complications occur.

*Reproduced, with permission, from Baxter JD, Tyrrell JB, in: *Endocrinology and Metabolism.* Felig P et al (editors). McGraw-Hill, 1981.

insufficiency scheduled for elective surgery require increased glucocorticoid coverage. This problem is most frequently encountered in patients with pituitary-adrenal suppression due to exogenous glucocorticoid therapy. The principles of management are outlined in Table 9–9. *Note:* Intramuscular cortisone acetate should not be used, for the reasons discussed above in the section on treatment of acute addisonian crisis.

PROGNOSIS OF ADRENOCORTICAL INSUFFICIENCY

Before glucocorticoid and mineralocorticoid therapy became available, primary adrenocortical insufficiency was invariably fatal, with death usually occurring within 2 years after onset. Survival now approaches that of the normal population, and most patients lead normal lives. In general, death from adrenal insufficiency now occurs only in patients with rapid onset of disease who may die before the diagnosis is established and appropriate therapy started.

Secondary adrenal insufficiency has an excellent prognosis with glucocorticoid therapy.

Adrenal insufficiency due to bilateral adrenal hemorrhage is still often fatal, with most cases being recognized only at autopsy.

CUSHING'S SYNDROME

Chronic glucocorticoid excess, whatever its cause, leads to the constellation of symptoms and physical features known as **Cushing's syndrome.** It is most commonly iatrogenic, resulting from chronic glucocorticoid therapy. "Spontaneous" Cushing's syndrome is caused by abnormalities of the pituitary or adrenal or may occur as a consequence of ACTH secretion by nonpituitary tumors **(ectopic ACTH syndrome). Cushing's disease** is defined as the specific type of Cushing's syndrome due to excessive pituitary ACTH secretion. This section will review the various

Table 9–10. Classification and etiology of Cushing's syndrome.*

	Percent
ACTH-dependent	
Cushing's disease	68
Ectopic ACTH syndrome	15
ACTH-independent	
Adrenal adenoma	9
Adrenal carcinoma	8
	100

*Reproduced, with permission, from Baxter JD, Tyrrell JB, in: *Endocrinology and Metabolism.* Felig P et al (editors). McGraw-Hill, 1981.

types of spontaneous Cushing's syndrome and discuss their diagnosis and therapy. (See also Chapter 4.)

Classification & Incidence

Cushing's syndrome is conveniently classified as either ACTH-dependent or ACTH-independent (Table 9–10).

The ACTH-dependent types of Cushing's syndrome—ectopic ACTH syndrome and Cushing's disease—are characterized by chronic ACTH hypersecretion, which results in hyperplasia of the adrenal zonae fasciculata and reticularis and therefore increased adrenocortical secretion of cortisol, androgens, and DOC.

ACTH-independent Cushing's syndrome is due to autonomous glucocorticoid-secreting adrenocortical adenomas or carcinomas; in these cases, the resulting cortisol excess suppresses pituitary ACTH secretion.

A. Cushing's Disease: This is the most frequent type of Cushing's syndrome and is responsible for about 70% of reported cases. Cushing's disease is much more common in women than in men (female:male ratio of about 8:1) and the age at diagnosis is usually between 20 and 40 years.

B. Ectopic ACTH Hypersecretion: This disorder is said to account for about 15% of cases of Cushing's syndrome. That figure is probably an underestimate, since it is likely that many patients are not diagnosed because they lack the classic features of hypercortisolism. In addition, severe hypercortisolism and rapid death are common. Ectopic ACTH secretion is most common with oat cell carcinoma of the lung; this tumor is responsible for about 50% of cases of the syndrome. Ectopic ACTH hypersecretion is estimated to occur in 0.5–2% of patients with this tumor. Other tumors are discussed below. The ectopic ACTH syndrome is more common in men, presumably because of their higher incidence of oat cell carcinoma. The female:male ratio is 1:3, and the peak incidence is at age 40–60 years.

C. Primary Adrenal Tumors: Primary adrenal tumors cause 17–19% of cases of Cushing's syndrome; adenoma and carcinoma occur with about equal frequency in adults. Glucocorticoid-secreting adrenal adenomas are more common in females. Adrenocortical carcinomas causing cortisol excess are also more common in females; however, if all types (including nonsecreting tumors) are considered, the overall incidence is higher in males. Adrenal carcinoma occurs in about 2 per million population per year; the mean age at diagnosis is 38 years; and 75% of cases occur in adults.

D. Childhood Cushing's Syndrome: Cushing's syndrome in childhood and adolescence is distinctly unusual; however, in contrast to the incidence in adults, adrenal carcinoma is the most frequent cause (51%), and adrenal adenomas are present in 14%. These tumors are more common in girls than in boys, and most occur between the ages of 1 and 8 years. Cushing's disease is more common in the adolescent population and accounts for 35% of cases; most of these patients are over 10 years of age at diagnosis, and the sex incidence is equal.

Pathology

A. Anterior Pituitary Gland:

1. Pituitary adenomas–Pituitary adenomas are present in over 90% of patients with Cushing's disease. These tumors are typically smaller than those secreting GH or PRL; 80– 90% are less than 10 mm in diameter (microadenomas), and 50% are 5 mm or less in diameter. A small group of patients have larger tumors (> 10 mm); these macroadenomas are frequently invasive, leading to extension outside the sella turcica. Malignant pituitary tumors occur rarely.

Microadenomas are located within the anterior pituitary; they are not encapsulated but surrounded by a rim of compressed normal anterior pituitary cells. With routine histologic stains, these tumors are composed of compact sheets of well-granulated basophilic cells in a sinusoidal arrangement. ACTH, β-LPH, and β-endorphin have been demonstrated in these tumor cells by immunocytochemical methods. Larger tumors may appear chromophobic on routine histologic study; however, they also contain ACTH and its related peptides. These ACTH-secreting adenomas typically show Crooke's changes (a zone of perinuclear hyalinization that is the result of chronic exposure of corticotroph cells to hypercortisolism). Electron microscopy demonstrates secretory granules that vary in size from 200 to 700 nm. The number of granules varies in individual cells; they may be dispersed throughout the cytoplasm or concentrated along the cell membrane. A typical feature of these adenomas is the presence of bundles of perinuclear microfilaments (average 7 nm in diameter) surrounding the nucleus; these are responsible for Crooke's hyaline changes visible on light microscopy.

2. Hyperplasia–Diffuse hyperplasia of corticotroph cells has been reported rarely in patients with Cushing's disease. These cases may be the consequence of excessive stimulation of the anterior pituitary by CRH. In an additional group of patients, adenomatous hyperplasia of the intermediate and posterior pituitary lobes has been described; these abnormal tissues also contained neural elements resembling those seen in normal posterior lobe tissue. The pathogenesis of these lesions is unclear.

3. Other conditions–In patients with adrenal tumors or ectopic ACTH syndrome, the pituitary corticotrophs show prominent Crooke hyaline changes and perinuclear microfilaments. The ACTH content of corticotroph cells is reduced consistent with their suppression by excessive cortisol secretion present in these conditions.

B. Adrenocortical Hyperplasia:
Bilateral hyperplasia of the adrenal cortex occurs with chronic ACTH hypersecretion. Three types have been described: simple, that associated with ectopic ACTH syndrome, and bilateral nodular hyperplasia.

1. Simple adrenocortical hyperplasia–This disorder is usually due to Cushing's disease. Combined adrenal weight (normal, 8– 10 g) is modestly increased, ranging from 12 to 24 g. On histologic study, there is equal hyperplasia of the compact cells of the zona reticularis and the clear cells of the zona fasciculata; consequently, the width of the cortex is increased. Electron microscopy reveals normal ultrastructural features.

2. Ectopic ACTH syndrome–In this disorder, the adrenals are frequently markedly enlarged; combined weights range from 24 g to more than 50 g. The characteristic microscopic feature is marked hyperplasia of the zona reticularis; columns of compact reticularis cells expand throughout the zona fasciculata and into the zona glomerulosa. The zona fasciculata clear cells are markedly reduced.

3. Bilateral nodular hyperplasia–This occurs in about 20% of cases of adrenocortical hyperplasia. The exact pathogenesis of this lesion is unclear; most cases appear to be secondary to pituitary ACTH excess, but in a minority of cases there may be autonomous function of the adrenals. The adrenals are enlarged; adrenal weight is increased and may be markedly so if large nodules are present. Grossly, there are multiple nodules within the adrenal cortices, with widening of the intervening cortex. The nodules are typically yellow and on histologic examination resemble the clear cells of the normal zona fasciculata. The adrenal cortex not involved by the nodules shows the histologic features of simple adrenocortical hyperplasia (see above). Adrenal carcinoma in association with nodular hyperplasia has been described in a few patients.

C. Adrenal Tumors:
Adrenal tumors causing Cushing's syndrome are independent of ACTH secretion and are either adenomas or carcinomas.

1. Glucocorticoid-secreting adrenal adenomas–These adenomas are encapsulated, weigh 10– 70 g, and range in size from 1 to 6 cm. Microscopically, clear cells of the zona fasciculata type predominate, although cells typical of the zona reticularis are also seen.

2. Adrenal carcinomas–Adrenal carcinomas usually weigh over 100 g and may exceed several kilograms. Thus, they are commonly palpable as abdominal masses. Grossly, they are encapsulated and highly vascular; necrosis, hemorrhage, and cystic degeneration are common, and areas of calcification may be present. The histologic appearance of these carcinomas varies considerably; they may appear to be benign or may exhibit considerable pleomorphism. Vascular or capsular invasion is predictive of malignant behavior, as is local extension. These carcinomas invade local structures (kidney, liver, and retroperitoneum) and metastasize hematogenously to liver and lung.

3. Uninvolved adrenal cortex–The cortex contiguous to the tumor and that of the contralateral gland are atrophic in the presence of functioning adrenal adenomas and carcinomas. The cortex is markedly thinned, whereas the capsule is thickened. Histologically, the zona reticularis is virtually absent; the remaining cortex is composed of clear fasciculata cells. The architecture of the zona glomerulosa is normal.

Etiology & Pathogenesis

A. Cushing's Disease: The causes and natural history of Cushing's disease are reviewed in Chapter 4. Current evidence is consistent with the view that spontaneously arising corticotroph-cell pituitary adenomas are the primary cause and that the consequent ACTH hypersecretion and hypercortisolism lead to the characteristic endocrine abnormalities and hypothalamic dysfunction. This is supported by evidence showing that selective removal of these adenomas by pituitary microsurgery reverses the abnormalities and is followed by return of the hypothalamic-pituitary-adrenal axis to normal.

Although these primary pituitary adenomas are responsible for the great majority of cases, a few patients have been described in whom pituitary disease has been limited to corticotroph-cell hyperplasia; these may be secondary to excessive hypothalamic CRH secretion.

B. Ectopic ACTH Syndrome: This syndrome arises when nonpituitary tumors synthesize and hypersecrete biologically active ACTH. The related peptides β-LPH and β-endorphin are also synthesized and secreted, as are inactive ACTH fragments. CRH-like activity has also been demonstrated in ectopic tumors secreting ACTH; however, CRH secretion into plasma has not been documented. Thus, whether CRH plays a role in pathogenesis is unclear.

Ectopic ACTH syndrome occurs predominantly in only a few tumor types (Table 9–11); oat cell carcinoma of the lung causes half of cases. Other tumors causing the syndrome are epithelial thymoma; pancreatic islet cell tumors; carcinoid tumors of lung, gut, pancreas, or ovary; medullary thyroid carcinoma; and pheochromocytoma and related tumors. Other rare miscellaneous tumor types have also been reported (see Chapter 24).

C. Adrenal Tumors: Glucocorticoid-producing adrenal adenomas and carcinomas arise spontaneously. They are not under hypothalamic-pituitary control and autonomously secrete adrenocortical steroids. Rarely, adrenal carcinomas develop in the setting of chronic ACTH hypersecretion in patients with either Cushing's disease and nodular adrenal hyperplasia or congenital adrenal hyperplasia.

Pathophysiology

A. Cushing's Disease: In Cushing's disease,

Table 9–11. Tumors causing the ectopic ACTH syndrome.*

Oat cell carcinoma of the lung (50% of cases)
Thymoma
Pancreatic islet cell tumors
Carcinoid tumors (lung, gut, pancreas, ovary)
Medullary carcinoma of the thyroid
Pheochromocytoma and related tumors

---

*Modified and reproduced, with permission, from Baxter JD, Tyrrell JB, in: *Endocrinology and Metabolism.* Felig P et al (editors). McGraw-Hill, 1981.

ACTH hypersecretion is random and episodic and causes cortisol hypersecretion with absence of the normal circadian rhythm. Feedback inhibition of ACTH (secreted from the pituitary adenoma) by physiologic levels of glucocorticoids is absent; thus, ACTH hypersecretion persists despite elevated cortisol secretion and results in chronic glucocorticoid excess. The episodic secretion of ACTH and cortisol results in variable plasma levels that may at times be within the normal range. However, measurement of the cortisol production rate, urine free cortisol, or sampling of multiple cortisol levels over 24 hours confirms cortisol hypersecretion (see sections on laboratory evaluation and diagnosis of Cushing's syndrome). In addition, because of the absence of diurnal variability, plasma ACTH and cortisol remain elevated throughout the day and night. This overall increase in glucocorticoid secretion causes the clinical manifestations of Cushing's syndrome; however, ACTH and β-LPH secretion are not usually elevated sufficiently to cause hyperpigmentation.

1. Abnormalities of ACTH secretion–Despite ACTH hypersecretion, stress responsiveness is absent; stimuli such as hypoglycemia or surgery fail to further elevate ACTH and cortisol secretion. This is probably due to suppression of hypothalamic function and CRH secretion by hypercortisolism, resulting in loss of hypothalamic control of ACTH secretion (see Chapter 4).

2. Effect of cortisol excess–Cortisol excess not only inhibits normal pituitary and hypothalamic function, affecting ACTH, thyrotropin, GH, and gonadotropin release, but also results in all the systemic effects of glucocorticoid excess described in previous sections and in the section on clinical features below.

3. Androgen excess–Secretion of adrenal androgens is also increased in Cushing's disease, and the degree of androgen excess parallels that of ACTH and cortisol. Thus, plasma levels of DHEA, DHEA sulfate, and androstenedione are moderately elevated in Cushing's disease; the peripheral conversion of these hormones to testosterone and dihydrotestosterone leads to androgen excess. In women, this causes hirsutism, acne, and amenorrhea. In men with Cushing's disease, cortisol suppression of LH secretion decreases testosterone secretion by the testis, resulting in decreased libido and impotence. The increased adrenal androgen secretion is insufficient to compensate for the decreased gonadal testosterone production.

B. Ectopic ACTH Syndrome: Hypersecretion of ACTH and cortisol is usually greater in patients with ectopic ACTH syndrome than in those with Cushing's disease. ACTH and cortisol hypersecretion is randomly episodic, and the levels are often greatly elevated. With few exceptions, ACTH secretion by ectopic tumors is not subject to negative-feedback control; ie, secretion of ACTH and cortisol is nonsuppressible with pharmacologic doses of glucocorticoids (see section on diagnosis).

Plasma levels, secretion rates, and urinary excretion of cortisol, the adrenal androgens, and DOC are often markedly elevated; despite this, the typical features of Cushing's syndrome are usually absent, presumably because of rapid onset of hypercortisolism, anorexia, and other manifestations of the associated malignant disease. However, features of mineralocorticoid excess (hypertension and hypokalemia) are frequently due to DOC and the mineralocorticoid effects of cortisol.

C. Adrenal Tumors:

1. Autonomous secretion–Primary adrenal tumors, both adenomas and carcinomas, autonomously hypersecrete cortisol. Circulating plasma ACTH levels are suppressed, resulting in cortical atrophy of the uninvolved adrenal. Secretion is randomly episodic, and these tumors are typically unresponsive to manipulation of the hypothalamic-pituitary axis with pharmacologic agents such as dexamethasone and metyrapone.

2. Adrenal adenomas–Adrenal adenomas causing Cushing's syndrome typically present solely with clinical manifestations of glucocorticoid excess, since they usually secrete only cortisol. Thus, the presence of androgen or mineralocorticoid excess should suggest that the tumor is an adrenocortical carcinoma.

3. Adrenal carcinomas–Adrenal carcinomas frequently hypersecrete multiple adrenocortical steroids and their precursors. Cortisol and androgens are the steroids most frequently secreted in excess; 11-deoxycortisol is often elevated, and there may be increased secretion of DOC, aldosterone, or estrogens. Plasma cortisol, urine free cortisol, and urine 17-hydroxycorticosteroids are often markedly increased; androgen excess is usually even greater than that of cortisol. Thus, high levels of plasma DHEA and DHEA sulfate and of urinary 17-ketosteroids typically accompany the cortisol excess. Clinical manifestations of hypercortisolism are usually severe and rapidly progressive in these patients. In women, features of androgen excess are prominent; virilism may occasionally occur. Hypertension and hypokalemia are frequent and most commonly result from the mineralocorticoid effects of cortisol; less frequently, DOC and aldosterone hypersecretion also contribute.

Clinical Features
(Table 9–12)

A. Symptoms and Signs:

1. Obesity–Obesity is the most common manifestation, and weight gain is usually the initial symptom. It is classically central, affecting mainly the face, neck, trunk, and abdomen, with relative sparing of the extremities. Generalized obesity with central accentuation is equally common, particularly in children.

Accumulation of fat in the face leads to the typical "moon facies," which is present in 75% of cases and is accompanied by facial plethora in most patients. Fat accumulation around the neck is prominent in the supraclavicular and dorsocervical fat pads; the latter is responsible for the "buffalo hump."

Obesity is absent in a handful of patients who do

Table 9–12. Clinical features of Cushing's syndrome.*

	Percent
Obesity	94
Facial plethora	84
Hirsutism	82
Menstrual disorders	76
Hypertension	72
Muscular weakness	58
Back pain	58
Striae	52
Acne	40
Psychologic symptoms	40
Bruising	36
Congestive heart failure	22
Edema	18
Renal calculi	16
Headache	14
Polyuria-polydipsia	10
Hyperpigmentation	6

*Reproduced, with permission, from Baxter JD, Tyrrell JB, in: *Endocrinology and Metabolism.* Felig P et al (editors). McGraw-Hill, 1981.

not gain weight; however, they usually have central redistribution of fat and a typical facial appearance.

2. Skin changes–Skin changes are frequent, and their presence should arouse a suspicion of cortisol excess. Atrophy of the epidermis and its underlying connective tissue leads to thinning (a transparent appearance of the skin) and facial plethora. Easy bruisability following minimal trauma is present in about 40%. Striae occur in 50–70%; these are typically red to purple, depressed below the skin surface secondary to loss of underlying connective tissue, and wider (not infrequently 0.5–2 cm) than the pinkish white striae that may occur with pregnancy or rapid weight gain. These striae are most commonly abdominal but may also occur over the breasts, hips, buttocks, thighs, and axillae.

Minor wounds and abrasions may heal slowly, and surgical incisions sometimes undergo dehiscence.

Mucocutaneous fungal infections are frequent, including tinea versicolor, involvement of the nails (onychomycosis), and oral candidiasis.

Hyperpigmentation of the skin is rare in Cushing's disease or adrenal tumors but is common in ectopic ACTH syndrome.

3. Hirsutism–Hirsutism is present in about 80% of female patients owing to hypersecretion of adrenal androgens. Facial hirsutism is most common, but increased hair growth may also occur over the abdomen, breasts, chest, and upper thighs. Acne and seborrhea usually accompany hirsutism. Virilism is unusual except in cases of adrenal carcinoma, in which it occurs in about 20%.

4. Hypertension–Hypertension is a classic feature of spontaneous Cushing's syndrome; it is present in about 75% of cases, and the diastolic blood pressure is greater than 100 mm Hg in over 50%. Hypertension and its complications contribute greatly to the morbidity and mortality rates in spontaneous Cushing's syndrome; in the series of Plotz et al, 40% of those dying with the syndrome did so as a direct result of hypertension or atherosclerosis.

5. Gonadal dysfunction–This is very common as a result of elevated androgens (in females) and cortisol (in males and to a lesser extent in females). Amenorrhea occurs in 75% of premenopausal women and is usually accompanied by infertility. Decreased libido is frequent in males, and some have decreased body hair and soft testes.

6. Psychologic disturbances–Psychologic disturbances occur in about 40% of patients. Mild symptoms consist of emotional lability and increased irritability. Anxiety, depression, poor concentration, and poor memory may also be present. Euphoria is frequent, and occasional patients manifest overtly manic behavior. Sleep disorders are present in most patients, with either insomnia or early morning awakening.

Severe psychologic disorders occur in a few patients and include severe depression, psychosis with delusions or hallucinations, and paranoia. Some patients have committed suicide.

7. Muscle weakness–This occurs in about 60% of cases; it is more often proximal and is usually most prominent in the lower extremities.

8. Osteoporosis–Osteoporosis is present in most patients; back pain is an initial complaint in 58% of cases. Pathologic fractures occur in severe cases involving the ribs and vertebral bodies. Compression fractures of the spine are demonstrable radiographically in 16–22%.

9. Renal calculi–Calculi secondary to glucocorticoid-induced hypercalciuria occur in approximately 15% of patients, and renal colic may occasionally be a presenting complaint.

10. Thirst and polyuria–Thirst and polyuria secondary to overt hyperglycemia and diabetes mellitus occur in about 10% of patients, whereas asymptomatic glucose intolerance is much more frequent. Diabetic ketoacidosis is rare, as are diabetic microvascular complications.

B. Laboratory Findings: Routine laboratory examinations are described here. Specific diagnostic tests to establish the diagnosis of Cushing's syndrome are discussed in the section on diagnosis.

High normal hemoglobin, hematocrit, and red cell counts are usual; polycythemia is rare. The total white count is usually normal; however, both the percentage of lymphocytes and the total lymphocyte count may be subnormal. Eosinophils are also depressed, and a total eosinophil count less than $100/\mu L$ is present in most patients. Serum electrolytes, with rare exceptions, are normal in Cushing's disease; however, hypokalemic alkalosis occurs when there is marked steroid hypersecretion with the ectopic ACTH syndrome or adrenocortical carcinoma.

Fasting hyperglycemia or clinical diabetes occurs in only 10–15% of patients; postprandial hyperglycemia is more common. Glycosuria is present in patients with fasting or postprandial hyperglycemia. Most patients have secondary hyperinsulinemia and abnormal glucose tolerance tests.

Serum calcium is normal; serum phosphorus is low normal or slightly depressed. Hypercalciuria is present in 40% of cases.

C. X-Ray Findings: Routine radiographs may reveal cardiomegaly due to hypertensive or atherosclerotic heart disease. Vertebral compression fractures, rib fractures, and renal calculi may be present.

D. Electrocardiographic Findings: Hypertensive, ischemic, and electrolyte-induced changes may be present on the ECG.

Features Suggesting a Specific Cause

A. Cushing's Disease: Cushing's disease typifies the classic clinical picture: female predominance, onset generally between ages 20 and 40, and a slow progression over several years. Hyperpigmentation and hypokalemic alkalosis are rare; androgenic manifestations are limited to acne and hirsutism. Secretion of cortisol and adrenal androgens is only moderately increased.

B. Ectopic ACTH Syndrome (Carcinoma): In contrast, this syndrome occurs predominantly in males, with the highest incidence between ages 40 and 60. The clinical manifestations of hypercortisolism are frequently limited to weakness, hypertension, and glucose intolerance; the primary tumor is usually apparent. Hyperpigmentation, hypokalemia, and alkalosis are common, as are weight loss and anemia. The hypercortisolism is of rapid onset, and steroid hypersecretion is frequently severe, with equally elevated levels of glucocorticoids, androgens, and DOC.

C. Ectopic ACTH Syndrome (Benign Tumor): A minority of patients with ectopic ACTH syndrome due to more "benign" tumors, especially bronchial carcinoids, present a more slowly progressive course, with typical features of Cushing's syndrome. These patients may be clinically identical with those having pituitary-dependent Cushing's disease, and the responsible tumor may not be apparent. Hyperpigmentation, hypokalemic alkalosis, and anemia are variably present. Further confusion may arise, since a number of these patients with occult ectopic tumors may have ACTH and steroid dynamics typical of Cushing's disease (see below).

D. Adrenal Adenomas: The clinical picture in patients with adrenal adenomas is usually that of glucocorticoid excess alone, and androgenic effects such as hirsutism are usually absent. Onset is gradual, and hypercortisolism is mild to moderate. Urinary 17-ketosteroids and plasma androgens are usually in the low normal or subnormal range.

E. Adrenal Carcinomas: In general, adrenal carcinomas have a rapid onset of the clinical features of excessive glucocorticoid, androgen, and mineralocorticoid secretion and are rapidly progressive. Marked elevations of both cortisol and androgens are usual; hypokalemia is common, as are abdominal pain, palpable masses, and hepatic and pulmonary metastases.

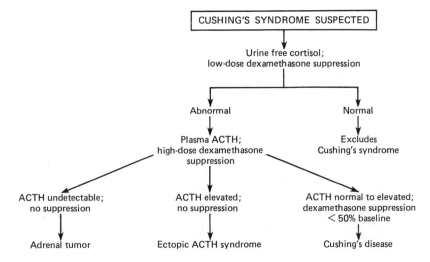

Figure 9–13. Diagnostic evaluation of Cushing's syndrome and procedures for determining the cause. Exceptions and diagnostic difficulties are discussed in the text. (Redrawn and reproduced, with permission, from Baxter JD, Tyrrell JB: The adrenal cortex. In: *Endocrinology and Metabolism.* Felig P et al [editors]. McGraw-Hill, 1981.)

Diagnostic Procedures
(Fig 9–13)

A. Diagnosis of Hypercortisolism (Cushing's Syndrome):

1. Overnight dexamethasone and urine free cortisol–Suspected hypercortisolism is investigated by means of the overnight 1-mg dexamethasone suppression test plus measurement of free cortisol in a 24-hour urine specimen collected on an outpatient basis. If the overnight suppression test is normal (plasma cortisol < 5 μg/dL), the diagnosis is very unlikely; if the urine free cortisol is also normal, Cushing's syndrome is excluded.

If these 2 tests are abnormal, hypercortisolism is present and the diagnosis of Cushing's syndrome can be considered established if conditions causing false-positive responses are excluded (see discussion below).

2. Two-day low-dose dexamethasone test–In patients with equivocal or borderline results, a 2-day low-dose dexamethasone suppression test is performed. Normal responses to this test are 17-hydroxycorticosteroid levels less than 4 mg/24 h (or 1 mg/g of creatinine) and free cortisol less than 25 μg/24 h. A normal response excludes Cushing's syndrome, and abnormal suppressibility is consistent with the diagnosis, since the incidence of false-positive responses is negligible.

3. Other tests–Other tests are less reliable in diagnosis and are no longer recommended; these include basal morning cortisol levels, afternoon or early evening cortisol, basal 24-hour urine 17-hydroxysteroids, 17-ketogenic steroids, or 17-ketosteroids, and responsiveness to either ACTH or metyrapone stimulation tests (see Laboratory Evaluation, above).

B. Differential Diagnosis of Hypercortisolism:

A number of factors may complicate the diagnosis of Cushing's syndrome. These include both rare false-negative results in patients with Cushing's syndrome and, more commonly, false-positive results in those who do not have the disorder.

1. False-negative responses–False-negative results occur rarely in Cushing's syndrome. In these patients, normal suppression of glucocorticoid secretion with low-dose dexamethasone may be due to delayed clearance of dexamethasone and thus higher than usual plasma levels. However, elevated urine free cortisol will establish the diagnosis. Periodic or episodic hormonogenesis in Cushing's syndrome also makes diagnosis difficult. In these unusual patients, hypercortisolism may be cyclic, with regular periodicity of days to weeks, or irregularly episodic; thus, cortisol secretion may be normal or nearly so between cycles or episodes. With spontaneously varying cortisol secretion, adrenal function may be normal at times, and dexamethasone administration during phases of normal secretion may appear to reveal normal suppressibility. In these patients, repeated evaluation is required to establish the diagnosis.

2. False-positive responses–False-positive results are more common:

a. Acute or chronic illness–Especially in hospitalized patients, acute or chronic illness may appropriately elevate glucocorticoid secretion. Patients may have elevated plasma cortisol and urine free cortisol and are frequently nonsuppressible with the 1-mg overnight dexamethasone test. If Cushing's syndrome is suspected, diagnostic evaluation should be repeated when acute stress has resolved.

b. Obesity–Obesity is the most common differential problem in Cushing's syndrome. Urinary 17-hydroxycorticosteroids and 17-ketogenic steroids are often elevated; furthermore, about 13% of obese patients do not adequately suppress plasma cortisol in response to the 1-mg overnight dexamethasone suppression test. However, urine free cortisol excretion is normal in simple obesity, as is normal suppressibility of urine corticosteroids with the 2-day low-dose suppression test.

c. High-estrogen states–Pregnancy, estrogen therapy, and oral contraceptives increase CBG and thus elevate total plasma cortisol levels to 40–60 μg/dL. The overnight 1-mg suppression test may be abnormal; however, urine free cortisol is normal, and there is normal suppressibility of urine steroids with the 2-day low-dose test.

d. Drugs–Various drugs, especially phenytoin, phenobarbital, and primidone, cause false-positive low-dose dexamethasone tests; however, urine free cortisol is normal.

e. Alcoholism–A number of alcoholic patients have both clinical and biochemical features of Cushing's syndrome (alcohol-induced pseudo-Cushing's syndrome) with elevated basal plasma cortisol levels, abnormal diurnal variation, increased cortisol production rate, increased urinary corticosteroid excretion, and abnormal dexamethasone suppressibility. These abnormalities revert to normal following abstinence from alcohol.

f. Depression–Endogenous depression frequently causes increased cortisol secretion with elevated plasma levels, absence of diurnal variation, increased urine free cortisol, increased urine 17-hydroxycorticosteroids, and impaired dexamethasone suppressibility in the overnight dexamethasone test. The abnormal steroid dynamics revert to normal upon psychologic recovery. These patients can be differentiated from those with true Cushing's syndrome, since patients with depression alone maintain normal cortisol responsiveness to insulin-induced hypoglycemia, whereas patients with Cushing's syndrome do not. In addition, depressed patients usually maintain normal responses to the 2-day low-dose dexamethasone test.

C. Differential Diagnosis of Cushing's Syndrome: When Cushing's syndrome is present, pituitary ACTH hypersecretion (Cushing's disease) must be differentiated from ectopic ACTH syndrome and primary adrenal tumors.

1. Procedures–The 2 most specific procedures are measurement of basal plasma ACTH levels and high-dose dexamethasone suppression testing (see Laboratory Evaluation, above). The combined results of these 2 tests will establish the correct diagnosis in most instances.

2. Results–

a. Cushing's disease–Patients with Cushing's disease have normal to modestly elevated plasma ACTH levels (Fig 9–14), and the presence of detectable levels is consistent with bilateral adrenocortical hyperplasia. Plasma ACTH levels in Cushing's disease range from 40 to 200 pg/mL (normal, 20–100 pg/mL), and about 50% of patients have values consistently within the normal range. Patients with Cush-

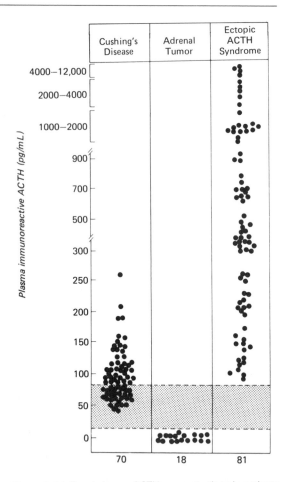

Figure 9–14. Basal plasma ACTH concentrations in patients with spontaneous Cushing's syndrome. (Reproduced, with permission, from Scott AP et al: Pituitary adrenocorticotropin and the melanocyte stimulating hormones. In: *Peptide Hormones.* Parsons JA [editor]. University Park Press, 1979.)

ing's disease characteristically maintain suppressibility of ACTH secretion; ie, cortisol secretion is suppressible to below 50% of basal levels with the high-dose dexamethasone tests.

b. Ectopic ACTH syndrome–In the ectopic ACTH syndrome, plasma ACTH levels are often markedly elevated (500–10,000 pg/mL) and are above 200 pg/mL in 65% of patients. However, since at lower levels these overlap with the range seen in Cushing's disease, dexamethasone suppression testing must also be used. Since hypothalamic control of ACTH secretion is absent, cortisol secretion is classically not suppressible with high-dose dexamethasone. In addition, the primary tumor is clinically evident in most patients.

c. Adrenal tumors–Glucocorticoid-secreting adrenal tumors function autonomously, and the resulting suppression of the normal hypothalamic-pituitary axis leads to undetectable plasma ACTH levels (< 20 pg/mL) and absent steroid suppression with high-dose dexamethasone.

3. Other tests—Preliminary results of CRH testing in Cushing's syndrome have revealed that the majority of patients with Cushing's disease respond to CRH, whereas those with ectopic ACTH syndrome do not. However, exceptions have already been reported in both entities, and thus the ultimate clinical utility of this procedure is not yet clear. Metyrapone testing and ACTH stimulation tests do not adequately distinguish the various causes of Cushing's syndrome and are of little diagnostic utility.

D. Problems in Making Etiologic Diagnoses:

1. Episodic hypercortisolism—Problems are encountered in rare patients with periodic, cyclic, or episodic hormonogenesis who may have either Cushing's disease, ectopic ACTH syndrome, or adrenal tumors. Variable responses to high-dose dexamethasone may be observed, and there may be apparent suppressibility if steroid secretion is declining spontaneously at the time of dexamethasone administration. When studied at other times, these patients may be nonsuppressible or even show paradoxic increases during high-dose dexamethasone treatment. Repeated evaluations and use of the localizing procedures described below may be necessary to establish the correct etiologic diagnosis in such patients.

2. Nonsuppressible Cushing's disease and nodular adrenal hyperplasia—About 10–30% of patients with Cushing's disease fail to suppress urinary 17-hydroxycorticosteroids with the standard 2-day high-dose dexamethasone suppression test. This incidence of inadequate suppressibility is less with the overnight 8-mg high-dose dexamethasone suppression test, and the overnight test is therefore preferred. Nonsuppressible Cushing's disease may occur with large pituitary tumors; however, it is also seen in patients with microadenomas and in patients without an obvious pituitary adenoma in whom ACTH is measurable; these findings falsely suggest the ectopic ACTH syndrome.

In these patients, additional procedures are required. Higher doses of dexamethasone (16 or 32 mg) may be administered, and if steroid suppression is demonstrated, Cushing's disease is suggested. The diagnosis is confirmed by demonstration of the pituitary adenoma using high-resolution CT scanning or the demonstration of pituitary ACTH hypersecretion by selective venous sampling. (See section on tumor localization, below.)

Some of these nonsuppressible patients have nodular adrenal hyperplasia, which is usually secondary to pituitary ACTH hypersecretion. This disorder frequently causes diagnostic difficulties, since about 75% of these patients are nonsuppressible with the standard 2-day high-dose dexamethasone suppression test. Plasma ACTH levels may be undetectable, normal, or elevated and may vary dramatically in the same patient. These patients should be evaluated with higher doses of dexamethasone (as described above) and pituitary localizing procedures to differentiate them from patients with either the ectopic ACTH syndrome or primary adrenal tumors. In addition, CT scanning of the adrenals may demonstrate nodular hyperplasia.

3. Ectopic ACTH syndrome—Although the ectopic ACTH syndrome is usually easily diagnosed by elevated ACTH levels and nonsuppressible steroid hypersecretion in the presence of an extrapituitary tumor, there are cases in which the tumor is occult, and in these, steroid secretion may be dexamethasone-suppressible and metyrapone-responsive. In addition, the tumor may not make its presence felt for a number of years following the onset of Cushing's syndrome. These occult tumors are usually carcinoids, and the plasma ACTH levels may be in the range of those seen with Cushing's disease. These findings may lead to a mistaken diagnosis of Cushing's disease and inappropriate pituitary therapy. Although it is not possible to make this differentiation with confidence in all cases, certain features should increase the suspicion of ectopic ACTH syndrome: male sex, rapid onset, severe hypercortisolism, hypokalemia, anemia, and weight loss. If ectopic ACTH syndrome is suspected but no tumor is obvious, selective venous ACTH sampling is helpful. Thus, the demonstration of a pituitary ACTH gradient establishes the diagnosis of Cushing's disease. In the absence of a pituitary gradient, ectopic ACTH syndrome is a likely diagnosis, and selective venous sampling may localize the ACTH-secreting ectopic tumor. If localization is not achieved by this method, additional diagnostic and radiologic procedures should be directed to the common sites of ACTH production, ie, the lungs, thymus, pancreas, thyroid, and adrenals.

E. Tumor Localization: The procedures described below are useful in the localization of tumors in Cushing's syndrome, but they should be preceded if possible by a definite biochemical diagnosis, since radiologic procedures may occasionally give misleading results. For example, nodular hyperplasia of the adrenals with a solitary or dominant nodule may be misinterpreted as an autonomous hyperfunctioning adenoma; or enlargement of the sella turcica may be due to the empty sella syndrome rather than to a pituitary tumor.

1. Neuroradiologic studies—In Cushing's disease, neuroradiologic procedures are utilized to localize the pituitary adenoma and to define sellar size, anatomy, and extrasellar tumor extension.

a. Macroadenomas—In patients with larger tumors (macroadenomas), CT scanning is used to document tumor size, suprasellar extension, lateral expansion, or the presence of a partially empty sella turcica. This procedure has replaced angiography and pneumoencephalography, which are rarely used at present.

b. Microadenomas—The problem of tumor localization in patients with Cushing's disease who have microadenomas has not been entirely solved, necessitating a secure biochemical diagnosis. Sellar polytomography has little utility and should not be used. High-resolution CT scanning is the current procedure

Figure 9–15. Adrenal CT scans in Cushing's syndrome. *A:* Patient with ACTH-dependent Cushing's syndrome. The adrenal glands are not detectably abnormal by this procedure. The curvilinear right adrenal (black arrow) is shown posterior to the inferior vena cava (V) between the right lobe of the liver and the right crus of the diaphragm. The left adrenal (white arrow) has an inverted Y appearance anteromedial to the left kidney (K). *B:* A 3-cm left adrenal adenoma (white arrow) is shown anteromedial to the left kidney (K). (Reproduced, with permission, from Korobkin MT et al: *Am J Roentgenol* 1979; **132:**231.)

of choice; however, because of the small size of pituitary adenomas in Cushing's disease, they are detected by CT scanning in only about 60% of patients. Patients with normal CT scans should undergo selective venous sampling.

2. Selective venous sampling for ACTH determination–This procedure is used when the source of ACTH hypersecretion is in doubt, eg, in patients in whom biochemical data suggest Cushing's disease but CT scanning does not localize the tumor. This procedure is also very useful in those with suspected dexamethasone-nonsuppressible Cushing's disease, nodular adrenal hyperplasia, or an occult ectopic ACTH-secreting tumor, as discussed above. In these circumstances, venous sampling may establish the pituitary as the source of ACTH and in some cases will localize an ectopic tumor. ACTH samples are obtained from the inferior petrosal sinuses (a major site of venous drainage of the anterior pituitary), from the jugular venous bulb, and from other sites and are compared with simultaneous peripheral vein samples. In patients with Cushing's disease, ACTH levels are higher in the inferior petrosal sinus samples than in the peripheral vein samples (ratios usually > 2:1). In patients with ectopic ACTH syndrome, no inferior petrosal-to-peripheral ACTH gradient is demonstrable, but selective venous sampling may localize the ectopic tumor.

3. Adrenal localizing procedures–CT scan (Fig 9–15), ultrasonography, and isotope scanning with iodocholesterol are used to define adrenal lesions. In patients with ACTH hypersecretion, these procedures exclude an adrenal tumor and confirm bilateral adrenal hyperplasia or nodular adrenal hyperplasia. These procedures also effectively localize adrenal tumors, since these tumors are usually over 2 cm in diameter. Invasive procedures such as arteriography and venography are rarely required.

Treatment

A. Cushing's Disease: The aim of treatment of Cushing's syndrome is to remove or destroy the basic lesion and thus correct hypersecretion of adrenal hormones without inducing pituitary or adrenal damage, which requires permanent replacement therapy for hormone deficiencies.

Treatment of Cushing's disease is currently directed at the pituitary to control ACTH hypersecretion; available methods include microsurgery, various forms of radiation therapy, and pharmacologic inhibition of ACTH secretion. Treatment of hypercortisolism per se by surgical or medical adrenalectomy is less commonly used. These methods are discussed in Chapter 4.

B. Ectopic ACTH Syndrome: Cure of ectopic ACTH syndrome is usually possible only in cases involving the more "benign" tumors such as thymomas, bronchial carcinoids, or pheochromocytomas. Treatment is made difficult by the presence of metastatic malignant tumors and accompanying severe hypercortisolism. Therapy directed to the primary tumor is usually unsuccessful, and other means must be used to correct the steroid-excess state.

Severe hypokalemia may require potassium replacement in large doses and spironolactone to block mineralocorticoid effects.

Drugs that block steroid synthesis (metyrapone and aminoglutethimide) are useful, but they may produce hypoadrenalism, and steroid secretion must be monitored and replacement steroids given if necessary.

Because of its slow onset of action, mitotane (o,p'-DDD) is less useful, and several weeks of therapy may be required to control cortisol secretion (see below).

Bilateral adrenalectomy is rarely required, but it may be necessary if hypercortisolism cannot otherwise be controlled.

C. Adrenal Tumors:

1. Adrenal adenomas–Patients with adrenal adenomas are successfully treated by unilateral adrenalectomy, and the outlook is excellent. Since the hypothalamic-pituitary axis and the contralateral adrenal are suppressed by prolonged cortisol secretion, these patients have postoperative adrenal insufficiency and require glucocorticoid therapy both during and following surgery until the remaining adrenal recovers.

2. Adrenal carcinomas–Therapy in cases of adrenocortical carcinoma is less satisfactory, since disease has already metastasized (usually to the retroperitoneum, liver, and lungs) by the time the diagnosis is made.

a. Operative treatment–Surgical cure is rare, but excision serves to reduce the tumor mass and the degree of steroid hypersecretion. Persisting nonsuppressible steroid secretion in the immediate postoperative period indicates residual or metastatic tumor.

b. Medical treatment–Mitotane (Lysodren; o,p'-DDD) is the drug of choice. The dosage is 6–12 g/d orally in 3 or 4 divided doses. The dose must often be reduced because of side effects in 80% of patients (diarrhea, nausea and vomiting, depression, somnolence). About 70% of patients achieve a reduction of steroid secretion, but only 35% achieve a reduction in tumor size. Since mitotane reduces urinary 17-hydroxycorticosteroid excretion by altering the hepatic metabolism of cortisol, these patients require follow-up by plasma cortisol or urine free cortisol assays.

Metyrapone and aminoglutethimide (singly or in combination) are useful in controlling steroid hypersecretion in patients who do not respond to mitotane.

Radiotherapy and conventional chemotherapy have not been useful in this disease.

Prognosis

A. Cushing's Syndrome: Untreated Cushing's syndrome is frequently fatal, and death may be due to the underlying tumor itself, as in the ectopic ACTH syndrome and adrenal carcinoma. However, in many cases, death is the consequence of sustained hypercortisolism and its complications, including hypertension, cardiovascular disease, stroke, thromboembolism, and susceptibility to infection. In older series, 50% of patients died within 5 years after onset.

B. Cushing's Disease: With current refinements in pituitary microsurgery and heavy particle irradiation, the great majority of patients with Cushing's disease can be treated successfully, and the operative mortality and morbidity rates that attended bilateral adrenalectomy are no longer a feature of the natural history of this disease. Although there are no current statistics on survival in these patients, it appears that it is considerably longer than in older series. Patients with Cushing's disease who have large pituitary tumors at the time of diagnosis have a much less satisfactory prognosis and may die as a consequence of tumor invasion or persisting hypercortisolism.

C. Adrenal Tumors: The prognosis in adrenal adenomas is excellent, although the mortality and morbidity rates associated with adrenalectomy must be considered in these patients. In adrenal carcinoma, the prognosis is almost universally poor, and the median survival from the date of onset of symptoms is about 4 years.

D. Ectopic ACTH Syndrome: Prognosis is also poor in patients with ectopic ACTH syndrome due to malignant tumors, and in these patients with severe hypercortisolism, survival is frequently only days to weeks. Some patients respond to tumor resection or chemotherapy. The prognosis is better in patients with benign tumors producing the ectopic ACTH syndrome.

HIRSUTISM & VIRILISM

Excessive adrenal or ovarian secretion of androgens or excessive conversion of androgens in peripheral tissues leads to these disorders. As previously discussed, the adrenal secretory products DHEA, DHEA sulfate, and androstenedione are weak androgens; however, the peripheral conversion to testosterone and dihydrotestosterone can result in a state of androgen excess. In most patients with hirsutism and in virtually all with virilism, plasma androgen concentrations are increased; a few have normal androgen and plasma concentrations but increased peripheral conversion or sensitivity.

Androgen excess in men may cause testicular atrophy but does not cause other manifestations. The clinical consequences of androgen excess in children are described in Chapter 13. In women, hirsutism is the usual clinical syndrome, and virilism due to markedly excessive androgen production is rare. Hirsutism in women is defined as excessive growth of hair in androgen-sensitive areas, most commonly resulting in increased facial hair. The severity ranges from a mild increase in the amount of hair on the upper lip and chin and at the sideburn areas to heavy facial growth requiring daily shaving. There may also be excessive hair in the pubic area, upper thighs, and lower abdomen (male pattern of hair growth) and on the lower back, chest, and breasts. These patients frequently have oily skin, acne, and menstrual irregularity or amenorrhea. Virilism results from marked androgen excess; in addition to hirsutism, these women have temporal recession of the hairline, male pattern baldness, clitoral enlargement, and masculine features, including increased muscle bulk, a male habitus, deepening of the voice, and amenorrhea. (See Chapter 14.)

Excessive androgen production is seen in both adrenal and ovarian disorders. Adrenal causes include Cushing's syndrome, adrenal carcinoma, and congenital adrenal hyperplasia (see previous sections and Chapter 15). Mild adult-onset cases of congenital adrenal enzyme deficiencies have been described; these appear to be relatively unusual. Ovarian causes include the polycystic ovary syndrome and, rarely, androgen-secreting tumors or stromal hyperthecosis (see Chapter 14). Polycystic ovary syndrome is the most common of these causes, and milder variants of this syndrome may be responsible for many cases of idiopathic hirsutism not accompanied by ovarian enlargement or menstrual irregularity. Idiopathic hirsutism is also common, and although most patients have demonstrable androgen hypersecretion, the site of abnormal androgen production is unclear. Thus, the ovary, adrenal, or both glands may contribute; current suppression and stimulation tests and even venous catheterization of the adrenals and ovaries have failed to resolve this controversy.

In children, androgen excess is usually due to congenital adrenal hyperplasia or adrenal carcinoma. In women, hirsutism accompanied by amenorrhea, infertility, ovarian enlargement, and elevated plasma LH levels is typical of the polycystic ovary syndrome, whereas in Cushing's syndrome hirsutism is accompanied by features of cortisol excess. Late-onset 21-hydroxylase deficiency is accompanied by elevated levels of plasma 17-hydroxyprogesterone. Virilism and severe androgen excess in adults are usually due to androgen-secreting adrenal or ovarian tumors; virilism is unusual in the polycystic ovary syndrome and rare in Cushing's disease. In the absence of these syndromes, hirsutism in women is usually idiopathic or due to milder forms of polycystic ovary syndrome.

Evaluation of possible androgen excess requires measurement of plasma androgens; one or more of these hormones are elevated in 85% of women with hirsutism. Urinary 17-ketosteroids are elevated in fewer than 20% of such patients. Although plasma assays are useful, certain guidelines are necessary in their use. First, androgen secretion is episodic and varies both with the circadian rhythm of ACTH and with the menstrual cycle. Thus, single plasma samples may not be diagnostic, and more reliable information is obtained by taking multiple samples that may be pooled before assay. Second, measurement of total plasma levels may not accurately reflect the biologically active free hormone concentration. This is of particular importance in states of androgen excess in which the circulating androgens reduce SHBG levels and binding capacity. Thus, in hirsutism, testosterone production, metabolic clearance, and free plasma testosterone concentration are usually increased; however, total plasma testosterone concentration is frequently normal. Therefore, measurement of the plasma free testosterone concentration, if available, is the most useful single measurement in these patients; it is elevated in 85% of patients. If free testosterone is normal or the test is not available, several measurements of the total androgen level should be done, since at least one of them will be elevated in almost every patient with hirsutism. The frequency of abnormal values is as follows: dihydrotestosterone, 75%; DHEA sulfate, 66%; testosterone, 60%; androstenedione, 45%; and DHEA, 45%. Androstanediol and its glucuronide, which are metabolic products of dihydrotestosterone, are elevated more frequently and are thus useful markers of androgen excess.

In the presence of excess androgens, the diagnosis of idiopathic hirsutism depends on exclusion of the other causes discussed above.

The therapy of hirsutism is discussed in Chapter 14.

REFERENCES

General

Baxter JD, Tyrrell JB: The adrenal cortex. In: *Endocrinology and Metabolism*. Felig P et al (editors). McGraw-Hill, 1981.

Besser GM, Rees LH: The pituitary-adrenocortical axis. *Clin Endocrinol Metab* 1985;**14**:765.

DeGroot LJ et al (editors): *Endocrinology*. 3 vols. Grune & Stratton, 1979.

Frohman LA: Diseases of the anterior pituitary. In: *Endocrinology and Metabolism*. Felig P et al (editors). McGraw-Hill, 1981.

James VHT (editor): *The Adrenal Gland*. Raven Press, 1979.

Nelson DH: *The Adrenal Cortex: Physiologic Function and Disease*. Saunders, 1980.

Embryology & Anatomy

Neville AM, O'Hare MJ: Aspects of structure, function and pathology. In: *The Adrenal Gland*. James VHT (editor). Raven Press, 1979.

Neville AM, O'Hare MJ: Histopathology of the human adrenal cortex. *Clin Endocrinol Metab* 1985;**14**:791.

Symington T: *Functional Pathology of the Human Adrenal Gland*. E&S Livingston, 1969.

Biosynthesis of Cortisol & Adrenal Androgens

Fehm HL et al: Differential and integral corticosteroid effects on ACTH secretion in hypoadrenocorticism. *J Clin Invest* 1979;**63**:247.

Gill GN: ACTH regulation of the adrenal cortex. In: *Pharmacology of Adrenal Cortical Hormones*. Gill GN (editor). Pergamon, 1979.

Jones MT: Control of adrenocortical hormone secretion. In: *The Adrenal Gland*. James VHT (editor). Raven Press, 1979.

Keller-Wood ME, Dallman MF: Corticosteroid inhibition of ACTH secretion. *Endocr Rev* 1984;**5**:1.

Kreiger DT: Plasma ACTH and corticosteroids. In: *Endocrinology*. DeGroot LJ et al (editors). Grune & Stratton, 1979.

Kreiger DT et al: Characterization of the normal temporal pattern of plasma corticosteroid levels. *J Clin Endocrinol Metab* 1971;**32**:266.

Nakanishi S et al: Nucleotide sequence of cloned cDNA for bovine corticotropin-beta-lipotropin precursor. *Nature* 1979;**278**:423.

Orth DN et al: Effect of synthetic ovine corticotropin-releasing factor: Dose response of plasma adrenocorticotropin and cortisol. *J Clin Invest* 1982;**71**:587.

Plumpton FS, Besser GM, Cole PV: Corticosteroid treatment and surgery. *Anaesthesia* 1969;**24**:3.

Ruhmann-Wennhold A, Nelson DH: Pituitary adrenocorticotrophin. In: *Endocrinology*. DeGroot LJ et al (editors). Grune & Stratton, 1979.

Schurmeyer TH et al: Human corticotropin-releasing factor in man: Pharmacokinetic properties and dose-response of plasma adrenocorticotropin and cortisol secretion. *Clin Endocrinol Metab* 1984;**59**:1103.

Vale W et al: Characterization of a 41-residue ovine hypothalamic peptide that stimulates secretion of corticotropin and β-endorphin. *Science* 1981;**213**:1394.

Vale W et al: Corticotropin-releasing factor. In: *Secretory Tumors of the Pituitary Gland*. Black PM et al (editors). Raven Press, 1984.

Yasuda N, Greer MA, Aizawa T: Corticotropin-releasing factor. *Endocr Rev* 1981;**3**:123.

Circulation & Metabolism of Cortisol & Adrenal Androgens

Abraham GE: Ovarian and adrenal contribution to peripheral androgens during the menstrual cycle. *J Clin Endocrinol Metab* 1974;**39**:340.

Ballard PL: Delivery and transport of glucocorticoids to target cells. In: *Glucocorticoid Hormone Action*. Baxter JD, Rousseau GG (editors). Springer-Verlag, 1979.

Bondy PK: The adrenal cortex. In: *Metabolic Control and Disease*. Bondy PK (editor). Saunders, 1979.

Brooks RV: Biosynthesis and metabolism of adrenocortical steroids. In: *The Adrenal Gland*. James VHT (editor). Raven Press, 1979.

Brown MS et al: Receptor-mediated uptake of lipoprotein-cholesterol and its utilization for steroid synthesis in the adrenal cortex. *Recent Prog Horm Res* 1979;**35**:215.

Finkelstein M, Shaefer JM: Inborn errors of steroid biosynthesis. *Physiol Rev* 1979;**59**:353.

Grant JK: An introductory review of adrenocortical steroid biosynthesis. In: *The Endocrine Function of the Human Adrenal Cortex*. James VHT et al (editors). Academic Press, 1978.

Habener JE: Hormone biosynthesis and secretion. In: *Endocrinology and Metabolism*. Felig P et al (editors). McGraw-Hill, 1981.

Migeon CJ: Adrenal androgens in man. *Am J Med* 1972; **53**:606.

Peterson RE: Metabolism of adrenal cortical steroids. In: *The Human Adrenal Cortex*. Christy NP (editor). Harper & Row, 1971.

Sandberg AA, Slaunwhite WR Jr: Physical state of adrenal cortical hormones in plasma. In: *The Human Adrenal Cortex*. Christy NP (editor). Harper & Row, 1971.

Siiteri PK: Qualitative and quantitative aspects of adrenal secretion of steroids. In: *The Human Adrenal Cortex*. Christy NP (editor). Harper & Row, 1971.

Biologic Effects

Baxter JD: Mechanisms of glucocorticoid inhibition of growth. *Kidney Int* 1978;**14**:330.

Baxter JD, Rousseau GG (editors): *Glucocorticoid Hormone Action*. Springer-Verlag, 1979.

Cahill GF: Action of adrenal cortical steroids on carbohydrate metabolism. In: *The Human Adrenal Cortex*. Christy NP (editor). Harper & Row, 1971.

Cahill GF, Owen OE: Metabolic effects of exogenous glucocorticoids in fasted man. *J Clin Invest* 1973;**52**:2596.

Craddock CG: Corticosteroid-induced lymphopenia, immunosuppression and body defense. *Ann Intern Med* 1978; **88**:564.

Fauci AS, Dale DC, Balow JE: Glucocorticoid therapy: Mechanisms of action and clinical considerations. *Ann Intern Med* 1976;**84**:304.

Findling JW et al: Vitamin D metabolites and parathyroid hormone in Cushing's syndrome: Relationship to calcium and phosphorus homeostasis. *J Clin Endocrinol Metab* 1982;**54**:1039.

Gaca G, Berend K: Plasma glucose, insulin and free fatty acids during long term corticosteroid treatment in children. *Acta Endocrinol* 1974;**77**:699.

Hahn TJ, Halstead LR, Teitelbaum SL: Altered mineral metabolism in glucocorticoid-induced osteopenia. *J Clin Invest* 1979;**64**:655.

Katt KJ, Dufau ML: Hormone action: Control of target-cell function by peptide, thyroid and steroid hormones. In: *Endocrinology and Metabolism*. Felig P et al (editors). McGraw-Hill, 1981.

Klein RG et al: Intestinal calcium absorption in exogenous hypercortisolism. *J Clin Invest* 1977;**60**:253.

Munch A, Guyre PM, Holbrook NJ: Physiologic functions of glucocorticoids in stress and their relation to pharmacological actions. *Endocr Rev* 1984;**5**:25.

Parillo JE, Fauci AS: Mechanisms of glucocorticoid action on immune processes. *Annu Rev Pharmacol Toxicol* 1979; **19**:179.

Tyrrell JB, Baxter JD: Glucocorticoid therapy. In: *Endocrinology and Metabolism*. Felig P et al (editors). McGraw-Hill, 1981.

Laboratory Evaluation

Abraham GE, Chakmakjian ZH: Plasma steroids in hirsutism. *Obstet Gynecol* 1974;**44**:171.

Besser GM et al: Immunoreactive corticotrophin levels in adrenocortical insufficiency. *Br Med J* 1971;**1**:374.

Burke CW, Beardwell CG: Cushing's syndrome: An evaluation of the clinical usefulness of urinary free cortisol and other urinary steroid measurements in diagnosis. *Q J Med* 1972;**42**:175.

Chrousos GP et al: The corticotropin-releasing factor stimulation test: An aid in the evaluation of patients with Cushing's syndrome. *N Engl J Med* 1984;**310**:622.

Crapo L: Cushing's syndrome: A review of diagnostic tests. *Metabolism* 1979;**28**:955.

Eddy RL et al: Cushing's syndrome: A prospective study of diagnostic methods. *Am J Med* 1973;**55**:621.

Givens JR: Normal and abnormal androgen metabolism. *Clin Obstet Gynecol* 1978;**21**:115.

Jacobs HS, Nabarro JDN: Tests of hypothalamic-pituitary-adrenal function in man. *Q J Med* 1969;**38**:475.

Krieger DT, Allen W: Relationships of bioassayable and immunoassayable plasma ACTH and cortisol concentrations in normal subjects and in patients with Cushing's disease. *J Clin Endocrinol Metab* 1975;**40**:675.

Liddle GW: Tests of pituitary adrenal suppressibility in the diagnosis of Cushing's syndrome. *J Clin Endocrinol Metab* 1960;**12**:1539.

Lindholm J et al: Reliability of the 30-minute ACTH test in assessing hypothalamic-pituitary-adrenal function. *J Clin Endocrinol Metab* 1978;**47**:272.

Maroulis GB, Manlimos FS, Abraham GE: Comparison between urinary 17-ketosteroids and plasma androgens in hirsute patients. *Obstet Gynecol* 1977;**49**:454.

Nelson JC, Tindall DJ: A comparison of the adrenal responses to hypoglycemia, metyrapone and ACTH. *Am J Med Sci* 1978;**275**:165.

Paulsen JD et al: Free testosterone concentrations in serum: Elevation is the hallmark of hirsutism. *Am J Obstet Gynecol* 1977;**128**:851.

Rosenfield RL: Plasma free androgen patterns in hirsute women and their diagnostic implications. *Am J Med* 1979;**66**:417.

Scott AP et al: Pituitary adrenocorticotrophin and the melanocyte stimulating hormones. In: *Peptide Hormones*. Parsons JA (editor). University Park Press, 1979.

Speckart PF, Nicoloff JT, Bethune JE: Screening for adrenocortical insufficiency with cosyntropin (synthetic ACTH). *Arch Intern Med* 1971;**128**:761.

Spiger M et al: Single dose metyrapone test: Review of a four-year experience. *Arch Intern Med* 1975;**135**:698.

Streeten DHP et al: The diagnosis of hypercortisolism: Biochemical criteria differentiating patients from lean and obese normal subjects and from females on oral contraceptives. *J Clin Endocrinol Metab* 1969;**29**:1191.

Streeten DHP et al: Normal and abnormal function of the hypothalamic-pituitary-adrenocortical system in man. *Endocr Rev* 1984;**5**:371.

Vermeulen A: Adrenal virilism. In: *The Adrenal Gland*. James VHT (editor). Raven Press, 1979.

Vermeulen A, Ando S: Metabolic clearance rate and interconversion of androgens and the influence of the free androgen fraction. *J Clin Endocrinol Metab* 1979;**48**:320.

Disorders of Adrenocortical Insufficiency

Amador E: Adrenal hemorrhage during anticoagulant therapy. *Ann Intern Med* 1965;**63**:559.

Irvine WJ, Barnes EW: Adrenocortical insufficiency. *Clin Endocrinol Metab* 1972;**10**:549.

Irvine WJ, Toft AD, Feek CM: Addison's disease. In: *The Adrenal Gland*. James VHT (editor). Raven Press, 1979.

Margaretten W, Nakai H, Landing BH: Septicemic adrenal hemorrhage. *Am J Dis Child* 1963;**105**:346.

Migeon CJ et al: Study of adrenal function in children with meningitis. *Pediatrics* 1967;**40**:163.

Nerup J: Addison's disease: Clinical studies. A report of 108 cases. *Acta Endocrinol* 1974;**76**:127.

Nerup J: Addison's disease: A review of some clinical, pathological and immunological features. *Dan Med Bull* 1974; **21**:201.

Nichols ML et al: Isolated deficiency of adrenocorticotropin (ACTH) and lipotropins (LPHs). *J Clin Endocrinol Metab* 1978;**47**:84.

Plumpton FS, Besser GM, Cole PV: Corticosteroid treatment and surgery. 2. The management of steroid cover. *Anaesthesia* 1969;**24**:12.

Thompson DG, Mason AS, Goodwin FJ: Mineralocorticoid replacement in Addison's disease. *Clin Endocrinol* 1979;**10**:499.

Xarli VP et al: Adrenal hemorrhage in the adult. *Medicine* 1978;**57**:211.

Cushing's Syndrome

Aron DC et al: Cushing's syndrome: Problems in diagnosis. *Medicine* 1981;**60**:25.

Aron DC et al: Cushing's syndrome: Problems in management. *Endocr Rev* 1982;**3**:229.

Azzopardi JG, Freeman F, Poole G: Endocrine and metabolic disorders in bronchial carcinoma. *Br Med J* 1970;**4**:528.

Azzopardi JG, Williams ED: Pathology of nonendocrine tumors associated with Cushing's syndrome. *Cancer* 1968;**22**:274.

Fehm HL, Voigt KH: Pathophysiology of Cushing's disease. *Pathobiol Annu* 1979;**9**:225.

Findling JW, Aron DC, Tyrrell JB: Cushing's disease. In: *The Pituitary*. Imura H (editor). Raven Press, 1985.

Findling JW et al: Selective venous sampling for ACTH in Cushing's syndrome. *Ann Intern Med* 1981;**94**:647.

Fitzgerald PA et al: Cushing's disease: Transient secondary adrenal insufficiency after selective removal of pituitary microadenomas: Evidence for a pituitary origin. *J Clin Endocrinol Metab* 1982;**54**:413.

Friedman M, Marshall-Jones P, Ross EJ: Cushing's syndrome: Adrenocortical activity secondary to neoplasms arising outside the pituitary-adrenal system. *Q J Med* 1966;**35**:193.

Hutter AM, Kayhoe DE: Adrenal cortical carcinoma: Clinical features of 138 patients. *Am J Med* 1966;**41**:572.

Korobkin M et al: Computed tomography in the diagnosis of adrenal disease. *Am J Roentgenol* 1979;**132**:231.

Krieger DT: Physiopathology of Cushing's disease. *Endocr Rev* 1983;**4**:22.

Lamberts SWJ, DeLange SA, Stefanko SZ: Adrenocorticotropin-secreting pituitary adenomas originate from the anterior or intermediate lobe in Cushing's disease: Differences in the regulation of hormone secretion. *J Clin Endocrinol Metab* 1982;**54**:286.

Linfoot JA: Heavy ion therapy: Alpha particle therapy of pituitary tumors. In: *Recent Advances in the Diagnosis and Treatment of Pituitary Tumors*. Raven Press, 1979.

McKeever PE et al: Refractory Cushing's disease caused by multinodular ACTH-cell hyperplasia. *J Neuropathol Exp Neurol* 1982;**41**:490.

Orth DN: The old and the new in Cushing's syndrome. *N Engl J Med* 1984;**310**:649.

Ross EJ, Marshall-Jones P, Friedman M: Cushing's syndrome: Diagnostic criteria. *Q J Med* 1966;**35**:149.

Singer W et al: Ectopic ACTH syndrome: Clinicopathological correlations. *J Clin Pathol* 1978;**31**:591.

Styne DM et al: Treatment of Cushing's disease in childhood and adolescence by transsphenoidal microadenomectomy. *N Engl J Med* 1984;**310**:889.

Tyrrell JB: Diagnosis of Cushing's disease. In: *Secretory Tumors of the Pituitary Gland*. Black PM et al (editors). Raven Press, 1984.

Tyrrell JB et al: Cushing's disease: Selective transsphenoidal resection of pituitary adenomas. *N Engl J Med* 1978;**298**:753.

Tyrrell JB et al: An overnight high-dose dexamethasone suppression test: Rapid differential diagnosis of Cushing's syndrome. *Ann Intern Med* 1986;**104**:180.

Urbanic RC, George JM: Cushing's disease: 18 years' experience. *Medicine* 1981;**60**:14.

Hirsutism & Virilism

Biffignandi P, Massucchetti C, Molinatti GM: Female hirsutism: Pathophysiological considerations and therapeutic implications. *Endocr Rev* 1984;**5**:498.

Chrousos GP et al: Late-onset 21-hydroxylase deficiency mimicking idiopathic hirsutism or polycystic ovarian disease. *Ann Intern Med* 1982;**96**:143.

Cumming DC et al: Treatment of hirsutism with spironolactone. *JAMA* 1982;**247**:1295.

Evron S, Shapiro G, Diamant YZ: Induction of ovulation with spironolactone (Aldactone) in anovulatory oligomenorrheic and hyperandrogenic women. *Fertil Steril* 1981;**36**:468.

Goldzieher JW: Polycystic ovarian disease. *Fertil Steril* 1981;**35**:39.

Hatch R et al: Hirsutism: Implications, etiology and management. *Am J Obstet Gynecol* 1981;**140**:815.

Horton R, Hawks D, Lobo R: $3\alpha,17\beta$-Adrostanediol glucuronide in plasma: A marker of androgen action in idiopathic hirsutism. *J Clin Invest* 1982;**69**:1203.

Lackelin GCL et al: Long term effects of nightly dexamethasone administration in patients with polycystic ovarian disease. *J Clin Endocrinol Metab* 1982;**55**:768.

Maroulis GB: Evaluation of hirsutism and hyperandrogenemia. *Fertil Steril* 1981;**36**:273.

10   Mineralocorticoids

Edward G. Biglieri, MD, & Claudio E. Kater, MD

The biosynthetic pathways of the mineralocorticoid hormones are shown in Fig 10–1 (see also Figs 9–4 and 9–5). The principal mineralocorticoid hormone is aldosterone. It is produced in the zona glomerulosa exclusively and is primarily controlled by the renin-angiotensin system. Other regulators include sodium and potassium levels, ACTH, and neural components of the adrenergic and dopaminergic systems. The precursors of aldosterone in this pathway normally contribute little to their peripheral concentrations—except for 18-hydroxycorticosterone. In the zona fasciculata, there are 2 steroid pathways—the glucocorticoid and mineralocorticoid pathways—both under control of ACTH. The glucocorticoid pathway results in the formation of cortisol. The major mineralocorticoid hormone of the zona fasciculata is deoxycorticosterone (DOC), but corticosterone and 18-hydroxydeoxycorticosterone are also produced in substantial amounts. The bulk of the circulating levels of DOC, 18-hydroxydeoxycorticosterone, and corticosterone originates from the zona fasciculata.

Activity of Aldosterone

The principal effects of aldosterone are on maintenance of normal sodium and potassium concentrations and extracellular volume. Aldosterone combines with an intracellular cytosol mineralocorticoid receptor. The active steroid-receptor complex moves into the nucleus of the target cell, where it initiates the transcription of RNA and subsequently induces a new protein providing the energy required for movement of sodium from the cell via the sodium pump. The major effect of this action quantitatively is to increase the difference in potential across the renal tubule. The increased luminal negativity affects tubular secretion of potassium and hydrogen (Fig 10–2). Tubular sodium, via the sodium pump, enters the extracellular fluid and helps maintain its normal composition and volume. All of these events occur in other secretory systems and can be measured in saliva, sweat, and feces. It is of interest that the increased difference in potential or increased luminal negativity noted in the kidney is also present in the gastrointestinal tract, and its measurement may be used to quantitate mineralocorticoid activity, eg, decreased stool sodium with increased serum potassium.

Acronyms Used in This Chapter

ACTH	Adrenocorticotropic hormone
CMO	Corticosterone methyloxidase
DHEA	Dehydroepiandrosterone
DOC	Deoxycorticosterone
DOCA	De[s]oxycorticosterone acetate
MCH	Mineralocorticoid hormone
RNA	Ribonucleic acid

Although renin and aldosterone move in concert in most situations, aldosterone is also influenced by ACTH, potassium balance and concentration, and probably other factors to maintain volume and electrolyte homeostasis. In the virtual absence of renin, as in patients with primary aldosteronism, circulating levels of aldosterone are modulated by variations in ACTH rhythm. Free aldosterone comprises 30–40% of its total concentration, whereas the free fractions of the steroids of the zona fasciculata comprise 5–10% of their total concentration. Aldosterone is *loosely* bound to corticosteroid-binding globulin, in contrast to the zona fasciculata steroids. Because it is the free hormone that combines with the mineralocorticoid receptor to initiate subsequent mineralocorticoid action, extremely high levels of DOC must be achieved to produce a mineralocorticoid effect.

Interactions of Hormones

The interactions of all circulating steroid hormones, the distribution between their free and bound forms, the influence of peptide hormones, and receptor availability determine their effectiveness as mineralocorticoids. For example, numerically normal levels of mineralocorticoid hormones can induce a state of hypermineralocorticoidism in situations in which synergistic or "facilitating" substances are also present that increase the receptor affinity for aldosterone. Cortisol itself, in high concentrations, can act as a mineralocorticoid in the presence of normal or even low levels of aldosterone or DOC.

Definition of Terms

Mineralocorticoid and **glucocorticoid hormones**

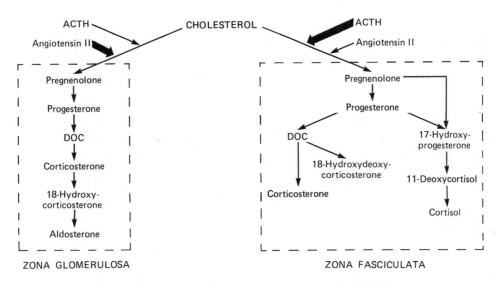

Figure 10–1. Biosynthetic pathways of the mineralocorticoids.

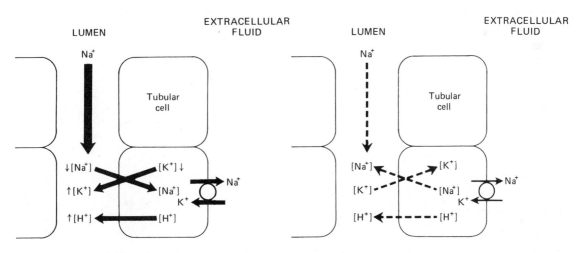

Figure 10–2. Mineralocorticoid action. On the left, high sodium intakes and high tubular sodium with increased mineralocorticoid action lead to K^+ and H^+ secretion and Na^+ movement into extracellular fluid. Similar amounts of mineralocorticoid are ineffective when tubular sodium is reduced (eg, by dietary sodium restriction).

have mineral- and carbohydrate-regulating activity, respectively. A mineralocorticoid is an adrenocortical steroid whose principal action is electrolyte regulation; it is not necessarily produced in the aldosterone biosynthetic pathway or even in the zona glomerulosa. A glucocorticoid hormone is an adrenocortical steroid whose predominant action is related to carbohydrate regulation, protein catabolism, ACTH suppression, and the immune system. Although some glucocorticoid activity can be produced in the zona glomerulosa, it is mainly formed in the zona fasciculata.

The terms **mineralocorticoid excess** and **mineralocorticoid deficiency** denote an absolute elevation and an absolute diminution, respectively, of the endogenous hormones as reflected by their plasma or urine levels. However, this is not necessarily related to the clinical manifestations of mineralocorticoid activity. A condition characterized by presumed increased mineralocorticoid activity, with salt retention, hypertension, hypokalemia, and metabolic alkalosis, is more appropriately called **hypermineralocorticoidism.** It can occur in the absence of any mineralocorticoid production, eg, in Liddle's syndrome or chronic ingestion of licorice. In contrast, in the mineralocorticoid resistance syndromes (receptor deficiency, pseudohypoaldosteronism), an excess of circulating mineralocorticoid cannot express its peripheral action and results in a clinical state of **hypomineralocorticoidism,** presenting with sodium loss, hypotension, hyperkalemia, and metabolic acidosis.

PRIMARY MINERALOCORTICOID EXCESS
(Table 10-1)

Disorders in this category are manifested by hypertension, hypokalemia, suppression of the renin system, and normal or low cortisol production. Although technically the mineralocorticoid hormones produced

in the 11β- and 17α-hydroxylase deficiency disorders are secondary to ACTH excess, their biochemical findings are those of primary mineralocorticoid excess.

PRIMARY ALDOSTERONISM

Recognition & Diagnosis

The increased production of aldosterone by abnormal zona glomerulosa tissue (adenoma or hyperplasia) initiates a series of events that result in the clinical abnormality known as primary aldosteronism. Aldosterone excess leads to increased sodium retention, expansion of the extracellular fluid volume, and increased total body sodium content. Although the effects on the kidney are greatest quantitatively, the other secretory tissues also participate in this event. Fecal excretion of sodium, for example, can be decreased to almost nil. The expanded extracellular fluid and plasma volumes are registered by stretch receptors at the juxtaglomerular apparatus and sodium flux at the macula densa, with resultant suppression of renin secretion, measured as suppressed plasma renin activity. These effects of aldosterone are further manifested by normal or elevated serum sodium concentration and reduced hematocrit. With primary increases in aldosterone production, the renin system is greatly suppressed. This is the hallmark of the disorder.

In addition to sodium retention, potassium depletion develops, decreasing the total body and plasma concentration of potassium and producing alkalosis. The extrusion of potassium from its intracellular position is followed by the intracellular movement of hydrogen ion, and along with increased renal secretion of hydrogen ion, alkalosis ensues. With moderate potassium depletion, decreased carbohydrate tolerance (shown by an abnormal glucose tolerance test) and resistance to antidiuretic hormone (vasopressin) occur. Severe potassium depletion blunts baroreceptor function.

Because aldosterone biosynthesis is intensified, the entire biosynthetic pathway becomes activated.

Table 10—1. Biochemical findings in primary hypermineralocorticoidism.

	Plasma		Aldos-terone	Other MCHs	Renin	Cortisol	ACTH	Hct	BUN/ Creatinine
	Na⁺	K⁺							
Aldosterone-producing adenoma	N or ↑	↓	↑↑	↑	↓↓	N	N	↓	N
Aldosterone-producing carcinoma	↑	↓	↑↑	↑↑	↓↓	N or ↑	N or ↓	↓	N
Hyperplasia									
Idiopathic hyperaldosteronism	N	↓	↑	N	↓	N	N	N or ↓	N
Indeterminate hyperaldosteronism	N	N or ↓	↑	N	↓	N	N	N or ↓	N
Glucocorticoid-remediable hyper- aldosteronism	N	↓	↑	N	↓	N	N	N or ↓	N
11β-Hydroxylase deficiency	N	N or ↓	↓	↑	N or ↓	N or ↓	↑	N or ↓	N
17α-Hydroxylase deficiency	N or ↑	↓	↓	↑↑	↓↓	↓	↑	N or ↓	N
Terminal steroid metabolic deficiency	N	↓	↓	N	↓	N	N	N	N

BUN, blood urea nitrogen; Hct, hematocrit; MCH, mineralocorticoid hormone; N, normal; ↑, increased; ↓ decreased; ↑↑, ↓↓, markedly increased, decreased.

Figure 10–3. Decision diagram for primary mineralocorticoidism.

Precursor steroids such as DOC, corticosterone, and 18-hydroxycorticosterone are present in increased amounts in the blood of persons with an aldosterone-producing adenoma (Fig 10–1). Primary aldosteronism is a disease of the zona glomerulosa. Cells of this zone do not have the capacity to make cortisol. There are no abnormalities in cortisol production, plasma cortisol level, or cortisol metabolism.

History & Physical Findings

Patients usually come to medical attention because of symptoms of hypokalemia or detection of previously unsuspected hypertension during the course of physical examination. The medical history reveals no characteristic symptoms—often only nonspecific complaints of tiredness, loss of stamina, weakness, nocturia, and lassitude—all symptoms of potassium depletion. If potassium depletion is more severe, with alkalosis, then increased thirst, polyuria (especially nocturnal), and paresthesias may be present. Headache is a frequent incidental complaint.

Excessive production of mineralocorticoids produces no characteristic physical findings. Blood pressure in patients with primary aldosteronism can range from borderline to severe hypertensive levels. The mean ± SEM blood pressure in the 136 patients reported by the Glasgow unit was 205 ± 21/123 ± 18 mm Hg, with no significant difference between the group with adenoma and that with hyperplasia. Accelerated (malignant) hypertension is extremely rare in patients with primary aldosteronism. Retinopathy is mild, and hemorrhages are rarely (if ever) present. Postural falls in blood pressure without reflex tachycardia are observed in the severely potassium-depleted patient because of blunting of the baroreceptors. Clinical edema is quite rare. A positive Trousseau or

Chvostek sign may be suggestive of alkalosis accompanying severe potassium depletion. The heart is usually only mildly enlarged if at all, and electrocardiographic changes are usually those of modest left ventricular hypertrophy and potassium depletion.

Initial Diagnosis
(Fig 10–3)

A. Hypokalemia: Determination of the presence or absence of hypokalemia is the most important initial screening procedure in patients with hypertension. Care must be taken to assess the state of sodium intake or balance in the patient before serum electrolytes are obtained. Serum potassium concentration is closely related to and determined to a great extent by sodium chloride intake. A low-sodium diet, by sparing potassium loss, can correct serum potassium abnormalities, thus masking total potassium depletion; as the amount of sodium ion available for reabsorption is reduced, potassium secretion is retarded in the distal tubule. In some series, up to 20% of patients with primary aldosteronism have had normal serum potassium concentrations, depending on criteria of dietary sodium and laboratory variability. In the presence of normal renal function and aldosterone excess, salt loading will unmask hypokalemia as a manifestation of potassium depletion. Normokalemic hyperaldosteronism under these conditions has been reported but is probably rare.

B. Salt Intake: In the USA, Japan, and many European countries, the average person consumes more than 110– 120 meq of sodium per day—enough to allow hypokalemia to become manifest. If a dietary history of high salt intake is obtained and potassium concentrations are normal, there is no need for further tests. A useful way to demonstrate hypokalemia is to have the patient ingest an unrestricted diet plus 1 g of sodium chloride (as a 1-g sodium chloride USP tablet, $^1/_5$ tsp of table salt, or packets containing 1 g of salt) with each meal for 4 days; blood samples for fasting electrolyte determinations should be obtained on day 5. The finding of a low serum potassium concentration warrants further study (Fig 10– 3).

C. Diuretic Therapy: Previous diuretic therapy always poses a problem in interpreting serum potassium concentrations and is the most common cause of hypokalemia in hypertension. The patient should discontinue use of diuretics for at least 3 weeks before potassium levels are measured.

In the absence of previous diuretic therapy, sodium concentrations less than 139 meq/L are rare in patients with primary aldosteronism, but they are common with diuretic therapy. Thus, any lower concentration should suggest secondary hyperaldosteronism. A high serum sodium concentration (139– 152 meq/L) in the presence of a reduced hematocrit (due to increased extracellular fluid and plasma volume from sodium retention) is presumptive evidence of mineralocorticoid excess. Additional clues to potassium depletion are failure to concentrate urine, an abnormal glucose tolerance test, and alkalosis.

If hypokalemia is documented, the renin-angiotensin system must be assessed. This is accomplished by a random plasma renin activity measurement. If plasma renin activity is normal or high in a patient who has been off diuretic therapy for 3 weeks, it is very unlikely that primary aldosteronism is present. If the random plasma renin activity is suppressed, primary aldosteronism is a likely diagnosis.

Measurement of Aldosterone & Other Steroids
(Table 10–2)

Assessment of aldosterone production can best be accomplished by measurement of urinary aldosterone excretion over a 24-hour period under the same conditions of sodium intake described for potassium measurement. Measurement of either the 18-glucuronide or the tetrahydroaldosterone metabolite is sufficient to assess the rate of total production. Blood samples must be obtained under proper conditions in order to yield reliable diagnostic information. Although the value obtained for plasma aldosterone concentration is the aldosterone level only at a given moment, in the properly prepared patient it can provide an excellent assessment of mineralocorticoid production. Both plasma and urinary aldosterone measurements should be performed while the patient is taking a high-salt diet with sodium chloride supplementation, as previously described. This is crucial, because with

Table 10–2. Simultaneous measurements (± SE) of plasma aldosterone, 18-hydroxycorticosterone, and plasma renin concentration in normal subjects and in primary aldosteronism during postural stimulation.

	Normal Subjects (n = 8)			Aldosterone-Producing Adenoma (n = 15)			Idiopathic Hyperaldosteronism (n = 14)		
	Aldosterone (ng/dL)	18-Hydroxycorticosterone (ng/dL)	Plasma Renin Concentration (ng/mL/h)	Aldosterone (ng/dL)	18-Hydroxycorticosterone (ng/dL)	Plasma Renin Concentration (ng/mL/h)	Aldosterone (ng/dL)	18-Hydroxycorticosterone (ng/dL)	Plasma Renin Concentration (ng/mL/h)
8 AM Recumbent	9.2 (± 0.7)	24.1 (± 3.4)	3.5 (± 0.9)	54.7 (± 9.5)	160.0 (± 29.9)	0.49 (± 0.11)	13.2 (± 1.2)	24.2 (± 3.7)	0.52 (± 0.08)
12 Noon Upright	24.5 (± 2.9)	49.9 (± 7.7)	8.7 (± 2.0)	49.8 (± 5.8)	136.9 (± 31.8)	0.61 (± 0.21)	32.5 (± 4.9)	49.0 (± 9.4)	1.13 (± 0.20)

any diminution of salt intake, plasma aldosterone concentration and aldosterone production normally increase. The plasma aldosterone concentration in a group of 47 patients with adenoma was over 20 ng/dL (61.8 ± 10.9 ng/dL); in 19 patients with idiopathic hyperaldosteronism (hyperplasia), it was less than 20 ng/dL (13.2 ± 1.2 ng/dL). The normal urinary aldosterone values are 5–20 μg/24 h. In one series, there were mean values for adenoma and hyperplasia of 37.6 ± 3 μg/24 h and 22.5 ± 1.5 μg/24 h, respectively. Although urinary measurements have been adequate for detecting abnormal production of aldosterone (and in fact superior to plasma aldosterone concentration measurement), it has not been possible to use daily excretion of aldosterone to discriminate between adenoma and hyperplasia.

Differentiation Between Aldosterone-Producing Adenoma & Adrenocortical Hyperplasia

It is important to distinguish between adenoma and hyperplasia, because surgery is indicated in the former but not in the latter.

Plasma Aldosterone, Deoxycorticosterone, Corticosterone, & 18-Hydroxycorticosterone Concentrations (Table 10–2)

The plasma aldosterone concentration provides not only diagnostic information about hyperaldosteronism but also differential diagnostic information about the pathologic process. After at least 4 days of sodium intake exceeding 120 meq daily and after overnight (at least 6 hours) recumbency, the 8 AM plasma aldosterone concentration can be used to distinguish patients with adenoma from those with hyperplasia. A plasma aldosterone concentration greater than 20 ng/dL indicates adenoma, and less than 20 ng/dL usually indicates hyperplasia. After 2 or 4 hours in the upright posture (which normally activates the renin system, with a rise in plasma aldosterone), plasma aldosterone concentration shows no significant change or diminution in 90% of patients with adenoma, but it almost always increases in patients with adrenocortical hyperplasia. This important differential maneuver is extremely accurate in identifying the pathogenetic mechanism. The difference is due to the profound suppression of the renin system by excessive aldosterone production caused by adenoma accompanied by a diminishing influence of ACTH from 8 AM to 12 noon. In contrast, in patients with adrenocortical hyperplasia, increased sensitivity of the hyperplastic gland to minute but measurable increases in renin that occur with assumption of the upright posture leads to an increased aldosterone level. The effectiveness of this maneuver depends on attention to the details of preparation described above.

Additional simultaneous measurements can be made of other precursor steroids and add significantly to the precision of diagnosis. Plasma DOC and corticosterone are frequently increased at 8 AM in patients with adenoma, whereas they are rarely if ever elevated in patients with hyperplasia. 18-Hydroxycorticosterone is invariably increased in patients with adenoma to levels greater than 85 ng/dL and shows no overlap with the normal or slightly high values of this steroid in patients with hyperplasia.

The procedures just discussed can identify primary aldosteronism and differentiate adenoma from hyperplasia in most cases; when uncertainty remains, 2 other tests, the desoxycorticosterone acetate (DOCA) maneuver and the saline infusion test, can be of further help. They can also be useful in further defining the type of hyperplasia.

The Desoxycorticosterone Acetate (DOCA) Maneuver

Patients should be hospitalized for the DOCA maneuver, which consists of administration of 10 mg of DOCA intramuscularly every 12 hours for 3 consecutive days accompanied by a salt intake of at least 7 g (120 meq/d). Fludrocortisone, 0.2 mg twice daily orally for 3–4 days, can be used with outpatients. On the third day of this regimen, either plasma aldosterone concentration or urinary aldosterone excretion is compared with pretreatment values. Aldosterone is suppressed minimally or not at all by DOCA in patients with adenoma. The lack of suppression of the 8 AM recumbent plasma aldosterone concentration or the urinary aldosterone excretion on the third day generally indicates the idiopathic hyperaldosteronism form of hyperplasia or adenoma, whereas suppression of either plasma aldosterone concentration or urinary aldosterone excretion establishes a second subset of hyperplasia patients, those with indeterminate hyperaldosteronism. Patients in the latter group present with milder degrees of hypokalemia, modest elevations of aldosterone production, and suppressed plasma renin concentration. Patients with adenoma do not respond by suppression of the already low plasma renin concentration.

Saline Infusion Test

Saline loading establishes aldosterone unresponsiveness to volume expansion and thereby identifies autonomy in patients with aldosterone-producing adenomas. As a rule, 2 L of isotonic saline is administered over a period of 2–4 hours, and blood samples are then obtained. This expansion of the extracellular fluid volume reduces plasma aldosterone concentration promptly in patients with "essential" hypertension but fails to suppress plasma aldosterone concentration into the normal range in patients with adenoma or idiopathic hyperplasia. However, the plasma aldosterone concentration is suppressed in the group with indeterminate hyperplasia.

The saline infusion test and the DOCA or fludrocortisone maneuver clearly distinguish hyperaldosteronism from essential hypertension. Response to upright posture identifies adenoma or hyperplasia. Suppression studies help determine the type of hyperplasia.

Glucocorticoid Treatment

The glucocorticoid-remediable form of hyperaldosteronism is rare, occurs primarily in young men, and is familial. It constitutes a remarkable subset of hyperaldosteronemic patients with hyperplasia in whom all of the biochemical abnormalities can be reversed after 2–3 weeks with the use of ACTH-suppressive doses of glucocorticoids (1–2 mg of dexamethasone daily). Patients with glucocorticoid-remediable hyperaldosteronism will maintain a normal blood pressure, plasma aldosterone, and other biochemical indices as long as the dexamethasone or other ACTH suppressant is administered. Plasma aldosterone concentration is only mildly elevated in these patients, and some still unidentified mineralocorticoid may also be operative.

Identification of Adrenocortical Carcinoma

Malignant tumors producing only aldosterone are extremely rare. The few patients reported have had large tumors with abundant precursor steroids and an absence of circadian rhythm.

Summary of Aldosterone-Producing Adenoma Versus Idiopathic Hyperaldosteronism

The most important disorder of the mineralocorticoid hormones is primary aldosteronism due to a solitary adenoma. As diagnostic precision increases, many cases of hypertension and hypokalemia with modest increases of aldosterone production have been identified and characterized as hyperaldosteronism due to hyperplasia. Whether this is a primary adrenal disorder or not is far from clear, but the weight of evidence suggests that it is not. During the course of diagnostic workups of patients with suspected adenoma, conditions involving other mineralocorticoid abnormalities have been found.

Defining the growing numbers of patients with adrenal hyperplasia and hyperaldosteronism is not as important clinically as identifying those patients with adenoma who can be cured. Hypokalemia in a hypertensive patient means hypermineralocorticoidism. The subsequent suppressed plasma renin activity confirms this.

The high urinary aldosterone level identifies the adrenal as the source of the disorder. If the urinary aldosterone level is low, another adrenal mineralocorticoid hormone is operative. Measurement of plasma aldosterone is perhaps the best means of discriminating between adenoma and hyperplasia by both the degree of elevation and the response to postural change.

Suppression studies in patients with increased aldosterone production help define the type of hyperplasia and autonomy of adenomas. Precursor steroids may be even more important in distinguishing hyperplasia from adenoma, because they are invariably normal in hyperplasia and elevated in adenoma. (18-Hydroxycorticosterone is almost always elevated, and DOC and corticosterone are elevated over half of the time.)

Location of Adenoma

Once the biochemical diagnosis is secure, lateralization procedures in patients with adenoma become extremely important in determining the surgical approach. A number of techniques have been developed: adrenal venography, ^{131}I iodocholesterol scanning, adrenal vein catheterization and bilateral sampling, and, more recently, CT scanning.

Adrenal venography was one of the first techniques used to locate tumors. However, a number of problems occurred, such as extravasation of dye, hemorrhage, and adrenal infarction, making this a potentially traumatic procedure. Tumors smaller than 7 mm cannot be located by this technique, and the success rate in identifying adrenal tumors has varied from 60 to 70%.

Scanning using intravenously administered ^{131}I iodocholesterol has located tumors in about 80% of patients. Again, size of tumor may be a limiting factor, because if tumors are less than 1 cm in diameter, the success rate drops considerably. The procedure is tedious and takes several weeks to accomplish. The use of 6β-iodomethyl-19-norcholesterol (NP59) reduces the interval between injection and scintiscanning to about 24 hours.

CT scanning, which is as effective as iodocholesterol scanning in locating adenomas, has proved to be even more useful, because it requires considerably less radiation than iodocholesterol scanning, and the diagnostic information is more readily available.

Adrenal vein catheterization to measure bilateral aldosterone levels continues to be useful in lateralizing tumors only after other lateralizing techniques fail and biochemical evidence still supports the diagnosis of adenoma.

Treatment

Treatment depends for the most part on the precision of diagnosis. In patients with an aldosterone-producing adenoma and no contraindication to operation, unilateral adrenalectomy is recommended. The degree of reduction of blood pressure and correction of hypokalemia achieved with spironolactone provides a surprisingly close approximation to the actual response to surgery; in fact, greater reduction often occurs postoperatively, presumably because of a greater reduction of extracellular fluid. The surgical cure rate of hypertension associated with adenoma is excellent—over 50% in several series—with reduction of hypertension in the remainder.

Preoperative Preparation

Patients should be treated preoperatively with spironolactone, 200–400 mg/d, until the blood pressure and serum potassium are entirely normal; this may take 1–3 months. This drug is particularly beneficial because of its unique mechanism of action as an antagonist—ie, it blocks steroid binding at the mineralocorticoid receptor level. Once both blood pressure and serum potassium levels are normal, the dose can be reduced gradually to a maintenance dose of approximately 100– 150 mg of spironolactone per day until the time of surgery. Spironolactone reduces the volume of the expanded extracellular fluid toward normal, restores normal serum potassium concentration, and promotes potassium retention. It often has the additional desirable effect of activating (after 1 or 2 months) the suppressed renin-angiotensin system. This will stimulate the suppressed zona glomerulosa of the nonadenomatous adrenal gland, so that postoperative hypoaldosteronism with hyperkalemia will be less likely, and the preoperative restoration of normal blood pressure is sustained. Preoperative treatment will also permit reversal to some extent of some of the changes in target organs that were produced by the hypertensive and hypokalemic states. Spironolactone is usually well tolerated; the side effects of rashes, gynecomastia, impotence, and epigastric discomfort are rare under the treatment program suggested.

The Surgical & Medical Treatment Periods

When the diagnosis and lateralization are certain, surgical removal of the adenoma is recommended. The transperitoneal (anterior) approach has been employed successfully for many years. However, if preoperative lateralization techniques identify the site of tumor, a unilateral posterior approach can be used with considerably less postoperative morbidity. If the tumor is identified at surgery, exploration of the contralateral adrenal is not indicated. If surgery is contraindicated or refused, indefinite treatment with spironolactone can be effective. The initial dose of 200– 400 mg of spironolactone per day must be continued for 4– 6 weeks before the full effect on blood pressure is realized. With prolonged treatment, aldosterone production does not increase even though potassium replenishment, decreased sodium and volume spaces, modest activation of the renin-angiotensin system, and a direct inhibiting effect on aldosterone synthesis occur.

Subtotal adrenalectomy will correct hypokalemia in patients with hyperplasia, but the blood pressure remains elevated. In some cases, removal of adrenal mass meliorates the hyperaldosterone-dependent hypertensive state. Preoperative identification of these cases is difficult. Primary adrenal hyperplasia appears to be a subtype of hyperaldosteronism, which accounts for cures following reduction of adrenal tissue mass. Biochemically, patients in this group are indistinguishable from those with tumor, but no lateralization of aldosterone production can be demonstrated. Therefore, other antihypertensive measures (which should include spironolactone) must be used to control hypertension in patients with hyperplasia.

In patients with aldosteronism of indeterminate type, spironolactone alone is usually effective in controlling both the hypertension and the potassium-depleted state. Because of the effectiveness of spirono-

lactone in these patients, other antihypertensive medications can often be discontinued.

Amiloride, a potassium-sparing diuretic, can also be used, in doses of 20– 40 mg/d, to manage primary aldosteronism.

Pathologic Findings

Over 50% of patients with primary aldosteronism who have undergone surgery have had unilateral adenoma. Bilateral tumors are rare. The characteristic adenoma is readily identified by its golden-yellow color. In addition, small satellite adenomas are often found, and distinction from micro- or macronodular hyperplasia is frequently difficult. In patients with adenoma, the contiguous adrenal gland can show hyperplasia throughout the gland. Hyperplasia is also present in the contralateral adrenal gland but is not associated with aldosterone abnormalities after removal of the primary adenoma.

DEOXYCORTICOSTERONE EXCESS SYNDROMES

Diagnosis

A. 11β-Hydroxylase Deficiency: 11β-Hydroxylase deficiency syndrome is usually recognized in infants and children because of virilization and the frequent presence of both hypertension and hypokalemia. Plasma 17α-hydroxyprogesterone, urinary pregnanetriol, and urinary 17-ketosteroids are increased. The defect is usually partial, so that some cortisol is produced, but it does not increase with further stimulation by ACTH. Blood levels and production rates of cortisol are usually within normal limits. A partial defect of 11β-hydroxylation results in increased production and blood levels of DOC, 11-deoxycortisol, and androgens (see Fig 9– 4). Hypertension results from excessive production of DOC by mechanisms previously described for aldosterone.

The blood levels and production rates of aldosterone are normal or reduced. Two mechanisms are proposed. One is that there is only partial inhibition of 11β-hydroxylation in the zona glomerulosa, which is a required biosynthetic step for aldosterone synthesis. The constancy of this block is supported by the fact that after normalization of DOC production and correction of the hypertension (by ACTH suppression), aldosterone production remains reduced and is not increased by sodium restriction. In fact, a sodium-losing state may be provoked by initial treatment. The other mechanism could be that suppression of renin by increased production of DOC might suppress the normal production of aldosterone in the zona glomerulosa. This notion is supported by the increase in renin and aldosterone production after suppression of ACTH and reduction of DOC production. It is still controversial whether the 11β-hydroxylating enzyme in the glomerulosa is the same as that of the fasciculata. The reduced levels of 18-hydroxydeoxycorticosterone (a zona fasciculata steroid) observed in this condition suggest that the 11β- and 18-hydroxylating enzymes may be similar.

B. 17α-Hydroxylase Deficiency: 17α-Hydroxylase deficiency syndrome is usually recognized at the time of puberty in young adults by the presence of hypertension, hypokalemia, and primary amenorrhea in the female or pseudohermaphroditism in the male. These features become more evident at this time because of the lack of increased sex steroid production associated with puberty. In contrast to the 11β-hydroxylation defect, there is no virilization or restricted growth. Patients often present with eunuchoid proportions and appearance. The virtual absence of 17α-hydroxyprogesterone, pregnanetriol, and ketosteroids is diagnostic of this type of hydroxylase deficiency (see Fig 9–4).

The key location of the 17α-hydroxylating system in the steroid biosynthetic pathway prevents normal production of androgens and estrogens. There has been no instance in which the adrenal defect has appeared without a concomitant gonadal defect. The defect seems to be in a single gene coding for the enzyme or in the expression of the gene. The diminution of cortisol production with this deficiency syndrome induces increased production of ACTH. Initially, the entire biosynthetic pathway of mineralocorticoids must be increased—namely, progesterone, DOC, corticosterone, 18-hydroxydeoxycorticosterone, and aldosterone. Progressive overproduction of the mineralocorticoids in both the zona glomerulosa and zona fasciculata pathways results in expansion of extracellular fluid and blood volumes, hypertension, and subsequent reduction and obliteration, in most cases, of plasma renin activity. Subsequent to this reduction, the plasma aldosterone concentration is virtually absent in most patients. Thus, the principal mineralocorticoid hormones present in great quantities are corticosterone, DOC, 18-hydroxycorticosterone, and 18-hydroxydeoxycorticosterone—all of them ACTH-dependent steroids of the zona fasciculata.

Treatment

Treatment of both of these disorders—11β-hydroxylase deficiency syndrome and 17α-hydroxylase deficiency syndrome—is similar to that of all non–sodium-losing forms of congenital adrenal hyperplasia. Treatment with replacement doses of glucocorticoid, such as hydrocortisone or dexamethasone, restores blood pressure to normal levels, corrects potassium depletion, reduces excessive DOC and corticosterone production in 17α-hydroxylase deficiency syndrome, and reduces DOC and 11-deoxycortisol production in 11β-hydroxylase deficiency syndrome. In 17α-hydroxylase deficiency syndrome, restoration of normal levels of DOC results in a return of plasma renin activity and aldosterone to normal values. A delay in return of the suppressed renin-aldosterone system toward normal can result in hypovolemic crises with the initial natriuresis and diuresis. It may take several years before the aldosterone and renin systems become normal. The amount of glucocorticoid administered must be carefully determined because of apparently exquisite tissue sensitivity to glucocorticoid hormones.

ABNORMALITY OF TERMINAL STEROID METABOLISM

An interesting subgroup of patients with hypertension, hypokalemia, and suppressed renin and aldosterone production has been described primarily in children. There is strong evidence that an unknown mineralocorticoid is active, although one has not been identified. Such a steroid responds to ACTH and intensifies the abnormalities. The hypertension is sodium-dependent and responds to treatment with spironolactone. The hallmark of this disorder is the reduced peripheral metabolism of cortisol. There is reduced production of tetrahydrocortisone relative to tetrahydrocortisol owing to reduced activity of 11β-hydroxysteroid oxidoreductase. This abnormality in metabolism of cortisol appears to be primarily a marker of the disorder, with probably little or no effect on the pathogenesis.

SECONDARY MINERALOCORTICOID EXCESS
(Table 10–3)

Activation of the zona glomerulosa by the renin-angiotensin system can lead to a variety of conditions in which increased aldosterone production occurs. Activation of the renin system can be accomplished by abnormalities such as sodium-wasting disease, laxative or diuretic abuse, decrease in intravascular volume, and direct overproduction of renin, such as in renovascular hypertension and renin-secreting tumors. This group can be subdivided into disorders with or without hypertension.

SECONDARY MINERALOCORTICOID EXCESS WITH HYPERTENSION

The following hypertensive disorders are for the most part renin-mediated, with hyperaldosteronism and hypokalemia as sequelae.

Renovascular Disease

Renovascular hypertension represents the most common cause of surgically reversible hypertension. It can be due to either atherosclerosis or fibromuscular hyperplasia. Other anatomic lesions may cause hypertension as well: renal infarction, solitary cysts, hydronephrosis, and other parenchymal lesions. Plasma renin activity in peripheral blood vessels is

Table 10–3. Biochemical findings in secondary hypermineralocorticoidism.

	Plasma		Aldos-terone	Other MCHs	Renin	Cortisol	ACTH	Hct	BUN/ Creatinine
	Na⁺	K⁺							
Without hypertension									
Sodium-wasting nephropathy	↓	↑ or ↓	↑↑	N or ↑	↑↑	N or ↑	N or ↑	↑	N or ↑
Bartter's syndrome	N	↓	↑	N	↑↑	N	N	N	N
Pseudohypoaldosteronism	N or ↓	↑	↑↑	N or ↑	↑↑	N	N	↑	N
Renal tubular acidosis	N	N or ↑	↑	N	↑	N	N	N or ↑	N
Diuretic/laxative abusers	N or ↓	↓	↑	N	↑	N	N	↑	N
With hypertension									
Renovascular hypertension	N or ↑	N or ↓	↑	N	↑	N	N	↑	N or ↑
Renin-secreting tumor	N or ↑	↓	↑↑	N	↑↑	N	N	↑	N
Accelerated hypertension	N	N or ↓	↑	N	↑	N	N	N or ↑	N or ↑
Estrogen therapy	N	N or ↓	↑	N	N or ↑	N or ↑	N	N or ↓	N

BUN, blood urea nitrogen; Hct, hematocrit; MCH, mineralocorticoid hormone; N, normal; ↑, increased; ↓, decreased; ↑↑, ↓↓, markedly increased, decreased.

within normal limits in half of the patients with renovascular hypertension. Hyperaldosteronism is not always apparent in these patients; it manifests itself when renin levels are elevated. It is important to appreciate that even though renin levels are within normal limits in the peripheral circulation, they may be inappropriate for the degree of sodium retention that may have occurred during the development of this hypertensive state.

Renin-Secreting Tumors

Renin-secreting tumors are extremely rare and can be mistaken for primary aldosteronism. This is because patients have high plasma levels of aldosterone, marked hypokalemia, and hypertension. The tumors are usually hemangiopericytomas containing elements of the juxtaglomerular cells. They are located by renal vein catheterization. Other tumors (Wilms' tumors, ectopic tumors) that secrete renin have been reported, including a pulmonary tumor that secreted excessive amounts of renin, producing hypertension and hypokalemia with secondary aldosteronism.

Accelerated Hypertension

Accelerated hypertension is characterized by marked elevations of diastolic blood pressure that can be abrupt in onset. This disorder is associated with progressive arteriosclerosis. The plasma levels of aldosterone are extremely high. It is believed that the intense vasospastic events that occur and the excessive renal cortical nephrosclerosis lead to hyperreninemia and accelerate the hypertensive process. Vigorous antihypertensive therapy usually mitigates the hyperaldosteronism.

Estrogen Therapy

Aldosterone levels are increased during replacement estrogen therapy or use of oral contraceptives. This is due to increases in plasma renin substrate and plasma renin activity. Angiotensin II levels are increased and thus stimulate aldosterone production. However, hypokalemia rarely occurs during estrogen administration.

SECONDARY MINERALOCORTICOID EXCESS WITHOUT HYPERTENSION

Sodium-Wasting Syndromes

In the preceding section we described primary renin overproduction due to direct and local diminution of volume to renin-secreting areas. The abnormalities discussed in this group of disorders are more systemic, resulting in major changes in extracellular fluid volume and affecting renin and aldosterone production accordingly. In patients with severe chronic renal insufficiency, sodium wasting can become a permanent effect, resulting in secondary hyperaldosteronism with hypo- or hypertension, hyponatremia, and hyper- or hypokalemia. Modest renal sodium wasting in patients with renal tubular acidosis may increase renin secretion and result in aldosterone excess, potassium depletion, and hypokalemia. Pseudohypoaldosteronism is a rare disease in which tubular resistance to mineralocorticoid hormones is present, presumably due to a deficiency of mineralocorticoid hormone receptors. Renal sodium wasting, volume depletion, and shock can occur; hyperkalemia is invariably present.

Diuretic abuse causes renal sodium wasting and thus secondary hyperaldosteronism by activation of the renin system. Similarly, surreptitious vomiting and laxative abuse can cause secondary aldosteronism and increase in renin secretion by depleting extracellular fluid volume via the gastrointestinal tract. Urinary chloride levels are low in this condition.

Edematous States

The classic edematous states associated with secondary aldosteronism are those of cirrhosis with ascites, nephrosis, and congestive heart failure. Activation of the renin system in patients with these diseases most likely results from changes in renal hemodynamics and redistribution of volume into extravascular tissues, so that the increase in the renin-aldosterone system may be looked upon as a homeostatic system. Although presumably a homeostatic mechanism, the hyperaldosteronism can further con-

Table 10—4. Biochemical findings in primary mineralocorticoid deficiency.

	Plasma		Aldos-terone	Other MCHs	Renin	Cortisol	ACTH	Hct	BUN/Creatinine
	Na+	K+							
Chronic adrenocortical deficiency	N or ↓	↑	↓	N or ↓	↑	↓	↑	↑	N or ↑
After unilateral adrenalectomy for aldosterone-producing tumor	N or ↓	N or ↑	↓	↓	↓↑	N	N	N or ↑	N
21-Hydroxylase deficiency (sodium-losing type)	↓	↑	↓	↓	↑	↓	↑	↑	N
Cholesterol desmolase deficiency	↓	↑	↓	↓	↑	↓	↑	↑	N
3β-Hydroxysteroid dehydrogenase deficiency	↓	↑	↓	↓	↑	↓	↑	↑	N
18-Hydroxylase deficiency (CMO type I)	↓	↑	↓	↑	↑	N	N	↑	N or ↑
18-Hydroxysteroid dehydrogenase deficiency (CMO type II)	↓	↑	↓	↑	↑	N	N	↑	N or ↑

BUN, blood urea nitrogen; Hct, hematocrit; MCH, mineralocorticoid hormone; N, normal; ↑, increased; ↓, decreased; ↑↑, ↓↓, markedly increased, decreased.

tribute to the edema. Hypokalemia is not a frequent finding in these patients unless intake of potassium is extremely low, because reabsorption of sodium in proximal nephron sites makes excessive potassium loss in the distal nephron and the collecting tubules less likely.

Bartter's Syndrome

Bartter's syndrome is a disorder characterized by hypokalemia, alkalosis, hyperreninemia, secondary hyperaldosteronism, increased renal prostaglandins, increased urinary levels of kallikreins, and resistance to pressor effects of angiotensin II. The defect seems to be primarily renal. Although its immediate cause has not been clearly identified, an initiating event may be the defect in chloride reabsorption in the ascending limb of Henle's loop.

PRIMARY MINERALOCORTICOID DEFICIENCY
(Table 10–4)

Disorders of primary mineralocorticoid deficiency consist of a group of adrenal diseases in which mineralocorticoid hormone production is subnormal or inadequate owing to a decrease in the mass of adrenocortical tissue or defective synthesis. As a consequence, variable degrees of sodium loss ensue, with hyponatremia, diminished effective blood volume, and hypotension. Potassium and hydrogen ion secretion are impaired in the renal tubule, resulting in hyperkalemia and metabolic acidosis. Renin activity, as a reliable index of sodium loss, is typically increased (Table 10–4).

Acute and chronic adrenocortical deficiencies are discussed in Chapter 9. Some problems relative to mineralocorticoids are reviewed here.

AFTER UNILATERAL ADRENALECTOMY FOR AN ALDOSTERONE-PRODUCING TUMOR

Patients who have had unilateral adrenalectomy for removal of an aldosterone-producing tumor usually have a transient period of relative hypomineralocorticoidism with negative sodium balance, potassium retention, and mild acidosis. Full recovery of the chronically unstimulated, contralateral zona glomerulosa usually takes place in 4–6 months following surgery, but sometimes it takes as long as 18–24 months. Restitution of the suppressed renin-angiotensin system to normal function usually precedes a completely normal adrenocortical response similar to the recovery of the pituitary-adrenal axis after removal of cortisol-producing adenoma (Cushing's syndrome). No specific treatment is necessary beyond adequate fluid intake and sodium supplementation, except when renal disease is present. A small percentage of patients (1%) do not have normal recovery of their renin-angiotensin-aldosterone system and require mineralocorticoid replacement therapy for life. Preexisting renal disease usually identifies this group.

CONGENITAL ADRENAL HYPOPLASIA & RELATED METABOLIC DISORDERS

Genetic disorders or congenital anomalies involving the adrenal glands have been reported rarely. Congenital adrenal hypoplasia, alone or in association with pituitary hypoplasia, was found at autopsy in a number of newborns who failed to thrive because of sodium loss and complications of hyperkalemia. Other infrequent metabolic disorders that usually involve the adrenal glands are Wolman's disease, cholesteryl ester storage disease, and adrenoleukodystrophy (X-linked Schilder's disease). Mineralocorticoid production is clearly deficient in patients with these diseases.

CONGENITAL ADRENAL HYPERPLASIA WITH RENAL SODIUM LOSS

In variants of congenital adrenal hyperplasia, cortisol synthesis is always impaired. ACTH is accordingly elevated, producing adrenal hyperplasia and stimulating ACTH-dependent steroid precursors.

The steroid biosynthetic pathways, both in the adrenal glands and the gonads, produce specific steroid hormones: cortisol, aldosterone, and testosterone or estradiol. These terminal products come from a single precursor, cholesterol, via a series of enzymatic reactions that introduce hydroxyl groups at specific sites (Fig 10– 1). Recessive autosomal inheritance is responsible for deficiencies in each of the enzymatic steps and results in several forms of the syndrome of deficient steroid production known generically as congenital adrenal hyperplasia. Synthesis of cortisol, aldosterone, and sex steroids is therefore involved in many different ways and combinations. The forms discussed here are those in which production of mineralocorticoid hormones is limited.

1. 21-HYDROXYLASE DEFICIENCY

The most common (95%) of the enzymatic abnormalities in steroid biosynthesis that cause congenital adrenal hyperplasia are due to a deficiency or defect in the enzymatic system responsible for 21-hydroxylation of steroids (see Fig 9– 4).

The incidence of this particular form of congenital adrenal hyperplasia in the USA is believed to be approximately 1:5000 live births. In almost two-thirds of these patients, sodium loss is not apparent, and aldosterone secretion or excretion is actually increased. The presence of elevated levels of progesterone, 17-hydroxyprogesterone, and probably other precursor steroids resulting from uninhibited ACTH stimulation of the adrenal cortex up to the level of the 21-hydroxylation block is probably responsible for the renin-mediated increase in aldosterone production, because these precursor steroids act as aldosterone antagonists at the distal tubule in the nephron and promote mild sodium loss. The ability to conserve sodium during periods of low-sodium intake in these patients is dependent, therefore, on how much aldosterone can be generated in the zona glomerulosa to counteract aldosterone antagonists. Because mild to moderate sodium loss can sometimes be demonstrated in the presence of increased aldosterone production, one has to assume that the high aldosterone levels are inadequate to promote sodium conservation. A wide range of clinical manifestations can be observed. The more severely affected patients, who represent approximately one-third of the whole group, have unquestionable deficiency in aldosterone production, with the 21-hydroxylation block unequivocally involving the zona glomerulosa biosynthetic pathway.

Diagnosis

Because 21-hydroxylase deficiency. is an inborn error of steroid metabolism, clinical manifestations are likely to occur early in infancy. The disorder should be suspected in any infant or child who has frequent and usually refractory episodes of dehydration and whose genitalia are ambiguous. Diagnosis can be confirmed by laboratory findings of electrolyte disturbance, low levels of urinary metabolites or plasma concentrations of cortisol and aldosterone, and elevated levels of steroid precursors such as 17-hydroxyprogesterone and its urinary metabolite pregnanetriol.

Treatment

Treatment must be instituted promptly, because the sodium and fluid losses result in severe dehydration, shock, and hyperkalemia and thus in usually fatal cardiac arrhythmias. Parenteral isotonic or even hypertonic saline and glucocorticoids (hydrocortisone, 25– 50 mg intravenously, and DOCA, 2– 5 mg intramuscularly) as required are lifesaving. Cationic resins (eg, sodium polystyrene sulfonate [Kayexalate]) may be used to lower extremely high potassium levels refractory to other treatment. Chronic treatment requires mineralocorticoid replacement and sodium chloride supplementation. In addition, patients achieve improvement in linear growth and experience decreased need for glucocorticoid hormones to suppress ACTH when small supplements of mineralocorticoids are given. For reasons not understood, sodium-retaining ability may improve with age, so that some patients are able to discontinue mineralocorticoid replacement, usually after puberty.

Patients with the "simple virilizing," non–sodium-losing type of 21-hydroxylase deficiency also have been shown to have elevated plasma renin levels. This elevation is presumably due to the increased production of precursor steroids with aldosterone-antagonistic properties, leading to higher plasma aldosterone levels. The level of plasma renin activity is accordingly an index for substitution therapy with added salt or fludrocortisone to correct this abnormality. These observations led some investigators to postulate that even in the non–sodium-losing type of 21-hydroxylase deficiency, a mild degree of sodium loss, usually manifested during stressful situations or low sodium intake, occurs as a consequence of inadequate aldosterone production even though the plasma concentration or urinary level of aldosterone may be elevated. Accordingly, the 21-hydroxylase deficiency should be considered as a single disorder with a wide spectrum of clinical manifestations related to sodium conservation instead of 2 separate disorders— the sodium-losing and non–sodium-losing forms.

2. CHOLESTEROL DESMOLASE DEFICIENCY

Prader in 1955 described a syndrome of sodium loss in which no steroid could be found in the urine.

Histologic and postmortem examination of patients showed a "lipoid" hyperplasia of adrenocortical tissue containing a high concentration of cholesterol-laden cells. A defect in cholesterol desmolase, the earliest step in steroid biosynthesis, that impeded the conversion of cholesterol to Δ^5-pregnenolone was proposed as the mechanism. Patients with this uncommon disorder cannot produce steroids from any source and present with a female phenotype and severe sodium loss; they frequently die in the first weeks of life, although a few survive with early recognition and treatment.

3. 3β-HYDROXYSTEROID DEHYDROGENASE & Δ⁴,⁵ ISOMERASE DEFICIENCY

3β-Hydroxysteroid dehydrogenase deficiency is a rare life-threatening form of congenital adrenal hyperplasia that was described by Bongiovanni in 1962. Pregnenolone (Δ^5) can be synthesized but not Δ^4 steroids derived from it, eg, progesterone (see Fig 9–4). The concomitant involvement of the gonads precludes production of sex steroids. Incomplete sexual differentiation is seen in males, whereas mild virilization is seen in females from weaker androgenic steroids derived from pregnenolone, ie, dehydroepiandrosterone (DHEA). Aldosterone, which is also derived from the Δ^4 steroid lineage, cannot be produced in adequate amounts, and sodium conservation is therefore poor. Recently, a mild or incomplete defect in this enzymatic step was reported in adults. Analysis of steroid metabolites in the urine or of plasma concentrations of steroids establishes the diagnosis, and treatment should consist of replacement of glucocorticoids, mineralocorticoids, and sex hormones.

4. DISORDERS OF TERMINAL ALDOSTERONE BIOSYNTHESIS

In contrast to congenital adrenal hyperplasia, specific enzymatic deficiencies can result in a syndrome of isolated mineralocorticoid deficiency. Two clinically similar sodium-losing syndromes have been described that present almost exclusively with sodium loss and some degree of growth retardation. The production of aldosterone from corticosterone is a 2-step reaction in which 18-hydroxycorticosterone is presumably formed as an intermediate precursor. However, Ulick proposed that aldosterone and 18-hydroxycorticosterone are both end products of the zona glomerulosa, being synthesized from corticosterone through a mixed function oxidation system. In so-called corticosterone methyloxidase (CMO) type I deficiency (18-hydroxylase deficiency), formation of aldosterone and 18-hydroxycorticosterone is blocked but not corticosterone formation. The salt loss and increased renin secretion stimulate the zona glomerulosa pathway and increase production of the 18-hydroxycorticosterone and aldosterone precursors cor-

ticosterone and DOC. In the second variant, corticosterone methyloxidase (CMO) type II deficiency (18-hydroxysteroid dehydrogenase deficiency), corticosterone and 18-hydroxycorticosterone are produced in increased amounts in the presence of reduced production of aldosterone. The accumulation of precursors in each case, however, is not sufficient to prevent sodium loss, hyperkalemia, and increased renin production. Both of these uncommon diseases are manifested early in infancy and have a tendency to improve with age. Early detection and treatment with mineralocorticoid and sodium supplements result in an excellent prognosis.

SECONDARY MINERALOCORTICOID DEFICIENCY (Table 10–5)

SECONDARY MINERALOCORTICOID DEFICIENCY WITHOUT HYPERTENSION

Secondary mineralocorticoid deficiency comprises a heterogeneous group of disorders in which endogenous mineralocorticoid secretion is abnormally low owing to suppressed or insufficient renin production. In the former situation, renin is suppressed by increased sodium retention and volume expansion resulting either from the presence of exogenous mineralocorticoids or mineralocorticoidlike substances or from a renal tubular defect. Hypertension, hypokalemia, and metabolic alkalosis are the usual manifestations. When renin production is insufficient to stimulate mineralocorticoid production, sodium loss, hyperkalemia, and metabolic acidosis occur.

Heparin & Heparinoids

Chronic administration of heparin and related compounds, either to humans or to experimental animals, is reportedly associated with decreased aldosterone production in some cases. The mechanism for impaired aldosterone synthesis is not clearly understood, although decreased sensitivity of the zona glomerulosa to renin-angiotensin stimulation is suspected. No evidence of any enzymatic defect induced by heparin has been demonstrated by measuring aldosterone precursors. Anatomic changes in the zona glomerulosa are nonspecific and seem to be reversible after heparin treatment is discontinued.

Hyporeninemic Hypoaldosteronism

An increasing number of patients have recently been reported in whom hyperkalemia and acidosis are present in association with variable degrees of renal failure in the course of diseases such as pyelonephritis, diabetes mellitus, and gout. The patients, usually men

Table 10–5. Biochemical findings in secondary mineralocorticoid deficiency.

	Plasma		Aldos-terone	Other MCHs	Renin	Cortisol	ACTH	Hct	BUN/Creatinine
	Na⁺	K⁺							
Without hypertension									
Heparin and heparinoids	N or ↓	N or ↑	N or ↓	N or ↓	N or ↑	N	N	N or ↑	N
Hyporeninemic hypoaldosteronism	N or ↓	↑	↓	N or ↓	↓	N	N	N or ↑	↑
Autonomic insufficiency	N or ↓	N or ↑	↓	N or ↓	↓	N	N	N	N
Renin blockers/angiotensin-converting enzyme inhibitors	N or ↓	N or ↑	↓	N or ↓	↓(↑)*	N	N	N	N or ↑
With hypertension									
Pseudohyperaldosteronism (Liddle's syndrome)	N or ↑	↓	↓	N or ↓	↓	N	N	↓	N
Arnold-Healy syndrome	N or ↑	↑	↓	N or ↓	↓	N	N	N or ↓	N
Synthetic MCH administration	N or ↑	↓	↓	↓†	↓	N	N	↓	N
Chronic ingestion of MCH-like sub-stances	N or ↑	↓	↓	↓†	↓	N	N	↓	N

*Angiotensin II or III is decreased; renin activity or concentration is increased by an artifact.

†Endogenous production of mineralocorticoid is decreased; high mineralocorticoid hormone activity results from exogenous administration.

BUN, blood urea nitrogen; Hct, hematocrit; MCH, mineralocorticoid hormone; N, normal; ↑, increased; ↓, decreased; ↑↑, ↓↓, markedly increased, decreased.

in the fifth to seventh decades of life, have an average decrease of 60% in renal function as evaluated by creatinine clearance, and the chronic renal insufficiency per se usually cannot account for the degree of hyperkalemia. Plasma sodium concentration is normal, but sodium conservation is frequently deficient. Plasma concentrations and urinary excretion of aldosterone are low and unresponsive to such stimulatory maneuvers as prolonged ACTH administration, upright posture, dietary sodium deprivation, furosemide administration, and angiotensin III ([des-Asp¹] angiotensin II) infusion. Plasma renin activity and concentration are consistently low and also unresponsive to stimulation. Cortisol- and ACTH-dependent steroids are normal and increase adequately in response to appropriate stimuli. The cause of the hyporeninemic state is presumably associated with chronic impairment of the juxtaglomerular apparatus. Potassium restriction, furosemide, alkali, and small doses of fludrocortisone (Florinef) (0.05 mg/d), singly or in combination, may be required to correct the acidosis and hyperkalemia.

Autonomic Insufficiency

This subset of hyporeninemic hypoaldosteronism can be further characterized by defective baroreceptor function, vasopressor sensitivity to vasopressin and norepinephrine, and mild sodium wasting.

Progressive degeneration and destruction of sympathetic nerve terminations leading to the juxtaglomerular apparatus and deficient neurotransmission in the afferent or efferent fibers associated with the synthesis and storage of renin granules are potential causes of secondary aldosterone deficiency. Stimuli such as upright posture or acute volume depletion, mediated by baroreceptors, do not effect normal responses in renin. Even stimuli mediated by the sodium concentration in the macula densa (ie, chemoreceptors) fail

to initiate a renin-aldosterone response. Aldosterone levels are low normal and subnormally responsive to sodium restriction in this condition. The classic manifestation of this disease is a moderate to severe postural fall in blood pressure. The impaired potassium excretion associated with the hypoaldosteronism can be further aggravated by the diminished renal blood flow, resulting in alarmingly high plasma levels of potassium. Doses of fludrocortisone (Florinef) in the range of 0.1–0.4 mg/d are usually necessary to maintain adequate blood volume, to ensure appropriate accommodation to postural changes, and to prevent potassium retention.

Prolonged Use of Renin Blockers or Angiotensin-Converting Enzyme Inhibitors

Several hypertensive states, especially those associated with high renin levels (angiotensinogenic hypertension)—eg, high-renin essential hypertension, renovascular hypertension, and accelerated hypertension—have recently been managed either by renin secretion inhibitors such as the beta-receptor blockers or a converting enzyme inhibitor of angiotensin II formation such as captopril. Although hormonal responses during treatment must be monitored, one can assume that chronic suppression of renin formation or release or continuous inhibition of the renin-angiotensin system cascade may induce varying degrees of aldosterone deficiency. Prostaglandin synthetase inhibitors (nonsteroidal anti-inflammatory agents) can reduce renin and aldosterone levels, and their use in a patient with impaired renal function may result in hyperkalemia.

SECONDARY MINERALOCORTICOID DEFICIENCY WITH HYPERTENSION

Pseudohyperaldosteronism (Liddle's Syndrome)

In 1963, Liddle et al studied a family in which the affected members had clinical manifestations resembling those of classic primary aldosteronism: hypertension, hypokalemia with renal potassium wasting, metabolic alkalosis, and suppressed plasma renin activity. However, aldosterone production was negligible. This unusual isolated finding suggested the possibility of excessive production of another unidentified mineralocorticoid hormone to explain the clinical manifestations. However, administration of spironolactone, a mineralocorticoid antagonist at the distal tubular receptor level, did not correct either the hypertension or the hypokalemia. Furthermore, the adrenocortical synthesis–blocking agent metyrapone, which inhibits 11β- and 18-hydroxylation of aldosterone precursors, also had no effect. In contrast, administration of triamterene, a diuretic agent with potassium-sparing activity acting at a proximal site in the nephron independently of mineralocorticoid hormones, was effective in correcting the abnormalities. The investigators proposed that a primary defect in sodium-potassium transport across membranes in the renal tubule was responsible for the syndrome, although the precise mechanism remains unclear.

Arnold-Healy Syndrome

Several patients have been reported in whom hypertension is present in association with hyperkalemia, impairment of potassium excretion, and hyperchloremic metabolic acidosis. A state of hyporeninemic hypoaldosteronism is well documented in the presence of normal renal function. The aldosterone response to stimulatory maneuvers appears to be adequate. Administration of large amounts of mineralocorticoids fails to produce a kaliuretic response and thus correct the hyperkalemia, suggesting a mineralocorticoid-resistant state. Impairment in renal potassium excretion was initially proposed as the primary defect. However, when patients were given a sodium bicarbonate or sulfate load, the increased distal delivery of sodium greatly facilitated potassium excretion and hyperkalemia was virtually corrected, suggesting that the proposed defect in potassium excretion was only secondary. The defect caused increases in chloride reabsorption proximal to the sodium- and mineralocorticoid-dependent driving forces for potassium secretion, resulting in hyperkalemia. By increasing proximal sodium reabsorption with consequent volume expansion, hypertension and suppression of renin and aldosterone production occurred. Abnormalities can be corrected in this syndrome by adding supplementary amounts of sodium bicarbonate or sulfate or hydrochlorothiazide.

Administration of Synthetic Mineralocorticoid Hormones

In several of the aforementioned mineralocorticoid deficiency syndromes, the appropriate therapy is mineralocorticoid replacement. The most commonly used synthetic mineralocorticoid is the 9α-fluoro derivative of hydrocortisone, 9α-fluorohydrocortisone (fludrocortisone [Florinef]). Its potent mineralocorticoid activity, which is similar to that of aldosterone, permits it to be used in amounts as small as 0.05 mg daily or every other day. Alternatively, DOCA in a long-acting preparation can be used intramuscularly. Because individual sensitivity to these preparations varies, blood pressure and plasma electrolyte panels should be monitored closely. When used in inappropriately high dosage or in the presence of increased sodium intake or inadequate metabolism, increased mineralocorticoid activity will occur and result in sodium retention, expansion of extracellular fluid volume, hypertension, and hypokalemia. Adjustment of the dosage easily controls undesirable side effects.

Chronic Ingestion of Mineralocorticoidlike Substances

Chronic ingestion of large amounts of substances containing mineralocorticoidlike activity—eg, certain candies, infusions, and some chewing tobaccos containing licorice—results in a syndrome of hypertension, hypokalemia, renal sodium retention, volume expansion, suppressed plasma renin activity, and metabolic alkalosis that is almost indistinguishable from primary hyperaldosteronism. Aldosterone secretion or excretion is, however, low or undetectable, as are other mineralocorticoid precursors in the aldosterone pathway. The responsible agents for this syndrome are certain substances, especially glycyrrhizinic acid and its metabolite glycyrrhizetic acid, that are present in certain commercially available products. Hypermineralocorticoidism can be induced by licorice and its derivatives—carbenoxolone (an anti–gastric ulcer drug), sodium hemisuccinate of 18β-glycyrrhizinic acid—and by other fluorinated steroids with powerful mineralocorticoidlike activity contained in some topical preparations such as nasal sprays and dermatologic creams. Electrolyte abnormalities and hypertension disappear within a few days or weeks upon discontinuation of licorice ingestion or carbenoxolone withdrawal.

REFERENCES

Biglieri EG, Baxter JD: The endocrinology of hypertension. Chapter 14 in: *Endocrinology and Metabolism*. Felig P et al (editors). McGraw-Hill, 1981.

Bravo EL, Tarazi RC, Dustan HP: The changing clinical spectrum of primary aldosteronism. *Am J Med* 1983;**303**:641.

Conn JW: Primary reninism. Pages 840–847 in: *Hypertension: Pathophysiology and Treatment*. Genest J, Koiw E, Kuchel O (editors). McGraw-Hill, 1977.

Conn JW, Rovner DR, Cohen E: Licorice induced pseudoaldosteronism: Hypertension, hypokalemia, aldosteronopenia, and suppressed plasma renin activity. *JAMA* 1968;**205**:492.

Ferriss JB et al: Treatment of low-renin ("primary") hyperaldosteronism. *Am Heart J* 1978;**96**:97.

Finkelstein M, Shaeffer JM: Inborn errors of steroid biosynthesis. *Physiol Rev* 1979;**59**:353.

Gill JR Jr: Bartter's syndrome. *Annu Rev Med* 1980;**31**:405.

Hunt TK, Schambelan M, Biglieri EG: Selection of patients and operative approach in primary aldosteronism. *Ann Surg* 1975;**182**:353.

Irvine WJ, Barnes EW: Adrenocortical insufficiency. *Clin Endocrinol Metab* 1972;**1**:549.

Lee PA et al (editors): *Congenital Adrenal Hyperplasia*. University Park Press, 1977.

Liddle GW, Bledsoe T, Coppage WS Jr: A familial renal disorder simulating primary aldosteronism but with negligible aldosterone secretion. *Trans Assoc Am Physicians* 1963;**76**:199.

Michelis MF, Murdaugh HV: Selective hypoaldosteronism: An editorial review revisited after 15 years. *Am J Med* 1975;**59**:1.

Peart WS: Renin-angiotensin system. *N Engl J Med* 1975;**292**:302.

Schambelan M, Perloff D: Renovascular and renal parenchymal hypertension. Pages 1719–1741 in: *The Kidney*. Brenner BM, Rector FC Jr (editors). Saunders, 1981.

Schambelan M, Sebastian A, Biglieri EG: Prevalence, pathogenesis and functional significance of aldosterone deficiency in hyperkalemic patients with chronic renal insufficiency. *Kidney Int* 1980;**17**:89.

Schambelan M et al: Circadian rhythm and effect of posture on plasma aldosterone concentration in primary aldosteronism. *J Clin Endocrinol Metab* 1976;**43**:115.

Ulick S et al: A syndrome of apparent mineralocorticoid excess associated with defects in peripheral metabolism of cortisol. *J Clin Endocrinol Metab* 1979;**49**:757.

Weinberger M et al: Primary aldosteronism: Diagnosis, localization, and treatment. *Ann Intern Med* 1979;**90**:386.

White EA et al: Use of computed tomography in diagnosing the cause of primary aldosteronism. *N Engl J Med* 1980;**303**:1503.

Wolff HP et al: Psychiatric disturbance leading to potassium depletion, sodium depletion, raised plasma renin concentration, and secondary hyperaldosteronism. *Lancet* 1968;**1**:257.

11

The Adrenal Medulla

Alan Goldfien, MD

The adrenal medulla was first distinguished from the adrenal cortex at the beginning of the 19th century. Its major secretory product, **epinephrine**, was isolated, purified, and synthesized a century later. **Norepinephrine** was synthesized in 1904, but not until 1946 was it recognized as a secretory product of the adrenal medulla and as the major neurotransmitter of the postganglionic sympathetic nerves. The adrenal medulla, a highly specialized part of the sympathetic nervous system, functions under stress or whenever marked deviations from normal homeostasis occur—in contrast to the rest of the sympathetic nervous system, which is involved in the minute-to-minute fine regulation of most physiologic processes.

ANATOMY

Embryology
(Fig 11–1)

The sympathetic nervous system arises in the fetus from the primitive cells of the neural crest (sympathogonia). At about the fifth week of gestation, these cells migrate from the primitive spinal ganglia in the thoracic region to form the sympathetic chain posterior to the dorsal aorta. They then begin to migrate anteriorly to form the remaining ganglia.

At 6 weeks, groups of these primitive cells migrate along the central vein and enter the fetal adrenal cortex to form the adrenal medulla, which is detectable by the eighth week. The adrenal medulla at this time is composed of sympathogonia and pheochromoblasts, which then mature into pheochromocytes. The cells appear in rosettelike structures, with the more primitive cells occupying a central position. Storage granules can be found in these cells by electron microscopy at 12 weeks. Pheochromoblasts and pheochromocytes also collect on both sides of the aorta to form the paraganglia. The principal collection of these cells is found at the level of the inferior mesenteric artery. They fuse anteriorly to form the organ of Zuckerkandl, which is quite prominent in fetal life. This organ is thought to be a major source of catecholamines during the first year of life, after which it begins to atrophy. Pheochromocytes (chromaffin cells) also are found scattered throughout the abdominal sympathetic plexuses as well as in other parts of the sympathetic nervous system.

Acronyms Used in This Chapter

ACTH	Adrenocorticotropic hormone
ATP	Adenosine triphosphate
cAMP	Cyclic adenosine monophosphate
COMT	Catechol-O-methyltransferase
DOMA	Dihydroxymandelic acid
DOPEG	Dihydroxyphenylglycol
MAO	Monoamine oxidase
MEN	Multiple endocrine neoplasia
MIBG	[^{131}I] Metaiodobenzylguanidine
PGE	Prostaglandin E
PNMT	Phenylethanolamine-N-methyltransferase
VMA	Vanillylmandelic acid (3-methoxy-4-hydroxymandelic acid)

Gross Structure

The anatomic relationships between the adrenal medulla and the adrenal cortex are different in different species. These organs are completely separate structures in the shark. They remain separate but in close contact in amphibians, and there is some intermingling in birds. In mammals, the medulla is surrounded by the adrenal cortex. In humans, the adrenal medulla occupies a central position in the widest part of the gland, with only small portions extending into the narrower parts. It constitutes approximately one-tenth of the weight of the gland, although the proportions vary from individual to individual. There is no clear demarcation between cortex and medulla. The central vein is usually surrounded by a cuff of adrenal cortical cells, and there may be islands of cortex elsewhere in the medulla.

Microscopic Structure

The **chromaffin cells,** or **pheochromocytes,** of the adrenal medulla are large ovoid columnar cells arranged in clumps or cords around blood vessels. They derive their name from the observation that their granules turn brown *(pheo-)* when stained with chromic acid. The color is due to the oxidation of epinephrine and norepinephrine to melanin. These cells have large nuclei and a well-developed Golgi apparatus. They contain large numbers of vesicles or granules containing catecholamines. Vesicles containing norepinephrine are darker than those containing epinephrine.

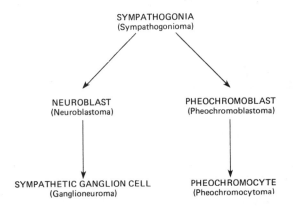

Figure 11–1. The embryonic development of adrenergic cells and tumors that develop from them. Sympathogonia are primitive cells derived from the neural crest. Neuroblasts are also called sympathoblasts; ganglion cells are the same as sympathocytes; and pheochromocytes are mature chromaffin cells.

vascular system arising from the capillaries in the cortex. There is also a capillary network of lymphatics that drain into a plexus around the central vein.

In mammals, the enzyme that catalyzes the conversion of norepinephrine to epinephrine (phenylethanolamine-N-methyltransferase, PNMT) is induced by adrenocortical steroids. The chromaffin cells containing epinephrine therefore receive most of their blood supply from the capillaries draining the cortical cells, whereas cells containing predominantly norepinephrine are supplied by the arteries that directly supply the medulla. (See Biosynthesis, below.)

On the right side, the central vein is short and drains directly into the vena cava, although some branches go to the surface of the gland and reach the azygos system. On the left, the vein is somewhat longer and drains into the renal vein.

HORMONES OF THE ADRENAL MEDULLA

The pheochromocytes may be arranged in nests, alveoli, or cords and are surrounded by a rich network of capillaries and sinusoids. The adrenal medulla also contains some sympathetic ganglion cells, singly or in groups. Ganglion cells are also found in association with the viscera, the carotid body, the glomus jugulare, and the cervical and thoracic ganglia.

Nerve Supply

The cells of the adrenal medulla are innervated by preganglionic fibers of the sympathetic nervous system, which release acetylcholine at the synapses. Most of these fibers arise from a plexus in the capsule of the posterior surface of the gland and enter the adrenal glands in bundles of 30–50 fibers without synapsing. They follow the course of the blood vessels into the medulla without branching into the adrenal cortex. Some reach the wall of the central vein, where they synapse with small autonomic ganglia. However, most fibers end in relationship to the pheochromocytes.

Blood Supply

The human adrenal gland derives blood from the superior, middle, and inferior adrenal branches of the inferior phrenic artery, directly from the aorta and from the renal arteries. Upon reaching the adrenal gland, these arteries branch to form a plexus under the capsule supplying the adrenal cortex. A few of these vessels, however, penetrate the cortex, passing directly to the medulla. The medulla is also nourished by branches of the arteries supplying the central vein and cuff of cortical tissue around the central vein. Capillary loops passing from the subcapsular plexus of the cortex also supply blood as they drain into the central vein. It would appear, then, that most of the blood supply to the medullary cells is via a portal

CATECHOLAMINES

Biosynthesis
(Fig 11–2)

Catecholamines are widely distributed in plants and animals. In mammals, **epinephrine** is synthesized mainly in the adrenal medulla, whereas **norepinephrine** is found not only in the adrenal medulla but also in the central nervous system and in the peripheral sympathetic nerves. **Dopamine,** the precursor of norepinephrine, is found in the adrenal medulla and in noradrenergic neurons. It is present in high concentrations in the brain, in specialized interneurons in the sympathetic ganglia, and in the carotid body, where it serves as a neurotransmitter. Dopamine is also found in specialized mast cells and in enterochromaffin cells.

The proportions of epinephrine and norepinephrine found in the adrenal medulla vary with the species (Table 11–1). In humans, the adrenal contains 15–20% norepinephrine.

Table 11–1. Approximate percentages of total adrenal medullary catecholamines present as norepinephrine in various species.

Whale	70	Horse	25
Chicken	70	Squirrel	25
Lion	55	Cow	25
Frog	50	Human	20
Pig	45	Guinea pig	15
Cat	40	Rat	15
Gazelle	35	Zebra	13
Sheep	35	Rabbit	5
Goat	35	Baboon	0
Dog	30		

Figure 11–2. Biosynthesis of catecholamines. The alternative pathways shown by the dashed arrows have not been found to be of physiologic significance in humans. PNMT, phenylethanolamine-N-methyltransferase.

A. Tyrosine as Precursor: The catecholamines are synthesized from **tyrosine,** which may be derived from ingested food or synthesized from phenylalanine in the liver. Tyrosine circulates at a concentration of 1–1.5 mg/dL of blood. It enters neurons and chromaffin cells by an active transport mechanism and is converted to **dihydroxyphenylalanine (dopa).** The reaction is catalyzed by **tyrosine hydroxylase,** which is transported via axonal flow to the nerve terminal. Tyrosine hydroxylase activity may be inhibited by a variety of compounds. Alpha-methylmetatyrosine is effective and is sometimes used in the therapy of malignant pheochromocytomas (see below). Substances that chelate iron or compete for the pteridine cofactor also inhibit the enzyme but are not useful clinically. Activity of this enzyme is a reliable marker of intact sympathetic nerve tissue and neurotransmitter synthesis.

B. Conversion of Dopa to Dopamine: Dopa is converted to dopamine by the enzyme aromatic

L-amino acid decarboxylase (dopa decarboxylase). This enzyme is found in all tissues, with the highest concentrations in liver, kidney, brain, and vas deferens. The various enzymes have different substrate specificities depending upon the tissue source. Competitive inhibitors of dopa decarboxylase such as methyldopa are converted to substances (an example is α-methylnorepinephrine) that are then stored in granules in the nerve cell and released in place of norepinephrine. These products (false transmitters) were thought to mediate the antihypertensive action of drugs at peripheral sympathetic synapses but are now believed to stimulate the alpha receptors of the inhibitory corticobulbar system, reducing sympathetic discharge peripherally.

C. Conversion of Dopamine to Norepinephrine: The conversion of dopamine to norepinephrine is catalyzed by dopamine β-hydroxylase, a mixed-function oxidase requiring oxygen and an external electron donor. The enzyme does not occur in tissues outside the neuron. Part of the biologic specificity of dopamine β-hydroxylase may result from its compartmentalization. Newly synthesized dopamine β-hydroxylase is incorporated directly into storage vesicles that take up, synthesize, and store the catecholamines. The membranes of these vesicles contain dopamine β-hydroxylase, ATPase, cytochrome P-561, and cytochrome P-561:NADH reductase. Dopamine β-hydroxylase is also found within the granule and is released with norepinephrine during secretion. Inhibitors of the enzyme, such as disulfuramic and picolinic acid, have no clinical importance.

D. Conversion of Norepinephrine to Epinephrine: PNMT catalyzes the N-methylation of norepinephrine to epinephrine, using S-adenosylmethionine as a methyl donor. It is found only in the adrenal medulla and in a few neurons in the central nervous system. The enzyme is found in the cytosol. Norepinephrine leaves the granule and after methylation reenters different granules. This enzyme is induced by the high levels of glucocorticoids (100 times the systemic concentration) found in the adrenal medulla. The conversion of dopamine to **epinine** is catalyzed by a nonspecific N-methyltransferase.

Catecholamine biosynthesis is coupled to secretion, so that the stores of norepinephrine at the nerve endings remain relatively unchanged even in the presence of marked nerve activity. In the adrenal medulla, it is possible to deplete stores with prolonged hypoglycemia. Biosynthesis appears to be increased during nerve stimulation by activation of tyrosine hydroxylase. Prolonged stimulation leads to the induction of increased amounts of this enzyme.

Storage

The catecholamines are found in the adrenal medulla and various sympathetically innervated organs, and their concentration reflects the density of sympathetic neurons. The adrenal medulla contains about 0.5 mg/g; the spleen, vas deferens, brain, spinal cord, and heart contain $1-5$ μg/g; liver, gut, and skeletal muscle contain $0.1-0.5$ μg/g. The catecholamines are stored in electron-dense granules approximately 1 μm in diameter that contain catecholamines and ATP

Figure 11–3. Rate of secretion of amines from one adrenal following injection of insulin. The percentage of the total released as norepinephrine is shown below.

in a 4:1 molar ratio, calcium, magnesium, and water-soluble proteins called **chromogranins.** The ratio of catecholamines to ATP is much higher in granules isolated from pheochromocytomas. The interior surface of the membrane contains dopamine β-hydroxylase and ATPase. The Mg^{2+}-dependent ATPase facilitates the uptake and inhibits the release of catecholamines by the granules. This activity is inhibited by reserpine.

Secretion

Adrenal medullary catecholamine secretion is increased by exercise, angina pectoris, myocardial infarction, hemorrhage, ether anesthesia, surgery, severe hypoglycemia, anoxia and asphyxia, and many other stressful stimuli. The rate of secretion of epinephrine increases more than that of norepinephrine in the presence of hypoglycemia and most other stimuli (Fig 11–3). However, anoxia and asphyxia produce a greater increase in adrenal medullary release of norepinephrine than is observed with other stimuli (Fig 11–4).

Secretion of the adrenal medullary hormones is mediated by the release of acetylcholine from the terminals of preganglionic fibers. The resulting depolarization of the axonal membrane triggers an influx

Table 11–2. Substances altering the release of norepinephrine at nerve endings by binding to specific presynaptic membrane receptors.

Increase	Decrease
Norepinephrine (beta receptor)	*Norepinephrine (alpha receptor)
Angiotensin	Serotonin
Epinephrine	Dopamine
	PGE₂
	Purines
	Metenkephalin
	Substance P
	Acetylcholine

*The alpha receptor–mediated inhibition of norepinephrine release is the dominant effect.

of calcium ion. The contents of the storage vesicles, including the chromogranins and soluble dopamine β-hydroxylase, are released by exocytosis by the calcium ion increase. Membrane-bound dopamine β-hydroxylase is not released. **Tyramine,** however, releases norepinephrine primarily from the free store in the cytosol. Cocaine and monoamine oxidase inhibitors inhibit the effect of tyramine but do not affect the release of catecholamines by nervous stimulation. The rate of release in response to nerve stimulation is increased or decreased by a wide variety of neurotransmitters acting at specific receptors on the presynaptic neuron. Norepinephrine has an important role in modulating its own release by activating the alpha receptors on the presynaptic membrane. Alpha receptor antagonists inhibit this reaction. Conversely, presynaptic beta receptors enhance norepinephrine release, whereas beta receptor blockers increase it. The effects of such substances are shown in Table 11–2. The accumulation of excess catecholamines that are not in the storage granules is prevented by the presence of intraneuronal monoamine oxidase.

Transport

When released into the circulation, the amines are bound to albumin or a closely associated protein with low affinity and high capacity (K_d 10^{-7}).

Metabolism & Inactivation

The actions of catecholamines are terminated rapidly by several mechanisms. These include reuptake by the sympathetic nerve ending, metabolism by the enzymes catechol-O-methyltransferase (COMT) and monoamine oxidase (Fig 11–5), conjugation with sulfate ion, and direct excretion by the kidney. Estimates of the metabolic clearance rates for epinephrine and norepinephrine are 4000–5000 L/d.

Uptake 1

A large proportion (85–90%) of the amines released at the synapse are taken up locally by the nerve endings from which they are released (uptake 1). Circulating amines can also be taken up by this mech-

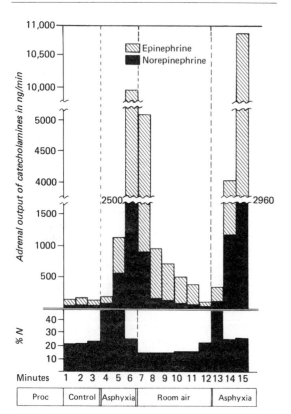

Figure 11–4. Rate of secretion of amines from one adrenal during asphyxia. The percentage of the total released as norepinephrine is shown below.

Figure 11–5. Metabolism of catecholamines by catechol-O-methyltransferase (COMT) and monoamine oxidase (MAO).

anism. However, this mechanism plays a less important role in the inactivation of circulating catecholamines. The axonal membrane uptake process is energy-requiring, saturable, stereoselective, and sodium-dependent. It is blocked by cocaine, other sympathomimetic amines such as metaraminol and amphetamine, and agents such as tricyclic antidepressants and phenothiazines. Neither calcium nor magnesium ion has any effect on uptake 1. There is also an uptake process for dopamine in neurons of the central nervous system, but this process is not inhibited by tricyclic antidepressants. After being taken up by the neuron, the amines are reutilized or deaminated by monoamine oxidase and the metabolites are released (Fig 11–6). The intraneuronal monoamine oxidase is a flavoprotein and is localized to the outer mitochondrial membrane. Its substrate specificity favors norepinephrine, which it oxidizes to dihydroxyphenylglycol (DOPEG) or dihydroxymandelic acid (DOMA). The major functions of monoamine oxidase are (1) to regulate dopamine and norepinephrine content of the neurons; (2) to destroy ingested amines; and (3) to metabolize the circulating catecholamines and their O-methyl metabolites. Progesterone increases the level of monoamine oxidase in women, whereas estrogens inhibit the enzyme.

Uptake 2

Extraneuronal tissues also take up catecholamines. This process, uptake 2, is saturable, is not specific for catecholamines, and is inhibited by various steroids, phenoxybenzamine, and normetanephrine but not by cocaine and other drugs that inhibit neuronal uptake.

At uptake 2, the catecholamines are metabolized to their O-methyl derivatives by COMT (Fig 11–6). This enzyme is found mainly in the soluble fraction of tissue homogenates, with the highest levels in the liver and kidney. S-Adenosylmethionine is the methyl donor, and divalent ions are required for the reaction. It is predominantly an extraneuronal enzyme and acts on circulating catecholamines as well as on the locally released norepinephrine. It is the most important enzyme in the metabolism of circulating amines. Approximately 70% of circulating epinephrine in humans is methoxylated, and about 24% is also deaminated. These enzymes also metabolize dopamine to homovanillic acid. Although normetanephrine is fairly active at the alpha receptor of the nictitating membrane, the metabolites of the catecholamines are generally devoid of biologic or physiologic activity.

Conjugation

The phenolic hydroxyl group of the catecholamines and their metabolites may be conjugated with sulfate or glucuronide. Liver and gut appear to be important sites of this reaction, and recent studies

Figure 11–6. Schematic diagram of the neuroeffector junction of the peripheral sympathetic nervous system. The nerves terminate in complex networks with varicosities or enlargements that form synaptic junctions with effector cells. The neurotransmitter at these junctions is norepinephrine, which is synthesized from tyrosine. Tyrosine uptake is linked to sodium uptake and transport into the varicosity where the secretory vesicles form. Tyrosine is hydroxylated by tyrosine hydroxylase to dopa, which is then decarboxylated by dopa decarboxylase to dopamine in the cytoplasm. Dopamine (DA) is transported into the vesicle by a carrier mechanism (②) that can be blocked by reserpine. The same carrier transports norepinephrine (NE) and several other amines into these granules. Dopamine is converted to norepinephrine through the catalytic action of dopamine β-hydroxylase (DβH). ATP is also present in high concentration in the vesicle. Release of transmitter occurs when an action potential is conducted to the varicosity by the action of voltage-sensitive sodium channels. Depolarization of the varicosity membrane opens voltage-sensitive calcium channels and results in an increase in intracellular calcium. The elevated calcium facilitates exocytotic fusion of vesicles with the surface membrane and expulsion of norepinephrine, ATP, and some of the dopamine β-hydroxylase. Release is blocked by drugs such as guanethidine and bretylium. Norepinephrine reaching either pre- or postsynaptic receptors modifies the function of the corresponding cells. Norepinephrine also diffuses out of the cleft, or it may be transported into the cytoplasm of the varicosity (uptake 1, blocked by cocaine, tricyclic antidepressants) or into the postjunctional cell (uptake 2). (Reproduced, with permission, from Katzung BG [editor]: *Basic & Clinical Pharmacology,* 2nd ed. Lange, 1984.)

suggest that circulating red blood cells are a significant site of sulfation in humans.

Connective tissue binds catecholamines by a process that is inhibited by oxytetracycline. The significance of this binding is unknown.

Receptors

The catecholamines exert their physiologic effects by binding to receptor molecules on the surfaces of target cells. The mechanism whereby binding of the hormone to the receptor activates the physiologic response is discussed in Chapter 1. Early studies of sympathetic activation suggested that there were 2 classes of responses designated as inhibitory or excitatory. Cannon and his colleagues in the 1930s pos-

tulated that this difference was produced by the release of different neurotransmitters: sympathin I and sympathin E. The discovery by von Euler and others that norepinephrine was the neurotransmitter released by peripheral sympathetic nerve endings and was responsible for both types of responses led to the proposal by Ahlquist in 1948 that there were 2 types of receptors that he designated alpha and beta, based on the relative potencies of a series of adrenergic agonists. The subsequent development of relatively specific antagonists confirmed this hypothesis and allowed the development of binding assays for the alpha, beta, and dopaminergic receptors. Subsequent pharmacologic and biochemical studies indicate that alpha, beta, and dopaminergic receptors can be further di-

Table 11–3. Characteristic interactions of agonists and antagonists at the adrenergic receptors.

Receptor	Agonist Potency*	Antagonist Potency	Agonist Effect on Adenylate Cyclase Activity
Alpha$_1$	Same for α_1 and α_2.	Prazosin > phentolamine > yohimbine.	None
Alpha$_2$	Epinephrine slightly > norepinephrine >> isoproterenol.	Phentolamine slightly > yohimbine >> prazosin.	Decrease
Beta$_1$	Isoproterenol > epinephrine ≅ norepinephrine.	Metoprolol > butoxamine.	Increase
Beta$_2$	Isoproterenol > epinephrine >> norepinephrine.	Butoxamine > metoprolol.	Increase

*These potencies are defined by studies of binding competition and pharmacologic response.

vided into subtypes. The characteristic interactions of these receptors with various agonists and antagonists are shown in Table 11–3.

A. Types of Receptors: The physiologic effects mediated by the alpha-adrenergic receptor are summarized in Table 11–4. Two subtypes of this receptor have been identified and designated α_1 and α_2. It was initially thought that the α_2 receptor was limited to the presynaptic nerve ending and, when activated, served to inhibit the release of norepinephrine. However, these receptors have been found in platelets and postsynaptically in combination with α_1 receptors in adipose tissue and smooth muscle. The physiologic

Table 11–4. Adrenergic responses of selected tissues.

Organ or Tissue	Receptor	Effect
Heart (myocardium)	β_1	Increased force of contraction Increased rate of contraction
Blood vessels	α	Vasoconstriction
	β_2	Vasodilatation
Kidney	β	Increased renin release
Gut	α, β	Decreased motility and increased sphincter tone
Pancreas	α	Decreased insulin release Decreased glucagon release
	β	Increased insulin release Increased glucagon release
Liver	α, β	Increased glycogenolysis
Adipose tissue	β	Increased lipolysis
Most tissues	β	Increased calorigenesis
Skin (apocrine glands on hands, axillae, etc)	α	Increased sweating
Bronchioles	β_2	Dilatation
Uterus	α	Contraction
	β_2	Relaxation

processes mediated by alpha receptors are dependent on the increased availability of intracellular calcium ion. However, the events leading to this increase have not been established. There is evidence that the α_2 receptor decreases the activity of adenylate cyclase, resulting in a reduction of cAMP formation. The activation of α_1 receptors enhances the phosphorylation and breakdown of phosphotidylinositol and may act by altering the phospholipid structure of the cell membrane. Selective α_1 and α_2 antagonists are shown in Table 11–3.

Two subtypes of the beta receptor, β_1 and β_2, have been identified. Beta$_1$ receptors appear to mediate the inotropic and chronotropic effects on cardiac muscle, whereas β_2 receptors mediate smooth muscle relaxation in the bronchi and vascular smooth muscle as well as the uterus and adipose tissue. Norepinephrine is a powerful agonist at the β_1 receptor but comparatively weak at the β_2 receptor, compared to epinephrine or isoproterenol. Relatively selective beta agonists have also been developed, as shown in Table 11–3. The role of cAMP as a second messenger of the beta-adrenergic response is discussed in Chapter 1.

Dopaminergic receptors are found in the central nervous system, pituitary, heart, renal and mesenteric vascular beds, and other sites. Two subtypes of the dopaminergic receptor, D_1 and D_2, have been identified. The effects of the D_1 receptor are mediated by the adenylate cyclase system and are found postsynaptically in the brain. Those in the pituitary are D_2 receptors.

B. Receptor as Site of Regulation: The receptor also serves as a site of regulation of adrenergic activity. As noted above, presynaptically, norepinephrine released during nerve stimulation binds to alpha receptors and reduces the amount of norepinephrine released. Nerve endings have also been found to have receptors for many other agents presynaptically (Table 11–2).

The number of receptors on the effector cell surface can be reduced by binding of agonist to receptor (antagonists do not have the same effect). This reduction is called "down-regulation." Thyroid hormone, on the other hand, has been shown to increase the number of beta receptors in the myocardium. Estrogen, which increases the number of alpha receptors in the myometrium, increases the affinity of some vascular alpha receptors for norepinephrine.

Although the receptors and areas of postreceptor events serve as sites of fine regulation, the major physiologic control is exerted by alterations in activity of the nervous system. The discovery of cAMP and elucidation of its role in controlling physiologic processes—and the finding that most cells in the body have adrenergic receptors—have led to an appreciation of the important regulatory role of the peripheral sympathetic nervous system. In contrast, the effects of the adrenal medulla are mediated via the circulating amines and, therefore, are much more generalized in nature. Furthermore, adrenal medullary secretion increases significantly only in the presence of stress or marked deviation from homeostatic or resting conditions. For example, a minor reduction in the available glucose leads to sympathetic activation of fat mobilization from adipose tissue, whereas the adrenal medulla may not release large amounts of epinephrine until the blood sugar falls to 40 mg/dL in normal individuals. A summary of physiologic effects of the catecholamines in various tissues is presented in Table 11–4.

Physiologic Effects

A. Cardiovascular Effects: Catecholamines increase the rate and frequency of contraction and increase the irritability of the myocardium by activating myocardial β_1 receptors. The contractile effects of the catecholamines on vascular smooth muscle are mediated via alpha receptors. Although beta receptors are present and cause dilatation, other mechanisms of vascular dilatation are probably more important. The release or injection of catecholamines can therefore be expected to increase heart rate and cardiac output and cause peripheral vasoconstriction—all leading to an increase in blood pressure. These events are modulated by reflex mechanisms, so that, as the blood pressure increases, reflex stimulation may slow the heart rate and tend to reduce cardiac output. Although norepinephrine in the usual doses will have these effects, the effect of epinephrine may vary depending on the smooth muscle tone of the vascular system at the time. For example, in an individual with increased vascular tone, the net effect of small amounts of epinephrine may be to reduce the mean blood pressure while increasing the heart rate and cardiac output. In an individual with a reduction in vascular tone, the mean blood pressure would be expected to increase. In addition to the reflex mechanisms, vascular output is integrated by the central nervous system, so that, under appropriate circumstances, one vascular bed may be dilated while others remain unchanged. The central organization of the sympathetic nervous system is such that its ordinary regulatory effects are quite discrete—in contrast to periods of stress, when stimulation may be rather generalized and accompanied by release of catecholamines into the circulation. The infusion of catecholamines leads to a rapid reduction in plasma volume, presumably to accommodate to the reduced volume of the arterial and venous beds (Fig 11–7).

B. Effects on Extravascular Smooth Muscle: The catecholamines also regulate the activity of smooth muscle in tissues other than blood vessels. These effects include relaxation and contraction of uterine myometrium, relaxation of intestinal and bladder smooth muscle, contraction of the smooth muscle in the bladder and intestinal sphincters, and relaxation of tracheal smooth muscle and pupillary dilatation.

C. Metabolic Effects: The catecholamines increase oxygen consumption and heat production. Although the effects appear to be mediated by the beta receptor, the mechanism is unknown. The catechol-

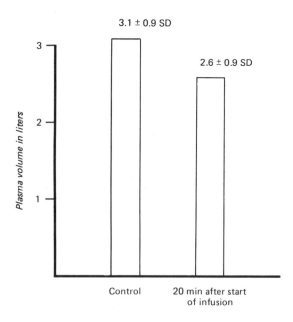

Figure 11–7. Changes in plasma volume produced by infusion of norepinephrine for 20 minutes in a dose sufficient to increase mean arterial pressure from 96 ± 10 mm Hg to 150 ± 16 mm Hg. (Data from Finnerty FA Jr, Buchholz JH, Guillaudeu RL: *J Clin Invest* 1958;**37**:425.)

amines also regulate glucose and fat mobilization from storage depots. Glycogenolysis in heart muscle and in liver leads to an increase in available carbohydrate for utilization. Stimulation of adipose tissue leads to lipolysis and the release of free fatty acids and glycerol into the circulation for utilization at other sites. In humans, these effects are mediated by the beta receptor.

The plasma levels of catecholamines required to produce some cardiovascular and metabolic effects in humans are shown in Table 11–5.

The catecholamines have effects on water, sodium, potassium, calcium, and phosphate excretion in the kidney. However, the mechanisms and the significance of these changes are not clear.

Table 11–5. Approximate circulating plasma levels of epinephrine and norepinephrine required to produce hemodynamic and metabolic changes during infusions of epinephrine and norepinephrine.* (Values are pg/mL.)

	Norepinephrine	Epinephrine
Systolic blood pressure	Increased at 2500	Increased at 500
Diastolic blood pressure	Increased at 2500	Decreased at 500
Pulse	Decreased at 2500	Increased at 250
Plasma glucose	Increased at 2500	Increased at 250–500

*Data from Silverberg AB et al: *Am J Physiol* 1978;**234**:E252; and from Clutter WE et al: *J Clin Invest* 1980;**66**:94.

The Role of Catecholamines in the Regulation of Hormone Secretion

The sympathetic nervous system plays an important role in the regulation and integration of hormone secretion at 2 levels. Centrally, norepinephrine and dopamine play important roles in the regulation of secretion of the anterior pituitary hormones. Dopamine, for example, has been identified as the prolactin-inhibiting hormone, and the hypothalamic releasing hormones appear to be under sympathetic nervous system control. Peripherally, the secretion of renin by the juxtaglomerular cells of the kidney is regulated by the sympathetic nervous system via the renal nerves and circulating catecholamines. The catecholamines release renin via a beta receptor mechanism. The B cell of the pancreatic islets is stimulated by activation of the beta receptors in the presence of alpha-adrenergic blockade. However, the dominant effect of norepinephrine or epinephrine is inhibition of insulin secretion, which is mediated by the alpha receptor. Similar effects have been observed in the secretion of glucagon by pancreatic A cells. The catecholamines have also been found to increase the release of thyroxine, calcitonin, parathyroid hormone, and gastrin by a beta receptor–mediated mechanism.

Plasma levels of catecholamines associated with various physiologic changes are shown in Table 11–5.

OTHER HORMONES

In addition to the catecholamines, the chromaffin cells of the adrenal medulla and peripheral sympathetic neurons synthesize and secrete opiatelike peptides, including met- and leu-enkephalin (see Chapter 4, Part I). They are stored in the large, dense-cored vesicles with the catecholamines in the adrenal medulla and at sympathetic nerve endings. These peptides are also found in the terminals of the splanchnic fibers that innervate the adrenal medulla. The observation that naloxone increases plasma catecholamine levels suggests that these peptides may inhibit sympathetic activity.

DISORDERS OF ADRENAL MEDULLARY FUNCTION

HYPOFUNCTION OF THE ADRENAL MEDULLA

Hypofunction of the adrenal medulla alone probably occurs only in individuals receiving adrenocor-

Figure 11–8. Plasma glucose, epinephrine, and norepinephrine levels after insulin administration in 14 normal subjects (●—●) and 7 patients with idiopathic orthostatic hypotension (○—○) with low or absent epinephrine responses. Results are expressed as mean ± SEM. (Reproduced, with permission, from Polonsky RJ et al: *J Clin Endocrinol Metab* 1980;**51**:1404.)

Table 11—6. Disorders associated with autonomic insufficiency.

Familial dysautonomia
Shy-Drager syndrome
Parkinson's disease
Tabes dorsalis
Syringomyelia
Cerebrovascular disease
Peripheral neuropathy due to diabetes
Idiopathic orthostatic hypotension
Sympathectomy
Drugs: antihypertensives, antidepressants

tical steroid replacement therapy following adrenalectomy. Such individuals with otherwise intact sympathetic nervous systems suffer no clinically significant disability. Patients with autonomic insufficiency, which includes deficiency of adrenal medullary epinephrine secretion, can be demonstrated to have minor defects in recovery from insulin-induced hypoglycemia (Fig 11–8). Patients with generalized autonomic insufficiency usually have orthostatic hypotension. The causes of disorders associated with autonomic insufficiency are listed in Table 11–6.

When a normal individual stands, a series of physiologic adjustments occur that maintain blood pressure and ensure adequate circulation to the brain. The initial lowering of the blood pressure stimulates the baroreceptors, which then activate central reflex mechanisms that cause arterial and venous constriction, increase cardiac output, and activate the release of renin and vasopressin. Interruption of afferent, central, or efferent components of this autonomic reflex results in autonomic insufficiency.

The treatment of symptomatic orthostatic hypotension is dependent upon maintenance of an adequate blood volume. If physical measures such as raising the head of the bed at night and using support garments do not alleviate the condition, pharmacologic measures may be used. Although agents producing constriction of the vascular bed, including ephedrine, phenylephrine, metaraminol, monoamine oxidase inhibitors, levodopa, propranolol, and indomethacin, have been used, volume expansion with fludrocortisone is the most effective treatment.

HYPERFUNCTION OF THE ADRENAL MEDULLA

The adrenal medulla is not known to play a significant role in essential hypertension. However, the role of the sympathetic nervous system in the regulation of blood flow and blood pressure has led to extensive investigations of its role in various types of hypertension. Some of the abnormalities observed, such as a resetting of baroreceptor activity, are thought to be secondary to the change in blood pressure. Others, such as the increased cardiac output found in early essential hypertension, have been thought by some investigators to play a primary role.

Catecholamines can increase blood pressure by increasing cardiac output, by increasing peripheral resistance through their vasoconstrictive action on the arteriole, and by increasing renin release from the kidney, leading to increased circulating levels of angiotensin II. Although many studies show an increase in circulating free catecholamine levels, evidence of increased sympathetic activity has not been a uniform finding in patients with essential hypertension.

PHEOCHROMOCYTOMA

Pheochromocytomas are tumors arising from chromaffin cells in the sympathetic nervous system. They release epinephrine or norepinephrine (or both)—and in some cases dopamine—into the circulation, causing hypertension and other signs and symptoms. It is estimated that 0.1% of patients with diastolic hypertension have pheochromocytomas. These tumors are found at all ages and in both sexes and are most commonly diagnosed in the fourth and fifth decades.

Although uncommon, this disorder is important to diagnose, because undiagnosed it may be fatal in pregnant women during delivery or in patients undergoing surgery for other disorders. However, with early diagnosis and proper management, almost all patients with benign tumors recover completely.

Clinical Manifestations

A. Symptoms and Signs: Although most patients with functioning tumors have symptoms most of the time, these vary in intensity and are perceived to be mainly episodic or paroxysmal by about half of the patients. Most patients with persistent hypertension also have superimposed paroxysms. A few patients are entirely free of symptoms and hypertension between attacks and give no evidence of excessive cate-

Table 11—7. Common symptoms in patients with hypertension due to pheochromocytoma.

Symptoms during or following paroxysms
Headache
Sweating
Forceful heartbeat with or without tachycardia
Anxiety or fear of impending death
Tremor
Fatigue or exhaustion
Nausea and vomiting
Abdominal or chest pain
Visual disturbances
Symptoms between paroxysms
Increased sweating
Cold hands and feet
Weight loss
Constipation

cholamine release during these intervals. In some instances, these tumors have been reported to occur with minimal clinical manifestations. Commonly reported symptoms and signs are listed in Table 11–7.

B. Description of an Attack: In patients with paroxysmal release of catecholamines, the symptoms resemble those produced by injections of epinephrine or norepinephrine, and the symptom complex is far more consistent than is suggested by the variability of patients' complaints. An episode usually begins with a sensation of something happening deep inside the chest, and a stimulus to deeper breathing is noted. The patient then becomes aware of a pounding or forceful heartbeat, caused by the β_1 receptor–mediated increase in cardiac output. This throbbing spreads to the rest of the trunk and head, causing headache or a pounding sensation in the head. The intense alpha receptor–mediated peripheral vasoconstriction causes cool, moist hands and feet and facial pallor. The combination of increased cardiac output and vasoconstriction causes marked elevation of the blood pressure when large amounts of catecholamines are released. The decreased heat loss and increased metabolism may cause a rise in temperature or flushing and lead to reflex sweating, which may be profuse and usually follows the cardiovascular effects that begin in the first few seconds after onset of an attack. The increased glycolysis and alpha receptor–mediated inhibition of insulin release cause an increase in blood sugar levels. Patients experience marked anxiety during all but the mildest attacks, and when episodes are prolonged or severe, there may be nausea, vomiting, visual disturbances, chest or abdominal pain, paresthesias, or seizures. A feeling of fatigue or exhaustion usually follows these episodes unless they are very mild or of short duration.

C. Frequency of Attacks: In patients with paroxysmal symptoms, attacks usually occur several times a week or oftener and last for 15 minutes or less though they may occur at intervals of months or as often as 25 times daily and may last from minutes to days. As time passes, the attacks usually increase in frequency but do not change much in character. They are frequently precipitated by activities that compress the tumor (eg, changes in position, exercise, lifting, defecation, or eating) and by emotional distress or anxiety.

D. Variability of Manifestations: Although the pattern of the manifestations described above can be elicited in almost all patients capable of clear communication, the variability of presenting complaints may be confusing and is sometimes misleading. Women whose episodes are first noted around the time of menopause may be thought to be experiencing "hot flushes." The diagnosis may only be made when hormonal therapy has failed to alleviate the "hot flush" or the episode is observed and the blood pressure taken during the attack. When a pheochromocytoma causes hypertension late in pregnancy, it may be confused with preeclampsia. Other causes of increased sympathetic activity must be distinguished from pheochromocytomas (see below) (Table 11–9).

E. Chronic Symptoms: Patients with persistently secreting tumors and chronic symptoms usually experience the symptom complex described above in response to transient increases in the release of catecholamines. In addition, in these patients the increased metabolic rate usually causes heat intolerance, increased sweating, and weight loss or (in children) lack of weight gain. The effects on glycogenolysis and insulin release can produce hyperglycemia and glucose intolerance, and patients may present with diabetes mellitus. Hypertension is usually present. Wide fluctuations of blood pressure are characteristic, and marked increases may be followed by hypotension and syncope. When pressure is elevated, postural hypotension is present. Typically, the hypertension does not respond to commonly used antihypertensive regimens, and such drugs as guanethidine and ganglionic blockers can induce paradoxic pressor responses. On examination, these patients, usually thin, have a forceful heartbeat that is often visible and easily palpable. They feel warm, may have pallor of the face and chest, perspire, have cool and moist hands and feet, and prefer a cool room. A mass may be palpable in the abdomen or neck, and deep palpation of the abdomen may produce a typical paroxysm. Chronic constriction of the arterial and venous beds leads to a reduction in plasma volume in most of these patients. The inability to further constrict this bed upon arising causes the postural hypotension that is characteristically observed.

Familial Syndromes & Other Tumors

Pheochromocytoma may also occur as a heritable disorder, either alone or more commonly in association with other endocrine tumors. In one syndrome, multiple endocrine neoplasia (MEN) type IIa (Sipple's syndrome), the patient may also have a calcitonin-producing adenoma of the thyroid, a parathyroid hormone–producing adenoma of the parathyroid, or a pituitary adenoma. In the other group (MEN type IIb), pheochromocytomas occur in association with mucosal neuromas, which are numerous and small and are found around the mouth. Transmission of these disorders follows the pattern of an autosomal dominant gene with incomplete penetrance.

Pheochromocytomas occurring as part of the familial syndromes appear to be the expression of an as yet unidentified stimulus to tumor formation. In MEN type IIa, bilateral adrenal tumors, frequently producing epinephrine, are common and may develop from hyperplasia of the adrenal medulla. Medullary carcinoma of the thyroid in these patients is commonly bilateral and associated with parafollicular or "C" cell hyperplasia. Multicentric tumors of the parathyroid gland are also quite typical and are found predominantly in patients with MEN type IIa and rarely in those with MEN type IIb. The thyroid tumors have been reported to secrete ACTH, serotonin, prostaglandins, and kallikreins, which may contribute to the clinical manifestations in these patients (see Chapter 1). Usually, the thyroid tumor (medullary carcinoma) is diagnosed by finding an elevated serum calcitonin level under basal conditions or after provocative testing with stimuli such as calcium or pentagastrin (see Chapters 7 and 8).

Pathology

A. Location of Tumor: Pheochromocytomas occur wherever chromaffin tissue is found (Fig 11–9). The adrenal medulla contains the largest collection of chromaffin cells. They are found in the organ of Zuckerkandl, which is very large in the fetus but is gradually replaced by fibrous tissue after delivery and is small in the adult. Chromaffin cells are also found in association with sympathetic ganglia, nerve plexuses, and nerves.

Over 95% of pheochromocytomas are found in the abdomen, and 85% of these are in the adrenal. Common extra-adrenal sites are near the kidney and in the organ of Zuckerkandl. Those found in the chest are in the posterior mediastinal area. The intracranial lesions reported are thought to be metastatic in origin. The tumors may be multicentric in origin, particularly when they are familial or part of the syndromes of multiple endocrine neoplasia and when they are seen in children. Although fewer than 10% of adults have multiple tumors, they are found in about one-third of affected children.

B. Size of Tumor: Pheochromocytomas vary in size from less than 1 g to several kilograms. However,

Figure 11–9. *Left:* Anatomic distribution of extra-adrenal chromaffin tissue in the newborn. *Right:* Locations of extra-adrenal pheochromocytomas reported before 1965. (Reproduced, with permission, from Coupland R: *The Natural History of the Chromaffin Cell.* Longmans, Green, 1965.)

Table 11–8. Causes of death in patients with unsuspected pheochromocytomas.

Myocardial infarction
Cerebrovascular accident
Arrhythmias
Irreversible shock
Renal failure
Dissecting aortic aneurysm

they are usually small, most weighing under 100 g. They are vascular tumors and commonly contain cystic or hemorrhagic areas. The cells tend to be large and contain typical catecholamine storage granules similar to those in the adrenal medulla. Multinucleated cells, pleomorphic nuclei, mitoses, and extension into the capsule and vessels are sometimes seen but do not indicate that the tumor is malignant. Fewer than 10% of pheochromocytomas are malignant, and these can be recognized either during surgery, by the finding of extensive local infiltration or metastases, or later, because of postsurgical local recurrence or metastases.

C. Adrenal Medullary Hyperplasia: This has also been described as the cause of an indistinguishable clinical picture and is found in the syndrome of multiple endocrine neoplasia (see above).

Complications

Patients with persistent symptoms and hypertension may develop hypertensive retinopathy or nephropathy. Postmortem studies indicate that there are a significant number of patients with pheochromocytomas who have myocarditis characterized by focal degeneration and necrosis of myocardial fibers with infiltration of histiocytes, plasma cells, and other signs of inflammation. Platelet aggregates and fibrin deposition are found in pulmonary arterioles. These changes may be associated with abnormal findings on the ECG but may not become apparent until the patient is exposed to marked cardiovascular stress and heart failure results. In patients harboring pheochromocytomas for long periods, the serious sequelae of hypertension are observed. Cerebrovascular accidents, congestive heart failure, and myocardial infarction have been observed. Some of the causes of death in unoperated patients are shown in Table 11–8.

Differential Diagnosis

The diagnosis of pheochromocytoma should be considered in all patients with paroxysmal symptoms; in children with hypertension; in adults with severe hypertension not responding to therapy; in hypertensive patients with diabetes or hypermetabolism; in patients with hypertension in whom symptoms resemble those described above or can be evoked by exercise, position change, emotional distress, or antihypertensive drugs such as guanethidine and ganglionic blockers; and in patients who become severely hypertensive or go into shock during anesthesia, surgery, or obstetric delivery. Patients who have disorders

Table 11–9. Disorders presenting with features of sympathetic discharge or hypermetabolism.

Angina due to coronary vasospasm
Severe anxiety states
Hypertension
Hypertensive crises associated with—
 Paraplegia
 Tabes dorsalis
 Lead poisoning
 Acute porphyria
Menopausal hot flushes
Autonomic epilepsy
Thyrotoxicosis
Hyperdynamic beta-adrenergic states

sometimes associated with pheochromocytomas (neurofibromatosis, mucosal adenomas, von Hippel's disease, medullary carcinoma of the thyroid) and those with first-degree relatives who have pheochromocytoma or other manifestations of MEN should be investigated. Other disorders associated with marked sympathetic stimulation are listed in Table 11–9. Plasma catecholamine levels at rest and with exercise and various disorders are shown in Table 11–10.

In these and other disorders in which elevated plasma catecholamine levels are under sympathetic nervous system control, it may be possible to reduce catecholamine release by autonomic blockade or sympathetic suppression. Pentolinium and clonidine have been used for this purpose. The reliability and safety of such procedures have not been established.

Ganglioneuromas (which are usually small, well-differentiated tumors arising from ganglion cells) and neuroblastomas (which are highly malignant tumors arising from more primitive sympathoblastic cells) can produce catecholamines and present a similar clinical picture. Dopamine is usually the major active catecholamine produced, and its production leads to elevated concentrations of homovanillic acid in urine.

Diagnostic Tests & Procedures

Assay of catecholamines and their metabolites has markedly simplified the diagnosis of this disorder. Operative exploration for pheochromocytoma should

Table 11–10. Range of plasma catecholamine levels observed in normal subjects and patients.

	Norepinephrine (pg/mL)	Epinephrine (pg/mL)
Normal subjects		
Basal	150–400	25–100
Ambulatory	200–800	30–150
Exercise	800–4000+	100–1000
Symptomatic hypoglycemia	200–1000	1000–5000
Patients		
Hypertension	200–500	20–100
Surgery	500–2000	100–500
Myocardial infarction	1000–2000	800–5000

Table 11–11. Maximal normal concentrations of the catecholamines and their metabolites in urine.* Substances interfering with their measurement are listed.

Compound	Excreted (mg/24 h)	Interfering Substances
Epinephrine	0.02	May be increased by highly fluorescent compounds such as tetracyclines and quinidine; by foods† and drugs containing catecholamines; and by levodopa, methyldopa, and ethanol.
Norepinephrine	0.08	
Dopamine	0.40	
Metanephrine	0.40	Increased by catecholamines, monoamine oxidase inhibitors, and others, depending on the method.
Normetanephrine	0.90	
Vanillylmandelic acid (VMA)	1.30	Increased by catecholamines, by foods containing vanillin, or by levodopa. Decreased by clofibrate, disulfiram, and monoamine oxidase inhibitors.
Homovanillic acid	7.00	

*Values may be higher under unusual stress, illness, or strenuous activity.
†For example, bananas contain significant amounts of norepinephrine.

not be done in the absence of chemical confirmation of the diagnosis. With currently available methods, it is possible to avoid unnecessary surgery and to successfully locate a tumor in almost all patients.

A. Hormone Assay: In patients with continuous hypertension or symptoms, levels of plasma or urine catecholamines and their metabolites are usually clearly increased. Therefore, in the selection of a particular assay, it is more important that the test be performed well by the laboratory than that a particular substance be measured. A reliable assay of the catecholamines, metanephrines, or vanillylmandelic acid (VMA) is usually sufficient to confirm the diagnosis. Patients with large tumors may excrete disproportionately greater amounts of catecholamine metabolites, because the amines can be metabolized by enzymes in the tumor cells prior to their release. Malignant tumors may release large amounts of dopamine, leading to the excretion of large amounts of homovanillic acid in the urine. It is important that the appropriate assay procedure be chosen to avoid misleading results and that drugs and foods that interfere with these assays be eliminated (Table 11–11).

In patients having brief and infrequent paroxysms with symptom-free intervals, confirmation of the diagnosis may be more difficult. Although large amounts of catecholamines are produced during the brief episode, the total amount excreted during the 24-hour urine collection period may not be clearly abnormal— in contrast to patients whose tumors secrete continuously. The latter group will accumulate larger amounts of catecholamines and metabolites in the urine even though secretion rates are lower and symptoms are less severe. Therefore, sampling of blood or timed urine collections during a carefully observed episode may be necessary to confirm the diagnosis.

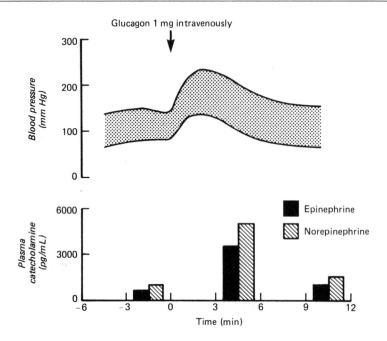

Figure 11–10. Blood pressure and plasma catecholamine levels following glucagon injection in a patient with a paroxysmally secreting pheochromocytoma. The blood sugar at 12 minutes was 180 mg/dL.

B. Glucagon Test: In patients with infrequent episodes, it may be useful to induce a paroxysm. This is not often necessary and should not be done in patients who have angina, visual changes, or other severe symptoms during spontaneous attacks, and phentolamine should be available to terminate the induced episode. Injection of 1 mg of glucagon intravenously will induce an attack in more than 90% of patients with pheochromocytoma. A typical response in such a patient is shown in Fig 11– 10. In those instances in which glucagon has failed to evoke a paroxysm and the clinical suspicion is very strong, histamine given intravenously in doses of 25– 50 μg may also be tried. However, histamine injection is associated with flushing and a brief but severe episode of headache. In general, the provoked episodes are no more severe than those occurring spontaneously. Provocative tests should be reserved for patients in whom it is necessary to rule out the presence of pheochromocytoma at the time they are seen (eg, prior to surgery or obstetric delivery).

C. Clonidine Suppression Test: In patients whose catecholamine levels are elevated because of neurogenic stimulation rather than release of catecholamine from a tumor, the administration of 0.3 mg of clonidine 2– 3 hours before sampling of blood may be useful in reducing plasma norepinephrine levels. This procedure can be used when it is not possible to obtain blood under resting conditions.

D. Trial of Phenoxybenzamine: In the occasional patient in whom the chemical tests are inconclusive, it may be useful or convenient to institute therapy with phenoxybenzamine over a period of 1– 2 months to observe effects both on the nature and frequency of attacks and on the blood pressure. A salutary effect will sometimes be observed for a few weeks but seldom longer than that in the absence of pheochromocytoma. A good response indicates the need for reappraisal of the patient.

Screening Patients for Pheochromocytoma

In addition to screening patients with typical clinical manifestations, assays for catecholamines and their metabolites can be used to screen other patients at

Table 11–12. Patients to be screened for pheochromocytoma.

Young hypertensives
Hypertensive patients with—
    Symptoms listed in Table 11—8
    Weight loss
    Seizures
    Orthostatic hypotension
    Unexplained shock
    Family history of pheochromocytoma or medullary carcinoma of thyroid
    Neurofibromatosis and other neurocutaneous syndromes
    Mucosal neuromas
    Hyperglycemia
Shock or severe pressor responses with—
    Induction of anesthesia
    Parturition
    Antihypertensive drugs

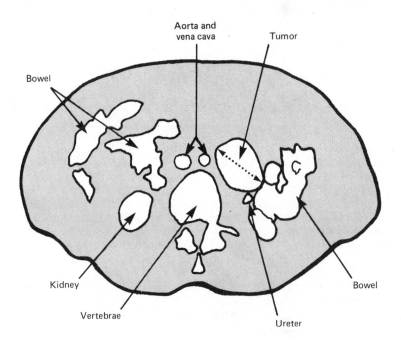

Figure 11–11. Left infrarenal pheochromocytoma shown by CT scanning. The lower diagram identifies many of the visible structures.

high risk. The indications for screening are listed in Table 11–12: When the presence of an undetected pheochromocytoma is particularly dangerous, as in pregnancy or prior to surgery, screening should be considered even when clinical manifestations are less typical.

Localization of Tumors

When the diagnosis has been established, the tumor must be located in order to facilitate its surgical removal. Although the larger tumors can usually be easily located by conventional radiographic proce-

dures (urography and arteriography) and sonography, the smallest tumors, particularly when located outside the adrenal, may require special techniques. CT scanning has given excellent results (Fig 11–11). Only the smallest tumors or those shielded by clips and other metal objects from previous surgery have been elusive.

Analysis of blood samples obtained via percutaneous venous catheterization can be of great value in locating small tumors in unusual locations. An example of the use of this technique is shown in Fig 11–12. Because of a small risk of complications and

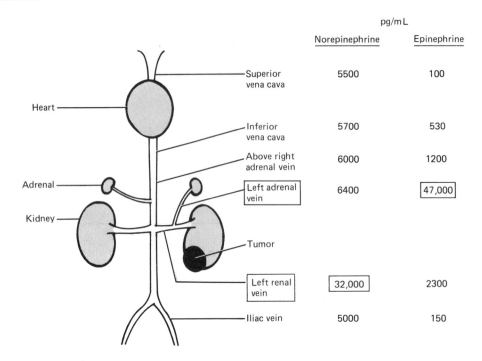

	Norepinephrine	Epinephrine
Superior vena cava	5500	100
Inferior vena cava	5700	530
Above right adrenal vein	6000	1200
Left adrenal vein	6400	47,000
Left renal vein	32,000	2300
Iliac vein	5000	150

pg/mL

Figure 11–12. Plasma norepinephrine and epinephrine levels in samples of blood obtained from the vena cava. Note that the level of epinephrine is very high in the left adrenal vein sample, distinguishing it from the drainage of the tumor, which secretes mainly norepinephrine. Note the relatively normal peripheral levels of epinephrine (as seen in the iliac vein or the superior vena cava).

the discomfort and cost of this procedure, it should be used only after simpler methods fail.

A scintigraphic procedure for the localization of pheochromocytomas has been described. [131I]Meta-iodobenzylguanidine (MIBG) is injected into the patient, resulting in detectable images 24–72 hours later. Very small tumors can be safely and conveniently located by this method. Although not all pheochromocytomas will produce detectable images, the specificity of the method seems high, and it has been possible to locate tumors not shown by CT scanning. MIBG is also taken up by some neuroblastomas.

Management

Optimal management of patients with pheochromocytomas requires an understanding of the pathophysiology produced by excessive catecholamines and an acquaintance with the action of adrenergic antagonists and other drugs used in the treatment of these patients.

A. Treatment With Adrenergic Antagonists: As soon as the diagnosis has been confirmed, therapy with adrenergic antagonists should be instituted. Treatment is directed toward reduction of symptoms, lowering of blood pressure, and amelioration of paroxysms occurring spontaneously or induced by studies undertaken to localize the tumors. Such treatment will allow expansion of the vascular bed and plasma volume and will reduce the amount of transfused blood required for maintenance of blood pressure during surgery.

Although only a few days of therapy are required for preoperative study and preparation of most patients for surgery, prolonged medical therapy is advantageous in patients who have had recent myocardial infarctions, those with electrocardiographic or clinical evidence of catecholamine cardiomyopathy, or those in the last trimester of pregnancy. They can be maintained on this regimen until the infant is delivered or the complication resolved, at which time the tumor can be removed.

Agents commonly used in therapy include phentolamine and phenoxybenzamine. Propranolol is occasionally helpful.

In patients with persistent hypertension or frequent paroxysms, **phenoxybenzamine** (Dibenzyline), a noncompetitive alpha-adrenergic antagonist with a prolonged effect, is indicated. Treatment is begun with doses of 20–40 mg/d orally and can be increased by 10–20 mg every 1–2 days until the desired effect is achieved. Postural hypotension may be marked at the beginning of therapy, and care should be taken to prevent syncope. Completely normal blood pressures (< 140/90 mm Hg) may not be achieved and are not required. A dose of 60–80 mg daily is usually adequate, but 2–3 times that amount may be necessary. When marked tachycardia or arrhythmias occur prior to or during surgery, small doses of **propranolol** may be required. Patients with infrequent paroxysms and an absence of interval manifestations can be treated in a similar manner.

Rapid titration of the dose may be difficult using phenoxybenzamine, because of its long half-life (36 hours). However, **prazosin** (Minipress), a recently introduced alpha antagonist with a shorter duration of activity, could prove to be useful in some patients. Prazosin is predominantly an α_1 antagonist and has not been found to be effective in all patients.

B. Preparation for Surgery: Preparation of the patient as described above minimizes the hazards of anesthesia and surgery. The patient's blood pressure and electrocardiographic patterns should be continuously monitored, and phentolamine, propranolol, and sodium nitroprusside can be used to reduce blood pressure if necessary. Suspected intra-abdominal tumors are usually approached through a transabdominal incision, since this allows exploration of the adrenals, sympathetic ganglia, bladder, and other pelvic structures. When bilateral adrenal tumors are found and the adrenals removed, adrenocortical steroid replacement is required (see Chapter 9).

C. Postoperative Care: When the tumor is removed, the blood pressure usually falls to about 90/60 mm Hg. Persistence of low blood pressures or poor peripheral perfusion may require blood volume expansion with whole blood, plasma, or other fluids as indicated. Pressor therapy is not usually required and should not be substituted for volume expansion.

Lack of a fall in pressure at the time of tumor removal (even in the presence of adrenergic blockade) indicates the presence of additional tumor tissue.

In patients with tumors producing persistent hypertension, the initial fall in blood pressure may be followed by an elevation of blood pressure in the postoperative period. However, the accompanying symptoms of sympathetic stimulation are gone, and the pressure returns to normal over the next few weeks. If the blood pressure remains elevated but the patient is otherwise asymptomatic, another cause for the el-

Table 11–13. Distribution of metastases in 41 cases of malignant pheochromocytoma.[*]

	Autopsy Cases (n = 26)	Nonautopsy Cases (n = 15)	Percentage
Skeleton	12	6	44
Liver	12	3	37
Lymph node	11	4	37
Lungs	9	2	27
Central nervous system	4	0	10
Pleura	4	0	10
Kidneys	2	0	5
Pancreas	1	0	2
Omentum	1	0	2

[*]Reproduced, with permission, from Schönebeck J: *Scand J Urol Nephrol* 1969;3:66.

evated blood pressure should be considered. Essential hypertension and renal vascular hypertension have been reported in several patients harboring pheochromocytomas.

D. Treatment of Malignant Tumors: Patients with nonresectable malignant tumors or metastases or those who for other reasons are not amenable to successful surgical treatment can be managed medically for prolonged periods. Phenoxybenzamine and perhaps prazosin can be used chronically as described above. Patients with malignant tumors have also benefited symptomatically from treatment with α-methylmetatyrosine, an inhibitor of tyrosine hydroxylase, the rate-limiting enzyme in the biosynthetic process. Although some patients with malignant pheochromocytomas die early because of disseminated disease, there are long-term survivors. Sites of metastases are shown in Table 11–13. The most common site of metastases is the skeleton, and bone lesions tend to respond well to radiation therapy. The use of combinations of chemotherapeutic agents such as cyclophosphamide, vincristine, and dacarbazine is effective in controlling soft tissue lesions in some patients.

REFERENCES

General

Blaschko H, Muscholl E (editors): *Catecholamines, Handbuch der Experimentellen Pharmakologie.* Vol 33. Springer, 1972.

Coupland RE: *The Natural History of the Chromaffin Cell.* Longmans, Green, 1965.

Cryer PE: Physiology and pathophysiology of the human sympathoadrenal neuroendocrine system. *N Engl J Med* 1980;**303**:436.

Iversen LL (editor): Catecholamines. *Br Med Bull* 1973;**29**:91.

Malmejhac J: Activity of the adrenal medulla and its regulation. *Phys Rev* 1964;**44**:186.

Hormones of the Adrenal Medulla

Ahlquist RP: A study of the adrenotropic receptors. *Am J Physiol* 1948;**153**:586.

Axelrod J: The metabolism, storage and release of catecholamines. *Recent Progr Horm Res* 1965;**21**:597.

Axelrod J: Relationship between catecholamines and other hormones. *Recent Progr Horm Res* 1975;**31**:1.

Baxter JD, Funder JW: Hormone receptors. *N Engl J Med* 1979;**301**:1149.

Bleasdale J, Eichberg J, Havser G (editors): *Inositol and Phosphoinositides.* Humana Press, 1985.

Clutter WE et al: Epinephrine plasma metabolic clearance rates and physiologic thresholds for metabolic and hemodynamic actions in man. *J Clin Invest* 1980;**66**:94.

Ganong WF, Reid IA: Role of the sympathetic nervous system and central alpha- and beta-adrenergic receptors in regulation of renin activity. *Am J Physiol* 1976;**230**:1733.

Goldfien A: Effects of glucose deprivation on the sympathetic outflow to the adrenal medulla and adipose tissue. *Pharmacol Rev* 1966;**18**:303.

Iversen LL: Uptake processes for biogenic amines. Pages 381–442 in: *Handbook of Psychopharmacology.* Section 1, Vol 3. Plenum Press, 1975.

Landsberg L, Young JB: Fasting, feeding and the regulation of the sympathetic nervous system. *N Engl J Med* 1978;**298**:1295.

Lefkowitz RJ: Direct binding studies of adrenergic receptors: Biochemical, physiologic, and clinical implications. *Ann Intern Med* 1979;**91**:450.

Murray E et al: Determination of norepinephrine apparent release rate and clearance in humans. *Life Sci* 1979;**25**:1461.

Silverberg AB et al: Norepinephrine: Hormone and neurotransmitter in man. *Am J Physiol* 1978;**234**:252.

Weiner N: Regulation of norepinephrine biosynthesis. *Annu Rev Pharmacol* 1970;**10**:273.

Woods SC, Porte D Jr: Neural control of the endocrine pancreas. *Physiol Rev* 1974;**54**:596.

Disorders of Adrenal Medullary Function; Pheochromocytoma

Bravo E, Gifford RW Jr: Pheochromocytoma: Diagnosis, localization and management. *N Engl J Med* 1984;**311**:1298.

Engelman K, Sjoerdsma A: Chronic medical therapy for pheochromocytoma. *Ann Intern Med* 1964;**61**:229.

Frohlich ED: The adrenergic nervous system and hypertension: State of the art. Second Pan American Symposium on Hypertension, Part 2. *Mayo Clin Proc* 1977;**52**:361.

Gagle RF et al: Natural history of the familial medullary thyroid carcinoma–pheochromocytoma syndrome and the identification of pre-neoplastic states by screening studies: A five-year report. *Trans Assoc Am Physicians* 1975; **88**:177.

Goldfien A: Pheochromocytoma: Diagnosis and anesthetic and surgical management. *Anesthesiology* 1963;**24**:462.

Goldstein DS: Plasma norepinephrine in essential hypertension. *Hypertension* 1981;**3**:48.

Hume DM: Pheochromocytoma in the adult and in the child. *Am J Surg* 1960;**99**:458.

Keiser HR et al: Treatment of malignant pheochromocytoma with combination chemotherapy. *Hypertension* 1985; **7(No. 3–Part 2)**:I18.

Kuchel O: Pseudopheochromocytoma. (Clinical Conference.) *Hypertension* 1985;**7**:151.

Landsberg L: Catecholamines and hyperthyroidism. *Clin Endocrinol Metab* 1977;**6**:697.

Manger WM, Gifford RW: *Pheochromocytoma.* Springer, 1977.

Modlin IM et al: Pheochromocytomas in 72 patients: Clinical and diagnostic features, treatment and long term results. *Br J Surg* 1979;**66**:456.

Moskowitz MA, Wurtman RJ: Catecholamines and neurologic diseases. *N Engl J Med* 1975;**293**:274.

Schenker JG, Chowers U: Pheochromocytoma and pregnancy: Review of 89 cases. *Obstet Gynecol Surv* 1971; **26**:739.

Schimke NR et al: Syndrome of bilateral pheochromocytoma, medullary thyroid carcinoma and multiple neuromas: A possible regulatory defect in the differentiation of chromaffin tissue. *N Engl J Med* 1968;**279**:1.

Sizemore GW, Heath H, Carney JA: Multiple endocrine neoplasia type 2. *Clin Endocrinol Metab* 1980;**9**:299.

Sjoerdsma A: Chronic medical therapy for pheochromocytoma. *Ann Intern Med* 1964;**61**:229.

Visser J, Axt R: Bilateral adrenal medullary hyperplasia: A clinicopathological entity. *J Clin Pathol* 1975;**28**:298.

Autonomic Insufficiency

Schatz IJ: Current management concepts in orthostatic hypotension. *Arch Intern Med* 1980;**140**:1152.

Schatz IJ: Orthostatic hypotension. *Arch Intern Med* 1984; **144**:733.

Renal Hormones

12

David J. Ramsay, DM, DPhil

The kidney is involved in 3 major hormonal systems in the body. First, it secretes **renin,** a proteolytic enzyme that initiates a chain of events leading to the production of the circulating peptide **angiotensin II,** which plays an important role in the regulation of salt and water metabolism and of blood pressure. Second, the kidney secretes **erythropoietin,** a glycoprotein that helps to control red cell production. Third, the final step in **activation of vitamin D** occurs in the kidney. The kidney takes up 25-hydroxychole-calciferol from the bloodstream and hydroxylates it to **1,25-dihydroxycholecalciferol.** This agent increases plasma calcium concentration by increasing its intestinal absorption and renal tubular reabsorption and by stimulating bone resorption. Metabolism of vitamin D and calcium is discussed in Chapter 8.

RENIN

In 1947, Goldblatt noted that reducing the flow of blood to the kidney in experimental animals was followed by an increase in blood pressure. This simple experiment, which implicated the kidney in the pathogenesis of hypertension, stimulated much of the research that led to elucidation of the **renin-angiotensin system** as we know it today.

As the afferent arteriole enters the glomerulus (Fig 12–1), the smooth muscle cells become modified to perform a secretory function. These cells, the **juxtaglomerular cells,** produce and secrete renin. Renin is a proteolytic enzyme with a molecular weight of approximately 40,000. There is evidence that the human kidney secretes both prorenin and renin into the bloodstream. **Prorenin,** which has a slightly higher molecular weight than renin, appears to be identical to the molecule previously termed inactive renin and can account for over 50% of total circulating renin. Prorenin can be converted into renin in vitro by a number of methods, but it is not clear if it is converted into renin in circulating plasma under physiologic conditions. Renin reaches the bloodstream, where it acts upon a circulating renin substrate, **angiotensinogen,** to form a decapeptide, **angiotensin I** (Fig 12–2). Angiotensin I, which is physiologically inert, is converted to **angiotensin II,** an octapeptide, by the action of **converting enzyme.** Angiotensin II accounts for the biologic activity. The half-life of angiotensin II in plasma is less than 1 minute as a result of the action of multiple angiotensinases located in most tissues of the body.

Angiotensinogen

Angiotensinogen (renin substrate) is an α_2-globulin secreted by the liver. It has a molecular weight of approximately 60,000 and is usually present in human plasma at a constant concentration of 1 μmol/L. Although the rate of production of angiotensin II is normally determined by changes in plasma renin concentration, the concentration of angiotensinogen is below the V_{max} for the reaction. Thus, if angiotensinogen concentration increases, the amount of angiotensin produced at the same plasma renin concentration will increase. Hepatic production of angiotensinogen is increased by glucocorticoids and by estrogens. Stimulation of angiotensinogen production by estrogen-containing contraceptive pills accounts

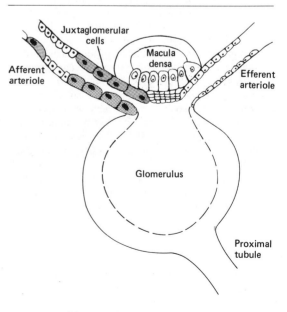

Figure 12–1. Diagram of glomerulus, showing juxtaglomerular apparatus and macula densa.

Figure 12–2. Sequence of formation of angiotensin II. Drugs that can be used to block various steps are shown in italics.

for some cases of hypertension encountered as a side effect of this treatment.

In situations such as sodium depletion, where there is a sustained high level of circulating angiotensin II, the rate of breakdown of substrate by renin in the plasma is greatly increased. Because the plasma concentration of angiotensinogen remains constant in these situations, hepatic production must increase to match the increased rate of breakdown. The mechanism of this increase is not clear, but it is of interest that angiotensin II itself is a stimulus to substrate production.

Converting Enzyme

Converting enzyme is found in most tissues in the body and circulates in plasma. Thus, theoretically, the conversion of angiotensin I to angiotensin II could take place anywhere in the circulatory system. However, there are particularly high activities of the enzyme in the lung such that on a single passage, 70–80% of angiotensin I is converted to angiotensin II. In the whole body, therefore, the lung is quantitatively the most important site of formation of angiotensin II.

Converting enzyme is a dipeptidyl carboxypeptidase, a glycoprotein of MW 130,000–160,000 that cleaves dipeptides from a number of substrates. In addition to angiotensin I, these include bradykinin, enkephalins, and substance P. Potent inhibitors of converting enzyme are available that prevent the formation of angiotensin II in the circulation and thus block its biologic effects (Fig 12–2). Captopril and enalapril (MK-421) are of particular importance because they are active when taken by mouth (see below). Because of the participation of converting enzyme in a number of peptide systems, blockade of the enzyme may not always exert its effects solely via the renin-angiotensin system.

Actions of Angiotensin II in the Periphery

Angiotensin II is a very potent pressor agent. It exerts its effects on peripheral arterioles to cause vasoconstriction and thus increases total peripheral resistance. Vasoconstriction occurs in all tissue beds, in-

cluding the kidney, and has been implicated in the phenomenon of renal autoregulation. There may also be an effect of angiotensin on the heart, causing increases in rate and strength of contraction, although this is less clear. The possible role of increased circulating levels of angiotensin II in the pathogenesis of hypertension is discussed below.

Angiotensin II acts directly on the adrenal cortex to stimulate aldosterone secretion. In fact, in many situations, angiotensin is the most important regulator of aldosterone secretion and thus plays a central role in the regulation of sodium balance. For example, during dietary sodium depletion, there is a contraction of extracellular fluid volume resulting from osmotic transfer of water to the intracellular fluid compartment. Subsequent stimulation of the renin-angiotensin system is important in 2 ways. The vasoconstrictor action of angiotensin helps to maintain blood pressure in the face of reduced extracellular fluid volume, whereas the action of angiotensin to stimulate aldosterone secretion and thus sodium retention allows volume to be conserved.

Angiotensin II modulates activity at sympathetic nerve endings in peripheral blood vessels and in the heart. It increases sympathetic activity partly by facilitating adrenergic transmitter release and partly by increasing the responsiveness of smooth muscle to norepinephrine. Angiotensin II also stimulates the release of catecholamines from the adrenal medulla.

Blockade of the peripheral effects of angiotensin II may be useful therapeutically. In low-output congestive cardiac failure, plasma levels of angiotensin II are high. These high circulating levels promote salt and water retention and—by constricting arterioles—raise peripheral vascular resistance, thus increasing cardiac afterload. Treatment with converting enzyme inhibitors such as captopril may result in peripheral vasodilatation, thereby improving tissue perfusion and cardiac performance as well as aiding renal elimination of salt and water.

Actions of Angiotensin on the Brain

In recent years, many actions of angiotensin on

Table 12–1. Actions of angiotensin on the brain.

Stimulates drinking.
Increases vasopressin secretion.
Stimulates ACTH secretion.
Raises blood pressure.
Increases salt appetite.

the central nervous system have been described. Angiotensin II is a polar peptide that does not cross the blood-brain barrier. Circulating angiotensin II, however, may affect the brain by acting through one or more of the circumventricular organs (see Chapter 3). These specialized regions within the brain lack a blood-brain barrier, so that receptive cells in these areas are sensitive to plasma composition. Of particular significance to the actions of angiotensin are the subfornical organ, the organum vasculosum of the lamina terminalis, and the area postrema.

It has been shown that tissues in the body other than the kidney may contain renin. Small amounts of renin have been identified in the brain. However, whether sufficient quantities of angiotensin can be generated within the central nervous system to bring about physiologic actions remains to be determined.

The major actions of angiotensin II on the brain are listed in Table 12–1. Angiotensin II is a potent dipsogen when injected directly into the brain or administered systemically. The major receptors for the dipsogenic action of circulating angiotensin II are located in the subfornical organ. Angiotensin II also stimulates vasopressin secretion, particularly in association with raised plasma osmolality. As such, the renin-angiotensin system may have an important part to play in the control of water balance, particularly during hypovolemia.

Angiotensin also acts on the brain to increase blood pressure, although its effects at this site seem to be less potent than those exerted directly in the systemic circulation. In most animals, the receptors are located in the area postrema.

Other central actions of angiotensin II include stimulation of adrenocorticotropic hormone (ACTH) secretion, suppression of plasma renin activity, and stimulation of sodium appetite, particularly in association with raised mineralocorticoid levels. The full implications of these (and other) central actions of angiotensin remain to be elucidated.

CONTROL OF RENIN SECRETION

The original experimental work that heralded the discovery of renin showed that a reduction of blood pressure to the kidney increases renin secretion. This led to the view that blood pressure is the major renin secretion control mechanism. However, the mechanism of the inverse relationship between blood pressure and renin secretion is not clear. There are 2 main theories. The **baroreceptor theory** argues that the

juxtaglomerular cells act as their own baroreceptors. Thus, if blood pressure increases, baroreceptors in the juxtaglomerular cells will be stretched, leading to a decrease in renin output. The second theory is that the **macula densa cells** contain different receptors sensitive to the sodium chloride load of the distal tubular fluid. The macula densa cells are in close contact with juxtaglomerular cells, so that a fall in sodium chloride load passing these cells in the distal tubule will be perceived by the macula densa cells and result in increased renin secretion. A third important stimulus to renin secretion is increased activity in renal sympathetic nerves.

In general, the important whole body stimulus that leads to renin secretion is **hypovolemia.** Hypovolemia causes a fall in blood pressure and thus, according to the baroreceptor theory, an increase in renin output. A fall in blood pressure will also reduce glomerular filtration rate and distal sodium and chloride load and thus, by the macula densa theory, stimulate renin secretion. Hypovolemic stimulation of renin secretion is enhanced by renal sympathetic nerves. Decreased discharge in atrial and pulmonary stretch receptors, as well as reduced arterial baroreceptor discharge, if present, leads to reflex augmentation of renin release via the renal nerves. The sympathetic nerves act directly on the juxtaglomerular cells as well as indirectly, by reducing blood flow through the kidney.

The significance of other effects on renin secretion is less well understood. Both vasopressin and angiotensin II decrease renin secretion, probably acting at the juxtaglomerular cells. These peptides have actions on renin secretion that can occur with variations of their plasma concentrations over the physiologic range, but the importance of their roles remains to be elucidated.

RENIN & HYPERTENSION

Since the original observation that impaired renal perfusion leads to secretion of renin and an increase in blood pressure, renin has been implicated in the etiology of hypertension. For many years, the evidence linking renin to hypertension was inconclusive, and many investigators discounted the participation of the renin-angiotensin system in all but a few forms of hypertension. For example, renal artery stenosis and coarctation of the aorta above the origin of the renal arteries are associated with hypertension and elevated plasma renin levels. Surgical correction of impaired renal perfusion leads to amelioration of hypertension. Similarly, malignant hypertension in end-stage renal disease is associated with increased plasma renin levels.

Recently, the connection between renin and hypertension has been rationalized largely by taking into account the fact that hypertension represents a mixture of clinical entities (Table 12–2). At one end of the spectrum lie various causes of hypertension that have in common intense peripheral vasoconstriction. Thus,

Table 12–2. Contribution of excessive arterial vasoconstriction and excessive blood volume in different types of hypertension. The diseases at the top show the greatest degree of vasoconstriction compared with volume excess; those at the bottom show the greatest degree of volume excess compared with arterial vasoconstriction.

Malignant hypertension.
Pheochromocytoma.
Unilateral renovascular hypertension.
High-renin essential hypertension.
Low-renin essential hypertension unresponsive to diuretics.
Normal-renin essential hypertension.
Bilateral renovascular hypertension.
Low-renin essential hypertension responsive to diuretics.
Primary aldosteronism.

increased activity of any **vasoconstrictor agent**—eg, angiotensin in renal vascular hypertension or catecholamines in pheochromocytomas—will cause arteriolar vasoconstriction and increase in total peripheral resistance and thus an increase in blood pressure. At the other end of the spectrum are increases in blood pressure due to expansion of **extracellular fluid volume.** Thus, any situation that leads to sodium or water retention can lead to an increase in blood pressure.

Most patients with hypertension are classified as having **essential hypertension.** A recent survey shows that 15% of such patients show high plasma renin levels, 55% normal levels, and 30% low levels. Patients with hypertension due to expansion of extracellular fluid volume would tend to have low plasma renin levels, because volume expansion exerts an inhibitory influence on renin secretion.

Much effort has been expended in defining a normal range for plasma renin activity. It is not easy to assess the state of the renin-angiotensin system from a single blood sample drawn for analysis of plasma renin activity, since the secretion rate may be affected by so many factors. Furthermore, assay methodology varies between laboratories in such important aspects as the pH of the incubation step. Of particular importance is the sodium content of the diet. One approach to this problem has been to correlate plasma renin activity with the sodium content of the diet as judged by 24-hour urine collection (Fig 12–3). Investigation of normal subjects has shown that in general, the higher the sodium content of the diet, the lower the plasma renin activity will be. However, widespread use of this renin ''profiling'' technique has not turned out to be practical. Also, the proof that low-renin hypertension is associated with expanded extracellular fluid and plasma volumes awaits confirmation. There is little doubt that changes in activity of the renin-angiotensin system are associated with most types of hypertension, although many of the causal relationships remain to be clarified.

From these statements, one might predict that patients with essential hypertension having high plasma renin activities should show a reduction in blood pressure if angiotensin levels in the plasma can be reduced or their effects blocked. Intravenous infusion of the angiotensin II receptor-blocking agent **saralasin** reduces blood pressure in patients with high-renin hypertension. More recently, the orally acting converting enzyme inhibitor **captopril** has been used. This drug decreases blood pressure in patients with high-renin or normal-renin hypertension; it has little or no effect in patients with essential hypertension who have low plasma renin levels. This correlates positively with experience with the beta-adrenergic blocking agent **propranolol,** which reduces blood pressure in 70% of patients with essential hypertension and especially those with high renin levels and most patients with normal renin levels. Propranolol markedly reduces plasma renin levels in these patients. However, the situation is complicated, since the ability of propranolol to reduce blood pressure does not always depend on a reduction in plasma renin levels.

Patients with essential hypertension caused by expansion of extracellular fluid volume in whom plasma renin levels are low would not be expected to respond to propranolol or captopril. On the other hand, it might be predicted that giving **diuretics** to cause excretion of the expanded volume would be more effective and that agents designed to cause peripheral **vasodilatation** would be less effective. This has generally turned out to be true.

Thus, in the treatment of hypertension, it is of first importance to investigate known causes of hypertension. If the ultimate diagnosis is essential hypertension, knowledge of plasma renin activity is

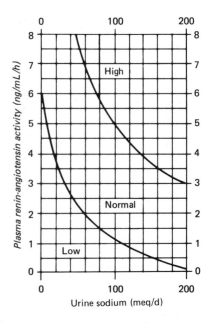

Figure 12–3. Correlation of plasma renin activity with 24-hour sodium excretion in human subjects. (Reproduced, with permission, from Laragh JH, Sealey JE: *Cardiovasc Med* 1977;2:1053.)

helpful in deciding whether the hypertension is of the high-volume or the vasoconstrictor type. This will allow rational decisions to be made about whether the major treatment strategy should be to use vasodilators, agents that block angiotensin formation, beta blockers, or diuretics. Identification of the type of hypertension will also affect prognosis, since it is patients with the vasoconstrictor type who are most liable to suffer serious sequelae of hypertension such as heart attacks and strokes.

Measurement of plasma renin activity is useful in helping to diagnose renin-secreting tumors. Although these are rare, it is important to spot them, since early detection is likely to improve the chances of surgical cure (see Chapter 10).

ERYTHROPOIETIN

It has long been realized that hypoxia is a potent stimulus to red cell production. Within a few hours after exposure of human subjects to hypoxia, there is an increase in reticulocyte count—denoting the presence of new red blood cells in the circulation—followed by an increase in circulating red cell mass. This is due to the increased production of a glycoprotein, erythropoietin. The kidney is the major source of this hormone, but it is also produced in the liver, particularly in fetuses. Day-to-day production of erythropoietin depends on the PO_2 of blood perfusing the kidneys.

The target cells for erythropoietin are the colony forming units–erythroid (CFU-E) cells in the bone marrow. Erythropoietin reacts with receptors on CFU-E cells, which leads to increased production of proerythroblasts and release of more erythrocytes into the circulation. Human erythropoietin cDNA has been cloned.

There is continuous secretion of erythropoietin even in the adult. Anephric patients generally have very low hematocrits, largely as a result of the absence of circulating erythropoietin in the plasma. The suppressed rate of formation of red blood cells due to lack of renal production of erythropoietin is a major problem in the treatment of patients with severe renal failure. Renal transplantation not only restores renal function to the anephric patient but also restores normal erythropoiesis.

Hypoxia is the most important stimulus to erythropoietin production. A number of pathologic conditions affecting the kidney, particularly those that reduce renal blood flow, may increase the rate of release of erythropoietin and inevitably increase red blood cell production. A few cases of erythropoietin-releasing tumors have been described in patients with very high hematocrits and hypertension resulting from the increased peripheral vascular resistance caused by high blood viscosity.

ATRIAL NATRIURETIC PEPTIDE

Extracts of atrial—but not ventricular—tissue cause marked natriuresis when injected into rats. The material is contained in densely staining granules in the atria of most mammalian species. A number of laboratories have sequenced and synthesized several natriuretic peptides containing between 22 and 28 amino acids, and rat and human atrial cDNA clones that encode atrial natriuretic peptides have been isolated and characterized. At present, it is not clear which of the peptides is normally secreted into the bloodstream, and a number of terms are in use, including atriopeptin, auriculin, cardionatrin, and atrial natriuretic factor. The major effects of administration of atrial natriuretic peptide are natriuresis and a fall in blood pressure. Although the peptide can cause relaxation of smooth muscle, the fall in blood pressure is due to depression of cardiac output in intact animals. The natriuresis is associated with a marked increase in filtration fraction without a sustained increase in renal blood flow, which suggests that the peptide may cause efferent arteriolar constriction. There is some evidence that glomerular membrane permeability may be increased. Thus, the natriuresis is due to glomerular rather than tubular factors. Atrial natriuretic peptide also inhibits secretion of renin, aldosterone, and vasopressin.

Recently, a number of radioimmunoassays for atrial natriuretic peptide have been developed. Although there are still questions concerning the specificity of these assays, it is clear that there are measurable levels of the material in normal plasma. Maneuvers that expand plasma volume and experiments that increase atrial pressure are associated with increased levels of radioimmunoassayable peptide in plasma. Thus, atrial natriuretic peptide may be involved in the control of sodium balance. When blood volume increases, the associated increase in atrial pressure and atrial stretch may trigger secretion of the peptide and lead to natriuresis and blood pressure reduction. However, the precise role (if any) that atrial natriuretic peptide plays in the control of sodium balance and blood volume under physiologic conditions is not clear.

REFERENCES

Currie MG et al: Purification and sequence analysis of bioactive atrial peptides (atriopeptins). *Science* 1984;**223**:67.

Davis JO, Freeman RH: Mechanisms regulating renin release. *Physiol Rev* 1976;**56**:1.

Fried W, Morley C: Update on erythropoietin. *Int J Artif Organs* 1985;**8**:79.

Hardman JA et al: Primary structure of the human renin gene. *DNA* 1984;**6**:457.

Huang CL et al: Renal mechanism of action of rat atrial natriuretic factor. *J Clin Invest* 1985;**75**:769.

Huang SL: Cloning and expression of human erythropoietic DNA in *Escherichia coli. Proc Natl Acad Sci USA* 1984;**81**:2708.

Laragh JH: Atrial natriuretic hormone, the renin-aldosterone axis, and blood pressure: Electrolyte homeostasis. *N Engl J Med* 1985;**313**:1330.

Laragh JH, Bühler FR, Seldin DW (editors): *Frontiers in Hypertension Research.* Springer-Verlag, 1981.

Laragh JH, Letcher RL, Pickering TG: Renin profiling for diagnosis and treatment of hypertension. *JAMA* 1979;**241**:151.

Maack T et al: Atrial natriuretic factor: Structure and functional properties. *Kidney Int* 1985;**27**:607.

Oikawa S et al: Cloning and sequence analysis of cDNA encoding a precursor for human atrial polypeptide. *Nature* 1984;**309**:724.

Ramsay DJ: The effects of circulating angiotensin II on the brain. Page 263 in: *Frontiers in Neuroendocrinology.* Vol 7. Ganong WF, Martini L (editors). Raven Press, 1982.

Reid IA, Morris BJ, Ganong WF: The renin-angiotensin system. *Annu Rev Physiol* 1978;**40**:377.

Seidah NG et al: Amino-acid sequence of homologous rat atrial peptides: Natriuretic activity of native and synthetic forms. *Proc Natl Acad Sci USA* 1984;**81**:2640.

Symposium: Biochemistry of the renin-angiotensin system. *Fed Proc* 1983;**42**:2272.

Yamanaka M et al: Clonic and sequence analysis of the cDNA for the rat atrial natriuretic factor precursor. *Nature* 1984;**309**:719.

The Testes

13

Glenn D. Braunstein, MD

The testes contain 2 major components, which are structurally separate and serve different functions. The **Leydig cells,** or **interstitial cells,** comprise the major endocrine component. The primary secretory product of these cells, testosterone, is responsible either directly or indirectly for embryonic differentiation along male lines of the external and internal genitalia, male secondary sexual development at puberty, and maintenance of libido and potency in the adult male. The **seminiferous tubules** comprise the bulk of the testes and are responsible for the production of approximately 30 million spermatozoa per day during male reproductive life (puberty to death).

Both of these testicular components are interrelated, and both require an intact hypothalamic-pituitary axis for initiation and maintenance of their function. In addition, several accessory genital structures are required for the functional maturation and transport of spermatozoa. Thus, disorders of the testes, hypothalamus, pituitary, or accessory structures may result in abnormalities of androgen or gamete production, infertility, or a combination of these problems.

ANATOMY & STRUCTURE-FUNCTION RELATIONSHIPS OF THE TESTES (Fig 13–1)

TESTES

The adult testis is a spheroid with a mean volume of 18.6 ± 4.8 mL (SD). The average length is 4.6 cm (range, 3.6–5.5 cm), and the average width is 2.6 cm (range, 2.1–3.2 cm). The testes are located within the scrotum, which not only serves as a protective envelope but also helps to maintain the testicular temperature approximately 2 °C below abdominal temperature. Three layers of membranes—visceral tunica vaginalis, tunica albuginea, and tunica vasculosa—comprise the testicular capsule. Extensions of the tunica albuginea into the testicle as fibrous septa

Acronyms Used in This Chapter

ACTH	Adrenocorticotropic hormone
cAMP	Cyclic adenosine monophosphate
DHEA	Dehydroepiandrosterone
FSH	Follicle-stimulating hormone
GnRH	Gonadotropin-releasing hormone
hCG	Human chorionic gonadotropin
LH	Luteinizing hormone
mRNA	Messenger ribonucleic acid
PRL	Prolactin
SHBG	Sex hormone–binding globulin

result in the formation of approximately 250 pyramidal lobules each of which contains coiled seminiferous tubules. Within each testis there are almost 200 m of seminiferous tubules, and these structures account for 80–90% of the testicular mass. The androgen-producing Leydig cells, as well as the blood and lymphatic vessels, nerves, and fibroblasts, are interspersed between the seminiferous tubules.

The blood supply to the testes is derived chiefly from the testicular arteries, which are branches of the internal spermatic arteries. After traversing a complicated capillary network, blood enters multiple testicular veins that form an anastomotic network, the pampiniform plexus. The pampiniform plexuses coalesce to form the internal spermatic veins. The right spermatic vein drains directly into the vena cava; the left enters the renal vein.

The seminiferous tubules in the adult average 165 μm in diameter and are composed of Sertoli cells and germinal cells. The Sertoli cells line the basement membrane and form tight junctions with other Sertoli cells. These tight junctions prevent the passage of proteins from the interstitial space into the lumen of the seminiferous tubules, thus establishing a "blood-testis barrier." Through extension of cytoplasmic processes, the Sertoli cells surround developing germ cells and provide an environment essential for germ cell differentiation. In addition, these cells have been shown to be responsible for the movement of germ cells from the base of the tubule toward the lumen and for the release of mature sperm into the lumen. These cells also actively phagocytose damaged germ

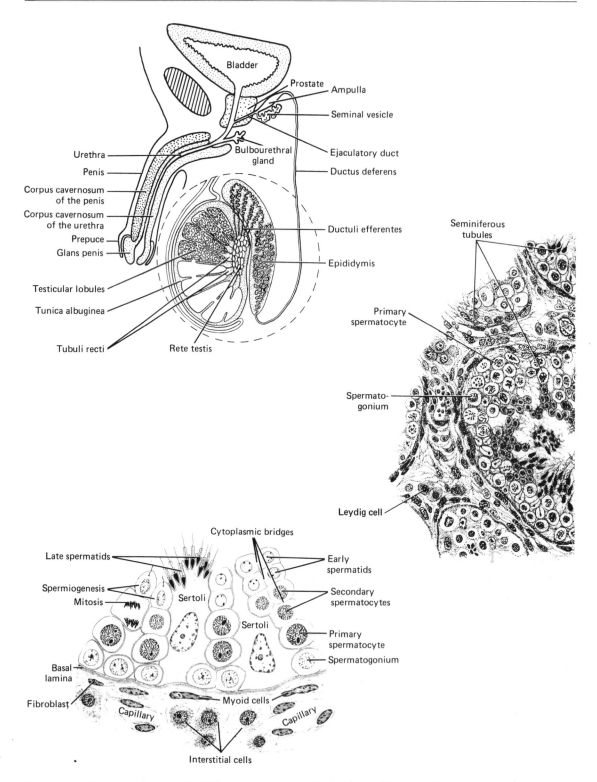

Figure 13–1. Male genital system. *Top:* The testis and the epididymis are in different scales from the other parts of the reproductive system. Observe the communication between the testicular lobules. *Bottom:* Structural organization of the human seminiferous tubule and interstitial tissue. This figure does not show the lymphatic vessels frequently found in the connective tissue. (Both illustrations reproduced, with permission, from Junqueira LC, Carneiro J: *Basic Histology,* 4th ed. Lange, 1983.) *At right:* Section of human testis. (Reproduced, with permission, from Ganong WF: *Review of Medical Physiology,* 12th ed. Lange, 1985.)

cells and residual bodies, which are portions of the germ cell cytoplasm not used in the formation of spermatozoa. Finally, in response to follicle-stimulating hormone (FSH) or testosterone, the Sertoli cells secrete androgen-binding protein, a molecule with high affinity for androgens. This substance, which enters the tubular lumen, provides a high concentration of testosterone to the developing germinal cells during the process of spermatogenesis.

More than a dozen different types of germ cells have been described in males. Broadly, they can be classified as spermatogonia, primary spermatocytes, secondary spermatocytes, spermatids, and spermatozoa. Spermatogenesis occurs in an orderly fashion, with the spermatocytes being derived from the spermatogonia via mitotic division. Through meiotic (or reduction) division, the spermatids are formed; they contain a haploid number of chromosomes (23). The interval from the beginning of spermatogenesis to release of mature spermatozoa into the tubular lumen is approximately 74 days. Although there is little variation in the duration of the spermatogenic cycle, a cross section of a seminiferous tubule will demonstrate several stages of germ cell development.

ACCESSORY STRUCTURES

The seminiferous tubules empty into a highly convoluted anastomotic network of ducts called the rete testis. Spermatozoa are then transported through efferent ductules and into a single duct, the epididymis, by testicular fluid pressure, ciliary motion, and contraction of the efferent ductules. During the approximately 12 days required for transit through the epididymis, spermatozoa undergo morphologic and functional changes essential to confer upon the gametes the capacity for fertilizing an ovum. The epididymis also serves as a reservoir for sperm. Spermatozoa stored in the epididymis enter the vas deferens, a muscular duct 35–50 cm long that propels its contents by peristaltic motion into the ejaculatory duct.

In addition to the spermatozoa and the secretory products of the testes, retia testis, and epididymides, the ejaculatory ducts receive fluid from the seminal vesicles. These paired structures, 10–20 cm long, are composed of alveolar glands, connective tissue, and muscle. They are the source of seminal plasma fructose, which provides nourishment to the spermatozoa. In addition, the seminal vesicles secrete phosphorylcholine, ergothioneine, ascorbic acid, flavins, and prostaglandins. About 60% of the total volume of seminal fluid is derived from the seminal vesicles.

The ejaculatory ducts terminate in the prostatic urethra. There additional fluid (approximately 20% of total volume) is added by the prostate, a tubuloalveolar gland with a fibromuscular stroma that weighs about 20 g and measures $4 \times 2 \times 3$ cm. The constituents of the prostatic fluid include spermine, citric acid, cholesterol, phospholipids, fibrinolysin, fibrinogenase, zinc, and acid phosphatase. Fluid is also added

to the seminal plasma by the bulbourethral (Cowper) glands and urethral (Littre) glands during its transit through the penile urethra.

PHYSIOLOGY OF THE MALE REPRODUCTIVE SYSTEM

GONADAL STEROIDS (Fig 13–2)

The 3 steroids of primary importance in male reproductive function are testosterone, dihydrotestosterone, and estradiol. From a quantitative standpoint, the most important androgen is testosterone. Over 95% of the testosterone is secreted by the testicular Leydig cells; the remainder is derived from the adrenals. In addition to testosterone, the testes secrete small amounts of the potent androgen dihydrotestosterone and the weak androgens dehydroepiandrosterone (DHEA) and androstenedione. The Leydig cells also secrete small quantities of estradiol, estrone, pregnenolone, progesterone, 17α-hydroxypregnenolone, and 17α-hydroxyprogesterone. The steps in testicular androgen biosynthesis are illustrated in Fig 13–2.

Dihydrotestosterone and estradiol are derived not only by direct secretion from the testes but also by conversion in peripheral tissues of androgen and estrogen precursors secreted by both the testes and the adrenals. Thus, about 80% of the circulating concentrations of these 2 steroids is derived from such peripheral conversion. Table 13–1 summarizes the approximate contributions of the testes, adrenals, and peripheral tissues to the circulating levels of several sex steroid hormones in men.

In the blood, androgens and estrogens exist in either a free (unbound) state or bound to serum proteins. Although about 38% of testosterone is bound to albumin, the major binding protein is sex hormone–binding globulin (SHBG), which binds 60% of the testosterone. This protein is distinct from the androgen-binding protein secreted by the Sertoli cells

Table 13–1. Relative contributions (approximate percentages) of the testes, adrenals, and peripheral tissues to circulating levels of sex steroids in men.

	Testicular Secretion	Adrenal Secretion	Peripheral Conversion of Precursors
Testosterone	95	<1	<5
Dihydrotestosterone	20	<1	80
Estradiol	20	<1	80
Estrone	2	<1	98
DHEA sulfate	<10	90	. . .

Figure 13–2. Pathways for testicular androgen and estrogen biosynthesis. Heavy arrows indicate major pathways. Circled numbers represent enzymes as follows: ① = 20,22-desmolase; ② = 3β-hydroxysteroid dehydrogenase and Δ⁵,Δ⁴-isomerase; ③ = 17-hydroxylase; ④ = 17,20-desmolase; ⑤ = 17-ketoreductase; ⑥ = 5α-reductase; ⑦ = aromatase.

Figure 13–3. Mechanisms of androgen action. T = testosterone; DHT = dihydrotestosterone; R_n = nuclear receptor; mRNA = messenger RNA.

toplasmic receptor protein (R_c in Fig 13–3) that is distinct from both androgen-binding protein and SHBG. After binding, the dihydrotestosterone-receptor complex is translocated into the nucleus, where it undergoes transformation (to R_n in Fig 13–3), allowing it to bind to the nuclear chromatin. Through presently obscure mechanisms, the interaction of the androgen-receptor complex with the chromatin results in the synthesis of messenger RNA (mRNA), which is eventually transported to the cytoplasm, where it directs the transcription of new protein synthesis and other changes that together constitute androgen action.

A variety of biologic effects of androgens have been defined in males. As discussed in Chapter 15, they are essential for appropriate differentiation of the internal and external male genital system during fetal development. During puberty, androgen-mediated growth of the scrotum, epididymis, vas deferens, seminal vesicles, prostate, and penis occurs. The functional integrity of these organs requires androgens. Androgens stimulate skeletal muscle growth and growth of the larynx, which results in deepening of the voice; and of the epiphyseal cartilaginous plates, which results in the pubertal growth spurt. Both ambisexual (pubic and axillary) hair growth and sexual (beard, mustache, chest, abdomen, and back) hair growth are stimulated, as is sebaceous gland activity. Other effects include stimulation of erythropoiesis and social behavioral changes.

and is synthesized in the liver. The serum concentrations of this protein are increased by estrogen or thyroid hormone administration, hyperthyroidism, and cirrhosis and are decreased by exogenous androgens or growth hormone, hypothyroidism, acromegaly, and obesity. About 2% of the circulating testosterone is not bound to serum proteins and is able to enter cells and exert its metabolic effects.

As noted below, testosterone may be converted to dihydrotestosterone within specific androgen target tissues. Most circulating testosterone is converted primarily by the liver into various metabolites such as androsterone and etiocholanolone, which, after conjugation with glucuronic or sulfuric acid, are excreted in the urine as 17-ketosteroids. However, it should be noted that only 20–30% of the urinary 17-ketosteroids are derived from testosterone metabolism. The majority of the 17-ketosteroids are formed from the metabolism of adrenal steroids. Therefore, 17-ketosteroid determinations do not reliably reflect testicular steroid secretion.

Testosterone leaves the circulation and rapidly traverses the cell membrane (Fig 13–3). In most androgen target cells, testosterone is enzymatically converted to the more potent androgen dihydrotestosterone by the microsomal enzyme 5α-reductase. Dihydrotestosterone then binds to a specific intracy-

CONTROL OF TESTICULAR FUNCTION

Hypothalamic-Pituitary–Leydig Cell Axis (Fig 13–4)

The hypothalamus synthesizes a decapeptide, gonadotropin-releasing hormone (GnRH), and secretes it in pulsatile fashion into the hypothalamohypophyseal portal blood. After reaching the anterior pituitary, GnRH binds to the gonadotropes and stimulates the release of both luteinizing hormone (LH) and, to a lesser extent, FSH into the general circulation. LH is taken up by the Leydig cells, where it binds to specific membrane receptors. This leads to activation of adenylate cyclase and generation of cAMP and other messengers that ultimately result in the secretion of androgens. In turn, the elevation of androgens inhibits the secretion of LH from the anterior pituitary through a direct action on the pituitary and an inhibitory effect at the hypothalamic level. The inhibitory effect of androgens on the hypothalamus is mediated principally by estradiol, which is formed locally in the hypothalamus from androgens.

Hypothalamic-Pituitary–Seminiferous Tubular Axis (Fig 13–4)

After stimulation by GnRH, the gonadotropes secrete FSH into the systemic circulation. This glycoprotein hormone binds to specific receptors in the

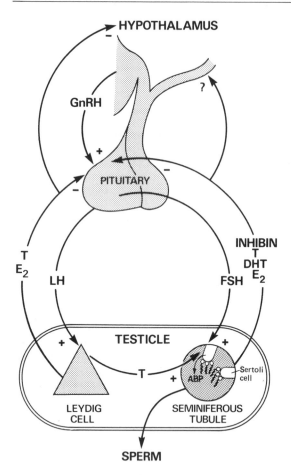

Figure 13–4. Hypothalamic-pituitary-testicular axis. GnRH = gonadotropin-releasing hormone; LH = luteinizing hormone; FSH = follicle-stimulating hormone; T = testosterone; DHT = dihydrotestosterone; ABP = androgen-binding protein; E_2 = estradiol; + = positive influence; − = negative influence.

Sertoli cells and stimulates the production of androgen-binding protein. FSH is necessary for the initiation of spermatogenesis. However, full maturation of the spermatozoa appears to require not only an FSH effect but also testosterone. Indeed, the major action of FSH on spermatogenesis may be via the stimulation of androgen-binding protein production, which allows a high intratubular concentration of testosterone to be maintained. In addition to androgen-binding protein, there is substantial evidence that another nonsteroid substance, **inhibin,** is also secreted by the Sertoli cells. This putative material appears to act principally at the pituitary level, where it selectively inhibits the secretion of FSH. It is not known whether inhibin also exerts a negative feedback control at a hypothalamic locus. Testosterone, dihydrotestosterone, and estradiol are also capable of inhibiting the secretion of FSH. However, it is not known if these steroids play a major role in the regulation of FSH secretion under normal physiologic conditions.

ERECTION & EJACULATION

The male sexual response may be divided into 4 distinct stages: excitement, plateau, orgasm, and resolution. Erotic stimuli result in increased blood pressure, increased cutaneous blood flow, and erection during the excitement stage. Penile erection occurs when blood flow to the penile erectile tissue (corpora cavernosa and spongiosum) increases as a result of dilatation of the urethral artery, the artery of the bulb of the penis, the deep artery of the penis, and the dorsal artery of the penis. Concurrent contraction of the ischiocavernosus muscle leads to compression of the veins draining the corpora cavernosa and spongiosum. This combination results in the distention, engorgement, and rigidity of the penis that constitute erection. Erection is an involuntary reflex that may occur via 2 different mechanisms. Psychogenic stimuli transmitted to the limbic system stimulate the thoracolumbar (T12–L2) parasympathetic nerves, and this in turn results in dilatation of the arteriolar vessels that supply the corpora cavernosa and spongiosum. In addition to the thoracolumbar center, sacral parasympathetic (S2–4) nerves may be activated by direct genital stimuli. The afferent limb for the spinal reflex arc is located within the pudendal nerves.

The plateau phase is the period between the initiation of erection and ejaculation. The duration of this phase is variable. While it lasts, mucus is secreted by Cowper's and Littre's glands.

Orgasm occurs in 2 stages. The first stage consists of reflex activity of the thoracolumbar sympathetic nerves, resulting in rhythmic contractions of the vas deferens, prostate, and seminal vesicles. These contractions propel sperm and seminal fluid into the posterior portion of the urethra (emission). Simultaneously, the bladder neck contracts by closure of the internal sphincter. The presence of semen in the urethral bulb leads to a feeling of impending or inevitable ejaculation. The second stage of the orgasmic phase is the ejaculatory reflex. Ejaculation is mediated through the pudendal nerves, which induce rhythmic contractions—at intervals of 0.8 second—of the bulbocavernosus and ischiocavernosus muscles. These contractions force semen out of the penis. During ejaculation, impulses are transmitted through the anterolateral tracts of the spinal cord to the cerebral cortex, where orgasm is perceived.

Following orgasm, the blood in the corpora cavernosa and spongiosum rapidly leaves the penis, resulting in a return to the flaccid state (resolution phase). A variable interval must elapse following the resolution phase before the sequence can be repeated (refractory period).

Table 13–2. Clinical findings in eunuchoidism.

Symptoms

    Deficient growth of axillary, pubic, facial, and body hair.

    Low or absent libido, erections, potency.

    Diminished strength and endurance compared with age mates.

Signs

    Failure to manifest pubertal growth spurt.

    Eunuchoid skeletal proportions (upper/lower segment ratio
      < 1; arm span/height ratio > 1).

    Sparse axillary, pubic, facial, and body hair.

    Poor muscle development.

    High-pitched (childish) voice.

    Small penis, testes, scrotum, and prostate.

    Osteoporosis with long-standing hypogonadism.

EVALUATION OF MALE GONADAL FUNCTION

CLINICAL EVALUATION

Effect of Age on Clinical Presentation

The clinical presentation of patients with deficient testosterone production or action depends upon the age at onset of hypogonadism. Androgen deficiency during the second to third months of fetal development results in varying degrees of ambiguity of the genitalia and male pseudohermaphroditism. These topics are covered in Chapters 15 and 16.

Prepubertal androgen deficiency leads to poor secondary sexual development and eunuchoid skeletal proportions (Table 13– 2). The penis fails to enlarge, the testes remain small, and the scrotum does not develop the marked rugae characteristic of puberty. The voice remains high-pitched and the muscle mass does not develop fully, resulting in less than normal strength and endurance. The lack of appropriate stimulation of sexual hair growth results in sparse axillary and pubic hair (which receive some stimulation from adrenal androgens) and absent or very sparse facial, chest, upper abdominal, and back hair. Although the androgen-mediated pubertal growth spurt will fail to take place, the epiphyseal plates of the long bones will continue to grow under the influence of somatomedins and other growth factors. Thus, the long bones of the upper and lower extremities will grow out of proportion to the axial skeleton. Normal white men have an average upper segment (crown to pubis) to lower segment (pubis to floor) ratio of > 1, whereas prepubertal hypogonadism results in a ratio of < 1. Similarly, the ratio of total arm span to total height averages 0.96 in white men. Because of the relatively

Figure 13–5. *A:* Hypogonadal habitus. Note absence of body and facial hair as well as feminine body distribution. *B:* Hypogonadal facies. Note absence of facial hair and fine wrinkles around the corners of the eyes and lips.

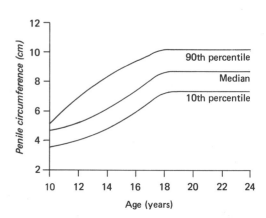

Figure 13–6. Penile length and circumference at various ages. *Left:* Normal values for stretched penile length. *Right:* Normal values for penile circumference. (Both redrawn and reproduced, with permission, from Schonfeld WA: *Am J Dis Child* 1943;**65**:535. Copyright © 1943 by the American Medical Association.)

greater growth in the upper extremities, the arm span of eunuchoid individuals exceeds height by 5 cm or more.

If testosterone deficiency develops after puberty, the patient may complain of decreased libido, impotence, and low energy. Patients with mild androgen deficiency or androgen deficiency of recent onset may not note a decrease in facial or body hair growth; it appears that although adult androgen levels must be achieved to *stimulate* male sexual hair growth, relatively low levels of androgens are required to *maintain* sexual hair growth. With long-standing hypogonadism, the growth of facial hair will diminish, and the frequency of shaving may also decrease (Fig 13– 5). In addition, fine wrinkles may appear in the corners of the mouth and eyes and, together with the sparse beard growth, result in the classic hypogonadal facies.

Genital Examination

Adequate assessment of the genitalia is essential in the evaluation of male hypogonadism. The examination should be performed in a warm room in order to relax the dartos muscle of the scrotum. The penis should be examined for the presence of hypospadias, epispadias, and chordee (abnormal angulation of the penis due to a fibrotic plaque), which may interfere with fertility. The fully stretched dorsal penile length should be measured in the flaccid state from the pubopenile skin junction to the tip of the glans. Penile circumference may also be measured in

the flaccid state. Both of these measurements may be compared to normal values (Fig 13– 6).

Assessment of testicular volume is also vital to the evaluation of hypogonadism. Careful measurement of the longitudinal and transverse axes of the testes may be made and testicular volume (V) calculated from the formula for a prolate spheroid: $V = 0.52 \times length \times width^2$. The mean volume for an adult testis is 18.6 ± 4.8 (SD) mL. The normal ranges

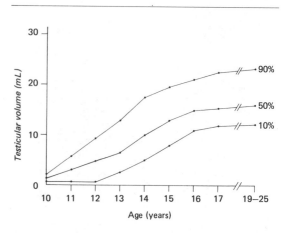

Figure 13–7. Normal values for testicular volume in relation to age. (Redrawn and reproduced, with permission, from Zachmann M et al: *Helv Paediatr Acta* 1974;**29**:61.)

Figure 13–8. Prader orchidometer.

for pre- and postpubertal individuals are shown in Fig 13–7. Alternatively, volume may be estimated with the Prader orchidometer, which consists of a series of plastic ellipsoids ranging in volume from 1 to 25 mL (Fig 13–8). Each testis is compared to the appropriate ellipsoid. Adults normally have volumes greater than 15 mL by this method.

Since 80–90% of testicular volume is composed of seminiferous tubules, decrease in volume indicates lack of tubular development or regression of tubular size. The consistency of the testicle should be noted. Small, firm testes are characteristic of hyalinization or fibrosis, as may occur in Klinefelter's syndrome. Small, rubbery testes are normally found in prepubertal males; in an adult, they are indicative of deficient gonadotropin stimulation. Testes with a mushy or soft consistency are characteristically found in individuals with postpubertal testicular atrophy.

The epididymis and vas deferens should also be examined. One of the most important parts of the examination is evaluation for the presence of varicocele resulting from incompetence of the internal spermatic vein. As will be discussed later, this is an important and potentially correctable form of male infertility. The patient should be examined in the upright position while performing the Valsalva maneuver. The examiner should carefully palpate the spermatic cords above the testes. A varicocele can be felt as an impulse along the posterior portion of the cord.

About 85% of varicoceles are located on the left side, and 15% are bilateral. A unilateral right varicocele is rare.

LABORATORY TESTS OF TESTICULAR FUNCTION

Semen Analysis

With some exceptions, a normal semen analysis excludes gonadal dysfunction. However, a single abnormal semen analysis is not a sufficient basis for a diagnosis of disturbance of testicular function, since marked variations in several of the parameters may be seen in normal individuals: At least 3 semen samples must be examined over a 2- to 3-month interval in order to evaluate this facet of male gonadal function. As noted above, approximately 3 months are required for completion of the spermatogenic cycle and movement of the mature spermatozoa through the ductal system. Therefore, when an abnormal semen sample is produced, one must question the patient about prior fever, trauma, drug exposure, and other factors that may temporarily damage spermatogenesis.

The semen should be collected by masturbation after 1–3 days of sexual abstinence. If the patient will not masturbate, a specially designed plastic condom (Mylex Corporation, Chicago) can be used during intercourse. Ordinary condoms cannot be used for this purpose, since they contain spermicidal chemicals. If neither of these methods is satisfactory, coitus interruptus may be used as long as the complete ejaculate is collected. It should be stressed to the patient that the greatest concentration of spermatozoa is in the first portion of the ejaculate and that this is the portion most often lost during coitus interruptus.

The specimen should be examined by an experienced technologist within 2 hours after collection. Normal values for semen analysis are given in Table 13–3.

Steroid Measurements

Each of the gonadal steroids may be measured by radioimmunoassay. Although single determinations may distinguish between normal individuals and pa-

Table 13–3. Normal values for semen analysis.

Liquefaction time: 3–25 minutes*
Volume: 1–6 mL
Concentration of sperm: $\geqslant 20 \times 10^6$/mL; $\geqslant 60 \times 10^6$ in total ejaculate
Motility of sperm: $\geqslant 2+$ on a scale of 1–4+
Morphology: $\geqslant 60\%$ normal or oval

*Following ejaculation, the semen forms a coagulum which is liquefied by proteolytic enzymes from the prostate.

0 = no motility; 1+ = sperm motile without forward progression; 2+ = sperm motile with slow forward progression; 3+ = sperm motile with forward progression at moderate to good rate of speed; 4+ = sperm motile, moving at high speed and in a straight line.

Table 13–4. Normal ranges for gonadal steroids, pituitary gonadotropins, and prolactin in men.

Testosterone	300–1100 ng/dL
Free testosterone	50–210 pg/mL
Dihydrotestosterone	60–300 ng/dL
Androstenedione	50–200 ng/dL
Estradiol	5–50 pg/mL
Estrone	30–170 pg/mL
FSH	2–15 mIU/mL
LH	2–15 mIU/mL
PRL	4–18 ng/mL

tients with severe hypogonadism, mild defects in androgen production may be missed. In normal individuals, there are frequent, rapid pulsatile changes in serum testosterone concentration as well as a slight nocturnal elevation. Therefore, at least 3 separate blood samples should be collected at 20- to 40-minute intervals during the morning for testosterone measurement. The testosterone may be measured in each of the serum samples, or equal aliquots of each of the 3 serum samples may be combined, mixed, and subjected to testosterone analysis. The latter procedure provides a savings in cost as well as a mean serum testosterone concentration that takes into account the pulsatile release of testosterone.

Androgen and estrogen radioimmunoassays measure total serum steroid concentrations. This is the sum of the free, biologically active hormone and the protein-bound moiety. Although in most circumstances it is not necessary to determine the actual quantity of free steroid hormones, in some situations alterations in the binding protein concentration may occur. Lowered concentrations of SHBG are seen in patients with hypothyroidism, obesity, and acromegaly. In these circumstances, the free testosterone concentration should be directly measured, since it may be normal when the total serum testosterone level is decreased. The normal male serum concentrations of gonadal steroids collected in the basal state are given in Table 13–4.

Gonadotropin & Prolactin Measurements

LH and, to a lesser extent, FSH are released in pulsatile fashion throughout the day. Therefore, as with testosterone, at least 3 blood samples should be obtained at 20- to 40-minute intervals during the day. FSH and LH may be measured in each of the samples or in a single pooled specimen. Although many laboratories give a numerical value for the lower limits of normal for gonadotropins, some normal males have concentrations of FSH and LH undetectable by presently available radioimmunoassay techniques. Furthermore, the concentrations of gonadotropins measured in one laboratory may not be directly comparable to those measured in another because of differences in the reference preparations used. The primary use

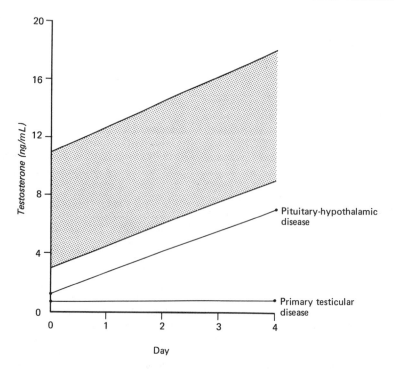

Figure 13–9. Testosterone response following stimulation with chorionic gonadotropin, 4000 IU/d intramuscularly, in normal males (shaded area) and in patients with primary and secondary hypogonadism.

of basal FSH and LH concentrations is to distinguish between hypergonadotropic hypogonadism, in which either or both of the gonadotropins are elevated, and hypogonadotropic hypogonadism, in which the gonadotropins are low or inappropriately normal in the presence of decreased androgen production.

Elevations of serum prolactin (PRL) may inhibit the normal release of pituitary gonadotropins, possibly through an effect on the hypothalamus. Thus, serum PRL measurements should be performed in any patient with hypogonadotropic hypogonadism. Serum PRL concentrations are generally stable throughout the day; therefore, measurement of this hormone in a single sample is usually sufficient. However, the patient should abstain from eating for 3 hours before the blood sample is obtained, since a protein meal may acutely stimulate the release of PRL from the pituitary. The normal ranges for serum PRL and gonadotropins are shown in Table 13–4.

Dynamic Tests

A. Chorionic Gonadotropin Stimulation Test: (Fig 13–9.) Human chorionic gonadotropin (hCG) is a glycoprotein hormone with biologic actions similar to those of LH. Following an injection of chorionic gonadotropin, this hormone binds to the LH receptors on the Leydig cells and stimulates the synthesis and secretion of testicular steroids. Therefore, the Leydig cells may be directly assessed by the intramuscular injection of 4000 IU of chorionic gonadotropin daily for 4 days. A normal response is a doubling of the testosterone level following the last injection. Alternatively, a single intramuscular dose of chorionic gonadotropin (5000 IU/1.7 m^2 in adults or 100 IU/kg in children) may be given, with blood samples taken for testosterone measurements 72 and 96 hours later. Patients with primary gonadal disease will have a diminished response following administration of chorionic gonadotropin, while patients with Leydig cell failure secondary to pituitary or hypothalamic disease will have a qualitatively normal response.

B. Clomiphene Citrate Stimulation Test: (Fig 13–10.) Clomiphene citrate (Clomid) is a nonsteroid compound with weak estrogenic activity. It binds to estrogen receptors in various tissues, including the hypothalamus. By preventing the more potent estrogen estradiol from occupying these receptors, the hypothalamus in effect "sees" less estradiol. As noted above, most if not all of the hypothalamic-pituitary feedback control by testicular androgens is mediated by estradiol, which is derived from the peripheral conversion of androgens. The apparent estradiol deficiency leads to an increase of GnRH release the net result of which is stimulation of the gonadotropes to secrete increased quantities of LH and FSH.

The test is performed by giving clomiphene citrate, 100 mg orally twice daily for 10 days. Three blood samples are collected at 20-minute intervals (see com-

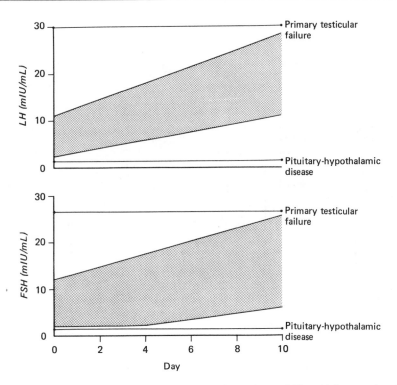

Figure 13–10. LH and FSH response following 10 days of clomiphene citrate, 200 mg/d, in normal males (shaded areas) and in patients with primary and secondary hypogonadism.

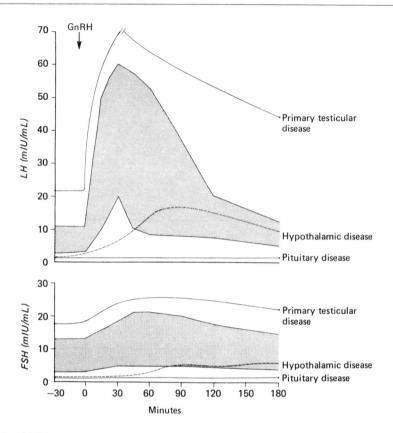

Figure 13–11. LH and FSH responses following a bolus injection of GnRH (gonadorelin; Factrel) in normal males (shaded areas) and in patients with primary testicular, hypothalamic, or pituitary disease. Note that patients with hypothalamic disorders may have a quantitatively normal but delayed rise. Some patients with hypothalamic disease show no response, while some patients with pituitary disease demonstrate a normal response.

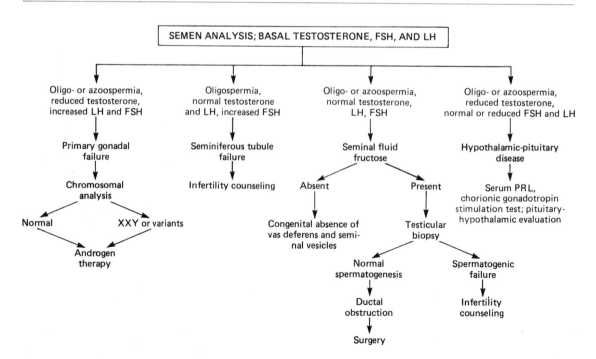

Figure 13–12. Scheme for evaluation of clinical hypogonadism.

ments above, under Steroid Measurements) 1 day before the drug is administered and again on days 9 and 10 of drug administration. LH, FSH, and testosterone should be measured in pooled aliquots from each of these samples. Normal men have a 50–250% increase in LH, a 30–200% increase in FSH, and a 30–220% increase in testosterone on day 10 of the test. Patients with pituitary or hypothalamic disease do not show a normal increment in LH or FSH.

C. Gonadotropin-Releasing Hormone Test: (Fig 13–11.) The decapeptide GnRH (gonadorelin; Factrel) directly stimulates the gonadotropes of the anterior pituitary to secrete LH and FSH. It was expected that measurement of LH and FSH following the administration of GnRH would be useful in distinguishing between hypothalamic and pituitary lesions, but this has not proved to be the case. Patients with destructive lesions of the pituitary and those with long-standing hypogonadism due to hypothalamic disorders may not show a response to a GnRH test. However, if the releasing factor is administered by repeated injections or by a programmable pulsatile infusion pump for 7–14 days, patients with hypothalamic lesions may have their pituitary responsiveness to GnRH restored, whereas patients with pituitary insufficiency do not. Conversely, a normal LH and FSH response to GnRH in a hypogonadal male does not eliminate hypopituitarism as the cause of the gonadal failure, since patients with mild hypogonadotropic hypogonadism may demonstrate a normal response.

The test is performed by administering 100 μg of gonadorelin by rapid intravenous bolus. Blood is drawn at −15, 0, 15, 30, 45, 60, 90, 120, and 180 minutes for LH and FSH measurements. Normal adult males have a 2- to 5-fold increase in LH over baseline concentrations and an approximately 2-fold rise of FSH. However, some normal males fail to have an increase in FSH following GnRH. Patients with primary testicular disease may respond with exaggerated increases in LH and FSH. If seminiferous tubule damage alone is present, abnormal FSH rise and normal LH response may be seen.

Testicular Biopsy

Testicular biopsy in hypogonadal men is primarily indicated in patients with normal-sized testes and azoospermia in order to distinguish spermatogenic failure and ductal obstruction. Although germinal aplasia, hypoplasia, maturation arrest, and other abnormalities of spermatogenesis may be diagnosed by examination of testicular tissue in oligospermic males, knowledge of the type of defect does not alter therapy. Therefore, testicular biopsy is not usually indicated for evaluation of mild to moderate oligospermia.

General Scheme for the Evaluation of Male Hypogonadism

Fig 13–12 outlines an approach to the diagnosis of male gonadal disorders. Semen analysis and determination of the basal concentrations of testosterone, FSH, and LH allow the clinician to distinguish patients with primary gonadal failure who have poor semen characteristics, low or normal testosterone, and elevated FSH or LH from those with secondary gonadal failure and abnormal semen analysis, decreased testosterone, and low or inappropriately normal gonadotropins.

In patients with elevations of gonadotropins resulting from primary testicular disease, chromosomal analysis will help to differentiate between genetic abnormalities and acquired testicular defects. Since no therapy exists that will restore spermatogenesis in an individual with severe testicular damage, androgen replacement is the treatment of choice. Patients with isolated seminiferous tubule failure may have normal or elevated FSH concentrations in association with normal LH and testosterone levels and usually severe oligospermia. Patients with azoospermia require evaluation for the possible presence of ductal obstruction, since this defect may be surgically correctable. Fructose is added to seminal plasma by the seminal vesicles, and an absence of fructose indicates that the seminal vesicles are absent or bilaterally obstructed. The combination of a poor semen analysis with low testosterone, FSH, and LH is indicative of a hypothalamic or pituitary defect. Such patients need further evaluation of anterior and posterior pituitary gland function with appropriate pituitary function tests, as well as neuroradiologic and neuro-ophthalmologic studies (see Chapter 4, Part I).

PHARMACOLOGY OF DRUGS USED TO TREAT MALE GONADAL DISORDERS

ANDROGENS

A variety of drugs are available for the treatment of androgen deficiency (Table 13–5). Preparations for sublingual and oral administration have the advantage of ease of administration but the disadvantages of erratic absorption, potential for cholestatic jaundice, and decreased effectiveness when compared to the intramuscular preparations. A new androgen, mesterolone (not available in the USA), has the advantage of oral administration without causing cholestatic jaundice; whether it will be as effective as the parenteral androgen preparations remains to be determined. Testosterone propionate is a short-acting androgen. Its main use is in initiating therapy in older men, whose prostate glands may be exquisitely sensitive to testosterone. Obstructive symptoms due to benign prostatic hypertrophy following therapy with this androgen usually resolve rapidly because of its short duration of action.

Table 13–5. Representative androgen preparations:
Dosages and routes of administration.

Oral administration	
Fluoxymesterone (Halotestin, Ora-Testryl)	5–10 mg daily
Mesterolone (Mestoranum, Pro-viron)*	30–60 mg daily
Sublingual (buccal) administration	
Methyltestosterone (Android, Metandren, Oreton Methyl, Testred)	25–50 mg daily
Subcutaneous administration	
Testosterone pellets	450 mg (6 pellets) every 4–6 months
Intramuscular administration	
Testosterone cypionate (Depo-Testosterone)	100–200 mg every 2–3 weeks
Testosterone enanthate (Delatestryl)	100–200 mg every 2–3 weeks
Testosterone propionate	50 mg 2–3 times a week

*Not available in the USA.

Androgen deficiency is best treated with testosterone enanthate or cyclopentylpropionate (cypionate) given intramuscularly. The duration of action of these preparations is usually 2 weeks, although some patients note an effect for up to 4 weeks. Unlike the oral androgen preparations, both of these agents are capable of completely virilizing the patients. Therapy may be initiated with 200 mg intramuscularly every 1–2 weeks for 1–2 years. After adequate virilization has been achieved, the androgen effect may be maintained by doses of 100–200 mg every 2–3 weeks. Testosterone pellets may be implanted subcutaneously for a longer duration of effect. However, this therapy has not enjoyed much popularity.

Androgen therapy is contraindicated in patients with known prostatic carcinoma. The adverse reactions that may occur during therapy are listed in Table 13–6. About 1–2% of patients receiving methyltestosterone and fluoxymesterone develop intrahepatic cholestatic jaundice that resolves when the drug is discontinued. Rarely, these methylated or halogenated

Table 13–6. Adverse effects of androgen therapy.

Prostatic hypertrophy
Cholestatic jaundice (methyltestosterone, fluoxymesterone)
Hepatoma (methyltestosterone, fluoxymesterone)
Premature epiphyseal fusion
Water retention with hypertension
Erythrocytosis
Inhibition of spermatogenesis
Gynecomastia
Priapism
Acne
Aggressive behavior
Alterations of thyroid and adrenal function tests

androgens have been associated with benign and malignant hepatocellular tumors.

Androgen therapy may also cause premature fusion of the epiphyses in an adolescent, and this may result in some loss of potential height. Therefore, androgen therapy is usually withheld until a hypogonadal male reaches 13 years of age. Water retention may be associated with hypertension or congestive heart failure in susceptible individuals. Since androgens stimulate erythropoietin production, erythrocytosis may occur during therapy. This is not usually clinically significant. Inhibition of spermatogenesis is mediated through suppression of gonadotropins by the androgens. Gynecomastia may develop during initiation of androgen therapy but usually resolves with continued administration of the drug. Priapism, acne, and aggressive behavior are dose-related adverse effects and generally disappear after reduction of dosage. Androgens decrease the production of thyroxine-binding globulin and corticosteroid-binding globulin by the liver. Therefore, total serum thyroxine and cortisone concentrations may be decreased though the free hormone concentrations remain normal.

GONADOTROPINS

In patients with hypogonadism due to inadequate gonadotropin secretion, spermatogenesis and virilization may be induced by exogenous gonadotropin injections. Since the gonadotropins are proteins with short half-lives, they must be administered parenterally 2–3 times a week. As previously noted, the spermatogenic cycle is approximately 3 months, and the drugs must therefore be administered for at least that length of time. The expense and inconvenience of this type of therapy preclude its routine use for the treatment of androgen deficiency. The 2 major indications for exogenous gonadotropins are treatment of cryptorchidism (see below) and induction of spermatogenesis in hypogonadal males who wish to father children. In order to induce spermatogenesis, 2000 IU of chorionic gonadotropin may be given intramuscularly 3 times a week. Menotropins (Pergonal), available in vials containing 75 IU each of FSH and LH, is administered in a dosage of 1–2 vials intramuscularly 3 times weekly. Adverse reactions with such therapy are minimal. Acne, gynecomastia, or prostatic enlargement may be noted due to excessive Leydig cell stimulation. Reduction of the chorionic gonadotropin dosage or a decrease in the frequency of chorionic gonadotropin injections generally results in resolution of the problem. GnRH, administered in a pulsatile fashion by portable infusion pumps, has recently been shown to be effective in stimulating the endogenous release of LH and FSH in hypogonadotropic hypogonadal patients. At present, this mode of therapy does not appear to offer any major advantage over the use of gonadotropins for induction of spermatogenesis or the use of testosterone enanthate or cypionate for virilization.

CLINICAL DISORDERS

Hypogonadism may be subdivided into 3 general categories (Table 13–7). A thorough discussion of the hypothalamic-pituitary disorders that cause hypogonadism is presented in Chapters 4 and 16. The defects in androgen biosynthesis and androgen action are described in Chapter 15. The following section emphasizes the primary gonadal abnormalities.

KLINEFELTER'S SYNDROME (XXY Seminiferous Tubule Dysgenesis)

Klinefelter's syndrome is the most common cause of male hypogonadism. An extra X chromosome is present in about 0.2% of live-born males. Sex chromosome surveys of mentally retarded males have revealed an extra X chromosome in 0.45–2.5% of such individuals. Patients with an XXY genotype have classic Klinefelter's syndrome; those with an XXXY, XXXXY, or XXYY genotype or with XXY/chromosomal mosaicism are considered to have variant forms of the syndrome (see below).

Etiology & Pathophysiology
The XXY genotype is usually due to maternal meiotic nondisjunction, which results in an egg with

Table 13–7. Classification of male hypogonadism.

Hypothalamic-pituitary disorders
  Panhypopituitarism
  Isolated LH deficiency (fertile eunuch)
  LH and FSH deficiency
    a. With normal sense of smell
    b. With hyposmia or anosmia (Kallmann's syndrome)
  Prader-Willi syndrome
  Laurence-Moon-Biedl syndrome
  Cerebellar ataxia
  Biologically inactive LH
Gonadal abnormalities
  Klinefelter's syndrome
  Other chromosomal defects (XX male, XY/XXY, XX/XXY, XXXY, XXXXY, XXYY, XYY)
  Bilateral anorchia (vanishing testes syndrome)
  Leydig cell aplasia
  Cryptorchidism
  Noonan's syndrome
  Myotonic dystrophy
  Adult seminiferous tubule failure
  Adult Leydig cell failure
  Defects in androgen biosynthesis
Defects in androgen action
  Complete androgen insensitivity (testicular feminization)
  Incomplete androgen insensitivity
    a. Type I
    b. Type II (5α-reductase deficiency)

two X chromosomes. Meiotic nondisjunction during spermatogenesis has also been documented. Both observations correlate positively with the epidemiologic findings that both the mother and the father tend to be older than average at the time of the patient's birth.

At birth there are generally no physical stigmas of Klinefelter's syndrome, and during childhood there are no specific signs or symptoms. The chromosomal defect is expressed chiefly during puberty. As the gonadotropins increase, the seminiferous tubules do not enlarge but rather undergo fibrosis and hyalinization, which results in small, firm testes. Obliteration of the seminiferous tubules results in azoospermia.

In addition to dysgenesis of the seminiferous tubules, the Leydig cells are also abnormal. They are present in clumps and appear to be hyperplastic upon initial examination of a testicular biopsy. However, the Leydig cell mass is not increased, and the apparent hyperplasia is actually due to the marked reduction in tubular volume. Despite the normal mass of tissue, the Leydig cells are functionally abnormal. The testosterone production rate is reduced, and there is a compensatory elevation in serum LH. Stimulation of the Leydig cells with exogenous chorionic gonadotropin results in a subnormal rise in testosterone. The clinical manifestations of androgen deficiency vary considerably from patient to patient. Thus, some individuals have virtually no secondary sexual developmental changes, whereas others are indistinguishable from normal individuals. The elevated LH concentrations also stimulate the Leydig cells to secrete increased quantities of estradiol and estradiol precursors. The relatively high estradiol:testosterone ratio is responsible for the variable degrees of feminization and gynecomastia seen in these patients. The elevated estradiol also stimulates the liver to produce SHBG. This may result in total serum testosterone concentrations that are within the low normal range for adult males. However, the free testosterone level may be lower than normal.

The pathogenesis of the eunuchoid proportions, personality, and intellectual deficits and associated medical disorders is presently unclear.

Testicular Pathology
Most of the seminiferous tubules are fibrotic and hyalinized, although occasional Sertoli cells and spermatogonia may be present in some sections. Absence of elastic fibers in the tunica propria is indicative of the dysgenetic nature of the tubules. The Leydig cells are arranged in clumps and appear hyperplastic, although the total mass is normal.

Clinical Features (Fig 13–13)
A. Symptoms and Signs: There are usually no symptoms before puberty other than poor school performance in some affected individuals. Puberty may be delayed, but not usually by more than 1–2 years. During puberty, the penis and scrotum undergo varying degrees of development, with some individuals

Figure 13–13. Klinefelter's syndrome in a 20-year-old man. Note relatively increased lower/upper body segment ratio, gynecomastia, small penis, and sparse body hair with a female pubic hair pattern.

appearing normal. Most patients (80%) have diminished facial and torso hair growth. The major complaint is often persistent gynecomastia, which is clinically present in over half of patients. The testes are uniformly small (< 2 cm in longest axis) and firm as a result of fibrosis and hyalinization. Other complaints include infertility or insufficient libido and potency. The patient may have difficulty putting into words his embarrassment in situations where he must disrobe in the presence of other men, and the subnormal development of the external genitalia along with gynecomastia may lead to feelings of inadequacy that may be partly responsible for the dyssocial behavior some patients exhibit.

Patients with Klinefelter's syndrome have abnormal skeletal proportions that are not truly eunuchoid. Growth of the lower extremities is relatively greater than that of the trunk and upper extremities; therefore, pubis-to-floor height is greater than crown-to-pubis height, and span is less than total height. Thus, the abnormal skeletal proportions are not the result of androgen deficiency per se (which results in span greater than height).

Intellectual impairment is noted in many patients with Klinefelter's syndrome, but the true proportion of affected individuals with subnormal intelligence is not known. Dyssocial behavior is common (see above). Patients generally show want of ambition, difficulties in maintaining permanent employment, and a tendency to ramble in conversations.

Medical disorders found to be associated with Klinefelter's syndrome with greater than chance frequency include chronic pulmonary disease (emphysema, chronic bronchitis), varicose veins, glucose intolerance, primary hypothyroidism, and breast cancer.

B. Laboratory Findings: Serum testosterone is low or normal; FSH and LH concentrations are elevated. Azoospermia is present. The buccal smear is chromatin-positive (> 20% of cells having a Barr body), and chromosomal analysis reveals a 47,XXY karyotype.

Differential Diagnosis

Klinefelter's syndrome should be distinguished from other causes of hypogonadism. Small, firm testes should suggest Klinefelter's syndrome. Hypothalamic-pituitary hypogonadism may be associated with small, rubbery testes if puberty has not occurred or atrophic testes if normal puberty has occurred. The consistency of the testes in Klinefelter's syndrome is also different from that noted in acquired forms of adult seminiferous tubular damage. The elevated gonadotropins place the site of the lesion at the testicular level, and chromosomal analysis confirms the diagnosis. Chromosomal analysis is also required to differentiate classic Klinefelter's syndrome from the variant forms.

Treatment

A. Medical Treatment: Androgen deficiency should be treated with testosterone replacement. Patients with personality defects should be virilized gradually to decrease the risk of aggressive behavior. Testosterone enanthate or cypionate, 100 mg intramuscularly, may be given every 2–4 weeks initially and increased to 200 mg every 2 weeks if well tolerated. Patients with low normal androgen levels may not require androgen replacement therapy.

B. Surgical Treatment: If gynecomastia presents a cosmetic problem, mastectomy may be performed.

Course & Prognosis

Patients generally feel better after androgen replacement therapy has begun. However, the personality defects do not improve, and these patients often require long-term psychiatric counseling. Life expectancy is not affected.

VARIANT KLINEFELTER'S SYNDROME & OTHER CHROMOSOMAL ABNORMALITIES

Several clinical and genotypic variants of Klinefelter's syndrome have been described. The salient

Table 13—8. Comparison of classic and variant forms of Klinefelter's syndrome.
(Approximate frequencies shown in parentheses if known.)
(0 = absent; 1+ = < 25%; 2+ = 25–50%; 3+ = 50–75%; 4+ = > 75%)

	Klinefelter's (47,XXY) (1:500)	XX Male* (1:9000)	XY/XXY† (1:1700)	XX/XXY	XXXY‡	XXXXY§	XXYY** (1:9000)	XYY†† (1:1000)
Small testes	4+	4+	3+	4+	4+	4+	4+	0
Azoospermia	4+	4+	3+	4+	4+	4+	4+	0
Deficient secondary sexual development	4+	4+	3+	4+	4+	4+	3+	0
Gynecomastia	2+	2+	2+	2+	3+	0	3+	0
Skeletal deformities	1+	0	1+	0	1+	4+	1+	1+
Mental retardation	1+	0	1+	1+	4+	4+	4+	1+
Cryptorchidism	1+	1+	0	1+	0	2+	1+	0
Increased gonadotropin levels	4+	4+	3+	4+	4+	4+	3+	1+

Other features:

*Normal skeletal proportions. Taller than XX female, shorter than XY male.

†May be fertile if gonads have XY; testes may have germinal aplasia.

‡Epicanthal folds, wide mouth.

§Peculiar facies, hypoplastic genitalia, congenital heart disease.

**Aggressive behavior; tall; varicose veins; acromegalic features.

††Antisocial behavior; macronodular acne; tall; electroencephalographic abnormalities; oligospermia.

clinical features are listed in Table 13– 8. In addition to small testes with seminiferous tubular hyalinization, azoospermia, deficient secondary sexual development, and elevated gonadotropins, patients with 3 or more X chromosomes uniformly have severe mental retardation. The presence of more than one Y chromosome tends to be associated with aggressive antisocial behavior and macronodular acne. Skeletal deformities such as radioulnar synostoses, flexion deformities of the elbows, and clinodactyly also are more commonly seen in Klinefelter variants. Patients with sex chromosome mosaicism (XX/XXY) may have only a few of the Klinefelter stigmas. These patients may have normal testicular size and may be fertile if their testes contain the XY genotype.

Phenotypic males with an XX chromosome composition have clinical features similar to those of Klinefelter's syndrome but tend to be shorter and maintain more normal skeletal proportions than patients with the classic syndrome. Mental retardation and behavioral abnormalities also are found less frequently in these patients. Although a Y chromosome is not evident in the karyotype of these patients, their cells do express the H-Y antigen, indicating that X-Y interchange occurs during paternal meiosis or that a Y chromosome–containing cell line was at one time present but was eliminated during development.

Patients with the XXXXY genotype have, in addition to small testes and hypogonadism, severe mental retardation, peculiar facies, and a variety of skeletal deformities. These include epicanthal folds, strabismus, hypertelorism, a broad, flat nose, a large mouth with prognathism, webbing of the neck, and large ears. Patients with the XXXY genotype have clinical features that are intermediate between those with XXXXY and typical Klinefelter's syndrome.

One of the most frequent sex chromosomal abnormalities in phenotypic males is the XYY genotype. In population surveys, this karyotype is found in approximately 1:1000 live male births. However, in penal institutions, the prevalence is 4 times greater; and in combined penal-mental institutions, the frequency is 20 times greater than in the general population. These patients are generally tall, and approximately half have macronodular acne. The aggressive social behavior noted in many of these individuals may in part represent a selection bias, since many of the subjects are identified in prisons. Although some individuals are clearly retarded, mental retardation is seen less frequently than in typical Klinefelter's syndrome. Testicular size is generally normal, and spermatogenesis may be normal or abnormal. Serum testosterone and gonadotropin levels are normal in most patients, although mild elevations of FSH have been noted in patients with the more severe degrees of spermatogenic maturation arrest.

BILATERAL ANORCHIA (Vanishing Testes Syndrome)

Approximately 3% of phenotypic boys undergoing surgery to correct unilateral or bilateral cryptorchidism are found to have absence of one testis, and in about 1% of cryptorchid males both testes are absent. Thus, bilateral anorchia is found in approximately one out of every 20,000 males.

Etiology & Pathophysiology (See also Chapters 15 and 16.)

Functional testicular tissue must be present during the first 14– 16 weeks of embryonic development in order for wolffian duct growth and müllerian duct regression to occur and for the external genitalia to differentiate along male lines. Absence of testicular function before this time will result in varying degrees of male pseudohermaphroditism with ambiguous genitalia. Prenatal testicular injury occurring after 16 weeks of gestation as a result of trauma, vascular insufficiency, infection, or other mechanisms may result in loss of testicular tissue in an otherwise normal phenotypic male; hence the term "vanishing testes syndrome."

Testicular Pathology
In most instances, no recognizable testicular tissue has been identified despite extensive dissections. Wolffian duct structures are generally normal, and the vas deferens and testicular vessels may terminate blindly or in a mass of connective tissue in the inguinal canal or scrotum.

Clinical Features
A. Symptoms and Signs: At birth, patients appear to be normal phenotypic males with bilateral cryptorchidism. Growth and development are normal until secondary sexual development fails to occur at puberty. The penis remains small; pubic and axillary hair does not fully develop despite the presence of adrenal androgens; and the scrotum remains empty. If the patient does not receive androgens, eunuchoid proportions develop. Gynecomastia does not occur.

An occasional patient will undergo partial spontaneous virilization at puberty. Although anatomically no testicular tissue has been identified in such patients, catheterization studies have demonstrated higher testosterone concentrations in venous blood obtained from the spermatic veins than in the peripheral venous circulation. This suggests that functional Leydig cells are present in some patients, although they are not associated with testicular germinal epithelium or stroma.

B. Laboratory Findings: Serum testosterone concentrations are generally quite low, and both LH and FSH are markedly elevated. Serum testosterone concentrations do not rise following a chorionic gonadotropin stimulation test. Chromosomal analysis discloses a 46,XY karyotype.

C. X-Ray Findings: Testicular artery arteriograms and spermatic venograms show vessels that taper and end in the inguinal canal or scrotum without an associated gonad.

D. Special Examinations: Thorough inguinal, abdominal, and retroperitoneal exploration may locate the testes. If testicular vessels and the vas deferens are identified and found to terminate blindly together, it may be assumed that the testis is absent.

Differential Diagnosis
Bilateral cryptorchidism must be differentiated from congenital bilateral anorchia. A normal serum testosterone concentration that rises following stimulation with chorionic gonadotropin is indicative of

functional Leydig cells and probable bilateral cryptorchidism. Elevated serum LH and FSH and a low testosterone that fails to rise after administration of exogenous chorionic gonadotropin indicate bilateral absence of functional testicular tissue.

Treatment
Androgen replacement therapy is discussed in the section on pharmacology (see Androgens, above).

Implantation of testicular prostheses for cosmetic purposes may be beneficial after the scrotum has enlarged in response to androgen therapy.

LEYDIG CELL APLASIA

Defective development of testicular Leydig cells is a rare cause of male pseudohermaphroditism with ambiguous genitalia.

Etiology & Pathophysiology
Testes are present in the inguinal canal and contain prepubertal-appearing tubules with Sertoli cells and spermatogonia without germinal cell maturation. The interstitial tissue has a loose myxoid appearance with an absence of Leydig cells. The binding of hCG or LH to testicular extracts from these patients is absent. It is not known whether this represents a primary defect in Leydig cell development due to an abnormality in the Leydig cell precursor cells or is the result of a deficiency of Leydig cell receptors for gonadotropins that may be responsible for inducing Leydig cell differentiation. The presence of a vas deferens and epididymis in these patients indicates that the local concentration of testosterone was high enough during embryogenesis to result in differentiation of the wolffian duct structures. However, the ambiguity of the genitalia indicates that the androgen concentration in these patients was insufficient to bring about full virilization of the external genitalia. The absence of müllerian duct structures is compatible with normal fetal secretion of müllerian duct inhibitory factor from the Sertoli cells.

Clinical Features
A. Symptoms and Signs: These patients may present in infancy with variable degrees of genital ambiguity, including a bifid scrotum, clitoral phallus, urogenital sinus, and blind vaginal pouch. Alternatively, they may appear as normal phenotypic females and escape detection until adolescence, when they present with primary amenorrhea, with or without normal breast development. The gonads are generally located in the inguinal canal. Axillary and pubic hair, although present, may be sparse.

B. Laboratory Findings: Serum gonadotropins are elevated, and testosterone levels are below normal limits for a male and within the low normal range for females. There is no increase in testosterone following chorionic gonadotropin administration.

Differential Diagnosis

Leydig cell aplasia should be differentiated from the vanishing testes syndrome, from testosterone biosynthetic defects, from disorders of androgen action, and from 5α-reductase deficiency. The differential diagnostic features of these disorders are discussed in Chapter 15.

Treatment

Patients with Leydig cell aplasia respond well to the exogenous administration of testosterone, and it would be anticipated that they would be fully virilized and even develop some degree of spermatogenesis with exogenous testosterone administration. However, since the few patients that have been reported have been discovered either late in childhood or as adolescents, it would be inappropriate to attempt a gender reversal at such a late period. Removal of the cryptorchid testes and feminization with exogenous estrogens would appear to be the most prudent course of therapy.

CRYPTORCHIDISM

Cryptorchidism is unilateral or bilateral absence of the testes from the scrotum because of failure of normal testicular descent from the genital ridge through the external inguinal ring. About 3% of full-term male infants have cryptorchidism. In most cases of cryptorchidism noted at birth, spontaneous testicular descent occurs during the first year of life, reducing the incidence to 0.2–0.8% by 1 year of age. Approximately 0.75% of adult males are cryptorchid. Unilateral cryptorchidism is 5–10 times more common than bilateral cryptorchidism.

Almost 50% of cryptorchid testes are located at the external inguinal ring or in a high scrotal position; 19% lie within the inguinal canal between the internal and external inguinal rings (canalicular); 9% are intra-abdominal; and 23% are ectopic, ie, located away from the normal pathway of descent from the abdominal cavity to the scrotum. Most ectopic testes are found in a superficial inguinal pouch above the external inguinal ring.

Etiology

Testicular descent usually occurs between the 12th week of fetal development and birth. Both mechanical and hormonal factors appear to be important for this process: Cryptorchidism is common in patients with congenital defects in androgen synthesis or action and in patients with congenital gonadotropin deficiency, and experimental studies have demonstrated that dihydrotestosterone is required for normal testicular descent. These observations suggest that prenatal androgen deficiency may be of etiologic importance in the development of cryptorchidism.

Testicular Pathology

Histologic studies on cryptorchid testes have demonstrated a decrease in the size of the seminiferous tubules and number of spermatogonia and an increase in peritubular tissue. The Leydig cells usually appear normal. It is unclear at what age these changes first appear. Abnormalities have been detected as early as 18 months to 2 years. It is well established that the longer a testis remains cryptorchid, the more likely it is to show pathologic changes. More severe changes are generally found in intra-abdominal testes than in canalicular testes.

Pathophysiology

It is not known whether pathologic changes in the testes are due to the effects of cryptorchidism or to intrinsic abnormalities in the gonad. Experimental studies in animals have shown that an increase in the temperature of the testes by 1.5–2 °C (the temperature differential between the abdomen and scrotum) results in depression of spermatogenesis. Serial testicular biopsies in cryptorchid patients have demonstrated partial reversal of the histologic abnormalities following surgical correction, suggesting that the extrascrotal environment is responsible for the observed pathologic abnormalities.

An intrinsic abnormality in the testes in patients with unilateral cryptorchidism is suggested by the observation that such patients are at increased risk for development of germ cell neoplasms in the scrotal testis. Similarly, the observation that adults with unilateral cryptorchidism surgically corrected before puberty had low sperm counts, high basal serum LH and FSH concentrations, and an exaggerated FSH response to GnRH suggests either that both testes are intrinsically abnormal or that the cryptorchid gonad somehow suppresses the function of the scrotal testis.

Clinical Features

A. Symptoms and Signs: There are usually no symptoms unless a complication such as testicular torsion, trauma, or malignant degeneration occurs. School-age children may have gender identity problems. Adults may complain of infertility, especially if they have a history of bilateral cryptorchidism.

Absence of one or both testes is the cardinal clinical finding. This may be associated with a small scrotum (bilateral cryptorchidism) or hemiscrotum (unilateral cryptorchidism). Signs of androgen deficiency are not present.

B. Laboratory Findings: Basal or stimulated serum FSH, LH, and testosterone concentrations are not helpful in evaluating prepubertal unilaterally cryptorchid males. However, serum FSH and LH concentrations and the testosterone response to exogenous chorionic gonadotropin are useful in differentiating cryptorchid patients from those with congenital anorchia. The latter have high basal gonadotropins, low serum testosterone, and absent or diminished testosterone rise following chorionic gonadotropin stimulation.

Postpubertal adults may have oligospermia, elevated basal serum FSH and LH concentrations, and an exaggerated FSH increase following GnRH stimulation. Such abnormalities are more prevalent in patients with a history of bilateral cryptorchidism than with unilateral cryptorchidism.

C. X-Ray Findings: Intravenous urography will disclose an associated abnormality of the upper urinary tract in 10% of cases—horseshoe kidney, renal hypoplasia, ureteral duplication, hydroureter, and hydronephrosis.

Differential Diagnosis

Retractile testis (pseudocryptorchidism) is due to a hyperactive cremasteric reflex, which draws the testicle into the inguinal canal. Cold temperature, fear, and genital manipulation commonly activate the reflex, which is most prominent between the ages of 5 and 6 years. The child should be examined with warm hands in a warm room. The testis can usually be "milked" into the scrotum with gentle pressure over the lower abdomen in the direction of the inguinal canal.

Bilateral anorchia is associated with elevated gonadotropins, decreased testosterone, and an absent or subnormal response to stimulation with chorionic gonadotropin.

The virilizing forms of congenital adrenal hyperplasia may result in prenatal fusion of the labial-scrotal folds and clitoral hypertrophy (see Chapter 15). Severely affected females have the appearance of phenotypic males with bilateral cryptorchidism. Because of the potentially disastrous consequences (acute adrenal insufficiency) if this diagnosis is missed, a buccal smear should be performed on bilaterally cryptorchid phenotypic male infants.

Complications & Sequelae

A. Hernia: Approximately 90% of cryptorchid males have associated ipsilateral inguinal hernia resulting from failure of the processus vaginalis to close. This is rarely symptomatic.

B. Torsion: Because of the abnormal connection between the cryptorchid testis and its supporting tissues, torsion may occur. This should be suspected in any patient with abdominal or pelvic pain and an ipsilateral empty scrotum.

C. Trauma: Testes that lie above the pubic tubercle are particularly susceptible to traumatic injury.

D. Neoplasms: A cryptorchid testis is 20–40 times more likely to undergo malignant degeneration than are normal testes. The incidence of such tumors is greater in patients with intra-abdominal testes than in patients with canalicular testes. Seminomas are the neoplasms most commonly associated with maldescended testes.

E. Infertility: Over 90% of untreated bilaterally cryptorchid males are infertile. About 30–50% of bilaterally cryptorchid patients who undergo prepubertal orchiopexy have been found to be fertile. About half of patients with untreated unilateral cryptorchidism are infertile, whereas infertility is found in less than one-fourth of such patients whose cryptorchidism is surgically repaired before puberty.

Prevention

Although cryptorchidism cannot be prevented, the complications can. It is clear that the adverse changes that take place in the testes are related in part to the location of the maldescended testis and the duration of the cryptorchidism. Most testes that are undescended at birth enter the scrotum during the first year of life. However, it is rare for a cryptorchid testis to descend spontaneously after the age of 1 year. Since adverse histologic changes have been noted around the age of 2 years, hormonal or surgical correction should be undertaken at or before that time.

Treatment

A. Medical Treatment:

1. Intramuscular chorionic gonadotropin therapy—Because growth of the vas deferens and testicular descent are at least partially dependent upon androgens, stimulation of endogenous testosterone secretion by chorionic gonadotropin may correct the cryptorchidism. Cryptorchidism is corrected in less than 25% of patients treated with a course of chorionic gonadotropin. Nevertheless, this therapy should be tried prior to orchiopexy, since it is innocuous and may avoid the need for surgery. For bilateral cryptorchidism, give a short course of chorionic gonadotropin consisting of 3300 units intramuscularly every other day over a 5-day period (3 injections). For unilateral cryptorchidism, give 500 units intramuscularly 3 times a week for 6½ weeks (20 injections).

2. Intranasal GnRH therapy—Recently, GnRH given 3 times a day for 28 days by nasal spray (Cryptolin) has been shown to be as effective as chorionic gonadotropin injections in correcting cryptorchidism. This preparation of GnRH has not yet been released for clinical use in the USA.

B. Surgical Treatment: Several procedures have been devised to place the maldescended testis into the scrotum (orchiopexy). The operation may be performed in one or 2 stages. Inguinal hernia should be repaired if present.

NOONAN'S SYNDROME
(Male Turner's Syndrome)

Phenotypic and genotypic males with many of the physical stigmas of classic Turner's syndrome have been described under a variety of names, including Noonan's syndrome, male Turner's syndrome, pseudo-Turner's syndrome, and Ullrich-Turner syndrome. The incidence and cause of this syndrome are unknown. It may occur sporadically or may be familial, inherited in an autosomal dominant fashion with variable penetrance. A number of pathologic features have been noted, including reduced seminiferous tubular size with or without sclerosis, diminished or absent germ cells, and Leydig cell hyperplasia.

Figure 13–14. Noonan's syndrome. Note ptosis and webbed neck. (Reproduced, with permission, from Bolton MR et al: *Ann Intern Med* 1974;**80**:626.)

Table 13–9. Clinical features of Noonan's syndrome.

Skin
Hyperelasticity
Dermatoglyphic abnormalities
Webbed neck
Nevi
Lymphedema
Low-set posterior hairline
Facial
Hypertelorism
Ptosis
Antimongoloid slant
Low-set ears
Misshapen auricles
Skeletal
Short stature
Short neck
Cubitus valgus
Pectus excavatum
Brachydactyly
High-arched palate
Dental malocclusion
Pes planus
Abnormal vertebrae
Cardiovascular
Pulmonary stenosis
Supravalvular pulmonary artery stenosis
Atrial septal defect
Coarctation of the aorta
Genitourinary
Cryptorchidism
Small testes
Horseshoe kidney
Miscellaneous
Mental retardation
Gynecomastia
Wide-spaced nipples

Clinical Features

A. Symptoms and Signs: (Fig 13– 14.) The most common clinical features are short stature, webbed neck, and cubitus valgus. Other somatic defects variably observed in these patients are listed in Table 13– 9. Congenital cardiac anomalies are common and involve primarily the right side of the heart—in contrast to patients with XO gonadal dysgenesis.

Cryptorchidism is frequently present. Although some affected individuals are fertile, with normal testes, most have small testes and mild to moderate hypogonadism.

B. Laboratory Findings: Serum testosterone concentrations are usually low or low normal, and serum gonadotropins are high. The karyotype is 46,XY.

Differential Diagnosis

The clinical features of Noonan's syndrome are sufficiently distinct so that confusion with other causes of hypogonadism is usually not a problem. However, a rare individual with XY/XO mosaicism may have similar somatic anomalies requiring chromosomal analysis for differentiation.

Treatment

If the patient is hypogonadal, androgen replacement therapy is indicated.

MYOTONIC DYSTROPHY

Myotonic dystrophy is one of the familial forms of muscular dystrophy. About 80% of affected males have some degree of primary testicular failure.

The disorder is transmitted in an autosomal dominant fashion, with marked variability in expression. The underlying cause is unknown, and no chromosomal abnormalities have been described.

Testicular histology varies from moderate derangement of spermatogenesis with germinal cell arrest to regional hyalinization and fibrosis of the seminiferous tubules. The Leydig cells are usually preserved and may appear in clumps.

The testes are normal in affected prepubertal individuals, and puberty generally proceeds normally. Testosterone secretion is normal, and secondary sexual characteristics develop. After puberty, seminiferous tubular atrophy results in a decrease in testicular size and change of consistency from firm to soft or mushy. Infertility is a consequence of disrupted spermatogenesis. If testicular hyalinization and fibrosis are extensive, Leydig cell function may also be impaired.

Figure 13–15. Myotonic dystrophy. Note myotonic facies with temporal baldness, ptosis, and wasting of the temporal and sternocleidomastoid muscles. (Reproduced, with permission, from Rimoin DL, Schimke RN: *Genetic Disorders of the Endocrine Glands.* Mosby, 1971.)

Clinical Features

A. Symptoms and Signs: (Fig 13–15.) The disease usually becomes apparent in adulthood. Progressive weakness and atrophy of the facial, neck, hand, and lower extremity muscles is commonly observed. Severe atrophy of the temporalis muscles, ptosis due to weakness of the levator muscles of the eye with compensatory wrinkling of the forehead muscles, and frontal baldness comprise the myopathic facies characteristic of the disorder. Myotonia is present in several muscle groups and is characterized by inability to relax the muscle normally after a strong contraction.

Testicular atrophy is not noted until adulthood, and most patients develop and maintain normal facial and body hair growth and libido. Gynecomastia is usually not present.

Associated features include mental retardation, cataracts, cranial hyperostosis, diabetes mellitus, and primary hypothyroidism.

B. Laboratory Findings: Serum testosterone is normal to slightly decreased. FSH is uniformly ele-

vated in patients with atrophic testes. LH is also frequently elevated, even in patients with normal serum testosterone levels. Leydig cell reserve is generally diminished, with subnormal increases in serum testosterone following stimulation with chorionic gonadotropin. An excessive rise in FSH and, to a lesser extent, LH is found following GnRH stimulation.

Differential Diagnosis

Myotonic dystrophy should be distinguished from forms of muscular dystrophy not associated with hypogonadism.

Treatment

There is no therapy that will prevent progressive muscular atrophy in this disorder. Testosterone replacement therapy is not indicated unless the serum testosterone levels are subnormal.

ADULT SEMINIFEROUS TUBULE FAILURE

Adult seminiferous tubule failure encompasses a spectrum of pathologic alterations of the seminiferous tubules that results in hypospermatogenesis, germinal cell arrest, germinal cell aplasia, and tubular hyalinization. Almost half of infertile males exhibit some degree of isolated seminiferous tubule failure.

Etiology, Pathology, & Pathophysiology

Etiologic factors in seminiferous tubule failure include mumps or gonococcal orchitis, leprosy, cryptorchidism, irradiation, uremia, alcoholism, paraplegia, lead poisoning, and therapy with antineoplastic agents such as cyclophosphamide, chlorambucil, vincristine, methotrexate, and procarbazine. Vascular insufficiency resulting from spermatic artery damage during herniorrhaphy, testicular torsion, or sickle cell anemia may also selectively damage the tubules. Similar pathologic changes may be found in oligospermic patients with varicoceles. In many patients, no etiologic factors can be identified, and the condition is referred to as "idiopathic."

The rapidly dividing germinal epithelium is more susceptible to injury than are the Sertoli or Leydig cells. Thus, pressure necrosis (eg, mumps or gonococcal orchitis), increased testicular temperature (eg, cryptorchidism and perhaps varicocele and paraplegia), and the direct cytotoxic effects of irradiation, alcohol, lead, and chemotherapeutic agents primarily injure the germ cells. Although the Sertoli and Leydig cells appear to be morphologically normal, severe testicular injury may result in functional alterations in these cells.

Several different lesions may be found in testicular biopsy specimens. The pathologic process may involve the entire testes or may appear in patches. The least severe lesion is hypospermatogenesis, in which all stages of spermatogenesis are present but there is a decrease in the number of germinal epithelial cells. Some degree of peritubular fibrosis may be present. Cessation of development at the primary spermatocyte or spermatogonial stage of the spermatogenic cycle is classified as germinal cell arrest. More severely affected testes may demonstrate a complete absence of germ cells with maintenance of morphologically normal Sertoli cells (Sertoli cell only syndrome). The most severe lesion is fibrosis or hyalinization of the tubules. This latter pattern may be indistinguishable from that seen in Klinefelter's syndrome.

Irrespective of the etiologic factors involved in damage to the germinal epithelium, the alterations in spermatogenesis result in oligospermia. If the damage is severe, as in the Sertoli cell only syndrome or tubular hyalinization, azoospermia may be present. Since testicular volume consists chiefly of tubules, some degree of testicular atrophy is often present in these patients. Some patients have elevations in basal serum FSH concentrations and demonstrate a hyper-responsive FSH rise following GnRH, suggesting that the Sertoli cells are functionally abnormal despite their normal histologic appearance.

Clinical Features

A. Symptoms and Signs: Infertility is usually the only complaint. Mild to moderate testicular atrophy may be present. Careful examination should be made for the presence of varicocele by palpating the spermatic cord during Valsalva's maneuver with the patient in the upright position. The patients are fully virilized, and gynecomastia is not present.

B. Laboratory Findings: Semen analysis shows oligospermia or azoospermia, and serum testosterone and LH concentrations are normal. Basal serum FSH levels may be normal or high, and an excessive FSH rise following GnRH may be present.

Differential Diagnosis

Patients with hypothalamic or pituitary disorders may have oligospermia or azoospermia and testicular atrophy. The serum FSH and LH concentrations are often in the low normal range, and the testosterone level is usually (not always) diminished. The presence of neurologic and ophthalmologic abnormalities, diabetes insipidus, anterior pituitary trophic hormone deficiencies, or an elevated serum PRL concentration distinguishes these patients from those with primary seminiferous tubule failure. Other causes of primary testicular failure are associated either with clinical signs and symptoms of androgen deficiency or with enough somatic abnormalities to allow differentiation from isolated seminiferous tubule failure.

Prevention

In many instances, damage to the seminiferous tubules cannot be prevented. Early correction of cryptorchidism, adequate shielding of the testes during diagnostic radiologic procedures or radiotherapy, and limitation of the total dose of chemotherapeutic agents may prevent or ameliorate the adverse effects.

Treatment

A. Medical Treatment: Attempts to treat oligospermia and infertility medically have included testosterone rebound therapy, low-dose testosterone, exogenous gonadotropins, thyroid hormone therapy, vitamins, and clomiphene citrate. None of these agents have been found to be uniformly beneficial, and several may actually lead to a decrease in the sperm count.

B. Surgical Treatment: Some of the pathologic changes in the testes have been reversed by early orchiopexy in cryptorchid individuals. If a varicocele is found in an oligospermic, infertile male, it should be ligated.

Course & Prognosis

Patients who have received up to 300 rads of testicular irradiation may show partial or full recovery of spermatogenesis months to years following exposure. The prognosis for recovery is better for individuals who receive the irradiation over a short interval than for those who are exposed over several weeks.

Recovery of spermatogenesis may also occur months to years following administration of chemotherapeutic agents. The most important factor determining prognosis is the total dose of chemotherapy administered.

Improvement in the quality of the semen is found in 60–80% of patients following successful repair of varicocele. Restoration of fertility has been reported in about half of such patients.

The prognosis for spontaneous improvement of idiopathic oligospermia due to infection or infarction is poor.

ADULT LEYDIG CELL FAILURE
(Male Climacteric Syndrome)

In contrast to the menopause in women, men do not experience an abrupt decline or cessation of gonadal function. However, a gradual diminution of testicular function does occur in many men as part of the aging process. It is not known how many men develop symptoms directly attributable to this phenomenon.

Etiology, Pathology, & Pathophysiology

There have been many studies of the relationships between age and testicular function, often with conflicting results. Several investigators have found that after age 50, there is a gradual decrease in the total serum testosterone concentration, although the actual values remain within the normal range. The levels of free testosterone decrease to a greater extent because of an increase in SHBG. The testosterone production rate declines, and Leydig cell responsiveness to hCG also decreases. A gradual compensatory increase in serum LH levels has also been noted. However, some studies on elderly men selected on the basis of their being in excellent physical health have shown no statistical changes in the basal levels of androgens and gonadotropins in comparison to younger healthy males.

Histologic studies of the aging testes have shown patchy degenerative changes in the seminiferous tubules with morphologically normal Leydig cells. The pathologic changes are first noted in the regions most remote from the arterial blood supply. Thus, microvascular insufficiency may be the etiologic basis for the histologic tubular changes and the decrease in Leydig cell function noted with aging. In addition, virtually all of the conditions that cause adult seminiferous tubule failure may lead to Leydig cell dysfunction if testicular injury is severe enough.

Clinical Features

A. Symptoms and Signs: A great many symptoms have been attributed to the male climacteric, including decreased libido and potency, emotional instability, fatigue, decreased concentrating ability, vasomotor instability (palpitations, hot flushes, diaphoresis), and a variety of diffuse aches and pains. There are usually no associated signs unless the testicular injury is severe. In such patients, a decrease in testicular volume and consistency may be present.

B. Laboratory Findings: Serum testosterone may be low or low normal; serum LH concentration is usually high normal or slightly high. Oligospermia is usually present.

C. Special Examinations: Because many men with complaints compatible with Leydig cell failure have testosterone and LH concentrations within the normal adult range, a diagnostic trial of testosterone therapy may be attempted. The test is best performed double-blind over an 8-week period. During the first or last 4 weeks, the patient receives testosterone enanthate, 200 mg intramuscularly per week; during the other 4-week period, placebo injections are administered. The patient is interviewed by the physician 2 weeks after the last course of injections. After the interview, the code is broken; if the patient notes amelioration of symptoms during the period of androgen administration but not during the placebo period, the diagnosis of adult Leydig cell failure is substantiated. If the patient experiences no subjective improvement following testosterone, or if improvement is noted following both placebo and testosterone injections, Leydig cell failure is effectively ruled out.

Differential Diagnosis

Impotence from vascular, neurologic, or psychologic causes must be distinguished from Leydig cell failure. A therapeutic trial of androgen therapy will not help impotence that is not due to androgen deficiency.

Treatment

Androgen replacement therapy is the treatment of choice for symptomatic Leydig cell failure.

IMPOTENCE

Impotence implies erectile dysfunction with or without associated disturbances of libido or ejaculatory ability. The overall prevalence of impotence in the general population is unknown, although it is likely that most men experience occasional episodes of impotence at some time during their lives.

Table 13–10. Organic causes of impotence.

Neurologic
  Anterior temporal lobe lesions
  Spinal cord lesions
  Autonomic neuropathy
Vascular
  Leriche's syndrome
  Pelvic vascular insufficiency
  Sickle cell disease
  Aging (?)
Endocrine
  Diabetes mellitus
  Hypogonadism
  Hyperprolactinemia
  Adrenal insufficiency
  Feminizing tumors
  Hypothyroidism
  Hyperthyroidism
Urogenital
  Trauma
  Castration
  Priapism
Systemic illness
  Cardiac insufficiency
  Cirrhosis
  Uremia
  Respiratory insufficiency
  Lead poisoning
Postoperative
  Aortoiliac or aortofemoral reconstruction
  Lumbar sympathectomy
  Perineal prostatectomy
  Retroperitoneal dissection
Drugs
  Alcohol
  Barbiturates
  Spironolactone
  Anticholinergics
  Estrogens
  Guanethidine
  Reserpine
  Methyldopa
  Ketoconazole
  Phenothiazines
  Butyrophenones
  Thiothixenes
  Tricyclic antidepressants
  Monoamine oxidase inhibitors
  Heroin
  Methadone
  Morphine
  Cocaine
  Amphetamines

Etiology & Pathophysiology

The physiology of erection and ejaculation is discussed in an earlier section of this chapter. Broadly speaking, erectile dysfunction may be divided into psychogenic and organic causes. Table 13–10 lists various pathologic conditions and drugs that may be associated with impotence. In many patients, however, impotence has a psychogenic basis. Fear, depression, anger, guilt, anxiety, and problems with interpersonal relationships may decrease libido and interfere with the ability to become sexually aroused or the ability to achieve and maintain an erection. Inhibition of sexual function is mediated through the central nervous system by poorly understood mechanisms.

Most organic causes of impotence result from disturbances in the neurologic pathways essential for the initiation and maintenance of erection (temporal lobe, spinal cord, peripheral and autonomic nerves) or in the blood supply to the penis (occlusion of the aortic bifurcation [Leriche's syndrome], pelvic vascular insufficiency, sickle cell disease, or microvascular insufficiency). Many of the endocrine disorders, systemic illnesses, and drugs associated with impotence affect libido, the autonomic pathways essential for erection, or the blood flow to the penis. Local urogenital disorders such as Peyronie's disease (idiopathic fibrosis of the covering sheath of the corpus cavernosum) may mechanically interfere with erection. In some patients, the cause of impotence is multifactorial. For example, some degree of erectile dysfunction is reported by over 50% of men with diabetes mellitus. The basis of the impotence is usually autonomic neuropathy. However, vascular insufficiency, antihypertensive medication, uremia, and depression may also cause or contribute to the problem in diabetics.

Clinical Features

A. Symptoms and Signs: Patients may complain of constant or episodic inability to initiate or maintain an erection, decreased penile turgidity, decreased libido, or a combination of these difficulties. Besides the specific sexual dysfunction symptoms, symptoms and signs of a more pervasive emotional or psychiatric problem may be elicited. If an underlying neurologic, vascular, or systemic disorder is the cause of impotence, additional symptoms and signs referable to the anatomic or metabolic disturbances may be present. A history of claudication of the buttocks or lower extremities should direct attention toward arteriovascular insufficiency.

The differentiation between psychogenic and organic impotence can usually be made on the basis of the history. Even though the patient may be selectively unable to obtain or maintain a satisfactory erection to complete sexual intercourse, a history of repeated normal erections at other times is indicative of psychogenic impotence. Thus, a history of erections that occur nocturnally, during masturbation, or during foreplay or with other sexual partners eliminates sig-nificant neurologic, vascular, or endocrine causes of impotence. Patients with psychogenic impotence often note a sudden onset of sexual dysfunction concurrently with a significant event in their lives such as loss of a friend or relative, an extramarital affair, or the loss of a job.

Patients with organic impotence generally note a more gradual and global loss of potency. They are unable to achieve a fully turgid erection under any circumstances. In contrast to patients with psychogenic impotence, patients with organic impotence generally maintain a normal libido. However, patients with systemic illness may have a concurrent diminution of libido and potency. Hypogonadism should be suspected in a patient who has never had an erection (primary impotence).

B. Laboratory Findings and Special Examinations: The integrity of the neurologic pathways and the ability of the blood vessels to deliver a sufficient amount of blood to the penis for erection to occur may be objectively examined by placement of a strain gauge behind the glans penis and at the base of the penis at the time the patient retires for sleep. The occurrence of nocturnal penile tumescence can thus be recorded. Normal men and those with psychogenic impotence have 3–5 erections a night associated with rapid eye movement (REM) sleep. Absence or reduced frequency of nocturnal tumescence indicates an organic lesion. A less cumbersome screening test can be carried out with a Snap-Gauge (Dacomed Corporation, Minneapolis, MN 55420), which consists of Velcro straps with 3 plastic connectors, each of which breaks at a defined tensile pressure.

Penile arterial blood pressure may be measured with a small pneumatic cuff wrapped around the base of the penis and connected to a manometer. Penile blood flow is monitored during inflation and deflation of the cuff by a Doppler ultrasound device. Comparison of ratio of penile systolic blood pressure with the brachial systolic blood pressure at rest and following exercise of the lower extremities is a useful technique for unmasking pelvic vascular insufficiency.

Neural innervation of the penis may be assessed by measurement of the bulbocavernosus reflex response latency period. This procedure is performed by electrical stimulation of the dorsal nerve to the penis, which evokes contraction of the bulbocavernosus muscle with a normal latency of 30–50 ms. Alternatively, since the autonomic pathways involved in erection and urination are the same, cystometrography with measurement of bladder capacity and residual urine may be used as an indirect measurement of penile innervation.

Serum PRL should be measured in all patients with cryptogenic organic impotence, since hyperprolactinemia, whether drug-induced or due to a pituitary or hypothalamic lesion, appears to inhibit the peripheral effects of androgens. In addition, testosterone measurements may uncover a mild and otherwise asymptomatic androgen deficiency. Because diabetes mellitus is a relatively common cause of impotence and impotence may be the presenting symptom of diabetes, fasting and 2-hour postprandial blood glucose measurements should be ordered. The choice of other laboratory tests depends upon associated organic symptoms or signs.

Treatment

A. Psychogenic Impotence: Simple reassurance and explanation, formal psychotherapy, and various forms of behavioral therapy have a reported 40–70% success rate. Androgen therapy should not be used in patients with psychogenic impotence, since androgens exert no more than a placebo effect and may focus the patient's attention on a nonexistent organic problem.

B. Organic Impotence: Discontinuation of an offending drug usually results in a return of potency. Similarly, effective therapy of an underlying systemic or endocrine disorder may cure the erectile dysfunction.

Patients with permanent impotence due to organic lesions that cannot be corrected should be counseled in noncoital sensate focus techniques. Alternatively, a penile prosthesis may be surgically implanted. Two major types of such prostheses have been developed. These include semirigid silicone rubber rods that are

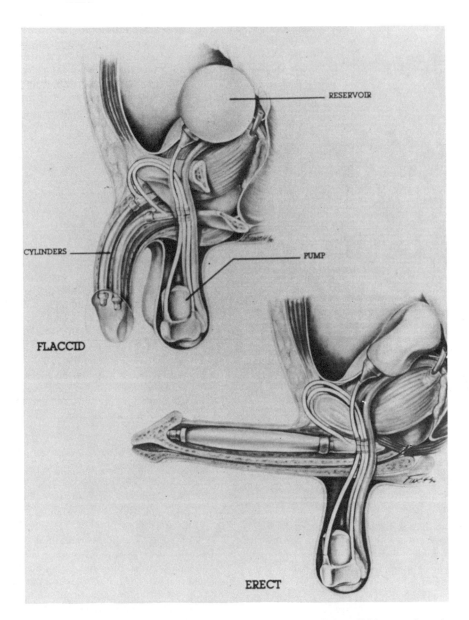

Figure 13–16. Inflatable penile prosthesis demonstrating position of 4 penile cylinders, fluid reservoir, and pump used for inflating or deflating the cylinders. (Courtesy of American Medical Systems, Inc., Minneapolis.)

implanted in the corpora (eg, Small-Carrion and Jonas protheses) or inflatable penile prostheses that allow the penis to remain flaccid until erection is desired (Fig 13–16). Both types of prostheses have given satisfactory results in 85–90% of cases.

MALE INFERTILITY

About 15% of married couples are unable to produce offspring. Female factors are responsible in about 40% of cases, male factors in about 40%, and couple factors in 20%.

Etiology & Pathophysiology

In order for conception to occur, spermatogenesis must be normal, the sperm must complete its maturation during transport through patent ducts, adequate amounts of seminal plasma must be added to provide volume and nutritional elements, and the male must be able to deposit the semen near the cervix. Any defect in this pathway can result in infertility, which is on the basis of a male factor problem. The spermatozoa must also be able to penetrate the cervical mucus and reach the uterine tubes, where conception takes place. These latter events may fail to occur if there are female reproductive tract disorders or abnormalities of sperm motility or fertilizing capacity.

Table 13–11 lists the identified causes of male infertility. About 9% of males evaluated for infertility have a disturbance of the hypothalamus, pituitary, adrenals, or thyroid. Sex chromosome abnormalities, cryptorchidism, and adult seminiferous tubule failure are found in 18% of infertile males. Almost 40% of cases of male infertility are associated with varicocele,

Table 13–11. Causes of male infertility.

Endocrine
    Hypothalamic-pituitary disorders
    Testicular disorders
    Defects of androgen action
    Hyperthyroidism
    Hypothyroidism
    Adrenal insufficiency
    Congenital adrenal hyperplasia
Systemic illness
Defects in spermatogenesis
    Immotile cilia syndrome
    Drug-induced
    Adult seminiferous tubule failure
Ductal obstruction
    Congenital
    Acquired
Seminal vesicle disease
Prostatic disease
Varicocele
Retrograde ejaculation
Antibodies to sperm or seminal plasma
Anatomic defects of the penis
Poor coital technique
Sexual dysfunction
Idiopathic

and 7% of patients have congenital or acquired ductal problems. Poor coital technique, sexual dysfunction, ejaculatory disturbances, and anatomic abnormalities such as hypospadias are etiologic factors in 8% of patients evaluated for infertility. Less common causes are autoimmune disturbances that lead to sperm agglutination and immobilization. Finally, in 5–6% of infertile males, no etiologic factor can be identified ("idiopathic").

Clinical Features

A. Symptoms and Signs: The clinical features of the hypothalamic-pituitary, thyroid, adrenal, testicular, and sexual dysfunctional disorders have been discussed in preceding sections of this chapter. Evaluation for the presence of varicocele has also been described.

Patients with immotile cilia syndrome have associated mucociliary transport defects in the lower airways that result in chronic pulmonary obstructive disease. Some patients with this disorder also have Kartagener's syndrome, with sinusitis, bronchiectasis, and situs inversus. Infections of the epididymis or vas deferens may be asymptomatic or associated with scrotal pain that may radiate to the flank, fever, epididymal swelling and tenderness, and urethral discharge. The presence of thickened, enlarged epididymis and vas is indicative of chronic epididymitis. Chronic prostatitis is usually asymptomatic, although a perineal aching sensation or low back pain may be described. A boggy or indurated prostate may be found on rectal palpation. A careful examination for the presence of penile anatomic abnormalities such as chordee, hypospadias, or epispadias should be made, since these defects may prevent the deposit of sperm in the vagina.

B. Laboratory Findings: A carefully collected and performed semen analysis is mandatory. A normal report indicates normal endocrine function and spermatogenesis and an intact transport system. Semen analysis should be followed by a postcoital test, which consists of examining a cervical mucus sample obtained within 2 hours after intercourse. The presence of large numbers of motile spermatozoa in mucus obtained from the internal os of the cervix rules out the male factor as a cause of infertility. If a postcoital test reveals necrospermia (dead sperm), asthenospermia (slow-moving sperm), or agglutination of sperm, examination of the female partner for the presence of sperm-immobilizing antibodies or cervical mucus abnormalities should be carried out.

If semen analysis shows abnormalities, at least 2 more specimens should be obtained at monthly intervals. Persistent oligospermia or azoospermia should be evaluated by studies outlined in Fig 13–12.

The wife should be thoroughly examined to verify patency of the uterus and uterine tubes, normal ovulation, and normal cervical mucus. This examination must be done even in the presence of a male factor abnormality, since infertility is due to a combination of male and female factors in about 20% of cases.

Treatment

A. Endocrine Disorders: Correction of hyperthyroidism, hypothyroidism, adrenal insufficiency, and congenital adrenal hyperplasia generally restores fertility. Patients with hypogonadotropic hypogonadism may have spermatogenesis initiated with gonadotropin therapy. Chorionic gonadotropin, 2000 units, and menotropins, 75 units, given intramuscularly 3 times a week, will restore spermatogenesis in most hypogonadotropic men. The sperm count following such therapy usually does not exceed 10 million/mL but may still allow impregnation. Patients with isolated deficiency of LH may respond to chorionic gonadotropin alone. There is no effective therapy for adult seminiferous tubule failure not associated with varicocele or cryptorchidism. However, if the oligospermia is mild (10–20 million/mL), cup insemination of the spouse with concentrates of semen may be tried. In vitro fertilization techniques are increasingly being utilized as a method for achieving pregnancy in couples in which the male is oligospermic.

B. Defects in Spermatogenesis: There is no treatment for immotile cilia syndrome or for chromosomal abnormalities associated with defective spermatogenesis. Drugs that interfere with spermatogenesis should be discontinued. These include the antimetabolites, phenytoin, marijuana, alcohol, monoamine oxidase inhibitors, and nitrofurantoin. Discontinuing use of these agents may be accompanied by restoration of normal sperm density.

C. Ductal Obstruction: Localized obstruction of the vas deferens may be treated by vasovasotomy. Sperms are detected in the ejaculate of 60–80% of patients following this procedure. However, the subsequent fertility rate is only 30–35%; the presence of antisperm antibodies that agglutinate or immobilize sperm probably accounts for the high failure rate.

Epididymovasostomy may be performed for epididymal obstruction. Sperm in the postoperative ejaculate have been found in approximately half of patients treated with this procedure, but subsequent fertility has been demonstrated in only 20% of cases.

D. Genital Tract Infections: Acute prostatitis may be treated with daily sitz baths, prostatic massage, and antibiotics. A combination of trimethoprim (400 mg) and sulfamethoxazole (2000 mg), twice a day for 10 days followed by the same dosage once a day for another 20 days, has been used with some success. Acute epididymitis may respond to injections of local anesthetic into the spermatic cord just above the testicle. Appropriate antibiotic therapy should also be given. The prognosis for fertility following severe bilateral chronic epididymitis or extensive scarring from acute epididymitis is poor.

E. Varicocele: The presence of varicocele in an infertile male with oligospermia is an indication for surgical ligation of the incompetent spermatic veins. Improvement in the semen is noted in 60–80% of treated patients, and about half are subsequently fertile.

F. Retrograde Ejaculation: Ejaculation of semen into the urinary bladder may occur following disruption of the internal bladder sphincter or with neuropathic disorders such as diabetic autonomic neuropathy. Normal ejaculation has been restored in a few patients with the latter problem following administration of phenylpropanolamine, 15 mg orally twice daily in timed-release capsules. Sperm can also be recovered from the bladder following masturbation for the purpose of direct insemination of the wife.

G. Antibodies to Sperm or Seminal Plasma: Antibodies in the female genital tract that agglutinate or immobilize sperm may be difficult to treat. One method that has enjoyed a modicum of success is condom therapy. Based on the assumption that women who have antibodies in their vaginal secretions have been transvaginally immunized against their husband's seminal plasma, it was postulated that removal of the antigenic stimulus would result in a decrease in the agglutinating or immobilizing factors. Condoms should be used during intercourse for 3–6 months while the wife maintains a basal body temperature chart. The couple then has unprotected intercourse at the time of the thermal (ovulatory) shift in basal body temperature. Pregnancy rates of about 50% have been reported with this regimen. Glucocorticoid therapy has also been associated with a decrease in antibodies to sperm and an increase in fertility.

H. Anatomic Defects of the Penis: Patients with hypospadias, epispadias, or severe chordee may collect semen by masturbation for use in insemination.

I. Poor Coital Technique: Couples should be counseled not to use vaginal lubricants or postcoital douches. In order to maximize the sperm count in cases of borderline oligospermia, intercourse should not be more frequent than every other day. Exposure of the cervix to the seminal plasma is increased by having the woman lie supine with her knees bent up for 20 minutes after intercourse.

Course & Prognosis

The prognosis for fertility depends upon the underlying cause. It is good for patients with nontesticular endocrine abnormalities, varicoceles, retrograde ejaculation, and anatomic defects of the penis. If fertility cannot be restored, the couple should be counseled regarding artificial donor insemination and adoption.

GYNECOMASTIA

Gynecomastia is common during the neonatal period and is present in about 70% of pubertal males. Clinically apparent gynecomastia has been noted at autopsy in almost 1% of adult males, and 40% of autopsied males have histologic evidence of gynecomastia.

Etiology & Pathophysiology

The causes of gynecomastia are listed in Table 13–12. Several mechanisms have been proposed to

Table 13–12. Causes of gynecomastia.

Physiologic
  Neonatal
  Pubertal
Drug-induced
  Amphetamines
  Androgens
  Chorionic gonadotropin
  Cimetidine
  Digitalis
  Estrogens
  Hydroxyzine
  Isoniazid
  Marijuana
  Meprobamate
  Methadone
  Methyldopa
  Phenothiazines
  Reserpine
  Spironolactone
Endocrine
  Primary hypogonadism with Leydig cell damage
  Hyperprolactinemia
  Hyperthyroidism
  Hypothyroidism
Systemic diseases
  Hepatic cirrhosis
  Uremia
  Recovery from malnourishment
Neoplasms
  Testicular germ cell or Leydig cell tumors
  Feminizing adrenocortical adenoma or carcinoma
  hCG-secreting nontrophoblastic neoplasms
Familial
Idiopathic

account for this disorder. All involve a relative imbalance between estrogen and androgen concentrations or action at the mammary gland level. Decrease in free testosterone may be due to primary gonadal disease or an increase in SHBG as is found in hyperthyroidism and some forms of liver disease (eg, alcoholic cirrhosis). Acute or chronic excessive stimulation of the Leydig cells by pituitary gonadotropins alters the steroidogenic pathways and favors excessive estrogen and estrogen precursor secretion relative to testosterone production. This mechanism may be responsible for the gynecomastia found with hypergonadotropic states such as Klinefelter's syndrome and adult Leydig cell failure. The rise of gonadotropins during puberty may lead to an estrogen-androgen imbalance by similar mechanisms. Patients who are malnourished or have systemic illness may develop gynecomastia during refeeding or treatment of the underlying disorder. Malnourishment and chronic illness are accompanied by a reduction in gonadotropin secretion, and during recovery the gonadotropins rise and may stimulate excessive Leydig cell production of estrogens relative to testosterone.

Excessive stimulation of Leydig cells may also occur in patients with hCG-producing trophoblastic or nontrophoblastic tumors. In addition, some of these tumors are able to convert estrogen precursors into estradiol. Feminizing adrenocortical and Leydig cell neoplasms may directly secrete excessive quantities of estrogens. The mechanisms by which PRL-secreting pituitary tumors and hyperprolactinemia produce gynecomastia are unclear. PRL may directly stimulate breast glandular development through its mammotropic action. Elevated serum PRL levels may also diminish the peripheral actions of testosterone, which may result in an excessive estrogen effect on the breast that is not counteracted by androgens.

Drugs such as phenothiazines, methyldopa, and reserpine may induce gynecomastia through elevations of PRL. Other drugs may reduce androgen production (eg, spironolactone), peripherally antagonize androgen action (spironolactone, cimetidine), or interact with breast estrogen receptors (spironolactone, digitalis, marijuana).

Finally, it has been proposed that patients with idiopathic and familial gynecomastia have breast glandular tissue that is inordinately sensitive to normal circulating levels of estrogens or excessively converts estrogen precursors to estrogens.

Pathology

Three histologic patterns of gynecomastia have been recognized. The florid pattern consists of an increase in the number of budding ducts, proliferation of the ductal epithelium, periductal edema, and a cellular fibroblastic stroma. The fibrous type has dilated ducts, minimal duct epithelial proliferation, no periductal edema, and a virtually acellular fibrous stroma. An intermediate pattern contains features of both types.

Although it has been proposed that different causes of gynecomastia are associated with either the florid or the fibrous pattern, it appears that the duration of gynecomastia is the most important factor in determining the pathologic picture. Approximately 75% of patients with gynecomastia of 4 months' duration or less exhibit the florid pattern, while 90% of patients with gynecomastia lasting a year or more have the fibrous type. Between 4 months and 1 year, 60% of patients have the intermediate pattern.

Clinical Features

A. Symptoms and Signs: The principal complaint is unilateral or bilateral concentric enlargement of breast glandular tissue. Nipple or breast pain is present in one-fourth of patients and objective tenderness in about 40%. A complaint of nipple discharge can be elicited in 4% of cases. Histologic examination has demonstrated that gynecomastia is almost always bilateral, although grossly it may be detected only on one side. The patient will often complain of discomfort in one breast despite obvious bilateral gynecomastia. Breast or nipple discomfort generally lasts less than 1 year. Chronic gynecomastia is usually asymptomatic, with the major complaint being the cosmetic one.

Symptoms and signs of underlying disorders may be present. Gynecomastia may be the earliest manifestation of an hCG-secreting testicular tumor; therefore, it is mandatory that careful examination of the testes be performed in any patient with gynecomastia. Enlargement, asymmetry, and induration of a testis may be noted in such patients.

B. Laboratory Findings: Serum hCG by the beta subunit radioimmunoassay method is the most sensitive test for detection of hCG-secreting neoplasms. Feminizing tumors of the adrenals or Leydig cells are associated with marked elevations of serum estradiol. However, most patients with gynecomastia not associated with these neoplasms have total serum estradiol levels within the normal range. Serum PRL and thyroid hormones should be measured to detect hyperprolactinemia and hyper- or hypothyroidism. If hyperprolactinemia is found in a patient who has been taking phenothiazines or other drugs that enhance PRL secretion, the drug should be withdrawn and the PRL concentration measured in 2–3 months.

C. X-Ray Findings: Chest x-ray may detect metastatic disease or an hCG-secreting primary lung neoplasm. CT scans of the pituitary-hypothalamic region should be performed if hyperprolactinemia is present. If gynecomastia is unilateral and especially if the "glandular" tissue is eccentric, mammograms should be taken to exclude breast carcinoma, which accounts for about 0.2% of all cancers in males.

D. Special Examinations: If small testes are found on physical examination, buccal smear or chromosomal analysis should be done, since Klinefelter's syndrome is one of the more common causes of persistent pubertal gynecomastia.

Differential Diagnosis

Gynecomastia should be differentiated from lipomas, neurofibromas, carcinoma of the breast, and obesity. Breast lipomas, neurofibromas, and carcinoma are usually unilateral, painless, and eccentric, whereas gynecomastia characteristically begins in the subareolar areas and enlarges concentrically. The differentiation between gynecomastia and enlarged breasts due to obesity may be difficult. The patient should be supine. Examination is performed by spreading the thumb and index fingers and gently palpating the breasts during slow apposition of the fingers toward the nipple. In this manner, a concentric ridge of tissue can be felt in patients with gynecomastia but not in obese patients without glandular tissue enlargement. The examination may be facilitated by applying soap and water to the breasts.

Complications & Sequelae

There are no complications other than possible psychologic damage from the cosmetic defect. Patients with gynecomastia may have a slightly increased risk of development of breast carcinoma.

Treatment

A. Specific Measures: The underlying disease should be corrected if possible, and offending drugs should be discontinued. Antiestrogens such as ta-

moxifen and clomiphene citrate have been found useful for relieving pain and reversing gynecomastia in a few patients. Whether this therapy will be useful in most patients with gynecomastia remains to be seen.

B. Surgical Treatment: Reduction mammoplasty should be considered for cosmetic reasons in any patient with long-standing gynecomastia that is in the fibrotic stage.

C. Radiation Therapy: Patients with prostatic carcinoma may receive low-dose radiation therapy (900 rads or less) to the breasts before initiation of estrogen therapy. This may prevent or diminish the gynecomastia that usually results from such therapy. Radiotherapy should not be given to other patients with gynecomastia.

Course & Prognosis

Pubertal gynecomastia usually regresses spontaneously over 1–2 years. Patients who develop drug-induced gynecomastia generally have complete or near-complete regression of the breast changes if the drug is discontinued during the early florid stage. Once gynecomastia from any cause has reached the fibrotic stage, little or no spontaneous regression occurs.

TESTICULAR TUMORS

Testicular neoplasms account for 1–2% of all male-related malignant neoplasms and 4–10% of all genitourinary neoplasms. They are the second most frequent type of cancer in men between 20 and 34 years of age. The incidence is 2–3 per 100,000 men in the USA and 4–6 per 100,000 men in Denmark. The incidence is lower in nonwhite than in white populations. Ninety-five percent of testicular tumors are of germ cell origin; 5% are composed of stromal or Leydig cell neoplasms.

Etiology

The cause of testicular tumors is not known. Predisposing factors include testicular maldescent and dysgenesis. About 4–12% of testicular tumors are found in association with cryptorchidism, and such a testicle has a 20- to 40-fold greater risk of developing a neoplasm than does a normally descended one. Almost 20% of testicular tumors associated with cryptorchidism arise in the contralateral scrotal testis, suggesting that testicular dysgenesis may be of etiologic importance in the development of germ cell neoplasms. Although trauma is frequently cited as an etiologic factor in testicular tumors, no causal relationship has been established. What is more likely is that testicular trauma serves to call the patient's attention to the presence of a testicular mass.

Pathology

A. Germ Cell Tumors: Seminomas account for 33–50% of all germ cell tumors. They are composed of round cells with abundant cytoplasm, prominent nuclei, and large nucleoli. The cells are arranged in cords and nests and have a thin delicate network of stromal connective tissue. Embryonal cell neoplasms comprise 20–33% of germ cell tumors. These tumors have multiple histologic patterns composed of cuboidal pleomorphic cells. One distinct pattern of cellular arrangement is the endodermal sinus tumor (yolk sac tumor), the most frequent germ cell neoplasm found in infants. Immunohistochemical techniques have localized alpha-fetoprotein to the embryonal cells. About 10% of germ cell tumors are teratomas, which are composed of well-differentiated cells derived from all 3 germ layers. When one or more of the teratoid elements are malignant or are mixed with embryonal carcinoma cells, the term teratocarcinoma is applied. These tumors account for one-tenth to one-third of germ cell neoplasms. Choriocarcinoma is the rarest form of germ cell tumor (2%) and is composed of masses of large, polymorphic, multinucleated syncytiotrophoblastic cells. Although pure choriocarcinoma is rare, many testicular tumors contain an occasional trophoblastic giant cell. Immunohistochemical techniques have shown that these cells are the source of hCG in such tumors.

B. Leydig Cell Tumors: Leydig cell (interstitial cell) tumors are rare. Most are benign and are composed of sheets of oval to polygonal cells arranged in lobules separated from one another by thin strands of connective tissue. Malignant Leydig cell tumor disseminates by both lymphatic and venous channels, with initial metastatic deposits being found in the regional lymph nodes, followed by metastases to liver, lung, and bone.

Pathophysiology

Bilateral gynecomastia is uncommon in patients who present with testicular cancer. It is generally associated with production of hCG by the trophoblastic elements in the tumor. The hCG stimulates the Leydig cells to produce excessive estrogens relative to androgen production, resulting in estrogen-androgen imbalance and gynecomastia. In addition, the trophoblastic tissue in some of the tumors may convert estrogen precursors to estrogens.

Clinical Features

A. Symptoms and Signs:

1. Germ cell tumors–Testicular tumors usually present as painless enlargement of a testicle with an associated feeling of fullness or heaviness in the scrotum. Thus, about 80% of patients note a testicular swelling or mass, whereas only 25% complain of testicular pain or tenderness. About 6–25% of patients give a history of testicular trauma that brought the testicular mass to their attention. Gynecomastia may be present initially in 2–4% of patients and develops subsequently in another 10%. About 5–10% of patients present with symptoms of distant metastatic disease, including backache, skeletal pains, gastrointestinal and abdominal pains, inguinal adenopathy, and neurologic dysfunction.

A testicular mass or generalized enlargement of the testis is often present on examination. In 5–10% of patients, a coexisting hydrocele may be present. In the presence of metastatic disease, supraclavicular and retroperitoneal lymph node enlargement may be present.

2. Leydig cell tumors–In children, Leydig cell tumors of the testes may produce sexual precocity, with rapid skeletal growth and development of secondary sexual characteristics. Adults with such tumors usually present with a testicular mass and occasionally gynecomastia. Decreased libido may also be present in such patients.

B. Laboratory Findings:

1. Germ cell tumors–The tumor markers hCG and alpha-fetoprotein should be measured in every male presenting with a testicular mass. hCG is found in the sera of 5–10% of males with seminoma, over half of patients with teratocarcinoma or embryonal cell carcinoma, and all patients with choriocarcinoma. hCG must be measured by the beta subunit radioimmunoassay method, since 44% of patients whose tumors produce hCG will not have detectable urinary hCG by the standard pregnancy tests. Elevated serum immunoreactive alpha-fetoprotein concentrations are found in almost 70% of patients with nonseminomatous forms of germ cell neoplasms. Both markers are elevated in over 50% of patients with nonseminomatous germ cell tumors, and at least one of the markers is elevated in 85% of such patients. These markers can also be used to monitor the results of therapy.

2. Leydig cell tumors–Urinary 17-ketosteroids and serum DHEA sulfate concentrations are increased. Both urinary and serum estrogen levels may also be increased. Serum testosterone concentrations tend to be low or within the normal adult range.

C. X-Ray Findings: Staging of testicular tumors requires several radiologic procedures, including chest tomograms, intravenous urograms, liver scans, gallium scans, and bipedal lymphangiography. CT scans of the abdomen and retroperitoneum have replaced lymphangiograms in many institutions.

Differential Diagnosis

Testicular tumors are sometimes misdiagnosed as epididymitis or epididymo-orchitis. An inflammatory reaction of the epididymis often involves the vas deferens. Therefore, both the vas and the epididymis will be thickened and tender on examination during the acute disease. Pyuria and fever also help to differentiate between epididymitis and testicular tumor. Because hydrocele may coexist with testicular tumor, the testes should be carefully examined following aspiration of the hydrocele.

Other conditions that can cause confusion with testicular tumors include inguinal hernia, hematocele, hematoma, torsion, spermatocele, varicocele, and (rarely) sarcoidosis, tuberculosis, and syphilitic gumma. Ultrasonic examination of the scrotum may help distinguish between testicular tumors and extra-testicular disease such as acute or chronic epididymitis, spermatocele, or hydrocele.

Benign Leydig cell tumors of the testes must be differentiated from adrenal rest tumors in patients with congenital adrenal hyperplasia. Since the testes and the adrenals are derived from the same embryologic source, ectopic adrenal tissue may be found to migrate with the testes. This tissue can enlarge under the influence of ACTH in patients with congenital adrenal hyperplasia or Cushing's disease. Adrenal rest tumors tend to be bilateral, whereas patients with Leydig cell tumors generally have unilateral disease. Both may be associated with elevated urine 17-ketosteroids and elevated serum DHEA sulfate concentrations. Elevated serum and urinary estrogen concentrations are found with both disorders. However, patients with congenital adrenal hyperplasia or Cushing's disease will have a decrease in 17-ketosteroids, DHEA sulfate, and estrogen concentrations, as well as a decrease in tumor size, following administration of dexamethasone.

Treatment

A. Germ Cell Tumors: Seminomas are quite radiosensitive, and disease localized to the testes is usually treated with orchiectomy and 2000–4000 rads of conventional radiotherapy delivered to the ipsilateral inguinal-iliac and bilateral para-aortic lymph nodes to the level of the diaphragm. For disease that has spread to the lymph nodes below the diaphragm, additional whole abdominal radiotherapy and prophylactic mediastinal and supraclavicular lymph node irradiation are usually given. Widely disseminated disease is generally treated with a combination of radiotherapy and chemotherapy, especially with alkylating agents.

Nonseminomatous tumors are treated with orchiectomy, retroperitoneal lymph node dissection, and, if necessary, radiotherapy or chemotherapy (or both). Although many chemotherapeutic agents have been used, combinations of vinblastine, bleomycin, and cisplatin currently appear to produce the best overall results. Patients with nonseminomatous tumors treated by these means should be monitored with serial measurements of serum hCG and alpha-fetoprotein.

B. Leydig Cell Tumors: Benign Leydig cell tumors of the testes are treated by unilateral orchiectomy. Objective remissions of malignant Leydig cell tumors have been noted following treatment with mitotane.

Course & Prognosis

A. Germ Cell Tumors: In patients with seminoma confined to the testicle, the 5-year survival rates after orchiectomy and radiotherapy are 98–100%. Disease in the lymph nodes below the diaphragm also has an excellent prognosis, with 5-year survival rates of 80–85%. Disease above the diaphragm and disseminated disease have 5-year survival rates as low as 18%.

In patients with nonseminomatous germ cell tumors, aggressive surgery and combination chemotherapy have raised the 5-year survival rates from less than 20% to 60–90%.

B. Leydig Cell Tumors: Removal of a benign Leydig cell tumor is accompanied by regression of precocious puberty in children or feminization in adults. The prognosis for malignant Leydig cell tumor is poor, with most patients surviving less than 2 years from the time of diagnosis.

REFERENCES

Anatomy & Structure-Function Relationships

Amelar RD, Dubin L, Walsh PC: *Male Infertility.* Saunders, 1977.

Fawcett DW: The cell biology of gametogenesis in the male. *Perspect Biol Med* 1979;**2:**S56.

Hafez ESE: *Human Semen and Fertility Regulation in Men.* Mosby, 1976.

Lipshultz LI, Howards SS (editors): *Infertility in the Male.* Churchill Livingstone, 1983.

Physiology

Brooks RV: Androgens. *Clin Endocrinol Metab* 1975;**4:**503.

deGroat WC, Booth AM: Physiology of male sexual function. *Ann Intern Med* 1980;**92(Part 2):**329.

James VHT, Serio M, Martini L: *The Endocrine Function of the Human Testis.* Vol 2. Academic Press, 1974.

Jeffcoate SL: The control of testicular function in the adult. *Clin Endocrinol Metab* 1975;**4:**521.

Newman HF, Reiss H, Northup JD: Physical basis of emission, ejaculation, and orgasm in the male. *Urology* 1982;**19:**341.

Odell WD, Swerdloff RS: Abnormalities of gonadal function in men. *Clin Endocrinol* 1978;**8:**149.

Steinberger E: Hormonal regulation of the seminiferous tubule function. *Curr Top Mol Endocrinol* 1975;**2:**337.

Weiss HD: The physiology of human penile erection. *Ann Intern Med* 1972;**76:**793.

Evaluation of Male Gonadal Function

Baker HWG, Hudson B: Male gonadal dysfunction. *Clin Endocrinol Metab* 1974;**3:**507.

Blasco L: Clinical tests of sperm fertilizing ability. *Fertil Steril* 1984;**41:**177.

Forest MG: How should we perform the human chorionic gonadotrophin (hCG) stimulation test? *Int J Androl* 1983;**6:**1.

Goldzieher JW et al: Improving the diagnostic reliability of rapidly fluctuating plasma hormone levels by optimized multiple-sampling techniques. *J Clin Endocrinol Metab* 1976;**43:**824.

Marshall JC: Investigative procedures. *Clin Endocrinol Metab* 1975;**4:**545.

Nieschlag E: Hormone diagnosis in male hypogonadism and infertility. *Horm Res* 1978;**9:**394.

Penny R: The testis. *Pediatr Clin North Am* 1979;**26:** 107.

Sandow J: Clinical applications of LHRH and its analogues. *Clin Endocrinol* 1983;**18:**571.

Schonfeld WA: Primary and secondary sexual characteristics: Study of their development in males from birth through maturity, with biometric study of penis and testes. *Am J Dis Child* 1943;**65:**535.

Zachmann M et al: Testicular volume during adolescence: Cross-sectional and longitudinal studies. *Helv Paediatr Acta* 1974;**29:**61.

Pharmacology of Drugs Used in Treatment

Davidson JM, Camargo CA, Smith ER: Effects of androgen on sexual behavior in hypogonadal men. *J Clin Endocrinol Metab* 1979;**48:**955.

Garcia CR et al (editors): *Current Therapy of Infertility 1984–1985*. D.C. Decker, 1984.

London DR: Medical aspects of hypogonadism. *Clin Endocrinol Metab* 1975;**4:**597.

Snyder PJ: Clinical use of androgens. *Annu Rev Med* 1984;**35:**207.

Steinberger E: Medical treatment of male infertility. *Andrologia* 1976;**8(Suppl 1):**77.

Klinefelter's Syndrome & Variants

Baghdassarian A et al: Testicular function in XXY men. *Johns Hopkins Med J* 1975;**136:**15.

de la Chapelle A: Analytic review: Nature and origin of males with XX sex chromosomes. *Am J Hum Genet* 1972;**24:**71.

Federman DD: *Abnormal Sexual Development: A Genetic and Endocrine Approach to Differential Diagnosis*. Saunders, 1968.

Ferguson-Smith MA: Sex chromatin, Klinefelter's syndrome and mental deficiency. Page 280 in: *The Sex Chromatin*. Moor KL (editor). Saunders, 1966.

Ishida H et al: Studies on pituitary-gonadal endocrine function in XYY men. *J Urol* 1979;**121:**190.

Ratcliffe SG: The sexual development of boys with the chromosome constitution 47,XXY (Klinefelter's syndrome). *Clin Endocrinol Metab* 1982;**11:**703.

Rimoin DL, Schimke RN: *Genetic Disorders of the Endocrine Glands*. Mosby, 1971.

Schiavi RC et al: Pituitary-gonadal function in XYY and XXY men identified in a population survey. *Clin Endocrinol* 1978;**9:**233.

Walzer S, Gerald PS, Shah SA: The XYY genotype. *Annu Rev Med* 1978;**29:**563.

Zuppinger K et al: Klinefelter's syndrome: A clinical and cytogenetic study in 24 cases. *Acta Endocrinol* 1967; **54(Suppl 113):**5.

Anorchia

Abeyaratne MR, Aherne WA, Scott JES: The vanishing testis. *Lancet* 1969;**2:**822.

Kirschner MA, Jacobs JB, Fraley EE: Bilateral anorchia with persistent testosterone production. *N Engl J Med* 1970;**282:**240.

Tosi SE, Morin LJ: The vanishing testis syndrome: Indications for conservative therapy. *J Urol* 1976;**115:**758.

Leydig Cell Aplasia

Lee PA et al: Leydig cell hypofunction resulting in male pseudohermaphroditism. *Fertil Steril* 1982;**37:**675.

Cryptorchidism

Getzoff PL: Surgical aspects of infertility. *Clin Endocrinol Metab* 1975;**4:**693.

Lipshultz LI: Cryptorchidism in the subfertile male. *Fertil Steril* 1976;**27:**609.

Rajfer J (editor): Cryptorchidism. *Urol Clin North Am* 1982;**9:**315.

Noonan's Syndrome

Collins E, Turner G: The Noonan syndrome: A review of the clinical and genetic features of 27 cases. *J Pediatr* 1973;**83:**941.

Schoen E: Diminished testicular function in "male Turner's syndrome." *J Clin Endocrinol Metab* 1965;**25:**101.

Myotonic Dystrophy

Febres F et al: Hypothalamic-pituitary-gonadal function in patients with myotonic dystrophy. *J Clin Endocrinol Metab* 1975;**41:**833.

Takeda R, Ueda M: Pituitary-gonadal function in male patients with myotonic dystrophy: Serum luteinizing hormone, follicle stimulating hormone, and testosterone levels and histological damage of the testis. *Acta Endocrinol* 1977;**84:**382.

Adult Seminiferous Tubule Failure

Abbasi AA et al: Gonadal function abnormalities in sickle cell anemia. *Ann Intern Med* 1976;**85:**601.

Ash PA: The influence of radiation on fertility in man. *Br J Radiol* 1980;**53:**271.

Braunstein GD, Dahlgren J, Loriaux DL: Hypogonadism in chronically lead-poisoned men. *Infertility* 1978;**1:**33.

de Kretser DM: The effects of systemic disease on the function of the testis. *Clin Endocrinol Metab* 1979;**8:**487.

Holdsworth S et al: The pituitary-testicular axis in men with chronic renal failure. *N Engl J Med* 1977;**296:**1245.

Johnsen SG, Agger P: Quantitative evaluation of testicular biopsies before and after operation for varicocele. *Fertil Steril* 1978;**29:**58.

Kikuchi TA et al: The pituitary-gonadal axis in spinal cord injury. *Fertil Steril* 1976;**27:**1142.

Morley JE, Melmed S: Gonadal dysfunction in systemic disorders. *Metabolism* 1979;**28:**1051.

Schilsky RL et al: Gonadal dysfunction in patients receiving chemotherapy for cancer. *Ann Intern Med* 1980;**93:**109.

Van Thiel DH, Lester R: The effect of chronic alcohol abuse on sexual function. *Clin Endocrinol Metab* 1979; **8:**499.

Adult Leydig Cell Failure

Baker HWG et al: Changes in the pituitary-testicular system with age. *Clin Endocrinol* 1976;**5:**349.

Hallberg MC et al: Impaired Leydig cell reserve and altered serum androgen binding in the aging male. *Fertil Steril* 1976;**27:**812.

Stearns EL et al: Declining testicular function with age: Hormonal and clinical correlates. *Am J Med* 1974;**57:**761.

Werner AA: The male climacteric: Report of two hundred and seventy-three cases. *JAMA* 1946;**132:**188.

Impotence

Blasco L: Clinical tests of sperm fertilizing ability. *Fertil Steril* 1984;**41:**177.

Ellenberg M: Sexual function in diabetic patients. *Ann Intern Med* 1980;**92(Part 2):**331.

Krane RJ, Siroky MB, Goldstein I (editors): *Male Sexual Dysfunction*. Little, Brown, 1983.

Reckless J, Geiger N: Impotence as a practical problem. *DM* (May) 1975;**3.**

Sacks SA: Evaluation of impotence: Comprehensive, compassionate approach. *Postgrad Med* (Oct) 1983;**74:**182.

Schiavi RC: Male erectile disorders. *Annu Rev Med* 1981; **32:**509.

Schurmeyer TH, Nieschlag E: Effect of ketoconazole and other imidazole fungicides on testosterone biosynthesis. *Acta Endocrinol* 1984;**105:**275.

Scott FB, Fishman IJ, Light JK: An inflatable penile prosthesis for treatment of diabetic impotence. *Ann Intern Med* 1980;**92(Part 2):**340.

Male Infertility

Cockett ATK, Takihara H, Cosentino MJ: The varicocele. *Fertil Steril* 1984;**41:**5.

Dubin L, Amelar RD: Etiologic factors in 1294 consecutive cases of male infertility. *Fertil Steril* 1971;**22:**469.

Eliasson R et al: The immotile-cilia syndrome: A congenital ciliary abnormality as an etiologic factor in chronic airway infections and male sterility. *N Engl J Med* 1977;**297:**1.

Howards SS et al: Symposium on male infertility. *Urol Clin North Am* 1978;**5:**433.

Jones WR: Immunologic infertility: Fact or fiction? *Fertil Steril* 1980;**33:**577.

Mathur S et al: Clinical significance of sperm antibodies in infertility. *Fertil Steril* 1981;**36:**486.

Ross LS: Diagnosis and treatment of infertile men: A clinical perspective. *J Urol* 1983;**130:**847.

Schill WB: Recent progress in pharmacological therapy of male subfertility: A review. *Andrologia* 1979;**11:**77.

Wong TW et al: Pathological aspects of the infertile testis. *Urol Clin North Am* 1978;**5:**503.

Gynecomastia

Bannayan GA, Hajdu SI: Gynecomastia: Clinicopathologic study of 351 cases. *Am J Clin Pathol* 1972;**57:**431.

Carlson HE: Gynecomastia. *N Engl J Med* 1980;**303:**795.

Chopra IJ et al: Alterations in circulating estradiol-17β in male patients with Graves' disease. *N Engl J Med* 1972;**286:**124.

Cook S, Rodriguez-Antunez A: Pre-estrogen irradiation of the breast to prevent gynecomastia. *Am J Roentgenol Radium Ther Nucl Med* 1973;**117:**662.

Jeffreys DB: Painful gynaecomastia treated with tamoxifen. *Br Med J* 1979;**2:**1119.

Nicolis SL, Modlinger RS, Gabrilove JL: A study of the histopathology of human gynecomastia. *J Clin Endocrinol Metab* 1971;**32:**173.

Williams MJ: Gynecomastia: Its incidence, recognition and host characterization in 447 autopsy cases. *Am J Med* 1963;**34:**103.

Wilson JD, Aiman J, McDonald PC: The pathogenesis of gynecomastia. *Adv Intern Med* 1980;**25:**1.

Testicular Tumors

Azer PC, Braunstein GD: Malignant Leydig cell tumor: Objective tumor response to *o,p'*-DDD. *Cancer* 1981;**47:**1251.

Braunstein GD et al: Germ cell tumors of the testes. *West J Med* 1977;**126:**362.

Catalona WJ: Current management of testicular tumors. *Surg Clin North Am* 1982;**62:**1119.

Damjanov I, Katz SM, Jewett MAS: Leydig cell tumors of the testis. *Ann Clin Lab Sci* 1979;**9:**157.

Einhorn LH, Williams SD: Chemotherapy of disseminated testicular cancer: A random prospective study. *Cancer* 1980;**46:**1339.

Hajdu SI: Pathology of germ cell tumors of the testis. *Semin Oncol* 1979;**6:**14.

Johnson DE: *Testicular Tumors*, 2nd ed. Medical Examination Publishing, 1976.

Peckham MJ, McElwain TJ: Testicular tumors. *Clin Endocrinol Metab* 1975;**4:**665.

Sample WF et al: Gray scale ultrasound of the scrotum. *Radiology* 1978;**127:**225.

Scardino PT et al: The value of serum tumor markers in the staging and prognosis of germ cell tumors of the testis. *J Urol* 1977;**118:**994.

The Ovaries

14

Alan Goldfien, MD, & Scott E. Monroe, MD

ANATOMY OF THE OVARIES

The mature ovaries are paired nodular structures $2.5-5 \times 2 \times 1$ cm, weighing from 4 to 8 g, the weight varying during the menstrual cycle. They are situated behind the peritoneum attached to the posterior surface of the broad ligament by a fold of the peritoneum called the mesovarium, which contains the blood vessels and nerves leading to the hilum. The ovaries are attached to the uterus by the ovarian ligament and lie in close association with the uterine tubes (oviducts, fallopian tubes) (Fig 14–1).

The ovaries develop from the genital ridges situated between the base of the dorsal mesentery and the mesonephros on either side of the coelomic cavity. The primordial germ cells that originate in the endoderm of the yolk sac at the third week begin to migrate through the hindgut to invade the genital ridges at about the sixth week. These primary oocytes are

Acronyms Used in This Chapter

ACTH	Adrenocorticotropic hormone
BSP	Bromsulphalein
CBG	Corticosteroid-binding globulin
DHEA	Dehydroepiandrosterone
EI	Eosinophilic index
FSH	Follicle-stimulating hormone
GH	Growth hormone
GnRH	Gonadotropin-releasing hormone
hCG	Human chorionic gonadotropin
HDL	High-density lipoprotein(s)
KPI	Karyopyknotic index
LDL	Low-density lipoprotein(s)
LH	Luteinizing hormone
MCR	Metabolic clearance rate
MI	Maturation index
mRNA	Messenger ribonucleic acid
PMN	Polymorphonuclear neutrophil
PRL	Prolactin
PTH	Parathyroid hormone
RNA	Ribonucleic acid
SGPT	Serum glutamic-pyruvic transaminase
SHBG	Sex hormone-binding globulin
TBG	Thyroid hormone-binding globulin
TSH	Thyroid-stimulating hormone (thyrotropin)
VLDL	Very low density lipoprotein(s)

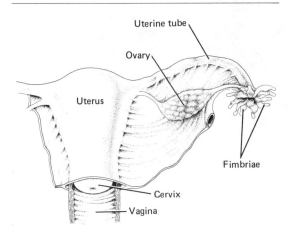

Figure 14–1. Internal organs of the female reproductive system: ovary, fimbriae of infundibulum, uterine tube, uterus, cervix, and vagina. (Reproduced, with permission, from Junqueira LC, Carneiro J: *Basic Histology,* 4th ed. Lange, 1983.)

surrounded by a layer of epithelium and mesenchymal cells that give rise to the primordial follicles. About 1700 germ cells are present before migration to the genital ridge begins; however, these multiply during the process of migration and within the genital ridge, reaching a peak of 7 million oocytes at mid gestation. The primordial germ cells increase in size early in their development and become oogonia. At mid gestation they begin the first meiotic division, becoming primary oocytes. This prophase lasts until just before ovulation, which may occur 12–40 years later. In this state, they are no longer capable of multiplication and in fact steadily decline in number (Fig 14–2). About 400 ova are lost through the process of ovulation during a woman's lifetime. The remainder undergo degeneration so that, by the time of the menopause, few are present.

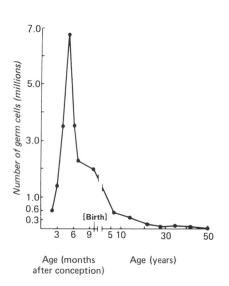

Figure 14–2. Total number of germ cells in the human ovary at different ages. (Reproduced, with permission, from Baker TG: *Reproduction in Mammals.* Austin CR, Short RV [editors]. Cambridge Univ Press, 1972.)

Blood Supply

The arterial vessels supplying the ovary are derived from branches of the ovarian and uterine arteries that enter through the mesovarium and divide into branches leading into the stroma of the medulla and then to the cortex. The small arteries of the ovary are characteristically spiral. The capillary blood gathers in veins that form a large, thin-walled plexus of vessels called the pampiniform plexus, leaving the ovary by way of the ovarian vein at the hilum. Lymphatics arise in the outer or cortical portion of the ovary and anastomose centrally, leaving through the hilum. Although the lymphatic channels are numerous in the theca externa, corpora lutea, and corpora albicantia, they are not seen in the theca interna, granulosa, or tunica albuginea.

Nerve Supply

The ovary has a rich autonomic innervation arising from the intermesenteric nerves and renal plexus; from the superior hypogastric plexus or presacral nerve and the hypogastric nerve; and from the inferior hypogastric plexus or pelvic plexus. The nerves appear to be mainly sympathetic in origin.

Microscopic Anatomy

As shown in Fig 14–3, the ovary consists of many

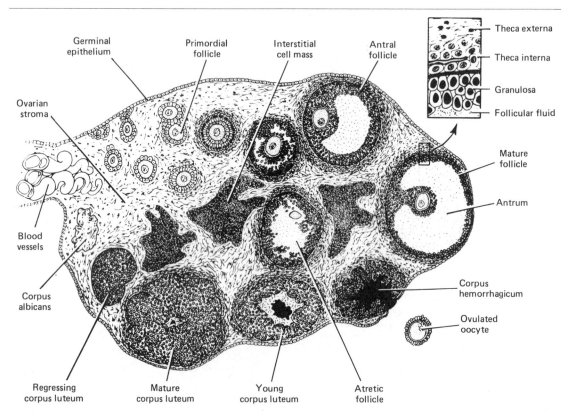

Figure 14–3. Diagram of a mammalian ovary, showing the sequential development of a follicle, formation of a corpus luteum, and, in the center, follicular atresia. A section of the wall of a mature follicle is enlarged at the upper right. The interstitial cell mass is not prominent in primates. (After Patten & Eakin. Reproduced, with permission, from Katzung BG [editor]: *Basic & Clinical Pharmacology,* 2nd ed. Lange, 1984.)

different structures. The mature ovary is covered by a layer of columnar cells that constitute the **germinal epithelium.** The dense layer of connective tissue under the epithelium is called the tunica albuginea. The remainder of the organ is divided into outer cortical and inner medullary portions, of which the cortex is the larger. The cortex contains follicular structures in all stages of development, surrounded by the connective tissue elements of the stroma and the hilar cells, a group of steroid-secreting cells that histologically resemble the Leydig, or interstitial, cells of the testes. The medulla consists of a connective tissue stroma containing elastic fibers, blood vessels, nerves, lymphatics, and smooth muscle fibers.

The follicular complex contains the ova as well as the cells responsible for production of the ovarian hormones and their precursors. Structural changes and hormonal activity that occur throughout the menstrual cycle are discussed below.

HORMONES OF THE OVARY

The mature ovary actively synthesizes and secretes a variety of hormones. Among these are the steroids, which include estrogens, progesterone, androgens, and their precursors. In addition, the ovary produces relaxin, prostaglandins, and other substances.

THE STEROID HORMONES

The ovary is normally the major source of estrogens, although the conversion of androgen precursors in other tissues is clinically important after the menopause and in some women with disorders of ovarian function. The ovary also produces and secretes large amounts of progesterone during the luteal phase of the cycle. It is also the source of small amounts of testosterone and other androgens that serve not only as precursors to estrogen synthesis but also are released into the circulation to act on peripheral tissues.

Biosynthesis of Steroid Hormones

The biochemical pathways, including the major enzymes and their intracellular localizations, are similar in the ovary, testis, and adrenal. The process in the ovary is outlined in Fig 14–4. The steroid hormones are synthesized from cholesterol, which is present in the gland both free and esterified to fatty acids (cholesteryl esters). Cholesterol derived either from circulating lipoproteins or from cholesteryl esters in the gland is converted to pregnenolone by removal of

Figure 14–4. Biosynthesis and metabolism of estrogens. (Reproduced, with permission, from Katzung BG [editor]: *Basic & Clinical Pharmacology,* 2nd ed. Lange, 1984.)

Table 14–1. Concentrations, metabolic clearance rates (MCR), production rates, and ovarian secretion rates of steroids in blood.*

	MCR (L/d)	Phase of Menstrual Cycle	Plasma Concentration (μg/dL)	Production Rate (mg/d)	Secretion Rate (Both Ovaries) (mg/d)
Estradiol	1350	Early follicular	0.006	0.081	0.07
		Late follicular	0.033–0.07	0.445–0.945	0.4–0.8
		Midluteal	0.02	0.27	0.25
Estrone	2210	Early follicular	0.005	0.11	0.08
		Late follicular	0.015–0.03	0.331–0.662	0.25–0.5
		Midluteal	0.011	0.243	0.16
Progesterone	2200	Follicular	0.095	2.1	1.5
		Luteal	1.13	25	24
Androstenedione	2010	...	0.159	3.2	0.8–1.6
Testosterone	690	...	0.038	0.26	...
Dehydroepiandrosterone	1640	...	0.49	8	0.3–3
Dihydrotestosterone	400	...	0.02	0.05	0.01–0.02

*Modified from Lipsett, MB: Steroid hormones. Page 84 in: *Reproductive Endocrinology.* Yen SSC, Jaffe RB (editors). Saunders, 1978.

a 6-carbon fragment, isocaproic acid. This reaction or group of reactions is the rate-limiting step in the biosynthetic process and is controlled by luteinizing hormone (LH) from the anterior pituitary.

Pregnenolone formed by this reaction may be converted either to progesterone or to 17α-hydroxypregnenolone. The conversion to progesterone requires the action of 3β-hydroxysteroid dehydrogenase and $\Delta^{5,4}$-ketosteroid isomerase, which shifts the double bond from the Δ^5 to the Δ^4 position. Progesterone is secreted by the corpus luteum in large amounts following ovulation (see below). However, it also serves as a precursor for androgen and estrogen, since it is a substrate for 17α-hydroxylase, which converts it to 17α-hydroxyprogesterone in the endoplasmic reticulum. Following 17α-hydroxylation, the 2-carbon (20–21) side chain may be cleaved by the C17,20-lyase enzyme to form androgens.

17α-Hydroxypregnenolone is converted by the lyase enzyme to dehydroepiandrosterone (DHEA). This compound can then be converted to androstenedione. The relative importance of these pathways to androgen production is not clear. Androstenedione is the major androgen secreted by the ovary, but small amounts of DHEA and testosterone are also released.

Estradiol, the major estrogen produced by the ovary, is synthesized by a group of enzymes known as the aromatase complex or system. The process involves 3 steps: hydroxylation of the methyl group at carbon 19, oxidation of this group, and hydroxylation at the 3α position. These steps are thought to occur in the microsomal fraction.

During the menstrual cycle, regulation of biosynthesis and release is controlled by the gonadotropins as well as by local factors.

Secretion of Steroid Hormones

The secretory activity of the steroid-producing granulosa and theca cells is closely coupled to their biosynthetic activity, since little hormone is stored in the cells. Direct measures of secretion rates in humans are difficult to obtain, because they require an accurate measure of the concentration of the hormone in the effluent blood from the gland and a measure of blood flow through the gland. Such samples and measurements are difficult to obtain without interfering with blood flow and normal gland activity. Therefore, indirect measures have been widely used. Some of the most useful information has been obtained by measuring the metabolic clearance rate (MCR) with an in vivo isotope dilution technique. Multiplying MCR by the concentration of the hormone in blood provides a total production rate for the hormone. However, the production rate also includes production of the hormone at other sites from circulating precursors, and it may therefore be greater than the amount secreted by the gland. The production rates, plasma levels, and MCRs of various ovarian steroids are shown in Table 14–1.

During pregnancy, the fetal-placental unit produces a large amount of steroid hormone. The placenta produces progesterone, which is released into the maternal circulation, and large amounts of pregnenolone, which is released into the fetal circulation. Enzymatic conversion of pregnenolone by the fetal adrenal and liver produces steroids, including 16-hydroxydehydroepiandrosterone sulfate, which are subsequently converted to estriol and other estrogens in the placenta and released into the maternal circulation (see Chapter 17).

Transport of Steroid Hormones

When released into the circulation, the gonadal steroids bind to plasma proteins. Estradiol binds avidly to a transport globulin called sex hormone–binding globulin (SHBG) and binds with less affinity to albumin. Progesterone binds strongly to corticosteroid-binding globulin (CBG) and weakly to albumin. The percentages of various steroids that bind to these carrier proteins are listed in Table 14–2. The concen-

Table 14—2. Total plasma concentration and percentage of steroid hormone that is free or bound to plasma transport proteins in normal women in the early follicular phase. During the luteal phase, the total concentrations of estradiol (0.72 nmol/L) and progesterone (38 nmol/L) are higher, but the distribution is the same.*

	Total Plasma Concentration (nmol/L)	Percentage Distribution of Steroid			
		Free	SHBG	CBG	Albumin
Estradiol	0.29	1.81	37.3	0.1	60.8
Estrone	0.23	3.58	16.3	0.1	80.1
Progesterone	0.65	2.36	0.63	17.7	79.3
Testosterone	1.3	1.36	66	2.26	30.4
Dihydrotestosterone	0.65	0.47	78.4	0.12	21
Androstenedione	5.4	7.54	6.63	1.37	84.5
Cortisol	400	3.77	0.18	89.7	6.33

*Data from Dunn JF, Nisula BC, Rodbard D: *J Clin Endocrinol Metab* 1981;**53**:58.

tration of these binding proteins is increased by estrogen and thyroxine and decreased by androgens and progestins. SHBG is synthesized in the liver, and because its synthesis is stimulated by estrogens and inhibited by androgen, levels are twice as high in women as in men. The proportions of free and bound estradiol do not vary significantly during the menstrual cycle. However, differences in binding may assume clinical importance after the menopause or in women with abnormal ovarian function.

Metabolism of Steroid Hormones

A. Progesterone: Progesterone is rapidly cleared from the circulation, having an initial half-life of about 5 minutes. As indicated by its high clearance rate (Table 14–1), it is rapidly converted to pregnanediol and conjugated to glucuronic acid in the liver. Pregnanediol glucuronide is excreted in the urine and may be used as an index of progesterone production. In addition, small amounts of 20α-hydroxyprogesterone are formed (Fig 14–5). This compound has one-fifth the activity of progesterone.

B. Estrogens: Circulating estradiol is rapidly converted in the liver to estrone by 17β-hydroxysteroid dehydrogenase (Fig 14–5). Some of the estrone reenters the circulation; however, most of it is further metabolized to 16α-hydroxyestrone (which is then converted to estriol) or to 2-hydroxyestrone. Much of the estrone is conjugated to form estrone sulfate. Estriol is converted largely to form estriol 3-sulfate-16-glucuronide before excretion by the kidney.

Physiologic Effects of Steroid Hormones

The biologic effects of the ovarian steroids are mediated by specific hormone receptors (see Chapter 1). The steroids enter cells by passive diffusion but only bind to specific receptor proteins in the cytoplasm of their target cells. These receptors, upon binding to the hormone, undergo transformation and move to the nucleus, where the complexes bind to specific sites on the chromosome. The hormone dissociates slowly from this binding site. This interaction with the gene

leads to the synthesis of specific messenger RNA (mRNA).

There are estimated to be between 5000 and 20,000 receptor molecules per cell. These receptors also serve as sites for regulation of hormonal activity. For example, estrogens induce development of increased numbers of estrogen receptors in some tissues and also stimulate the synthesis of progesterone receptors. By contrast, progesterone may cause a reduction in the number of estrogen and progesterone receptors.

Although it is clear that these intracellular receptors mediate many of the important effects of steroid hormones, some effects, such as the anesthetic effect of progesterone and the stimulatory effect of estrogens on uterine blood flow, suggest that these steroids also act at the cell membrane.

A. Estrogens: Estrogens are required for the normal maturation of the female. They stimulate the development of the vagina, uterus, and uterine tubes as well as the secondary sex characteristics. They stimulate stromal development and ductal growth in the breast and are responsible for the accelerated growth phase and the closing of the epiphyses of the long bones that occurs at puberty. They alter the distribution of body fat so as to produce typical female body contours, including some accumulation of body fat around the hips and breasts. Larger quantities also stimulate development of pigmentation in the skin, most prominently in the region of the nipples and areolae and in the genital region.

In addition to its effects on growth of uterine muscle, estrogen also plays an important role in development of the endometrial lining. Continuous exposure to estrogens for prolonged periods leads to an abnormal hyperplasia of the endometrium that is usually associated with abnormal bleeding patterns. When estrogen production is properly coordinated with the production of progesterone during the normal human menstrual cycle, regular periodic bleeding and shedding of the endometrial lining occur.

Estrogens have a number of important metabolic effects. They seem to be partially responsible for maintenance of the normal structure of the skin and

Figure 14–5. Metabolism of ovarian steroid hormones.

blood vessels in women. Estrogens decrease the rate of resorption of bone by antagonizing the effect of parathyroid hormone (PTH) on bone; they do not stimulate bone formation. Estrogens may have important effects on intestinal absorption, because they reduce the motility of bowel. In addition to stimulating the synthesis of enzymes leading to uterine growth, they alter the production and activity of many other enzymes in the body. In the liver, there is an increase in the synthesis of binding or transport proteins, including those for estrogen, testosterone, and thyroxine.

Estrogens enhance the coagulability of blood. Many changes in factors influencing coagulation have been reported, including increased circulating levels of factors II, VII, IX, and X. Increased plasminogen levels and decreased platelet adhesiveness have been reported.

Alterations in the composition of the plasma lipids caused by estrogens include an increase in high-density lipoproteins (HDL), a slight reduction in low-density lipoproteins (LDL), and a reduction in plasma cholesterol levels. Plasma triglyceride levels are increased.

Estrogens have many other effects. They are responsible for estrous behavior in animals and influence libido in humans. They facilitate the loss of intravascular fluid into the extracellular space, producing edema. The resulting decrease in plasma volume causes a compensatory retention of sodium and water by the kidney. Estrogens also modulate sympathetic nervous system control of smooth muscle function.

B. Progesterone: The effects of progesterone on reproductive organs include the glandular development of the breasts and the cyclic glandular development of the endometrium described below (see Menstrual Cycle) and are critical for successful reproduction. However, progesterone exhibits important metabolic effects in other organs and tissues. It effects changes in carbohydrate, protein, and lipid metabolism.

A dose of 50 mg of progesterone intramuscularly daily can lead to increased insulin levels and decreased response of blood glucose levels to insulin as observed in normal pregnancy.

Progesterone can compete with aldosterone at the renal tubule, causing a decrease in Na^+ reabsorption. This leads to an increased secretion of aldosterone by the adrenal cortex—eg, in pregnancy. Progesterone increases the body temperature in humans. The mechanism of this effect is not known, but an alteration of the temperature-regulating centers in the hypothalamus has been suggested. Progesterone also alters the function of the respiratory centers. The ventilatory response to CO_2 is increased, leading to a measurable reduction in arterial and alveolar P_{CO_2} during pregnancy and in the luteal phase of the menstrual cycle. Synthetic progestins with an ethinyl group do not have these respiratory effects. Progesterone and related steroids also have hypnotic effects on the brain.

C. Androgens: The normal ovary produces small amounts of androgens, including testosterone, dihydrotestosterone, androstenedione, Δ^5-androstenediol, and DHEA. Only testosterone and dihydrotestosterone have significant biologic activity, although androstenedione is converted to testosterone in peripheral tissues. The normal woman produces less than 300 μg of testosterone in 24 hours, and about one-fourth of this is probably formed in the ovary directly. The physiologic significance of these small amounts of androgens is not established, but they may be partly responsible for normal hair growth at puberty and may have other important metabolic effects. Androgen production by the ovary may be markedly increased in some abnormal states (usually in association with amenorrhea), and weakly active precursors may be converted to active hormones in target tissues such as the hair follicle.

RELAXIN

Relaxin is a polypeptide that has been extracted from the ovary. In certain animal species, it appears to play an important role at the time of parturition, causing relaxation of the pelvic ligaments and softening of the uterine cervix. The 3-dimensional structure of relaxin is similar to that of insulin and related growth-promoting polypeptides, although the amino acid sequences are different. It consists of 2 chains linked by disulfide bonds, cleaved from a prohormone. It is found in the ovary, placenta, and uterus and in the blood. Relaxin synthesis has been demonstrated in luteinized granulosa cells of the corpus luteum. In addition to changing the mechanical properties of tissues such as the cervix and pubic ligaments, it increases glycogen synthesis and water uptake by the myometrium and decreases its contractility. It may also have mammotropic effects.

In women, relaxin has been measured by immunoassay. During the menstrual cycle, levels were highest immediately after the LH surge and during menstruation. Circulating levels of relaxin are reported to be 25% higher by the end of the first trimester than during the second and third trimesters. Relaxin has not been shown to be clinically useful in patients with dysmenorrhea or premature labor or during prolonged labor.

OTHER OVARIAN HORMONES

The ovary also produces one or more substances that may decrease the pituitary release of follicle-stimulating hormone (FSH) in a manner similar to inhibin produced by the testis. This activity has been found in follicular fluid, but its structure, activity, and distribution remain to be defined.

THE MENSTRUAL CYCLE

The female reproductive system undergoes a series of regular cyclic changes termed the menstrual cycle. The most obvious of these changes is periodic vaginal bleeding, resulting from shedding of the endometrial lining of the uterus. Normal menstrual function results from the interaction of the hypothalamus, pituitary, and ovaries and associated changes in the target tissues of the reproductive tract. Although each component is essential for normal reproductive function, the ovary plays a central role in this process, since it appears to be responsible for regulating both the cyclic changes and the length of the menstrual cycle. In most women in the middle reproductive years, menstrual bleeding recurs every 25–35 days, with a median cycle length of 28 days (Fig 14–6). In women with ovulatory cycles, the interval from the onset of menses to ovulation—the proliferative (follicular) phase—is variable in duration and accounts for the range of cycle lengths observed in ovulating women. The interval from ovulation to the onset of menstrual bleeding—the secretory (luteal) phase—is relatively constant and averages 14 ± 2 days in most women. The greatest variability in cycle length is found in the first few years after menarche and the years immediately preceding the menopause. There is a high incidence of anovulatory vaginal bleeding at these times.

HORMONAL PROFILES DURING THE MENSTRUAL CYCLE

Pituitary Gonadotropins

Luteinizing hormone (LH) and follicle-stimulating hormone (FSH) are glycoproteins with molecular weights of about 28,000 and 33,000, respectively. Each hormone is composed of an alpha subunit and a beta subunit. The alpha subunits have essentially the same amino acid sequences. The beta subunits, however, are unique and are responsible for the characteristic biologic activities of each hormone. The initial plasma half-life of LH is 30 minutes, whereas the half-life of FSH is 3 hours. The profiles of LH and FSH throughout the menstrual cycle are illustrated in Fig 14–7. Because of the diversity of standards

used to quantitate gonadotropins, the LH and FSH values for the same serum sample reported by different laboratories may vary 2- or 3-fold. The clinician must therefore be aware of the laboratory's upper and lower limits of normal. Serum FSH levels persistently greater than 40 mIU/mL (milli-International Units of the Second International Reference Preparation of Human Menopausal Gonadotropin; mIU-2nd IRP-HMG) usually indicate declining or absent ovarian follicular activity.

In the normal menstrual cycle, serum concentrations of both LH and FSH begin to increase a few days prior to menses. FSH concentrations initially increase more rapidly than those of LH and attain maximum levels during the first half of the follicular phase. FSH levels gradually decline in the latter half of the follicular phase and, with the exception of a brief peak at midcycle, continue to fall until the lowest concentrations in the cycle are reached during the second half of the luteal phase. The preovulatory decline in serum concentrations of FSH is a consequence

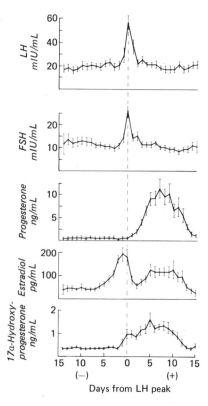

Figure 14–7. Mean values of LH, FSH, progesterone, estradiol, and 17α-hydroxyprogesterone in daily serum samples from 9 women during ovulatory menstrual cycles. Data from different cycles have been combined using the day of the midcycle LH peak as the reference day (day 0). The vertical bars represent one standard error of the mean. (Reproduced, with permission, from Thorneycroft IH et al: *Am J Obstet Gynecol* 1971;**111**:947.)

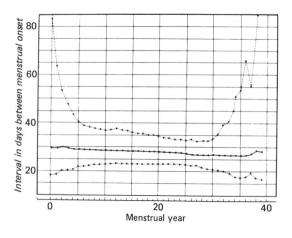

Figure 14–6. Median lengths of menstrual cycles (solid line) throughout reproductive life in women from menarche (year 0) to menopause (year 40). Ninety percent of all cycles fall within the upper and lower dotted lines. (After Treolar AE et al. Reproduced, with permission, from Yen SSC, Jaffe RB [editors]: *Reproductive Endocrinology.* Saunders, 1978.)

of the rising concentration of estradiol in this period. LH levels increase gradually throughout the follicular phase. At midcycle, there is a large peak in serum concentration of LH (midcycle LH surge) lasting 1–3 days. Subsequently, LH levels gradually decline, also reaching their lowest concentrations late in the luteal phase. Frequent measurements of serum gonadotropin levels in individual women indicate that gonadotropin secretion—particularly LH—is pulsatile, with intervals of 1–4 hours between pulses depending on the phase of the menstrual cycle. These pulses are also dependent upon the pulsatile secretion of GnRH by the hypothalamus.

Prolactin (PRL)

In contrast to LH and FSH profiles, there are no consistent cyclic changes in individual PRL profiles during the normal menstrual cycle. In studies of large numbers of women, however, mean PRL levels in the preovulatory and luteal phases of the menstrual cycle may be slightly higher than in the follicular phase. There is also a significant diurnal variation in plasma concentrations of PRL, with peak levels during the night and early morning hours. Laboratories vary in their reporting of PRL levels (as they do also in reporting gonadotropin levels) because of the use of standards with different biologic and immunologic potencies. The upper limit of normal may thus vary from 15 ng/mL to 30 ng/mL, depending upon the laboratory.

Ovarian Steroids

The ovary secretes progestins, androgens, and estrogens. Many of these steroids are also secreted by the adrenal gland or can be formed by peripheral conversion of other steroid precursors; consequently, plasma concentrations of these hormones may not directly reflect ovarian steroidogenic activity. Table 14–1 summarizes the plasma concentrations, metabolic clearance rates, and production rates of the major steroids secreted by the ovary in normal women.

A. Estrogens: Estradiol (E_2) is perhaps the most important secretory product of the ovary, because of its biologic potency and diverse physiologic effects on peripheral target tissues. Plasma concentrations of estradiol during the first half of the follicular phase are low, generally less than 50 pg/mL (Fig 14–7). About 1 week prior to the midcycle gonadotropin surge, estradiol concentrations begin to increase rapidly, and peak levels of approximately 200–300 pg/mL are attained on the day preceding—or, less commonly, the day of—the LH surge. The rise in plasma estradiol levels correlates closely with the increase in size of the preovulatory follicle. After the LH surge, serum estradiol levels fall rapidly for several days. There is a secondary increase in plasma estradiol levels in the midportion of the luteal phase, reflecting estrogen secretion by the corpus luteum. Plasma patterns of estrone during the menstrual cycle are similar to those of estradiol, but the changes in concentrations are less than those of estradiol; thus, the ratio of

estrone to estradiol varies throughout the cycle. The ratio is highest at the time of menses, when estradiol secretion is minimal, and lowest in the preovulatory period, when estradiol secretion is maximal. While most of the estradiol in the peripheral circulation results from direct ovarian secretion, a significant fraction of the circulating estrone arises from estradiol and the peripheral conversion of androstenedione. Catheterization studies have shown that increased plasma concentrations of estradiol in the preovulatory and midluteal phases of the cycle principally reflect secretion from the ovary containing the dominant or preovulatory follicle, which later becomes the corpus luteum.

B. Progesterone: Throughout the follicular phase, serum concentrations of progesterone are low—less than 1 ng/mL. At the time of the LH surge, there is a small increase in plasma concentrations of progesterone, followed by a rise over the next 4–5 days (Fig 14–7). Progesterone levels reach a plateau at concentrations between 10 and 20 ng/mL during the midportion of the luteal phase. Thereafter, progesterone levels decline rapidly, reaching concentrations of about 1 ng/mL by the first day of menses. Although catheterization studies have shown that progesterone is secreted by both ovaries during the first half of the follicular phase, most of the circulating progesterone at this time appears to be derived from the extraglandular conversion of the adrenal steroids, pregnenolone and pregnenolone sulfate, and from the direct secretion of small amounts of progesterone by the adrenal glands. During the luteal phase of the cycle, virtually all of the circulating progesterone arises by direct secretion from the corpus luteum. Measurement of plasma concentrations of progesterone is widely used to monitor ovulation. Concentrations greater than 4 or 5 ng/mL suggest that ovulation has occurred. To fully assess corpus luteum function and to exclude an inadequate luteal phase in women with unexplained infertility, several progesterone determinations throughout the luteal phase may be required.

C. Androgens: In normal women, circulating androgens can be derived from secretion by the ovaries and the adrenal glands and also by peripheral conversion of steroid precursors of ovarian and adrenal origin. The plasma profiles of androstenedione and testosterone throughout the menstrual cycle are summarized in Fig 14–8. In normal women, testosterone is secreted in small quantities by the ovaries and adrenal glands. About 50–70% of the circulating testosterone, however, arises primarily from the peripheral conversion of androstenedione. Mean plasma concentrations of testosterone range from 0.2 ng/mL to 0.4 ng/mL during most of the follicular and luteal phases and increase slightly in the preovulatory phase. Androstenedione arises primarily from direct secretion by the ovaries and adrenal glands. Only a small percentage (about 10%) is formed by peripheral conversion. Secretion of androstenedione by the adrenal does not vary significantly during different phases of the menstrual cycle, although there is a diurnal variation

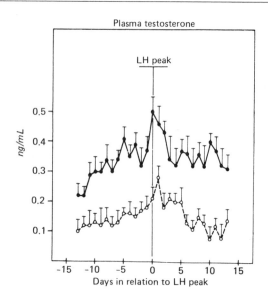

Figure 14–8. Patterns and levels (mean ± SEM) of plasma androstenedione (at left) and plasma testosterone (at right) during 2 consecutive menstrual cycles in 6 women. The women received no treatment during the first cycle (control; solid dots connected by solid lines). The adrenal cortex was suppressed by dexamethasone (open dots connected by dashed lines) during the second cycle. (Reproduced, with permission, from Abraham GE: *J Clin Endocrinol Metab* 1974;**39**:340.)

in adrenal secretion of androstenedione similar to that of cortisol. Ovarian secretion of androstenedione, however, fluctuates throughout the menstrual cycle, and the pattern of secretion resembles that of estradiol. Serum concentrations of androstenedione increase in the late follicular phase of the cycle and are maximal at the time of the midcycle gonadotropin surge. There is a small secondary peak of androstenedione during the midluteal phase. Plasma concentrations of both DHEA and DHEA sulfate vary independently of the phase of the menstrual cycle. Both hormones, especially DHEA sulfate, are secreted primarily by the adrenal gland.

THE OVARIAN CYCLE

Ovarian Structure

Throughout adult reproductive years, the structural composition and hormonal activity of the ovary are continually changing (Figs 14–3 and 14–9). These changes in composition and activity are responsible for many of the physiologic events in the normal menstrual cycle. The 2 major functions of the adult ovary—the synthesis and secretion of sex steroids and the release of a mature ovum every 28–30 days—normally progress in concert with one another and are closely interrelated. The basic reproductive unit of the ovary is the small **primordial follicle,** consisting of (1) a small oocyte (< 25 μm in diameter) arrested in the diplotene stage of meiotic prophase; (2) a few or a complete ring of poorly differentiated granulosa cells;

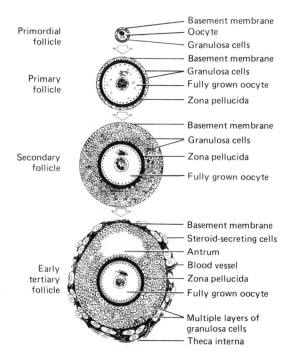

Figure 14–9. Morphologic changes that occur in ovarian follicles during growth and development. (Reproduced, with permission, from Erickson GF: Follicular growth and development. Chapter 12 in: *Gynecology and Obstetrics.* Vol 5. Sciarra JJ [editor]. Harper & Row, 1981.)

and (3) a basement membrane that surrounds the granulosa cells, separating them from the adjacent ovarian stroma. Primordial follicles are found principally in the outer cortex just beneath the fibrous capsule of the ovary. These primordial follicles constitute an inactive or resting pool from which all ovulatory follicles will eventually develop. During late fetal life and throughout the prepubertal years, a small percentage of these small, inactive follicles are continually resuming growth. At an early stage of development and prior to antrum formation, however, growth is arrested and the follicles undergo atresia. Although ovulation does not occur, the continual process of limited growth and atresia in the prepubertal ovary depletes a large portion of the small primordial follicles, so that only about 400,000 primordial follicles remain at puberty (Fig 14–2). Of these follicles, only about 400 will reach full development and release an oocyte during ovulation in the adult.

The earliest morphologic change indicating that the primordial follicle has left the pool of resting follicles and resumed the process of growth is an increase in size of the oocyte. As the oocyte enlarges, the zona pellucida, a membrane that will eventually surround the oocyte, begins to form. The flat, poorly differentiated granulosa cells, which form a single layer, assume a cuboid shape as the oocyte approaches its maximum size of 80–100 μm. At this stage of development, the follicular unit is known as a **primary follicle.** Subsequently, the granulosa cells rapidly proliferate, forming a multilayered covering around the oocyte. Small patches of fluid form between the granulosa cells. Blood vessels, however, do not penetrate the basement membrane surrounding the granulosa cells, and the granulosa layer remains avascular until after ovulation has occurred. As the follicle continues to enlarge, cells that are indistinguishable from mesenchymal fibroblasts align themselves concentrically outside the basement membrane. These cells form the thecal layer and complete the formation of the **secondary follicle (preantral follicle).** As the granulosa cells continue to multiply, there is further production and accumulation of fluid within the granulosa cell layer, leading to the formation of a follicular cavity, or **antrum.** The oocyte and a portion of the surrounding granulosa cells (cumulus cells) are gradually displaced to one side of the follicular cavity, and a **tertiary follicle (antral follicle)** is formed. There is both a rapid accumulation of follicular fluid and additional growth of granulosa cells, causing further enlargement of the **preovulatory (graafian) follicle.** The follicle reaches a diameter of 2–2.5 cm shortly before ovulation. Following ovulation, the antrum fills with blood and lymph fluid (Fig 14–3). The wall of the follicle collapses and becomes convoluted, and vessels from the thecal layer invade the granulosa layer. The appearance of the granulosa cells changes markedly after ovulation, and they become luteinized. In conjunction with the contiguous thecal layer or adjacent stromal cells, the luteinized granulosa layer forms the corpus luteum. If pregnancy does not follow ovulation, the corpus luteum lasts about 14 days and is gradually replaced by fibrous tissue, forming a **corpus albicans.** The mechanisms responsible for regression (luteolysis) of the corpus luteum after 14 days in women are unknown. In nonprimates, prostaglandins appear to play an important role in luteolysis.

Control of Growth & Steroidogenesis in Ovarian Follicles

The factors that stimulate resting primordial follicles to resume growth and development are unknown. Pituitary gonadotropins, however, are not involved in initiating these events. Cohorts of primordial follicles in prepubertal girls—in whom LH and FSH levels are undetectable—and in hypophysectomized laboratory animals are continually leaving the large pool of inactive primordial follicles and resuming growth. Development beyond the preantral or early antral stage, however, depends upon the interaction of pituitary gonadotropins, ovarian steroids, and other local factors within the follicle.

Receptors for FSH have been found only in granulosa cells. Each cell is estimated to contain about 1000 receptors. The binding of FSH to its receptor stimulates the synthesis of enzymes which have aromatase activity and which convert androgen precursors to estrogens. Estradiol, in turn, plays a critical role in follicular growth and development both by a local effect on granulosa cells and via positive and negative feedback regulation of FSH and LH secretion (see below). In small follicles, estradiol induces the proliferation of granulosa cells. In the absence of FSH, estradiol per se can stimulate follicular growth to the preantral stage, but further development is dependent upon gonadotropin stimulation. FSH and estradiol, working in concert, also induce the formation of LH receptor in granulosa cells. In contrast to FSH receptors, which are restricted to granulosa cells, LH receptors also have been found in theca, interstitial, and luteal cells.

The cellular origin of estradiol in large ovarian follicles in primates remains controversial. In the rat, granulosa cells lack the enzymes 17α-hydroxylase and C17,20 lyase and thus are unable to directly synthesize androgens or estrogens from C21 precursors—eg, progesterone or pregnenolone. Therefore, estradiol production by granulosa cells is dependent upon the availability of C19 androgenic precursors (testosterone and androstenedione), which can be aromatized to estrogens. These observations have led to the formation of the "2-cell theory" to explain estradiol formation within the follicular complex (Fig 14–10). According to this hypothesis, LH stimulates the synthesis of androgenic precursors, primarily androstenedione and to a lesser extent testosterone, by the theca cells. The androgens diffuse across the basement membrane that separates the theca and granulosa cells. Some of the androstenedione and testosterone enters the antral fluid, while the remainder is converted to estradiol by the granulosa cells. Studies in primates, however, have shown that both the thecal layer and the granulosa

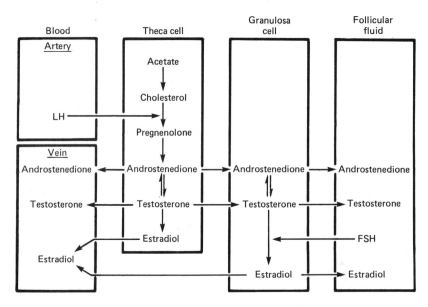

Figure 14–10. Pathways involved in the synthesis and secretion of androgens and estradiol by the preovulatory follicle. In primates, it is not known if the theca cells or granulosa cells are the major source for estradiol in plasma. (Reproduced, with permission, from Peters H, McNatty KP: *The Ovary: A Correlation of Structure and Function in Mammals.* Granada Publishing, 1980.)

cells of antral follicles are able to synthesize estradiol; consequently, it is unclear whether it is the theca cells or the granulosa cells that are the principal site of estradiol synthesis in the mid and late follicular phases of the menstrual cycle. A study in the rhesus monkey suggested that most of the estradiol production in the preovulatory period was of theca cell—not granulosa cell—origin. It is possible that most of the estradiol produced by the granulosa cells remains within the follicular fluid, while estradiol in the serum arises primarily from the thecal layer.

In the normal ovary, androgens produced by the thecal layer—particularly androstenedione—serve, in part, as precursors of estrogen synthesis by granulosa cells. Androgens utilized in this fashion thus indirectly facilitate follicular growth via estradiol stimulation. However, high concentrations of testosterone or dihydrotestosterone—or increased ratios of androgen to estrogen—have been found in follicles undergoing atresia, and this suggests an inhibitory action of androgens on follicular development. This could explain, in part, the lack of normal follicular development in polycystic ovary syndrome. In this disorder, high levels of LH may promote excessive androgen production by the thecal layer. Since FSH levels are low, granulosa cells may have a reduced capacity to convert these androgens to estrogens. High local levels of androstenedione and testosterone in the polycystic ovary may impede normal follicular growth and increase the rate of atresia, resulting in the formation of numerous small cystic follicles. (See Polycystic Ovary Syndrome, below.)

All of the developing follicles within the ovary are initially exposed to similar concentrations of FSH and LH. Since fewer than 1% of these follicles will eventually reach full maturity and ovulate, local factors must play a critical role in selection of the dominant preovulatory follicle. There are significant differences in the concentrations of protein and steroid hormones in the antral fluid of follicles of differing sizes and at differing stages of the menstrual cycle. The presence of this fluid-filled cavity provides a mechanism by which the granulosa cells and oocyte of one developing follicle can be exposed to a unique microenvironment that differs from that of the other developing follicles within the ovary. Studies have shown that it is the concentrations of pituitary gonadotropins and ovarian steroids within the follicular fluid rather than the serum concentrations of these hormones that correlate most closely with both the mitotic and synthetic activity of the granulosa cells as well as with the future viability of the oocyte. The highest concentrations of FSH and LH in antral fluid are found in the largest follicles during the late follicular phase of the menstrual cycle. Prolactin (PRL) levels, in contrast, are highest in small follicles and lowest in large follicles in the late follicular phase. The concentrations of LH and FSH in follicular fluid are generally lower than corresponding serum levels, but the concentrations of ovarian steroids—androstenedione, testosterone, dihydrotestosterone, and estradiol—may be 10–40,000 times greater than their serum levels. Although androgen concentrations do not differ greatly in follicular fluid from either small or large follicles, mean estradiol concentrations in antral fluid increase markedly, reaching levels in excess of 1500 ng/mL in large follicles in the late follicular phase of the menstrual cycle. It is not known at present whether these increases in the absolute concentration of estradiol and the ratio of estradiol to androgen in antral fluid are a consequence of follicular growth and development or play an important role in the process that leads to selection of a single preovulatory follicle.

HORMONE INTERACTION & REGULATION DURING THE MENSTRUAL CYCLE

Gonadotropin-Releasing Hormone (GnRH)

GnRH (also referred to as luteinizing hormone–releasing hormone [LHRH]; luteotropin-releasing hormone [LRH]; and luteotropin-releasing factor [LRF]) is a decapeptide synthesized by neurosecretory cells located primarily within the hypothalamus. It regulates the secretion of LH and FSH and is essential for their synthesis and release. LH and FSH cannot be detected in serum from peripheral blood of women with congenital absence of hypothalamic GnRH. Ovarian sex steroids are not essential for the synthesis of LH and FSH, but they modulate release of these hormones by altering either gonadotrope response to GnRH or secretion of hypothalamic GnRH. Concentrations of GnRH in serum from peripheral blood are very low, and the pattern of GnRH secretion throughout the menstrual cycle in women has not been accurately characterized. Preliminary studies suggest that GnRH secretion may be increased in the preovulatory period. GnRH has been measured in pituitary portal blood of rhesus monkeys. In these nonhuman primates, GnRH is secreted in a pulsatile fashion with an interval of 1–3 hours between pulses. Concentrations of GnRH in portal blood during the follicular phase of the menstrual cycle range from undetectable (< 10 pg/mL) to a maximum of 200 pg/mL. Continuous infusions of GnRH initially increase the secretion of LH and FSH. After several hours or days of continuous infusion, densensitization and receptor "down-regulation" occur, and the pituitary gland becomes refractory to further stimulation by GnRH.

In both rhesus monkeys and women, intermittent pulses of GnRH every 60–90 minutes stimulate indefinitely the release of LH and FSH. In rhesus monkeys, changes in the frequency of the GnRH pulses can selectively increase or decrease the serum concentration of either LH or FSH. This observation suggests a mechanism by which a single releasing hormone, GnRH, can alter the ratio of LH to FSH in serum and further supports the concept that GnRH is the only hypothalamic hormone required for the regulation of both LH and FSH secretion.

Effects of Ovarian Steroids on Gonadotropin Secretion

A. Negative Feedback: Under most conditions, ovarian steroids limit or reduce the secretion of pituitary gonadotropins. Serum concentrations of both FSH and LH increase markedly following ovariectomy or in postmenopausal women, whereas the administration of estrogen (or estrogen and progesterone) lowers serum gonadotropin levels. Throughout most of the normal menstrual cycle, the negative feedback effects of ovarian steroids predominate and plasma gonadotropin concentrations remain below 25 mIU/mL.

B. Positive Feedback: Estradiol and progesterone, under certain conditions, can induce the release of LH and FSH. During the menstrual cycle, rising concentrations of estradiol in the latter part of the follicular phase initiate the preovulatory surge of LH via this mechanism. This increase in LH secretion in turn stimulates a small but significant increase in the secretion of progesterone that further augments the LH surge and, coupled with estradiol, initiates the midcycle surge of FSH. Although the negative feedback action of ovarian steroids may become apparent within a few hours, positive feedback develops more slowly, and 48–72 hours of sustained estrogen stimulation is generally required before an increase in LH secretion is observed. It is probable that the negative and positive feedback actions of ovarian sex steroids result from both (1) a direct effect of the steroids on the pituitary gonadotropes that alters their sensitivity to GnRH and (2) modulation of the frequency and magnitude of the pulses of hypothalamic GnRH.

Neural Regulation of the Menstrual Cycle

In nonhuman primates—and perhaps in women as well—the neural components that control both the tonic and surge secretion of gonadotropins are located within the medial basal hypothalamus. When the medial basal hypothalamus, which includes the median eminence, the arcuate nucleus, and portions of the ventromedial nucleus, was surgically isolated from the remainder of the brain without disrupting the hypothalamic-pituitary-portal vasculature, gonadotropin secretion in rhesus monkeys was not significantly altered. Both the negative and positive feedback actions of estradiol remained intact, and many monkeys continued to have spontaneous ovulatory menstrual cycles. It is probable, however, that other neural areas outside the hypothalamus (eg, limbic structures) normally modify gonadotropin secretion.

Recent studies suggest that GnRH plays primarily a permissive, though still essential, role in the regulation of LH and FSH secretion throughout the menstrual cycle. Pulsatile administration of exogenous GnRH every 60–90 minutes induced ovulatory menstrual cycles in monkeys with hypothalamic lesions or in women with congenital absence of hypothalamic GnRH. In these cycles, the serum profiles of pituitary gonadotropins and ovarian steroids were within normal limits. These observations suggest that the cyclic nature of the menstrual cycle in primates is regulated by the ovary and not by the brain. The length of the menstrual cycle thus is determined by both the time required for development of a mature follicle and by the functional life span of the corpus luteum. Following luteolysis, follicular development resumes, and a new menstrual cycle begins.

CYCLIC CHANGES IN THE FEMALE REPRODUCTIVE TRACT

As a consequence of the changing rates of secretion of estrogen and progesterone throughout the menstrual cycle, the female reproductive tract undergoes a series of regular and cyclic changes. These changes can be recognized by histologic study of the endometrium, the composition and appearance of the cervical mucus, and the cytologic features of the vaginal epithelium. The end of each cycle is marked by vaginal bleeding that continues for 3–7 days.

HISTOLOGY OF THE ENDOMETRIUM THROUGHOUT THE MENSTRUAL CYCLE

The endometrium consists of 2 distinct layers or zones differing in both histologic appearance and functional responsiveness to hormonal stimulation: a **basal layer** and a **functional layer.** The basal layer is in direct contact with the myometrium, undergoes little change throughout the menstrual cycle, and is not sloughed during menses. The functional layer arises from the basal layer and eventually surrounds the entire lumen of the uterine cavity. The functional layer can be subdivided further into 2 components: a thin superficial **compact layer** and a deeper **spongiosa layer,** of which most of the secretory or fully developed endometrium is composed. The blood supply of the endometrium consists of a highly specialized network of arterial and venous channels. The **spiral arteries** arise within the myometrium from branches of the uterine artery, pass through the basal endometrial layer, and extend into the functional zone. The proximal portion of the spiral artery, the **straight artery,** distributes blood to tissues of the basal layer and is not influenced by changes in estrogen and progesterone secretion. The spiral arteries, however, undergo cyclic regeneration and degeneration during each menstrual cycle in response to hormonal changes.

The endometrial cycle can be subdivided into 3 major phases: proliferative, secretory, and menstrual. The morphologic changes of the endometrium that occur during the normal menstrual cycle have been described in great detail and are summarized in Fig 14–11. For convenience, the changes described in this figure and the following discussion are based on a hypothetical menstrual cycle of 28 days, in which the follicular and luteal phases are each approximately 14 days in length.

Proliferative Phase

When menstrual flow ceases, a thin layer of basal endometrial tissue remains. This tissue, consisting of the remnants of glands and stroma, grows rapidly. Epithelial cells from the glands proliferate and cover the raw stromal surfaces with a layer of simple columnar epithelium. In the early proliferative phase, most of the glands are straight, short, and narrow. The glandular epithelium exhibits increasing mitotic activity. Throughout the proliferative phase, there is continued and rapid growth of both the epithelial and stromal components of the endometrium. By the late proliferative phase of the menstrual cycle, the surface of the endometrium is somewhat undulant. The glands are becoming tortuous and are lined by tall columnar cells with basal nuclei. Pseudostratification of nuclei is prominent. The stroma at this time is moderately dense, with many mitotic figures.

Secretory Phase

During the secretory phase, histologic changes occur very rapidly. During the first half of this phase, the appearance of the glandular epithelium is most useful in precise dating of the endometrium, whereas in the second half, accurate dating depends largely on the characteristics of the stroma. On the 16th day of the cycle (second postovulatory day), subnuclear glycogen-rich vacuoles become prominent in the glandular epithelium. The vacuoles push the epithelial cell nuclei into a central position within the cells. By the 19th day (fifth postovulatory day), few vacuoles remain within the cells. Acidophilic intraluminal glandular secretory material is most apparent on day 21. Stromal edema, which is variable during the proliferative phase, also becomes prominent at this time and peaks on day 22. By day 24, pseudodecidual or predecidual changes begin to appear within the stroma. These changes are initially most apparent near the spiral arteries and eventually encompass large areas of the stroma. Lymphocytic infiltration of the stroma increases markedly in conjunction with the appearance of pseudodecidual changes, and by day 26, PMN invasion also is apparent.

Menstrual Phase

In the absence of pregnancy, changes in the endometrium secondary to declining hormone production by the corpus luteum can be observed by day 24. The functional layer of the stroma begins to shrink, and the endometrial glands become more tortuous and saw-toothed in appearance. Intermittent constriction of the spiral arteries leads to stasis within the capillaries of the functional layer, tissue ischemia, and extravasation of blood into the stroma with formation of small hematomas. Eventually, desquamation and sloughing of the entire functional layer of the endometrium occurs.

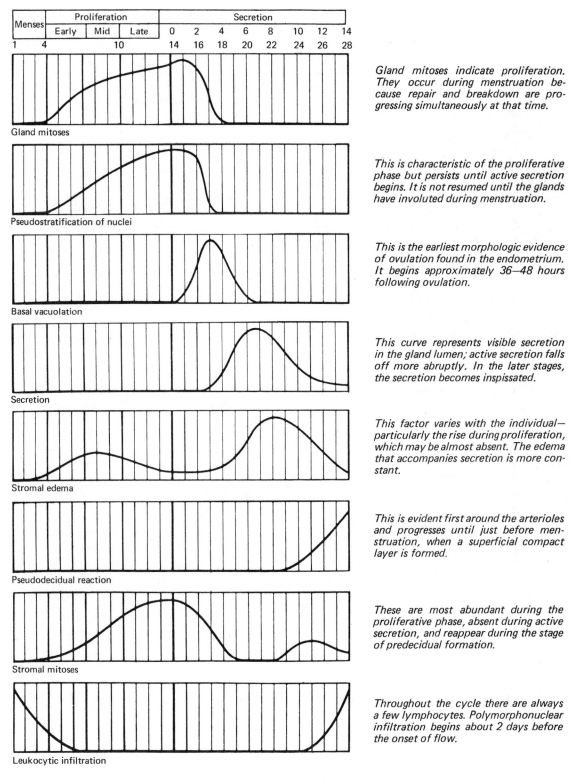

Figure 14–11. Morphologic changes in the endometrium that are useful in determining the stage of the menstrual cycle. (After Noyes, Hertig, & Rock. Reproduced, with permission, from Benson RC [editor]: *Current Obstetric & Gynecologic Diagnosis & Treatment,* 5th ed. Lange, 1984.)

Endometrial biopsy has been used extensively in the past to assess progesterone secretion in women with menstrual dysfunction and infertility. With the widespread availability of reliable radioimmunoassays to measure serum concentrations of progesterone, the need for endometrial biopsy is limited. Endometrial biopsy is most informative when performed a few days before the anticipated menstrual period. At this time, sufficient tissue for adequate histologic examination can usually be obtained, and the response of the endometrium to prior estradiol and progesterone stimulation can be assessed most accurately. Although biopsy late in the luteal phase may potentially interrupt a pregnancy if conception has occurred, the risk is minimal.

CERVICAL MUCUS

Cervical mucus is a complex secretion produced by the glands of the endocervix. It is composed of 92–98% water and approximately 1% inorganic salts, of which NaCl is the main constituent. The mucus also contains free simple sugars, polysaccharides, proteins, and glycoproteins. Its pH is usually alkaline and ranges from 6.5 to 9.0. Several physical characteristics of cervical mucus can be evaluated readily by the clinician. Since these characteristics are influenced by serum estrogen and progesterone levels, it is often possible to gain an approximate assessment of the hormonal status of a patient by examination of cervical mucus. Estrogen stimulates the production of copious amounts (up to 700 mg/d) of clear, watery mucus through which sperm can penetrate most readily. Progesterone, however, even in the presence of high plasma levels of estrogen, reduces the secretion of mucus. Both during the luteal phase of the menstrual cycle and during pregnancy, the mucus is scant, viscous, and cellular. During most of the menstrual cycle, 20–60 mg of mucus is produced each day.

Fig 14–12 summarizes those characteristics of cervical mucus that the clinician can readily determine and correlates them with the day of the menstrual cycle.

Spinnbarkeit is the property that allows cervical mucus to be stretched or drawn into a thread. Spinnbarkeit can be estimated by stretching a sample of mucus between 2 glass slides and measuring the maximum length of the thread before it breaks. At midcycle, spinnbarkeit usually exceeds 10 cm. **Ferning,** or **arborization,** refers to the characteristic microscopic pattern cervical mucus forms when dried on a slide (Fig 14–13). Ferning results from the crystallization of inorganic salts around small and optimal amounts of organic material present in cervical mucus. As serum concentrations of estradiol increase, the composition of cervical mucus changes, so that dried mucus begins to demonstrate ferning in the latter part of the follicular phase. In the periovulatory interval, when estradiol levels are maximal and prior to sig-

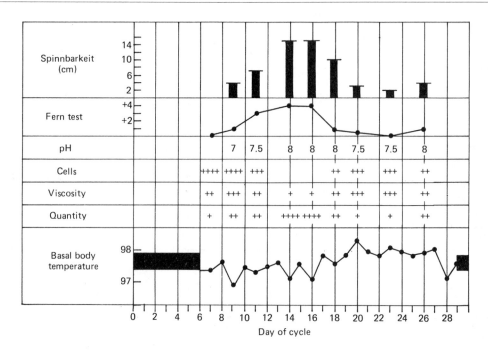

Figure 14–12. Changes in the composition and properties of cervical mucus throughout the menstrual cycle. (Modified and reproduced, with permission, from Moghissi KS: Composition and function of cervical secretion. Chapter 31 in: *Handbook of Physiology,* Section 7: Endocrinology, Vol 2, Part 2. Greep RO [editor]. American Physiological Society, 1973.)

Normal cycle, 14th day

·Midluteal phase, normal cycle

Anovulatory cycle with estrogen present

Figure 14–13. Patterns formed when cervical mucus is smeared on a slide, permitted to dry, and examined under the microscope. Progesterone makes the mucus thick and cellular. In the smear from a patient who failed to ovulate *(bottom)*, there is no progesterone to inhibit the estrogen-induced fern pattern. (Reproduced, with permission, from Ganong WF: *Review of Medical Physiology,* 12th ed. Lange, 1985.)

nificant progesterone secretion, ferning is most prominent and the mucus is thin, watery, and contains few cells. As serum progesterone concentrations increase following ovulation, the quality of the mucus changes and ferning disappears. The absence of ferning can reflect either inadequate stimulation of endocervical glands by estrogen or inhibition by increased secretion of progesterone. Persistent ferning throughout the menstrual cycle suggests anovulatory cycles or insufficient progesterone secretion.

VAGINAL EPITHELIUM

The vaginal mucosa is composed of a stratified squamous epithelium and does not contain glands. Cells in the outer layer during the reproductive years are flattened and may contain keratohyaline granules, but true cornification does not normally occur. The epithelial cells of the vagina, like other tissues of the female reproductive tract, respond to changing levels of ovarian sex steroids. Estrogen stimulates the proliferation and maturation of the epithelial cells, resulting in a thickening of the vaginal mucosa and increased glycogen content of the epithelial cells. This glycogen is fermented to lactic acid by the normal

bacterial flora of the vagina, thus accounting for the mildly acid pH of vaginal fluid. The histologic and cytologic changes of the vaginal epithelium of women during the normal menstrual cycle are less marked than those occurring in the estrous cycle of rodents.

Cytologists describe 3 types of exfoliated vaginal epithelial cells—superficial, intermediate, and basal-parabasal—which do not refer to the locations of the cells within the epithelium but to their degree of cellular maturity or differentiation. Exfoliated cells, obtained by light scrapings from the midportion of the lateral vaginal wall, are most useful for cytohormonal assessment.

Superficial cells are mature, flat, usually polygonal, squamous epithelial cells with pyknotic, hyperchromatic nuclei. These cells develop in response to high levels of unopposed estrogen stimulation.

Intermediate cells are relatively mature squamous epithelial cells with eosinophilic or cyanophilic cytoplasm and a vesicular, nonpyknotic nucleus. The appearance of the nucleus is the critical factor in differentiating intermediate cells from superficial cells. Intermediate cells predominate in endocrinologic states in which progesterone levels are high, such as in pregnancy or in the midluteal phase of the menstrual cycle.

Basal-parabasal cells are thick, small, oval or round, immature cells with large vesicular nuclei and cyanophilic cytoplasm. Parabasal cells usually indicate estrogen deficiency and are the predominant cell type in the prepubertal and postmenopausal periods.

Among the various indices that describe the ratio or percentage of superficial, intermediate, and basal-parabasal cells are (1) the karyopyknotic index (KPI), the ratio of superficial cells to intermediate cells; (2) the eosinophilic index (EI), the ratio of mature eosinophilic cells to mature cyanophilic cells; and (3) the maturation index (MI), the percentage of parabasal, intermediate, and superficial cells present, in that order. Since only MI includes as a factor the presence of all 3 cell types, it may provide more information than the other 2 indices.

In general, only 2 diagnostic patterns of vaginal epithelial cells are clinically useful. When the vaginal epithelium has been stimulated by estrogen, MI may range from (0/40/60) at midcycle, when estradiol concentrations are highest, to (0/70/30) late in the luteal phase, when progesterone effects are most prominent. A finding of parabasal cells with a few intermediate cells and no superficial cells indicates that the vaginal epithelium has received little or no estrogen stimulation. The MI in this instance may be (100/0/0) or (80/20/0). The vaginal smear can be used to provide a qualitative assessment of estrogen production in women with amenorrhea.

EXTRAGENITAL SYMPTOMS ASSOCIATED WITH NORMAL MENSTRUAL FUNCTION

PREMENSTRUAL SYNDROME

The premenstrual syndrome designates a wide variety of symptoms commonly associated with the normal menstrual cycle. Common symptoms are described below, but the particular pattern of symptoms varies in different women. They are severe enough to be noticeable in about half of women, although many of those not consciously aware of symptoms are able to recognize that their menses are about to begin before the bleeding starts. In rare instances, the symptoms may be completely disabling and even require hospitalization. The symptoms usually begin a few days to a week before the onset of menses and cease abruptly or are markedly ameliorated with the onset of menstrual flow. However, patterns vary greatly, and in some women symptoms may be more severe during the first few days of bleeding.

The transitory increase in water content of body tissues contributes to weight gain, edema, bloating, and breast tenderness. These appear to be predominantly the result of estrogen secretion, which facilitates the loss of electrolytes and fluid into the extravascular tissues. The resulting hypovolemia causes a secondary increase in aldosterone and antidiuretic hormone release, resulting in retention of sodium and water by the kidney. These symptoms frequently respond to diuretic therapy.

Neurologic and behavioral symptoms are often the most difficult to manage. Women frequently become nervous, irritable, agitated, and depressed. In severe cases, these disturbances frequently disrupt family and other personal relationships. The cause of the symptoms is unknown but is probably related to the central nervous system effects of the hormones as well as social, cultural, and psychologic factors.

Treatment is symptomatic. In many women, this symptom complex can be abolished by treatment with oral contraceptives or with medroxyprogesterone acetate, 150 mg intramuscularly every 3 months. In some women, treatment with oral medroxyprogesterone or other progestational agents for the week before menses is helpful.

DYSMENORRHEA

Dysmenorrhea unrelated to any identifiable disorder almost always begins before age 20 but seldom within the first year or so after menarche. It is one of the most important causes of lost working hours and failure to attend school. The pain is colicky in nature and thought to be related to uterine contractions caused by prostaglandins released at the time of endometrial breakdown. When severe, the pain may radiate from the pelvic region to the back and thighs and is frequently accompanied by nausea and in some women vomiting and diarrhea. Treatment with aspirin before the onset of pain is effective in milder cases; however, the nonsteroidal anti-inflammatory compounds that are active inhibitors of prostaglandin synthesis are more effective when the pain is severe. Naproxen (Naprosyn), 250 mg twice daily, and ibuprofen (Motrin), 400 mg 3 times daily, are useful for this purpose, as is indomethacin (Indocin), 25 mg 3–4 times daily, or mefenamic acid (Ponstel), 250 mg 4 times daily. These compounds are often more effective if started before the pain begins. Since dysmenorrhea rarely accompanies bleeding in the absence of ovulation, suppression of ovulation with oral contraceptives is also effective treatment.

DISORDERS OF OVARIAN FUNCTION

Abnormal ovarian endocrine function is manifested by (1) inappropriate evidence of estrogen secretion (eg, precocious puberty); (2) deficient estrogen secretion (eg, delayed puberty); (3) disturbances of the menstrual cycle in mature women; or (4) evidence of excessive androgen production by the ovary. Emphasis will be placed on disorders occurring in postpubertal adults, since these comprise the vast majority of disorders encountered and because disorders of development and differentiation are described in Chapters 5 and 15 and pituitary disorders in Chapter 4.

The pattern of menstrual bleeding with regard to the frequency, duration, and amount of flow tends to be fairly consistent in most normal women. Periodic, regular menstrual cycles are usually ovulatory. However, there are a wide variety of organic and functional disturbances of menstrual flow. In general, when the basic pattern of bleeding is undisturbed and there are superimposed episodes of spotting or bleeding, the cause is likely to be a local organic lesion or hematologic disorder. When the basic pattern of bleeding is changed, it is more often due to lack of ovulation and disturbances in the pattern of hormone secretion. Table 14–3 sets forth the terms frequently used to describe abnormalities of menses, their definitions, and some common causes.

The great majority of disorders of ovarian function causing amenorrhea occur without known or identifiable structural changes in the components of the complex system required for normal ovulatory cycles. They can result from abnormalities in function of the central mechanism that regulates the pulsatile secretion of GnRH; from abnormalities in feedback; or from

Table 14–3. Types of abnormal vaginal bleeding.

	Definition	Causes
Hypermenorrhea (menorrhagia)	Cyclic bleeding in excessive amount.	Uterine myomas and endometrial polyps, hyperplasia, adenomyosis, endometritis, von Willebrand's disease.
Hypomenorrhea	Cyclic bleeding in abnormally small amount.	Cervical obstruction, synechia of endometrium, tuberculosis of endometrium.
Polymenorrhea	Frequent periods (cycle length of <21 days).	Shortening of follicular phase, luteal insufficiency, frequent anovulatory bleeding.
Oligomenorrhea	Infrequent periods (cycle length of >35 days).	Anovulation, systemic disturbances.
Amenorrhea	More than 6 months since last menstrual period.	Anovulation, absence or destruction of endometrium.
Metrorrhagia	Bleeding between normal cycles.	Except for ovulatory bleeding or spotting, this symptom usually indicates disease of the vagina, cervix, or uterus.

changes in intraovarian regulatory mechanisms. Environmental changes, physical and emotional stress, extreme weight loss, and drugs seem to be able to interfere with the functioning of the hypothalamic centers and their control of GnRH secretion. In such cases, a variety of hormonal abnormalities may be identified. In some patients, follicle stimulation by FSH is insufficient to produce adequate estrogen to induce the release of LH required for ovulation. Failure of the preovulatory LH surge to occur may have the same result even though follicles have developed and produced estrogen. On the other hand, the continuous secretion of somewhat larger amounts of LH in the absence of normally developing follicles may result in overproduction of androgens and lead to amenorrhea and hirsutism (eg, polycystic ovary syndrome). The role of estrogens, androgens, and other local hormones in the ovary is not presently well delineated, but these hormones may be responsible for abnormalities in ovarian function in some patients. Abnormalities of gonadotropin secretion leading to anovulation are sometimes associated with the release of increased amounts of PRL in the absence of any demonstrable lesion of the pituitary. In such patients, amenorrhea may be associated with galactorrhea.

Treatment of these disorders depends to some extent on their causes and manifestations. However, the desired outcome is the critical consideration. It would be fruitless, for example, to treat hirsutism secondary to excess production of ovarian androgens by suppressing the ovary with oral contraceptives in a patient whose main objective was to achieve a pregnancy.

In considering the possible causes of amenorrhea in a given patient, it is useful to review the requirements for normal cyclic ovarian function: (1) a normal outflow tract, (2) normal ovaries, (3) a normal pituitary gland, and (4) a normal central nervous system. Each of these systems can be examined by means of the history, direct observation, and appropriate tests or procedures. The problem may be moderately complicated in young women without evidence of sexual maturation and normal menstrual function. On the other hand, in others the process may require little in the way of testing. By the time one has begun to speak to the patient, certain observations have been made. The approximate age, appearance, stature, and sexual development have been noted; the diagnostic process has begun; and some direction is given to the taking of the history.

AMENORRHEA IN THE ABSENCE OF SEXUAL MATURATION

The diagnostic considerations for a young, immature woman are quite different from those for a mature woman with secondary amenorrhea. In the normal but sexually immature patient over 16 years of age, the first question that arises is whether puberty is late but will otherwise be normal. This question can sometimes be answered by finding a normal level of gonadotropins and a history of late puberty in the family. No conclusion can be drawn if the levels are low. In these patients, LH and FSH responses to testing with GnRH may help to differentiate delayed puberty from a more serious disorder. However, elevated concentrations of FSH and LH indicate unresponsiveness or absence of functioning ovarian tissue. If the patient is short in stature and has obvious stigmas of Turner's syndrome (gonadal dysgenesis), the gonadotropins will be elevated. Chromosomal analysis will confirm the diagnosis, determine the genotype, and indicate the need for gonadectomy if a Y chromosome mosaicism is found. If the patient is of normal height or has relatively longer arms and legs compared with the length of the trunk (eunuchoid proportions), gonadal absence or agenesis must be differentiated from selective hypogonadotropism. FSH will be elevated in the former and low in the latter. If height and stature are normal and gonadotropins are low, one must also consider a central nervous system defect such as Kallmann's syndrome. These patients have anosmia, which can be determined by the history or by testing the ability to smell.

Patients with amenorrhea and hypogonadism in whom the levels of gonadotropins are normal or lower than normal may be experiencing a delay in onset of puberty. However, after age 16, this is sufficiently unusual to warrant further investigation. When the cause is craniopharyngioma or pituitary tumor, there is commonly an interference with growth secondary to deficient GH secretion. Clinical or laboratory evidence of thyroid or adrenal insufficiency or decreased reserve also may be present. These and other pituitary disorders causing amenorrhea are discussed in Chapter 4, Part I.

AMENORRHEA IN PATIENTS WITH NORMAL SECONDARY SEX CHARACTERISTICS

The evaluation of women with amenorrhea but otherwise normal sexual development can be done by taking a competent history and performing a physical examination plus a few laboratory tests (Fig 14–14). This evaluation will localize the underlying cause of the amenorrhea to dysfunction of either the outflow tract, the ovary, or the hypothalamic-pituitary complex. In most cases, further diagnostic procedures will not be required. The medical history should include a complete description of prior menstrual patterns, the presence or absence of breast discharge, and any changes that might suggest increased androgen secretion. The possibility of pregnancy should always be considered.

The initial evaluation consists of a qualitative assessment of the patient's endogenous estrogen level and determination of the serum PRL concentration. The presence of endogenous estrogens can be established by attempting to induce withdrawal uterine bleeding by administering progesterone. An oral progestin with no estrogenic activity—eg, medroxyprogesterone, 10 mg daily for 5–7 days—or a single intramuscular injection of 200 mg of progesterone in oil may be used. The presence of vaginal bleeding within 7 days after conclusion of the progesterone treatment indicates that the outflow tract is intact and that the patient is producing sufficient estrogen to stimulate endometrial growth. If the serum PRL concentration also is within normal limits, a pituitary tumor is very unlikely. These patients can be considered to be anovulatory, and in most cases no further evaluation is required.

Failure to induce menstrual bleeding by exogenous progestin indicates either a defect at the level of the outflow tract with normal estrogen production or insufficient estrogen production secondary to hypothalamic-pituitary-ovarian dysfunction. To differentiate between these possibilities in women with normal PRL levels, oral estrogen (1.25–2.5 mg of conjugated estrogens [Premarin, etc] or 50 μg of ethinyl estradiol per day) is given daily for 21 days. A progestin should be added during the last 5 days of treatment. Lack of withdrawal bleeding following treatment usually indicates an abnormality of the outflow tract. In most instances, however, bleeding will occur and the outflow tract is found to be normal.

The next step in evaluation is to differentiate between ovarian failure and hypothalamic-pituitary dysfunction. Since exogenous estrogens and progestins will alter basal levels of FSH and LH, it is necessary to wait several weeks before determining serum gonadotropin concentrations after treatment with these steroids. This may unnecessarily delay completion of the evaluation, and for the sake of efficiency, FSH and LH measurement often are obtained prior to assessment of the outflow tract with estrogen. If ovarian failure is the primary cause of amenorrhea, serum FSH and LH levels will be elevated because of the loss of negative feedback by ovarian sex steroids. If serum concentrations of FSH and LH are low or low normal, radiologic examination of the pituitary gland is indicated to rule out a pituitary tumor. Therapy for these disorders is discussed below.

Abnormalities of the Outflow Tract

Patients with amenorrhea in whom gonadal tissue is presumed to be present because they have undergone normal sexual maturation may have abnormalities of the outflow tract. Patients who cannot be induced to bleed by treatment with a progestational agent and who fail to bleed following administration of estrogens in conjunction with a progestational agent after several attempts can be presumed to have an abnormality of the outflow tract. In these patients, the presence or absence of ovulation can be determined by following the basal body temperature over a month or more or by measuring serum progesterone levels once a week for several weeks.

A. Müllerian Defects: In women with no history of vaginal bleeding, developmental abnormalities of the müllerian tube must be considered. These abnormalities range from the presence of an imperforate hymen to the total absence of müllerian structures. In the presence of a uterus lined with endometrium, interruption of the outflow tract by an abnormal cervix, interruptions of the vaginal canal, or imperforate hymen may be accompanied by collection of the menstruum proximal to the point of obstruction. This leads to pain and distention of the proximal structures or accumulation of blood in the peritoneal cavity. **Absence of the vagina,** with varying degrees of uterine development associated with normal ovarian function, is one of the more common abnormalities of müllerian development (Mayer-Rokitansky-Küster-Hauser syndrome). Affected patients commonly have developmental abnormalities of the urinary and skeletal systems. Surgical creation of an artificial vagina is indicated when there is evidence that a functioning uterus exists and that fertility might be restored. Otherwise, progressive dilatation by the use of vaginal dilators can be used to form a functional vagina.

B. Testicular Feminization: This disorder in its classic form is characterized by primary amenorrhea, an absent uterus, and the absence of pubic and axillary hair. Affected patients are male pseudohermaphrodites with testes and an XY karyotype. Incomplete forms of this disorder have also been described. They are discussed in detail in Chapter 15.

C. Asherman's Syndrome (Uterine Synechia): In women in whom menses have once been established, destruction of the endometrial cavity by chronic infections such as tuberculosis or destruction of the endometrium by curettage can lead to amenorrhea. Such scarring (Asherman's syndrome) is uncommon and can sometimes be treated by careful dilatation under hysteroscopic view, followed by insertion of a small Foley catheter or other device to prevent adhe-sions from recurring. Treatment should include the use of broad-spectrum antibiotics for 10 days follow-ing the procedure and cyclic stimulation of endo-metrial development with large doses of estrogen plus a progestin.

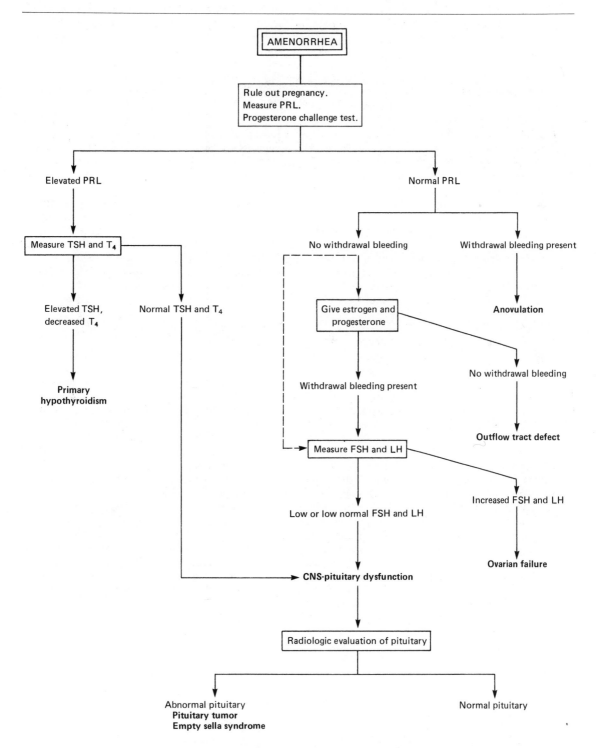

Figure 14–14. Diagnostic evaluation of amenorrhea.

Primary Ovarian Disorders

In patients with amenorrhea and a normal outflow tract, abnormal ovarian function may result from disorders of the ovary itself or disorders of the controlling mechanisms. A plasma FSH of more than 40 mIU/mL accompanied by high levels of LH is evidence of failure of the ovary to function hormonally. This is a very serious diagnosis, not only because of the hormone deficiency, which is correctable, but also—and more importantly from the patient's point of view—because lack of a functioning follicular apparatus results in sterility. For this reason, it is worth repeating the test to be sure there is no error. In women near menopause, elevated gonadotropin levels are sometimes found in the presence of ovulatory cycles. However, a misdiagnosis in this group of patients is rarely clinically important unless the patient is pregnant.

A. Gonadal Agenesis: Hypogonadism may result from absent or incomplete development of the ovary. This abnormality could result from environmentally induced abnormalities in development early in pregnancy (see Chapter 15).

B. Turner's Syndrome (Gonadal Dysgenesis): Turner's syndrome and related variants of gonadal dysgenesis are the most common cause of congenital hypogonadism. The karyotype in affected patients is 45,X, showing an absence of the second X chromosome. Clinical features, in addition to the lack of sexual maturation, include short stature, webbed neck, shield chest, and valgus deformity of the elbow. This syndrome is described in detail in Chapter 15. Gonadal dysgenesis may also occur in the presence of multiple cell lines with varying chromosomal composition. This is called "mosaicism." Many patients with mosaicism have typical phenotypic characteristics of Turner's syndrome, and the diagnosis may be made before puberty. A karyotype should be performed on all of these patients to determine whether or not a Y chromosome is present. Patients having Y chromosomes require laparotomy and excision of the gonadal area to prevent development of gonadoblastomas. It should also be noted that patients having an XX constituent to their mosaicism may have functional ovarian tissue. In some of these, normal puberty (including menses) occurs, and they are able to reproduce. These individuals frequently experience premature menopause.

C. Resistant Ovary Syndrome: Rare individuals have been found to exhibit amenorrhea and elevated gonadotropin levels in the presence of potentially functioning ovarian follicles. It may be possible to induce follicular growth and estrogen secretion in these patients by administration of large amounts of exogenous gonadotropins. However, it may be difficult or impossible to induce ovulation and subsequent pregnancy in these patients. Although this disorder can only be diagnosed with certainty by ovarian biopsy, the infrequency of the disorder and the poor prognosis dictate that ovarian biopsy not be done in every patient with high gonadotropins and normal karyotype. Although guidelines from reliable studies are not available, it may be possible as a practical matter to rule out this diagnosis by establishing the absence of increased estrogen levels following administration of large doses of menotropins.

D. Premature Ovarian Failure: Ovarian failure following spontaneous sexual maturation is occasionally encountered in women under the age of 35. Women with premature ovarian failure may have experienced the effects of only a few years or less of estrogen secretion or normal ovulatory menses for 20 years. In some patients, ovarian failure is associated with ovarian autoantibodies and is probably due to autoimmune destruction of the ovary. It is frequently associated with autoantibodies to other glands such as the thyroid and adrenal (Schmidt's syndrome) (see Chapters 7, 9, and 25). In other patients, the ovaries show a few primordial follicles, and in some they resemble menopausal ovaries. In the presence of viable follicles, it has been possible to induce ovulation with menopausal gonadotropins. However, pregnancy is rarely, if ever, achieved.

E. Other Causes of Hypergonadotropic Hypogonadism or Amenorrhea: The findings of hypogonadism and the presence of elevated levels of gonadotropin can be found in patients with 17α-hydroxylase deficiency, a rare form of congenital adrenal hyperplasia in which there is impaired conversion of pregnenolone and progesterone to cortisol and to androgens and estrogens. The impairment leads to increased production of deoxycorticosterone and corticosterone, resulting in hypokalemia and hypertension (see Chapter 10). Hypogonadism may also occur with the absence of only one of the gonadotropins. Amenorrhea and elevated gonadotropin levels have also been described with tumors, particularly lung cancer and ovarian tumors of embryonic origin.

F. Functioning Ovarian Tumors: Hormone-producing tumors of the ovary presenting clinically as endocrine disorders are uncommon. Classification of these tumors is made difficult by the uncertainty of embryonic origin in some and the lack of correlation between the functional and morphologic characteristics. However, it is convenient to divide them into broad morphologic categories, keeping in mind that the diagnostic approach will be based on the clinical presentation. Detection of androgen-producing tumors is considered in the section on amenorrhea with excess androgen production (see below). The estrogen-producing tumors cause amenorrhea or anovulatory bleeding in premenopausal women, irregular bleeding after the menopause, and precocious puberty in children. A classification of these tumors is presented in Table 14–4.

1. Germ cell tumors—

a. Germinomas (dysgerminoma, seminoma, gonocytoma, embryonal carcinoma)—These tumors of the ovary are usually found on routine examination in young women. They are generally small and asymptomatic unless associated with teratomatous elements that produce hCG. When hCG is produced, the patient will develop amenorrhea and other signs and symptoms of early pregnancy.

Table 14—4. Classification and clinical features of functioning ovarian tumors.

	Hormones*	Usual Age at Onset	Percent Palpable	Percent Bilateral	Percent Malignant
Germ cell tumors					
Germinomas-teratomas					
Struma ovarii	Thyroxine	10—40	90	10	Rare
Carcinoid tumors	Serotonin	10—40	90	10	Rare
Choriocarcinomas	Chorionic gonadotropin	6—15	100	Rare	100
Gonadoblastomas	Androgens, estrogens	10—30		40	50
Sex cord–mesenchymal tumors					
Granulosa–theca cell tumors	Estrogens, androgens, progestins	30—70	90	10	20
Sertoli–Leydig cell tumors (arrhenoblastomas)	Androgens, estrogens	20—50	80	Rare	20
Hilar cell tumors	Androgens, estrogens	45—75	50	Rare	Rare

*Steroid-producing tumors may produce estrogens or androgens. The usual hormone released is listed first.

b. Gonadoblastomas–These rare tumors arise in dysgenetic gonads. They are typically seen in phenotypic females with a Y chromosome. They are morphologically similar to germinomas but also have cells of mesenchymal or sex cord origin. The latter may differentiate into Leydig or granulosa cells and secrete androgens or estrogens. Prophylactic removal of the dysgenetic gonads is recommended in patients with a Y chromosome (see Chapter 15).

c. Teratomas–Teratomas arising in gonadal tissue are common. Although rarely active hormonally, they may contain hormone-secreting elements. Tumors containing thyroid tissue (struma ovarii) can release thyroxine. Carcinoid tumors producing serotonin have also been reported.

Choriocarcinoma of the ovary is usually secondary to uterine choriocarcinoma and very rarely arises within the ovary. It is composed of trophoblastic tissue, usually with extensive hemorrhage and necrosis. These tumors produce large amounts of hCG. The elevated plasma levels of this hormone are useful in diagnosing the tumor and in monitoring treatment. Treatment is similar to that of tumors of trophoblastic origin in the uterus. However, the prognosis is less favorable.

2. Sex cord–mesenchymal tumors–
a. Granulosa–theca cell tumors–These tumors constitute 5– 10% of ovarian neoplasms. They are usually associated with some clinical or pathologic evidence of estrogen secretion. Androgen-producing tumors of this type have been reported but are rare. Granulosa cell tumors are unilateral in 90% of patients. They are usually solid and vary in appearance from mature granulosa cells arranged in circumferential rows around spaces ("Call-Exner bodies") to immature cells with a sarcomatous appearance. The cells may take on the polyhedral appearance of the luteinized granulosa cells of the corpus luteum. Although the prognosis following removal of these tumors is better than for ovarian carcinomas, about 20% recur in 5 years and about 40% in 10 years. The recurrences may be circumscribed and can be quite sensitive to radiation.

b. Sertoli–Leydig cell tumors (arrhenoblastoma, androblastoma)–This group of tumors, as noted above, may cause feminization. They more commonly produce virilization and under these circumstances are commonly called arrhenoblastomas or androblastomas. They are not common, accounting for fewer than 5% of ovarian tumors. They vary in size and, although usually small, may become large. The histologic pattern varies from that of well-differentiated testicular tubules (Pick's adenoma) to an undifferentiated sarcomatous appearance and mixtures of both.

Typically, the first manifestation of an androgen-producing tumor is amenorrhea, followed by hirsutism, acne, and breast atrophy; clitoral hypertrophy, balding, and deepening of the voice occur later. Plasma androgen levels are usually in the normal male range and cannot be suppressed by administration of estrogens or estrogen-containing oral contraceptives. Removal of the tumor is followed by a return of menses and partial or complete loss of abnormal hair. The tumors are seldom bilateral and usually benign.

3. Hilar cell (lipoid cell) tumors–These androgen-producing tumors usually occur in older patients and cause severe masculinization, including hirsutism, balding, clitoral enlargement, and deepening of the voice. They are usually small and less likely to be palpated than other ovarian tumors. Histologically, they are typical steroid-producing cells and contain Reinke crystalloids, which are characteristically found in the interstitial cells of the testis. They are almost always benign and are treated by extirpation, which reverses the hirsutism, baldness, and metabolic changes, though clitoral enlargement and voice changes persist.

Disorders of the Pituitary

The anterior pituitary gland plays a key role in normal ovarian function. In adults, the loss of pituitary gonadotropic activity is usually noted before the loss of other pituitary trophic functions when the organ is damaged by vascular, inflammatory, or neoplastic processes.

A. Pituitary Tumors: Most patients with amenorrhea and low gonadotropin levels have a regulatory disorder due to abnormalities of central nervous system activity. However, the presence of a pituitary tumor must be considered. Although amenorrhea may be the only clue to a nonfunctioning tumor, it may be associated with galactorrhea when the normal tonic inhibition of PRL is lost. Galactorrhea is found in about 50% of patients with PRL-secreting adenomas (see Chapter 4, Part I), whereas GH-secreting tumors are associated with clinical signs of acromegaly. Although the latter is an unusual cause of amenorrhea, it is important to consider the diagnosis in appropriate clinical circumstances, since early diagnosis and treatment can prevent the permanently disfiguring effects of excessive GH. Amenorrhea may also be the presenting symptom in patients with Cushing's syndrome due to a pituitary tumor (Cushing's disease).

B. Empty Sella Syndrome: The finding of amenorrhea and galactorrhea may occur in the presence of empty sella syndrome (see Chapter 4, Part I). In this condition, there appears to be an extension of the subarachnoid space into the fossa, which leads to flattening of pituitary tissue against the wall of the sella and may lead to its enlargement. The disorder is found in 5% of patients at autopsy. It is benign and requires no treatment unless associated abnormalities of pituitary function are present. This condition can be differentiated from tumor by CT scanning.

Disorders Due to Central Nervous System Abnormalities of Regulation of Gonadotropin Secretion

A. Hypothalamic Amenorrhea: This term is used to describe amenorrhea due to functional abnormalities in the central regulation of ovulatory function. Young women commonly fail to ovulate at times of stress such as may be occasioned by changes (eg, relocation of the family to a different city) or during illness, and these events may mark the onset of prolonged periods of amenorrhea.

The treatment of hypothalamic amenorrhea is dependent upon the expectations of the patient. If she wishes to become pregnant, induction of ovulation by clomiphene would be the initial treatment. If this does not induce ovulation, treatment with clomiphene plus chorionic gonadotropin, with menotropins (Pergonal), or with pulsatile administration of GnRH will be required. If pregnancy is not desired, consideration of the estrogenic status of the patient will help to determine treatment. Women who have a negative progesterone challenge test (no withdrawal bleeding) may have significant loss of calcium with the eventual development of osteoporosis secondary to low levels of estrogen. In these patients, treatment with estrogen and a cyclic progestin should be considered to prevent these changes. Women who have a positive progesterone challenge test (withdrawal bleeding) have either normal or only moderately reduced levels of estrogen. Cyclic treatment with a progestational agent will prevent endometrial hyperplasia in these women.

B. Amenorrhea in Athletes: Menstrual abnormalities are sufficiently common in female athletes to suggest a causal relationship between vigorous physical effort and amenorrhea. About one-third of long-distance runners experience amenorrhea or oligomenorrhea. The incidence appears to vary with the degree of stress and effort in other activities. The incidence of amenorrhea correlates directly with the amount of weight lost and inversely with the percentage of body weight as fat. It is less frequent in multiparous women. No consistent changes in plasma estradiol, testosterone, or gonadotropin levels have been reported. In general, these menstrual abnormalities disappear with a reduction of physical activity and a return to the individual's natural weight and proportion of body weight as fat. Some of these women with prolonged amenorrhea show excessive bone loss in spite of their intense physical activity, and appropriate therapy should be instituted.

C. Anorexia: Anorexia nervosa in its classic form is a serious but uncommon disorder characterized by extreme malnutrition and hypogonadotropism. It is considered to be a severe behavioral disorder, with endocrine changes secondary to both psychologic and nutritional disturbances. Amenorrhea may precede weight loss. Malnutrition may result from refusal to eat, induced vomiting (bulimia), and excessive use of laxatives. Psychiatric treatment is required, and hospitalization may be necessary to prevent death from starvation, suicide, or intercurrent illnesses. Milder forms of malnutrition and amenorrhea are more commonly seen in formerly overweight women with an abnormal fear of regaining weight lost by dieting.

D. Post-Pill Amenorrhea: Although it has not been possible to clearly demonstrate a reduction in the fertility rate of women following the use of oral contraceptives, studies are available that show a moderate increase in the incidence of amenorrhea in such women. Furthermore, the syndrome of amenorrhea with galactorrhea (see below) is more common in women treated with oral contraceptives. The nature of this relationship is not established. However, it is clear that most women who develop amenorrhea following the use of contraceptive pills would probably have developed amenorrhea without them, and the disorder must be investigated as in other women.

E. Hypogonadotropism and Anosmia: This syndrome, similar to Kallmann's syndrome in the male, is a rare cause of amenorrhea. Patients fail to mature at the expected time for puberty and are found to have low gonadotropins, normal stature, anosmia, and a female karyotype. The disorder is believed to involve failure of development of the olfactory lobe and a deficiency of GnRH. Ovulation can be induced by injection of menopausal gonadotropins and by pulsatile injection of GnRH.

Amenorrhea With Galactorrhea

Galactorrhea may be induced by a wide variety of stimuli ranging from local irritation or stimulation of the chest wall to ingestion of drugs that interfere with the hypothalamic release of dopamine or its binding to the pituitary lactotrophs (see Chapter 4). The expression of even 1 drop of fluid from the nipple is clinically significant and is rarely seen in normal women who have not taken contraceptives or who have not been recently pregnant or exposed to drugs such as phenothiazines (which cause galactorrhea) or to excessive breast stimulation. In women with amenorrhea, an attempt should be made to elicit such a secretion by gentle manual pressure at the base of the breast, working toward the nipple. The secretion may be present in only one breast at any given time.

While there is no universal agreement about the best approach to patients presenting with amenorrhea and galactorrhea, it must be kept in mind that a significant proportion of these patients have tumors of the pituitary, which are often quite small. Patients with tumors often have markedly elevated levels of serum PRL. Although the clinical findings may precede the detectable presence of a tumor by many years, it is useful to obtain a CT scan of the sella turcica in any patient in whom PRL levels are more than minimally elevated. Studies of pituitary function, including the gonadotropin response to GnRH and the effect of levodopa and other drugs on PRL secretion, do not reliably identify patients with pituitary tumors. However, these and other tests of pituitary function are useful in assessing residual pituitary function. CT scanning will detect microadenomas as small as 3–5 mm in size. Bulging and demineralization of the sella turcica usually occur when the tumor exceeds 1 cm in diameter, and larger tumors are usually found in patients presenting with visual field defects.

Criteria for the selection of patients with tumors for surgical treatment or medical treatment with bromocriptine have not been firmly established and may be expected to change over the next few years. About 10–20% of women examined at autopsy show small pituitary adenomas. The natural history of the disorder is not well understood.

Although clomiphene or gonadotropins may induce ovulation in many of these patients, bromocriptine is more effective. Bromocriptine mesylate (Parlodel) is an ergot alkaloid that acts by binding to the dopaminergic receptors in the pituitary, resulting in inhibition of PRL secretion. In 90% or more of these patients, treatment leads to the onset of menses in 3–5 weeks. The usual dose is 2.5 mg 2 or 3 times a day. Since there are side effects of nausea and mild dizziness, it is useful to start with a small dose, such as 2.5 mg daily—or half that amount in sensitive patients—and increase to 2.5 mg twice daily. PRL levels should be depressed to normal if treatment is adequate.

The long-term use of bromocriptine to induce regression of pituitary tumors is under study. Preliminary results indicate that at least in some patients tumors can be shown to regress. Even incomplete regression may be useful in patients whose tumors are too large to favor the transsphenoidal approach to the removal of the tumor. As noted above, the indications for surgery in patients with small tumors have not been established. Transsphenoidal tumor removal will restore normal gonadal function and normal PRL levels in the large majority of these patients. However,

others have been followed for many years without evidence of tumor enlargement. In any case, patients must be followed carefully with PRL levels. Patients with tumors require x-ray reevaluation of the sella every 1–2 years. (See Chapter 4, Part I.)

Amenorrhea With Androgen Excess

The presence of excessive amounts of androgen is usually associated with oligomenorrhea or amenorrhea. The causes of androgen excess are shown in Table 14–5.

A. Polycystic Ovary Syndrome: Polycystic ovary (Stein-Leventhal) syndrome is a complex of varying symptoms ranging from amenorrhea to anovulatory bleeding often associated with obesity and hirsutism. The term has been used to describe such a variety of symptom complexes (Table 14–6) that it is almost a barrier to communication. In the most characteristic form of the disorder, the term denotes an absence of ovulation in association with continuous stimulation of the ovary by disproportionately high levels of LH. The chronic stimulation leads to increases in androgen secretion by the ovary and characteristic morphologic changes in the ovaries. The ovaries are usually (not always) enlarged and may reach several times normal size. One ovary may be significantly larger than the other. The ovaries are typically glistening white in appearance, because of a thickened capsule, and show many small follicles in various stages of development and atresia at the surface. The theca cells are often hyperplastic and luteinized. The syndrome is also associated with changes in adrenal androgen production in some patients. Estrogen production in these patients is variable but is sometimes sufficient to produce endometrial hyperplasia, eventually leading to the occurrence of adenocarcinoma of the endometrium.

1. Etiology–The cause of this syndrome is unknown, and it is possible that there are several causes. Each of the functional changes that occur tends to maintain the cycle of functional abnormalities as shown in Fig 14–15. It has been suggested that in some patients this disorder may be initiated by excessive

Table 14–5. Causes of increased androgen production, hirsutism, or both.

Ovarian causes
   Polycystic ovary syndrome
   Hyperthecosis
   Androgen-producing tumors
   Virilization of pregnancy (luteoma)
Adrenal causes
   Congenital or adult-onset adrenal hyperplasia
   Androgen-producing tumors
Combined ovarian-adrenal dysfunction: polycystic ovary syndrome
Cushing's syndrome
Idiopathic or familial hirsutism
Postmenopausal state
Incomplete testicular feminization
Iatrogenic (eg, phenytoin, diazoxide, danazol, minoxidil)

Table 14–6. Incidence of various clinical findings in women with polycystic ovary syndrome. Data are derived from 187 references comprising a total of 1079 cases.*

	Incidence (%)	
	Mean	Range
Infertility	74	35–94
Hirsutism	69	17–83
Amenorrhea	51	15–77
Obesity	41	16–49
Functional bleeding	29	6–65
Dysmenorrhea	23	
Corpus luteum at surgery	22	0–71
Virilization	21	0–28
Biphasic basal body temperature	15	12–40
Cyclic menses	12	7–28

*Reproduced, with permission, from Goldzieher JW: Polycystic ovarian disease. In: *Progress in Infertility*, 2nd ed. Behrman SH, Kistner RW (editors). Little, Brown, 1975.

adrenal androgen production at the time of puberty or by a stress-induced increase in adrenal androgen secretion. The peripheral conversion of androgen to estrogen could facilitate the secretion of increased amounts of LH, leading to increased ovarian androgen production and impaired follicular maturation. In some patients, there is a strong family history, and the pattern of inheritance suggests that the trait is dominant and may be linked to the X chromosome. A group of patients have also been found in whom amenorrhea and androgen excess are associated with acanthosis nigricans and insulin resistance.

This syndrome could also result from central nervous system abnormalities, leading to inappropriate secretion of hypothalamic GnRH. This, in turn, could increase the secretion of LH and reduce the secretion of FSH. High levels of LH may promote excessive androgen production by the thecal layer. Since FSH

levels also are low, granulosa cells may have a reduced capacity to convert these androgens to estrogens. High local levels of androstenedione and testosterone in the polycystic ovary may impede normal follicular growth and increase the rate of atresia, resulting in the formation of numerous small cystic follicles. Serum levels of estrone and free estradiol are elevated secondarily to increased peripheral aromatization of the ovarian androgens. The elevated levels of estrogen, in turn, further sensitize the pituitary gland to hypothalamic GnRH, sustaining the abnormality.

Although androgen production is quite variable, it seldom reaches the levels seen in the presence of androgen-producing ovarian tumors. As a result, the vast majority of women show hirsutism and increased activity of the sebaceous glands often associated with acne. Signs of more severe virilization, such as male pattern (bitemporal) balding, clitoral hypertrophy, and voice changes, are rare. In general, there is a good correlation between levels of free testosterone and clinical evidence of androgen excess.

2. Management–The major manifestations of polycystic ovary syndrome are hirsutism secondary to androgen excess and failure of ovulation causing amenorrhea and infertility. The goals of therapy in the individual patient are of prime importance in determining the appropriate therapeutic program. For example, the treatment of hirsutism by ovarian suppression would not allow an infertile patient to conceive; conversely, ovulation induction does not usually reduce androgen secretion. Some obese patients have been reported to resume ovulation and reduce androgen secretion on a program of weight reduction alone. Hirsutism can be treated by suppression of ovarian androgen production or by antiandrogen therapy, as discussed in the section on treatment of hirsutism (see below).

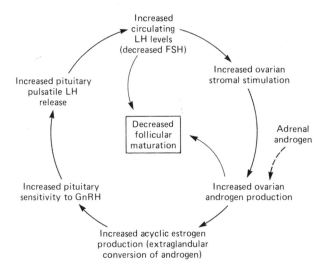

Figure 14–15. Pathophysiology of chronic anovulation in women with polycystic ovary syndrome. (Reproduced, with permission, from Yen SSC, Jaffe RB [editors]: *Reproductive Endocrinology.* Saunders, 1978.)

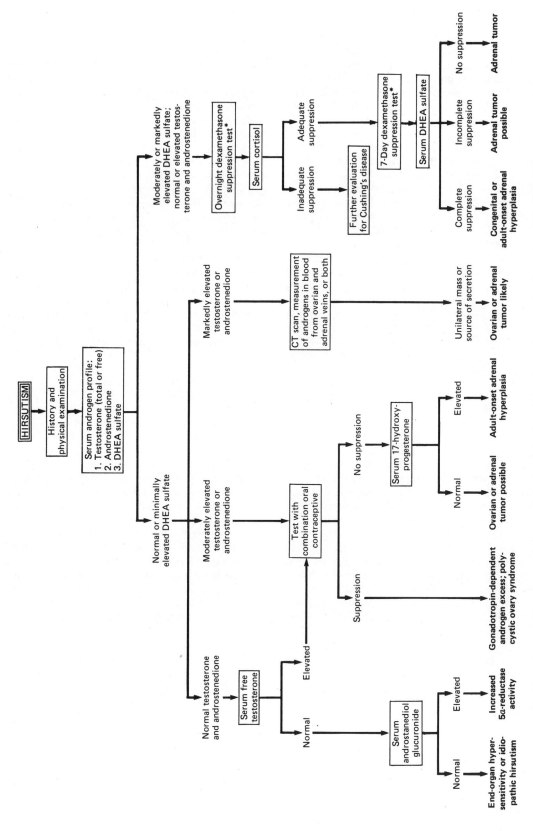

Figure 14–16. A guide to the use of hormone measurements in the evaluation of hirsutism. *See text for discussion of dexamethasone suppression tests.

Induction of ovulation is required for anovulatory patients who wish to conceive. These patients have also been treated by wedge resection of the ovaries. This procedure is associated with resumption of ovulation in many patients but does not usually lead to a reduction in androgen production. The effect is often temporary, and the procedure should be reserved for patients in whom simpler methods have failed and who wish to become pregnant immediately following the procedure.

In patients who have amenorrhea but do not wish to become pregnant, treatment may not be required. However, in patients producing moderate to large amounts of estrogen continuously, endometrial hyperplasia with consequent bleeding and even endometrial carcinoma may develop. In such patients, the cyclic administration of a progestational agent may be required (see Anovulatory Bleeding).

B. Other Causes of Androgen Excess: Excessive production of androgens is far more commonly of ovarian than adrenal origin. However, it is important that the diagnosis be established in order to rule out androgen-producing adrenal and ovarian tumors, Cushing's syndrome, and mild forms of congenital adrenal hyperplasia. Other causes of androgen excess are shown in Table 14–5. The general clinical approach to the evaluation of patients is discussed below and summarized in Fig 14–16.

HIRSUTISM

Hair can be classified as either vellus or terminal. Vellus hairs are fine, soft, and nonpigmented. They are found over most of the body and predominate prior to puberty. They are often so fine that they are barely visible. Terminal hairs are coarse and pigmented. Before puberty, terminal hairs normally are found only on the scalp and eyebrows. Under the influence of increasing levels of androgen at puberty, vellus hairs are transformed into terminal hairs. In women, this conversion to terminal hairs involves principally the axillary and pubic regions and to a lesser extent the extremities. Under conditions of excessive androgen production or increased 5α-reductase activity (which increases conversion of testos-

terone to dihydrotestosterone), there is increased conversion of vellus to terminal hairs. Terminal hairs may thus develop in body regions where such hair growth is normally considered to be a male secondary sex characteristic. The presence of increasing numbers of terminal hairs on the face, chest, back, lower abdomen, and inner thighs is referred to as hirsutism and suggests either increased androgen secretion from the ovaries or adrenals or increased 5α-reductase activity. In many women, hirsutism is accompanied by menstrual dysfunction (usually oligomenorrhea but sometimes amenorrhea). Rarely, abnormal androgen production increases to levels normally found only in men. In such instances, the high circulating levels of androgen also produce somatic changes referred to as virilization. These changes include frontal balding, deepening of the voice, breast atrophy, clitoral enlargement, increased muscle mass, and loss of normal female body contours. The clinical assessment and treatment of women with mild to moderate hirsutism may be complicated by the difficulty in determining if the pattern of hair growth is secondary to an increase in androgen production or utilization or is merely a normal familial trait. The availability of specific and sensitive radioimmunoassays to estimate androgen production, however, may facilitate this difficult differential diagnosis.

Production & Metabolism of Serum Androgens

The major circulating androgens in women are testosterone, dihydrotestosterone, androstenedione, dehydroepiandrosterone (DHEA), and DHEA sulfate. The relative androgenic activity, serum concentrations, and sources of these androgens are summarized in Table 14–7. Testosterone is the principal circulating androgen in normal women. Both the ovaries and the adrenals normally secrete testosterone. Approximately 50% of the testosterone in serum, however, is derived from the peripheral conversion of steroid precursors, principally androstenedione and to a lesser extent DHEA. Testosterone can directly stimulate most androgen-sensitive tissues without prior conversion to dihydrotestosterone. However, in many androgen-sensitive tissues, such as hair follicles, the enzyme 5α-reductase converts testosterone to di-

Table 14–7. Circulating androgens and their relative androgenic activity, serum concentration, and site of formation in women.

Hormone	Relative Androgenic Activity*	Serum Concentration† (ng/mL)	Source of Circulating Hormone (Percentage of Total)		
			Adrenal	Ovary	Peripheral Conversion
Testosterone	100	0.2–0.7	5–25	5–25	50–70
Dihydrotestosterone	250	0.05–0.3	. . .	. . .	100
Androstenedione	10–20	0.5–2.5	30–45	45–60	10
DHEA	5	1.3–9.8	80	20	. . .
DHEA sulfate	Minimal	400–3200	>95	<5	. . .

*Testosterone has been assigned a potency of 100. Values are approximate and may vary depending upon the biologic system in which the hormones are evaluated.

†Normal ranges will vary in different laboratories.

hydrotestosterone. It is believed that dihydrotestosterone per se (and not testosterone) is mainly responsible for stimulating hair growth in many areas of the body. Virtually all of the dihydrotestosterone in the circulation is formed in androgen-dependent peripheral tissues by 5α-reductase conversion of testosterone. Most of the dihydrotestosterone formed in these target tissues is metabolized further to androstanediols. Circulating androstenedione, in contrast to testosterone and dihydrotestosterone, is derived primarily from direct secretion by the ovaries and adrenals. Approximately 5–10% of the circulating androstenedione may also be derived from peripheral conversion of DHEA. Although androstenedione is a relatively weak androgen, possessing only 10–20% of the biologic activity of testosterone, it can be converted to testosterone in androgen-sensitive target tissues. Increased production and secretion of androstenedione thus may play a role in promoting the development of hirsutism in many women. DHEA is a very weak androgen with little biologic activity. More than 80% of the circulating DHEA is of adrenal origin. DHEA sulfate has little or no androgenic activity. Virtually all of the DHEA sulfate in the serum is derived from the adrenal glands. Measurement of serum DHEA sulfate is useful in assessing adrenal function and may reflect adrenal androgen production.

Pathophysiology of Hirsutism

A. Increased Androgen Production: Studies in which women with mild to moderate hirsutism have been evaluated with sensitive and specific androgen assay techniques (eg, assessment of free testosterone concentrations) have shown that most women with excessive hair growth have increased serum androgen levels or increased 5α-reductase activity. Thus, fewer women are currently classified as having "idiopathic" hirsutism. The source (adrenal, ovarian, or both) of the increased production of androgens in women with mild to moderate hirsutism is sometimes difficult to establish by means of suppression and stimulation tests. Many published reports support a combined adrenal-ovarian source for the increased serum levels of androgens, with the ovary as the major contributor in most instances. Approximately 1–5% of women with mild hirsutism have elevated serum levels of 17-hydroxyprogesterone and are thought to have increased androgen production secondary to adult-onset adrenal hyperplasia.

B. Serum Binding Proteins and the Serum Transport of Androgens: As reviewed earlier (Table 14–2), circulating steroid hormones are bound, to varying degrees, to plasma proteins, eg, albumin and specific transport proteins. In normal women, approximately 65% of the circulating testosterone is tightly bound to SHBG, while most of the remaining hormone is loosely bound to albumin. Only 1–2% of the total testosterone is free (not bound to protein). In contrast to testosterone, less than 10% of the circulating androstenedione is bound to SHBG, and nearly 85% is bound to albumin. It is generally thought that

Table 14–8. Conditions affecting SHBG synthesis and therefore the percentage of plasma testosterone that is free.

	SHBG Synthesis
Hypothyroidism Androgen therapy Corticosteroid therapy Obesity Acromegaly	Decreased
Hyperthyroidism Pregnancy Estrogen therapy Cirrhosis	Increased

free steroid hormones are biologically active at target tissues. Factors that can alter the serum concentration of SHBG are shown in Table 14–8. Hirsute women often have reduced serum concentrations of SHBG. Thus, a small increase in total testosterone, accompanied by a decrease in the concentration of SHBG, may result in a significant increase in free or biologically active hormone. The measurement of free testosterone levels in serum is a more sensitive indicator of androgen activity. Most clinical studies have shown that a greater proportion of women with mild to moderate hirsutism have elevated concentrations of free—as compared to total—plasma testosterone.

C. Androgen Metabolism in Skin and Hair Follicles: Factors that alter the activity of 5α-reductase can influence the androgenic activity of testosterone. In vitro studies utilizing skin biopsies from hair-bearing regions have demonstrated increased 5α-reductase activity in hirsute women; thus, many women presently thought to have idiopathic hirsutism may actually have increased formation of dihydrotestosterone in hair follicles. This mechanism also is suggested by the high percentage of women with hirsutism and normal levels of testosterone who have been found to have increased serum levels of androstanediol glucuronide, a major metabolite of dihydrotestosterone.

Evaluation of Women With Hirsutism

The common causes of increased androgen production and hirsutism are listed in Table 14–5. The initial assessment of hirsute women should include a thorough history and physical examination. Hirsutism is usually secondary to a mild increase in androgen activity. The increase in body hair occurs gradually and may be accompanied by other symptoms of mild androgen excess such as acne, oily skin, and oligomenorrhea or amenorrhea. The sudden appearance of rapid hair growth and amenorrhea associated with virilization, however, suggests an ovarian or adrenal androgen-producing tumor (see Chapter 9 and Table 14–4). The physical examination should detect signs of associated endocrine dysfunction, such as Cushing's syndrome or virilization. The degree and extent of growth of terminal hairs should be carefully recorded. This will help the physician decide if further endocrine investigation is warranted and help assess the effects of any future therapy. A pelvic examination also should be included in the initial evaluation of the patient, especially if she has oligomenorrhea or amenorrhea.

The laboratory evaluation of women with hirsutism is important for ruling out a serious underlying disease process such as an ovarian or adrenal androgen-producing tumor, steroid enzymatic defect (eg, partial 21-hydroxylase deficiency), or Cushing's syndrome. Once therapy has been initiated, measurement of serum androgen levels also can be used to determine if serum concentrations of testosterone (total and free), androstenedione, or androstanediol glucuronide have been reduced. Suppression of androgen production or action at the hair follicle will, in most women, reduce the extent of excessive hair growth.

A general approach to the hormonal evaluation of women with hirsutism who are suspected of having either increased production of androgens or increased formation of dihydrotestosterone in peripheral target tissues is shown in Fig 14–16. The rate of ovarian and adrenal androgen secretion can be estimated initially by measuring the serum concentrations of testosterone, androstenedione, and DHEA sulfate. In many women with hirsutism, serum testosterone or androstenedione will be somewhat elevated. Patients with raised levels of these hormones and normal or minimally increased levels of DHEA sulfate can be evaluated further by administering a combination oral contraceptive to suppress pituitary LH and FSH secretion. If the excess production of androgen is gonadotropin-dependent and of ovarian origin (eg, as in polycystic ovary syndrome), serum androgen levels (especially free testosterone levels) also will be suppressed after a 1-month trial of oral contraceptives. Failure of serum androgens to suppress indicates that the excessive production is either of adrenal origin (eg, a tumor or enzyme defect) or secondary to an ovarian neoplasm. Women with adult-onset adrenal hyperplasia secondary to a 21-hydroxylase deficiency will have elevated serum levels of 17-hydroxyprogesterone, which are readily suppressed by dexamethasone.

Women in whom serum levels of total testosterone and androstenedione initially are found to be normal can be evaluated further by measuring free testosterone. If free testosterone levels are within normal limits, 5α-reductase activity can be estimated by measuring serum levels of androstanediol glucuronide. Only a small percentage of hirsute women eventually will be found to have both normal androgen production and 5α-reductase activity. These women can be classified as having idiopathic hirsutism.

Women with signs or symptoms of virilization generally will have greatly elevated testosterone levels (> 3 ng/mL), androstenedione levels above 10 ng/mL, or both. These women are most likely to have an androgen-producing *ovarian* tumor if DHEA sulfate levels are normal or an androgen-producing *adrenal* tumor if DHEA sulfate levels are elevated. Rarely, an androgen-secreting adrenal tumor can be found in the presence of normal serum DHEA sulfate levels. Further evaluation of women with virilization should include suppression tests (dexamethasone for adrenal suppression and an oral contraceptive for ovarian suppression) as well as CT scans of the adrenals and ovaries. If the androgens are not suppressible, surgical exploration is required. A few patients have been found to have tumors with LH-dependent androgen secretion.

Moderately to markedly elevated serum levels of DHEA sulfate indicate increased adrenal androgen secretion resulting from excessive stimulation (eg, Cushing's disease) or indicate adrenal hyperplasia secondary to an enzyme defect, stress, or a tumor. In these cases, serum testosterone and androstenedione levels may vary from minimally to markedly elevated. Initially, women in this group should be evaluated by an overnight dexamethasone suppression test (1 mg of dexamethasone given at bedtime, and serum cortisol levels measured in the morning) to rule out Cushing's syndrome. Suppression of serum cortisol levels to less than 5 μg/dL excludes this disorder. If suppression to this level is not achieved, further assessment of adrenal function, as described in Chapter 9, is required. An overnight dexamethasone suppression test, however, is inadequate to assess adrenal androgen production as reflected by levels of DHEA sulfate, since this hormone has a long plasma half-life. In women who have elevated levels of DHEA sulfate but in whom Cushing's syndrome has been excluded, dexamethasone (2 mg/d) given for 4–7 days will differentiate an adrenal tumor (no suppression) from other causes of increased adrenal androgen production.

Treatment of Hirsutism

Medical therapies directed at reducing the production of ovarian or adrenal androgens are effective primarily in reducing or preventing the formation of new hair growth. For the most part, such treatment has limited effect on terminal hairs previously formed, since the cycle of hair growth ordinarily occurs only every 6 months to 2 years. Consequently, an effective approach to the management of hirsutism usually consists of both medical and cosmetic treatment.

A. Suppression of Androgen Production: The reduction of serum levels of androgens by trials with combination oral contraceptives, progestins, or glucocorticoids should provide a rational basis for choosing one or another of these various forms of therapy. However, most women with hirsutism have only slightly increased androgen production, and its precise source or sources cannot be identified readily. In these patients, estrogen-containing oral contraceptives are generally more effective and are most often the initial form of treatment.

1. Oral contraceptives or progestins—Oral contraceptives containing both an estrogen and a progestin suppress the secretion of LH and FSH and reduce LH-dependent ovarian androgen production. The progestin component also increases the metabolic clearance rate of testosterone, while the estrogen component stimulates the production of SHBG. Although treatment with a progestin alone (ie, oral or injectable medroxyprogesterone acetate) suppresses the secretion of LH and increases the metabolic clearance rate of androgens, there is no concomitant increase in SHBG levels. Progestins are therefore generally less effective than combination oral contraceptives. They may be useful when estrogens are contraindicated.

The available combination oral contraceptives are listed in Table 14–11. In selecting a particular contraceptive for the treatment of hirsutism, the physician should avoid compounds containing the more androgenic progestins, particularly norgestrel. Contraceptives containing a minimum of 35–50 μg of ethinyl estradiol may increase serum concentrations of SHBG and reduce the levels of both total and free testosterone in most patients. If significant clinical improvement— eg, a decrease in acne, skin oiliness, and rate of hair growth—is not apparent after 3 months of treatment, serum androgen levels should be reevaluated to make certain that adequate suppression of ovarian function has occurred. Treatment with oral contraceptives is discussed in a subsequent section of this chapter.

2. Glucocorticoids–If increased androgen production is predominantly or entirely of adrenal origin—such as occurs in adult-onset adrenal hyperplasia—treatment with glucocorticoids is indicated. In these cases, dexamethasone, 0.5–0.75 mg/d, or prednisone, 5–7.5 mg/d, has been used to reduce the production of adrenal androgens. In most women with hirsutism, however, excess androgen secretion is generally of ovarian origin, and glucocorticoids are not effective.

3. Antiandrogens–Cyproterone acetate was the first antiandrogen to be employed extensively for the treatment of hirsutism. Clinical studies with this drug in Europe have resulted in a high rate of improvement. Cyproterone acetate is a derivative of the progestin chlormadinone acetate and possesses both progestational and antiandrogenic activity. It suppresses the secretion of LH, with a subsequent decrease in ovarian androgen production, and blocks the binding of androgens to receptors in the hair follicles. Estrogen is usually administered concurrently, since endogenous estrogen production also is reduced during treatment. Although few serious side effects have been reported, cyproterone acetate is not available in the USA. A commonly used dosage is 2 mg of cyproterone acetate plus 50 μg of ethinyl estradiol daily on days 5–20 of each menstrual cycle.

Spironolactone, a competitive inhibitor of aldosterone, has been shown to possess antiandrogenic properties and competes with dihydrotestosterone for androgenic receptors in target tissues. It also decreases 17α-hydroxylase activity and thus reduces serum levels of testosterone and androstenedione. Doses ranging from 50 to 200 mg/d have been used to treat hirsutism. Spironolactone is especially useful for therapy in women in whom oral contraceptives are contraindicated or ineffective.

B. Cosmetic Therapy: The initial response to medical treatment is generally slow, and 3–6 months of therapy may be required before there is noticeable improvement in hirsutism. During the initial period of treatment, the patient can either continue with or start a simple and inexpensive method for the temporary removal of hair, eg, shaving or use of a depilatory or hot wax. After several months of medical treatment, the rate of formation of new terminal hairs will be reduced markedly, and permanent hair removal by electrolysis can be initiated, if desired. If permanent hair removal is tried prior to adequate medical treatment, the results will be transient, since new terminal hairs will continue to be formed.

ANOVULATORY BLEEDING

In the absence of ovulatory cycles, the pattern of bleeding (Table 14–3) is dependent upon the amount and timing of estrogen secretion, since the bleeding is due to estrogen stimulation of the endometrium. When estrogen secretion is low, there is usually no bleeding. On the other hand, the heaviest bleeding is observed in association with continuous secretion of substantial amounts of estrogen. In these instances, the estrogen produces proliferation of the endometrium, leading to hyperplasia or adenomatous hyperplasia. In some of these women, endometrial carcinoma will develop over long periods. When the level of estrogen fluctuates, bleeding will occur during periods of reduced secretion. However, when the secretion is continuous and maturation is not synchronized by progesterone, the tissue is subject to spontaneous breakdown and bleeding of differing portions of the endometrium at different times. Furthermore, local factors such as the coiling and contraction of the spiral vessels do not contribute to the hemostasis, and bleeding may be severe. Such bleeding is more common in postpubertal teenagers and in the premenopausal period in older women. It is also seen in some patients in association with polycystic ovary syndrome and in women receiving estrogen therapy.

OVULATION INDUCTION

CLOMIPHENE CITRATE

Clomiphene citrate (Clomid) is a weak estrogen that effectively inhibits the action of stronger estrogens and stimulates the secretion of gonadotropins; it is used for the treatment of anovulatory patients in whom ovulation is desired. In general, a single ovulation is induced by a single course of therapy, and the patient must be treated repeatedly until pregnancy is achieved. The compound is of no use in the treatment of ovarian or pituitary failure.

The recommended initial dose of clomiphene citrate is 50 mg/d for 5 days. If ovulation occurs, this same course may be repeated until pregnancy is achieved. If ovulation does not occur, the dose is doubled to 100 mg/d for 5 days. If ovulation and menses occur, the next course can be started on the fifth day of the cycle. About 80% of patients with anovulatory disorders or amenorrhea can be expected to respond to this treatment by having ovulatory cycles. Approximately half of these patients will become pregnant. In patients in whom pregnancy is achieved, the incidence of early abortion seems to be slightly increased, as is the occurrence of multiple pregnancy (10%). Although a variety of congenital defects have been described in the offspring of these pregnancies, the incidence does not appear to be greater than that of the general population. Ovulation can be induced in some of the patients not responding to 50 or 100 mg of clomiphene daily for 5 days by using larger doses (up to 200 mg/d) for longer periods or by injecting 5000 units of chorionic gonadotropin at the time of expected ovulation. The combination of clomiphene and bromocriptine has also been reported to be successful in some patients with normal PRL levels. Clomiphene has also been used in combination with menotropins to reduce the amount of the latter required to induce ovulation.

The effective use of clomiphene is associated with some stimulation of the ovaries and usually with ovarian enlargement. The degree of enlargement tends to be greater and its incidence higher in patients who have enlarged ovaries at the beginning of therapy.

The most common side effects in patients treated with this drug are hot flushes, which resemble those experienced by menopausal patients. These tend to be mild and disappear when the drug is discontinued. There have been occasional reports of visual disturbances consisting of intensification and prolongation of afterimages. These are generally of short duration. Headache, constipation, allergic skin reactions, and reversible hair loss have been reported occasionally.

HUMAN MENOPAUSAL GONADOTROPINS (Menotropins)

Human menopausal gonadotropins, or menotropins (Pergonal), in conjunction with chorionic gonadotropin, are used to stimulate ovulation in patients who do not ovulate but who have potentially functional ovarian tissue. Patients with ovarian failure should not be considered for therapy. This treatment has induced ovulation in patients with hypopituitarism and other defects of gonadotropin secretion. It has also been used in patients with amenorrhea or anovulatory cycles and in those in whom ovulatory disturbances are associated with galactorrhea or hirsutism. Menotropins are generally used only after less complicated therapies, such as clomiphene citrate or bromocrip-

Table 14–9. Results of treatment with menotropins.

Pregnancy achieved: 25–40%
Multiple births
Twins, 10–20%
Triplets, etc, 5–10%
Abortions, 20%
Hyperstimulation syndrome: 0.5–1.5%

tine, have been unsuccessful. Since therapy is difficult and expensive, it is also important to exclude other factors that might preclude pregnancy (eg, obstruction of the uterine tubes or abnormalities in sperm production by the husband) prior to initiating treatment. The possibility of multiple births must be acceptable to the patient.

Contraindications & Cautions

The most common problem encountered is excessive ovarian stimulation. Ovarian enlargement is common. When marked, as in the ovarian hyperstimulation syndrome, it may be accompanied by pain, ascites, and pleural effusion. A few patients experience fever and swelling along with discomfort at the injection site. Undesirable results of therapy include a high incidence of multiple pregnancy and abortion. The frequency of birth defects has not been increased in the offspring of patients who have succeeded in carrying their pregnancies to term.

The typical outcome of therapy in properly selected patients treated by experienced physicians is shown in Table 14–9. Menotropins are potentially dangerous and should be administered by physicians with experience in endocrine disturbances and problems of reproductive function. This mode of therapy is complicated, time-consuming, and expensive and should not be undertaken unless simpler therapeutic measures have failed.

Dosages

Human menopausal gonadotropins (menotropins, Pergonal) are supplied in lyophilized form in ampules containing 75 units each of FSH and LH and 10 mg of lactose. The usual dosage is one or more ampules intramuscularly daily until estrogen production is optimal—ie, plasma levels of 600–1000 pg/mL. Growth of ovarian follicles can also be monitored by ultrasonography to assist in determining the optimal dosage and duration of treatment with menotropins. Chorionic gonadotropin (see Chapter 17) in doses of 5000–10,000 units intramuscularly is then administered on one or more occasions; if estrogen production becomes excessive, chorionic gonadotropin should be withheld to avoid the ovarian hyperstimulation syndrome. Patients must be examined frequently (daily or on alternate days) for 2 weeks following the last injection to detect signs of overstimulation and should be advised to have intercourse at least every other day near the time of expected ovulation.

GONADOTROPIN-RELEASING HORMONE

The induction of ovulation by GnRH has been under study. The pulsatile administration of this hormone in doses of $1-10$ μg at 60- to 120-minute intervals will induce ovulation in patients with amenorrhea due to hypothalamic dysfunction or deficiency. GnRH can be given intravenously or subcutaneously using a peristaltic pump. Although the method is cumbersome, ovarian hyperstimulation is less likely to occur.

BROMOCRIPTINE

Although bromocriptime is occasionally effective in treating patients with amenorrhea in the absence of elevated serum levels of PRL, its use is generally reserved for patients with hyperprolactinemia or galactorrhea. Its use in such patients is described elsewhere in this chapter.

THERAPEUTIC USE OF OVARIAN HORMONES & THEIR SYNTHETIC ANALOGS

Estrogens are used in combination with progestins by more than 40 million women for contraception and are widely used after the menopause. Estrogens are also used to limit the height of tall girls and to replace absent or deficient endogenous hormone in patients with hypogonadism or after gonadectomy. It is therefore important to understand the effects of these agents and problems engendered by their use.

TREATMENT OF PRIMARY HYPOGONADISM

Treatment of primary hypogonadism is usually begun at $11-13$ years of age in order to stimulate the development of secondary sex characteristics and menses and to promote optimal growth. Treatment consists mainly of the administration of estrogens and progestins. Androgens and anabolic agents have also been used in these patients to stimulate growth, but no further increase in final height was achieved. Furthermore, acne, hirsutism, clitorimegaly, and premature closure of the epiphyses have occurred as unwanted effects of androgens and anabolic agents. Progestins are advisable in conjunction with estrogens, because long-term replacement therapy, even when used cyclically in modest doses, has been associated with an increase in the incidence of endometrial hyperplasia and endometrial carcinoma. Oral contraceptives have also been used for replacement therapy.

OVARIAN SUPPRESSION

Estrogen-progestin combinations (oral contraceptives) are used to suppress ovarian function in patients with LH-dependent excess androgen production or endometriosis and are discussed elsewhere in this chapter.

Progestational hormones alone are used to produce long-term ovarian suppression when estrogens are contraindicated. When used parenterally in large doses—eg, medroxyprogesterone acetate, 150 mg intramuscularly every 90 days—prolonged anovulation and amenorrhea are produced. This procedure has been employed in the treatment of dysmenorrhea, endometriosis, hirsutism, and bleeding disorders. The major problem encountered with this regimen is the prolonged time required for ovulatory function to return after cessation of therapy in some patients. Irregular spotting also occurs. This treatment should not be used for patients planning a pregnancy in the near future.

THREATENED ABORTION

Progestins do not appear to have any place in the therapy of threatened or habitual abortion. Early reports of the usefulness of these agents were based on the unwarranted assumption that after several abortions the likelihood of repeated abortions was over 90%. When progestational agents were administered to patients with previous abortions, a salvage rate of 80% was achieved. It is now recognized that similar patients abort only 20% of the time even when untreated.

In some patients with "threatened" abortion, progesterone production is decreased. It is likely that the decrease in progesterone reflects damage to the placenta or fetus and is a result of events leading to abortion rather than a cause of the abortion. Administration of progesterone in these circumstances does not appear to be useful and may allow retention of the dead fetus, thus delaying recognition of an abortion that has occurred. Prolonged postpartum bleeding has also been reported in some patients treated with repository medroxyprogesterone or hydroxyprogesterone caproate.

INADEQUATE LUTEAL PHASE

Progesterone and medroxyprogesterone have been used in the treatment of women who have difficulty in conceiving and who demonstrate a slow rise in basal body temperature. Some investigators believe that these patients suffer from a relative luteal insufficiency, and progesterone or related compounds are given to replace the deficiency. There is no convincing evidence that this treatment is effective. In the absence of satisfactory controls, the successes reported are impossible to distinguish from placebo effects.

DIAGNOSTIC USES

Progesterone is also used as a test of estrogen secretion. A single intramuscular injection of 200 mg of progesterone in oil or a course of medroxyprogesterone, 10 mg/d for 5–7 days, is followed by withdrawal bleeding in amenorrheic patients only when the endometrium has been stimulated by estrogens. In the absence of withdrawal bleeding, a combination of estrogen and progestin can be given to test the responsiveness of the endometrium in patients with amenorrhea.

INHIBITORS OF OVARIAN FUNCTION

GONADOTROPIN-RELEASING HORMONE ANALOGS

As noted above, GnRH administered in a pulsatile manner will induce ovulation in patients with amenorrhea. However, when large amounts are administered continuously, inhibition of gonadotropin release occurs. This property has been exploited by the development of highly potent agonist analogs, such as buserelin and nafarelin. These analogs can be administered intranasally or subcutaneously on a daily basis. High-dose suppression is useful when marked gonadotropin suppression is required, such as in cases of precocious puberty, endometriosis, and hormone-dependent tumors. Smaller doses may be useful for contraception.

TAMOXIFEN

Tamoxifen is a nonsteroidal competitive inhibitor of estradiol at its receptor. It can be given orally and is being used in the palliative treatment of advanced breast cancer in postmenopausal women (see Chapter 23). Peak plasma levels are reached in a few hours. It has an initial half-life of 7–14 hours in the circulation and is predominantly excreted by the liver. It is dispensed as the citrate in the form of tablets (Nolvadex) containing the equivalent of 10 mg of tamoxifen. It is used in doses of 10–20 mg twice daily. Hot flushes and nausea and vomiting occur in 25% of patients, and many other adverse effects have been reported.

DANAZOL

Danazol (Danocrine), an isoxazole derivative of ethisterone (17α-ethinyl testosterone) with weak progestational and androgenic activities, is used to suppress ovarian function. It inhibits the midcycle surge of LH and FSH and can prevent the compensatory increase in LH and FSH following castration in animals, but it does not significantly lower or suppress basal LH or FSH levels in normal women. Danazol binds to androgen, progesterone, and glucocorticoid receptors and can translocate the androgen receptor into the nucleus to initiate androgen-specific RNA synthesis. It does not bind to intracellular estrogen receptors, but it does bind to SHBG and CBG. It inhibits the cholesterol-cleaving enzyme, 3α-hydroxysteroid dehydrogenase, 17α-hydroxysteroid dehydrogenase, 17,21-lyase, 17α-hydroxylase, 11α-hydroxylase, and 21-hydroxylase, but it does not inhibit aromatase. It increases the mean clearance rate of progesterone, probably by displacing the hormone from binding proteins, and may have similar effects on other active steroid hormones. Ethisterone, a major metabolite, has both progestational and mild androgenic effects.

Danazol has been employed as an inhibitor of gonadal function and has found its major use in the treatment of endometriosis. For this purpose, it is usually administered at a starting dose of 400 mg/d, and in patients who do not respond, the dose can be increased to 600 or 800 mg/d. In most patients requiring the larger doses, the dosage can be reduced after several months of therapy without a return of symptoms.

The major side effects are weight gain, edema, decreased breast size, acne and oily skin, mild hirsutism, deepening of the voice, headache, hot flushes, changes in libido, and muscle cramps. Although mild side effects are very common, it is seldom necessary to discontinue the drug because of them.

Danazol should be used with great caution in patients with hepatic dysfunction, since it has been reported to produce mild to moderate hepatocellular damage in some patients, as evidenced by enzyme changes. It is also contraindicated during pregnancy and breast feeding, as it can produce urogenital abnormalities in the offspring.

Danazol has also been used for the treatment of fibrocystic disease of the breast. It has been effective in some patients for the relief of severe cyclic breast pain and tenderness but should be reserved for use in patients in whom analgesics and other drugs have failed.

ANTIANDROGENS

The possibility of using antiandrogens to treat hirsutism and other disorders due to excessive amounts of testosterone has led to a search for effective drugs via 2 approaches that have met with limited success experimentally. Several compounds have been developed that inhibit the 17-hydroxylation of progesterone or pregnenolone, thereby preventing the action of the side chain–splitting enzyme and the further transformation of these steroid precursors to active androgens. A few of these compounds have been tested clinically but have been too toxic for prolonged use. Another approach has been the development of steroids that are chemically similar and act as competitive inhibitors. A few of them have been tried in patients on a limited basis.

Cyproterone and **cyproterone acetate** are effective antiandrogens that inhibit the action of the androgens at the target organ. The acetate form has a marked progestational effect that suppresses LH and FSH, thus leading to a more effective antiandrogen effect. These compounds have been used to decrease excessive sexual drive in disturbed individuals and are being studied in other conditions in which reduction of androgenic effects would be useful. In Europe, they are used in the treatment of hirsutism. They are not available in the USA.

THE MENOPAUSE

The menopause begins with the last episode of menstrual bleeding induced by the cyclic endogenous secretion of ovarian hormones. It normally occurs between the ages of 42 and 60 years. It occurs prematurely as a result of surgical removal, irradiation, or abnormalities of the ovaries.

HORMONAL CHANGES

The changes in endocrine function are not abrupt in women undergoing spontaneous menopause. The circulating levels of gonadotropins begin to increase several years before ovulation ceases. Production of estrogen and progesterone decreases, and irregular cycles and anovulatory bleeding are not uncommon (Table 14–10). The increase in FSH is greater than that of LH and reflects the lack of feedback inhibition by estrogen. The stromal cells of the ovary respond

Table 14–10. Serum concentrations (mean ± SEM) of steroids in premenopausal and postmenopausal women.*

Steroid	Premenopausal† (ng/mL)	Postmenopausal (ng/mL)
Progesterone	0.47 ± 0.03	0.17 ± 0.02
DHEA	4.2 ± 0.5	1.8 ± 0.2
DHEA sulfate	1600 ± 350	300 ± 70
Androstenedione	1.5 ± 0.1	0.6 ± 0.01
Testosterone	0.32 ± 0.02	0.25 ± 0.03
Estrone	0.08 ± 0.01	0.029 ± 0.002
Estradiol	0.05 ± 0.005	0.013 ± 0.001

*Reproduced, with permission, from Benson RC (editor): *Current Obstetric & Gynecologic Diagnosis & Treatment,* 5th ed. Lange, 1984.
†Follicular phase concentrations.

to increased LH stimulation by producing more androstenedione but only tiny amounts of estrogen.

The average production rate of estradiol falls to 12 μg/24 h, and the clearance rate is reduced. Since very little estradiol is found in ovarian or adrenal veins, most of the circulating estradiol is derived from estrone, which in itself is produced by the peripheral conversion of androstenedione. The average production rate for estrone is 55 μg/24 h, and there is a 20% reduction in its clearance.

Progesterone levels are approximately 30% of the concentration seen in young women during the follicular phase. The source of this progesterone appears to be the adrenal.

Androgen levels are also reduced postmenopausally. Androstenedione falls to about half of the concentration found in young women, and most of that apparently comes from the adrenal, as suggested by its peak concentrations at 8 AM and nadir concentrations at 3–4 PM. The clearance rate does not change. The average production rate is about 1.5 mg/24 h. About 20% of it is thought to come from the ovary. Testosterone production rates are approximately 150 μg/24 h, as compared to about 200 μg/24 h in younger women. This fall is less than that seen after ovariectomy, indicating that testosterone is produced by conversion of androstenedione as well as being secreted by the adrenal and ovary. It is of interest that DHEA and DHEA sulfate also fall with age, although almost all of these steroids come from the adrenal gland.

CLINICAL MANIFESTATIONS OF MENOPAUSE

Menstrual Changes

The interval prior to the menopause is usually characterized sequentially by cycles with a shortening of the follicular phase, an interval of very irregular cycles, and an interval of anovulatory bleeding. Fertility is usually very low during this time. Although menses may cease abruptly, usually there is a gradual diminution in the amount of menstrual flow as well as its duration. However, if secretion of estrogen is prolonged in the absence of ovulation, endometrial hyperplasia may occur and cause heavy bleeding. It is sometimes difficult to clinically distinguish this type of bleeding from that produced by organic diseases, including endometrial carcinoma. Any bleeding that occurs more than a year after the last previous period is likely to be an indication of organic disease.

Vasomotor Symptoms

The most common menopausal complaint is hot flushes, which occur in 75% of women at the menopause. They are due to declining estrogen levels rather than to estrogen deficiency per se. Women with estrogen deficiency from childhood do not develop hot flushes unless they have been treated with exogenous estrogens and treatment is interrupted. Episodes of flushing are associated with periodic increases in core temperature, causing reflex peripheral vasodilatation, a small increase in pulse rate, and sweating. They are synchronous with the pulsatile release of LH and appear to be linked to the central mechanism controlling the release of GnRH. These symptoms occur most frequently in a warm environment and are common at night, contributing to insomnia.

The hot flush often starts with a sensation of pressure in the head, followed by a feeling of warmth in the head and neck and upper thorax. It may be associated with palpitations and gradually spreading waves of heat over the entire body. The feeling of warmth and flushing is quickly followed by sweating. The sweating and vasodilatation lead to heat loss and a decrease in core temperature of approximately 0.2 °C. These episodes last 10–20 minutes.

In 20% of patients, hot flushes are a transient phenomenon lasting for less than 1 year, but 25–50% of women experience them for more than 5 years. Estrogen therapy is remarkably effective in controlling hot flushes in over 90% of patients.

Atrophic Changes in the Genitourinary System

The decline in estrogen production results in reduction in mucus secretion and gradual atrophy of the vaginal and urethral epithelium. The rugae progressively disappear with thinning of the epithelium. The surface may appear vascular at first but then becomes pale. These changes lead to itching, dyspareunia, and burning. Similar changes in the urinary tract may give rise to atrophic cystitis, with symptoms of urgency, incontinence, and frequency. The cervix decreases in size, and the mucus secretion diminishes. The endometrium and myometrium also undergo atrophy. Myomas become smaller and endometriosis less symptomatic. The adverse symptoms can be treated by administration of estrogens locally as well as systemically (see below).

Osteoporosis

Osteoporosis results from a combination of in-

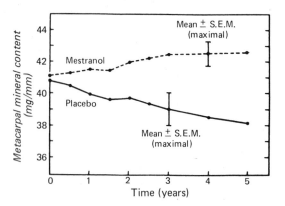

Figure 14–17. Metacarpal mineral content in postmenopausal women treated with mestranol or placebo for 5 years. Note loss of bone density in placebo but not mestranol treatment group. (Reproduced, with permission, from Lindsay R et al: Long-term prevention of postmenopausal osteoporosis by oestrogen. *Lancet* 1976;1:1038.)

creased bone resorption and decreased bone formation. It is predominantly a disease of trabecular bone. Affected patients show increased calcium loss from bone, which could account for the slight elevation of plasma Ca^{2+}, reduction of $1,25(OH)_2D_3$, and reduction in the intestinal absorption of Ca^{2+} found in this disorder. The problem is enhanced in winter months because of decreased activity and decreased exposure to sunlight and by the difficulty of maintaining calcium balance at normal levels of intake.

During the first few years following menopause, women lose an average of about 2.5% of their bone mass per year (Fig 14–17), and the percentage gradually decreases to about 0.75% per year for the rest of their lives. It is the initial rapid bone loss which is inhibited by estrogen. Loss of bone mass leads to reduced skeletal strength and susceptibility to fractures. There is, for example, a 10-fold increase in the

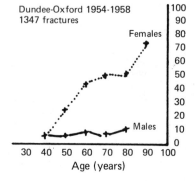

Figure 14–18. Indices of Colles' fracture in relation to age in Malmö, Dundee, and Oxford. (Reproduced, with permission, from Cope E: Physical changes associated with post-menopausal years. Page 4 in: *Management of the Menopause and Post-Menopause Years.* Campbell S [editor]. MTP Press Ltd, 1976.)

incidence of Colles' fractures in women between the ages of 35 and 55, although a similar increase is not seen in men (Fig 14–18). Hip fractures, which are ultimately fatal in about one-third of patients and disable others for life, also occur more frequently.

The availability of a method for assessing bone density has led to a better understanding of the disorder and its response to therapy. Studies indicate that bone density decreases in women as the years advance. However, the loss is accelerated at menopause. Other studies indicate that estrogen therapy started at that time can prevent the loss (Fig 14–17). If estrogens are administered subsequently, the process can be arrested. However, when treatment is delayed for 5–6 years, little effect is noted. Treatment with estrogen decreases plasma Ca^{2+} and increases plasma PTH and $1,25(OH)_2D_3$, which, in turn, increases calcium absorption. The risk for osteoporosis is highest in smokers who are thin, Caucasian, inactive, and have a low calcium intake and a strong family history of osteoporosis. (See also Chapter 8.)

Skin & Hair

At the time of the menopause, changes in the skin due to aging are noticeable. There is some thinning and wrinkling. Although estrogen creams are widely used cosmetically, it is not clear that they have any effects other than enhancement of the dermal water content. Changes in hair include loss of some underarm and pubic hair and occasionally replacement of vellus hair on the chin and upper lip by terminal hairs.

Emotional Changes

Anxiety, depression, and irritability are commonly reported around the time of the menopause. There is no good evidence that these symptoms are directly related to estrogen deficiency. However, sleep disturbances caused by hot flushes may contribute to the irritability. The majority of women treated with estrogens report some improvement in their sense of well-being and relief of insomnia and other symptoms produced by estrogen deficiency.

MANAGEMENT OF THE MENOPAUSAL PATIENT

Hormonal Therapy

The major indications for hormonal therapy in menopausal patients are the treatment of hot flushes and atrophic vaginitis and the prevention of osteoporosis in patients at high risk for development of that disorder. Estrogens should be used in the smallest dose consistent with relief of symptoms. In women with a uterus, estrogen therapy should be given for the first 21–25 days of each month and a progestational agent administered during the last 10–14 days of estrogen administration. The recommended daily dosage of estrogen is 0.3–1.25 mg of conjugated estrogens or 0.01–0.02 mg of ethinyl estradiol. Doses in the middle of these ranges have been shown to be maximally effective in preventing the decrease in bone density occurring at the menopause. In order to prevent osteoporosis, it is important to begin therapy as soon as possible after the menopause. Studies indicate that addition of 10 mg medroxyprogesterone acetate orally daily for the last 10–14 days of estrogen therapy markedly reduces the risk of endometrial carcinoma.

Patients at low risk for development of osteoporosis with only mild atrophic vaginitis can be treated with local vaginal preparations. This route of application is also useful in treatment of urinary tract symptoms. It is important to realize, however, that locally administered estrogens are almost completely absorbed into the circulation and should be used intermittently.

In patients in whom estrogen replacement therapy is contraindicated (eg, those with estrogen-sensitive tumors), relief of vasomotor symptoms may be obtained by the use of progestational agents. Medroxyprogesterone acetate, 150 mg intramuscularly once a month, norgestrel, 250 μg orally daily, or medroxyprogesterone, 10 mg orally daily, can be useful. Mild tranquilizers and clonidine are also effective in some patients, as are atropine-barbiturate mixtures. Calcium carbonate supplements (eg, Os-Cal) are useful in bringing the total daily calcium intake up to 1500 mg. Vitamin D therapy may be useful when calcium intake is less than optimal. Preliminary studies show that fluoride in adequate amounts can increase bone density, but the effects on bone strength have not been assessed.

Adverse Effects of Therapy

Therapeutic use of estrogens is accompanied by adverse effects of varying degrees of severity (see Hormonal Contraception, below).

Estrogen therapy has now become the major cause of postmenopausal bleeding. Unfortunately, vaginal bleeding at this time of life may be due to carcinoma of the endometrium, and many women are being subjected to dilatation and curettage of the uterus unnecessarily. In order to avoid this complication, patients should be treated with the smallest effective amount of estrogen, given cyclically, with addition of a progestational agent in the last 10 days of estrogen in each cycle. This will usually produce regular and predictable withdrawal bleeding.

Nausea and breast tenderness are common and can be minimized by using the smallest effective dose. These symptoms may be more marked at the beginning of therapy. The presence of cystic mastitis or fibroids that increase in size during treatment may also interfere with the use of estrogen. Hyperpigmentation also occurs. Estrogen therapy is associated with an increase in frequency of migraine headaches as well as cholestasis, hypertension, and gallbladder disease.

The relationship of estrogen therapy to cancer continues to be the subject of active investigation. It has not been possible to establish that there is an increased risk in the incidence of breast cancer. However, it is not clear that it is safe to use estrogen in patients at high risk for development of this tumor. The risk of endometrial carcinoma is increased in patients taking estrogens and varies with the dose and duration of treatment. It increases 15 times in patients taking large doses of estrogen for 5 or more years but only 2–4 times in patients receiving lower doses for 2 years. The concomitant use of a progestin not only prevents this increased risk but actually reduces the incidence of endometrial cancer below that in the general population.

HORMONAL CONTRACEPTION
(Oral Contraceptives)

A large number of oral contraceptives containing estrogens or progestins (or both) are now available for clinical use (Table 14–11). These preparations vary in chemical composition and, as might be expected, have many properties in common, but there are also differences. Two types of preparations are used for oral contraception: (1) monophasic, biphasic, and triphasic combinations of estrogens and progestins; and (2) progestins without concomitant administration of estrogens.

PHARMACOLOGIC EFFECTS OF ESTROGENS & SYNTHETIC PROGESTINS

Mechanisms of Contraceptive Action

Estrogens and progestin combinations inhibit gonadotropin secretion, which prevents ovulation. They also change the cervical mucus, the endometrium, and tubal motility and secretion, all of which decrease the likelihood of conception and implantation. Continuous use of progestins alone does not inhibit ovulation, and the other effects play a major role in prevention of pregnancy when these agents are used.

Genital Effects of Oral Contraceptives

Chronic use of estrogen-progestin combinations depresses ovarian function. The ovary shows minimal follicular development and an absence of corpora lutea, larger follicles, stromal edema, and other morphologic features normally seen in ovulating women. Estrogen production is decreased, and progesterone secretion is minimal. Although cystic follicles have been described in patients taking oral contraceptives, the ovaries usually become smaller even when previously enlarged.

Cytologic findings on vaginal smears vary depending on the preparation used. However, with almost all of the combined drugs, a midzone maturation index is found because of the presence of progestational agents.

Effects on the uterus include hypertrophy of the cervix and polyp formation after prolonged use. The cervical mucus becomes thick and less copious and contains much cellular debris. Initially, there may be some stimulation of the uterine muscle, resulting in softening. Stromal deciduation occurs toward the end of the cycle. The agents containing 19-nortestosterone derivatives combined with smaller amounts of estrogen tend to produce more glandular atrophy and less bleeding than agents containing progestins that stimulate glandular development.

Although studies in humans are not available, experiments in animals indicate that alterations in the transport of the gamete through the uterine tube are produced by estrogens and progestins. The effect on germ cell transport is thought by some to be an important mechanism for the impairment of fertility, particularly with the use of low-dosage continuous progestin therapy.

Stimulation of the breasts occurs in most patients receiving estrogen-containing agents. Some enlargement is generally noted. These agents tend to suppress lactation, but when the doses are small, the effects on breast feeding are not appreciable. Preliminary studies of transport of oral contraceptives into the breast milk suggest that only small amounts of these compounds are found and they have not been considered to be of importance.

Extragenital Effects of Oral Contraceptives

It is important to understand the extragenital effects of oral contraceptives, because of the large and growing number of normal individuals using them.

A. Central Nervous System Effects: The effects of the oral contraceptives on the central nervous system have not been well studied in humans. In animals, estrogens tend to lower the threshold of excitability in the brain, whereas progesterone tends to increase it. In addition, the increased respiration and thermogenic actions of progesterone and some of the synthetic progestins are thought to be due to effects on the central nervous system. The suppression of ovarian function results in part from inhibition of GnRH secretion by the hypothalamus.

It is very difficult to evaluate any behavioral or emotional effects of these compounds. Although there is a low incidence of pronounced changes in mood, affect, and behavior in most studies, milder changes are common. Behavioral changes are variable and therefore difficult to evaluate. However, it is possible that the changes in neuronal activity and thresholds produced by these drugs may lead to changes conditioned by psychologic, social, and environmental factors.

B. Effects on Endocrine Function: The combined agents inhibit the secretion of pituitary gonadotropins, as mentioned above. Estrogens increase the plasma concentration of CBG. This increases plasma cortisol concentrations but does not lead to chronic alteration in the rate of cortisol secretion. It has also been observed that the ACTH response to the administration of metyrapone (see Chapter 4) is attenuated by estrogens and the oral contraceptives.

These preparations alter the angiotensin-aldosterone system, increasing plasma renin activity and therefore aldosterone secretion. The relationship between these alterations and the hypertension that oc-

curs in some patients taking oral contraceptives is not clear.

TBG is increased, resulting in higher circulating thyroxine levels. However, the free thyroxine level in these patients is normal.

C. Hematologic Effects: Serious thromboembolic phenomena occurring in women taking oral contra-

Table 14–11. Oral contraceptive agents in use. The estrogen-containing compounds are arranged in order of increasing content of estrogen (ethinyl estradiol and mestranol have similar potencies). The relative progestational potencies are shown in the last column.*

	Estrogen (mg)		Progestin (mg)		PP†
Monophasic combination tablets					
Loestrin 1/20	Ethinyl estradiol	0.02	Norethindrone acetate	1.0	4
Loestrin 1.5/30	Ethinyl estradiol	0.03	Norethindrone acetate	1.5	6
Lo/Ovral	Ethinyl estradiol	0.03	dl-Norgestrel	0.3	18
Nordette	Ethinyl estradiol	0.03	L-Norgestrel	0.15	18
Brevicon Modicon	Ethinyl estradiol	0.035	Norethindrone	0.5	1
Demulen 1/35	Ethinyl estradiol	0.035	Ethynodiol diacetate	1.0	30
Norinyl 1/35 Ortho-Novum 1/35	Ethinyl estradiol	0.035	Norethindrone	1.0	2
Ovcon 35	Ethinyl estradiol	0.035	Norethindrone	0.4	0.8
Demulen 1/50	Ethinyl estradiol	0.05	Ethynodiol diacetate	1.0	30
Norlestrin 1/50	Ethinyl estradiol	0.05	Norethindrone acetate	1.0	4
Norlestrin 2.5/50	Ethinyl estradiol	0.05	Norethindrone acetate	2.5	10
Ovcon 50	Ethinyl estradiol	0.05	Norethindrone	1.0	2
Ovral	Ethinyl estradiol	0.05	dl-Norgestrel	0.5	30
Norinyl 1/50 Ortho-Novum 1/50	Mestranol	0.05	Norethindrone	1.0	2
Enovid 5	Mestranol	0.075	Norethynodrel	5.0	11
Norinyl 1/80 Ortho-Novum 1/80	Mestranol	0.08	Norethindrone	1.0	2
Enovid E	Mestranol	0.1	Norethynodrel	2.5	6
Norinyl-2 Ortho-Novum-2	Mestranol	0.1	Norethindrone	2.0	4
Ovulen	Mestranol	0.1	Ethynodiol diacetate	1.0	30
Biphasic combination tablets					
Ortho-Novum 10/11					
Days 1–10	Ethinyl estradiol	0.035	Norethindrone	0.5	1
Days 11–21	Ethinyl estradiol	0.035	Norethindrone	1.0	2
Triphasic combination tablets					
Triphasil					
Days 1–6	Ethinyl estradiol	0.03	L-Norgestrel	0.05	2
Days 7–11	Ethinyl estradiol	0.04	L-Norgestrel	0.075	3
Days 12–21	Ethinyl estradiol	0.03	L-Norgestrel	0.125	5
Ortho-Novum 7/7/7					
Days 1–7	Ethinyl estradiol	0.035	Norethindrone	0.5	1
Days 8–14	Ethinyl estradiol	0.035	Norethindrone	0.75	1.5
Days 15–21	Ethinyl estradiol	0.035	Norethindrone	1.0	2
Tri-Norinyl					
Days 1–7	Ethinyl estradiol	0.035	Norethindrone	0.5	1
Days 8–16	Ethinyl estradiol	0.035	Norethindrone	1.0	2
Days 17–21	Ethinyl estradiol	0.035	Norethindrone	0.5	1
Daily progestin tablets					
Micronor		. . .	Norethindrone	0.35	0.7
Nor-QD		. . .	Norethindrone	0.35	0.7
Ovrette		. . .	dl-Norgestrel	0.075	3

*Modified and reproduced, with permission, from Katzung BG (editor): *Basic & Clinical Pharmacology,* 2nd ed. Lange, 1984.
†Progestational potency.

ceptives have stimulated a great many studies of their effects on blood coagulation. A clear picture of such effects has not yet emerged. The oral contraceptives do not consistently alter bleeding or clotting times. Conflicting information has arisen from studies of effects of these agents on the clotting factors. However, in general they indicate that the changes observed are similar to those reported in pregnancy and include an increase in factors VII, VIII, IX, and X. Increased amounts of coumarin derivatives are required to produce a reduction in prothrombin time in patients taking oral contraceptives. The platelet aggregation response to catecholamines is also increased.

Significant alterations in the cellular components of blood have not been reported with any consistency. Oral contraceptives inhibit the conversion of polyglutamic folate found in food to the monoglutamic folate that is absorbed in the gastrointestinal tract, thereby causing folic acid–deficiency anemias, which can be reversed by folic acid supplementation or by discontinuing oral contraceptives.

D. Hepatic Effects: The liver plays an important role in the metabolism of the estrogens and progestins used in oral contraceptives. These hormones also affect liver function. (See Adverse Effects of Oral Contraceptives, below.)

Estrogens increase the synthesis of the various transport globulins and fibrinogen and decrease the synthesis of serum haptoglobins.

Important alterations in drug excretion and metabolism also occur in the liver. Estrogens in the amounts present during pregnancy or ingested in oral contraceptive agents delay the clearance of sulfobromophthalein (Bromsulphalein, BSP) and reduce bile flow.

Oral contraceptives increase the saturation of cholesterol in bile, and the ratio of cholic acid to chenodeoxycholic acid is increased. These changes may cause the observed increase in cholelithiasis associated with use of these agents.

E. Effects on Lipid Metabolism: Estrogens increase plasma high-density lipoproteins (HDL) and very low density lipoproteins (VLDL) while lowering low-density lipoproteins (LDL). In young women with normal lipids, this results in higher circulating triglyceride and free and esterified cholesterol levels. In older women with higher cholesterol levels, a reduction is usually observed because of the reduction of LDL. Phospholipid levels are increased. Although the effects are marked with doses of 100 μg of mestranol or ethinyl estradiol, doses of 50 μg or less have minimal effects. The progestins—particularly the 19-nortestosterone derivatives—tend to antagonize the effects of estrogen. Preparations containing small amounts of estrogen and a progestin may slightly decrease triglycerides and high-density lipoproteins.

F. Effects on Carbohydrate Metabolism: The administration of oral contraceptives produces alterations in carbohydrate metabolism similar to those observed in pregnancy (see Chapter 17). There is a reduction in the rate of absorption of carbohydrates from the gastrointestinal tract. These agents antagonize the effects of insulin, causing decreases in glucose tolerance or increased secretion of insulin following administration of glucose. Studies in experimental animals indicate that estrogens enhance islet cell function, whereas progesterone interferes with insulin action. The changes in glucose tolerance are reversible on discontinuing medication.

G. Cardiovascular Effects: These agents cause small increases in cardiac output associated with slightly higher systolic and diastolic blood pressure and heart rate. Pathologic increases in blood pressure occur in a small number of patients, in whom the pressure slowly returns to normal when treatment is terminated. It is important that blood pressure be followed in each patient.

Venous engorgement has been reported. Changes in connective tissue in the arteries of rodents have been reported, but their significance is not known. Plasma from women taking oral contraceptives stimulates growth of arterial smooth muscle in tissue culture, and it is postulated that this effect could enhance the atherosclerotic process.

H. Effects on the Skin: Oral contraceptives have been noted to increase pigmentation of the skin (chloasma). This effect seems to be enhanced in women with dark complexions and by exposure to ultraviolet light. Agents with larger amounts of androgenlike progestins may increase the production of sebum and cause acne. However, estrogen-dominant oral contraceptive preparations usually decrease sebum production by suppressing the ovarian production of androgens.

CLINICAL USES OF ORAL CONTRACEPTIVES

The most important use of the estrogen and progestin compounds is for prevention of pregnancy. Many preparations are available, and they are packaged to provide for ease of administration. When these agents are taken according to directions, the risk of conception is estimated to be about 0.5– 1 per 100 woman years.

These compounds are also used in the treatment of endometriosis. When severe dysmenorrhea is the major symptom of this disorder, suppression of ovulation with estrogen may be followed by painless periods. However, in most patients, long-term continuous administration of large doses of progestins or estrogen-progestin combinations to prevent cyclic breakdown of the endometrial tissue leads to endometrial fibrosis and prevents the reactivation of implants for prolonged periods.

As is true with most hormonal preparations, many of the side effects are physiologic or pharmacologic effects of the drug that are objectionable only because they are not pertinent to the situation for which they are being used. Therefore, the product containing the smallest amounts of hormones should be selected for use.

The differences between preparations can be used to advantage for individualized treatment. These preparations differ in amounts and types of estrogen and progestin (Table 14–11). Preparations containing larger amounts of estrogen tend to produce more withdrawal bleeding, nausea, and mastalgia. Preparations containing 19-nortestosterone derivatives tend to reduce the amount of withdrawal bleeding and have more anabolic or androgenic effects.

ADVERSE EFFECTS OF ORAL CONTRACEPTIVES

The incidence of serious known side effects associated with the use of these drugs is low. There are a number of reversible changes in intermediary metabolism. However, the long-term effects of the metabolic alterations are not well understood. Minor side effects are frequent but transient. Although it is not often necessary to discontinue taking the pills because of these side effects, one-third of patients started on oral contraception discontinue therapy for reasons other than a desire to become pregnant. Common minor problems may respond to simple changes in pill formulation.

Mild Side Effects

Breakthrough bleeding is the most common problem in use of progestational agents alone for contraception, occurring in as many as 25% of patients. It also occurs in patients taking combined agents and is more common with preparations containing less than 50 μg of ethinyl estradiol (or equivalent). The newer biphasic and triphasic formulations containing 35 μg of ethinyl estradiol and varying doses of progestin (Table 14–11) appear to be associated with less breakthrough bleeding without increasing the total amount of hormone administered during a cycle.

Nausea, mastalgia, excessive withdrawal bleeding, and edema are more common with larger amounts of estrogen and can often be alleviated by a shift to a preparation containing smaller amounts of estrogen or more potent progestational compounds.

Psychologic changes are often transient and are not predictable with any of the preparations. In general, most patients "feel better" because they are relieved of anxiety about becoming pregnant. Some patients experience symptoms of irritability and depression throughout the cycle. Depression and fatigue may respond to a reduction in progestin content.

Withdrawal bleeding sometimes fails to occur and may cause confusion with regard to pregnancy. If this is disturbing to the patient, a preparation with higher estrogenic or lower progestational potency may be tried or another method of contraception used. Increased estrogen potency can also reduce early and midcycle spotting.

Moderately Severe Side Effects

Any of the following may require discontinuation of oral contraceptives:

Mild and transient headaches may occur. Migraine is often made worse and is associated with an increased frequency of cerebrovascular accidents. Therefore, when migraine becomes more severe or has its onset during therapy with these agents, treatment should be discontinued.

Weight gain is more common with the combination agents containing more potent progestins. It can usually be controlled by shifting to preparations with less progestin effect or by dieting.

Increased skin pigmentation occurs in 5% of women at the end of the first year and about 40% after 8 years. It is thought to be exacerbated by vitamin B deficiency. The condition improves upon discontinuance of medication, but pigmentation may disappear very slowly.

Acne may be exacerbated by agents containing androgenic progestins, whereas agents containing large amounts of estrogen frequently cause marked improvement in acne in women with androgen excess.

Hirsutism may be aggravated by the 19-nortestosterone derivatives. This effect is seldom seen, because the suppression of ovarian androgens usually causes a net reduction in androgen effect.

Ureteral dilatation similar to that observed in pregnancy has been reported, and bacteriuria is more frequent.

Vaginal infections are more common and more difficult to treat in patients who are receiving oral contraceptives.

When therapy is terminated, the great majority of patients return to normal menstrual patterns. About 75% will ovulate in the first posttreatment cycle and 97% by the third posttreatment cycle. Patients with a history of irregular cycles more commonly develop amenorrhea following cessation of therapy.

About 2% of patients remain amenorrheic for up to several years after stopping the pills, and the prevalence of amenorrhea, often with galactorrhea, is higher in women who have used this form of contraception.

Severe Side Effects

A. Vascular Disorders: Thromboembolism was one of the earliest of the serious unanticipated effects to be reported and has been the most thoroughly studied. Studies were devised to determine whether the case reports represented coincidental occurrences or an increased risk due to treatment with these preparations. By use of case control and cohort studies, it has been possible in most cases to determine the incidence of a disorder in oral contraceptive users compared to that in nonusers and in some instances to determine whether this disorder occurs rarely or commonly. It should be kept in mind that almost all of these studies have been conducted in Great Britain, the USA, and Scandinavia and that effects in other populations might be somewhat different. During the past 15 years, the amounts of estrogen used in these preparations have been reduced, and this decline has been associated with a reduction in frequency of many of these effects. The most important adverse side effect of the oral contraceptives is the increased risk of cardiovascular disease, including venous thromboembolism, myocardial infarction, and stroke.

1. Venous thromboembolic disease–Epidemiologic studies indicate that about one patient per 1000 woman years not using oral contraceptives will develop superficial or deep thromboembolic disease. The overall incidence of these disorders in patients taking oral contraceptives is about 3 per 1000 woman years. Data obtained by studying changes in plasma fibrinogen or by ^{125}I fibrinogen uptake studies suggest that subclinical thrombosis occurs much more frequently than overt disease. An incidence of one episode per person per year lasting about 1 month is found in healthy nonpregnant women of reproductive age; in patients using oral contraceptives who are otherwise comparable, it is approximately 3 per year. The risk for this disorder is increased during the first month of contraceptive use and remains constant for several years or more. The risk returns to normal within a month when treatment is discontinued. The risk of venous thrombosis or pulmonary embolism among women with predisposing conditions may be higher than that in normal women.

The incidence of this complication is related to the estrogen content of oral contraceptives. A reduction from 100– 150 μg to 50– 80 μg reduced the incidence of pulmonary embolism by 50% or more. The most recent studies employing contraceptives containing 30 μg of estrogen indicate that the risk of death from pulmonary embolism is even lower. There is no clear relationship between progestin content and the incidence of this complication. The risk of superficial or deep thromboembolic disease in patients treated with oral contraceptives is not related to age, parity, mild obesity, or cigarette smoking. However, the risk of idiopathic deep venous thromboembolic disease in women with blood types A, B, or AB is twice as great as in those with blood type O who are not taking contraceptives and 3 times as great in type O women using these compounds. These studies indicate a genetic susceptibility to this disorder and suggest that oral contraceptives magnify the effect. Decreased venous blood flow, endothelial proliferation in veins and arteries, and increased coagulability of blood due to changes in platelet coagulation and fibrinolytic systems contribute to the increased incidence of thrombosis. In general, these changes are similar to those seen in pregnancy. It has been proposed that the main factor responsible is a decrease in the ability to halt the progression of intravenous coagulation by inhibitory effects on the thrombin system or an inhibition of fibrin clot dissolution. The major plasma inhibitor of thrombin is antithrombin 3, which is substantially decreased during oral contraceptive use. This change occurs in the first month of treatment and lasts as long as treatment persists.

Current information, therefore, suggests that oral contraceptives increase both the risk of overt venous thromboembolic disease and the occurrence of subclinical venous thromboembolic disease, primarily by increasing the size of the intravenous clots formed in response to endothelial injury or other stimuli that lead to thrombin formation. This effect appears to be primarily due to the estrogenic component of the oral contraceptives and appears to involve decreased antithrombin 3 activity.

2. Myocardial infarction–Myocardial infarction occurs more frequently in oral contraceptive users but is unrelated to the duration of use. The attributable risk of myocardial infarction is about 5– 7 per 100,000 current user years at age 30– 39, rising to approximately 60 at age 40– 44. The risk is related to the dose of estrogen and is significantly lower in women using low-dose estrogen compounds. There are also data indicating that the risk is increased in women using oral contraceptives containing 3– 4 mg, as compared to 1 or 2 mg, of the progestin norethindrone acetate.

The use of oral contraceptives is associated with a higher risk of myocardial infarction in women who smoke 15 or more cigarettes a day, who have a history of preeclampsia or hypertension, or who have type II hyperlipoproteinemia or diabetes. Since 40% of women 20– 50 years of age smoke 15 or more cigarettes a day, this becomes clinically very important. The risk attributable to oral contraceptives in women 30– 39 years of age who do not smoke is about 4 cases per 100,000 users per year, as compared to 185 cases per 100,000 among women 40– 44 who smoke heavily. The pathogenesis of myocardial infarction is thought to be related to acceleration of atherogenesis, decreased levels of HDL, and increased platelet aggregation. However, the facilitation of coronary arterial spasm may play a role in some of these patients. The progestational component of oral contraceptives decreases HDL cholesterol, whereas the estrogenic component increases it. The net difference, therefore, will depend entirely on the specific composition of the pill used and the patient's susceptibility to the particular effects. Preparations containing norgestrel, 0.5 mg, or norethindrone acetate, 2.5 mg, have been reported to have strong antiestrogenic effects and to decrease HDL cholesterol, while some of the others have no effect.

3. Cerebrovascular disease–The risk of stroke is concentrated in women over 35. It is increased in current users but not in past users. However, the incidence of subarachnoid hemorrhage is increased among both current and past users and may increase with time. The risk of thrombotic or hemorrhagic stroke attributable to oral contraceptives is about 37 cases per 100,000 users per year. Ten percent of these strokes are fatal, and most of them are due to subarachnoid hemorrhage. Insufficient data are available on which to base an assessment of the effects of smoking and other risk factors. However, it is thought that the pattern of risk is similar to that seen for myocardial infarction.

Elevations in blood pressure may also increase the risk, since there is a 3- to 6-fold increase in the incidence of overt hypertension in women taking oral contraceptives.

In summary, the information available indicates that oral contraceptives increase the risk of various cardiovascular disorders at all ages and among both smokers and nonsmokers. However, this risk appears to be concentrated in women 35 years of age or older who are heavy smokers. It is clear that the presence of these risk factors must be considered in each individual patient for whom oral contraceptives are considered.

B. Gastrointestinal Disorders: Many cases of cholestatic jaundice have been reported in patients taking progestin-containing drugs. The differences in incidence of these disorders from one population to another suggest that genetic factors are involved. The jaundice caused by these agents is similar to that produced by other 17-alkyl–substituted steroids. It is most often observed in the first 3 cycles and is particularly common in women with a history of cholestatic jaundice during pregnancy. Liver biopsies from such women show bile thrombi in the canaliculi and occasional areas of focal necrosis. Serum alkaline phosphatase and SGPT are increased. The BSP retention and serum enzyme changes observed in some patients may indicate liver damage. Jaundice and pruritus disappear 1–8 weeks after the drug is discontinued.

These agents have also been found to increase the incidence of symptomatic gallbladder disease, including cholecystitis and cholangitis. This is probably the result of alterations in bile secretion and content.

It also appears that the incidence of hepatic adenomas is increased in women taking oral contraceptives. Ischemic bowel disease secondary to thrombosis of celiac and superior and inferior mesenteric arteries and veins has also been reported in women using these drugs.

C. Depression: Depression severe enough to require stopping the pills occurs in about 6% of patients taking some preparations.

D. Other Disorders: In addition to the above effects, a number of other adverse reactions have been reported for which a causal relationship has not been established. These include alopecia, erythema multiforme, erythema nodosum, and other skin disorders.

NONCONTRACEPTIVE ADVANTAGES OF HORMONAL CONTRACEPTION

The advent of oral contraceptives with low hormone content has significantly reduced the incidence of serious adverse effects. Furthermore, it has become apparent that their use is associated with important health benefits such as less risk of developing endometrial cancer, iron deficiency anemia, benign breast disease, functional ovarian cysts, premenstrual tension syndrome, and dysmenorrhea.

These and other benefits make hormonal contraception with low-dose, low-potency combination pills an excellent contraceptive method for younger women who do not smoke.

CONTRAINDICATIONS & CAUTIONS

Oral contraceptives are contraindicated in patients with thrombophlebitis, thromboembolic phenomena, and cerebrovascular disorders or a past history of these conditions. They should not be used to treat vaginal bleeding when the cause is unknown. They should be avoided in patients known or suspected to have a tumor of the breast or other estrogen-dependent neoplasm. They are contraindicated in adolescents in whom epiphyseal closure has not yet been completed, because they may prevent attainment of normal adult height.

Since these preparations have caused aggravation of preexisting disorders, they should be avoided or used with caution in patients with liver disease, hypertriglyceridemia, asthma, eczema, migraine, diabetes, hypertension, congestive heart failure, optic neuritis, retrobulbar neuritis, or convulsive disorders.

Estrogens may increase the rate of growth of fibroids. Therefore, for women with these tumors, agents with the smallest amounts of estrogen and the most potent progestins should be selected. The use of progestational agents alone for contraception might be especially useful in such patients (see below).

CONTRACEPTION WITH PROGESTINS

Small doses of progestins administered orally can be used for contraception (Table 14–11). They are particularly suited for patients who should not take estrogens. They are about as effective as intrauterine devices or combination pills containing 20–30 μg of ethinyl estradiol. There is a high incidence of abnormal bleeding. Giving infrequent injections of long-acting progestins such as medroxyprogesterone acetate has also found limited usefulness. Progesterone has also been incorporated into an intrauterine device.

POSTCOITAL CONTRACEPTIVES

Pregnancy can be prevented following coitus by the administration of estrogens alone or in combination with progestins. Insertion of an intrauterine device within 5 days has also been effective.

Table 14–12. Schedules for use of postcoital contraceptives.

Conjugated estrogens: 10 mg 3 times daily for 5 days
Ethinyl estradiol: 2.5 mg twice daily for 5 days
Diethylstilbestrol: 50 mg daily for 5 days
Norgestrel, 0.5 mg, with ethinyl estradiol, 0.05 mg: 2 tablets and 2 in 12 hours

A variety of schedules have been tested and found effective, and these are shown in Table 14–12. When treatment is begun within 72 hours, the failure rate is less than 1%. Since 40% of patients treated experience nausea or vomiting, antiemetics are recommended. Headache, dizziness, breast tenderness, and abdominal and leg cramps have also been reported as side effects. Because these compounds have serious teratogenic effects early in pregnancy and because vaginal adenosis and cancer, cervical abnormalities, and impairment of reproductive function have been found in the offspring of women treated with diethylstilbestrol during gestation, voluntary termination of pregnancy is advised when conception occurs in these patients.

INFERTILITY

Infertility is usually defined as failure of conception by a couple who have been having regular intercourse for 1 year or more without contraception. The intensity of the patients' concern varies, and a physician may be consulted after only a few months or many years of trying to become pregnant. Semen abnormalities are responsible for infertility in about half of cases. Some of the more common problems encountered are listed in Table 14–13.

SEMEN ABNORMALITIES

Semen analysis is usually obtained early in the investigation of infertile couples, because male factors are a common cause of infertility and because the test is relatively simple and inexpensive; furthermore, sperm abnormalities may compound the problem in women who fail to ovulate or have other problems reducing fertility. The characteristics of normal semen and sperm are discussed in Chapter 13. One of the most common causes of male infertility is varicocele of the left internal spermatic vein. Correction of this disorder usually results in marked improvement in sperm motility, and even when lower than normal sperm counts remain, pregnancy is achieved about half the time. The quality and concentration of sperm can also be improved in some men by the use of split ejaculates. In about 90% of men, the first few drops of semen contain a higher concentration of sperm with better motility than the remainder of the ejaculate. The combination of this technique with artificial insemination increases the chances of pregnancy in some couples.

OVULATORY DISORDERS

Absent or infrequent ovulation accounts for about 15% of infertility problems. Whether ovulation is completely absent or occurs infrequently, the opportunity for conception is diminished, and the patient should be treated by ovulation induction.

Women who have menstrual bleeding at regular intervals preceded by recognizable symptoms or who have dysmenorrhea almost always ovulate regularly. The occurrence of ovulation can be confirmed by the finding of a progesterone level greater than 4 ng/mL. However, it is useful to obtain daily basal body temperatures in order to determine the length of the luteal phase and to find out whether coitus has occurred at the time of ovulation. The timing of coitus is important, since the egg is fertilizable for only 12–24 hours, and sperm retain their ability to fertilize for 24–48 hours. Ideally, coitus should occur every other day for the 3 days preceding and following ovulation.

INFERTILITY IN THE PRESENCE OF OVULATION

When conception has not occurred in spite of a normal sperm analysis in the man and regular ovulation in the woman, a postcoital test of cervical mucus should be done near the time of expected ovulation as indicated by basal body temperature charts, length of cycle, or the patient's observation of increased amounts of clear mucus at an appropriate time of the cycle. The cervical mucus at this time is under the influence of high estrogen levels and is clear and abundant. It can be stretched between a slide and cover slip as much as 10 cm at this time ("spinnbarkeit"). When the mucus is dried on the slide, the interaction of the electrolytes and protein results in a crystalline pattern called "ferning" (Fig 14–13). This mucus contains chains of glycoproteins that form channels

Table 14–13. Causes of infertility.

Male (40–50%)	Female (50–60%)
Abnormalities of sperm	Tubal disease (20%)
Infection (mumps)	Anovulation (15%)
Failure to liquefy	Cervical factors (5%)
Agglutination	Unknown (10–20%)
Chronic infection (epididymitis, prostatitis)	Immunologic abnormalities*
High scrotal temperature	
Varicocele	
Baths	
Jockey shorts	
Prolonged sitting	
Radiation exposure	
Drugs (cimetidine, sulfasalazine, nitrofurantoin, etc)	
Retrograde ejaculation	
Severe allergic reactions (rare)	
Endocrine disorders	
Immunologic abnormalities*	

*Failure of conception correlates best with agglutinating antibodies to sperm in the male and with agglutinating and immobilizing antibodies in the female.

through which the sperm can migrate. In order to perform the test, mucus is obtained from the cervix following intercourse, preferably within 8 hours. If the mucus is thick and cloudy, the specimen may have been obtained too late in the cycle, and the test should be repeated. Absence of spermatozoa in the specimen indicates the need for a more careful study of the semen specimen, as does the presence of dead sperm cells without motility. The presence of 20 or more motile sperm per high dry field is associated with a higher fertility rate than when few sperm are found. However, pregnancies occur even when no motile sperm cells are found in this test. The finding of dead cells suggests the use of spermicidal lubricants or may indicate the need for sperm antibody testing.

Tests of Tubal Patency

When there is a history of pelvic infection or pelvic surgery, tubal patency should be examined. Such examinations are also indicated in patients in whom other factors have not been identified that might explain the infertility. Rubin's test (insufflation with carbon dioxide) has been used for this purpose because of its convenience and because irradiation is not required. However, the test is quite uncomfortable and sometimes produces tubal spasm, giving erroneous readings. Hysterosalpingography is generally preferable except in the presence of allergy to the radiopaque dye. It is best performed a few days following cessation of menstrual flow, thus avoiding the disruption of an early pregnancy. It is contraindicated in the presence of active pelvic inflammatory disease, as indicated by the presence of pelvic masses, tenderness, or an elevated sedimentation rate. Radiation should be minimized by the use of image intensification fluoroscopy and by taking the minimum number of films. An increased number of conceptions has been reported following this procedure when oil-based dye

is used. The increase has been attributed to various mechanical and chemical effects of lavage with an iodine-containing and possibly bacteriostatic substance.

When semen analysis and the above tests are found to be normal in the infertile couple, the possibility of endometriosis should be considered even in the absence of typical signs and symptoms such as severe dysmenorrhea, dyspareunia, thickening of the broad ligament, nodularity and tenderness, or fixation of the uterus on pelvic examination. In these instances, laparoscopy may detect the presence and indicate the extent of any intrapelvic disease. Surgical treatment of minimal endometriosis established in this manner is followed by conception in half of women so treated. Hormonal treatment can be used in some patients.

IN VITRO FERTILIZATION

In vitro fertilization and transfer of the fertilized ovum into the uterus is now a therapeutic option to achieve pregnancy. After thorough fertility evaluation and study of the patient's menstrual cycles, the patient is given clomiphene citrate, menotropins, or both to increase the number of large mature follicles. Just before ovulation, several ova are obtained by laparoscopy or percutaneously under ultrasound guidance. The ova are incubated for several hours, and washed sperm are added to the culture medium. After 2–3 days of incubation, a 4- to 6-cell conceptus is transferred to the uterus via the cervix.

Seventy to 80% of mature ova obtained can be fertilized. Early abortion is frequent, and the overall success rate is less than 30% even in experienced hands. The process is very expensive, lengthy, and time-consuming. However, the risks of fetal abnormalities and maternal complications are low.

REFERENCES

General

Catt KJ, Pierce JG: Gonadotropic hormones of the adenohypophysis (FSH, LH and prolactin). Chapter 2 in: *Reproductive Endocrinology*. Yen SSC, Jaffe RB (editors). Saunders, 1978.

Hodgen GD: The dominant ovarian follicle. *Fertil Steril* 1982;**38**:281.

Hseuh AJ et al: Hormonal regulation of the differentiation of cultured ovarian granulosa cells. *Endocr Rev* 1984;**5**:76.

Peters H, McNatty KP: *The Ovary: A Correlation of Structure and Function in Mammals*. Granada Publishing, 1980.

Siiteri PK, MacDonald PC: Role of extraglandular estrogen in human endocrinology. Chapter 28 in: *Handbook of Physiology*. Section 7: Endocrinology. Vol 2, Part 1. Geiger SR, Astwood EB, Greep RO (editors). American Physiological Society, 1973.

Speroff L, Glass RH, Kase NG: *Clinical Gynecologic Endocrinology and Infertility,* 3rd ed. Williams & Wilkins, 1982.

Van Wagenen G, Simpson ME: *Embryology of the Ovary and Testis: Homo Sapiens and Macaca Mulatta*. Yale Univ Press, 1965.

Menstrual Cycle

Abraham GE: The normal menstrual cycle. Part I in: *Endocrine Causes of Menstrual Disorders*. Givens JR (editor). Year Book, 1978.

Abraham GE: Ovarian and adrenal contribution to peripheral androgens during the menstrual cycle. *J Clin Endocrinol Metab* 1974;**39**:340.

Erickson GF: Normal ovarian function. *Clin Obstet Gynecol* 1978;**21**:31.

Jaffe RB, Monroe SE: Hormone interaction and regulation during the menstrual cycle. Chapter 8 in: *Frontiers in Neuroendocrinology*. Vol 6. Martin L, Ganong W (editors). Raven Press, 1980.

Knobil E: On the control of gonadotropin secretion in the rhesus monkey. *Recent Prog Horm Res* 1974;**30**:1.

Knobil E: The neuroendocrine control of the menstrual cycle. *Recent Prog Horm Res* 1980;**36**:53.

McNatty KP et al: Concentrations of oestrogens and androgens in human ovarian venous plasma and follicular fluid through the menstrual cycle. *J Endocrinol* 1976;**71**:77.

Midgley AR Jr, Jaffe RB: Regulation of human gonadotropins. 4. Correlation of serum concentrations of follicle stimulating and luteinizing hormones during the menstrual cycle. *J Clin Endocrinol Metab* 1968;**28**:1699.

Moghissi KS: Composition and function of cervical secretion. Chapter 31 in: *Handbook of Physiology.* Section 7: Endocrinology. Vol 2, Part 2. Greep RO (editor). American Physiological Society, 1973.

Noyes RW, Hertig AT, Rock J: Dating the endometrial biopsy. *Fertil Steril* 1950;**1**:3.

Papanicolaou GN et al: *The Epithelia of Women's Reproductive Organs.* Commonwealth, 1948.

Richards JS: Maturation of ovarian follicles: Actions and interactions of pituitary and ovarian hormones on follicular cell differentiation. *Physiol Rev* 1980;**60**:51.

Wied GL, Bibbo M: Evaluation of endocrinologic condition by exfoliative cytology. Chapter 12 in: *Gynecologic Endocrinology,* 3rd ed. Gold JJ, Josimovich JB (editors). Harper & Row, 1981.

Yen SSC: The human menstrual cycle (integrative function of the hypothalamic-pituitary-ovarian-endometrial axis). Chapter 7 in: *Reproductive Endocrinology.* Yen SSC, Jaffe RB (editors). Saunders, 1978.

Disorders of Ovarian Function

Bardin CW, Lipsett MB: Testosterone and androstenedione blood production rates in normal women and women with idiopathic hirsutism or polycystic ovaries. *J Clin Invest* 1967;**46**:891.

Fries H, Nillius SF, Pettersson F: Epidemiology of secondary amenorrhea. *Am J Obstet Gynecol* 1974;**118**:473.

Goldzieher JW: Polycystic ovarian disease. Chapter 15 in: *Progress in Infertility.* Behrman SJ, Kistner RW (editors). Little, Brown, 1968.

Griffin JE, Wilson JD: The syndromes of androgen resistance. *N Engl J Med* 1980;**302**:198.

Judd HL: Endocrinology of polycystic ovary disease. *Clin Obstet Gynecol* 1978;**21**:99.

Kleinberg DL et al: Galactorrhea: A study of 235 cases, including 48 with pituitary tumor. *N Engl J Med* 1977;**296**:589.

Malkasian GD Jr et al: Functioning tumors of the ovary in women under 40. *Obstet Gynecol* 1965;**26**:669.

Ross GT, Vande Wiele RL, Frantz AG: The ovaries and the breasts. Chapter 7 in: *Textbook of Endocrinology.* Williams RH (editor). Saunders, 1981.

Warren MP, Vande Wiele RL: Clinical and metabolic features of anorexia nervosa. *Am J Obstet Gynecol* 1973;**117**:435.

Hirsutism

Cummings DC et al: Treatment of hirsutism with spironolactone. *JAMA* 1982;**247**:1295.

Ferriman D, Gallwey JD: Clinical assessment of body hair growth in women. *J Clin Endocrinol Metab* 1961;**21**:1440.

Givens JR: Hirsutism and hyperandrogenism. *Adv Intern Med* 1976;**21**:221.

Horton R, Hawks D, Lobo R: $3\alpha,17\beta$-Androstanediol glucuronide in plasma: A marker of androgen action in idiopathic hirsutism. *J Clin Invest* 1982;**69**:1203.

Kirschner M et al: Idiopathic hirsutism: An ovarian abnormality. *N Engl J Med* 1976;**294**:637.

Mahesh VB, Greenblatt RB (editors): *Hirsutism and Virilism: Pathogenesis, Diagnosis and Management.* John Wright, PSG Inc., 1983.

Molinatti GM, Martini L, James VHT (editors): *Androgenization in Women: Pathophysiology and Clinical Aspects.* Raven Press, 1983.

Raj SG et al: Normalization of testosterone levels using a low estrogen-containing oral contraceptive in women with polycystic ovarian syndrome. *Obstet Gynecol* 1982;**60**:15.

Therapeutic Use of Ovarian & Hypothalamic Hormones & Inhibitors

Dmowski WP: Endocrine properties and clinical application of danazol. *Fertil Steril* 1979;**31**:237.

Hammond CS et al: Effects of long-term estrogen replacement therapy. *Am J Obstet Gynecol* 1979;**133**:525.

Ory SJ: Clinical uses of luteinizing hormone–releasing hormone. *Fertil Steril* 1983;**39**:577.

Voss HE, Oertel G: Androgens II and antiandrogens. In: *Handbook of Experimental Pharmacology.* Vol 35, Part 2. Springer, 1974. [New series.]

Yen SSC: Clinical applications of gonadotropin-releasing hormone and gonadotropin-releasing hormone analogs. *Fertil Steril* 1983;**39**:257.

Menopause

Cann CE et al: Spinal mineral loss by quantitative computed tomography in oophorectomized women. *JAMA* 1980; **244**:2056.

Judd HL: Hormonal dynamics associated with the menopause. *Clin Obstet Gynecol* 1976;**19**:775.

Lindsay R et al: Bone response to termination of oestrogen treatment. *Lancet* 1978;**1**:1325.

Meema S, Bunker ML, Meema HE: Preventive effect of estrogen on postmenopausal bone loss. *Arch Intern Med* 1975;**135**:1436.

Sherman BM, West JH, Korenman SG: The menopausal transition: Analysis of LH, FSH, estradiol, and progesterone concentrations during menstrual cycles of older women. *J Clin Endocrinol Metab* 1976;**42**:629.

Van Keep PA, Lauritzen C (editors): Frontiers of hormone research. In: *Ageing and Estrogens.* Vol 2. Karger, 1973.

Hormonal Contraception

Bradley BD et al: Serum high-density-lipoprotein cholesterol in women using oral contraceptives, estrogen and progestins. *N Engl J Med* 1978;**299**:17.

Royal College of General Practitioners: *Oral Contraceptives and Health.* Pitman, 1974.

Salhanick HA, Kipnis DM, Vande Wiele RL (editors): *Metabolic Effects of Gonadal Hormones and Contraceptive Steroids.* Plenum Press, 1969.

Infertility

Glass RH: Infertility. Chapter 19 in: *Reproductive Endocrinology.* Yen SSC, Jaffe RB (editors). Saunders, 1978.

Abnormalities of Sexual Differentiation*

15

Felix A. Conte, MD, & Melvin M. Grumbach, MD

Advances in cytogenetics, experimental embryology, steroid biochemistry, and methods of evaluation of the interaction between the hypothalamus, pituitary, and gonads have helped to clarify problems of sexual differentiation. Such anomalies may occur at any stage of intrauterine maturation and can lead to gross ambisexual development or to subtle abnormalities that do not become manifest until sexual maturity is achieved.

NORMAL SEX DIFFERENTIATION

Chromosomal Sex

The normal human diploid cell contains 22 autosomal pairs of chromosomes and 2 sex chromosomes (two X or one X and one Y). Arranged serially and numbered according to size and centromeric position, they are known as a karyotype. Advances in the techniques of staining chromosomes (Fig 15–1) permit positive identification of each chromosome by its unique "banding" pattern. Bands can be produced in the region of the centromere (C bands), with the fluorescent dye quinacrine (Q bands), and with Giemsa's stain (G bands). Fluorescent banding (Fig 15–2) is particularly useful because the Y chromosome stains so brightly that it can be identified easily in both interphase and metaphase cells. The standard nomenclature for describing the human karyotype is shown in Table 15–1.

Studies in patients with abnormalities of sexual differentiation indicate that the sex chromosomes (the X and Y chromosomes) and possibly the autosomes carry genes that influence sexual differentiation by causing the bipotential gonad to develop either as a testis or as an ovary. Two intact and normally func-

*This chapter is modified slightly from the authors' Chapter 33 in Smith DR: *General Urology*, 11th ed. Lange, 1984. Figs 15–1 to 15–4, Figs 15–6 to 15–10, Fig 15–14, and Tables 15–1, 15–2, 15–4, and 15–5 are reproduced, with permission, from Grumbach MM, Conte FA: Disorders of sex differentiation. Chap 9, pp 423–514, in: *Textbook of Endocrinology*, 6th ed. Williams RH (editor). Saunders, 1981.

Acronyms Used in This Chapter

ACTH	Adrenocorticotropic hormone
DHEA	Dehydroepiandrosterone
DHT	Dihydrotestosterone
DNA	Deoxyribonucleic acid
DOC	Deoxycorticosterone
DOCA	De[s]oxycorticosterone acetate
FSH	Follicle-stimulating hormone
GH	Growth hormone
GnRH	Gonadotropin-releasing hormone
hCG	Human chorionic gonadotropin
HLA	Human leukocyte antigen
LH	Luteinizing hormone
RNA	Ribonucleic acid
TSH	Thyroid-stimulating hormone (thyrotropin)

Figure 15–1. A normal 46,XY karyotype stained with Giemsa's stain to produce G bands. Note that each chromosome has a specific banding pattern.

Figure 15–2. Metaphase chromosomes stained with quinacrine and examined through a fluorescence microscope. Note the bright fluorescence of the distal arms of the Y chromosome, which can also be seen in interphase cells ("Y body" at right).

tioning X chromosomes, in the absence of a Y chromosome (and the genes for testicular organogenesis), lead to the formation of an ovary.

Careful examination of the karyotype in humans reveals a marked discrepancy in size between the X and Y chromosomes. There is evidence that gene dosage compensation is achieved in all persons with 2 or more X chromosomes in their genetic constitution by inactivation of all X chromosomes except one. This phenomenon is thought to be a random process that occurs in each cell in the late blastocyst stage of embryonic development. The result of this process is formation of a sex chromatin body (Barr body) in the interphase cells of persons having 2 or more X chromosomes (Fig 15–3).

Recent data indicate that the distal portion of the short arm of the X chromosome escapes inactivation. Several genes have been localized to this region, including steroid sulfatase, the Xg^a red cell antigen, and a locus influencing the expression of H-Y antigen. Furthermore, it is this segment of the X chromosome that pairs with the Y chromosome during meiosis.

In buccal mucosal smears of 46,XX females, a sex chromatin body is evident in 20–30% of the nuclei examined, whereas in normal 46,XY males, a comparable sex chromatin body is absent. In patients with more than two X chromosomes, the maximum number of sex chromatin bodies in any diploid nucleus is one less than the total number of X chromosomes. By utilizing sex chromatin and Y fluorescent staining (Figs 15–3 and 15–4), one can determine indirectly the sex chromosome complement of any individual (Table 15–2).

H-Y Antigen

In 1955, Eichwald and Silmser showed that among inbred strains of mice, most male-to-female skin grafts were rejected, whereas male-to-male and female-to-female grafts survived. This phenomenon was attributed to a specific Y-linked histocompatibility locus, the H-Y antigen.

Utilizing a sperm cytotoxicity test to test for this antigen, Wachtel et al expanded the study of H-Y antigen from inbred mice to rats, guinea pigs, rabbits,

Table 15–1. Nomenclature for describing the human karyotype pertinent to designating sex chromosome abnormalities.

Paris Conference	Description	Former Nomenclature
46,XX	Normal female karyotype	XX
46,XY	Normal male karyotype	XY
47,XXY	Karyotype with 47 chromosomes including an extra X chromosome	XXY
45,X	Monosomy X	XO
45,X/46,XY	Mosaic karyotype composed of 45,X and 46,XY cell lines	XO/XY
p	Short arm	p
q	Long arm	q
46,X,del (X) (qter → p21:)	Deletion of the short arm of the X distal to band Xp21	XXp−
46,X,del (X) (pter → q21:)	Deletion of the long arm of the X distal to band Xq21	XXq−
46,X,i (Xq)	Isochromosome of the long arm of X	XXqi
46,X,i (Xp)	Isochromosome of the short arm of X	XXpi
46,X,r (X)	Ring X chromosome	XXr
46,X,t (Y;7) (q11;q36)	Translocation of the distal fluorescent portion of the Y chromosome to the long arm of chromosome 7	46,XYt (Yq−7q+)

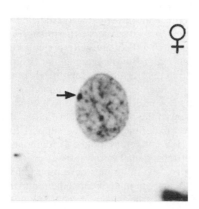

Figure 15–3. X chromatin body in the nucleus of a buccal mucosal cell from a normal female.

Figure 15–4. An interphase nucleus stained with quinacrine and examined by fluorescence microscopy. This cell reveals a "Y body" and an X chromatin body. The patient has a 47,XXY karyotype.

and humans. They demonstrated the association of H-Y antigen with the heterogametic sex (usually the male) in a wide range of vertebrates. In mammals, H-Y antigen is expressed in the heterogametic male but not usually in the homogametic XX female.

Wachtel and Ohno and their associates noted the striking conservation throughout evolution of this ubiquitous minor cross-reacting plasma membrane histocompatibility antigen, its appearance early in embryonic development (in the 8-cell male mouse embryo), and its association with heterogametic sex. These observations led them to suggest that this phylogenetically conserved antigen is the factor responsible for inducing testicular organogenesis of the bipotential fetal gonads. They examined their hypothesis by testing patients with testicular tissue who had XX

karyotypes, eg, XX males and XX true hermaphrodites. Despite the absence of a Y chromosome in these patients, H-Y antigen was detected in all patients tested (although it is usually at lower levels than that observed in control 46,XX females). In addition, the gonad of the bovine freemartin (the intersex XX twin of a male fetus) is positive for H-Y antigen. Further evidence indicates that even in the absence of a discrete Y chromosome, or karyotypic evidence of a Y-to-X chromosome, or Y-to-autosome translocation or insertion, the presence of testicular tissue is invariably associated with a positive test for H-Y antigen. The chromosome sites of the structural and regulatory genes for the expression of H-Y antigen are uncertain. Evidence suggests that there are sites in the pericentromeric region of the Y chromosome, on the short arm of the X chromosome, and possibly on autosomes that affect the synthesis and action of H-Y antigen.

According to Ohno, biologically active H-Y antigen is a protein (MW 16,000–18,000) composed of hydrophobic peptide units that are linked by intersubunit disulfide bonds. The only gonadal cell known to disseminate H-Y antigen is the primitive Sertoli cell. H-Y antigen has been detected on all cell membranes from normal XY males except those of immature germ cells. Apparently, cells have 2 receptors for H-Y antigen. Ohno has proposed that one receptor is nonspecific and ubiquitous and represents the stable cell membrane anchorage sites for H-Y antigen on all male cells; this anchorage site is conceived as an association of "major histocompatibility complex" cell surface antigens (HLA) with β_2-microglobulin. The second receptor is found only on gonadal cells, both male and female, and binds free H-Y antigen with a greater affinity than do the nonspecific anchorage sites.

A hypothesis for the organogenesis of the indifferent embryonic gonad as testis can be summarized

Table 15–2. Sex chromosome complement correlated with X chromatin and Y bodies in somatic interphase nuclei.*

Sex Chromosomes	Maximum Number in Diploid Somatic Nuclei	
	X Bodies	Y Bodies
45,XO	0	0
46,XX	1	0
46,XY	0	1
47,XXX	2	0
47,XXY	1	1
47,XYY	0	2
48,XXXX	3	0
48,XXXY	2	1
48,XXYY	1	2
49,XXXXX	4	0
49,XXXXY	3	1
49,XXXYY	2	2

*The maximum number of X chromatin bodies in diploid somatic nuclei is one less than the number of Xs, whereas the maximum number of Y fluorescent bodies is equivalent to the number of Ys in the chromosome constitution.

Figure 15–5. Interaction of H-Y antigen, germ cells, and somatic elements of the primordial gonad in testicular differentiation.

as follows: The pericentromeric region of the Y chromosome contains a locus (or loci) that either codes for H-Y antigen or regulates its expression. H-Y antigen is disseminated by Sertoli cells in the gonadal blastema, binds to gonad-specific H-Y receptors, and induces differentiation of the primitive gonad as a testis by the seventh week of gestation (Fig 15– 5). In the absence of H-Y antigen and in the presence of 2 structurally normal X chromosomes, an ovary will develop. Indirect evidence suggests the presence of a specific ovarian organizing antigen.

All of the evidence discussed previously in support of the testis-organizing function of H-Y antigen is indirect and circumstantial. However, in vitro experimental data provide more direct evidence for this hypothesis. In a series of experiments, Ohno and Zenzius and their associates have reported cell dissociation and reaggregation experiments on newborn rat and mouse gonads (Fig 15– 6). The Moscona technique was used to obtain a suspension of single cells from newborn mouse or rat testes. The free cell suspension was exposed to excess anti–H-Y serum and incubated in rotation culture. Untreated testicular cells reorga-

nized as "seminiferous tubule–like structures," whereas H-Y antibody–treated dissociated testicular cells did not. In a subsequent experiment (Fig 15– 6), Ohno et al purified H-Y antigen from culture medium of a human male, Burkitt lymphoma cell line, which lacks the putative β_2-microglobulin H-Y anchorage site. Bovine fetal XX indifferent gonads and human embryonic XX indifferent gonads exhibited testicular organization in the presence of purified H-Y antigen. Thus, these experiments provide support for the capacity of H-Y antigen to induce differentiation of the indifferent fetal gonad into a testis.

Recently, several groups have reported the detection of H-Y antigen in unexplained circumstances, ie, patients with Turner's syndrome (XO and XXqi). Questions of the specificity, reproducibility, and quantification of these technically difficult serologic assays for H-Y antigen must be addressed before one can interpret these discrepancies between a putative immunoreactive H-Y antigen and gonadal and chromosomal sex. (See Ohno, 1985.)

TESTICULAR & OVARIAN DIFFERENTIATION

Until the 12-mm stage (approximately 42 days of gestation), the embryonic gonads of males and females are indistinguishable. By 42 days, 300– 1300 primordial germ cells have seeded the undifferentiated gonad. These large cells later become oogonia and spermatogonia, and lack of these cells is incompatible with further ovarian differentiation. Under the influence of the genes that code for the H-Y antigen, the gonad will begin testicular differentiation by 43– 50 days of gestation. Leydig cells are apparent by about 60 days, and differentiation of male external genitalia occurs by 65– 77 days of gestation.

In the gonad destined to be an ovary, the lack of

Figure 15–6. Diagrammatic scheme summarizing experimental evidence supporting H-Y antigen as the inducer of the testis in gonadal organogenesis.

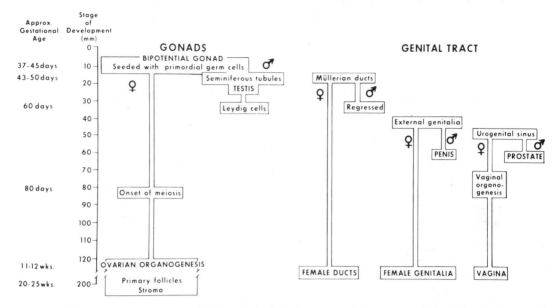

Figure 15–7. Schematic sequence of sexual differentiation in the human fetus. Note that testicular differentiation precedes all other forms of differentiation.

differentiation persists. At 77–84 days, long after differentiation of the testis in the male fetus, a significant number of germ cells enter meiotic prophase to characterize the transition of oogonia into oocytes, which marks the onset of ovarian differentiation from the undifferentiated gonads (Fig 15–7).

Differentiation of Genital Ducts (Fig 15–8)

By the seventh week of intrauterine life, the fetus is equipped with the primordia of both male and female genital ducts. The müllerian ducts, if allowed to persist, form the uterine (fallopian) tubes, the uterus, the cervix, and the upper third of the vagina. The wolffian ducts, on the other hand, have the potential for differentiating into the epididymis, vas deferens, seminal vesicles, and ejaculatory ducts of the male. In the presence of a functional testis, the müllerian ducts involute under the influence of "müllerian duct inhibitory factor," a nonsteroid macromolecule secreted by Sertoli cells. This substance acts "locally" to cause müllerian duct repression ipsilaterally. The differentiation of the wolffian duct is stimulated by testosterone secretion from the testis. In the presence of an ovary or in the absence of a functional fetal testis, müllerian duct differentiation occurs, and the wolffian ducts involute.

Differentiation of External Genitalia (Fig 15–9)

Up to the eighth week of fetal life, the external genitalia of both sexes are identical and have the capacity to differentiate into the genitalia of either sex. Female sex differentiation will occur in the presence of an ovary or streak gonads or if no gonad is present

(Fig 15–10). Differentiation of the external genitalia along male lines depends on the action of testosterone and particularly dihydrotestosterone, the 5α-reduced metabolite of testosterone. In the male fetus, testosterone is secreted by the Leydig cells, possibly autonomously at first, thereafter under the influence of hCG, and then by stimulation from fetal pituitary LH. Masculinization of the external genitalia and urogenital sinus of the fetus results from the action of dihydrotestosterone, which is converted from testosterone in the target cells by the enzyme 5α-reductase. Dihydrotestosterone is bound to a cytosol receptor (binding protein) in the target cell. It is then translocated to the nucleus of the cell, where chromatin binding occurs, which initiates DNA-directed, RNA-mediated transcription and results in androgen-induced differentiation and growth of the cell. The gene that codes for the cytosol androgen-binding protein is located on the X chromosome. Thus, an X-linked gene controls the androgen response of all somatic cell types by specifying the cytosol/nuclear androgen receptor protein.

As in the case of the genital ducts, there is an inherent tendency for the external genitalia and urogenital sinus to develop along female lines. Differentiation of the external genitalia along male lines requires androgenic stimulation early in fetal life. The testosterone metabolite dihydrotestosterone and its specific cytosol/nuclear receptor must be present to effect masculinization of the external genitalia of the fetus. Dihydrotestosterone stimulates growth of the genital tubercle, fusion of the urethral folds, and descent of the labioscrotal swellings to form the penis and scrotum. Androgens also inhibit descent and growth of the vesicovaginal septum and differentiation

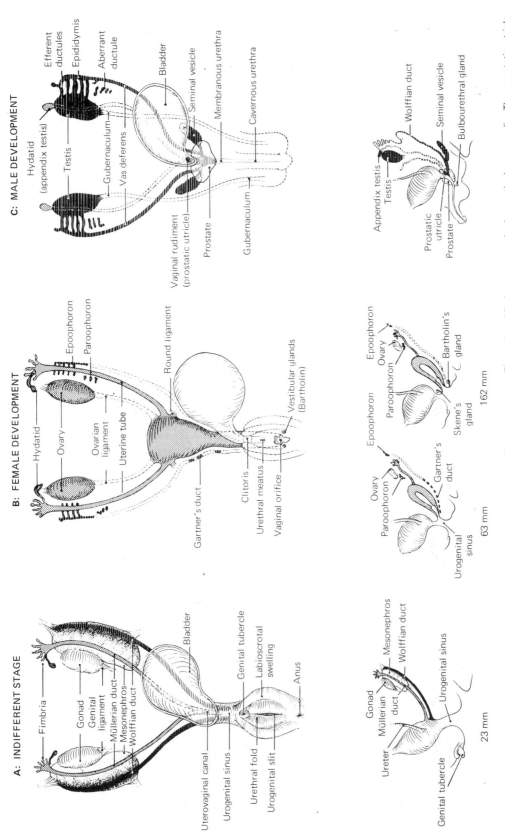

Figure 15–8. Embryonic differentiation of male and female genital ducts from wolffian and müllerian primordia. *A:* Indifferent stage showing large mesonephric body. *B:* Female ducts. Remnants of the mesonephros and wolffian ducts are now termed the epoophoron, paroophoron, and Gartner's duct. *C:* Male ducts before descent into scrotum. The only müllerian remnant is the testicular appendix. The prostatic utricle (vagina masculina) is derived from the urogenital sinus. (Redrawn from Corning & Wilkins.)

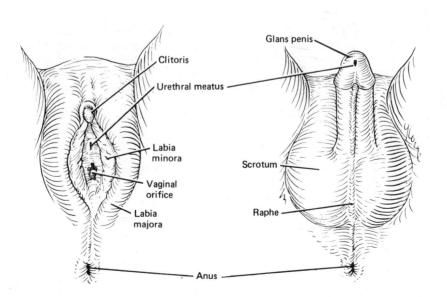

Figure 15–9. Differentiation of male and female external genitalia from bipotential primordia.

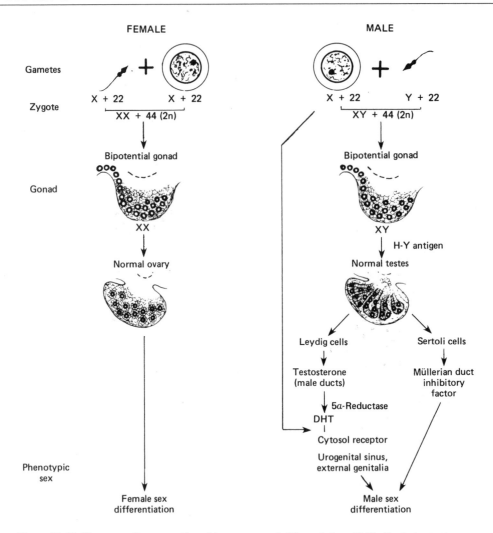

Figure 15–10. Diagrammatic summation of human sexual differentiation. DHT, dihydrotestosterone.

of the vagina. There is a critical period for action of the androgen. After about the 12th week of gestation, fusion of the labioscrotal folds will not occur even under intense androgen stimulation, although phallic growth can be induced. Impairment in the synthesis or secretion of fetal testosterone or in its conversion to dihydrotestosterone, deficient or defective androgen receptor activity, or defective production and local action of müllerian duct inhibitory factor leads to incomplete masculinization of the male fetus (Fig 15–10). Exposure of the female fetus to abnormal amounts of androgens from either endogenous or exogenous sources, especially before the 12th week of gestation, can result in virilization of the external genitalia.

PSYCHOSEXUAL DIFFERENTIATION

Psychosocial differentiation may be classified into 4 broad categories: (1) gender identity, defined as the identification of self as either male or female; (2) gender role, ie, those aspects of behavior in which males and females differ from one another in our culture at this time; (3) gender orientation, which is the choice of erotic partner; and (4) cognitive differences.

Studies in individuals who have been reared in a sex opposite to their chromosomal or gonadal sex—as well as prenatally androgenized females with virilizing adrenal hyperplasia—provide strong evidence that gender identity is not coded for primarily by sex chromosomes or prenatal sex steroid exposure. Rather, it is imprinted postnatally by words, attitudes, and comparisons of one's body with that of others. Generally, gender identity agrees with the sex of assignment in the intersex patient, provided the child is raised *unambiguously* and appropriate surgical and hormonal therapy is instituted so that the child has an unambiguous male or female phenotype. Under these circumstances, gender identity is usually established by 18–30 months of age. If at puberty discordant

Table 15—3. Classification of anomalous sexual development.

Disorders of Gonadal Differentiation
- A. Seminiferous tubule dysgenesis (Klinefelter's syndrome).
- B. Syndrome of gonadal dysgenesis and its variants (Turner's syndrome).
- C. Complete and incomplete forms of XX and XY gonadal dysgenesis.
- D. True hermaphroditism.

Female Pseudohermaphroditism
- A. Congenital virilizing adrenal hyperplasia.
- B. Androgens and synthetic progestins transferred from maternal circulation.
- C. Malformations of intestine and urinary tract (nonadrenal female pseudohermaphroditism).
- D. Other teratologic factors.

Male Pseudohermaphroditism
- A. Testicular unresponsiveness to hCG and LH (Leydig cell agenesis or hypoplasia).
- B. Inborn errors of testosterone biosynthesis:
  - 1. Enzyme defects affecting synthesis of both corticosteroids and testosterone (variants of congenital adrenal hyperplasia).
    - a. Cholesterol desmolase complex deficiency (congenital lipoid adrenal hyperplasia).
    - b. 3β-Hydroxysteroid dehydrogenase deficiency.
    - c. 17α-Hydroxylase deficiency.
  - 2. Enzyme defects primarily affecting testosterone biosynthesis by the testes.
    - a. 17,20-Desmolase (lyase) deficiency.
    - b. 17β-Hydroxysteroid oxidoreductase deficiency.
- C. Defects in androgen-dependent target tissues:
  - 1. End-organ resistance to androgenic hormones (androgen receptor and postreceptor defects).
    - a. Syndrome of complete androgen resistance and its variants (testicular feminization and its variant forms).
    - b. Syndrome of incomplete androgen resistance and its variants (Reifenstein's syndrome).
    - c. Androgen resistance in infertile men.
  - 2. Defects in testosterone metabolism by peripheral tissues; 5α-reductase deficiency (pseudovaginal perineoscrotal hypospadias).
- D. Dysgenetic male pseudohermaphroditism:
  - 1. X chromatin–negative variants of the syndrome of gonadal dysgenesis (eg, XO/XY,XYp–).
  - 2. Incomplete form of XY gonadal dysgenesis.
  - 3. Associated with degenerative renal disease.
  - 4. "Vanishing testes" (embryonic testicular regression; XY agonadism → XY gonadal agenesis → rudimentary testes → anorchia).
- E. Defects in synthesis, secretion, or response to müllerian duct inhibitory factor: Female genital ducts in otherwise normal men—"uteri herniae inguinale"; persistent müllerian duct syndrome.
- F. Maternal ingestion of estrogens and progestogens.

Unclassified Forms of Abnormal Sexual Development
- A. In males:
  - 1. Hypospadias.
  - 2. Ambiguous external genitalia in XY males with multiple congenital anomalies.
- B. In females: Absence or anomalous development of the vagina, uterus, and uterine tubes (Rokitansky-Küster syndrome).

secondary sexual characteristics are allowed to develop and persist, some intersex individuals may develop doubts about their gender identity and request a change of sex.

Thus, it appears that gender identity may be more plastic than previously thought and that at puberty sex steroids as well as socialization play a role in the function and maintenance of gender identity. However, the weight of evidence still strongly supports environmental factors as the principal determinant of gender identity in our culture.

ABNORMAL SEX DIFFERENTIATION

Classification of Errors in Sex Differentiation (Table 15–3)

Disorders of sexual differentiation are the result of abnormalities in the complex processes of sexual differentiation, which originate in genetic information on the X and Y chromosomes as well as on the autosomes. A true hermaphrodite is defined as a person who possesses both ovarian and testicular tissue. A male pseudohermaphrodite is one whose gonads are exclusively testes but whose genital ducts or external genitalia, or both, exhibit incomplete masculinization. A female pseudohermaphrodite is a person whose gonadal tissue is exclusively ovarian but whose genital development exhibits an ambiguous or male appearance.

SEMINIFEROUS TUBULE DYSGENESIS: CHROMATIN-POSITIVE KLINEFELTER'S SYNDROME & ITS VARIANTS

Klinefelter's syndrome is one of the most common forms of primary hypogonadism and infertility in males (see also Chapter 13). Affected patients usually have an XXY sex chromosome constitution and an X chromatin–positive buccal smear, although patients with a variety of sex chromosome constitutions, including mosaicism, have been described. Virtually all of these variants have in common the presence of at least two X chromosomes and a Y chromosome, except for the rare group in which only an XX sex chromosome complement is found.

Surveys of the prevalence of XXY fetuses by karyotype analysis of unselected newborn infants indicate an incidence of one per 1500 newborn males. The invariable clinical features of Klinefelter's syndrome in adults are a male phenotype; small, firm testes less than 3 cm in length; and azoospermia. Prepubertally, the disorder is characterized by small testes, disproportionately long legs, personality and behavioral disorders, and a lower verbal IQ score when compared to controls but no significant difference in full-scale IQ. Gynecomastia and other signs of androgen deficiency such as diminished facial and body hair, a small phallus, poor muscular development, and a eunuchoid body habitus occur postpubertally in affected patients. Adult males with an XXY karyotype tend to be taller than average, mainly because of the disproportionate length of their legs. They also have an increased incidence of mild diabetes mellitus, varicose veins, chronic pulmonary disease, and carcinoma of the breast. Sexual precocity due to an hCG-secreting extragonadal polyembryoma has recently been described in six XXY males.

The testicular lesion appears to be progressive and gonadotropin-dependent. It is characterized in the adult by extensive seminiferous tubular hyalinization and fibrosis, absent or severely deficient spermatogenesis, and pseudoadenomatous clumping of the Leydig cells. Although hyalinization of the tubules is usually extensive, it varies considerably from patient to patient and even between testes in the same patient. Spermatogenesis is rarely found, and patients who have been reported to be fertile have been XY/XXY mosaics.

Advanced maternal age and meiotic nondisjunction have been found to play a role in the genesis of the XXY karyotype. Pedigree studies indicate that both X chromosomes are of maternal origin in 67% of XXY patients.

The diagnosis of Klinefelter's syndrome is suggested by the classic phenotype and hormonal changes. It is confirmed by the finding of an X chromatin–positive buccal smear and demonstration of an XXY karyotype in blood, skin, or gonads. After puberty, levels of serum and urinary gonadotropins, especially FSH, are raised. The testosterone production rate, the total and free levels of testosterone, and the metabolic clearance rates of testosterone and estradiol tend to be low, while plasma estradiol levels are normal or high. Testicular biopsy reveals the classic findings of hyalinization of the seminiferous tubules, severe deficiency of spermatogonia, and pseudoadenomatous clumping of Leydig cells.

Treatment of patients with Klinefelter's syndrome is directed toward androgen replacement, if necessary. Testosterone enanthate in oil, 200 mg intramuscularly every 2 weeks, is recommended as a replacement dose in adults. Gynecomastia is not amenable to hormone therapy but can be surgically corrected if it is severe or psychologically disturbing to the patient.

Variants of Chromatin-Positive Seminiferous Tubule Dysgenesis

A. XY/XXY Mosaicism: This is the second most common chromosome complement associated with the Klinefelter phenotype. Mosaicism with any XY cell line may modify the clinical syndrome and result in less severe gynecomastia, as well as a lesser degree of testicular pathology. Some affected patients are fertile. Mean testosterone levels tend to be higher in XY/XXY patients than in XXY patients. In order to rule out XY/XXY mosaicism, cultures for karyotype analysis should be obtained from 2 or more tissues, and a sufficient number of cells (50 or more) should be examined from each tissue. Therapy depends on the severity of the clinical and gonadal aberrations associated with the XXY cell line.

B. XXYY: Patients with this karyotype comprise 3% of chromatin-positive males. In addition to exhibiting the usual characteristics of Klinefelter's syndrome, they tend to be tall, and almost all reported patients have been mentally retarded. Therapy with testosterone is similar to that in patients with XXY Klinefelter's syndrome.

C. XXXY and XXXYY: All patients with these karyotypes have had significant mental retardation; developmental anomalies (short neck, epicanthal folds, radioulnar synostosis, and clinodactyly) are present in half of patients.

D. XXXXY: Patients with this karyotype are more severely affected than those with a lesser number of X chromosomes. In addition to severe mental retardation, they exhibit radioulnar synostosis, hypoplastic external genitalia, and cryptorchid testes. Other anomalies such as congenital heart disease, cleft palate, strabismus, and microcephaly may be present. The facies is characteristic, with prognathism, hypertelorism, and myopia.

E. XX Males: Over 150 phenotypic males with a 46,XX karyotype have been described since 1964. In general, they have a male phenotype, male psychosocial gender identity, and testes with histologic features similar to those observed in patients with an XXY karyotype. At least 10% of patients have had hypospadias or ambiguous external genitalia. XX males have normal body proportions and a mean final height that is shorter than patients with an XXY karyotype or normal males but taller than normal females. As in XXY males, testosterone levels are low or low normal, gonadotropins are elevated, and spermatogenesis is impaired. Gynecomastia is present in approximately one-third of the patients.

The presence of testes and male sexual differentiation in 46,XX individuals has been a perplexing problem. However, the paradox has been clarified by the discovery that XX males are H-Y antigen–positive.

Three theories have been advanced to explain this rare example of sex reversal: (1) the presence of hidden sex chromosome mosaicism in an XX male with an undetected cell line containing a Y chromosome; (2) interchange or translocation between a Y and an X chromosome or an autosome that results in relocation of masculinizing genes from the Y chromosome onto an X chromosome or an autosome; and (3) a putative mutant autosomal gene that leads to the differentiation of testes in an XX embryo, as in the "Saanen" goat. Several lines of evidence support a Y-to-X interchange in at least some XX males. Karyotypic heteromorphism has been found involving the short arms of the X chromosome in XX males, suggesting a Y-to-X translocation. Furthermore, XX sex-reversed mice have been found to have a nonreciprocal crossover involving the Y and X chromosomes. Finally, 3 of four XX males studied with a Y-specific DNA probe were shown to have Y-specific material in their genomes. There is also evidence to support the other possibilities in the pathogenesis of this abnormality, and all would lead to an XX individual who is H-Y antigen–positive. The presence of XX males and true hermaphrodites in the same family in mammals suggests that the pathogenesis of these conditions is similar.

SYNDROME OF GONADAL DYSGENESIS: TURNER'S SYNDROME & ITS VARIANTS

Turner's Syndrome: XO Gonadal Dysgenesis

One in 10,000 newborn females has an XO sex chromosome constitution. The cardinal features of XO gonadal dysgenesis are a variety of somatic anomalies, sexual infantilism at puberty secondary to gonadal dysgenesis, and short stature. (See also Chapter 14.) Patients with an XO karyotype can be recognized in infancy usually because of lymphedema of the extremities and loose skin folds over the nape of the neck. In later life, the typical patient is often recognizable by her distinctive facies, in which micrognathia, epicanthal folds, prominent low-set ears, a fishlike mouth, and ptosis are present to varying degrees. The chest is shieldlike and the neck short, broad, and webbed (40% of patients). Additional anomalies associated with Turner's syndrome include coarctation of the aorta (10%), hypertension, renal abnormalities (50%), pigmented nevi, cubitus valgus, a tendency to keloid formation, puffiness of the dorsum of the hands, short fourth metacarpals, and recurrent otitis media. Routine intravenous urography is indicated for all patients to rule out a surgically correctable renal abnormality. The internal ducts as well as the external genitalia of these patients are female.

Short stature is an invariable feature of the syndrome of gonadal dysgenesis. Mean final height in XO patients is 142 cm, with a range of 133– 153 cm. Current data suggest that the short stature found in patients with the syndrome of gonadal dysgenesis is not due to a deficiency of growth hormone, somatomedin, sex steroids, or thyroid hormone. No significant increase in final height has been documented in these patients after therapy with growth hormone, anabolic steroids, and estrogens.

Gonadal dysgenesis is another feature of patients with an XO sex chromosome constitution. The gonads are typically streaklike and usually contain only fibrous stroma arranged in whorls. Longitudinal studies of both basal and GnRH-evoked gonadotropin secretion in patients with gonadal dysgenesis indicate a lack of feedback inhibition of the hypothalamic-pituitary axis by the dysgenetic gonads in affected infants and children (Fig 15– 11). Thus, plasma and urinary gonadotropin levels, particularly FSH levels, are high, especially during early infancy and after 10 years of age. Since ovarian function is impaired, puberty does not usually ensue spontaneously; thus, sexual infantilism is a hallmark of this syndrome.

A variety of disorders are associated with this syndrome, including obesity, diabetes mellitus, Hashimoto's thyroiditis, rheumatoid arthritis, and inflammatory bowel disease.

Phenotypic females with the following features should have a buccal smear for sex chromatin and a karyotype analysis: (1) short stature (> 2.5 SD below the mean value per age); (2) somatic anomalies associated with the syndrome of gonadal dysgenesis; and (3) delayed adolescence and increased concentration of plasma gonadotropins. In normal XX females, 20– 30% of the nuclei are sex chromatin–positive. Although a buccal smear for sex chromatin is useful, karyotype analysis should be performed for definitive diagnosis.

Therapy is directed toward the institution of estrogen therapy in order to produce secondary sexual characteristics and menarche at an age commensurate with normal peers. A successful regimen is to initiate therapy at age 12– 13 years with conjugated estrogens (0.3 mg or less) or ethinyl estradiol (5 μg); either agent is given orally for the first 21 days of the calendar month. Thereafter, the dose of estrogen is gradually increased over the next 2– 3 years to 0.6– 1.25 mg of conjugated estrogens daily or 10 μg of ethinyl estradiol daily. The patient is maintained on the minimum dose of estrogen necessary to maintain secondary sexual characteristics and menses. Medroxyprogesterone acetate, 5 mg daily, is given on the 12th– 21st days of the cycle to ensure physiologic menses and to try to reduce the risk of endometrial carcinoma associated with sustained estrogen stimulation.

X Chromatin–Positive Variants of the Syndrome of Gonadal Dysgenesis

Patients with structural abnormalities of the X chromosome (deletions and additions) and mosaicism with XX cell lines may manifest the somatic as well as the gonadal features of the syndrome of gonadal

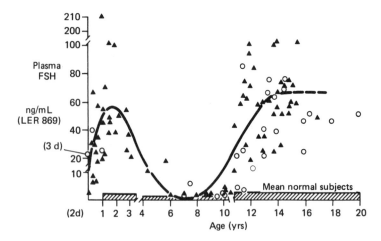

Figure 15–11. Diphasic variation in basal levels of plasma FSH (ng/mL-LER 869) in patients with an XO karyotype (solid triangles) and patients with structural abnormalities of the X chromosome, and mosaics (open circles). Note that mean basal levels of plasma FSH in patients with gonadal dysgenesis are in the castrate range before 4 years and after 10 years of age. (Reproduced, with permission, from Grumbach MM, Conte FA, Kaplan SL: *J Clin Endocrinol Metab* 1975;**40**:670.)

dysgenesis (Table 15–4). Evidence suggests that genes on both the long and short arms of the X chromosome control gonadal differentiation, whereas genes on the short arms of the X prevent the short stature and somatic anomalies that are seen in XO patients. In general, mosaicism with an XX cell line in association with an XO cell line will modify the phenotype toward normal and can even result in normal gonadal function.

X Chromatin–Negative Variants of the Syndrome of Gonadal Dysgenesis

Patients usually have mosaicism with an XO- and a Y-bearing cell line—XO/XY, XO/XYY, XO/XY/XYY—or perhaps a structurally abnormal Y chromosome. They range from phenotypic females with the features of Turner's syndrome through patients with ambiguous genitalia to (rarely) completely virilized males with a few stigmas of Turner's syndrome.

The gonadal differentiation varies from bilateral streaks to bilateral dysgenetic testes, along with asymmetric development, ie, a streak on one side and a dysgenetic testicle (or, rarely, a normal testis) on the other side, sometimes called "mixed gonadal dysgenesis." The development of the external genitalia as well as the internal ducts correlates well with the degree of testicular differentiation and, presumably, the capacity of the fetal testes to secrete müllerian duct inhibitory factor and testosterone.

The risk of development of gonadal tumors is greatly increased in patients with XO/XY mosaicism, and prophylactic removal of streak gonads or dysgenetic undescended testes in this syndrome is indicated. Breast development at or after the age of puberty in these patients is commonly associated with a gonadal neoplasm, usually a gonadoblastoma. Pelvic sonography as well as CT scanning may be useful in screening for neoplasms in these patients. Gonadoblastomas

Table 15–4. Relationship of structural abnormalities of the X and Y to clinical manifestations of the syndrome of gonadal dysgenesis.

Type of Sex Chromosome Abnormality	Karyotype	Phenotype	Sexual Infantilism	Short Stature	Somatic Anomalies of Turner's Syndrome
Loss of an X or Y	XO	Female	+	+	+
*Deletion of short arm of an X	XXqi	Female	+ (occ. ±)	+	+
	XXp−	Female	+, ±, or −	+ (−)	+ (−)
*Deletion of long arm of an X	XXpi	Female	+	−	− or (±)
	XXq−	Female	+	− (+)	− or (±)
Deletion of ends of both arms of an X	XXr	Female	− or +	+	+ or (±)
Deletion of short arm of Y	XYp−	Ambiguous	+	+	+

*In Xp− and Xq−, the extent and site of the deleted segment are variable.

Xqi = isochromosome for long arm of an X; Xp− = deletion of short arm of an X; Xpi = isochromosome for short arm of an X; Xq− = deletion of long arm of an X; Xr = ring chromosome derived from an X.

are calcified, so that they may be visible even on a plain film of the abdomen.

The diagnosis of XO/XY mosaicism can be established by the demonstration of both XO and XY cells in blood, skin, or gonadal tissue. The decision as to the sex of rearing of the child should be based on the age at diagnosis and the potential for normal function of the external genitalia. In patients assigned a female gender role, the gonads should be removed and the external genitalia repaired. Estrogen therapy should be initiated at the age of puberty, as in patients with an XO karyotype (see above). In affected infants who are assigned a male gender role, all gonadal tissue except that which appears histologically normal and is in the scrotum should be removed. Removal of the müllerian structures and repair of hypospadias are also indicated. At puberty, depending on the functional integrity of the retained gonad, androgen replacement therapy may be indicated in doses similar to those for patients with XY gonadal dysgenesis (see below).

XX & XY GONADAL DYSGENESIS

The terms XX and XY gonadal dysgenesis have been applied to XX or XY patients who have bilateral streak gonads, a female phenotype, and no stigmas of Turner's syndrome. After puberty, they exhibit sexual infantilism, castrate levels of plasma and urinary gonadotropins, normal or tall stature, and eunuchoid proportions.

XX Gonadal Dysgenesis

Familial and sporadic cases of XX gonadal dysgenesis have been reported. Pedigree analysis of familial cases is consistent with autosomal recessive inheritance. In 3 families, XX gonadal dysgenesis was associated with deafness of the sensorineural type. In several affected groups of siblings, a spectrum of clinical findings occurred, eg, varying degrees of ovarian function, including breast development and menses followed by secondary amenorrhea. The diagnosis of XX gonadal dysgenesis should be suspected in phenotypic females with sexual infantilism and normal müllerian structures who lack the somatic stigmas of the syndrome of gonadal dysgenesis (Turner's syndrome). Karyotype analysis reveals only 46,XX cells. As in Turner's syndrome, gonadotropin levels are high, estrogen levels are low, and treatment consists of cyclic estrogen replacement.

Sporadic cases of XX gonadal dysgenesis may represent a heterogeneous group of patients from a pathogenetic point of view. XX gonadal dysgenesis should be distinguished from ovarian failure due to infections such as mumps, antibodies to gonadotropin receptors, biologically inactive FSH, and gonadotropin-insensitive ovaries as well as errors in steroid (estrogen) biosynthesis.

XY Gonadal Dysgenesis

XY gonadal dysgenesis occurs both sporadically and in familial aggregates. Patients with the complete form of this syndrome have female external genitalia, normal or tall stature, bilateral streak gonads, müllerian duct development, sexual infantilism, eunuchoid habitus, and a 46,XY karyotype. Clitorimegaly is quite common, and in familial cases, a continuum of involvement ranging from the complete syndrome to ambiguity of the external genitalia has been described. The phenotypic difference between the complete form of XY gonadal dysgenesis and the incomplete form is due to the degree of differentiation of the testicular tissue and its functional capacity to produce testosterone and müllerian duct inhibitory factor. Postpubertally, plasma and urinary gonadotropin levels are markedly elevated.

Analysis of familial cases suggests that XY gonadal dysgenesis is transmitted as an X-linked recessive or sex-limited autosomal dominant trait. Both H-Y antigen–positive and H-Y antigen–negative forms of this syndrome have been described and reflect the genetic heterogeneity of this syndrome. XY gonadal dysgenesis may result from a mutant gene that affects the expression of H-Y antigen (H-Y negative); from a defect in the gonad-specific H-Y antigen receptor (H-Y positive); or possibly from the production of a serologically reactive but abnormal H-Y antigen that lacks affinity for H-Y antigen receptors on gonadal cells (H-Y antigen–positive). Sporadic cases may represent teratologic defects in gonadal morphogenesis.

Therapy for patients with XY gonadal dysgenesis who have female external genitalia involves prophylactic gonadectomy and estrogen substitution at puberty. In the incomplete form of XY gonadal dysgenesis, assignment of a male gender role may be possible. It depends upon the degree of ambiguity of the genitalia and the potential for normal function. Prophylactic gonadectomy must be considered, since fertility is unlikely and there is an increased risk of malignant gonadal transformation in these patients. Recent studies have suggested a relationship between the development of gonadal tumors and H-Y antigen serotype; 95% of those found to have gonadal tumors are H-Y antigen–positive. Prosthetic testes should be implanted at the time of gonadectomy, and androgen substitution therapy is instituted at the age of puberty. Testosterone enanthate in oil is utilized, beginning with 50 mg intramuscularly monthly and gradually increasing the dose over 3–4 years to a full replacement dose of 200 mg intramuscularly every 2 weeks.

TRUE HERMAPHRODITISM

True hermaphrodites have both ovarian and testicular tissue present in either the same or opposite gonads. Differentiation of the internal and external genitalia is highly variable. The external genitalia may simulate those of a male or female, but most often they are ambiguous. Cryptorchidism and hypospadias are common. In all cases, a uterus is present. The differentiation of the genital ducts usually follows that of the ipsilateral gonad. The ovotestis is the most common gonad found in true hermaphrodites, followed by the ovary and, least commonly, the testis. At puberty, breast development is usual in the untreated patients, and menses occur in over 50% of cases. Whereas the ovary or the ovarian portion of an ovotestis may function normally, the testis or testicular portion of an ovotestis is almost always dysgenetic.

Sixty percent of true hermaphrodites have a 46,XX karyotype, 20% have 46,XY, and about 20% have mosaicism or XX/XY chimerism. True hermaphroditism may result from (1) sex chromosome mosaicism or chimerism, (2) Y-to-autosome or Y-to-X chromosome translocation or interchange, and (3) an autosomal mutant gene. There is evidence to support each of these possibilities in the pathogenesis of this clinically and anatomically heterogeneous syndrome, and all could lead to the serologic expression of H-Y antigen.

The diagnosis of true hermaphroditism should be considered in all patients with ambiguous genitalia. The finding of an XX/XY karyotype or a bilobed gonad compatible with an ovotestis in the inguinal region or labioscrotal folds suggests the diagnosis. If all other forms of male and female pseudohermaphroditism have been excluded, laparotomy and histologic confirmation of both ovarian and testicular tissue establish the diagnosis. The management of true hermaphroditism is contingent upon the age at diagnosis and a careful assessment of the functional capacity of the gonads, genital ducts, and external genitalia.

Gonadal Neoplasms in Dysgenetic Gonads

While gonadal tumors are rare in patients with Klinefelter's syndrome and XO gonadal dysgenesis, the prevalence of gonadal neoplasms is greatly increased in patients with certain types of dysgenetic gonads. Gonadoblastomas, dysgerminomas, seminomas, and teratomas are found most frequently. The frequency is increased (1) in XO/XY mosaicism and

in patients with a structurally abnormal Y chromosome and (2) in XY gonadal dysgenesis, either with a female phenotype or with ambiguous genitalia. Prophylactic gonadectomy is advised in these 2 categories as well as in individuals with gonadal dysgenesis who manifest signs of virilization, regardless of karyotype.

The gonad should be preserved in patients who are being raised as males only if it is a relatively normal testicle that can be relocated in the scrotum. The fact that a gonad is palpable in the scrotum does not preclude malignant degeneration and spread, since seminomas tend to metastasize at an early stage before a local mass is obvious.

FEMALE PSEUDOHERMAPHRODITISM

Affected individuals have normal ovaries and müllerian derivatives associated with ambiguous external genitalia. In the absence of testes, a female fetus will be masculinized if subjected to increased circulating levels of androgens derived from an extragonadal source. The degree of masculinization depends upon the stage of differentiation at the time of exposure (Fig 15–12). After 12 weeks of gestation, androgens will produce only clitoral hypertrophy. Rarely, ambiguous genitalia that superficially resemble those produced by androgens are the result of teratogenic malformations.

Congenital Adrenal Hyperplasia (Fig 15–13)

There are 6 major types of congenital adrenal hyperplasia, all transmitted as autosomal recessive disorders. (See also Chapter 10.) The common denominator of all 6 types is a defect in the synthesis of cortisol that results in an increase in ACTH and then in adrenal hyperplasia. Both males and females can be affected, but males are rarely diagnosed at birth unless they have ambiguous genitalia or are salt losers

Figure 15–12. Female pseudohermaphroditism induced by prenatal exposure to androgens. Exposure after the 12th fetal week leads only to clitoral hypertrophy (diagram on left). Exposure at progressively earlier stages of differentiation (depicted from left to right in drawings) leads to retention of the urogenital sinus and labioscrotal fusion. If exposure occurs sufficiently early, the labia will fuse to form a penile urethra. (Reproduced, with permission, from Grumbach MM, Ducharme J: *Fertil Steril* 1960;**11**:757.)

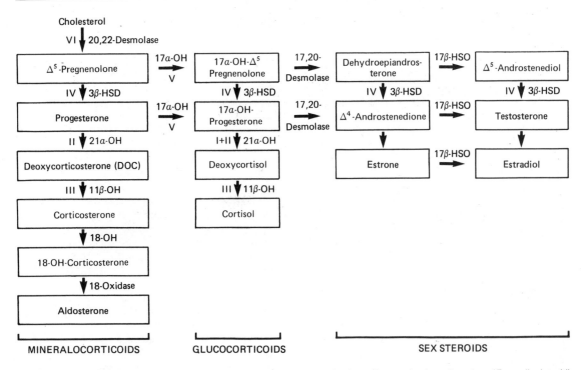

Figure 15–13. A diagrammatic representation of the steroid biosynthetic pathways in the adrenal and gonads. I to VI correspond to enzymes whose deficiency results in congenital adrenal hyperplasia. OH, hydroxy or hydroxylase; 3β-HSD, 3β-hydroxysteroid dehydrogenase; 17β-HSO, 17β-hydroxysteroid oxidoreductase. (Slightly modified and reproduced, with permission, from Conte FA, Grumbach MM: Pathogenesis, classification, diagnosis, and treatment of anomalies of sex. Chapter 106 in: *Endocrinology.* DeGroot L [editor]. Grune & Stratton, 1979.)

and manifest adrenal crises. Defects of types I–III are confined to the adrenal gland and produce virilization. Defects of types IV–VI have in common blocks in cortisol and sex steroid synthesis, in both the adrenals and the gonads. The latter 3 types produce primarily incomplete masculinization in the male and little or no virilization in the female (Table 15–5). Consequently, these will be discussed primarily as forms of male pseudohermaphroditism.

A. Type I–C21-Hydroxylase Deficiency Primarily Affecting C21-Hydroxylation in the Zona Fasciculata (Simple Virilization): This is the most common type of congenital adrenal hyperplasia, with a prevalence of 1:5000 to 1:10,000 live births in Caucasians. Recent data indicate that the locus for the gene which codes for 21-hydroxylation is on the short arm of chromosome No. 6 in close proximity to the locus for C4 (complement) between HLA-B and HLA-D. Thus,

Table 15–5. Clinical manifestations of the various types of congenital adrenal hyperplasia.

Enzymatic Defect	Cholesterol Desmolase System (Cholesterol 20α-Hydroxylase)		3β-Hydroxysteroid Dehydrogenase		17α-Hydroxylase		11β-Hydroxylase		21α-Hydroxylase	
Type	VI		IV		V		III		II and I	
Chromosomal	XX	XY	XX	XY	XX	XY	XX	XY	XX	XY
External genitalia	Female	Female	Female (clitorimegaly)	Ambiguous	Female	Female or ambiguous	Ambiguous	Male	Ambiguous*	Male
Postnatal virilization	— (Sexual infantilism at puberty)		±	Mild to moderate	— (Sexual infantilism at puberty)		+		+	
Addisonian crises	+		±		—		—		+ in 40% (type II)	
Hypertension	—		—		+		+		—	

*Normal female in late-onset and "cryptic" forms.

the gene for 21-hydroxylase deficiency is closely linked to the HLA supergene complex. In addition, certain specific HLA subtypes are found to be statistically increased in patients with 21-hydroxylase deficiency. These include B5 in the simple virilizing form and Bw47 in the salt-losing form.

A defect in 21-hyroxylase activity in the zona fasciculata of the adrenal cortex results in impaired cortisol synthesis, increased ACTH levels, and increased adrenal androgen and androgen precursor production. Prior to 12 weeks of gestation, high fetal androgen levels lead to a varying degree of labioscrotal fusion and clitoral enlargement in the female fetus; exposure to androgen after 12 weeks induces clitorimegaly alone. In the male fetus, no structural abnormalities in the external genitalia are evident at birth, but the phallus may be enlarged. These patients produce sufficient amounts of aldosterone to prevent the signs and symptoms of mineralocorticoid deficiency. Recently, the heterogeneity of 21-hydroxylase deficiency has been demonstrated by the finding that "classic" adrenal hyperplasia, acquired (late-onset) adrenal hyperplasia, and "cryptic" adrenal hyperplasia are all HLA-linked and thus represent forms of 21-hydroxylase deficiency with a wide range of clinical and biochemical severity. The "nonclassic" variants of 21-hydroxylase deficiency are postulated to be due to allelic variants at a single locus on chromosome No. 6.

B. Type II–C21-Hydroxylase Deficiency Affecting C21-Hydroxylation in the Zona Fasciculata and Zona Glomerulosa (Virilization With Salt Wasting): The salt-losing variant of 21-hydroxylase deficiency involves a more severe deficit of 21-hydroxylase in the zona fasciculata and zona glomerulosa of the adrenal cortex, which leads to impaired secretion of both cortisol (fasciculata) and aldosterone (glomerulosa). This results in electrolyte and fluid losses after the fifth day of life which are manifested as hyponatremia, hyperkalemia, acidosis, dehydration, and vascular collapse. Masculinization of the external genitalia of affected females tends to be more severe than that found in patients with simple 21-hydroxylase deficiency.

The diagnosis of 21-hydroxylase deficiency should always be considered (1) in patients with ambiguous genitalia who have an XX karyotype and are thus female pseudohermaphrodites; (2) in apparent cryptorchid males; (3) in any infant who presents with shock, hypoglycemia, and chemical findings compatible with adrenal insufficiency; and (4) in males and females with signs of virilization prior to puberty, including premature adrenarche. In the past, the diagnosis of 21-hydroxylase deficiency was based on the finding of elevated levels of 17-ketosteroids and pregnanetriol in the urine. Although still valid and useful, urinary steroid determinations have been replaced by the measurement of plasma 17-hydroxyprogesterone. The concentration of plasma 17-hydroxyprogesterone is elevated in umbilical cord blood but rapidly decreases into the range of 100–200 ng/

dL by 24 hours after delivery. In premature infants and in stressed full-term newborns, the levels of 17-hydroxyprogesterone are higher than those observed in nonstressed full-term infants. In patients with 21-hydroxylase deficiency, the 17-hydroxyprogesterone values usually range from 3000 to 40,000 ng/dL, depending on the age of the patient and the severity of 21-hydroxylase deficiency. Patients with mild 21-hydroxylase deficiency, ie, late-onset and "cryptic" forms, may have borderline basal 17-hydroxyprogesterone values, but they can be distinguished from heterozygotes on the basis of a more augmented 17-hydroxyprogesterone response to the administration of ACTH. Salt losers can be ascertained clinically, usually by chemical evidence of hyponatremia and hyperkalemia on a regular or low-salt diet. In these patients, aldosterone levels in both plasma and urine are low in relation to the serum electrolyte pattern, while plasma renin activity is elevated. HLA typing and measurement of amniotic fluid 17-hydroxyprogesterone levels have been utilized in the prenatal diagnosis of affected infants. Heterozygosity has been ascertained by HLA typing in informative families and by the use of ACTH-induced rises in plasma 17-hydroxyprogesterone levels.

C. Type III–C11-Hydroxylase Deficiency (Virilization With Hypertension): A defect in hydroxylation at C11 leads to the hypersecretion of 11-deoxycorticosterone and 11-deoxycortisol in addition to adrenal androgens. Marked heterogeneity in the clinical and hormonal manifestations of this defect have also been described. Patients with this form of adrenal hyperplasia exhibit virilization secondary to increased androgen production and hypertension caused by increased 11-deoxycorticosterone secretion. The hypertension is not obligatory and may appear in late childhood or adolescence.

Recent data suggest that the defect in 11β-hydroxylation may be primarily in the zona fasciculata. The 11β-hydroxylase gene is not linked to the HLA complex. As in other forms of congenital adrenal hyperplasia, mild forms of 11β-hydroxylase deficiency may not become manifest until adolescence or early adulthood.

The diagnosis of 11β-hydroxylase deficiency can be confirmed by demonstration of elevated plasma levels of 11-deoxycortisol and 11-deoxycorticosterone and increased excretion of their metabolites in urine (mainly tetrahydro 11-deoxycortisol).

D. Type IV–3β-Hydroxysteroid Dehydrogenase Deficiency (Male or Female Pseudohermaphroditism and Adrenal Insufficiency): See below.

E. Type V–17α-Hydroxylase Deficiency (Male Pseudohermaphroditism, Sexual Infantilism, Hypertension, and Hypokalemic Alkalosis): See below.

F. Type VI–Cholesterol Desmolase Complex Deficiency (Congenital Lipoid Adrenal Hyperplasia, Male Pseudohermaphroditism, Sexual Infantilism, and Adrenal Insufficiency): See below.

Treatment

Treatment of patients with adrenal hyperplasia may be divided into acute and chronic phases. In acute adrenal crises, a deficiency of both cortisol and aldosterone results in hypoglycemia, hyponatremia, hyperkalemia, hypovolemia, and shock. An infusion of 5% glucose in isotonic saline should be started immediately. In the first hour, if the patient is in shock, a saline infusion of 20 mL/kg may be given; thereafter, fluid and electrolyte replacement is calculated on the basis of deficits and standard maintenance requirements. Hydrocortisone sodium succinate, 50 mg/m², should be given as a bolus and another 50–100 mg/m² added to the infusion fluid over the first 24 hours of therapy. If profound hyponatremia and hyperkalemia are present, desoxycorticosterone acetate (DOCA), 1–2 mg, may be given every 12–24 hours intramuscularly. The amount of DOCA and the concentration and amount of saline solution must be adjusted according to the results of frequent electrolyte determinations, assessment of the state of hydration, and blood pressure measurements. Excess DOCA and salt can result in hypokalemia, hypertension, congestive heart failure, and hypertensive encephalopathy, whereas too little salt and DOCA will fail to correct the electrolyte imbalance.

Once the patient is stabilized and a definitive diagnosis with appropriate steroid studies has been made, the patient should receive maintenance doses of glucocorticoids to permit normal growth, development, and bone maturation (hydrocortisone, approximately 18 mg/m²/d by mouth in 3 divided doses). Salt losers need treatment with mineralocorticoid (fludrocortisone, 0.05–0.1 mg/d by mouth) and added dietary salt. The dose of mineralocorticoid should be adjusted so that plasma renin activity is maintained in the normal range.

Patients with ambiguous external genitalia should have plastic repair of the external genitalia before age 1 year. Clitoral recession or clitoroplasty rather than clitoridectomy is preferred. Of major importance to the family with an affected child is the assurance that their child will grow and develop into a normal functional adult. In patients with the most common form of adrenal hyperplasia—21-hydroxylase deficiency—fertility in males and feminization, menstruation, and fertility in females can be expected with adequate treatment. Long-term psychologic guidance and support for the patient and family by the physician is essential.

Aberrant adrenal rests are common in males with adrenal hyperplasia and may be mistaken for either adult testicular maturation or testicular neoplasms. These adrenal rests are often bilateral and are made up of cells that appear indistinguishable from Leydig cells histologically except for the fact that they lack Reinke crystalloids. The rests are usually seen in noncompliant or undertreated patients. To prevent this complication as well as the risk of adrenal crisis, pituitary hyperplasia, and adrenal carcinoma, continuous treatment with a glucocorticoid (and, if indicated, a mineralocorticoid) is recommended even in adult males.

MATERNAL ANDROGENS & PROGESTOGENS

Masculinization of the external genitalia of a female infant can occur if the mother ingested testosterone or synthetic progestational agents during the first trimester of pregnancy. After the 12th week of gestation, exposure results in clitorimegaly only. Norethindrone, ethisterone, norethynodrel, and medroxyprogesterone acetate have all been implicated in masculinization. Recently, several reports have appeared of female pseudohermaphroditism as a consequence of the maternal ingestion of danazol, the 2,3-*d*-isoxazole derivative of 17α-ethinyl testosterone. In rare instances, masculinization of a female fetus may be secondary to an ovarian or adrenal tumor, adrenal hyperplasia, or luteoma of pregnancy.

The diagnosis of female pseudohermaphroditism arising from transplacental passage of androgenic steroids is based on exclusion of other forms of female pseudohermaphroditism and a history of drug exposure. Surgical correction of the genitalia, if needed, is the only therapy necessary. Nonadrenal female pseudohermaphroditism can be associated with imperforate anus, renal anomalies, and other congenital anomalies of the lower intestine and urinary tract. Sporadic as well as familial cases have been reported.

MALE PSEUDOHERMAPHRODITISM

Male pseudohermaphrodites have gonads that are testes, but the genital ducts or external genitalia are not completely masculinized. Male pseudohermaphroditism can result from deficient testosterone secretion as a consequence of (1) failure of testicular differentiation, (2) failure of secretion of testosterone or müllerian duct inhibitory factor, (3) failure of target tissue response to testosterone or dihydrotestosterone, and (4) failure of conversion of testosterone to dihydrotestosterone.

Testicular Unresponsiveness to hCG & LH

Male sexual differentiation is dependent upon the production of testosterone by fetal Leydig cells. Data indicate that Leydig cell testosterone secretion is under the influence of placental hCG during the critical period of male sexual differentiation, and, thereafter, fetal pituitary LH during gestation.

The finding of normal male sexual differentiation in XY males with anencephaly, apituitarism, or congenital hypothalamic hypopituitarism suggests that male sex differentiation can occur independently of the secretion of fetal pituitary gonadotropins.

Absence, hypoplasia, or unresponsiveness of Leydig cells to hCG-LH would result in deficient testosterone production and, consequently, male pseudohermaphroditism. The extent of the genital ambiguity is a function of the degree of testosterone deficiency. A small number of patients with absent, hypoplastic, or unresponsive Leydig cells (attributed to a lack of receptor activity for hCG-LH) have been reported, as well as an animal model—the ''vet'' rat. In most of the patients thus far reported, the defect resulted in female-appearing genitalia. Müllerian duct regression was complete. Basal gonadotropin levels as well as GnRH-evoked responses were elevated in postpubertal patients. Plasma 17α-hydroxyprogesterone, androstenedione, and testosterone levels were low, and hCG elicited little or no response in testosterone or its precursors.

Inborn Errors of Testosterone Biosynthesis

Fig 15–14 demonstrates the major pathways in testosterone biosynthesis in the gonads; each step is associated with an inherited defect that results in testosterone deficiency and, consequently, male pseudohermaphroditism. (See also Chapter 13.) Steps 1, 2, and 3 are enzymatic deficiencies that occur in both the adrenals and gonads and result in defective synthesis of both corticosteroids and testosterone. Thus, they represent forms of congenital adrenal hyperplasia.

(1) 20,22-Desmolase deficiency, cholesterol desmolase complex defect, type VI adrenal hyperplasia, congenital lipoid adrenal hyperplasia (male pseudohermaphroditism, sexual infantilism, and adrenal insufficiency): This is a very early defect in the synthesis of all steroids and results in severe adrenal and gonadal insufficiency. Affected males have female (or, rarely, ambiguous) external genitalia with a blind vaginal pouch and hypoplastic male genital ducts but no müllerian derivatives; the genitalia of affected females are normal. Large lipid-laden adrenals that displace the kidneys downward may be demonstrated by intravenous urography, abdominal ultrasonography, or CT scanning. Death in early infancy from adrenal insufficiency is not uncommon. The diagnosis is confirmed by the lack of or low levels of all steroids in plasma and urine and an absent response to ACTH stimulation.

(2) 3β-Hydroxysteroid dehydrogenase deficiency, type IV congenital adrenal hyperplasia (male or female pseudohermaphroditism and adrenal insufficiency): 3β-Hydroxysteroid dehydrogenase deficiency is an early defect in steroid synthesis that results in inability of the adrenals and gonads to convert 3β-hydroxy-Δ⁵ steroids to 3-keto-Δ⁴ steroids. This defect in its complete form results in a deficiency of aldosterone, cortisol, testosterone, and estradiol. Males with this defect are incompletely masculinized, and females have mild clitorimegaly. Salt loss and adrenal crises usually occur in early infancy in affected patients. As in other forms of congenital adrenal hyperplasia, mild or ''nonclassical'' cases with normal genitalia and normal mineralocorticoid activity have been described. In these cases, patients usually present with premature pubarche or hirsutism.

The diagnosis of 3β-hydroxysteroid dehydrogenase deficiency is based on finding elevated concentrations of 17α-hydroxy-Δ⁵ pregnenolone, dehydro-

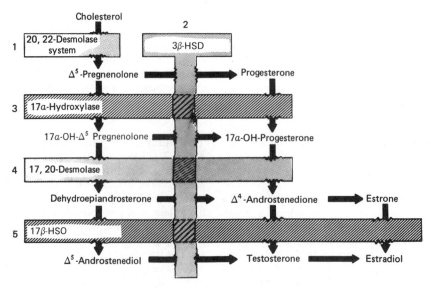

Figure 15–14. Enzymatic defects in the biosynthetic pathway for testosterone. All 5 of the enzymatic defects cause male pseudohermaphroditism in affected males. Although all of the blocks affect gonadal steroidogenesis, those at steps 1, 2, and 3 are associated with major abnormalities in the biosynthesis of glucocorticoids and mineralocorticoids in the adrenal. OH, hydroxy; 3β-HSD, 3β-hydroxysteroid dehydrogenase; 17β-HSO, 17β-hydroxysteroid oxidoreductase.

epiandrosterone (DHEA) and its sulfate, and other 3β-hydroxy-Δ^5 steroids in the plasma and urine of patients with a consistent clinical picture. Suppression of the increased plasma and urinary 3β-hydroxy-Δ^5 steroids by the administration of dexamethasone distinguishes 3β-hydroxysteroid dehydrogenase deficiency from a virilizing adrenal tumor.

(3) 17α-Hydroxylase deficiency, type V congenital adrenal hyperplasia (male pseudohermaphroditism, sexual infantilism, hypertension, and hypokalemic alkalosis): A defect in 17α-hydroxylation in the zona fasciculata of the adrenal and in the gonads results in impaired synthesis of 17α-hydroxyprogesterone and 17α-hydroxypregnenolone and, consequently, cortisol and sex steroids. The secretion of large amounts of corticosterone and deoxycorticosterone (DOC) leads to hypertension, hypokalemia, and alkalosis. Increased DOC secretion with resultant hypertension produces suppression of renin and consequently aldosterone secretion.

The clinical manifestations result from the adrenal and gonadal defect. XX females have normal development of the internal ducts and external genitalia but manifest sexual infantilism with elevated gonadotropin concentrations at puberty. XY males have impaired testosterone synthesis by the fetal testes, which results in female or ambiguous genitalia. At adolescence, sexual infantilism and hypertension are the hallmarks of this defect.

The diagnosis of 17α-hydroxylase deficiency should be suspected in XY males with female or ambiguous genitalia or XX females with sexual infantilism, who also manifest hypertension associated with hypokalemic alkalosis. High levels of progesterone, Δ^5-pregnenolone, DOC, and corticosterone in plasma and increased excretion of their urinary metabolites establish the diagnosis. Plasma renin activity and aldosterone secretion are markedly diminished in these patients.

The following errors affect testosterone and estrogen biosynthesis in the gonads primarily:

(4) 17,20-Desmolase (lyase) deficiency: This is a rare defect in sex steroid synthesis that affects the conversion of the C21 steroids 17α-hydroxyprogesterone and 17α-hydroxy-Δ^5 pregnenolone to the C19 steroids androstenedione and DHEA. Patients described with 17,20-desmolase deficiency have been male pseudohermaphrodites with either female or ambiguous genitalia and inguinal or intra-abdominal testes. Müllerian derivatives are absent, presumably as a result of the secretion of müllerian duct inhibitory factor. At puberty, incomplete virilization without gynecomastia may occur.

Patients with 17,20-desmolase deficiency have low circulating levels of testosterone, androstenedione, DHEA, and estradiol. The diagnosis can be confirmed by demonstration of an increased ratio of 17α-hydroxy C21 steroids to C19 steroids (testosterone, DHEA, Δ^5-androstenediol, and androstenedione) after stimulation with ACTH or chorionic gonadotropin.

(5) 17β-Hydroxysteroid oxidoreductase deficiency: The last step in testosterone and estradiol biosynthesis by the gonads involves the reduction of androstenedione to testosterone and estrone to estradiol. At birth, males with a deficiency of the enzyme 17β-hydroxysteroid oxidoreductase have female or mildly ambiguous external genitalia resulting from testosterone deficiency during male differentiation. They have male duct development, absent müllerian structures with a blind vaginal pouch, and inguinal or intra-abdominal testes. At puberty, progressive virilization with clitoral hypertrophy occurs, often associated with the concurrent development of gynecomastia. Plasma gonadotropin, androstenedione, and estrone levels are markedly elevated, whereas testosterone and estradiol concentrations are relatively low.

17β-Hydroxysteroid oxidoreductase deficiency should be included in the differential diagnosis of (1) male pseudohermaphrodites with absent müllerian derivatives who have no abnormality in glucocorticoid or mineralocorticoid synthesis and (2) male pseudohermaphrodites who virilize at puberty, especially if gynecomastia is present. The diagnosis of 17β-hydroxysteroid oxidoreductase deficiency can be confirmed by the demonstration of inappropriately high plasma levels of estrone and androstenedione and increased ratios of plasma androstenedione to testosterone and estrone to estradiol before and after stimulation with chorionic gonadotropin.

Management of the patients, as with other forms of male pseudohermaphroditism, depends on the age at diagnosis and the degree of ambiguity of the external genitalia. In the patient assigned a male gender identity, plastic repair of the genitalia and testosterone replacement therapy at puberty will be necessary. In patients reared as females (the usual case), the appropriate treatment is castration, followed by estrogen replacement therapy at puberty.

Defects in Androgen-Dependent Target Tissues

The complex mechanism of action of steroid hormones at the cellular level has recently been clarified (Fig 15–15).

Free testosterone enters the target cells and undergoes 5α reduction to dihydrotestosterone, which in turn is bound to a receptor protein; the receptor protein complex is translocated into the nucleus of the target cell. In the nucleus, the receptor-dihydrotestosterone complex binds to chromatin and initiates transcription. Messenger RNA is synthesized, modified, and exported to the cytoplasm of the cell, where ribosomes translate mRNA into new proteins that have an androgen effect on the cell. A lack of androgen effect at the end organ and consequently male pseudohermaphroditism may result from abnormalities in 5α-reductase activity, dihydrotestosterone receptor activity, translocation of the steroid-receptor complex, nuclear binding, transcription, exportation, or translation. (See also Chapter 13.)

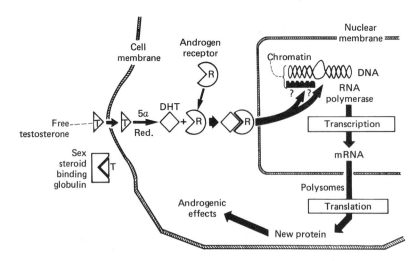

Figure 15–15. A simplified diagrammatic representation of the mechanism of action of testosterone at the target organ. 5α-Red., 5α-reductase; DHT, dihydrotestosterone. (Reproduced, with permission, from Conte FA, Grumbach MM: Pathogenesis, classification, diagnosis, and treatment of anomalies of sex. Chapter 106 in: *Endocrinology.* DeGroot L [editor]. Grune & Stratton, 1979.)

End-Organ Resistance to Androgenic Hormones (Androgen Receptor & Postreceptor Defects)

A. Syndrome of Complete Androgen Resistance and Its Variants (Testicular Feminization): The syndrome of complete androgen resistance (testicular feminization) is characterized by a 46,XY karyotype, bilateral testes, female-appearing external genitalia, a blind vaginal pouch, and absent müllerian derivatives. At puberty, female secondary sexual characteristics develop, but menarche does not ensue. Pubic and axillary hair is usually sparse and in one-third of patients totally absent. Some patients have a variant form of this syndrome and exhibit slight clitoral enlargement. At puberty, these patients may exhibit mild virilization in addition to the development of breasts and a female habitus.

Androgen resistance during embryogenesis prevents masculinization of the external genitalia and differentiation of the wolffian ducts. Secretion of müllerian duct inhibitory factor by the fetal Sertoli cells leads to regression of the müllerian ducts. Thus, affected patients are born with female external genitalia and a blind vaginal pouch. At puberty, androgen resistance results in augmented LH secretion with subsequent increases in testosterone and estradiol. Estradiol arises from conversion of testosterone and androstenedione as well as from direct secretion by the testes. Androgen resistance coupled with increased estradiol secretion results in the development of female secondary sexual characteristics at puberty.

Data on rodents as well as mammals indicate that androgen resistance is modulated, at least in part, by abnormalities in androgen receptor activity in androgen-sensitive tissues. Studies utilizing fibroblasts cultured from genital skin indicate that patients with complete androgen resistance are genetically heterogeneous. Patients have been described who have (1) an undetectable or low amount of androgen receptor activity, (2) a qualitatively abnormal (thermolabile, unstable, or both) androgen receptor, and (3) a normal amount of androgen receptor activity (a presumed postreceptor defect). Inheritance in all forms appears to be X-linked.

The diagnosis of complete androgen resistance can be suspected from the clinical features. Prepubertally, testislike masses in the inguinal canal or labia in a phenotypic female suggest the diagnosis. Postpubertally, the patients present with primary amenorrhea, normal breast development, and absent or sparse sexual hair. Characteristically, the concentrations of LH and testosterone are markedly elevated. This latter finding is an important hormonal feature of androgen resistance. The family history, phenotype, endocrine evaluation, androgen receptor studies, and, if necessary, the metabolic response to testosterone will help confirm the diagnosis.

Therapy of patients with complete androgen resistance involves affirmation and reinforcement of their female gender identity. Castration, either prior to or after puberty, is indicated because of the increased risk of gonadal neoplasms with age.

B. Syndrome of Incomplete Androgen Resistance and Its Variants (Reifenstein's Syndrome): Patients with incomplete androgen resistance manifest a wide spectrum of phenotypes as far as masculinization is concerned. The external genitalia at birth can range from ambiguous, with a blind vaginal pouch, to hypoplastic male genitalia. Müllerian duct derivatives are absent and wolffian duct derivatives present, but they are usually hypoplastic. At puberty, virilization is poor; pubic and axillary hair as well as gynecomastia are usually present. The testes remain small and exhibit azoospermia as a consequence of germinal cell arrest. As in the case of patients with complete androgen resistance, there are high levels of plasma LH, testosterone, and estradiol. However, the degree of feminization in these patients despite high estradiol levels is less than that found in the syndrome of complete androgen resistance.

Androgen receptor studies in these patients have primarily revealed (1) a partial deficiency of androgen receptor activity and (2) a qualitatively abnormal androgen receptor. As in the syndrome of complete androgen resistance, inheritance appears to be X-linked.

Androgen Resistance in Infertile Men

Partial androgen resistance has been described in a group of infertile men who have a normal male phenotype but may exhibit gynecomastia. Unlike other patients with androgen resistance, some of these patients have normal plasma LH and testosterone levels. Infertility in otherwise normal men may be the only clinical manifestation of androgen resistance, and thus infertility represents one extreme of the highly variable phenotypic expression of androgen resistance in patients with a comparable deficiency of androgen receptor activity as determined by in vitro studies.

Defects in Testosterone Metabolism by Peripheral Tissues; 5α-Reductase Deficiency (Pseudovaginal Perineoscrotal Hypospadias)

The defective conversion of testosterone to dihydrotestosterone produces a unique form of male pseudohermaphroditism (Fig 15–16). At birth, ambiguous external genitalia are manifested by a small hypospadiac phallus bound down in chordee, a bifid scrotum, and a urogenital sinus that opens onto the perineum. A blind vaginal pouch is present. The testes are either inguinal or labial. The müllerian structures are absent, and the wolffian structures are well differentiated. At puberty, affected males virilize; the voice deepens, muscle mass increases, and the phallus enlarges. The bifid scrotum becomes rugate and pigmented. The testes enlarge and descend into the labioscrotal folds, and spermatogenesis may ensue. Gynecomastia is notably absent in these patients. Of

note also is the absence of acne, temporal hair recession, and hirsutism. A remarkable feature of this form of male pseudohermaphroditism has been the reported change in gender identity from female to male at puberty, primarily in affected individuals living in rural communities in the Dominican Republic.

After the onset of puberty, patients with 5α-reductase deficiency have normal to elevated testosterone levels and elevated plasma concentrations of LH. As expected, plasma dihydrotestosterone is low and the testosterone/dihydrotestosterone ratio is abnormally high. Apparently, lack of 5α reduction of testosterone to dihydrotestosterone in utero during the critical phases of male sex differentiation results in incomplete masculinization of the external genitalia, while testosterone-dependent wolffian structures are normally developed. The marked virilization that occurs at puberty in these patients is in sharp contrast to that which occurs in utero and is as yet not well explained. Since the androgen receptor binds both dihydrotestosterone and testosterone (but with a lower affinity), the sustained high levels of circulating testosterone attained at puberty may be a factor in the virilization achieved. In addition, the enzyme defect is incomplete, and at puberty the plasma concentration of dihydrotestosterone, while low, is detectable. Also, the hormonal environment is markedly different at puberty in that large quantities of competitive steroids (estrogens and progestins) are not present as they are in utero. In particular, high concentrations of progesterone may have a marked effect on 5α-reductase activity in utero, whereas at puberty progesterone levels are low in males. 5α-Reductase deficiency is inherited as an autosomal recessive, and the enzymatic defect exhibits genetic heterogeneity.

5α-Reductase deficiency should be suspected in male pseudohermaphrodites with a blind vaginal pouch. The diagnosis can be confirmed by demonstration of an abnormally high plasma testosterone/dihydrotestosterone ratio, either under basal conditions or after hCG stimulation. Other confirmatory findings include an increased 5β/5α ratio of urinary C19 steroid metabolites of testosterone, a decreased level of 5α-reductase activity in genital skin in vitro, and decreased conversion of infused testosterone to dihydrotestosterone in vivo.

Figure 15–16. Metabolism of testosterone.

The early diagnosis of this condition is particularly critical. In view of the natural history of this disorder, affected males can be assigned a male gender identity, treated with dihydrotestosterone, and have appropriate plastic repair of their external genitalia. In patients who are diagnosed after infancy, in whom gender identity is unequivocally female, prophylactic orchiectomy and estrogen substitution therapy may still be considered the treatment of choice until further experience with this biochemical entity and sex reversal in our culture is available.

Dysgenetic Male Pseudohermaphroditism (Ambiguous Genitalia Due to Dysgenetic Gonads)

Defective gonadogenesis results in ambiguous development of the genital ducts, urogenital sinus, and external genitalia. Patients with XO/XY mosaicism, structural abnormalities of the Y chromosome, and forms of XY gonadal dysgenesis manifest defective gonadogenesis and thus defective virilization. These disorders are classified under disorders of gonadal differentiation but also are included as a subgroup of male pseudohermaphroditism.

A. Ambiguous Genitalia Associated With Degenerative Renal Disease: Several cases are recorded of male pseudohermaphroditism associated with degenerative renal disease and hypertension as well as with Wilms' tumor. In this syndrome, both the kidneys and the testes are dysgenetic, and a predisposition for renal neoplasms exists.

B. Vanishing Testes Syndrome (Embryonic Testicular Regression Syndrome; XY Agonadism; Rudimentary Testes Syndrome; Congenital Anorchia): Cessation of testicular function during the critical phases of male sex differentiation can lead to varying clinical syndromes depending on when testicular function ceases. At one end of the clinical spectrum of these heterogeneous conditions are the XY patients in whom testicular functional deficiency occurred prior to 8 weeks of gestation, which results in female differentiation of the internal and external genitalia. At the other end of the spectrum are the patients with "anorchia" or "vanishing testes." These patients have perfectly normal male differentiation of their internal and external structures, but gonadal tissue is absent. The diagnosis of anorchia should be considered in all cryptorchid males. Administration of chorionic gonadotropin, 1000–2000 units injected intramuscularly every other day for 2 weeks (total of 7 injections), is a useful test of Leydig cell function. In the presence of normal Leydig cell function, there will be a rise in plasma testosterone from concentrations of less than 20 ng/dL to over 200 ng/dL in prepubertal males. In infants under 4 years of age and children over 10 years of age, plasma FSH levels are a sensitive index of gonadal integrity. The gonadotropin response to a 100-μg bolus injection of GnRH can also be utilized to diagnose the absence of gonadal feedback on the hypothalamus and pituitary. In agonadal children, GnRH will elicit a rise in LH and FSH levels that is greater than that achieved in prepubertal children with normal gonadal function. Patients with high gonadotropin levels and no testosterone response to chorionic gonadotropin are usually found to lack recognizable gonadal tissue at laparotomy.

Defects in the Synthesis, Secretion, or Response to Müllerian Duct Inhibitory Factor

A small number of patients have been described in whom normal male development of the external genitalia has occurred but in whom the müllerian ducts persist. The retention of müllerian structures can be ascribed to failure of the Sertoli cells to synthesize müllerian duct inhibitory factor or to a defect in the response of the duct to that factor. This condition appears to be transmitted as an autosomal recessive trait. Therapy involves removal of the müllerian structures.

UNCLASSIFIED FORMS OF ABNORMAL SEXUAL DEVELOPMENT IN MALES

Hypospadias

Hypospadias occurs as an isolated finding in one per 1000 newborn males. On an embryologic basis, deficient virilization of the external genitalia implies subnormal Leydig cell function in utero, end-organ resistance, or improper chronologic correlation between hormone level and critical time for tissue response. Although in most patients there is little reason to suspect these mechanisms, recent reports in a small number of patients have suggested that simple hypospadias is associated with an abnormality in androgen receptor activity, nuclear localization, or an aberration in the maturation of the hypothalamic-pituitary-gonadal axis. Further studies are necessary to determine the role of these factors in the pathogenesis of simple hypospadias. Nonendocrine factors that affect differentiation of the primordia may be found in a variety of genetic syndromes. Aarskog prospectively studied 100 patients with hypospadias and found one patient to be a genetic female with congenital adrenal hyperplasia, 5 with sex chromosome abnormalities, and one with the incomplete form of XY gonadal dysgenesis. Nine patients were from pregnancies in which the mother had taken progestational compounds during the first trimester. Thus, a pathogenetic mechanism was found in 15% of these patients.

Microphallus

Microphallus can result from a heterogeneous group of disorders, but by far the most common is fetal testosterone deficiency. In the human male fetus, testosterone synthesis by the fetal Leydig cell during the critical period of male differentiation (8–12 weeks) is under the influence of placental hCG. After midgestation, fetal pituitary LH seems to modulate fetal

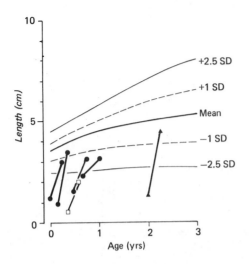

Figure 15–17. The response in phallic length to a 3-month course of testosterone in 6 patients with microphallus. Patients were under 2 years of age. Each patient was given 25 mg of testosterone enanthate in oil intramuscularly monthly for 3 months. Δ, □ indicate 2 patients who subsequently underwent a second course of testosterone therapy. (Reproduced, with permission, from Burstein S, Grumbach MM, Kaplan SL: Early determination of androgen-responsiveness is important in the management of microphallus. *Lancet* 1979;2:983.)

testosterone synthesis by the Leydig cell and, consequently, growth of the phallus. GH also appears to play a role in growth of the phallus. Thus, males with congenital hypopituitarism as well as isolated gonadotropin deficiency and "late" testicular failure can present with normal male differentiation and microphallus at birth (phallus < 2 cm in length). Patients with hypothalamic hypopituitarism or pituitary aplasia may also have midline defects, hypoglycemia, and giant cell hepatitis. After appropriate evaluation of anterior pituitary function (ie, GH, ACTH, cortisol, TSH, and gonadotropins) and stabilization of the patient with hormone replacement, if necessary, an hCG stimulation test should be performed. Thereafter, a trial of testosterone therapy should be administered to all patients with microphallus before definitive gender assignment is made. Patients with fetal testosterone deficiency as a cause of their microphallus respond to 25–50 mg of testosterone enanthate intramuscularly monthly for 3 months with a mean increase of 2 cm in phallic length (Fig 15–17). If a trial of testosterone therapy does not result in a reasonable increase in phallic size, castration and assignment of a female gender may then be a prudent course to follow in the management of patients with microphallus.

UNCLASSIFIED FORMS OF ABNORMAL SEXUAL DEVELOPMENT IN FEMALES

Congenital absence of the vagina occurs in one per 5000 female births. It can be associated with müllerian derivatives that vary from normal to absent. Ovarian function is usually normal. Therapy involves plastic repair of the vagina, if indicated.

MANAGEMENT OF PATIENTS WITH INTERSEX PROBLEMS

Choice of Sex

The goal of the physician in the management of patients with ambiguous genitalia is to establish a diagnosis and to assign a sex for rearing that is most compatible with a well-adjusted life and sexual adequacy. Once the sex for rearing is assigned, the gender role is reinforced by the use of appropriate surgical, hormonal, or psychologic measures. Except in female pseudohermaphrodites, ambiguities of the genitalia are caused by lesions that almost always make the patient infertile. In recommending male sex assignment, the adequacy of the size of the phallus should be the most important consideration.

Differential Diagnosis

The steps in the diagnosis of intersexuality are delineated in Fig 15–18.

Reassignment of Sex

Reassignment of sex in infancy and childhood is always a difficult psychosocial problem for the patient, the parents, and the physicians involved. While easier in infancy than after 2 years of age, it should always be undertaken with much deliberation and with provision for long-term medical and psychiatric supervision and counseling.

Reconstructive Surgery

It is desirable to initiate plastic repair of the external genitalia prior to 6–12 months of age. In children raised as females, the clitoris should be salvaged, if possible, by clitoroplasty or clitoral recession. Reconstruction of a vagina, if necessary, can be deferred until adolescence.

Removal of the gonads in children with the variant forms of gonadal dysgenesis should be performed at the time of initial repair of the external genitalia, because gonadoblastomas, seminomas, and dysgerminomas have been reported to occur during the first decade.

In a patient with testicular feminization, the gonads may be left in situ (provided they are not situated in the labia majora) to provide estrogen until late adolescence. The patient may then undergo prophylactic castration, having had her female identity reinforced by normal feminization at puberty.

Diagnosis of Intersexuality

1. History: Family, pregnancy.
2. Physical examination: Palpation of inguinal region, labioscrotal folds, and rectal examination.
3. Initial studies: X chromatin pattern, karyotype analysis, serum electrolytes, 17-hydroxyprogesterone, androstenedione, dehydroepiandrosterone, testosterone, and dihydrotestosterone. Sonogram of kidneys, ureters, and pelvic contents.
4. Provisional diagnosis: "Abnormal" external genitalia—proceed as shown below.

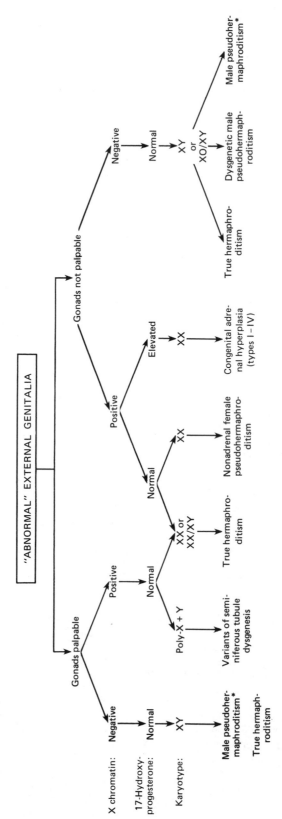

Figure 15–18. Steps in the diagnosis of intersexuality in infancy and childhood. *The 17-hydroxyprogesterone levels may be modestly elevated in patients with 3β-hydroxysteroid dehydrogenase deficiency (type IV) and are "low" in patients with 17α-hydroxylase deficiency (type V) and cholesterol desmolase deficiency (type VI). (Modified, with permission, from Grumbach MM: In: *Pediatrics*, 13th ed. Holt LE Jr, McIntosh R, Barnett HL [editors]. Appleton-Century-Crofts, 1962.)

In patients with incomplete testicular feminization reared as females or in patients with errors of testosterone biosynthesis in whom some degree of masculinization occurs at puberty, gonadectomy should be performed prior to puberty.

Hormonal Substitution Therapy

Cyclic estrogen and progestin are used in individuals reared as females in whom a uterus is present. In males, virilization is achieved by the administration of repository testosterone.

Psychologic Management

Sex is not a single biologic entity but the sum-mation of many morphogenetic, functional, and psychologic potentialities. There must never be any doubt in the mind of the parent or child as to the child's true sex. Chromosomal and gonadal sex are secondary matters; the sex of rearing is paramount. With proper surgical reconstruction and hormone substitution, the individual whose psychosexual gender is discordant with chromosomal sex need not have any psychologic catastrophes as long as the sex of rearing is accepted with conviction by the family and others during the critical early years. These individuals should reach adulthood as well-adjusted men or women capable of normal sexual interaction, albeit usually not of procreation.

REFERENCES

Austin CR, Edwards RB (editors): *Mechanisms of Sex Differentiation in Animals and Man.* Academic Press, 1981.

Bandmann HJ, Breit R, Perwein E (editors): *Klinefelter's Syndrome.* Springer-Verlag, 1984.

Conte FA, Grumbach MM: Pathogenesis, classification, diagnosis, and treatment of anomalies of sex. Chapter 106 in: *Endocrinology.* DeGroot L (editor). Grune & Stratton, 1979.

Griffen JE, Wilson JD: The syndrome of androgen resistance. *N Engl J Med* 1980;**302:**198.

Grumbach MM, Conte FA: Disorders of sex differentiation. In: *Williams' Textbook of Endocrinology,* 7th ed. Wilson JD, Foster DW (editors). Saunders, 1985.

Hamerton JL: *Human Cytogenetics.* Vols 1 and 2. Academic Press, 1971.

Imperato-McGinley JL et al: Androgens and the evolution of male-gender identity among male pseudohermaphrodites with 5α-reductase deficiency. *N Engl J Med* 1979;**300:**1233.

Lee PA et al (editors): *Congenital Adrenal Hyperplasia.* University Park Press, 1977.

McKusick VA: *Mendelian Inheritance in Man,* 6th ed. Johns Hopkins Univ Press, 1983.

Money J, Ehrhardt AA: *Man and Woman, Boy and Girl: The Differentiation and Dimorphism of Gender Identity From Conception to Maturity.* Johns Hopkins Univ Press, 1972.

New MI, Levine LS: Steroid 21-hydroxylase deficiency. Pages 83–94 in: *Adrenal Diseases in Childhood.* New MI, Levine LS (editors). Karger, 1984.

New MI et al: Congenital adrenal hyperplasia and related conditions. In: *The Metabolic Basis of Inherited Disease,* 5th ed. Stanbury JB et al (editors). McGraw-Hill, 1983.

Ohno S: *Major Sex Determining Genes.* Springer-Verlag, 1979.

Ohno S: The Y-linked testis determining gene and H-Y plasma membrane antigen gene: Are they one and the same? *Endocr Rev* 1985;**6:**421.

Peters H, McNulty KP: *The Ovary.* Univ of California Press, 1980.

Peterson RE et al: Male pseudohermaphrodism due to steroid 5α-reductase deficiency. *Am J Med* 1977;**62:**170.

Rosenfield RL, Lucky AW, Allen TD: The diagnosis and management of intersex. *Curr Probl Pediatr* 1980;**10:**7. [Entire issue.]

Serio M et al (editors): *Sexual Differentiation: Basic and Clinical Aspects.* Vol 11 of: *Serono Symposia.* Raven Press, 1984.

Simpson JL: *Disorders of Sexual Differentiation: Etiology and Clinical Delineation.* Academic Press, 1976.

Simpson JL, Photopulos G: The relationship of neoplasia to disorders of abnormal sexual differentiation. *Birth Defects* 1976;**12(Suppl 1):**15.

Singh L, Jones KW: Sex reversal in the mouse *(Mus musculus)* is caused by a recurrent nonreciprocal crossover involving the X and an aberrant Y chromosome. *Cell* 1982;**28:**205.

Vallet HL, Porter IH (editors): *Symposium on Genetic Mechanisms of Sexual Development.* Academic Press, 1979.

Van Niekerk WA: *True Hermaphrodism.* Harper & Row, 1974.

Wachtel SS: *H-Y Antigen and the Biology of Sex Determination.* Grune & Stratton, 1983.

Wilson JD et al: The androgen resistance syndromes. In: *The Metabolic Basis of Inherited Disease,* 5th ed. Stanbury JB et al (editors). McGraw-Hill, 1983.

16

Puberty

Dennis M. Styne, MD

Puberty is one stage in the continuing process of growth and development that begins during gestation and continues until the end of reproductive life. After an interval of childhood quiescence, hypothalamic-pituitary-gonadal activity intensifies in the peripubertal period, leading to increased secretion of gonadal sex steroids that cause secondary sexual development, the pubertal growth spurt, and fertility. Historical records show a lowering of the age at onset of certain stages of puberty in boys and girls in Western countries since about 1850; this is probably due to improvement in socioeconomic conditions, nutrition, and general health during that period. There is no evidence that this trend has continued during the past 4 decades.

Many factors can alter age at onset of puberty. Moderate obesity may be associated with an earlier onset of puberty, while severe, morbid obesity may delay puberty. Chronic illness and malnutrition may delay puberty. There is a significant concordance of age at menarche between mother-daughter pairs and within ethnic populations, indicating an influence of genetic factors.

Physical Changes Associated With Puberty

Descriptive standards proposed by Tanner for assessing pubertal development in males and females are in wide use. They focus attention on specific details of the examination and make it possible to objectively record subtle progression of secondary sexual development that may otherwise be overlooked.

A. Female Changes: In the female, breast development (Fig 16–1) is stimulated chiefly by ovarian estrogen secretion, although other hormones also play a part. The size and shape of the breasts may be determined by genetic and nutritional factors, but the characteristics of the stages in Fig 16–1 are the same in all females. Other estrogenic features include enlargement of the labia minora and majora, dulling of the vaginal mucosa, and production of a clear or slightly whitish vaginal secretion prior to menarche. Pubic hair development (Fig 16–2) is determined primarily by adrenal and ovarian androgen secretion. Breast development and growth of pubic hair usually proceed at similar rates, but because discrepancies in rates of advancement are possible, it is best to stage breast development separately from pubic hair progression.

Acronyms Used in This Chapter

AASH	Adrenal androgen–stimulating hormone
ACTH	Adrenocorticotropic hormone
DHEA	Dehydroepiandrosterone
FSH	Follicle-stimulating hormone
GH	Growth hormone
GnRH	Gonadotropin-releasing hormone
hCG	Human chorionic gonadotropin
hGH	Human growth hormone
LH	Luteinizing hormone
PRL	Prolactin
SHBG	Sex hormone–binding globulin
TSH	Thyroid-stimulating hormone (thyrotropin)

B. Male Changes: The first sign of normal puberty in boys is usually an increase in the size of the testes to greater than 2.5 cm in the longest diameter, excluding the epididymis. Most of the increase in testicular size is due to seminiferous tubular development secondary to stimulation by FSH. Pubic hair development is caused by adrenal and testicular androgens and is classified separately from genital development, as noted in Fig 16–3.

C. Age at Onset: The limits of onset of normal secondary sexual development in 98.8% of North American children (ie, mean ± 2.5 SD) are 8–13 years for girls and 9–14 years for boys. A graphic representation of the stages of pubertal development for British children is shown in Fig 16–4; North American and British boys develop at about the same ages, but 6 months should be subtracted from these figures to correct for North American girls. Black boys develop comparably to white boys, but black girls develop earlier than white girls. Late development may indicate hypothalamic, pituitary, or gonadal failure. The time from onset of puberty to complete adult development is also of importance; delays in reaching subsequent stages may indicate hypogonadism. Girls complete secondary sexual development in 1.5–6 years, with a mean of 4.2 years; and boys in 2–4.5 years, with a mean of 3.5 years.

The striking increase in growth velocity in puberty (pubertal growth spurt) is under complex endocrine

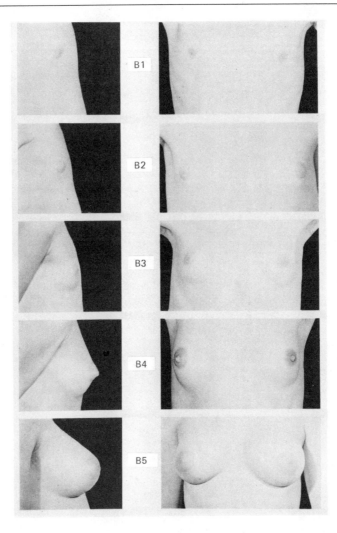

Figure 16–1. Stages of breast development, according to Marshall and Tanner. (Photographs from van Wieringen JC et al, 1971; with permission.) *Stage B1:* Preadolescent; elevation of papilla only. *Stage B2:* Breast bud stage; elevation of breast and papilla as a small mound, and enlargement of areolar diameter. *Stage B3:* Further enlargement of breast and areola, with no separation of their contours. *Stage B4:* Projection of areolar and papilla to form a secondary mound above the level of the breast. *Stage B5:* Mature stage; projection of papilla only, owing to recession of the areola to the general contour of the breast. (Reproduced, with permission, from Marshall WA, Tanner JM: *Arch Dis Child* 1969;**44**:291.)

control. GH and sex steroids appear to be of major importance; when either or both are absent, the growth spurt is decreased or absent. The pubertal growth spurt occurs before menarche and is thus an early to mid pubertal event in girls, whereas it occurs toward the end of puberty in boys. Total height attained during the growth spurt in girls is about 25 cm; in boys, it is about 28 cm. The mean adult height differential of 10 cm between men and women is due in part to heights already attained before the onset of the pubertal growth spurt and in part to the height gained during the spurt.

D. Changes in Body Composition: Changes in body composition are also prominent during pubertal development. Prepubertal boys and girls start with equal lean body mass, skeletal mass, and body fat, but at maturity men have approximately 1.5 times the lean body mass, skeletal mass, and muscle mass of women, while women have twice as much body fat as men. Using statistical analysis of age at menarche compared to height and weight at menarche, Frisch and Revelle have postulated that menarche is related to attainment of a critical body weight or to changes in body fat percentage. These theories have been criticized as being too general to be predictive in one individual.

Endocrine Changes From Fetal Life to Puberty

A. Fetal Life: The concept of the continuum of development between the fetus and the adult is well

Figure 16–2. Stages of female pubic hair development, according to Marshall and Tanner. (Photographs from van Wieringen JC et al, 1971; with permission.) *Stage P1:* Preadolescent; the vellus over the pubes is no further developed than that over the anterior abdominal wall, ie, no pubic hair. *Stage P2:* Sparse growth of long, slightly pigmented, downy hair, straight or only slightly curled, appearing chiefly along the labia. This stage is difficult to see on photographs. *Stage P3:* Hair is considerably darker, coarser, and curlier. The hair spreads sparsely over the junction of the pubes. *Stage P4:* Hair is now adult in type, but the area covered by it is still considerably smaller than in most adults. There is no spread to the medial surface of the thighs. *Stage P5:* Hair is adult in quantity and type, distributed as an inverse triangle of the classic feminine pattern. Spread is to the medial surface of the thighs but not up the linea alba or elsewhere above the base of the inverse triangle. (Reproduced, with permission, from Marshall WA, Tanner JM: *Arch Dis Child* 1969;**44**:291.)

illustrated by the changes that occur in the hypothalamic-pituitary-gonadal axis. Gonadotropins are demonstrable in fetal pituitary glands during the first trimester, and serum FSH and LH can be measured by 12 weeks of gestation. The pituitary content of gonadotropins rises to a plateau at mid gestation. Serum concentrations of LH and FSH increase to a peak at mid gestation and then gradually decrease until term. During the first half of gestation, an increase in hypothalamic GnRH content is also noted, and the hypophyseal-portal circulation achieves anatomic maturity. These data are compatible with a general theory of early unrestrained GnRH secretion stimulating pi-

tuitary gonadotropin secretion, followed by the appearance of factors that inhibit GnRH release and decrease gonadotropin secretion at mid gestation. Since male fetuses have measurable serum testosterone concentrations but have lower serum gonadotropin concentrations than female fetuses, negative feedback inhibition of gonadotropin secretion by testosterone appears operative after mid gestation.

B. Changes at Birth: At term, plasma gonadotropin concentrations are suppressed, but with postnatal clearing of high circulating estrogen concentrations, negative inhibition is reduced and postnatal peaks of LH and FSH are measurable several months after

G1

G2

G3

G4

G5

Figure 16–3. Stages of male genital development and pubic hair development, according to Marshall and Tanner. (Photographs from van Wieringen JC et al, 1971; with permission.) **Genital:** *Stage G1:* Preadolescent. Testes, scrotum, and penis are about the same size and proportion as in early childhood. *Stage G2:* The scrotum and testes have enlarged, and there is a change in the texture and some reddening of the scrotal skin. *Stage G3:* Growth of the penis has occurred, at first mainly in length but with some increase in breadth; further growth of testes and scrotum. *Stage G4:* Penis further enlarged in length and girth with development of glans. Testes and scrotum further enlarged. The scrotal skin has further darkened. *Stage G5:* Genitalia adult in size and shape. No further enlargement takes place after stage G5 is reached. **Pubic hair:** *Stage P1:* Preadolescent. The vellus over the pubes is no further developed than that over the abdominal wall, ie, no pubic hair. *Stage P2:* Sparse growth of long, slightly pigmented, downy hair, straight or only slightly curled, appearing chiefly at the base of the penis. *Stage P3:* Hair is considerably darker, coarser, and curlier and spreads sparsely over the junction of the pubes. *Stage P4:* Hair is now adult in type, but the area it covers is still considerably smaller than in most adults. There is no spread to the medial surface of the thighs. *Stage P5:* Hair is adult in quantity and type, distributed as an inverse triangle. Spread is to the medial surface of the thighs but not up the linea alba or elsewhere above the base of the inverse triangle. Most men will have further spread of pubic hair. (Modified and reproduced, with permission, from Marshall WA, Tanner JM: *Arch Dis Child* 1970;**45**:13.)

birth. Elevated testosterone may be noted for several months after birth in males: early to mid pubertal plasma concentrations of testosterone have been documented. While episodic peaks of plasma gonadotropins may occur until 2 years of age, serum gonadotropin concentrations are low during later years in normal childhood.

C. Mid Childhood Nadir of Gonadotropin Secretion: Patients with gonadal failure—such as in the syndrome of gonadal dysgenesis (Turner's syndrome)—have an exaggeration of the normal pattern of gonadotropin secretion, with exceedingly high concentrations of LH and FSH during the first 2–4 years of life (see Chapter 15). Such patients show that neg-

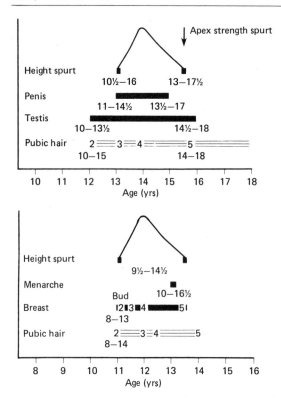

Figure 16–4. Sequence of secondary sexual development in British males *(top)* and females *(bottom)*. The range of ages is indicated. (Reproduced, with permission, from Marshall WA, Tanner JM: *Arch Dis Child* 1970;**45**:13.)

Figure 16–5. Plasma LH and testosterone measured during a 24-hour period in a 14-year-old boy in pubertal stage 2. Samples collected at night are displayed with electroencephalographic sleep stages. (Reproduced, with permission, from Boyar RM et al: *J Clin Invest* 1974;**54**:609.)

ative feedback inhibition is active during childhood; without sex steroid secretion to exert inhibition, gonadotropin values are greatly elevated. Absence of inhibin probably also allows elevated FSH values in such patients. During mid childhood, normal individuals and patients with primary hypogonadism have lower gonadotropin levels than in the neonatal period, but the range of gonadotropin concentrations in hypogonadal patients during mid childhood is still higher than that found in normal children of the same age. The decrease in gonadotropin concentrations in hypogonadal children during mid childhood is incompletely understood but has been attributed to an increasing central nervous system inhibition of gonadotropin secretion during these years. (See Fig 15–11.)

D. Peripubertal Gonadotropin Increase: During the peripubertal period of endocrine change prior to secondary sexual development, a decrease of sensitivity to negative feedback inhibition occurs. Episodic secretion of gonadotropins becomes evident during sleep (Fig 16–5). As puberty progresses, the peaks of LH and FSH occur more often during waking hours, and, finally, in late puberty, the peaks occur at all times. Thus, daytime samples of plasma for gonadotropin concentrations are of less value during early puberty because nighttime peaks would be missed.

E. Sex Steroid Secretion: Sex steroid secretion is correlated with development of gonadotropin secretion. During the postnatal period of episodic gonadotropin secretion, elevated plasma concentrations of gonadal steroids occur. This indicates potential for secretory activity in the neonatal gonad. Later, when gonadotropin secretion decreases in mid childhood, gonadal activity decreases, but testes can still be stimulated by LH or hCG and ovaries by FSH, with resulting secretion of gonadal steroids. With the onset of puberty, plasma gonadal steroid concentrations progressively increase (Fig 16–6). As sex steroids remain elevated hours after gonadotropin stimulation, random daytime sex steroid determinations may be useful indications of the stage of pubertal development; however, as noted above, gonadotropin values may be less helpful.

Most (97–99%) of the circulating estradiol and testosterone is associated with sex hormone–binding globulin (SHBG). The free hormone is the active fraction, but SHBG modulates the activity of the total testosterone and estradiol. Boys and girls have equal concentrations of SHBG, but adult men have only half the concentration of SHBG that adult women have. While adult men have 20 times the amount of plasma testosterone that adult women have, the amount of free testosterone is actually 40 times higher in men than in women.

F. GnRH Stimulation: The use of intravenous GnRH has further clarified the pattern of pubertal development (Fig 16–7). When GnRH is administered to children under 2 years of age, pituitary secretion of LH and FSH increases markedly. During the period of low basal gonadotropin secretion (age 2 to age 9 or 10 years), exogenous GnRH has less

Figure 16–6. Mean plasma LH, FSH, and estradiol (girls) or testosterone (boys) correlated with stage of puberty and bone age. LER 869 and LER 960 are the reference standards for FSH and LH, respectively. The values reported here in ng/mL would be reported as mIU/mL in most laboratories. The conversion factors are as follows: for FSH (LER 869), 1 ng = 3 mIU; for LH (LER 960), 1 ng = 7.8 mIU. (Reproduced, with permission, from Grumbach MM: Onset of puberty. In: *Puberty.* Berenberg SR [editor]. H.E. Stenfert Kroese. Copyright © 1975 by Martinus Nijhoff.)

effect on LH release. By the peripubertal period, 100 µg of intravenous GnRH induces a rise in LH of greater than 15.6 mIU/mL* in boys and girls, and this response continues until adulthood. There is no significant change in the magnitude of FSH secretion after GnRH with the onset of puberty, although females at all ages release more FSH than males.

Gonadotropins are released in secretory spurts in response to endogenous GnRH, which itself is secreted episodically about every 90–120 minutes in response to a central nervous system "pulse generator." GnRH has been administered to patients in boluses every 90 minutes, mimicking the natural secretory episodes. A prepubertal subject without significant gonadotropin peaks in the basal state will demonstrate the normal pubertal pattern of episodic secretion of gonadotropins after only a few days of GnRH boluses. Hypogonadotropic patients, who in

*This would be reported as 2 ng/mL (LER 960) in some laboratories. See Fig 16–6 legend.

Figure 16–7. The changes in plasma FSH *(top)* and LH *(bottom)* after GnRH was administered in prepubertal, pubertal, and adult subjects. LER 869 and LER 960 are the reference standards for FSH and LH, respectively. See legend for Fig 16–6 for conversion of ng/mL to mIU/mL. (Reproduced, with permission, from Grumbach MM et al: *Control of the Onset of Puberty.* Grumbach MM, Grave GD, Mayer FE [editors]. Wiley, 1974.)

Table 16–1. Mean serum concentrations of DHEA sulfate during childhood.*

	Boys (µg/dL)	Girls (µg/dL)
Chronologic age (years)		
1–6	15.4 ± 6.8	24.7 ± 11.1
6–8	18.8 ± 4.1	30.4 ± 7.6
8–10	58.6 ± 10.1	117.3 ± 41.7
10–12	126.4 ± 28.0	112.7 ± 16.4
12–14	133.4 ± 22.2	168.9 ± 19.3
14–16	264.3 ± 19.4	253.5 ± 41.3
16–20	264.1 ± 61.8	232.5 ± 49.8
Bone age (years)		
1–6	16.6 ± 6.1	2.5 ± 2.5
6–8	36.3 ± 6.7	27.2 ± 9.6
8–10	57.4 ± 8.5	–
10–12	125.0 ± 22.7	112.9 ± 27.6
12–14	214.9 ± 30.1	159.7 ± 26.3
14–16	403.4 ± 99.4	261.0 ± 45.0
16–20	–	145.3 ± 32.2

*Modified and reproduced, with permission, from Reiter EO, Fuldauer LG, Root AW: *J Pediatr* 1977;90:766.

the basal state do not have secretory episodes of gonadotropin release, have also been restored to normal episodic gonadotropin secretion and normal fertility by this method of pulsatile GnRH administration. Varying the timing of pulsatile GnRH administration can regulate the ratio of FSH to LH; the frequency of hypothalamic GnRH release shifts during the menstrual cycle to naturally change the ratio. If GnRH is continuously administered or if superactive analogs of GnRH are given, a brief period of increased gonadotropin secretion is followed by LH and FSH suppression.

Menarche

The last stage in hypothalamic-pituitary development is the onset of positive feedback. After mid puberty, estrogen is capable of stimulating gonadotropin release. The frequency of pulsatile GnRH release changes during the normal menstrual cycle and varies the ratio of LH to FSH secretion. This stimulates the ovary to produce estrogen and leads to the midcycle LH surge. Even if the midcycle surge of gonadotropins is operative, ovulation may not occur during the first menstrual cycles; 90% of all menstrual cycles are anovulatory in the first year after menarche. In the USA, the mean age at menarche is 12.8 years (± 1.2 years SD). Menarche is closely correlated with a skeletal age of 13 years (see Chapter 5).

Adrenarche

While the hypothalamic-pituitary axis has been well characterized in recent years, our understanding of the mechanism of control of adrenal androgen secretion is still somewhat rudimentary. The adrenal cortex secretes the weak androgens dehydroepiandrosterone (DHEA), dehydroepiandrosterone sulfate (DHEA sulfate), and androstenedione in increasing amounts at an average age of 6–7 years in girls and 7–8 years in boys (Table 16–1). A continued rise in adrenal androgen secretion persists until late puberty. Thus, adrenarche (the secretion of adrenal androgens) occurs years before gonadarche (the secretion of gonadal sex steroids). It is postulated that an adrenal androgen–stimulating hormone (AASH) secreted by the pituitary gland is responsible for adrenarche. An alternative explanation is that primary intra-adrenal changes modulate the release of androgens. The observation that patients with Addison's disease, who do not secrete adrenal androgens, and patients with premature adrenarche, who secrete increased amounts of adrenal androgens at an early age, usually enter gonadarche at a normal age suggests that age at adrenarche does not significantly influence age at gonadarche. It is important to note that measurements of urinary 17-ketosteroids reflect principally adrenal androgen secretion and not secretion of testosterone or its metabolites. Thus, urinary 17-ketosteroid levels rise at adrenarche.

DELAYED SECONDARY SEXUAL DEVELOPMENT (Delayed Puberty)

Any boy of 14 or girl of 13 years of age with no signs of pubertal development falls more than 2.5 SD below the mean and is considered to have delayed puberty (Table 16–2). By this definition, 0.6% of the normal population are classified as having constitutional delay in growth and adolescence. These patients

Table 16–2. Classification of delayed puberty.

Constitutional delay in growth and adolescence
Hypogonadotropic hypogonadism
    Central nervous system disorders
        Tumors
        Other acquired disorders
        Congenital disorders
    Isolated gonadotropin deficiency
    Multiple pituitary hormonal deficiencies
    Miscellaneous disorders
        Prader-Willi syndrome
        Laurence-Moon-Biedl syndrome
        Chronic disease
        Weight loss
        Anorexia nervosa
        Increased physical activity in female athletes
        Hypothyroidism
Hypergonadotropic hypogonadism
    Klinefelter's syndrome
    Other forms of primary testicular failure
    Anorchia or cryptorchidism
    Turner's syndrome
    Other forms of primary ovarian failure
    Pseudo-Turner's syndrome
    XX and XY gonadal dysgenesis

need reassurance rather than treatment and will ultimately progress through the normal stages of puberty, albeit later than their peers. It is the duty of the examining physician to decide which patients are constitutionally delayed and which truly have organic disease.

Constitutional Delay in Growth & Adolescence

A patient with delayed onset of secondary sexual development who has a history of always being shorter than age-matched peers but who consistently maintains a normal growth velocity for bone age and whose skeletal development is more than 2 SD less than the mean is likely to have constitutional delay in puberty (Fig 16– 8). There is often a family history of a similar pattern in a parent or sibling. The subject is usually thin. These patients are at the older end of the distribution curve of age at onset of puberty. In many cases, even if they show no physical signs of puberty at the time of examination, the initial elevation of gonadal sex steroids has already begun, or their plasma LH response to intravenous GnRH is pubertal (a rise in LH of > 15.6 mIU/mL). These results suggest that secondary sexual development will commence within 6 months. However, in some cases, observation for endocrine or physical signs of puberty must continue for a period of months or years before the diagnosis is made. Generally, signs of puberty will appear after the patient reaches a skeletal age of 12 years (boys) or 11 years (girls). Patients with constitutional delay in adolescence will almost always manifest secondary

Figure 16–8. Girl 13 $^4/_{12}$ years old with constitutional delay in growth and puberty. History revealed a normal growth rate but short stature at all ages. Physical examination revealed a height of 138 cm (−4.5 SD) and a weight of 28.6 kg (−3 SD). The patient had early stage 2 breast development, with 1 cm of glandular tissue on the right breast and 2 cm on the left breast. The vaginal mucosa was dulled, and there was no pubic hair. Karyotype was 46,XX. Bone age was 10 years. After administration of GnRH, LH rose from 14.8 to 37.4 mIU/mL and FSH from 11.7 to 20.1 mIU/mL. Estradiol was 40 pg/mL. She has since spontaneously progressed through pubertal development. (Reproduced, with permission, from Styne DM, Kaplan SL: *Pediatr Clin North Am* 1979;**26**:123.)

sexual development by 18 years of chronologic age. Adrenarche is characteristically delayed, along with gonadarche.

Hypogonadotropic Hypogonadism

The absent or decreased ability of the hypothalamus to secrete GnRH or of the pituitary to secrete LH and FSH leads to hypogonadotropic hypogonadism. This classification denotes an irreversible condition requiring replacement therapy. If the deficiency is limited to gonadotropins, patients are usually of normal height for age, in contrast to the shorter patients with constitutional delay. Of course, if GH deficiency accompanies gonadotropin deficiency, severe short stature will result.

A. Central Nervous System Disorders:

1. Tumors–A tumor involving the hypothalamus or pituitary gland has the potential for interfering with hypothalamic-pituitary-gonadal function as well as the control of GH, ACTH, TSH, PRL, and vasopressin secretion. Thus, delayed puberty may be a manifestation of a central nervous system tumor accompanied by any or all of the following: GH deficiency, sec-

ondary hypothyroidism, secondary adrenal insufficiency, hyperprolactinemia, or diabetes insipidus. The combination of anterior and posterior pituitary deficiencies acquired after birth is an especially ominous sign, pointing to the likelihood of a hypothalamic-pituitary tumor.

Craniopharyngioma is the most common type of hypothalamic-pituitary tumor leading to delay or absence of pubertal development. This neoplasm originates in Rathke's pouch but may develop into a suprasellar tumor. The peak age incidence of craniopharyngioma is between 6 and 14 years. Presenting symptoms may include headache, visual deficiency, growth failure, polyuria, and polydipsia; presenting signs may include visual defects, optic atrophy or papilledema, and clinical manifestations of gonadotropin, thyroid, and GH deficiency. Laboratory evaluation may reveal any type of anterior or posterior pituitary deficiencies. Bone age may be retarded at the time of presentation.

Calcification in the suprasellar region is the hallmark of craniopharyngiomas; 80% of cases will have calcifications on lateral skull x-ray, and a higher per-

Figure 16–9. Boy 15 $^{10}/_{12}$ years old with Kallmann's syndrome. His testes were originally undescended, but they descended into the scrotum after human chorionic gonadotropin treatment was given. His height was 163.9 cm (−1.5 SD), and the upper to lower segment ratio was 0.86 (eunuchoid). The penis was 6.3 × 1.8 cm. Each testis was 1 × 2 cm. Plasma LH was not detectable and rose to 5.5 mIU/mL after administration of 100 μg of GnRH; FSH rose from 3.6 mIU/mL to 7.2 mIU/mL. Testosterone did not change from 17 ng/dL. He had no ability to smell standard odors. (Reproduced, with permission, from Styne DM, Grumbach MM: *Reproductive Endocrinology.* Yen SSC, Jaffe RB [editors]. Saunders, 1978.)

centage will show this on CT scan. The tumor often presents a cystic appearance on CT scan. Small intrasellar tumors may be resected by transsphenoidal surgery; larger ones are best treated by partial resection and radiation therapy (see Chapter 4).

Extrasellar tumors that involve the hypothalamus and produce sexual infantilism include germinomas, gliomas (sometimes with neurofibromatosis), and astrocytomas. Intrasellar tumors such as chromophobe adenomas are quite rare in children.

2. Other acquired central nervous system disorders–Other acquired central nervous system disorders may lead to hypothalamic-pituitary dysfunction. Hand-Schüller-Christian disease (histiocytosis X), when involving the hypothalamus, most frequently leads to diabetes insipidus, but any other hypothalamic defect may also occur. Tuberculous or sarcoid granulomas, other postinfectious inflammatory lesions, vascular lesions, and trauma more rarely cause hypogonadotropic hypogonadism.

3. Developmental defects–Developmental defects of the central nervous system may cause hypogonadotropic hypogonadism or other types of hypothalamic dysfunction. Optic dysplasia is associated with small, dysplastic optic disks and, in some patients, absence of the septum pellucidum on pneumoencephalography or CT scanning; associated hypothalamic deficiencies are often present. It is essential to differentiate optic hypoplasia or dysplasia from optic atrophy. Both anterior and posterior pituitary deficiencies may occur with this defect. Cleft palate or other midline anomalies may also be associated with hypothalamic dysfunction.

4. Radiation therapy–Central nervous system radiation therapy involving the hypothalamic-pituitary area can lead to hypogonadotropic hypogonadism with onset at 6–18 months (or sometimes longer) after treatment.

B. Isolated Hormonal Deficiency: Patients who have isolated deficiency of gonadotropins but normal GH secretion tend to be of normal height for age. They will have eunuchoid proportions of increased span for height and decreased upper to lower segment ratios. Their skeletal development will be delayed for chronologic age during the teen years.

Kallmann's syndrome is the most common form of isolated gonadotropin deficiency (Fig 16–9). Gonadotropin deficiency in these patients is associated with hypoplasia or aplasia of the olfactory lobes and hyposmia or anosmia; remarkably, they may not notice that they have no sense of smell, although olfactory testing will reveal it. This is a familial syndrome of variable manifestations in which anosmia may occur with or without hypogonadism in a given member of a kindred. Kallmann's syndrome was at first believed to have an X-linked inheritance pattern, but recent reports show autosomal dominant or autosomal recessive patterns as well.

Other cases of hypogonadotropic hypogonadism may occur sporadically or via an autosomal recessive pattern without anosmia. Some patients lack only LH

secretion and have spermatogenesis without testosterone production (fertile eunuch syndrome); others lack only FSH.

C. Idiopathic Hypopituitary Dwarfism: Patients with congenital GH deficiency have early onset of growth failure (Fig 16–10); this feature separates them from patients with GH deficiency due to hypothalamic tumors, who usually have late onset of growth failure. Even without associated gonadotropin deficiency, untreated GH-deficient patients often have delayed onset of puberty associated with their delayed bone ages.

Figure 16–10. Twenty-year-old male with congenital deficiency of GH, GnRH, TSH, and ACTH. Height was 8 SD below the mean, and the phallus was 2 × 1 cm. Bone age was 10 years, and the sella turcica was small on lateral skull x-ray. LH was 1.6 mIU/mL and rose only to 4.7 mIU/mL after administration of 100 μg of GnRH. Testosterone was less than 10 ng/dL and did not rise after administration of GnRH. (Reproduced, with permission, from Styne DM, Grumbach MM: *Reproductive Endocrinology.* Yen SSC, Jaffe RB [editors]. Saunders, 1978.)

With appropriate hGH therapy, however, onset of puberty occurs at a normal age. Patients who have combined GH and gonadotropin deficiency do not undergo puberty even when bone age reaches the pubertal stage.

Idiopathic hypopituitarism most often is sporadic but may follow an autosomal recessive or X-linked inheritance pattern. Birth injury or breech delivery is a common feature of the neonatal history of patients with idiopathic hypopituitarism.

The syndrome of microphallus (due to congenital gonadotropin deficiency) and neonatal hypoglycemic seizures (due to congenital ACTH deficiency, GH deficiency, or both) must be diagnosed and treated early to avoid mental retardation. Patients with this syndrome will not undergo spontaneous pubertal development. Testosterone in low doses (testosterone enanthate, 25 mg intramuscularly every month for 3 doses) can increase the size of the penis in such patients without significantly advancing bone age. Males with isolated GH deficiency can also have microphallus; the penis will enlarge to some degree with hGH therapy in these patients. It is important to note that microphallus due to hypopituitarism is medically treatable, and sex reversal usually need not be considered.

D. Miscellaneous Disorders:

1. Prader-Willi syndrome–Prader-Willi syndrome occurs sporadically and is associated with fetal and infantile hypotonia, short stature, massive obesity, characteristic facies, small hands and feet, mental retardation, and emotional instability in patients of either sex, delayed menarche in females, and micropenis and cryptorchidism in males. Recently, the syndrome has been associated with deletion or translocation of chromosome 15.

2. Laurence-Moon-Biedl syndrome–This autosomal recessive condition is characterized by polydactyly, obesity, short stature, mental retardation, and retinitis pigmentosa. Hypogonadotropic hypogonadism and primary hypogonadism have also been reported in affected patients.

3. Chronic disease and malnutrition–A delay in sexual maturation may be due to chronic disease or malnutrition. Weight loss to less than 80% of ideal weight caused by disease or voluntary dieting may result in gonadotropin deficiency; increase in weight toward the ideal usually restores gonadotropin function. Delayed puberty and short stature have been reported to occur in healthy individuals who voluntarily diet because of "fear of obesity."

4. Anorexia nervosa–Anorexia nervosa involves weight loss associated with significant psychologic disorder. Patients are usually girls who have a disturbed body image, avoid food, and often induce regurgitation after ingestion. Weight loss may be so severe as to cause a fatal complication such as immune dysfunction, fluid and electrolyte imbalance, or circulatory collapse. Primary or secondary amenorrhea is a classic finding in these patients and has been correlated with the degree of weight loss. Weight gain

to the normal range for height, however, does not ensure immediate resumption of menses. Functional amenorrhea may also occur in women of normal weight, some of whom demonstrate evidence of psychologic stress.

5. Increased physical activity–Girls who regularly participate in strenuous athletics or ballet dancing may have delayed thelarche, delayed menarche, and irregular or absent menstrual periods; since some affected girls are of normal weight, this effect is not always related to less than ideal weight. It was reported that one patient resumed menses while her activity was decreased as a result of being temporarily bedridden.

6. Hypothyroidism–Hypothyroidism can delay all aspects of growth and maturation, including puberty and menarche. Conversely, severe hypothyroidism may advance the age at onset of pubertal signs in some patients (Van Wyk–Grumbach syndrome); galactorrhea may also occur in such patients.

Hypergonadotropic Hypogonadism

Primary gonadal failure is heralded by elevated gonadotropins due to the absence of negative feedback effects of gonadal sex steroids. The most common causes of hypergonadotropic hypogonadism are associated with karyotypic and somatic abnormalities, but isolated gonadal failure can also present with delayed puberty without other physical findings.

A. Syndrome of Seminiferous Tubule Dysgenesis (Klinefelter's Syndrome): (See Chapters 13 and 15.) The most common form of primary testicular failure is Klinefelter's syndrome (XXY karyotype), with an incidence of 1:1000 males. Before puberty, patients have decreased upper to lower segment ratios, increased arm span, small testes, and an increased incidence of mental retardation and personality disorders. Onset of puberty is not usually delayed, because Leydig cell function is characteristically less affected than seminiferous tubule function. Gonadotropin levels rise after the onset of puberty; the testes become firm and are rarely larger than 3.5 cm in diameter. After the onset of puberty, there are histologic changes of seminiferous tubule hyalinization and fibrosis, adenomatous changes of the Leydig cells, and impaired spermatogenesis. Gynecomastia is common, and variable degrees of male secondary sexual development are found.

Other forms of male hypergonadotropic hypogonadism are found with XX/XXY, XXYY, XXXY, and XXXXY karyotypes. Phenotypic males have been described with XX karyotypes and some physical features of Klinefelter's syndrome.

B. Other Forms of Primary Testicular Failure: The "Sertoli cell only" syndrome (germinal cell aplasia) is a congenital form of testicular failure with azoospermia and elevated FSH but generally normal secondary sexual characteristics, normal testosterone concentrations, and no other anomalies.

C. Cryptorchidism or Anorchia: Phenotypic males with an XY karyotype but no palpable testes have either cryptorchidism or anorchia. Cryptorchid males should be able to produce a rise in testosterone 72 hours after 2000 units of chorionic gonadotropin is given intramuscularly, and the testes may descend during 2 weeks of treatment with 2000 units given 3 times a week. Patients with increased plasma testosterone in response to chorionic gonadotropin but no testicular descent should have the testes surgically brought into the scrotum to decrease the likelihood of undetected tumor formation. Anorchia is diagnosed in a phenotypic sexually infantile male if no testosterone is measurable in serum before or after treatment with chorionic gonadotropin. Except for absent testes, these patients have normal male genital development, including wolffian duct formation and müllerian duct regression. The testes were presumably present in early fetal life during sexual differentiation but degenerated after the 13th week of gestation for unknown reasons ("vanishing testes syndrome").

D. Syndrome of Gonadal Dysgenesis (Turner's Syndrome): (See Chapters 14 and 15.) 45,X gonadal dysgenesis is associated with short stature, female phenotype with sexual infantilism, and a chromatin-negative buccal smear. Patients have "streak" gonads consisting of fibrous tissue without germ cells. Other classic but variable phenotypic features include micrognathia, "fish" mouth, ptosis, low-set or deformed ears, a broad shieldlike chest, hypoplastic areolae, a short neck with low hairline and webbing (pterygium colli), short fourth metacarpals, cubitus valgus, structural anomalies of the kidney, extensive nevi, hypoplastic nails, and cardiovascular anomalies of the left side of the heart (most commonly coarctation of the aorta). The medical history of patients with gonadal dysgenesis will often reveal small size at birth, lymphedema of the extremities, and loose posterior cervical skin folds. (The terms Bonnevie-Ullrich syndrome and infant Turner syndrome have been applied to this neonatal appearance.) Affected patients often have a history of frequent otitis media with conductive hearing loss. Patients have no pubertal growth spurt and reach a mean final height of 142 cm. Short stature is a classic feature of Turner's syndrome but not of other forms of hypergonadotropic hypogonadism that occur without karyotypic abnormalities. GH function is normal in Turner's syndrome, and the cause of short stature is not known. However, preliminary studies suggest that hGH treatment may improve growth rate in certain affected girls; it is not known if final height can be improved by administration of hGH. Pubic hair may appear late and is usually sparse in distribution.

Serum gonadotropin concentrations in Turner's syndrome are high between birth and age 4 years. They decrease toward the normal range in prepubertal patients and then rise to castrate levels after age 10 years. (See Chapter 15.)

Sex chromatin–positive variants of gonadal dysgenesis include XO/XX, XO/XXX, and XO/XX/XXX mosaicism with chromatin-positive buccal smears.

Patients with these karyotypes may resemble patients with the classic syndrome of gonadal dysgenesis, or they may have fewer manifestations and have normal or nearly normal female phenotypes. Streak gonad formation is not invariable; some patients have had secondary sexual development, and menarche and (rarely) even pregnancy have been reported.

Sex chromatin–negative variants of the syndrome of gonadal dysgenesis have karyotypes revealing XO/XY mosaicism. Physical features vary; some patients have the features of classic Turner's syndrome, while others may have ambiguous genitalia or even the features of phenotypic males. Gonads are dysgenetic but vary from streak gonads to functioning testes. These patients are at risk for gonadoblastoma formation. Since gonadoblastomas may secrete androgens or estrogens, patients with a gonadoblastoma may virilize or feminize as though they had functioning gonads. Gonadoblastomas may demonstrate calcification on abdominal x-ray. Malignant germ cell tumors may arise in dysgenetic testes, and orchiectomy is generally indicated.

E. Other Forms of Primary Ovarian Failure: Radiation therapy, chemotherapy, and premature menopause may cause primary ovarian failure. Patients with Addison's disease may have autoimmune oophoritis as well as adrenal failure. Primary amenorrhea will occur in phenotypic females with an XY genotype and androgen resistance (syndrome of feminizing testes) (see Chapter 15). A sex steroid biosynthetic defect due to 17α-hydroxylase deficiency will be manifested as sexual infantilism and primary amenorrhea in a phenotypic female (regardless of genotype) with hypokalemia and hypertension.

F. Pseudo-Turner's Syndrome (Noonan's Syndrome, Ullrich's Syndrome, Male Turner's Syndrome): Pseudo-Turner's syndrome is associated with manifestations of Turner's syndrome such as webbed neck, ptosis, short stature, cubitus valgus, and lymphedema, but other clinical findings such as a normal karyotype, triangular-shaped facies, pectus excavatum, right-sided heart disease, a normal karyotype, and an increased incidence of mental retardation should differentiate these patients from those with Turner's syndrome. Males may have undescended testes and variable degrees of germinal cell and Leydig cell dysfunction. Pseudo-Turner's syndrome follows an autosomal dominant pattern of inheritance with incomplete penetrance.

G. Familial and Sporadic Forms of XX or XY Gonadal Dysgenesis: These forms of gonadal dysgenesis are characterized by structurally normal chromosomes and streak gonads or partially functioning gonads. If there is some gonadal function, XY gonadal dysgenesis may present with ambiguous genitalia or virilization at puberty. If no gonadal function is present, patients appear as phenotypic sexually infantile females. Patients with XY gonadal dysgenesis and dysgenetic testes should undergo gonadectomy to eliminate the possibility of malignant germ cell tumor formation.

Table 16–3. Differential diagnosis of delayed puberty.

	Serum Gonadotropins	Serum Gonadal Steroids	Miscellaneous
Constitutional delay in growth and adolescence	Prepubertal (low)	Low	Patient usually has short stature for chronologic age but appropriate height and growth rate for bone age. Adrenarche and gonadarche are delayed.
Hypogonadotropic hypogonadism	Prepubertal (low)	Low	Patient may have anosmia (Kallmann's syndrome) or other associated pituitary hormone deficiencies. If gonadotropin deficiency is isolated, patient usually has normal height and growth rate. Adrenarche may be normal in spite of absent gonadarche (serum DHEA sulfate may be pubertal).
Hypergonadotropic hypogonadism	Elevated	Low	Patient may have abnormal karyotype and stigmas of Turner's or Klinefelter's syndrome.

Differential Diagnosis of Delayed Puberty (Table 16–3)

Young people who do not begin secondary sexual development by age 14 (boys) or age 13 (girls) and patients who do not progress through development on a timely basis (boys should have reached stage 5 pubertal development 4½ years after onset; girls should menstruate within 5 years after breast budding) may have some form of hypogonadism.

If the diagnosis is not obvious on the basis of physical or historical features, the differential diagnostic process begins with determination of whether plasma gonadotropins are (1) elevated owing to primary gonadal failure or (2) decreased owing to secondary or tertiary hypogonadism or constitutional delayed puberty. If plasma gonadotropins are low, the differential diagnosis is between hypogonadotropic hypogonadism and constitutionally delayed puberty. A patient with constitutional delay may have a characteristic history of short stature for age with normal growth velocity for bone age and a family history of delayed but spontaneous puberty. The patient's mother may have had late onset of menses, or the father may have begun to shave late. Not all patients with constitutional delay are classic, and gonadotropin-deficient patients may have some features similar to those of constitutional delay in adolescence. The determination of rise in LH after administration of GnRH is helpful in differential diagnosis. Frequent nighttime sampling (every 20 minutes through an indwelling catheter) for peaks of LH secretion during sleep is an alternative to GnRH testing. Patients with constitutional delay should have peaks of LH demonstrable at an age when their LH response to GnRH becomes pubertal; the onset of physical pubertal changes usually follows this endocrine conversion by 6 months. Other methods of differential diagnosis between constitutional delay and hypogonadotropic hypogonadism have been proposed but are complex or suffer from overlap in the response between the groups; eg, most patients with hypogonadotropic hypogonadism have lower prolactin concentrations after protirelin or chlorpromazine administration than do patients with constitutional delay.

Clinical observation for signs of pubertal development and laboratory evaluation for the start of rising sex steroids may have to continue until the patient is 18 years of age or older before the diagnosis is definite. In most cases, if spontaneous pubertal development is not noted by 18 years of age, the diagnosis is gonadotropin deficiency. Of course, the presence of neurologic impairment or other endocrine deficiency should immediately lead to investigation for central nervous system tumor or congenital defect in a patient with delayed puberty. CT scanning may be helpful in this situation.

Treatment of Sexual Infantilism

A. Constitutional Delay in Growth and Adolescence:

1. Psychologic support–Patients with constitutional delay in growth and adolescence should be counseled that normal pubertal development will occur spontaneously. Peer pressure and teasing can be oppressive. Severe depression must be treated seriously, since short patients with pubertal delay have become suicidal.

2. Sex steroids–The teenager who is so embarrassed about his or her short stature and lack of sexual development as to have significant psychologic problems may require special help. The following treatment can be given: (1) for girls, a 3-month course of conjugated estrogens (0.3 mg) or ethinyl estradiol (5–10 μg) given orally each day for 21 days a month; or (2) for boys, a 3-month course of testosterone enanthate (100 mg) given intramuscularly once every 28 days. This treatment will elicit gratifyingly noticeable secondary sexual development and slight increase in stature without seriously compromising skeletal age development or final height. The short course of therapy may also improve patients' psychologic outlook and allow them to await spontaneous pubertal development with greater ease. Continuous gonadal steroid replacement in these patients is not indicated, as it will advance bone age and lead to epiphyseal fusion and a decrease in ultimate stature.

B. Permanent Hypogonadism: Once the diagnosis of delayed puberty due to permanent hypogonadism, either primary or secondary, is made, replacement therapy must be considered.

Males with hypogonadism may be treated with testosterone enanthate intramuscularly every month, gradually increasing the dosage from 100 to 300 mg a month. Frequent erections may occur if the higher dose is used initially but are less likely to occur if the dose is built up over several months. Alternatively, oral testosterone propionate or halogenated testosterone may be administered daily; methylated testosterone is usually not recommended, because there is a risk of hepatocellular carcinoma or cholestatic jaundice.

Females may be treated with ethinyl estradiol (increasing from 5 to 10–20 μg/d depending upon results) or conjugated estrogens (0.3–0.625 mg/d) on days 1–21, with 5 mg of medroxyprogesterone acetate added on days 12–21. Neither hormone is administered from day 22 to the end of the month.

C. Coexisting GH Deficiency: Patients with coexisting GH deficiency require consideration of bone age and amount of growth left before epiphyseal fusion; if adequate treatment with growth hormone has not been received, sex steroid therapy may be delayed to optimize final adult height.

D. Gonadal Dysgenesis: In the past, patients with the syndrome of gonadal dysgenesis were frequently not given estrogen replacement until after age 13 years, for fear of compromising final height. It has now been demonstrated that low-dose estrogen therapy (5–10 μg of ethinyl estradiol orally) can be used to allow feminization at 12–13 years of age without decreasing final height in these patients.

SEXUAL PRECOCITY

The appearance of secondary sexual development before the age of 8 years in girls and 9 years in boys is greater than 2.5 SD below the mean age at onset of puberty and constitutes precocious sexual development (Table 16–4). When the cause is premature activation of the hypothalamic-pituitary axis, the diagnosis is complete (true) precocious puberty; if ectopic gonadotropin secretion occurs in boys or autonomous sex steroid secretion occurs in either sex, the diagnosis is incomplete precocious puberty. In all forms of sexual precocity, there is an increase in height velocity, somatic development, and skeletal maturation. A major concern is that rapid epiphyseal development may lead to tall stature during the early phases of the disorder until epiphyseal fusion causes cessation of growth and short final stature. Plasma somatomedin values may be elevated for age in the untreated state.

Complete (True) Isosexual Precocity (Fig 16–11)

A. Constitutional Complete (True) Precocious Puberty: Children who demonstrate isosexual precocity at an age more than 2.5 SD below the mean may simply represent the lower reaches of the distribution curve of age at onset of puberty; often there is a familial tendency toward early puberty. True precocious puberty may rarely be due to an autosomal recessive or (in males) sex-limited autosomal dominant trait.

B. Idiopathic Complete (True) Precocious Puberty: Other affected children with no familial tendency toward early development and no organic disease are considered to have idiopathic precocious puberty. Electroencephalographic abnormalities may be found in these patients. Patients may follow the normal course of pubertal development or may have a waxing and waning course. Gonadotropin and sex steroid concentrations and response to GnRH are similar to those found in normal pubertal subjects. In idiopathic true precocious puberty, as in all forms of true isosexual precocity, testicular enlargement in boys should be the first sign; in girls, either breast development or pubic hair appearance may be first. Girls present with idiopathic precocious puberty more commonly than boys.

C. Central Nervous System Disorders:

1. Tumors–Central nervous system tumor as a cause of precocious puberty is more common in boys than in girls. Optic gliomas or hypothalamic gliomas (isolated or with neurofibromatosis), astrocytomas, ependymomas, and other central nervous system tumors may cause precocious puberty by interfering with neural pathways inhibiting GnRH secretion. Hamartomas of the tuber cinereum have been reported to contain GnRH and neurosecretory cells such as are found in the median eminence; they may cause precocious puberty by secreting GnRH. Most tumors of the hypothalamus that cause precocious puberty are in critical areas of the brain and are not amenable to surgical excision; medical therapy is the treatment of choice. Germinomas are sensitive to radiation therapy.

2. Other causes of true precocious pu-

Table 16–4. Classification of sexual precocity.

Complete (true) precocious puberty
    Constitutional
    Idiopathic
    Central nervous system disorders
    Severe hypothyroidism
    Following androgen exposure
Incomplete precocious puberty
    Males
        Gonadotropin-secreting tumors
        Excessive androgen production
        Premature Leydig and germinal cell maturation
    Females
        Ovarian cysts
        Estrogen-secreting neoplasms
Sexual precocity due to gonadotropin or sex steroid exposure
Variation in pubertal development
    Premature thelarche
    Premature pubarche
    Adolescent gynecomastia

Figure 16–11. Boy 2 5/12 years of age with idiopathic true precocious puberty. By 10 months of age, he had pubic hair and phallic and testicular enlargement. At 1 year of age, his height was 4 SD above the mean; the phallus was 10 × 3.5 cm; each testis was 2.5 × 1.5 cm. Plasma LH was 14.8 mIU/mL and rose to 65.5 mIU/mL after administration of 100 μg of GnRH. Plasma testosterone was 416 ng/dL. At the time of the photograph, he had been treated with medroxyprogesterone acetate for 1½ years, with reduction of his rapid growth rate and decreased gonadotropin and testosterone secretion. His height was 95.2 cm (> 2 SD above mean height for his age); plasma testosterone was 7 ng/dL, and after 100 μg of GnRH, plasma LH rose from 7 mIU/mL to 17.9 mIU/mL. (Reproduced, with permission, from Styne DM, Grumbach MM: *Reproductive Endocrinology.* Yen SSC, Jaffe RB [editors]. Saunders, 1978.)

long bones with cysts, and precocious puberty. However, cases have been reported in which there was an additional finding of hyperthyroidism, adrenal nodules, or autonomous functioning ovarian cysts in girls. Thus, precocious puberty may be complete or incomplete.

E. Hypothyroidism: Severe untreated hypothyroidism can be associated with sexual precocity and galactorrhea (Van Wyk–Grumbach syndrome); treatment with thyroxine will correct hypothyroidism, halt precocious puberty and galactorrhea, and lower PRL levels. The cause of this syndrome is postulated to be increased gonadotropin secretion associated with the massive increase in TSH secretion.

F. Virilizing Syndromes: Patients with long-untreated virilizing adrenal hyperplasia who have an advanced bone age may manifest precocious puberty after the adrenal hyperplasia is controlled. Children with virilizing tumors or long-term androgen therapy may follow the same pattern when the androgen source is removed. Advanced maturation of the hypothalamic-pituitary-gonadal axis appears to occur with excessive androgen conditions along with advanced skeletal age.

Incomplete Sexual Precocity

A. Males: Male patients may manifest premature sexual development in the absence of hypothalamic pituitary maturation from either (1) ectopic or autonomous secretion of hCG or LH or iatrogenic administration of chorionic gonadotropin, which can stimulate Leydig cell production of testosterone; or (2) autonomous secretion of androgens from the testes or adrenal glands or from iatrogenic administration of exogenous androgens.

1. Gonadotropin-secreting tumors–These include hepatomas or hepatoblastomas of the liver as well as teratomas or chorionepitheliomas of the mediastinum, gonads, retroperitoneum, or pineal gland and germinomas of the central nervous system. (In females, secretion of hCG will not by itself cause secondary sexual development.)

2. Autonomous androgen secretion–Secretion can occur because of inborn errors of adrenal enzymes, as in 21-hydroxylase deficiency or 11β-hydroxylase deficiency, virilizing adrenal carcinomas, interstitial cell tumors of the testes, or premature Leydig and germinal cell maturation.

In all forms of incomplete male isosexual precocity, FSH is not elevated, and since the seminiferous tubules are not stimulated, the testes do not enlarge as much as in complete sexual precocity. If incomplete sexual precocity is due to a testicular tumor, the testes may be large, asymmetric, and irregular in contour. Symmetric bilateral moderate enlargement of the testes suggests gonadotropin-independent premature maturation of Leydig and germinal cells, which is a sex-limited dominant condition. The testes are somewhat smaller in this condition than in true precocious puberty but are still greater than 2.5 cm in diameter. In boys with premature Leydig and germinal cell matura-

berty–Infectious or granulomatous conditions such as encephalitis, brain abscess, postinfectious (or postsurgical or congenital) suprasellar cysts, sarcoidosis, tuberculous granulomas of the hypothalamus, and head trauma have been reported to cause true precocious puberty. Epilepsy and mental retardation have also been associated with precocious puberty, without anatomic lesions of the central nervous system.

D. McCune-Albright Syndrome: McCune-Albright syndrome is classically manifested as a triad of irregular café au lait spots, fibrous dysplasia of tion, plasma testosterone is in the pubertal range but plasma gonadotropins and the LH response are in the prepubertal range because the autonomous testosterone secretion suppresses GnRH release. The differential diagnosis rests between a testosterone-secreting tumor of the adrenal, a testosterone-secreting Leydig cell neoplasm, and premature Leydig and germinal cell maturation.

B. Females: Female patients with incomplete isosexual precocity have a source of excessive estrogens. In all cases of autonomous estrogen secretion or ingestion, serum LH and FSH should be low.

1. Follicular cysts–If follicular cysts are large enough, they can secrete sufficient estrogen to cause breast development and even vaginal withdrawal bleeding; some girls have recurrent cysts that lead to several episodes of vaginal bleeding. Patients with cysts may have levels of serum estrogen so high as to mimic a tumor.

2. Granulosa or theca cell tumors–These tumors of the ovaries secrete estrogen and are palpable in 80% of cases. Gonadoblastomas found in streak gonads, lipoid tumors, cystadenomas, and ovarian carcinomas are rare ovarian sources of estrogens or androgens.

3. Exogenous estrogen administration–Ingestion of estrogen-containing substances or even cutaneous absorption of estrogen from cosmetics can cause feminization in children. Recent epidemics of gynecomastia and precocious thelarche in Puerto Rico and Italy appear to be linked to ingestion of estrogen-contaminated food or estrogens in the environment.

Variations in Pubertal Development

A. Premature Thelarche: The term "premature thelarche" denotes unilateral or bilateral breast enlargement without other signs of androgen or estrogen secretion of puberty. Patients are usually under 3 years of age; the breast enlargement may regress within months or remain until actual pubertal development occurs at a normal age. Nipple development and vaginal mucosal signs of estrogen effect are usually absent. The cause of premature thelarche may be brief episodes of estrogen secretion from ovarian cysts. Plasma estrogens are usually low in this disorder, possibly because blood samples are drawn after the initiating secretory event.

B. Premature Adrenarche: The term "premature adrenarche" denotes the early appearance of pubic or axillary hair without other signs of virilization or puberty. This nonprogressive disorder is compatible with a normal age at onset of other signs of puberty. It is more common in girls than in boys and usually is found in children over 6 years of age. Plasma DHEA sulfate and urinary 17-ketosteroids are elevated to stage 2 pubertal levels, which are higher than normally found in this age group. Bone age and height age may be slightly advanced for chronologic age. Patients may have abnormal electroencephalographic tracings without other signs of neurologic dysfunction.

C. Adolescent Gynecomastia: This may be uni-lateral or bilateral and usually begins in boys in stage 2–3 of puberty, regressing about 2 years later. Plasma estrogen and testosterone concentrations are normal, but the estradiol/testosterone ratio may be elevated and SHBG concentrations may be high. Reassurance is usually all that is required, but some severely affected patients with extremely prominent breast development will require reduction mammoplasty if psychologic distress is extreme. Some pathologic conditions such as Klinefelter's and Reifenstein's syndromes and the incomplete syndrome of androgen resistance are also associated with gynecomastia; these disorders should be clearly differentiated from the gynecomastia of normal puberty in males.

Differential Diagnosis of Sexual Precocity

The history and physical examination should be directed toward eliciting pertinent findings that may confirm one of the diagnostic possibilities discussed above. Gonadotropin and sex steroid concentrations should be determined in order to distinguish between gonadotropin-mediated secondary sexual development (gonadotropins and sex steroids elevated) or autonomous secretion or exogenous administration of gonadal steroids (gonadotropins suppressed and sex steroids elevated). If plasma LH (or hCG) is quite high in a boy or a pregnancy screening test is positive, the likely diagnosis is an extrapituitary hCG-secreting tumor. If no abdominal source of hCG is found, a CT scan of the head to evaluate the possibility of a germinoma of the pineal is indicated. If plasma sex steroids are very high and gonadotropins low, an autonomous source of gonadal steroid secretion must be assumed. If plasma gonadotropin and sex steroid values are in the pubertal range, the most likely diagnosis is complete precocious puberty. In such patients, the GnRH test will usually result in a rise in LH compatible with normal puberty and will thus confirm the diagnosis (Table 16–5).

The presence of true or complete precocious puberty may be a marker for the presence of a hypothalamic tumor. Boys more often than girls have central nervous system tumors associated with complete precocious puberty. Skull x-rays are not usually helpful, but CT scanning is indicated in children with true precocious puberty. The present generation of CT scanners can make thin cuts through the hypothalamic-pituitary area with good resolution; small hypothalamic hamartomas are now being diagnosed more frequently.

Treatment

A. Complete Precocious Puberty:

1. Medroxyprogesterone–In the USA, medical treatment of true precocious puberty was most commonly accomplished with medroxyprogesterone acetate, a progestational agent that reduces gonadotropin secretion by negative feedback. In girls, medroxyprogesterone will stop menses and breast development; in boys, it will decrease testicular size, decrease

Table 16–5. Differential diagnosis of sexual precocity.

	Serum Gonadotropin Concentrations	LH Response to GnRH	Serum Sex Steroid Concentrations	Gonadal Size	Miscellaneous
Complete (true) precocious puberty	Pubertal.	Pubertal pattern.	Pubertal values.	Normal pubertal enlargement of testes in males.	CT scan of head useful to rule out a central nervous system tumor.
Incomplete precocious puberty **Males** Gonadotropin-secreting tumor	High hCG or LH (positive pregnancy test).	High basal LH that does not rise with GnRH.	High or pubertal values.	Slight to moderate enlargement of testes.	Hepatic tumor must be considered. CT scan of head if gonadotropin-secreting central nervous system tumor suspected.
Leydig cell tumor	Prepubertal (low).	Prepubertal or suppressed pattern.	Extremely high testosterone.	Irregular asymmetric enlargement of testes.	
Gonadotropin-independent sexual precocity with premature Leydig and germinal cell maturation	Prepubertal (low).	Prepubertal or suppressed pattern.	Pubertal or higher values.	Testes larger than 2.5 cm but smaller than expected for stage of pubertal development.	Often found in sex-limited dominant patterns.
Females Granulosa cell tumor (follicular cysts may be similar in presentation)	Prepubertal (low).	Prepubertal or suppressed pattern.	Extremely high estradiol.	Ovarian enlargement on physical, CT, or sonographic examination.	Granulosa cell tumor is usually palpable on rectal examination.
Follicular cyst	Prepubertal (low).	Prepubertal pattern of LH. FSH secretion may rise above normal range.	Estradiol may be normally low or quite high, depending upon the stage of cyst formation or regression.	Cysts may be visible on sonogram.	Withdrawal bleeding may occur when estrogen levels decrease. Cysts may recur.

erections, and modify aggressive behavior. Growth velocity and skeletal maturation may also be reduced with adequate dosage. In animal studies, medroxyprogesterone has caused breast nodules in beagles; in humans, no conclusive case of breast cancer associated with medroxyprogesterone administration has been noted. Since medroxyprogesterone has glucocorticoidlike effects, ACTH and corticosteroid suppression occurs with its use, and, with larger doses, a cushingoid appearance may develop. Medroxyprogesterone has not yet been approved for use in precocious puberty, so the preparation must be considered experimental treatment for this disorder. The dosage is 10– 20 mg orally twice daily or 100 mg/m² intramuscularly weekly or fortnightly.

2. Gonadotropin-releasing hormone agonists–A new experimental approach to the treatment of precocious puberty resulting from a central nervous system lesion is now under study. Chronic use of highly potent and long-acting analogs of GnRH has been shown to down-regulate GnRH receptors and reduce pituitary gland response to GnRH, thereby causing decreased secretion of gonadotropins and sex steroids. Reversal of the suppressive effect occurs after discontinuation of therapy. This treatment has led to the rapid cessation of progression of signs of sexual precocity in numerous children studied at several centers. Treatment of precocious puberty that is idiopathic or caused by hamartomas of the tuber cinereum, neoplasms of the central nervous system, or long-term androgen exposure has been successful, but mixed results were obtained when McCune-Albright syndrome was treated with GnRH agonists, probably owing to the heterogeneous nature of the syndrome. The GnRH agonists are given daily subcutaneously or by intranasal insufflation. In the USA, GnRH agonists have been approved for treatment of prostatic carcinoma but are currently available only on a research basis for treatment of precocious puberty. They promise to become the preferred treatment for true precocious puberty.

3. Supportive measures–Psychologic management is of great importance in patients with sexual precocity. The somatic changes or menses will frighten some children and may make them the object of ridicule. These patients do not experience social maturation to match their physical development, although their peers, teachers, and relatives will tend to treat them as if they were older because of their large size. Thus, supportive counseling must be offered to both patient and family.

B. Incomplete Sexual Precocity: Treatment of the disorders discussed above under incomplete precocious puberty is directed toward the underlying tumor or abnormality rather than toward the signs of precocious puberty. If the primary cause is controlled, signs of sexual development will be halted in progression or may even regress.

Males with familial Leydig cell maturation will not respond to GnRH agonist therapy, but some have improved with medroxyprogesterone acetate. Recently, 4 boys were successfully treated with ketoconazole, which can block 17-20 lyase and therefore decrease testosterone production. Girls with recurrent ovarian cyst formation may have a decreased incidence of cysts with medroxyprogesterone acetate therapy.

REFERENCES

General

Styne DM, Grumbach MM: Puberty in the male and female: Its physiology and disorders. Pages 313–384 in: *Reproductive Endocrinology*, 2nd ed. Yen SSC, Jaffe RB (editors). Saunders, 1986.

Styne DM, Kaplan SL: Normal and abnormal puberty in the female. *Pediatr Clin North Am* 1979;**26:**123.

Wilkins L: *The Diagnosis and Treatment of Endocrine Disorders in Childhood and Adolescence*, 2nd ed. Thomas, 1965.

Physical Changes Associated With Puberty

Bayley N, Pinneau SF: Tables for predicting adult height from skeletal age: Revised for use with the Greulich-Pyle standards. *J Pediatr* 1952;**40:**423.

Greulich WW, Pyle SI: *Radiographic Atlas of Skeletal Development of the Hand and Wrist*, 2nd ed. Stanford Univ Press, 1959.

Harlan WR, Harlan EA, Grillo GP: Secondary sex characteristics of girls 12 to 17 years of age: The U.S. Health Examination Survey. *J Pediatr* 1980;**96:**1074.

Harlan WR et al: Secondary sex characteristics of boys 12 to 17 years of age: The U.S. Health Examination Survey. *J Pediatr* 1979;**95:**293.

Marshall JC, Kelch RP: Low dose pulsatile gonadotropin-releasing hormone in anorexia nervosa: A model of human pubertal development. *J Clin Endocrinol Metab* 1979;**49:**712.

Marshall WA, Tanner JM: Variations in the pattern of pubertal changes in boys. *Arch Dis Child* 1970;**45:**13.

Marshall WA, Tanner JM: Variations in the pattern of pubertal changes in girls. *Arch Dis Child* 1969;**44:**291.

McKusick VA: Pages 73–74 in: *Heritable Disorders of Connective Tissue*, 4th ed. Mosby, 1972.

Tanner JM et al: The adolescent growth spurt of boys and girls of the Harpenden Growth Study. *Ann Hum Biol* 1976;**3:**109.

Van Wieringen JC et al: *Growth Diagrams 1965 Netherlands: Second National Survey on 0–24 Year Olds.* Groningen, Netherlands Institute for Preventive Medicine TNO Leiden, Wolters-Noordhoff Publishing, 1971.

Endocrine Changes From Fetal Life to Puberty

August GP, Grumbach MM, Kaplan SL: Hormonal changes in puberty. 3. Correlation of plasma testosterone, LH, FSH, testicular size and bone age with male pubertal development. *J Clin Endocrinol Metab* 1972;**34:**319.

Boyar RM et al: Simultaneous augmented secretion of luteinizing hormone and testosterone during sleep. *J Clin Invest* 1974;**54:**609.

Burr IM et al: Hormonal changes in puberty. 1. Correlation of serum luteinizing hormone and follicle-stimulating hormone with stages of puberty, testicular size and bone age in normal boys. *Pediatr Res* 1970;**4:**25.

Corley KP et al: Estimation of GnRH pulse amplitude during pubertal development. *Pediatr Res* 1981;**15:**157.

Faiman C, Winter JSD: Gonadotropins and sex hormone patterns in puberty: Clinical data. Pages 32–61 in: *Control of the Onset of Puberty.* Grumbach MM, Grave GD, Mayer FE (editors). Wiley, 1974.

Forest MG, de Peretti E, Bertrand J: Hypothalamic-pituitary-gonadal relationships in man from birth to puberty. *Clin Endocrinol* 1976;**5:**551.

Grumbach MM: The neuroendocrinology of puberty. *Hosp Pract* (March) 1980;**51:**60.

Grumbach MM: Onset of puberty. Pages 1–21 in: *Puberty.* Berenberg SR (editor). H.E. Stenfert Kroese B.V., 1975.

Grumbach MM et al: Hypothalamic-pituitary regulation of puberty in man: Evidence and concepts derived from clinical research. Pages 115–166 in: *Control of the Onset of Puberty.* Grumbach MM, Grave GD, Mayer FE (editors). Wiley, 1974.

Harris DA et al: Somatomedin-C in normal puberty and in true precocious puberty before and after treatment with a potent LRF-agonist: Evidence for an effect of estrogen and testosterone on somatomedin-C concentrations. *J Clin Endocrinol Metab* 1985;**61:**152.

Jenner MR et al: Hormonal changes in puberty. 4. Plasma estradiol, LH, and FSH in prepubertal children, pubertal females, and in precocious puberty, premature thelarche, hypogonadism, and in a child with a feminizing ovarian tumor. *J Clin Endocrinol Metab* 1972;**34:**521.

Kaplan SL, Grumbach MM, Aubert ML: The ontogenesis of pituitary hormones and hypothalamic factors in the human fetus: Maturation of central nervous system regulation of anterior pituitary function. *Recent Prog Horm Res* 1976;**32**:161.

Kelch RP, Kaplan SL, Grumbach MM: Suppression of urinary and plasma follicle-stimulating hormone by exogenous estrogens in prepubertal and pubertal children. *J Clin Invest* 1973;**52**:122.

Luna AM et al: Somatomedins in adolescence: A cross-sectional study of the effect of puberty on plasma insulin-like growth factor I and II levels. *J Clin Endocrinol Metab* 1983;**57**:268.

Reame N et al: Pulsatile gonadotropin secretion during the human menstrual cycle: Evidence for altered frequency of gonadotropin-releasing hormone secretion. *J Clin Endocrinol Metab* 1984;**59**:328.

Reiter EO et al: Responsivity of pituitary gonadotropes to luteinizing hormone–releasing factor in idiopathic precocious puberty, precocious thelarche, and precocious adrenarche. *Pediatr Res* 1975;**9**:111.

Rosenfield RI, Furlanetto RW, Bock D: Relationship of somatomedin-C concentrations to pubertal changes. *J Pediatr* 1983;**103**:723.

Roth JC, Grumbach MM, Kaplan SL: Effect of synthetic luteinizing hormone–releasing factor on serum testosterone and gonadotropins in prepubertal, pubertal and adult males. *J Clin Endocrinol Metab* 1973;**37**:680.

Roth JC et al: FSH and LH response to luteinizing hormone–releasing factor on serum testosterone and gonadotropins in prepubertal, pubertal and adult males. *J Clin Endocrinol Metab* 1972;**35**:926.

Sizonenko PC et al: Hormonal changes in puberty. 2. Correlation of serum luteinizing hormone and follicle-stimulating hormone with stages of puberty and bone age in normal girls. *Pediatr Res* 1970;**4**:36.

Wildt L, Marshall G, Knobil E: Experimental induction of puberty in the infantile female rhesus monkey. *Science* 1980;**207**:1373.

Adrenarche

Grumbach MM et al: Clinical disorders of adrenal function and puberty: An assessment of the role of the adrenal cortex in normal and abnormal puberty in man and evidence for an ACTH-like pituitary adrenal androgen stimulating hormone. In: *The Endocrine Function of the Human Adrenal Cortex*. Serio M (editor). Academic Press, 1977.

Reiter EO, Fuldauer VG, Root AW: Secretion of the adrenal androgen, dehydroepiandrosterone sulfate, during normal infancy, childhood, and adolescence, in sick infants and in children with endocrinologic abnormalities. *J Pediatr* 1977;**90**:766.

Sklar CA, Kaplan SL, Grumbach MM: Evidence for dissociation between adrenarche and gonadarche: Studies in patients with idiopathic precocious puberty, gonadal dysgenesis, isolated gonadotropin deficiency, and constitutionally delayed growth and adolescence. *J Clin Endocrinol Metab* 1980;**51**:548.

Delayed Puberty & Sexual Infantilism

Connors MH, Styne DM: Familial functional anorchism: A review of etiology and management. *J Urol* 1985;**133**:1049.

Conte FA, Grumbach MM: Pathogenesis, classification, diagnosis and treatment of anomalies of sex. In: *Metabolic Basis of Endocrinology*. DeGroot L et al (editors). Grune & Stratton, 1977.

Frisch RE, Wyshak G, Vincent L: Delayed menarche and amenorrhea in ballet dancers. *N Engl J Med* 1980; **303**:17.

Hoffman AR, Crowley WR: Induction of puberty in men by long-term pulsatile administration of low-dose gonadotropin-releasing hormone. *N Engl J Med* 1982;**307**:1237.

Kaplan SL, Grumbach MM, Hoyt WF: A syndrome of hypopituitary dwarfism, hypoplasia of optic nerves, and malformation of prosencephalon: Report of 6 patients. *Pediatr Res* 1970;**4**:480.

Patton ML, Woolf PD: Hyperprolactinemia and delayed puberty: A report of three cases and their response to therapy. *Pediatrics* 1983;**71**:572.

Pugliese MT et al: Fear of obesity: A cause of short stature and delayed puberty. *N Engl J Med* 1983;**309**:513.

Schwabe AD et al: Anorexia nervosa. *Ann Intern Med* 1981;**94**:371.

Sklar CA et al: Hormonal and metabolic abnormalities associated with central nervous system germinoma in children and adolescents and the effect of therapy: Report of 10 patients. *J Clin Endocrinol Metab* 1981;**52**:9.

Thomsett MJ et al: Endocrine and neurologic outcome in childhood craniopharyngioma: Review of effect of treatment in 42 patients. *J Pediatr* 1980;**97**:728.

Valk TW et al: Hypogonadotropic hypogonadism: Hormonal responses to low-dose pulsatile administration of gonadotropin-releasing hormones. *J Clin Endocrinol Metab* 1980;**51**:730.

Warren MP, Vande Wiele RL: Clinical and metabolic features of anorexia nervosa. *Am J Obstet Gynecol* 1973;**117**:435.

Sexual Precocity

Bongiovanni AM: An epidemic of premature thelarche in Puerto Rico. *J Pediatr* 1983;**103**:245.

Cacciari E et al: How many cases of true precocious puberty in girls are idiopathic? *J Pediatr* 1983;**102**:357.

Crowley WF et al: Therapeutic use of pituitary desensitization with a long-acting LHRH agonist: A potential new treatment for idiopathic precocious puberty. *J Clin Endocrinol Metab* 1981;**52**:370.

Egli CA et al: Pituitary gonadotropin-independent male-limited autosomal dominant sexual precocity in nine generations: Familial testotoxicosis. *J Pediatr* 1985;**106**:33.

Hochman HI, Judge DM, Reichlin S: Precocious puberty and hypothalamic hamartoma. *Pediatrics* 1981;**67**:236.

Holland FJ et al: Ketoconazole in the management of precocious puberty not responsive to LHRH-analogue therapy. *N Engl J Med* 1985;**312**:1023.

Judge DM et al: Hypothalamic hamartoma: A source of luteinizing hormone–releasing factor in precocious puberty. *N Engl J Med* 1977;**296**:7.

Leyendecker G, Wildt L, Hansmann M: Pregnancies following chronic intermittent (pulsatile) administration of GnRH by means of a pulsatile pump (''Zyklomat''): A new approach to the treatment of infertility in hypothalamic amenorrhea. *J Clin Endocrinol Metab* 1980;**51**:1214.

Luder AS et al: Intranasal and subcutaneous treatment of central precocious puberty in both sexes with a long-acting analog of luteinizing hormone–releasing hormone. *J Clin Endocrinol Metab* 1984;**58**:966.

Mills JL et al: Premature thelarche: Natural history and etiologic investigation. *Am J Dis Child* 1981;**135**:743.

Pescovitz OH et al: True precocious puberty complicating congenital adrenal hyperplasia: Treatment with a luteinizing hormone–releasing hormone analog. *J Clin Endocrinol Metab* 1984;**58**:847.

Reiter EU et al: Male-limited familial precocious puberty in three generations. *N Engl J Med* 1984;**311**:515.

Rosenthal SM, Grumbach MM, Kaplan SL: Gonadotropin-independent familial sexual precocity with premature Leydig and germinal cell maturation (familial testotoxicosis): Effects of a potent luteinizing hormone–releasing factor agonist and medroxyprogesterone acetate therapy in four cases. *J Clin Endocrinol Metab* 1983;**57**:571.

Schwedewie K et al: Testicular Leydig cell hyperplasia as a cause of familial sexual precocity. *J Clin Endocrinol Metab* 1981;**52**:271.

Sklar CA et al: Human chorionic gonadotropin–secreting pineal tumor: Relation to pathogenesis and sex limitation of sexual precocity. *J Clin Endocrinol Metab* 1981;**53**:656.

Styne DW et al: Treatment of true precocious puberty with a potent luteinizing hormone–releasing factor agonist: Effect on growth, sexual maturation, pelvic sonography, and the hypothalamic-pituitary-gonadal axis. *J Clin Endocrinol Metab* 1985;**61**:142.

Van Wyk JJ, Grumbach MM: Syndrome of precocious menstruation and galactorrhea in juvenile hypothyroidism: An example of hormonal overlap in pituitary feedback. *J Pediatr* 1960;**57**:416.

Wierman ME et al: Puberty without gonadotropins. *N Engl J Med* 1985;**312**:65.

17　The Endocrinology of Pregnancy

Mary C. Martin, MD, & Philip G. Hoffman, Jr., MD, PhD

Throughout pregnancy, the fetal-placental unit secretes protein and steroid hormones into the mother's bloodstream, and these apparently or actually alter the function of every endocrine gland in her body. Both clinically and in the laboratory, pregnancy can mimic hyperthyroidism, Cushing's disease, pituitary adenoma, diabetes mellitus, and polycystic ovary syndrome.

The endocrine changes associated with pregnancy are adaptive, allowing the mother to nurture the developing fetus. Although maternal reserves are usually adequate to tolerate the expenditure, occasionally, as in the case of gestational diabetes or hypertensive disease of pregnancy, a woman may develop overt signs of disease as a direct result of pregnancy.

Aside from creating a satisfactory maternal environment for fetal development, the placenta serves as a fetal endocrine gland as well as a respiratory, alimentary, and excretory organ. Measurements of fetal-placental products in the maternal serum provide one means of assessing the health of the developing fetus. This chapter will consider the changes in maternal endocrine function in pregnancy as well as fetal endocrine development. The chapter concludes with a discussion of some endocrine disorders complicating pregnancy.

CONCEPTION & IMPLANTATION

Fertilization

In fertile women, ovulation occurs approximately 12–16 days after the onset of the previous menses. The ovum must be fertilized within 24–48 hours if conception is to result. For about 48 hours around ovulation, cervical mucus is copious, nonviscous, and slightly alkaline—an ideal environment for sperm. Following intercourse, sperm that are to survive penetrate the cervical mucus within minutes and can remain viable there until the mucus character changes, approximately 24 hours following ovulation. Sperm begin appearing in the outer third of the uterine tube (the ampulla) 5–10 minutes after coitus and continue to migrate to this location from the cervix for about 24–48 hours. Fertilization normally occurs in the ampulla.

Acronyms Used in This Chapter

ACTH	Adrenocorticotropic hormone
cAMP	Cyclic adenosine monophosphate
CBG	Corticosteroid-binding globulin
CST	Contraction stress test
DHEA	Dehydroepiandrosterone
DOC	Deoxycorticosterone
FSH	Follicle-stimulating hormone
GH	Growth hormone
GnRH	Gonadotropin-releasing hormone
hCG	Human chorionic gonadotropin
hCGnRH	Human chorionic gonadotropin–releasing hormone
hCS	Human chorionic somatomammotropin
hGH	Human growth hormone
hPL	Human placental lactogen
hPRL	Human prolactin
LATS	Long-acting thyroid stimulator
LH	Luteinizing hormone
L/S	Lecithin/sphingomyelin (ratio)
NST	Nonstress test
PRL	Prolactin
SHBG	Sex hormone–binding globulin
TBG	Thyroid hormone–binding globulin
TRH	Thyrotropin-releasing hormone
TSH	Thyroid-stimulating hormone (thyrotropin)
TSI	Thyroid-stimulating immunoglobulin

Implantation

Implantation in the uterus does not occur until 6 or 7 days later, when the conceptus is a blastocyst of 1000–10,000 cells. In most pregnancies, the dates of ovulation and implantation are not known. Weeks of gestation ("gestational age") are by convention calculated from the first day of the last menstrual period. Within 24 hours after implantation, or at about 3 weeks of gestation, human chorionic gonadotropin (hCG) is detectable in maternal serum. Under the influence of hCG, the corpus luteum, which otherwise regresses within 7 days, continues to secrete steroid hormones in increasing quantities.

Symptoms of Pregnancy

Breast tenderness, fatigue, nausea, absence of menstruation, softening of the uterus, and a sustained elevation of basal body temperature are all attributable to hormone production by the corpus luteum.

Ovarian Hormones of Pregnancy

The hormones produced by the corpus luteum include progesterone, 17-hydroxyprogesterone, and estradiol. The indispensability of the corpus luteum in early pregnancy has been demonstrated by ablation studies, in which luteectomy or oophorectomy before 42 days of gestation results in precipitous decreases in levels of serum progesterone and estradiol, followed by abortion. Exogenous progesterone will prevent abortion, proving that progesterone alone is required for maintenance of early pregnancy. After about the seventh gestational week, the corpus luteum can be removed without subsequent abortion, owing to increasing progesterone production by the placenta.

Because the placenta does not produce appreciable amounts of 17-hydroxyprogesterone, this steroid provides a marker of corpus luteum function. As shown in Fig 17–1, the serum concentrations of estrogens and total progesterone exhibit a steady increase, but the concentration of 17-hydroxyprogesterone rises and then declines to low levels that persist for the duration of the pregnancy. The decline of corpus luteum function occurs despite the continued production of hCG; in fact, corpus luteum production of 17-hydroxyprogesterone declines while hCG is still rising to maximal levels.

Another marker of corpus luteum function is the polypeptide hormone relaxin, a dipeptide with a molecular weight of about 6000. It is similar in its tertiary structure to insulin. Relaxin becomes detectable at about the same time as hCG begins to rise, and it maintains a maximum maternal serum concentration of about 1 ng/mL during the first trimester. The serum concentration then falls approximately 20% and is constant for the remainder of the pregnancy.

Pharmacologically, relaxin ripens the cervix, softens the pubic symphysis, and acts synergistically with progesterone to inhibit uterine contractions. A major physiologic role for relaxin in human gestation, however, is doubtful, since luteectomy after 7 weeks of gestation does not interfere with gestation in spite of undetectable relaxin levels. Extraluteal production of relaxin by the decidua or placenta has been postulated but not proved.

FETAL-PLACENTAL-DECIDUAL UNIT

The placenta is responsible for establishing effective communication between the mother and the developing fetus while maintaining the immune and genetic integrity of both individuals. Initially, the placenta functions autonomously. By the end of the first trimester, however, the fetal endocrine system is sufficiently developed to influence placental function and to provide some hormone precursors to the placenta. From this time, it is useful to consider the conceptus as the fetal-placental unit.

The placenta and the fetal-placental unit will be considered in 3 separate but related categories: as sources of secretion of protein and steroid hormones into the maternal circulation; as participants in the control of fetal endocrine function, growth, and development; and as selective barriers governing the interaction between fetal and maternal systems.

Seven days after fertilization, implantation begins. The trophoblast invades the endometrium, and 2 layers of developing placenta can be demonstrated. The mature syncytiotrophoblast adjacent to the endometrium is derived from the precursor cytotrophoblast. The syncytiotrophoblast is the major source of hormone production, containing the cellular machinery needed for synthesis, packaging, and secretion of both steroid and polypeptide hormones. It is in direct contact with the maternal circulation and the decidua.

The decidua is the endometrium of pregnancy. Recent investigation has shown that the decidual cells are capable of synthesizing a variety of polypeptide hormones, the best-studied being prolactin (PRL). The importance of the role of the decidua as an endocrine organ has not been established, but its role as a source of prostaglandins during labor is certain (see Endocrine Control of Parturition, below).

POLYPEPTIDE HORMONES

Human Chorionic Gonadotropin

The first measurable product of the placenta is chorionic gonadotropin (hCG). hCG is a glycoprotein consisting of about 237 amino acids. It is quite similar in structure to the pituitary glycoproteins in that it consists of 2 chains: an alpha chain, which is species-specific; and a beta chain, which determines receptor interaction and ultimate biologic effect. The alpha chain is almost identical in sequence to the alpha chains of the hormonal glycoproteins TSH, FSH, and LH. The beta chain has significant sequence homology with LH but is not identical; of the 145 amino acids in β-hCG, 97 (67%) are identical to those of β-LH. In addition, the placental hormone has a carboxy-terminal segment of 30 amino acids not found in the pituitary LH molecule. Carbohydrate constitutes approximately 30% by weight of each subunit. Sialic acid alone accounts for 10% of the weight of the molecule and confers a high degree of resistance to degradation.

In the early weeks of pregnancy, the concentration of hCG doubles every 1.7–2 days, and serial measurements provide a sensitive index of early trophoblast function. Maternal plasma hCG peaks at about 100,000 mIU/mL during the 10th gestational week and then declines gradually to about 10,000 mIU/mL in the third trimester.

These characteristics of hCG all contribute to the possibility of diagnosing pregnancy several days before any symptoms occur or a menstrual period has been missed. Without the long plasma half-life of hCG (approximately 24 hours), the tiny mass of cells comprising the blastocyst, which are less than 1 μL in volume, could not produce sufficient hormone to be detected in the peripheral circulation within 24 hours

SYSTEM	HORMONE	PATTERN	AVERAGE PEAK CONCENTRATION (TIME)	
Progestins	Progesterone	Rises to term.	190 ng/mL (term)	
	17-Hydroxy-progester-one	Peaks at 5 weeks, then declines.	6 ng/mL (5 weeks)	
Adrenal	Cortisol	Increases to 3 times prepregnancy values at term.	300 ng/mL (term)	
	Aldosterone	Plateaus at 34 weeks with small rise near term.	100 ng/mL	
	DOC	Increases to 10 times prepregnancy value at term.	1200 pg/mL (term)	
Thyroid	Total T_4	Increases during first trimester, then plateaus.	150 ng/mL	
	Free T_4	Unchanged.	30 pg/mL	
	Total T_3	Increases during first trimester, then plateaus.	2 ng/mL	
	Free T_3	Unchanged.	4 pg/mL	

Figure 17–1. Maternal serum hormone changes during pregnancy.

SYSTEM	HORMONE	PATTERN	AVERAGE PEAK CONCENTRATION (TIME)
Anterior pituitary	GH	Unchanged.	
	LH, FSH	Low, basal levels.	
	ACTH	Unchanged.	
	TSH	Unchanged.	
	PRL	Rise to term.	≃ 200 ng/mL (term)
Placenta	hCG	Peaks at 10 weeks, then decreases to a lower plateau.	5 μg/mL (end of first trimester)
	hCS	Rises with placental weight.	5–25 μg/mL (term)
Estrogens	Estradiol	Increases to term.	15–17 ng/mL (term)
	Estriol	Increases to term.	12–15 ng/mL (term)
	Estrone	Increases to term.	5–7 ng/mL (term)
	Estetrol	Increases to term.	4–5 ng/mL (term)
Androgens	Testosterone	Rises to 10 times prepregnancy values.	≃ 2000 pg/mL (term)
	DHEA	Falls during pregnancy.	5 ng/mL (prepregnancy)
	Androstenedione	Small increase.	2.6 ng/mL (term)

Figure 17–1 (cont'd). Maternal serum hormone changes during pregnancy.

of implantation. The unique β-carboxy–terminal segment of hCG has been isolated, and an antibody has been raised against it in rabbits. The beta subunit assay for hCG that uses this antibody does not cross-react significantly with any of the pituitary glycoproteins. As little as 5 mIU/mL (1 ng/mL) of hCG in plasma can be detected without interference from the higher levels of LH, FSH, and TSH. The reliable sensitivities of commonly available pregnancy tests are summarized in Table 17–1.

Like its pituitary counterpart LH, hCG is luteotropic, and the corpus luteum has high-affinity receptors for hCG. The stimulation of increased amounts of progesterone production by corpus luteum cells can be demonstrated in vitro and is believed to be mediated by the cAMP system. hCG has been shown to enhance placental conversion of precursors to pregnenolone and progesterone. The hCG molecule also demonstrates TSH-like activity, but the biologic significance of this activity in normal pregnancy is modest, because hCG has only 1/4000 the potency of TSH.

The concentration of hCG in the fetal circulation is less than 1% of that found in the maternal compartment. However, there is evidence that fetal hCG is an important regulator of the development of the fetal adrenal and gonad during the first trimester.

hCG is also produced by trophoblastic neoplasms such as hydatidiform mole or choriocarcinoma, and the concentration of hCG or its beta subunit is used both as a tumor marker and as an indication of the success or failure of chemotherapy in these disorders. Women with very high hCG levels due to trophoblastic disease may become clinically hyperthyroid and revert to euthyroidism as hCG is reduced during chemotherapy.

Somatomammotropin

A second placental polypeptide hormone, also with homology to a pituitary protein, is termed placental lactogen (hPL) or chorionic somatomammotropin (hCS). hCS is detectable in the early trophoblast, but detectable serum concentrations are not reached until 4–5 gestational weeks. hCS is a protein of about 190 amino acids whose primary, secondary, and tertiary structures are similar to those of human growth hormone (hGH). The 2 molecules cross-react in immunoassays and in some receptor and bioassay systems. However, hCS has only some of the biologic activities of hGH. Like hGH, hCS is diabetogenic, but it has minimal growth-promoting activity as measured by standard hGH bioassays. hCS also shares many structural features with human prolactin (hPRL) and is a potent stimulator of pigeon crop sac growth. hCS appears to have greater intrinsic lactogenic activity than hGH.

The physiologic role of hCS during pregnancy remains controversial. Although not clearly shown to be a mammotropic agent, hCS contributes to altered glucose metabolism and mobilization of free fatty acids; causes a hyperinsulinemic response to glucose loads; and contributes to the peripheral insulin resistance characteristic of pregnancy. Factors that regulate the synthesis or release of hCS have not been fully determined, but prolonged fasting and insulin-induced hypoglycemia raise hCS concentrations. hCS production is roughly proportionate to placental mass. Actual production rates may reach as much as 1–1.5 g/d. The disappearance curve shows multiple components but yields a serum half-life of 15–30 minutes. Serum hCS concentration has been proposed as an indicator of the continued health of the placenta and has been used to monitor intrauterine growth retardation and fetal jeopardy. It was hoped that chronically low hCS or acute drops in its concentrations would be clinically useful in predicting placental compromise in pregnancies complicated by chronic hypertension, preeclampsia, intrauterine growth retardation, or postmaturity. Concentrations of hCS are indeed low in verified placental insufficiency, but the range of normal values is wide, and serial determinations are necessary. hCS determinations have largely been replaced by fetal heart rate monitoring, which is a more sensitive indicator of fetal jeopardy. In conditions such as diabetes, in which fetal jeopardy occurs with normal placental function, serum concentrations of hCS are of no predictive value.

Other Chorionic Peptide Hormones

Other chorionic peptides have been identified, but their functions have not yet been defined. One of these proteins is a glycoprotein with partial sequence and functional homology to TSH. Its existence as a separate entity from hCG has been debated in the literature, with some reports suggesting that chorionic TSH is a protein with a molecular weight of about 28,000, structurally different from hCG, with weak thyrotropic activity. Similarly, ACTH-like, lipotropinlike, and endorphinlike peptides have been isolated from placenta, but they have low biologic potency and undetermined physiologic roles. A chorionic FSH–like protein has also been isolated from placenta but has not yet been detected in plasma. Good evidence now exists that the cytotrophoblast produces a human chorionic gonadotropin–releasing hormone (hCGnRH) that is biologically and immunologically indistinguishable from the hypothalamic GnRH. The

Table 17–1. Relative sensitivity of various pregnancy tests.

Test	Sensitivity (mIU/mL)	Time Required (hours)	Reliable Detection After Ovulation (days)
Agglutination inhibition			
Slide test	1500–3000	0.5	28–30
Tube test	200–1000	2	14–30
Radioimmunoassay	5–50	1–36	8–14
Radioreceptor assay	200	1–3	14–17

release of hCG from the syncytiotrophoblast is apparently under the direct control of this factor, in a fashion analogous to the hypothalamic control of anterior pituitary secretion of gonadotropins. Preliminary evidence is also available for similar paracrine control of syncytiotrophoblastic release of TSH, somatostatin, and corticotropin by analogous cytotrophoblastic releasing hormones.

STEROID HORMONES

In contrast to the impressive synthetic capability exhibited in the production of placental proteins, the placenta does not appear to have the capability to synthesize steroids de novo. All steroids produced by the placenta are derived from maternal or fetal precursor steroids.

No tissue, however, even remotely approaches the syncytiotrophoblast in its capacity to efficiently interconvert steroids. This activity is demonstrable even in the preimplantation blastocyst, and by the seventh gestational week, when the corpus luteum has undergone relative senescence, the placenta becomes the dominant source of steroid hormones.

Progesterone

The placenta relies on maternal cholesterol as its substrate for progesterone production. Fetal death has no immediate influence on progesterone production, suggesting that the fetus is a negligible source of substrate. The placenta cleaves the cholesterol side chain, yielding pregnenolone, which in turn is partially isomerized to progesterone; 250–350 mg of progesterone is produced daily by the third trimester, and most enters the maternal circulation. The maternal plasma concentration of progesterone rises progressively throughout pregnancy and appears to be independent of factors that normally regulate steroid synthesis and secretion. Whereas exogenous hCG increases progesterone production in pregnancy, hypophysectomy has no effect. Administration of ACTH or cortisol does not influence progesterone concentrations, nor does adrenalectomy or oophorectomy do so after 7 weeks.

Progesterone is necessary for establishment and maintenance of pregnancy. Insufficient corpus luteum production of progesterone may contribute to failure of implantation, and luteal phase deficiency is implicated in some cases of infertility. Furthermore, progesterone is indispensable to a relatively quiescent state of the myometrium. In some animals, such as the rabbit or sheep, labor is heralded by a decrease in progesterone concentration, and the administration of progesterone in these species can delay labor indefinitely. Progesterone is also active as an immunosuppressive agent in some systems and inhibits T cell–mediated tissue rejection. Thus, high local concentrations of progesterone may contribute to immunologic tolerance by the uterus of invading embryonic trophoblast tissue.

Estrogens

Estrogen production by the placenta also depends on circulating precursors, but in this case both fetal and maternal steroids are important sources. Most of the estrogens are derived from fetal androgens, primarily dehydroepiandrosterone sulfate (DHEA sulfate). Fetal DHEA sulfate, produced mainly by the fetal adrenal, is converted by placental sulfatase to the free dehydroepiandrosterone (DHEA) and then, through enzymatic pathways common to steroid-producing tissues, to androsterone and testosterone. These androgens are finally aromatized by the placenta to estrone and estradiol, respectively.

The greater part of fetal DHEA sulfate is metabolized to produce a third estrogen: estriol. While serum estrone and estradiol concentrations are increased during pregnancy about 50-fold over their maximal prepregnancy values, estriol increases approximately 1000-fold. The key step in estriol synthesis is 16α-hydroxylation of the steroid molecule (see Fig 14–4). The substrate for the reaction is primarily fetal DHEA sulfate, and the vast majority of the production of 16α-hydroxy-DHEA sulfate occurs in the fetal adrenal and liver, not in maternal or placental tissues. The final steps of desulfation and aromatization to estriol occur in the placenta. Maternal serum or urinary estriol measurements, unlike measurements of progesterone or hCS, reflect fetal as well as placental function. Normal estriol production, therefore, reflects the integrity of fetal circulation and metabolism as well as adequacy of the placenta. Rising serum or urinary estriol concentrations are the best available biochemical indicator of fetal well-being. When estriol is assayed daily, a significant drop ($> 50\%$) often is a more sensitive early indicator of fetal jeopardy than are changes in fetal heart rate variability.

There are many circumstances in which altered estriol production does not signal fetal compromise but is instead the result of congenital derangements or iatrogenic intervention. Maternal estriol remains low in pregnancies with placental sulfatase deficiency and in cases of fetal anencephaly. In the first case, DHEA sulfate cannot be hydrolyzed; in the second, little fetal DHEA is produced because fetal adrenal stimulation by ACTH is lacking. Administration of glucocorticoids inhibits fetal ACTH and lowers maternal estriol. Administration of DHEA to the mother during a healthy pregnancy increases estriol production. Antibiotic therapy can reduce estriol by interfering with maternal reabsorption of estriol from the gut.

Estetrol, an estrogen with a fourth hydroxyl at the 15 position, is unique to pregnancy, but at present it is not clear that determinations of estetrol offer any clinical advantage over estriol measurements.

MATERNAL ADAPTATION TO PREGNANCY

Like a successful parasite, the fetal-placental unit

manipulates the maternal ''host'' for its own gain but normally avoids imposing excessive stress that would jeopardize the ''host'' and thus the ''parasite'' itself. The prodigious production of polypeptide and steroid hormones by the fetal-placental unit directly or indirectly results in physiologic adaptations of virtually every maternal organ system. These alterations are summarized in Fig 17–2. Most of the commonly measured maternal endocrine function tests are radically changed. In some cases, true physiologic alteration has occurred; in others, the changes are due to increased production of specific serum binding proteins by the liver or to decreased serum levels of albumin. Additionally, some hormonal changes are mediated by altered clearance rates owing to increased glomerular filtration, decreased hepatic excretion of anions, or metabolic clearance of steroid and protein hormones by the placenta. The changes in endocrine function tests are summarized in Table 17–2. Failure to recognize normal pregnancy-induced alterations in endocrine function tests can lead to unnecessary diagnostic tests and therapy that may be seriously detrimental to mother and fetus.

Maternal Pituitary Gland

The mother's anterior pituitary gland hormones have little influence on pregnancy after implantation has occurred. The gland itself enlarges by about one-third, with the major component of this increase being hyperplasia of the lactotrophs in response to the high plasma estrogens. PRL, the product of the lactotrophs, is the only anterior pituitary hormone that rises progressively during pregnancy. In spite of the high serum concentrations, pulsatile release of PRL and nocturnal and food-induced increases persist. Hence, the normal neuroendocrine regulatory mechanisms appear to be intact. Pituitary ACTH and TSH secretion remain unchanged. Serum FSH and LH fall to the lower limits of detectability and are unresponsive to GnRH stimulation. hGH concentrations are not significantly different from nonpregnant levels, but pituitary response to provocative testing is markedly altered. hGH response to hypoglycemia and arginine infusion is enhanced but thereafter becomes depressed. Established pregnancy can continue in the face of hypophysectomy, and in women hypophysectomized prior to pregnancy, induction of ovulation and normal pregnancy can be achieved with appropriate replacement therapy. In cases of pituitary hyperfunction, the fetus is not affected.

Maternal Thyroid Gland

The thyroid becomes palpably enlarged during the first trimester, and a bruit may be present. [131]I uptake and thyroid iodide clearance are increased. These changes are due in large part to the increased renal clearance of iodide, which causes a relative iodine deficiency. While total serum thyroxine is elevated as a result of increased thyroid hormone–binding globulin (TBG), free thyroxine and triiodothyronine are normal (Fig 17–1).

Table 17–2. Effect of pregnancy on endocrine function tests.

	Test	Result
Pituitary		
FSH, LH	GnRH stimulation	Unresponsive from third gestational week until puerperium.
GH	Insulin tolerance test	Response increases during the first half of pregnancy and then is blunted until the puerperium.
	Arginine stimulation	Hyperstimulation during the first and second trimesters, then suppression.
TSH	TRH stimulation	Response unchanged.
Pancreas		
Insulin	Glucose tolerance	Peak glucose increases, and glucose concentration remains elevated longer.
	Glucose challenge	Insulin concentration increases to higher peak levels.
	Arginine infusion	Insulin response is blunted in mid to late pregnancy.
Adrenal		
Cortisol	ACTH infusion	Exaggerated cortisol and 17-hydroxycorticosterone responses.
	Metyrapone	Diminished response.
Mineralo-corticoids	ACTH infusion	No DOC response.
	Dexamethasone suppression	No DOC response.

Maternal Parathyroid Gland

The net calcium requirement imposed by fetal skeletal development is estimated to be about 30 g by term. This is met by hyperplasia of the parathyroid glands and elevated serum levels of parathyroid hormone. The maternal serum calcium concentration declines to a nadir at 28–32 weeks, largely owing to the hypoalbuminemia of pregnancy. Ionized calcium is maintained at normal concentrations.

Maternal Pancreas

The nutritional demands of the fetus require alteration of maternal metabolic homeostatic control, which results in both structural and functional changes in the maternal pancreas. The size of pancreatic islets increases, and insulin-secreting B cells undergo hyperplasia. Basal levels of insulin are lower or unchanged in early pregnancy but increase during the second trimester. Thereafter, pregnancy is a hyperinsulinemic state, with resistance to the peripheral metabolic effects of insulin. The increased concentration of insulin has been shown to be a result of increased secretion rather than decreased metabolic clearance. The measured half-life for insulin is unchanged in pregnant women. The effects of pregnancy on the pancreas can be mimicked by appropriate treatment with estrogen, progesterone, hCS, and corticosteroids.

Pancreatic production of glucagon remains responsive to usual stimuli and is suppressed by glucose loading, although the degree of responsiveness has not been well evaluated.

The major role of insulin and glucagon is the control of concentrations of nutrients, specifically glucose, amino acids, and fatty acids. These concentrations are regulated during pregnancy for fetal needs, and the pre- and postfeeding levels cause pancreatic responses that act to support the fetal economy. Insulin is not transported across the placenta but rather exerts its effects on transportable metabolites. Peak insulin secretion in response to meals is accelerated, and glucose tolerance curves are characteristically altered. Fasting glucose levels are maintained at slightly lower levels but within normal limits. Excess carbohydrate is converted to fat, and fat is readily mobilized during decreased caloric intake.

Amino acid metabolism is also altered during pregnancy, at the expense of maternal needs. Hypoglycemia, hypoinsulinemia, and hyperketonuria do not cause an augmented hepatic gluconeogenesis. The key amino acid substrate, alanine, is diminished by mechanisms as yet unknown.

The normal result of pregnancy, then, is to reduce glucose levels modestly but to reserve glucose for fetal needs while maternal energy requirements are met increasingly by the peripheral metabolism of fatty acids. The changes in energy metabolism are beneficial to the fetus and innocuous to the mother with an adequate diet. Even modest fasting, however, causes ketosis, which is potentially injurious to the fetus.

Maternal Adrenal Cortex

A. Glucocorticoids: Plasma cortisol concentrations increase to 3 times nonpregnant levels by the third trimester. Most of the increase can be accounted for by a doubling of corticosteroid-binding globulin (CBG). In spite of cortisol concentrations approaching those found in Cushing's syndrome, diurnal variation in plasma cortisol is maintained. The increased estrogen levels of pregnancy account for the increase in CBG, which, in turn, is sufficient to account for decreased catabolism of cortisol by the liver. The result is a doubling of the half-life of plasma cortisol. The actual production of cortisol by the zona fasciculata is reduced by about 20%. The net effect of these changes, however, is an increase in plasma free cortisol, which is approximately doubled by late pregnancy. Whether this increase is mediated through ACTH or by other mechanisms is not known. The elevated free cortisol probably contributes to the insulin resistance of pregnancy and possibly to the appearance of striae, but most signs of hypercortisolism do not occur in pregnancy. It is possible that high progesterone levels act as a glucocorticoid antagonist and prevent some cortisol effects.

B. Mineralocorticoids and the Renin-Angiotensin System: Serum aldosterone is markedly elevated in pregnancy. The increase is due to an 8- to 10-fold increased production of aldosterone by the zona glomerulosa and not to increased binding or decreased clearance. The peak in aldosterone pro-

duction is reached by mid pregnancy and is maintained until delivery. Renin substrate is increased owing to the influence of estrogen on hepatic synthesis, and renin also is increased.

The increases in both renin and renin substrate inevitably lead to increases in renin activity and angiotensin. In spite of these dramatic changes, normal pregnant women show few signs of hyperaldosteronism. There is no tendency to hypokalemia or hypernatremia, and blood pressure at mid pregnancy—when changes in the aldosterone-renin-angiotensin system are maximal—tends to be lower than in the nonpregnant state. It has been suggested that edema of late pregnancy is due to these changes, but hyperaldosteronism in nonpregnant women leads to hypertension, not edema.

Although the quantitative aspects of this apparent paradox are not fully understood, a qualitative explanation is possible. Progesterone is a reasonably effective competitive inhibitor of mineralocorticoids in the distal renal tubules. Exogenous progesterone (but not synthetic progestins) is natriuretic and potassium-sparing in intact humans, whereas it has no effect in adrenalectomized subjects not receiving mineralocorticoids. Progesterone also blunts the response of the kidney to exogenous aldosterone—thus, the increases in renin and aldosterone may simply be an appropriate response to the high gestational levels of progesterone. The concomitant increase in angiotensin II as a result of increased plasma renin activity apparently does not result in hypertension, because of diminished sensitivity of the maternal vascular system to angiotensin. Even during the first trimester, exogenous angiotensin provokes less of a rise in blood pressure than in the nonpregnant state.

It is clear that the high levels of renin, angiotensin, and aldosterone in pregnant women are subject to the usual feedback controls, because they respond appropriately to changes in posture, dietary sodium, and water loading and restriction in qualitatively the same way as they do in nonpregnant women. Finally, in patients with pregnancy-induced hypertension in the second half of pregnancy, serum renin, aldosterone, and angiotensin levels are lower than in normal pregnancy, thus ruling out any primary role for the renin-angiotensin system in this disorder.

Production of the mineralocorticoid 11-deoxycorticosterone (DOC) rises throughout pregnancy, and plasma levels 6–10 times "normal" are achieved by term. In contrast to the nonpregnant state, DOC production in pregnancy is unaffected by ACTH or glucocorticoid administration. The source of DOC appears to be conversion of progesterone to DOC in peripheral tissue. DOC is not elevated in hypertensive disorders of pregnancy.

C. Androgens: In normal pregnancy, the adrenal and ovarian production of androgens is slightly increased. The most important determinant of plasma levels of specific androgens, however, appears to be whether or not the androgen binds to sex hormone–binding globulin (SHBG). Testosterone, which binds

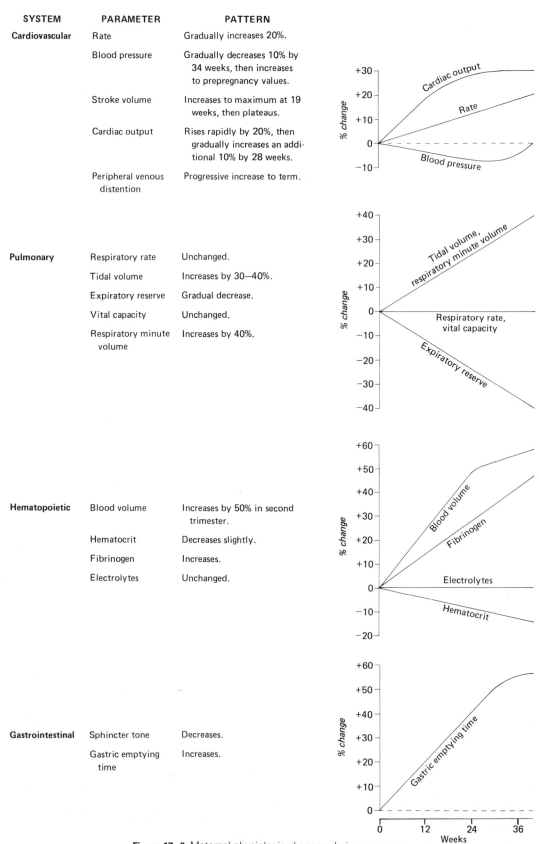

SYSTEM	PARAMETER	PATTERN
Cardiovascular	Rate	Gradually increases 20%.
	Blood pressure	Gradually decreases 10% by 34 weeks, then increases to prepregnancy values.
	Stroke volume	Increases to maximum at 19 weeks, then plateaus.
	Cardiac output	Rises rapidly by 20%, then gradually increases an additional 10% by 28 weeks.
	Peripheral venous distention	Progressive increase to term.
Pulmonary	Respiratory rate	Unchanged.
	Tidal volume	Increases by 30–40%.
	Expiratory reserve	Gradual decrease.
	Vital capacity	Unchanged.
	Respiratory minute volume	Increases by 40%.
Hematopoietic	Blood volume	Increases by 50% in second trimester.
	Hematocrit	Decreases slightly.
	Fibrinogen	Increases.
	Electrolytes	Unchanged.
Gastrointestinal	Sphincter tone	Decreases.
	Gastric emptying time	Increases.

Figure 17–2. Maternal physiologic changes during pregnancy.

SYSTEM	PARAMETER	PATTERN	
Renal	Renal flow	Increases 25–50%.	
	Glomerular filtration rate	Increases early, then plateaus.	
Weight	Uterine weight	Increases from about 60–70 g to about 900–1200 g.	
	Body weight	Average 11-kg (25-lb) increase.	

Figure 17–2 (cont'd). Maternal physiologic changes during pregnancy.

avidly to SHBG, increases to the normal male range by the end of the first trimester, but free testosterone levels are actually lower than in the nonpregnant state. Dehydroepiandrosterone sulfate (DHEA sulfate) does not bind to SHBG, and plasma concentrations of DHEA sulfate actually decrease during pregnancy. The desulfation of DHEA sulfate by the placenta and the conversion of DHEA sulfate to estrogens by the fetal-placental unit are also important factors in its increased metabolic clearance.

FETAL ENDOCRINOLOGY

Because of the inaccessibility of the fetus, much of our information about fetal endocrinology is derived indirectly. Most early studies of fetal endocrinology relied upon observations of infants with congenital disorders or inferences from ablation studies or acute experiments in mammals. The development of effective cell culture methods and sensitive radiolabeled assay systems and the ability to achieve stable preparations of chronically catheterized monkey fetuses have increased our understanding of the dynamics of intrauterine endocrine events.

Study of the fetal endocrine system is further complicated by the multiplicity of sources of the various hormones. The fetus is exposed to maternal and placental hormones as well as to those it produces itself. Amniotic fluid contains a variety of hormones of mixed fetal and maternal origin, and these hormones are of uncertain importance. Study of the isolated fetus, even if possible, would thus be of little physiologic relevance.

A final pitfall in the study of fetal endocrine systems relates to the process of development itself. Inferences from the behavior of adult endocrine systems are not transferable to the fetus, because target organs, receptors, modulators, and regulators develop at different times. Thus, the role of a particular hormone in the fetal economy at any one point in gestation may

bear little or no relationship to its role in postnatal life.

Dating of events in fetal development is usually given in "fetal weeks," which begin at the time of ovulation. Thus, fetal age is always 2 weeks less than gestational age.

Fetal Anterior Pituitary Hormones

The characteristic anterior pituitary cell types are discernible as early as 8–10 fetal weeks, and all of the hormones of the adult anterior pituitary are extractable from the fetal adenohypophysis by 12 weeks. Similarly, the hypothalamic hormones thyrotropin-releasing hormone (TRH), gonadotropin-releasing hormone (GnRH), and somatostatin are present by 8–10 weeks. The direct circulatory connection between hypothalamus and pituitary develops later, with capillary invasion initially visible at about 16 weeks.

The role of the fetal pituitary in organogenesis of various target organs during the first trimester appears to be negligible. None of the pituitary hormones are released into the fetal circulation in large quantities until after 20 fetal weeks. Even growth hormone (GH) appears not to be influential, and in fact total absence of GH is consistent with normal development at birth. Development of the gonads and adrenals during the first trimester appears to be directed by hCG rather than by fetal trophic hormones, and the development of the thyroid glands during the first trimester occurs independently of TSH production by the fetus.

During the second trimester, there is a marked increase in secretion of all of the anterior pituitary hormones, which coincides with maturation of the hypophyseal portal system. Observations include a marked rise in production of GH and an increase in fetal serum TSH, with a concomitant increase in fetal thyroidal iodine uptake. Gonadotropin production also increases, with the female achieving higher FSH levels in both pituitary and serum than does the male. The fetal gonadotropins do not direct the events of organogenesis but are essential for normal development of the differentiated gonads and external genitalia. ACTH rises significantly during the second trimester and assumes an increasing role in directing the maturation of the differentiated adrenal, as shown by the anencephalic fetus, in which the fetal zone of the adrenal undergoes atrophy after 20 weeks. Fetal PRL secretion also increases after the 20th fetal week, but the functional significance of this hormone, if any, is unknown.

During the third trimester, maturation of feedback systems modulating hypothalamic release signals causes serum concentrations of all of the pituitary hormones except PRL to decline.

Fetal Posterior Pituitary Hormones

Vasopressin and oxytocin are demonstrable by 12–18 weeks in the fetal posterior pituitary gland and correlate with the development of their sites of production, the supraoptic and paraventricular nuclei. The hormone content of the gland increases to term, with no evidence of feedback control.

During labor, umbilical artery oxytocin is higher than umbilical vein oxytocin. Dawood et al have suggested that the fetal posterior pituitary may contribute to the onset or maintenance of labor.

Fetal Thyroid Gland

The thyroid gland develops at about the same stage in development as the pituitary. Initial first-trimester development occurs in the absence of detectable TSH, and by 12 weeks the thyroid is capable of iodine-concentrating activity and thyroid hormone synthesis.

During the second trimester, TRH, TSH, and free T_4 all begin to rise. The maturation of feedback mechanisms is suggested by the subsequent plateau of TSH at about 20 fetal weeks. Fetal T_3 and reverse T_3 do not become detectable until the third trimester. The hormone produced in largest amount throughout fetal life is T_4, with the metabolically active T_3 and its inactive derivative, reverse T_3, rising in parallel to T_4 during the third trimester. At birth, conversion of T_4 to T_3 becomes demonstrable.

The development of thyroid hormones occurs independently of maternal systems, and very little placental transfer of thyroid hormone occurs in physiologic concentrations. This prevents maternal thyroid disorders from affecting the fetal compartment but also prevents effective therapy for fetal hypothyroidism through maternal supplementation. Goitrogenic agents such as propylthiouracil are transferred across the placenta and may induce fetal hypothyroidism and goiter.

The function of the fetal thyroid hormones appears crucial to somatic growth and for successful neonatal adaptation.

Fetal Parathyroid Gland

The fetal parathyroid is capable of synthesizing parathyroid hormone by the end of the first trimester. However, the placenta actively transports calcium into the fetal compartment, and the fetus remains relatively hypercalcemic throughout gestation. This contributes to a suppression of parathyroid hormone, and fetal serum levels in umbilical cord have been reported to be low or undetectable. Fetal serum calcitonin levels are elevated, enhancing bone accretion. Fetal vitamin D levels reflect maternal levels but do not appear to be significant in fetal calcium metabolism.

Fetal Adrenal Cortex

The fetal adrenal differs anatomically and functionally from its adult state. The cortex is identifiable as early as 4 weeks of fetal age, and by the seventh week, steroidogenic activity can be detected in the inner zone layers.

By 20 weeks, the adrenal cortex has increased to a mass that is considerably larger than its relative postnatal size. During gestation, it occupies as much as 0.5% of total body volume, and most of this tissue is composed of a unique fetal zone that subsequently regresses or is transformed into the definitive (adult) zone during the early neonatal period. The inner fetal zone is responsible for the majority of steroids produced during fetal life and comprises 80% of the mass of the adrenal. During the second trimester, the inner fetal zone continues to grow, while the outer zone remains relatively undifferentiated. At about 25 weeks, the definitive (adult) zone develops more rapidly and begins to produce steroids, ultimately assuming the principal role in steroid synthesis during the early postnatal weeks. This transfer of function is accompanied by involution of the fetal zone, which is completed during the first months of neonatal life.

Fetal Gonads

The testis is a detectable structure by about 6 fetal weeks. The interstitial cells, which synthesize fetal testosterone, are functional at this same stage. The maximal production of testosterone coincides with the maximal production of hCG by the placenta; binding of hCG to fetal testes with stimulation of testosterone release has been demonstrated. Other fetal testicular products of importance are the reduced testosterone metabolite dihydrotestosterone and müllerian duct inhibitory factor. Dihydrotestosterone is responsible for development of the external genital structures, whereas müllerian duct inhibitory factor prevents development of female internal structures.

Little is known about fetal ovarian function. By 7–8 weeks of intrauterine life, the ovaries become recognizable, but their importance in the fetal economy has not been established, and the significance of the steroids produced by the ovaries remains unclear.

ENDOCRINE CONTROL OF PARTURITION

During the last few weeks of normal pregnancy, 2 processes herald approaching labor. Uterine contractions, usually painless, become increasingly frequent, and the lower uterine segment and cervix become softer and thinner, a process known as efface-ment, or "ripening." Although false alarms are not uncommon, the onset of true labor is usually fairly abrupt, with the establishment of regular contractions every 2–5 minutes, leading to delivery in less than 24 hours. There is a huge literature describing the physiologic and biochemical events that occur during human labor, but the key inciting event has eluded detection. For sheep, it is the fetus that controls the onset of labor. The initial measurable event is an increase in fetal plasma cortisol, which, in turn, alters placental steroid production, resulting in a drop in progesterone. Cortisol reliably induces labor in sheep, but in humans, glucocorticoids do not induce labor and there is no drop in plasma progesterone prior to labor. Exogenous progesterone does not prevent labor in humans.

The difficulty in identifying a *single* initiating event in human labor may simply be that there is more than one. Approaching the matter in a different way, one could ask: What are the factors responsible for main-tenance of pregnancy, and how can they fail?

Sex Steroids

Progesterone is essential for maintenance of early pregnancy, and withdrawal of progesterone leads to termination of pregnancy. In the rabbit, the corpus luteum (rather than the placenta) is the primary source of progesterone throughout pregnancy.

Oophorectomy of the pregnant rabbit initiates la-bor, even near term, unless exogenous progesterone is given. Progesterone causes hyperpolarization of the myometrium, decreasing the amplitude of action po-tentials and preventing effective contractions. In var-ious experimental systems, progesterone decreases al-pha-adrenergic receptors, stimulates cAMP produc-tion, and inhibits oxytocin receptor synthesis. Progesterone also inhibits estrogen receptor synthesis, promotes the storage of prostaglandin precursors in the decidua and fetal membranes, and stabilizes the lysosomes containing prostaglandin-synthesizing en-zymes. Estrogen opposes progesterone in these actions and may have an independent role in ripening the uterine cervix and promoting uterine contractility. Thus, the estrogen:progesterone ratio may be an im-portant parameter. In small series of patients, an in-crease in the estrogen:progesterone ratio has been shown to precede labor. Thus, for some individuals, a drop in progesterone or an increase in estrogen may initiate labor. The cause of the change in steroids may be placental maturation or a signal from the fetus, but there are no data to support either thesis. A recent finding in experimental animals that an increase in the estrogen:progesterone ratio increases the number of myometrial gap junctions may explain the coor-dinate, effective contractions that characterize true labor as opposed to the nonpainful, ineffective con-tractions of false labor.

Oxytocin

Oxytocin infusion is commonly used to induce or augment labor. Both maternal and fetal oxytocin levels increase during labor, but neither has been convinc-ingly shown to increase prior to labor. Data in animals suggest that oxytocin's role in initiation of labor is due to increased sensitivity of the uterus to oxytocin rather than increased plasma concentrations of the hormone. Even women with diabetes insipidus are able to deliver without oxytocin augmentation; thus, the hormone is not indispensable—at least not ma-ternal oxytocin.

Prostaglandins

Prostaglandin $F_{2\alpha}$ intra-amniotically or intrave-nously is an effective abortifacient as early as 14 weeks of gestation. Prostaglandin E_2 by vagina will induce labor in most women in the third trimester. The am-nion and chorion contain high concentrations of arachidonic acid, and the decidua contains active pros-taglandin synthetase. Prostaglandins are almost cer-tainly involved in maintenance of labor once it is established. They also probably are important in ini-tiating labor in some circumstances, such as in am-nionitis or when the membranes are "stripped" by the physician. They probably are part of the "final common pathway" in labor.

Prostaglandin synthetase inhibitors abolish pre-mature labor, but their clinical usefulness has been restricted by their simultaneous effect of closing the ductus arteriosus, leading to fetal pulmonary hyper-tension.

Catecholamines

Catecholamines with α_2-adrenergic activity cause uterine contractions, whereas β_2-adrenergics inhibit labor. Progesterone increases the ratio of beta recep-tors to alpha receptors in myometrium, thus favoring continued gestation. There is no evidence that changes in catecholamines or their receptors initiate labor, but it is likely that such changes help sustain labor once initiated. The beta-adrenergic drug ritodrine has proved to be a valuable agent in the management of premature labor. Alpha-adrenergic agents are not useful in in-ducing labor, because of their cardiovascular side ef-fects.

ENDOCRINOLOGY OF THE PUERPERIUM

Extirpation of any active endocrine organ leads to compensatory changes in other organs and systems. Delivery of the infant and placenta causes both im-mediate and long-term adjustment to loss of the preg-nancy hormones. The sudden withdrawal of fetal-placental hormones at delivery permits determination of their serum half-lives and some evaluation of their function during pregnancy.

Physiologic & Anatomic Changes

Some of the physiologic and anatomic adjustments

that take place after delivery are hormone-dependent, whereas others are themselves responsible for hormonal changes. For example, major readjustments of the cardiovascular system occur in response to the normal blood losses associated with delivery and to loss of the low-resistance placental shunt. By the third postpartum day, blood volume is estimated to decline to about 84% of predelivery values. The cardiovascular changes influence renal and liver clearance of hormones.

Reproductive Tract Changes

The uterus decreases progressively in size at the rate of about 500 g/wk and continues to be palpable abdominally until about 2 weeks postpartum, when it reoccupies its position entirely within the pelvis. Nonpregnant size and weight (50– 80 g) are reached by 6 weeks. The reversal of myometrial hypertrophy occurs with a decrease in size of individual myometrial cells rather than by reduction in number. Uterine discharge also changes progressively during this period, with the mixture of fresh blood and decidua becoming a serous transudate and then ceasing in 3– 6 weeks.

The uterine surface, which is sloughed at the time of delivery, regenerates rapidly; by the seventh day, there is restoration of surface epithelium, except at the placental site. By the second week after delivery, the endometrium resembles normal proliferative-phase endometrium, except for the characteristic hyalinized decidual areas. The earliest documented appearance of a secretory endometrium occurred on day 44 in one series of daily biopsies. These rapid regenerative changes do not apply to the area of placental implantation, which requires much longer for restoration and retains pathognomonic histologic evidence of placentation indefinitely.

The cervix and vagina also recover rapidly from the effects of pregnancy, labor, and delivery. The cervix regains tone over the first week; by 6 weeks postpartum, it usually exhibits complete healing of lesions sustained at the time of delivery. Histologically, involution may continue beyond 6 weeks, with stromal edema, leukocytic infiltration, and glandular hyperplasia still apparent. Similarly, the vagina regains muscular tone following delivery, and rugae appear as early as 3 weeks. However, in women who nurse, the vaginal mucosa may remain atrophic for months, causing dyspareunia and a watery discharge.

Endocrine Changes

A. Steroids: With expulsion of the placenta, the steroid levels decline precipitously, their half-lives being measured in minutes or hours. As a consequence of continued low-level production by the corpus luteum, progesterone does not reach basal prenatal levels as rapidly as does estradiol. Plasma progesterone falls to luteal-phase levels within 24 hours after delivery but to follicular-phase levels only after several days. Removal of the corpus luteum results

in a fall to follicular levels within 24 hours. Estradiol reaches follicular-phase levels within 1– 3 days after delivery.

B. Pituitary Hormones: The pituitary gland, which enlarges during pregnancy owing primarily to an increase in lactotrophs, does not diminish in size until after lactation ceases. Secretion of FSH and LH continues to be suppressed during the early weeks of the puerperium, and stimulus with bolus doses of GnRH results in subnormal release of LH and FSH. Over the ensuing weeks, responsiveness to GnRH gradually returns to normal, and most women exhibit follicular-phase serum levels of LH and FSH by the third or fourth postpartum week.

C. Prolactin: Serum prolactin (PRL), which rises throughout pregnancy, falls with the onset of labor and then exhibits variable patterns of secretion depending upon whether breast feeding occurs. Delivery is associated with a surge in PRL, which is followed by a rapid fall in serum concentrations over 7– 14 days in the nonlactating mother.

In nonlactating women, the return of normal cyclic function and ovulation may be expected as soon as the second postpartum month, with the initial ovulation occurring at an average of 9– 10 weeks postpartum. In lactating women, PRL usually causes a persistence of anovulation. Surges of PRL are believed to act on the hypothalamus to inhibit GnRH secretion. Administration of exogenous GnRH during this time induces normal pituitary responsiveness, and occasional ovulation may occur spontaneously even during lactation. The average time for ovulation in women who have lactated for at least 3 months is about 17 weeks. The percentage of nonlactating women who have resumed menstruation increases linearly up to 12 weeks, by which time 70% will have restored menses. In contrast, the linear increase for lactating women exhibits a much shallower slope, and 70% of lactating women will have menstruated by about 36 weeks.

Lactation

Development of the breast alveolar lobules occurs throughout pregnancy. This period of mammogenesis requires the concerted participation of estrogen, progesterone, PRL, GH, and glucocorticoids. hCS may also play a role but is not indispensable. Milk secretion in the puerperium is associated with further enlargement of the lobules, followed by synthesis of milk constituents such as lactose and casein.

Lactation requires PRL, insulin, and adrenal steroids. It does not occur until unconjugated estrogens fall to nonpregnant levels at about 36– 48 hours postpartum.

PRL is essential to milk production. Its action involves induced synthesis of large numbers of PRL receptors; these appear to be autoregulated by PRL, since PRL increases receptor levels in cell culture and since bromocriptine, a PRL inhibitor, causes a decrease in both PRL and its receptors. In the absence of PRL, milk secretion does not take place; but even in the presence of high levels of PRL during the third trimester, milk secretion does not take place until after delivery, owing to the blocking effect of high levels of estrogen.

Galactopoiesis, or the process of continued milk secretion, is also dependent upon the function and integration of several hormones. Evidence from GH-deprived dwarves and hypothyroid patients suggests that GH and thyroid hormone are not required.

Milk secretion requires the additional stimulus of emptying of the breast. A neural arc must be activated for continued milk secretion. Milk ejection occurs in response to a surge of oxytocin, which induces a contractile response in the smooth muscle of the gland ductules. Oxytocin release is occasioned by stimuli of a visual, psychologic, or physical nature that prepare the mother for suckling.

INHIBITION OF LACTATION

There are relatively few contraindications to breast feeding. Among these are inverted nipples; mastitis; breast cancer; and ingestion of medications such as chemotherapeutic agents or radioactive iodide, which might be harmful to the fetus and are secreted in breast milk. The major indication for suppression of lactation is personal preference on the part of mothers unwilling or unable to breast-feed. Methods of suppression of lactation include avoidance of breast stimulation; use of estrogens, androgens, or both; and use of dopamine agonists to inhibit PRL. If avoidance of breast stimulation is used alone, about 50% of women will have significant engorgement and pain. This discomfort led to the practice of seeking pharmacologic means of preventing engorgement. Estrogen, combinations of estrogen and androgen, and synthetic antiestrogens such as clomiphene have all been promoted for this use. Their mechanism of action is not established but is believed to be at the level of the breast as opposed to the pituitary or hypothalamus. Estrogens alone are only slightly more effective than placebo. Problems associated with the administration of large doses of estrogen compounds include the increased risk of thromboembolic complications in patients already at risk due to parturition itself and occasional rebound lactation following therapy. Estrogen-androgen combinations may act at the pituitary level as well, and results of controlled studies suggest they may provide greater relief than placebo or estrogen alone. These steroids must be given at the time of delivery, because effectiveness diminishes after even 1 or 2 hours have elapsed. Rebound lactation may occur. Virilization has not been reported despite the use of large doses of androgens. Clomiphene and tamoxifen have been reported to provide relief in more than 90% of cases, with minimal side effects; these drugs are believed to act primarily by reducing serum PRL. Bromocriptine mesylate, a dopamine agonist that effectively inhibits PRL secretion, is 97% effective in inhibiting both engorgement and secretion. A 14-day course of 2.5

mg orally twice daily is recommended. A third week of 2.5 mg daily is suggested by some. Only 3% of patients have sufficient side effects (nausea or dizziness) to require early cessation of therapy. Mild rebound lactation requiring only supportive therapy or an additional 7-day course of the drug occurs in one out of 4 patients.

In summary, where suppression of lactation is required, avoidance of stimulation will be effective in 60–70% of women. A single injection of a combination of testosterone and estradiol valerate given immediately at delivery has a high success rate, but there is a risk of rebound lactation. Inhibition of PRL with dopamine agonists can be initiated either immediately postpartum or after lactation has begun but requires at least 2 weeks of therapy.

ENDOCRINE DISORDERS & PREGNANCY

PREGNANCY & PITUITARY ADENOMAS

In women of reproductive age, small tumors of the anterior pituitary are not uncommon (see also Chapter 4). While most are nonfunctional and asymptomatic, the most common symptom of pituitary microadenomas is amenorrhea, frequently accompanied by galactorrhea. In the past, few affected women became pregnant, but now most can be made to ovulate and to conceive with the aid of clomiphene citrate, menotropins and hCG, or bromocriptine. Before ovulation is induced in any patient, serum PRL should be determined. If it is elevated, the sella turcica should be evaluated by high-resolution CT scanning with contrast. About 10% of women with secondary amenorrhea will be found to have adenomas, while 20–50% of women with amenorrhea and galactorrhea will have detectable tumors. Once pregnancy is achieved, the normal gestational increase in PRL makes the modest increases observed with small adenomas undetectable, and radiographic procedures become undesirable.

The effect of pregnancy on pituitary adenomas depends on the size of the adenoma. Among 215 women with microadenomas (< 10 mm in diameter), fewer than 1% developed progressive visual field defects, 5% developed headaches, and none experienced more serious neurologic sequelae. Of 60 patients who had macroadenomas and became pregnant, 20% developed abnormal changes in their visual fields or other neurologic signs, usually in the first half of their pregnancies. Many of these required therapy.

Visual disturbances are usually experienced as "clumsiness" and are objectively found to be due to visual field changes. The most frequent finding is bitemporal hemianopia, but in advanced cases the defect can progress to concentric contraction of fields and enlargement of the blind spot.

Since the pituitary normally increases in size during pregnancy, headaches are common and bitemporal hemianopia not uncommon. These changes almost always revert to normal after delivery, so that aggressive therapy for known pituitary adenomas is not indicated except in cases of rapidly progressive visual loss.

Management

Management of the pregnant woman with a small adenoma includes early ophthalmologic consultation for formal visual field mapping and repeat examinations once a month or every other month throughout pregnancy.

If visual field disturbances are minimal, pregnancy may be allowed to proceed to term. If symptoms become progressively more severe and the fetus is mature, labor should be induced. If symptoms are severe and the fetus is immature, management may consist of transsphenoidal resection of the adenoma or medical treatment with bromocriptine. While bromocriptine inhibits both fetal and maternal pituitary PRL secretion, it does not affect decidual PRL secretion. At present, bromocriptine appears not to be teratogenic, and no adverse fetal effects have been reported. It should, of course, be used with caution in pregnancy, but in most cases it is probably preferable to surgery. Radiation therapy should not be used.

Management of PRL-secreting tumors in women who want to become pregnant is controversial. Surgical resection by surgeons with experience in transsphenoidal procedures results in reduction of PRL levels and resumption of normal ovulation in 60– 80% of women with microadenomas and 30– 50% of women with macroadenomas. The incidence of recurrence is at least 10– 15% and will probably increase with further follow-up. Bromocriptine is usually well tolerated and is successful in achieving normal menstrual cycles and lowering PRL levels in 40– 80% of patients. Bromocriptine also causes a marked decrease in tumor size, but the original size of the tumor is usually regained within days or weeks after discontinuing therapy. In the case of large tumors, combined medical and surgical management may often be appropriate. Radiation therapy has an important role in arresting growth of tumors that are resistant to other management, particularly large tumors that involve the cavernous sinuses and tumors that secrete both GH and PRL.

Prognosis & Follow-Up

There appears to be no increase in obstetric complications associated with adenomas, and no fetal jeopardy. The rate of prematurity increases in women with tumors requiring therapy, but this is probably due to aggressive intervention rather than to spontaneous premature labor.

The postpartum period is characterized by rapid relief of even severe symptoms, with less than 4% of untreated tumors developing permanent sequelae. In some cases, tumors improve following pregnancy, with normalization or lowering of PRL relative to prepregnancy values. Management should include radiography and assessment of PRL levels 4– 6 weeks after delivery. There is no contraindication to breast feeding.

PREGNANCY & BREAST CANCER

Breast cancer complicates one in 1500– 5000 pregnancies. Only one-sixth of breast cancers occur in women of reproductive age, but of these, one in 7 is diagnosed during pregnancy or the puerperium. Pregnancy and breast cancer have long been considered such an ominous combination that only one in 20 young women who have had breast cancer have later become pregnant. It now appears, however, that pregnancy has little effect on growth of breast cancer, though it presents problems of detection and management of the cancer (see Chapter 23).

Influence of Pregnancy on Breast Cancer

Pregnancy is not an etiologic factor in breast cancer. Indeed, there is good evidence that pregnancy at an early age actually reduces the risk of developing mammary cancer, and multiple pregnancies may also make the disease less likely. Moreover, contemporary concepts of the rate of tumor growth suggest that a tumor becomes clinically evident only 8– 10 years after its inception. Thus, a tumor cannot arise and be discovered during the same pregnancy. In view of the increased glandular proliferation and blood flow and marked increase in lymph flow that occur during pregnancy, it could be argued that pregnancy accelerates the appearance of previously subclinical diseases, but this has not been demonstrated.

Probably the most important influence of pregnancy on breast cancer is the delay it may cause in making the diagnosis and starting therapy. In some series, the interval between initial symptoms and treatment was 6– 7 months longer than in the absence of pregnancy. The increased density of the breasts in pregnancy makes small masses less apparent; and even when masses are found, both the patient and the physician are apt to attribute them to expected physiologic changes in pregnancy. Larger tumors may be misdiagnosed as galactoceles, and inflammatory carcinoma in the puerperium is liable to be misdiagnosed as mastitis.

At the time of diagnosis, 60% of pregnancy-associated breast cancers have metastasized to regional lymph nodes, and an additional 20% have distant metastases. Stage for stage, however, salvage rates following appropriate therapy are comparable to those achieved in nonpregnant patients. Termination of pregnancy, either by abortion or by early delivery, does not influence maternal survival.

Pregnancy After
Treatment for Cancer

Pregnancy following definitive treatment of breast cancer has no adverse effect on survival. Indeed, women who become pregnant following stage I or II breast cancer have a somewhat better 5-year survival rate than matched controls who did not become pregnant but who survived at least as long as their match before becoming pregnant.

Women who have had breast cancer are frequently advised to avoid pregnancy for 5 years. Because most fertile women with breast cancer are in their mid 30s, such a plan virtually precludes pregnancy. Because pregnancy is not known to influence the rate of cancer recurrence, the only reasons for proscribing pregnancy are to avoid the possibility that management of a recurrence will be complicated by the pregnancy or to avoid the problem of producing motherless children. For a couple strongly desiring pregnancy, these risks may become acceptable in a much shorter time than 5 years, especially if the original lesion was small and the spread of disease minimal.

Estrogen in Cancer

Determinations of cytoplasmic estrogen and progesterone receptors are frequently used in breast cancer to predict whether the tumor is likely to respond to endocrine therapy. There is also evidence that the presence of significant estrogen receptor is correlated with a lower risk of early recurrence. In the pregnant patient, however, high progesterone levels inhibit estrogen and progesterone receptor synthesis, and high levels of both hormones cause translocation of their receptors out of the cytoplasm and into the nucleus. Thus, all breast cancers arising in pregnancy appear to be receptor-negative, making such measurements in pregnancy at best worthless and at worst dangerously misleading.

Early Diagnosis

It is clear that early diagnosis of breast cancer in pregnancy gives the best chance of improved survival. Self-examination should be encouraged in spite of the anxiety it will cause, and thorough breast examinations should be performed periodically throughout pregnancy, not just at the initial examination. Even mildly suspicious lesions should be investigated if they persist for 1–2 weeks; waiting for a lesion to grow before further investigation is not acceptable practice. If a woman has discovered a small mass, her assessment should be accepted even if the physician cannot feel the mass by the usual techniques. Small lesions that would otherwise be missed can often be felt if soap and water are used for lubrication. Cytologic examination of fine-needle aspirates is probably the best technique for investigating small discrete lesions. If any question persists, ultrasonography or low-dose mammography should be employed. Unless one is very experienced with evaluating early breast carcinomas, consultation with a surgical oncologist is always in order.

Treatment of Breast Cancer
in Pregnancy

Once the diagnosis of cancer is made, the patient must be treated surgically without delay. In view of the large percentage of patients with positive nodes, the procedure should be one that provides adequate sampling of the axillary nodes, such as modified radical mastectomy. Simple mastectomy with axillary irradiation should be avoided. Therapeutic abortion is not routinely indicated. If, on the basis of surgical staging, adjuvant therapy is considered advisable, the decision must be made either to terminate the pregnancy by abortion or early delivery or to postpone therapy. Since delay in treatment is the principal known reason for the poorer prognosis of breast cancer in pregnancy, delivery should be accomplished as soon as there is a substantial probability of good fetal outcome—usually at 32–34 weeks. Most forms of cytotoxic therapy are absolutely contraindicated in pregnancy. Radiation can be given with appropriate shielding, but the dose to the fetus will not be negligible.

HYPERTENSIVE DISORDERS
OF PREGNANCY

Traditionally, gestational edema–proteinuria–hypertensive disorders have been termed preeclampsia or eclampsia, depending on whether the patient has had seizures. More recently, there is a trend toward classifying gestational hypertension according to the severity of diastolic hypertension, the degree of proteinuria, and the severity and cause of any underlying hypertensive disorder present before conception. The incidence of gestational hypertension is about 7%. Women at highest risk include primigravidas under 18 years old, multiparous women over 35 years old, black women, and women with twin gestations, diabetes, hydramnios, or prepregnancy hypertension. About half of women with prepregnancy hypertension develop exacerbations of hypertension in the third trimester.

Course of Hypertension in Pregnancy

In normal pregnancies, as well as those complicated by mild essential hypertension, diastolic blood pressure decreases 10–15 mm Hg in the second trimester. Hypertensive patients first seen at that time may be mistakenly identified as having pure gestational hypertension when the blood pressure again increases in the third trimester. Clinically, gestational hypertension usually appears after the 32nd week of gestation and, most frequently, during labor. In severe cases, especially those complicated by essential hypertension, acute rises in blood pressure may occur as early as 26 weeks. If hypertension appears in the first or early second trimester, it is associated either with gestational trophoblastic disease or an underlying disorder such as an acute flare-up of lupus nephritis. Occasionally, the onset of hypertension is recognized during the 24 hours following delivery.

In normal pregnancies, all of the components of the renin-angiotensin-aldosterone system are markedly elevated. In pregnancies complicated by essential hypertension or gestational hypertension, these components are reduced toward normal nonpregnant levels, reflecting an appropriate feedback response. The most consistent finding in women with hypertension in pregnancy is the increased sensitivity to angiotensin, in contrast to reduced sensitivity to angiotensin that is characteristic of normal pregnancy. Arteriolar constriction in response to angiotensin is diminished during normal pregnancy from the first trimester until delivery. In pregnancies destined to be complicated by hypertension, there is a gradual *increase* in arteriolar response to angiotensin that becomes statistically significant by 18–22 weeks of gestation—long before changes in blood pressure are detectable. The cause of this increase in vascular sensitivity to angiotensin is not known. It appears more likely that the unknown effector responsible for hyporesponsiveness to angiotensin in normal pregnancy is simply diminished in hypertensive pregnancies than that some uterine or placental "toxin" causes increased vascular responsiveness to angiotensin.

Symptoms & Signs

Signs of gestational hypertension include edema, a rise in diastolic blood pressure by 15 mm Hg or more over *first* trimester values, and proteinuria ranging from 1 to 10 g daily. Symptoms include headaches, visual disturbances, and epigastric pain. Eclampsia may occur even with mild to moderate hypertension and is associated with a maternal mortality rate as high as 10%, with deaths occurring most frequently from cerebral hemorrhage but also from renal failure, disseminated intravascular coagulopathy, acute pulmonary edema, or hepatic failure. The fetal perinatal mortality rate is in excess of 30%, and the risk of perinatal morbidity due to hypoxia is even higher.

Treatment of Gestational Hypertension

The only definitive therapy for gestational hypertension is delivery. If a modest increase in blood pressure first occurs in association with proteinuria at 32–36 weeks of gestation, bed rest, preferably in the left lateral decubitus position, is frequently effective in temporarily inducing diuresis and controlling progression of the disease, thus gaining time for the developing fetus. If labor occurs or induction of labor is attempted, parenteral magnesium sulfate should be used to prevent seizures and should be continued for 24 hours following delivery. Moderate hypertension need not be treated with antihypertensive agents; however, diastolic blood pressure above 120 mm Hg must be controlled to reduce the risk of intracranial hemorrhage. The agent of choice is hydralazine, 5 mg intravenously at 15- to 20-minute intervals, until the diastolic pressure is approximately 100 mm Hg. If hydralazine is unsuccessful, diazoxide or nitroprusside may be used, but these agents are almost never required.

Treatment of Essential Hypertension

Women with essential hypertension who become pregnant require special management. Chesley's recommendations are probably the best:

(1) Diastolic pressures under 100 mm Hg should not be treated. However, if a woman is receiving antihypertensive therapy when first seen in pregnancy, therapy should be continued. If she is taking propranolol, consideration may be given to switching to a more specific β_1-antagonist such as metoprolol or atenolol. The rare patient who has been taking ganglionic blockers should receive another form of therapy instead. Owing to a transient decrease in blood volume and placental perfusion associated with thiazide diuretics, use of these agents should usually not be initiated during pregnancy; however, if a woman is already receiving such therapy, it may be continued.

(2) Diastolic pressures above 100 mm Hg discovered during pregnancy call for antihypertensive management. Initial therapy should be with methyldopa, 250 mg orally at bedtime. This may be increased to 1 g twice daily as required. If unacceptable drowsiness lasting more than 2–3 days occurs, the dosage may be reduced, and hydralazine, beginning at 10 mg orally twice daily and increasing up to 100 mg twice daily, may be added. If hydralazine is not tolerated, prazosin may be gradually added to the methyldopa therapy.

(3) Accelerated hypertension at any stage of gestation should be managed with bed rest and, if necessary, intravenous hydralazine. Unless diastolic pressure can be reduced to 110 mm Hg promptly, delivery should be performed regardless of gestational age.

Prognosis

The prognosis for hypertensive cardiovascular disease in later life in women with gestational hypertension depends on the patient's age and parity. Gestational hypertension in the young primigravida is not associated with an increased risk of hypertension in later pregnancies or in later life. Hypertension in later pregnancies is associated with an increased risk of essential hypertension in later life. However, if the hypertensive pregnancy was complicated by multiple gestation or trophoblastic disease, there is no increased risk of later hypertension.

HYPERTHYROIDISM IN PREGNANCY

Pregnancy mimics hyperthyroidism. There is thyroid enlargement, increased cardiac output, and peripheral vasodilatation. Owing to the increase in thyroid hormone–binding globulin (TBG), total serum thyroxine is in the range expected for hyperthyroidism. Free thyroxine, the free thyroxine index, and TSH levels, however, remain in the normal range (see Chapter 7).

Hyperthyroidism complicates one or 2 per 1000 pregnancies. The most common form of hyperthyroidism during pregnancy is Graves' disease. Hyperthyroidism is associated with an increased risk of premature delivery (11–25%) and may modestly increase the risk of early abortion. In Graves' disease, thyroid-stimulating immunoglobulin (TSI), also known as long-acting thyroid stimulator (LATS), a 7S globulin, crosses the placenta and may cause fetal goiter and transient neonatal hyperthyroidism, but these effects do not seriously jeopardize the fetus.

Treatment

The treatment of maternal hyperthyroidism is complicated by pregnancy. Radioiodides are strictly contraindicated. Iodide therapy can lead to huge fetal goiter and is contraindicated except as acute therapy to prevent thyroid storm before thyroid surgery. All antithyroid drugs cross the placenta and may cause fetal hypothyroidism and goiter or cretinism in the newborn. However, propylthiouracil in doses of 300 mg/d or less has been shown to be reasonably safe, although even at low doses about 10% of newborns will have detectable goiter. Propranolol has been used to control maternal cardiovascular symptoms but may result in fetal bradycardia, growth retardation, premature labor, and neonatal respiratory depression. Partial or total thyroidectomy, especially in the second trimester, is a reasonably safe procedure except for the risk of premature labor.

A. Propylthiouracil: A reasonable plan of management is to begin therapy with propylthiouracil in doses high enough to bring the free T_4 index into the mildly hyperthyroid range and then to taper the dose gradually. Giving thyroxine along with propylthiouracil in the hope that it will cross the placenta in sufficient quantities to prevent fetal hypothyroidism is not effective and serves only to increase the amount of propylthiouracil required. If the maintenance dose of propylthiouracil is above 300 mg/d, serious consideration should be given to partial thyroidectomy.

B. Propranolol: Propranolol may be used transiently to ameliorate cardiovascular symptoms while control is being achieved.

Management of Newborn

Newborns should be observed carefully. In infants of mothers given propylthiouracil, even equivocal evidence of hypothyroidism is an indication for thyroxine replacement therapy. Neonatal Graves' disease requires intensive therapy (see Chapter 7).

HYPOTHYROIDISM IN PREGNANCY

Hypothyroidism is uncommon in pregnancy, since most women with the untreated disorder are oligo-ovulatory. As a practical matter, women taking thyroid medication at the time of conception should be maintained on the same dose throughout pregnancy, whether or not the obstetrician believes thyroid replacement was originally indicated. Physiologic doses of thyroid are innocuous, but maternal hypothyroidism may be hazardous to the developing fetus. The correlation between maternal and fetal thyroid status is poor, and hypothyroid mothers frequently deliver euthyroid infants. The strongest correlation between maternal and newborn hypothyroidism occurs in areas where endemic goiter due to iodide deficiency is common. In these regions, dietary iodide supplementation in addition to thyroid hormone treatment of the mother may be of the greatest importance in preventing cretinism.

DIABETES MELLITUS & PREGNANCY
John L. Kitzmiller, MD

Hormone & Fuel Balance During Normal Pregnancy

Pregnancy produces major changes in the homeostasis of all metabolic fuels and in this way affects the management of diabetes. Plasma concentrations of glucose in the **postabsorptive state** decline as pregnancy advances, because of increasing placental uptake of glucose and a probable limitation on hepatic glucose output. Therefore, fasting hypoglycemia is more common during pregnancy. Gluconeogenesis could be limited by a relative lack of the major substrate alanine. The plasma concentration of alanine has been shown in some studies to be lower during pregnancy, probably as a result of placental uptake and a restraint on proteolysis. Although fat deposition is accentuated in early pregnancy, lipolysis is enhanced by human placental lactogen (hPL) later in gestation, and more glycerol and free fatty acids are released in the postabsorptive state. Ketogenesis is thus accentuated in the postabsorptive state during pregnancy, probably secondary to increased provision of substrate free fatty acids and hormonal effects on the maternal liver cells.

The balance of metabolic fuels is also different in the **fed state** during pregnancy. Despite hyperinsulinism in normal pregnancy, the disposal of glucose is impaired, producing somewhat higher maternal blood levels. The contra-insulin effects of gestation have been related to hPL, progesterone, and cortisol. The disappearance in plasma of administered insulin is not greater during pregnancy, despite the presence of placental insulin receptors and degrading enzymes. Glucagon is well suppressed by glucose during pregnancy, and secretory responses of glucagon to amino acids are not increased above nonpregnant levels. After meals, more glucose is converted to triglyceride in pregnant compared with nonpregnant animals, which would tend to conserve calories and enhance fat deposition. Insulin resistance during pregnancy apparently does not extend to the lipogenic and antilipolytic effects of the hormone.

Overview of Diabetes During Pregnancy

Diabetic pregnant women have been classified on the basis of duration and severity of diabetes (Table 17–3). A classification system (White) was originally used for prognosis of perinatal outcome and to de-

Table 17—3. Classification of diabetes during pregnancy (Priscilla White).

Class	Characteristics	Implications
Gestational diabetes	Abnormal glucose tolerance during pregnancy; postprandial hyperglycemia during pregnancy.	Diagnosis before 30 weeks' gestation important to prevent macrosomia. Treat with diet adequate in calories to prevent maternal weight loss. Goal is postprandial blood glucose <130 mg/dL at 1 hour or <105 mg/dL at 2 hours. If insulin is necessary, manage as in classes B, C, and D.
A	Chemical diabetes diagnosed before pregnancy; managed by diet alone; any age at onset.	Management as for gestational diabetes.
B	Insulin treatment or oral hypoglycemic agent used before pregnancy; onset at age 20 or older; duration <10 years.	Some endogenous insulin secretion may persist. Fetal and neonatal risks same as in classes C and D, as is management; can be type I or II.
C	Onset at age 10—20, or duration 10—20 years.	Insulin-deficient diabetes of juvenile onset; type I.
D	Onset before age 10, or duration >20 years, or chronic hypertension (not preeclampsia), or background retinopathy (tiny hemorrhages).	Fetal macrosomia or intrauterine growth retardation possible. Retinal microaneurysms, dot hemorrhages, and exudates may progress during pregnancy, then regress after delivery.
F	Diabetic nephropathy with proteinuria.	Anemia and hypertension common; proteinuria increases in third trimester, declines after delivery. Fetal intrauterine growth retardation common; perinatal survival about 85% under optimal conditions; bed rest necessary.
H	Coronary artery disease.	Serious maternal risk.
R	Proliferative retinopathy.	Neovascularization, with risk of vitreous hemorrhage or retinal detachment; laser photocoagulation useful; abortion usually not necessary. With active process of neovascularization, prevent bearing-down efforts.

termine obstetric management. Because the perinatal mortality rate has declined dramatically for many reasons in women in all classes, the system is now used mainly to describe and compare populations of diabetic pregnant women. However, certain characteristics of patients are still pertinent. The risk of complications is minimal if gestational diabetes is well controlled by diet alone, and these patients may be otherwise managed as normal pregnant women. Class B patients, whose insulin dependence is of recent onset, will probably have residual islet B cell function, and control of hyperglycemia may be easier than in class C or D patients; however, fetal and neonatal risks are generally equivalent. Finally, the most complicated and difficult pregnancies occur in women with renal, retinal, or cardiovascular disease.

The hormonal and metabolic effects of pregnancy are associated with increased risks of both hypoglycemic reactions and ketoacidosis. Increasing amounts of insulin are usually required to control hyperglycemia throughout gestation.

If diabetes is poorly controlled in the first weeks of pregnancy, the risks of spontaneous abortion and congenital malformation of the infant are increased. Later in pregnancy, polyhydramnios is also common in women with poorly controlled diabetes and may lead to preterm delivery. Fetal distress may develop in the third trimester, especially if diabetic control has been inadequate. Careful fetal monitoring must be used to prevent stillbirths. The high incidence of fetal macrosomia (birth weight > 90th percentile for gestational age) increases the potential for traumatic vaginal delivery; primary cesarean deliveries are more common in these cases. Fetal intrauterine growth retardation may occur in diabetic women with vascular disease.

Other neonatal risks include respiratory distress syndrome, hypoglycemia, hyperbilirubinemia, hypocalcemia, and poor feeding; however, these problems are limited to the first days of life, and childhood development is usually normal. Despite these possible complications, diabetic women now have a 97–98% chance of delivering a healthy child if they adhere to a program of careful management and surveillance.

In the following sections, the convention used for designating the number of weeks of gestation is the number of weeks from the last menstrual period.

Gestational Diabetes

The hormonal and metabolic changes of pregnancy result in the diagnosis of glucose intolerance during the second half of gestation in 2–3% of pregnant women. Criteria for diagnosis are given in Table 17–4. It is unclear whether gestational diabetes results from inadequate insulin response to carbohydrate load, from excessive resistance to the action of insulin, or from both. Once the diagnosis has been made, the patient should be placed on a diabetic diet modified for pregnancy: 25–35 kcal/kg ideal weight, 40–55% carbohydrate, 20% protein, and 25–40% fat. Calories are distributed over 3 meals and 3 snacks (Table 17–5). The goal of therapy is not weight reduction but prevention of both fasting and postprandial hyperglycemia. If 1-hour or 2-hour postprandial glucose values are consistently greater than 130 or 105 mg/dL, respectively, it is necessary to determine if the "hyperglycemia" will persist on the same diet given in the hospital. If the diet fails to prevent hyperglycemia, therapy is begun with human insulin, and the patient is managed as if insulin-dependent.

The risk of developing overt diabetes later in life is influenced by body weight. Follow-up studies in-

Table 17–4. Diagnosis of gestational diabetes.

Screening with glucose loading test:

Indications: (1) Screen all gravidas **or** (2) screen all gravidas who are overweight* or over 25 years of age (misses 10% of cases) **plus** all gravidas with glycosuria, a family history of diabetes (in parents, siblings, aunts, or uncles), or a history of stillbirth or macrosomic infant (misses 40% of cases).

Procedure: Give 50 g of glucose by mouth at 24–26 weeks' gestation. Measure plasma glucose 1 hour later. If value exceeds 140 mg/dL, give the oral glucose tolerance test.

Oral glucose tolerance test:

Procedure: Give 100 g of glucose by mouth. Normal values for plasma or serum glucose† are as follows:

fasting, 105 mg/dL
1 hour, 190 mg/dL
2 hours, 165 mg/dL
3 hours, 145 mg/dL

Results are abnormal if 2 values are elevated above limits listed.

Caution: Glucose should not be given if fasting blood glucose is > 130 mg/dL.

*Overweight = height under 165 cm with weight over 68 kg (< 5 ft 5 in, > 150 lb) in first trimester; height over 165 cm with weight over 81 kg (> 5 ft 5 in, > 180 lb) in first trimester.
†Criteria of National Diabetes Data Group (NIH). (See *Diabetes* 1979;**28**:1039.)

dicate that 5–15% of nonobese gestational diabetics will need treatment in 5–20 years, compared to 35–50% of gestational diabetic women with a body weight greater than 120% of ideal. This suggests the possibility of preventive benefits of achieving weight loss after pregnancy and lactation.

Insulin Management

The goal of insulin therapy during pregnancy is to prevent both fasting and postprandial hyperglycemia and to avoid debilitating hypoglycemic reactions. The level of glucose control that will yield the least maternal and perinatal morbidity has not yet been established. However, most experts believe that one should aim for fasting plasma glucose levels below 105 mg/dL and postprandial levels below 140 mg/dL. Self-monitoring of capillary blood glucose at home with glucose oxidase strips and portable reflectance colorimeters has proved a reliable means of helping patients monitor the course of therapy. Since glycosylated hemoglobin correlates with mean daily capillary blood glucose over a few weeks during pregnancy, sequential measurement will provide another indicator of long-term control. Yet because insulin dosage must be frequently adjusted up or down during the metabolically dynamic state of pregnancy, capillary blood glucose must be measured several times each day to assist in the "fine-tuning" of insulin management.

Most pregnant insulin-dependent patients will require at least 2 injections of about a 1:2 mixture of regular and intermediate insulin each day in order to prevent fasting and postprandial hyperglycemia. The usual practice is to give two-thirds of the insulin before breakfast and one-third before supper (Table 17–6). More stringent regimens of administering regular subcutaneous insulin 4–6 times each day or continuously with a portable insulin pump are under investigation.

Hypoglycemic reactions are more frequent and sometimes more severe in early pregnancy. Therefore, patients must keep glucagon on hand, and a member of the household must be instructed in the technique of injection. Hypoglycemic reactions have not been associated with fetal death or congenital anomalies.

Fetal Development & Growth

Major congenital anomalies are those which may severely affect the life of the individual or require major surgery for correction. The incidence of major congenital anomalies in infants of diabetic mothers is 6–12%, compared with 2% in infants of a nondiabetic population. While perinatal deaths due to stillbirth and respiratory distress syndrome have declined in pregnancies complicated by diabetes, the proportion of fetal and neonatal deaths ascribed to congenital anomalies has risen to 50–80%. The types of anomalies most common in infants of diabetic mothers and their presumed time of occurrence during embryonic development are listed in Table 17–7. It is apparent that any intervention to reduce the incidence of major congenital anomalies must be applied very early in pregnancy. The additional finding that the excess risk of anomalies is associated with the group of diabetic women with elevated glycosylated hemoglobin early in pregnancy suggests that poor diabetic control is related to the risk of major congenital anomalies in infants of diabetic mothers. Protocols of intensive diabetic management instituted prior to conception and continued through early pregnancy have resulted in significant reduction in the frequency of anomalies. This means that primary care physicians treating women of reproductive age must evaluate them for the possibility of becoming pregnant and inform them

Table 17–5. Management of diet for patients with gestational diabetes.

(1) Assess present pattern of food consumption.
(2) Balance calories with optimal weight gain.
   (a) Caloric intake: 25–35 kcal/kg ideal weight.
   (b) Weight gain: 0.45 kg (1 lb) per month during the first trimester; 0.2–0.35 kg (0.5–0.75 lb) per week during the second and third trimesters.
(3) Distribute calories and carbohydrates over 3 meals and 3 snacks; evening snack to include complex carbohydrate and at least one meat exchange.
(4) Use food exchanges to assess the amount of carbohydrate, protein, and fat:
   (a) Carbohydrate: 40–55% of calories or ≥ 150 g/d.
   (b) Protein: 20% of calories or ≥ 74 g/d.
   (c) Fat: 25–40% of calories.
(5) Emphasize high-fiber, complex carbohydrate foods.
(6) Identify individual glycemic responses to certain foods.
(7) Tailor eating plans to personal needs.

Table 17–6. Illustration of use of home blood glucose monitoring to determine insulin dosage during pregnancy.

Self-Monitored Capillary Blood Glucose		Insulin Doses
Fasting blood glucose	148 mg/dL	14 units regular, 28 units intermediate
1 h after breakfast	206 mg/dL	
1 h after lunch	152 mg/dL	
1 h after supper	198 mg/dL	9 units regular, 10 units intermediate
2–4 AM	142 mg/dL	

Suggested changes based on pattern of blood glucose values over 2–3 days: slight increases in presupper intermediate insulin to control fasting blood glucose next day, in morning regular insulin to control postbreakfast glucose, and in presupper regular insulin to control postsupper hyperglycemia. Dose of morning intermediate insulin is adequate to control early afternoon blood glucose. When dose of presupper intermediate insulin is increased, patient should test to detect and prevent nocturnal hypoglycemia. One-hour postprandial testing is advised to detect the probable peaks of glycemic excursions. Patient should also test when symptoms of hypoglycemia appear.

of the risks related to the level of hyperglycemia.

Ultrasonography in the first half of pregnancy may detect neural tube defects (anencephaly, meningomyelocele) that occur with a higher than normal incidence in infants of diabetic mothers. The physician should also screen all insulin-dependent pregnant women for elevated serum alpha-fetoprotein levels at 14–16 weeks of gestation to detect other cases of neural tube defects. Later in pregnancy, sophisticated ultrasonographic examinations may detect congenital heart defects or other anomalies.

The initial ultrasonographic examination at 18–20 weeks confirms the dating of gestation, and subsequent examinations at 26 and 36 weeks measure fetal growth. Many of these infants are large for dates, ie, macrosomic infants with increased fat stores, increased length, and increased abdomen-to-head or thorax-to-head ratios. The hypothesis that fetal macrosomia results from the causal chain of maternal hyperglycemia → fetal hyperglycemia → fetal hyperinsulinemia → fetal macrosomia has long been debated. Excess insulin increases fetal fat deposition. Macrosomic infants of diabetic mothers have significantly higher concentrations of C peptide in their cord sera or amniotic fluid (representing endogenous insulin secretion) than do infants of diabetic mothers with birth weights appropriate for gestational age. The determinants of fetal hyperinsulinemia throughout pregnancy may not be simply maternal hyperglycemia, however. Other metabolic substrates that cross the placenta and are insulinogenic (eg, branched-chain amino acids) may play a role in fetal macrosomia, and transplacental lipids could contribute to fat deposition.

The degree of maternal glycemia is related to birth weights of infants of diabetic mothers, as adjusted for gestational age. This suggests that prevention of maternal hyperglycemia throughout pregnancy may re-

duce the incidence of macrosomia. Pilot studies of highly selected patients have shown this to be the case in many but not all instances. The metabolic and nutritional determinants of birth weights of infants of diabetic mothers other than maternal glucose are under study.

Polyhydramnios is an excess volume of amniotic fluid (> 1000 mL, often > 3000 mL). It may cause severe discomfort or premature labor and is most often associated with fetal macrosomia. The excess volume of amniotic fluid was not related to the concentration of glucose or other solutes in amniotic fluid or to excess fetal urine output as measured by change in bladder size by means of ultrasonography in one study. Additional possible factors in causation of polyhydramnios in diabetic pregnancies include fetal swallowing, decidual and amniotic fluid PRL, and as yet unknown determinants of the complicated multicompartmental intrauterine transfer of water. However, diuretics do little to mobilize excessive amniotic fluid. Polyhydramnios is rare in women with well-controlled diabetes.

In contrast to fetal macrosomia, the fetus of a woman with diabetes of long duration and vascular disease may suffer intrauterine growth retardation. This problem is apparently related to inadequate uteroplacental perfusion. All body diameters may be below normal on ultrasonographic measurements; oligohydramnios is common; and after 30 weeks of gestation, maternal plasma or urinary estriol levels are usually below the 95% confidence limits for stage of gestation.

Table 17–7. Congenital malformations in infants of diabetic mothers.*

	Ratio of Incidences Diabetic vs Control Group	Latest Gestational Age for Occurrence (Weeks After Menstruation)
Caudal regression	252	5
Anencephaly	3	6
Spina bifida, hydrocephalus, or other central nervous system defects	2	6
Cardiac anomalies	4	
Transposition of great vessels		7
Ventricular septal defect		8
Atrial septal defect		8
Anal/rectal atresia	3	8
Renal anomalies	5	
Agenesis	6	7
Cystic kidney	4	7
Ureter duplex	23	7
Situs inversus	84	6

*Modified and reproduced, with permission, from Kucera J: Rate and type of congenital anomalies among offspring of diabetic women. *J Reprod Med* 1971;**7**:61; and Mills JL, Baker L, Goldman AS: Malformations in infants of diabetic mothers occur before the seventh gestational week: Implications for treatment. *Diabetes* 1979;**28**:292.

Obstetric Management

Not long ago, the incidence of apparently sudden intrauterine fetal demise in the third trimester of diabetic pregnancies was at least 5%. Since the risk increased as pregnancies approached term, preterm delivery was instituted but risk of neonatal death from respiratory distress syndrome increased. Curiously, the cause of stillbirth was usually not obvious. The risk was greater with poor diabetic control, and the incidence of fetal death exceeded 50% with ketoacidosis. Some instances of fetal demise were associated with preeclampsia, which is a common complication of diabetic pregnancy. Fetal death was also associated with pyelonephritis, which is now largely prevented by screening for and treating asymptomatic bacteriuria. Other than these known risk factors, one can speculate that fetal distress was related to (1) a combination of relative fetal hypoxia and hyperglycemia or (2) fetal myocardial dysfunction.

Advances during the past decade have led to techniques for detecting fetal distress and preventing stillbirth. The infrequency of fetal movement as noted in fetal activity determinations (< 4/h) may indicate fetal jeopardy. More quantitative studies of fetal activity patterns using ultrasonography are under investigation.

Maternal estriol assays were also used for fetal evaluation, based on the knowledge that placental production of estriol is dependent on precursors from the fetal adrenals. It has been demonstrated that the maternal 24-hour urine estriol level correlates with the mass of the fetal-placental unit and that a 40% or greater drop in maternal plasma or urinary estriol level usually precedes fetal demise in pregnancies complicated by diabetes. However, owing to the rapid changes in estriol production, maternal estriol levels must be measured daily to be of any value in anticipating and preventing stillbirth.

The primary mode of fetal assessment is antepartum fetal heart rate monitoring. The presence of fetal heart rate accelerations and good long-range variability on the nonstress test (NST) and the absence of late decelerations (lower rate persists after the contraction subsides) on the contraction stress test (CST) almost always suggest that the fetus is well oxygenated and has a low risk of dying within several days. However, the predictive value of normal test results is only valid for a short duration in diabetic women with unstable metabolic control or hypertension. Generally, the NST and CST are sensitive screening tests, and abnormal results in these tests of fetal heart monitoring will overestimate the diagnosis of fetal distress. Therefore, some authorities require that additional evidence of fetal distress (by estriol assay or by biophysical ultrasonographic assessment) be obtained before intervention in preterm pregnancies can be recommended.

Insulin-dependent diabetic patients were usually admitted to the hospital at 36 weeks' gestation or earlier for fetal monitoring and careful control of diabetes. However, normotensive women achieving very good control (fasting blood glucose about 100 mg/dL, 1-hour postprandial blood glucose < 140 mg/dL) with self-monitoring of blood glucose levels have no excess risk of fetal distress and do not require antepartum admission to the hospital.

Unless maternal or fetal complications arise, the goal for the termination of pregnancy should be 38 weeks or even later, in order to reduce neonatal morbidity from preterm deliveries. On the other hand, the obstetrician may wish to induce labor before 38 weeks if he or she is concerned about increasing fetal weight. Before the delivery decision is made, fetal pulmonary maturity should be determined. The standard test for pulmonary maturity is the lecithin/sphingomyelin (L/S) ratio, in which a value greater than 2 indicates a low risk for respiratory distress syndrome. However, in pregnancies complicated by diabetes, many authors have reported a false-positive rate of 6–12% with L/S values between 2 and 3. The reason for the discrepancy is unknown, but the lowest risk for respiratory distress syndrome is attained by delaying delivery (if possible) until the L/S ratio becomes abnormally high (> 3.5). The false-negative rate for L/S ratios of 1.5–2.0 is at least 50% in nondiabetic pregnancies (ie, delivery occurs within 72 hours, but respiratory distress syndrome does not develop). Other amniotic fluid assays (eg, measurement of phosphatidylglycerol) can be used to evaluate the risk for respiratory distress syndrome. If phosphatidylglycerol is present in the amniotic fluid, the risk is low even if the L/S ratio is below 3.5.

Once fetal lung maturity is likely, the route of delivery must be selected based on the usual obstetric indications. If the fetus seems large on clinical and ultrasonographic examination (> 4000 g), primary cesarean section probably should be performed because of the possibility of shoulder dystocia. Otherwise, induction of labor is reasonable, because maternal and peripartum risks are fewer following vaginal delivery. Once labor is under way, continuous fetal heart rate monitoring (with scalp pH backup measurements) must be performed.

Traditional insulin management for labor and delivery has been to give only one-third to one-half the prepregnancy dose in the morning. The diabetic parturient may be unusually sensitive to insulin during active labor and delivery, and insulin shock is possible if delivery occurs sooner than anticipated. Protocols for continuous low-dose intravenous insulin administration during labor or prior to cesarean delivery are being appraised to determine whether stringent control of blood glucose will reduce the incidence of intrapartum fetal distress and neonatal metabolic problems. A cord blood glucose level at delivery correlates positively with the higher maternal levels, and there does not seem to be an upper limit on placental transfer of glucose. During labor, maternal plasma glucose can usually be kept below 100 mg/dL with 1–2 units of regular insulin and 7.5 g of dextrose given intravenously every hour. If cesarean section is necessary, insulin management is similar, and infants do equally well with general, spinal, or epidural anesthesia. Nonetheless, the anesthesiologist should be cautioned against the administration of copious glucose-containing intravenous solutions.

Neonatal Morbidity

Planning for the care of infants of diabetic mothers should begin prior to delivery, with participation by the neonatologist in decisions about timing and management of delivery. The pediatrician must be in attendance to know of antenatal problems, to assess the need for resuscitation, and to determine major congenital anomalies.

Infants of diabetic mothers have an increased risk of respiratory distress syndrome compared with infants of matched nondiabetic mothers. Possible reasons include abnormal production of pulmonary surfactant or connective tissue changes leading to decreased pulmonary compliance. The relationship of fetal metabolic characteristics to pulmonary abnormalities in the environment of maternal diabetes is not yet clear. However, in recent years, the incidence of respiratory distress syndrome has declined from 24% to 5%, probably related to use of the L/S ratio and delivery of most infants at term (see above). The diagnosis of respiratory distress syndrome is based on clinical signs (grunting, retraction, respiratory rate > 60/min), typical findings on chest x-ray (diffuse reticulogranular pattern and air bronchogram), and an increased oxygen requirement (to maintain the P_aO_2 at 50–70 mm Hg) for more than 48 hours with no other identified cause of respiratory difficulty (heart disease, infection). Survival of infants with respiratory distress syndrome has dramatically improved as a result of advances in ventilation therapy.

Hypoglycemia is common in the first 48 hours after delivery and is defined as blood glucose below 30 mg/dL regardless of gestational age. The symptomatic infant may be lethargic rather than jittery, and hypoglycemia may be associated with apnea, tachypnea, cyanosis, or seizures. Hypoglycemia has been related to elevated fetal insulin levels during and after delivery. Nevertheless, infants of diabetic mothers may also have deficient catecholamine and glucagon secretion, and the hypoglycemia may be related to diminished hepatic glucose production and oxidation of free fatty acids. The neonatologist attempts to prevent hypoglycemia in "well" infants with early feedings of 10% dextrose in water by bottle or gavage by 1 hour of age. If this is not successful, treatment with glucagon injections or intravenous dextrose solutions is indicated. Rigid control of diabetes to prevent fetal hyperglycemia may reduce the incidence of neonatal hypoglycemia. There are usually no long-term sequelae of episodes of neonatal hypoglycemia.

Other frequent problems in infants of diabetic mothers include hypocalcemia (< 7 mg/dL), hyperbilirubinemia (> 15 mg/dL), polycythemia (central hematocrit > 70%), and poor feeding. Further investigation is necessary to determine the cause of these problems. Better control of the maternal diabetic state in the future should reduce their incidence.

REFERENCES

General

Burrow GN, Ferris TF (editors): *Medical Complications During Pregnancy*, 2nd ed. Saunders, 1982.

Chez RA (editor): Fetal and placental endocrinology. *Clin Obstet Gynecol* 1980;**23**:719.

Goebelsmann U: Protein and steroid hormones in pregnancy. *J Reprod Med* 1979;**23**:166.

Jaffe RB: Endocrine-metabolic alterations induced by pregnancy. Chap 24–26, pp 735–788, in: *Reproductive Endocrinology: Physiology, Pathophysiology, and Clinical Management*, 2nd ed. Yen SSC, Jaffe RB (editors). Saunders, 1986.

Milne JA (editor): The physiologic response to pregnancy in health and disease. Proceedings of a symposium arranged by the Department of Obstetrics and Gynaecology, University of Cambridge, Sept 15–16, 1978. *Postgrad Med J* 1979;**55**:293. [Entire issue.]

Tulchinsky D, Ryan KJ (editors): *Maternal-Fetal Endocrinology*. Saunders, 1980.

Chorionic Proteins & Pregnancy Tests

Derman R, Edelman DA, Berger GS: Current status of immunologic pregnancy tests. *Int J Gynaecol Obstet* 1979; **17**:190.

Fisher DA: Maternal-fetal thyroid function in pregnancy. *Clin Perinatol* 1983;**10**:615.

Harada A et al: Comparison of thyroid stimulators and thyroid hormone concentrations in the sera of pregnant women. *J Clin Endocrinol Metab* 1979;**48**:793.

Healy DL, Hodgen GD: The endocrinology of human endometrium. *Obstet Gynecol Surv* 1983;**38**:509.

Horne CHW, Nisbet AD: Pregnancy proteins: A review. *Invest Cell Pathol* 1979;**2**:217.

Hsueh AJW, Jones PBC: Gonadotropin-releasing hormone: Extrapituitary actions and paracrine control mechanisms. *Annu Rev Physiol* 1983;**45**:83.

Siler-Khodr TM: Hypothalamic-like releasing hormones of the placenta. *Clin Perinatol* 1983;**10**:533.

Weiss G: Relaxin. *Annu Rev Physiol* 1984;**46**:43.

Steroid Hormones

Bammann BL, Coulam CB, Jiang NS: Total and free testosterone during pregnancy. *Am J Obstet Gynecol* 1980; **137**:293.

Buster JE: Gestational changes in steroid hormone biosynthesis, secretion, metabolism, and action. *Clin Perinatol* 1983;**10**:527.

Laatikainen T et al: Fetal and maternal serum levels of steroid sulfates, unconjugated steroids and prolactin at term pregnancy and in early spontaneous labor. *J Clin Endocrinol Metab* 1980;**50**:489.

Lind T: Clinical chemistry of pregnancy. *Adv Clin Chem* 1980;**21**:1.

Nolten WE, Holt LH, Rueckert PA: Desoxycorticosterone in normal pregnancy. 3. Evidence of a fetal source of desoxycorticosterone. *Am J Obstet Gynecol* 1981;**139**:477.

Parker CR et al: Hormone production during pregnancy in the primigravid patient. 2. Plasma levels of desoxycorticosterone throughout pregnancy of normal women and women who developed pregnancy-induced hypertension. *Am J Obstet Gynecol* 1980;**138**:626.

Siiteri PK et al: Progesterone and maintenance of pregnancy: Is progesterone nature's immunosuppressant? *Ann NY Acad Sci* 1977;**286**:384.

Fetal Endocrinology

Jaffe RB: Fetoplacental endocrine and metabolic physiology. *Clin Perinatol* 1983;**10**:669.

Serón-Ferré M, Jaffe RB: The fetal adrenal gland. *Annu Rev Physiol* 1981;**43**:141.

Parturition

Challis JRG: Endocrinology of late pregnancy and parturition. In: *Reproductive Physiology, III. International Review of Physiology*. Vol 22. Greep RO (editor). University Park Press, 1980.

Fuchs AR: Hormonal control of myometrial function during pregnancy and parturition. *Acta Endocrinol [Suppl]* 1978;**89**:1.

Garfield RE et al: Hormonal control of GAP junction formation in sheep myometrium during parturition. *Biol Reprod* 1979;**21**:999.

Liggins GC: Initiation of parturition. *Br Med Bull* 1979;**35**:145.

Liggins GC et al: Control of parturition in man. *Biol Reprod* 1977;**16**:39.

Ryan KJ: New concepts in hormonal control of parturition. *Biol Reprod* 1977;**16**:88.

Thorburn G, Challis JRG: Endocrine control of parturition. *Physiol Rev* 1979;**59**:863.

Puerperium & Lactation

Duchesne C, Leke R: Bromocriptine mesylate for prevention of postpartum lactation. *Obstet Gynecol* 1981;**57**:464.

Harrison RG: Suppression of lactation. *Semin Perinatol* 1979;**3**:287.

Monheit AG, Cousins L, Resnick R: The puerperium, anatomic and physiologic readjustments. *Clin Obstet Gynecol* 1980;**23**:973.

Tucker HA: Endocrinology of lactation. *Semin Perinatol* 1979;**3**:199.

Vance ML, Evans WS, Thorner MO: Bromocriptine. *Ann Intern Med* 1984;**100**:78.

Vorherr H: Hormonal and biochemical changes of pituitary and breast during pregnancy. *Semin Perinatol* 1979;**3**:193.

Pituitary Adenomas

Barbieri RL, Ryan KJ: Bromocriptine: Endocrine pharmacology and therapeutic applications. *Fertil Steril* 1983;**39**:727.

Johnston DG et al: Hyperprolactinemia: Long-term effects of bromocriptine. *Am J Med* 1983;**75**:868.

Marshall JR: Pregnancy in patients with prolactin-producing pituitary tumors. *Clin Obstet Gynecol* 1980;**23**:453.

Breast Cancer & Pregnancy

Cooper DR, Butterfield J: Pregnancy subsequent to mastectomy for cancer of the breast. *Ann Surg* 1970;**171**:429.

Donegan WL: Breast cancer and pregnancy. *Obstet Gynecol* 1977;**50**:244.

Hochman A, Schreiber H: Pregnancy and cancer of the breast. *Obstet Gynecol* 1953;**2**:268.

Holleb AI, Farrow JH: The relation of carcinoma of the breast and pregnancy in 283 patients. *Surg Gynecol Obstet* 1962;**115**:65.

Wynder EL, Bross IJ, Hirayama T: A study of the epidemiology of cancer of the breast. *Cancer* 1960;**13**:559.

Zinns JS: The association of pregnancy and breast cancer. *J Reprod Med* 1979;**22**:297.

Hypertensive Disorders

Carr BR, Gant NF: The endocrinology of pregnancy-induced hypertension. *Clin Perinatol* 1983;**10**:737.

Chesley LC: The control of hypertension in pregnancy. *Obstet Gynecol Annu* 1981;**10**:67.

Roberts JM: Pregnancy-related hypertension. Pages 703–752 in: *Maternal-Fetal Medicine: Principles and Practice*. Creasy RK, Resnick R (editors). Saunders, 1984.

Sullivan JM: The hypertensive diseases of pregnancy and their management. *Adv Intern Med* 1982;**27**:407.

Symonds EM: The renin-angiotensin system in pregnancy. *Obstet Gynecol Annu* 1981;**10**:45.

Wilson M et al: Blood pressure, the renin-aldosterone system and sex steroids throughout normal pregnancy. *Am J Med* 1980;**68**:97.

Worley AJ et al: Vascular responsiveness to pressor agents during human pregnancy. *J Reprod Med* 1979;**23**:115.

Hyperthyroidism in Pregnancy

Burrow GN: Hyperthyroidism during pregnancy. *N Engl J Med* 1978;**298**:150.

Cheron RG et al: Neonatal thyroid function after propylthiouracil therapy for maternal Graves' disease. *N Engl J Med* 1981;**304**:525.

Stoffer SS, Hamburger JI: Inadvertent ^{131}I therapy for hyperthyroidism in the first trimester of pregnancy. *J Nucl Med* 1976;**17**:146.

Sugrue D, Drury MI: Hyperthyroidism complicating pregnancy: Results of treatment by antithyroid drugs on 77 pregnancies. *Br J Obstet Gynaecol* 1980;**87**:970.

Diabetes Mellitus & Pregnancy

Algert S, Shragg P, Hollingsworth DR: Moderate caloric restriction in obese women with gestational diabetes. *Obstet Gynecol* 1985;**65**:487.

Cheney C, Shragg P, Hollingsworth D: Demonstration of heterogeneity in gestational diabetes by a 400-kcal breakfast meal tolerance test. *Obstet Gynecol* 1985;**65**:17.

Cousins L et al: Glycosylated hemoglobin as a screening test for carbohydrate intolerance in pregnancy. *Am J Obstet Gynecol* 1984;**150**:455.

Dibble CM et al: Effect of pregnancy on diabetic retinopathy. *Obstet Gynecol* 1982;**59**:699.

Eriksson UJ: Congenital malformations in diabetic animal models: A review. *Diabetes Res* 1984;**1**:57.

Fuhrmann K et al: Prevention of congenital malformations in infants of insulin-dependent diabetic mothers. *Diabetes Care* 1983;**6**:219.

Gabbe SG et al: Management and outcome of class A diabetes mellitus. *Am J Obstet Gynecol* 1977;**127**:465.

Gabbe SG et al: Management and outcome of pregnancy in diabetes mellitus, classes B to R. *Am J Obstet Gynecol* 1977;**129**:723.

Jovanovic L, Peterson CM: Optimal insulin delivery for the pregnant diabetic patient. *Diabetes Care* 1982;**5(Suppl)**:24.

Kitzmiller JL: The endocrine pancreas and maternal metabolism. Pages 56–83 in: *Maternal-Fetal Endocrinology*. Tulchinsky DT, Ryan KJ (editors). Saunders, 1980.

Kitzmiller JL et al: Diabetic nephropathy and perinatal outcome. *Am J Obstet Gynecol* 1981;**141**:741.

Kitzmiller JL et al: Diabetic pregnancy and perinatal morbidity. *Am J Obstet Gynecol* 1978;**131**:560.

Merkatz IR, Adam PAJ: *The Diabetic Pregnancy: A Perinatal Perspective.* Grune & Stratton, 1979.

Miller E et al: Elevated maternal hemoglobin A_{1C} in early pregnancy and major congenital anomalies in infants of diabetic mothers. *N Engl J Med* 1981;**304**:1331.

Mills JL, Baker L, Goldman AS: Malformations in infants of diabetic mothers occur before the seventh gestational week: Implications for treatment. *Diabetes* 1979;**28**:292.

Miodovnik M et al: Elevated maternal glycohemoglobin in early pregnancy and spontaneous abortion among insulin-dependent diabetic women. *Am J Obstet Gynecol* 1985;**153**:439.

Moloney JBM, Drury MI: The effect of pregnancy on the natural course of diabetic retinopathy. *Am J Ophthalmol* 1982;**93**:745.

Mueller-Heubach E et al: Lecithin/sphingomyelin ratio in amniotic fluid and its value for the prediction of neonatal respiratory distress syndrome in pregnant diabetic women. *Am J Obstet Gynecol* 1978;**130**:28.

O'Sullivan JB: Body weight and subsequent diabetes mellitus. *JAMA* 1982;**248**:949.

O'Sullivan JB et al: Medical treatment of the gestational diabetic. *Obstet Gynecol* 1974;**43**:817.

Pedersen J: *The Pregnant Diabetic and Her Newborn,* 2nd ed. Williams & Wilkins, 1977.

Roversi GD et al: The intensive care of perinatal risk in pregnant diabetics: A new therapeutic scheme for the best control of maternal disease. *J Perinatal Med* 1973;**1**:114.

White P: Diabetes mellitus in pregnancy. *Clin Perinatol* 1974;**1**:331.

Ylinen K et al: Risk of minor and major fetal malformations in diabetics with high haemoglobin A_{1C} values in early pregnancy. *Br J Med* 1984;**289**:345.

Regulatory Peptides of the Gut

18

Clifford W. Deveney, MD, & Lawrence W. Way, MD

The gastrointestinal tract is the largest endocrine organ in the body. It secretes more hormones than any other organ and perhaps more than the combined total of all other organs. Unlike other endocrine organs, which are solid masses of glandular tissue, the endocrine cells of the gastrointestinal tract are scattered throughout the pancreas and the mucosa of the stomach, small intestine, and colon. Target organs are made up of other cells that may either be remote from or near to the hormone-secreting cell. The principal stimulus for gastrointestinal hormonal secretion is food in the lumen of the gut, but hormone release may also be affected by neural mechanisms and by other hormones.

Mode of Gastrointestinal Hormone Action (Fig 18–1)

Gastrointestinal hormones regulate the digestive process by influencing gastrointestinal secretion, absorption, motility, and blood flow. These hormones may function in 3 different ways: Some are released into the circulation to affect a distant cell **(endocrine function)**, and some are released into the interstitial fluid to affect cells proximal to the releasing cell **(paracrine function)**. Still others act as neurotransmitters or neuromodulators **(neurocrine function)**. Because of these various functions, it may be preferable to refer to these peptides as ''regulatory peptides'' rather than as ''hormones.'' (See also Fig 3–1.)

The Gastrointestinal Hormones

Formerly, when gastrointestinal hormones were thought to function only through release into the bloodstream, a substance had to satisfy the following criteria before earning hormonal status: (1) postprandial release, as demonstrated by measuring a rise in blood levels; and (2) elicitation of physiologic response of the target organ by infusing exogenous hormone at a rate that reproduced postprandial blood levels. At present, only 4 polypeptides completely satisfy these criteria: (1) gastrin (for gastric acid and pepsin secretion), (2) secretin (for pancreatic bicarbonate secretion), (3) cholecystokinin (CCK) (for gallbladder contraction and pancreatic enzyme secretion), and (4) gastric inhibitory polypeptide (GIP) (for insulin release). Motilin (for the interdigestive mi-

Acronyms Used in This Chapter

ACTH	Adrenocorticotropic hormone
APUD	Amine precursor uptake and decarboxylation
BLI	Bombesinlike immunoreactivity
CCK	Cholecystokinin
DNA	Deoxyribonucleic acid
GH	Growth hormone
GIP	Gastric inhibitory polypeptide
GLI	Glucagonlike immunoreactivity
GRP	Gastrin-releasing peptide
5-HIAA	5-Hydroxyindoleacetic acid
MEN	Multiple endocrine neoplasia
MSH	Melanocyte-stimulating hormone
NSE	Neuronal-specific enolase
PP	Pancreatic polypeptide
PRL	Prolactin
PTH	Parathyroid hormone
PYY	Peptide YY
VIP	Vasoactive intestinal polypeptide
WDHA	Watery diarrhea, hypokalemia, and achlorhydria

gratory motor complex) and pancreatic polypeptide (for inhibition of pancreatic bicarbonate and protein secretion) probably also function as circulating hormones.

Proof that hormones act in a neurocrine or paracrine manner requires different criteria. It is not possible at present to confirm the hormonal status of locally acting hormones and to comprehensively define their physiologic actions. In the future, experiments that characterize specific peptide receptor sites on cells and involve specific peptide antagonists will be used to learn more about local release of peptides.

Although gastrin and secretin were identified in the early years of the 20th century, over 50 years passed before their existence was confirmed; it was not until the late 1950s that biochemical techniques became sophisticated enough to isolate, measure, and synthesize these substances. In the early 1960s, Gregory et al isolated gastrin, and a short time later they elucidated its structure and synthesized the molecule. Concurrently, Mutt and Jorpes isolated secretin and CCK from hog intestine and deciphered their amino acid sequences. Radioimmunoassay, developed in the

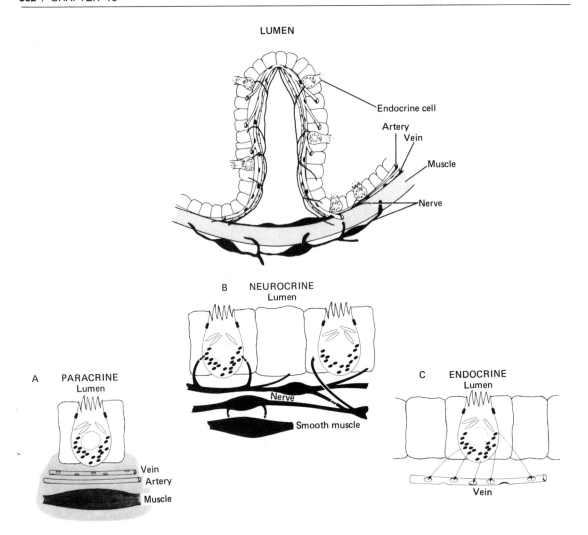

Figure 18–1. Schematic representation of the wall of the small intestine. Note the close proximity of endocrine cells and nerves to mucosal cells, blood vessels, and smooth muscle. Anatomically, local release of hormone by endocrine cells or nerves could affect secretion and absorption (mucosal cells), motility (muscle), and blood flow (blood vessels). *A:* Paracrine function—release of a messenger locally to affect adjacent cells. *B:* Neurocrine function—release of messenger by nerves to affect mucosal cells, other endocrine cells, or smooth muscle of both small intestine and blood vessels. *C:* Endocrine function—release of messenger into the blood to act as a circulating hormone.

1950s by Yalow and Berson for measurement of circulating insulin, has subsequently become the principal means of measuring serum concentrations of gastrointestinal hormones. Since these breakthroughs of the early 1960s, many new gut peptides have been isolated, identified, and synthesized. The synthesis of pure peptides is the only way to provide sufficient material necessary to perform biologic studies and to develop radioimmunoassays.

Structure of Gastrointestinal Hormones

All of the gastrointestinal hormones with 2 possible exceptions (serotonin [5-hydroxytryptamine] and melatonin) are polypeptides and can be extracted from gut mucosa and purified using similar techniques. The initial steps in extraction involve exposure to solvents

(eg, short-chain aliphatic alcohols, acids, salts, and boiling water). The extract is subsequently purified by fractional precipitation with acids and salts; gel filtration (size separation); and anion exchange chromatography (charge separation). Because several different peptides may be found in the same portion of the gut, an initial extract may contain several hormones. If the extract is not pure, biologic actions that seem to be a property of the hormone may in fact be due to an impurity. To determine with certainty the physiologic effects of a hormone, it is essential to have a pure preparation, and the purest preparations are the synthetic hormones.

The amino acid sequence is known for at least 10 gastrointestinal hormones and is partially known for several others (Table 18–1). Most gastrointestinal

Table 18–1. Gastrointestinal hormones.

	Mechanism of Action*			Major Action
	E	N	P	
Gastrin	+	(+)	−	Gastric acid and pepsin secretion.
Cholecystokinin (CCK)	(+)	(+)	−	Pancreatic amylase secretion.
Secretin	+	−	−	Pancreatic bicarbonate secretion.
Gastric inhibitory polypeptide (GIP)	+	−	−	Enhances glucose-mediated insulin release. Inhibits gastric acid secretion.
Vasoactive intestinal polypeptide (VIP)	−	+	(−)	Smooth muscle relaxation. Stimulates pancreatic bicarbonate secretion.
Motilin	(+)	−	−	Initiates interdigestive intestinal motility.
Somatostatin	−	+	(+)	Numerous inhibitory effects.
Pancreatic polypeptide (PP)	(+)	−	(+)	Inhibits pancreatic bicarbonate and protein secretion.
Enkephalins	−	+	(+)	Opiatelike actions.
Substance P	−	+	(+)	Physiologic actions uncertain.
Gastrin-releasing peptide (GRP)†	−	+	(+)	Stimulates release of gastrin and CCK.
Neurotensin	−	+	(+)	Physiologic actions unknown.
Enteroglucagon	(+)	(+)	(+)	Physiologic actions unknown.
Peptide YY (PYY)	(+)	(−)	(+)	Inhibits pancreatic bicarbonate and protein secretion.

*E = endocrine; N = neurocrine; P = paracrine; ( ) = suggested but not proved; + = yes; − = no.
†Gastrin-releasing peptide (GRP) is probably the mammalian form of bombesin and is responsible for bombesinlike immunoreactivity (BLI).

hormones occur in several forms of different molecular weights, all of which contain the same active peptide segment—an arrangement which suggests that large precursor peptides are initially synthesized in the cell of origin and are subsequently cleaved to produce the active hormone. Secretin, glucagon, VIP, and GIP share structural similarities and overlapping biologic activities and represent one hormonal family. CCK and gastrin have the same carboxy-terminal 5 amino acids, share many biologic activities, and comprise a second family (Fig 18–2). The remaining hormones are structurally different.

Concentration of Hormones

The concentration of peptide hormones in blood is in the picomolar (10^{-12} mol/L) to nanomolar (10^{-9} mol/L) range. Radioimmunoassay is the only method available at present that is sensitive enough to measure these concentrations. A substantial amount of pure hormone is needed to develop a radioimmunoassay.

The gastrin-cholecystokinin family

Figure 18–2. Gastrin and cholecystokinin possess identical carboxy-terminal pentapeptides. However, the tyrosine is 7 amino acids from the carboxyl end of CCK and must be sulfated for maximal potency. The tyrosine is 6 positions from the carboxyl end in gastrin and need not be sulfated for maximal potency. R_1 and R_2 represent the amino terminal sequences for gastrin and CCK.

Once antibodies are generated and the radioimmunoassay is available, the hormone can be further characterized by cellular localization and by physiologic events that cause changes in serum levels (ie, hormone release). Although radioimmunoassays have been developed for many hormones, only a few are reliable enough to be used clinically.

Endocrine Cells

Gut endocrine cells are scattered singly throughout the mucosa of the gastrointestinal tract and are distinguished by a clear cytoplasm and prominent acidophilic granules at the base of the cell. Most of these cells have a broad base and a narrow apex with a brush border that faces the intestinal lumen. They probably act as chemoreceptors, with the luminal brush border detecting changes in luminal contents and the hormone being released from the granules in response (Fig 18–3). Those gastrointestinal endocrine cells that lack a luminal brush border are presumably affected by nerves or other endocrine (paracrine) cells.

Stains containing silver salts may be used to separate these cells into enterochromaffin (argentaffin) or argyrophil types. The enterochromaffin cells take up silver salts and deposit silver on their granules, whereas the argyrophil cells require the presence of a reducing agent before they take up silver. Most gastrointestinal hormone–producing cells are of the argyrophil type.

Proof that these cells store specific peptides may be adduced by incubating tissue sections with antibodies that bind specific hormones. The hormone-antibody complex within the cell may be made visible on light or electron microscopy by attaching a label directly to the antibody beforehand or by reacting the hormone-antibody complex with a second labeled antibody. Fluorescein is commonly used as a label for light microscopy and peroxidase for both light and electron microscopy. Thus, to demonstrate gastrin within G cells, the cells are first exposed to antigastrin antibody and then to a labeled second antibody directed at the antigastrin antibody. Although the concept is simple, development of these techniques has

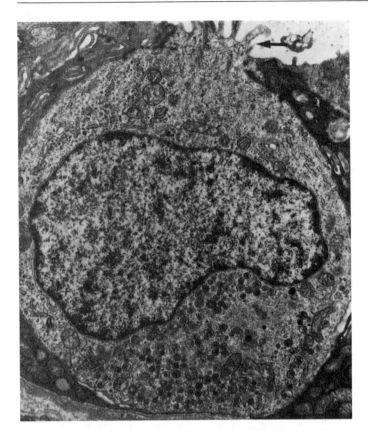

Figure 18–3. Typical endocrine cell of the gut. The arrow points to the brush border, which is at the cell apex and is open to the lumen of the gut. Granules at the cell base contain a peptide messenger, which in this cell is gastrin (G cell). (Reproduced, with permission, from Lechago J: Endocrine cells of the gastrointestinal tract and their pathology. *Pathol Annu* 1978;**13**:329.)

been difficult, because it depends on the discovery of methods of tissue fixation that do not denature polypeptides.

Many different endocrine cells exist in the gut and the pancreas. Ten hormones made by different gut cells and 4 made by cells in the pancreas have been identified (Table 18–2). (Insulin made by the B cell is not included in Table 18–2.) It appears that with one exception, each kind of cell makes and stores only one peptide hormone. Substance P is found in an enterochromaffin cell that also makes serotonin.

Receptors

Cellular membrane receptors can be characterized by using in vitro cell or membrane suspensions and radioiodinated hormone. Biologic activity (eg, acid secretion for the parietal cell and amylase secretion for the acinar cell) can be measured as a function of the amount of hormone bound, and binding affinities of the hormone and analogs can be calculated. Pancreatic acinar cells and gastric parietal cells have been most extensively studied. Gallbladder smooth muscle cells have CCK binding sites. The detection of binding sites, which enables one to determine precisely which cell the hormone directly affects, should be particularly valuable for studying peptides that are thought to have only paracrine or neurocrine functions.

APUD Concept

The cytochemical and ultrastructural characteristics of the gastrointestinal endocrine cells were described by Pearse in 1966. These cells were similar in their ability to produce peptide hormones and biogenic amines (epinephrine, norepinephrine, dopamine, and serotonin) and to actively absorb amine precursors and convert them to amines. It was speculated that the uptake of 5-hydroxytryptophan and conversion to 5-hydroxytryptamine (serotonin) was linked to the production of peptide hormones. Most of the cells possessing these characteristics are found in the gut or central nervous system (hypothalamus, pituitary axis, and pineal gland), but they are also present in the thyroid (calcitonin cell), parathyroid, and placenta. Pearse referred to them as APUD cells from their characteristic amine handling (**amine precursor uptake and decarboxylation**). It was postulated that APUD cells originated from the primitive neural crest.

Whether all APUD cells actually come from the neural crest is not known. Studies using quail and chick embryos have disputed the claim that the APUD cells of the gastrointestinal tract originate from neural ectoderm. However, the endocrine cells of the gastrointestinal tract and pancreas contain an enzyme specific to neural cells (neuronal-specific enolase, NSE), which supports the postulate of a common neural origin. Regardless of their origin, it is clear that the endocrine cells of the gut are remarkably similar to other cells of the hypothalamic-pituitary axis and to neurons within the gut wall, and the gut en-

Table 18–2. Distribution of gastrointestinal hormones.*

	Endocrine Cell†	Localization	Localized in Gut Nerves
Gastrin	G	Gastric antrum, duodenum	No
CCK	I	Duodenum, jejunum	Yes
Secretin	S	Duodenum, jejunum	No
GIP	K	Small bowel	No
VIP	D_1	Pancreas	Yes
Motilin	EC_2	Small bowel	No
Substance P	EC_1	Entire gastrointestinal tract	Yes
Neurotensin	N	Ileum	No
Somatostatin	D	Stomach, duodenum, pancreas	Yes
Enkephalins	. . .	Stomach, duodenum, gallbladder	Yes
GRP	P	Stomach, duodenum	Yes
PP	D_2F	Pancreas	No
Enteroglucagon	A	Pancreas	No
	L	Small intestine	
PYY	. . .	Small intestine, colon	No

*Note that several peptides are found both in nerves and in endocrine cells. VIP has been found only in nerves and is probably not present in endocrine cells.
†Endocrine cells identified with a specific hormone are identified by a letter. EC = enterochromaffin cell. The cells containing enkephalins and PYY have yet to be named.

Table 18–3. Peptides found in gut and central nervous system.

Isolated from both brain and gut:
　Substance P
　Neurotensin
　Secretin
　Somatostatin
　CCK
　GRP
Isolated from either brain or gut: immunoreactivity found in the other organ:
　VIP
　PP and motilin
　Enkephalins and endorphins
　Insulin
　Glucagon

docrine cells are considered to be "neuroendocrinologically" programmed.

The APUD concept assumes that all cells that produce and release peptide hormones have a common embryologic origin. Even though its validity has been challenged, the concept is appealing because it posits a common origin for gut and central nervous system cells with almost identical cytochemical characteristics (storage of peptides) and cellular functions (release of peptide messengers). It helps clarify why identical peptides are synthesized, stored, and released by gut epithelial cells, neurons of the gastrointestinal tract, and nerve cells in the central nervous system. Peptide-releasing neurons and peptide-releasing epithelial cells actually have the same function—release of a chemical messenger.

The Peptidergic Nervous System

When substance P was isolated from brain and gut in 1933, it was believed that this peptide acted as a neurotransmitter. At present, at least 13 peptides are known to exist in both gut and brain (Table 18–3), and all of them probably serve as neurotransmitters. The nerves emitting these transmitters are called **peptidergic nerves.**

There is abundant indirect evidence that the nervous system of the gut contains many neurons that are neither adrenergic nor cholinergic. For example, stimulation of the vagus nerve produces contractions

in the isolated rabbit jejunum that are not inhibited by atropine, implicating the presence of a parasympathetic neurotransmitter other than acetylcholine. Other gut responses to nerve stimulation—such as release of bicarbonate from the pancreas, relaxation of the antral musculature, and vasodilatation—are resistant to adrenergic and cholinergic blockade. Although many of the gut peptides have been found in the central nervous system (Table 18–3), substance P, VIP, the enkephalins, somatostatin, GRP, and CCK have been identified in nerves of the gut and are candidate neurotransmitters (Table 18–2).

In most gut nerves, the nerve cell bodies are located within the gut wall, either in the submucosal or myenteric plexus. The proximity of nerve cell fibers to mucosa, smooth muscle, and blood vessels suggests that they exert local or segmental control over intestinal absorption, secretion, motility, and blood flow.

There is indirect evidence that several of the gut hormones are unable to act through the systemic circulation and may be confined to a role as neurotransmitter or paracrine hormone. For example, somatostatin, VIP, and substance P are so rapidly destroyed in the circulation (their half-life is < 3 minutes) that they would not be effective as circulating hormones. In addition, the action of these peptides when given intravenously is so diffuse that it is difficult to envision a physiologic purpose for them in the circulation.

GASTRIN

In 1905, Edkins discovered a potent gastric acid secretagogue in extracts of antral mucosa and named it gastrin. However, he could not exclude the possibility that the extract contained histamine, and for many years it was not known whether Edkins' gastrin was truly different from histamine. The existence of gastrin was firmly established in the early 1960s when Gregory et al isolated the peptide, identified its amino acid sequence, and synthesized the hormone. Because of the availability of pure synthetic gastrin and the relative ease with which physiologic concentrations can be measured by radioimmunoassay, gastrin is the best-studied gastrointestinal hormone.

Biochemistry & Distribution

There are presently 3 known biologically active forms of the gastrin molecule: a 14-amino-acid (G14), a 17-amino-acid (G17), and a 34-amino-acid (G34) peptide. They are also known as "mini gastrin," "little gastrin," and "big gastrin." Their 14 carboxy-terminal residues are identical, and G34 also contains the entire G17 sequence. In each form of gastrin, the tyrosine moiety in the sixth position from the carboxyl terminus may be sulfated or unsulfated, an alteration with no effect on range of action or potency. Digestion of big gastrin (G34) with trypsin cleaves 2 lysyl residues and releases little gastrin (G17). A molecule larger than G34, called component I or "big big gastrin," has also been discovered. Although the structure of component I has not been completely deciphered, tryptic digestion of this compound also releases G17, suggesting that component I consists of G17 joined at the N terminus with basic amino acids to a larger peptide.

G17 accounts for most of the gastrin in antral G cells; G34 predominates in serum, however, because it has a longer half-life. G17 is presumed to be the physiologically most important form of gastrin. The significance of the larger forms is not known, but it appears that many peptide hormones may be synthesized as a larger molecule containing the active fragment and that the precursor molecule is cleaved at positions where basic amino acids occur. A similar process occurs with proinsulin and insulin.

The carboxyl terminus of gastrin is responsible for its biologic activity. In fact, the carboxy-terminal tetrapeptide alone (gastrin tetrapeptide) displays the full range of actions, although it is only about one-sixth as potent on a molar basis as G17 for stimulation of acid secretion. G17 is about 3 times more potent than G34.

Gastrin and CCK have 5 identical carboxy-terminal amino acids (Fig 18–2). For CCK, 7 carboxy-terminal peptides are necessary for full biologic activity, whereas for gastrin, only the 4 carboxy-terminal amino acids are necessary. The effects of gastrin and CCK are similar to the extent that both hormones stimulate gastric acid and pancreatic enzyme secretion and contraction of the gallbladder. However, their potency for eliciting these responses differs considerably. Gastrin is a strong stimulant of acid secretion and a weak stimulant of enzyme secretion and gallbladder contraction, while the relative potency of CCK for these actions is reversed. These differences are determined by the position of the tyrosine molecule located near the carboxyl end of the molecule. In gastrin, tyrosine is the sixth amino acid from the carboxyl end, while in CCK it is the seventh. For CCK-like activity, the tyrosine must be sulfated, but whether or not the tyrosine is sulfated does not affect the activity of gastrin.

Gastrin is synthesized and stored in the G cell.

Ninety percent of gastrointestinal gastrin is found in the gastric antrum, and most of the remainder is in the duodenum. Under normal conditions, there is virtually no gastrin in the pancreas, although pancreatic endocrine tumors often produce gastrin.

Measurement & Release

Serum concentrations of gastrin range from 10 to 50 pmol/L. The concentration is often expressed as picograms of G17 per milliliter, since G17 is used as the standard. Because gastrin is present in other forms in serum, however, this is not entirely precise. Owing to the molecular heterogeneity of gastrin, antibodies used for immunoassay must measure G17 and G34 both in the sulfated and in the nonsulfated forms. Clinical laboratories use an antibody that recognizes all forms of gastrin, and the results are expressed as total gastrin in serum.

Serum gastrin concentrations increase by 20–40 pmol/L 30–60 minutes postprandially. Partially digested proteins, peptides, and amino acids in the antrum release gastrin, while carbohydrates and fats do not. The half-life in the circulation for G17 is 3–6 minutes and for G34 about 15 minutes.

Gastrin release is inhibited by antral acidification. Substantial inhibition occurs at pH 2.5, and release is abolished at pH 1. Secretin, glucagon, VIP, GIP, calcitonin, and somatostatin inhibit the release of meal-stimulated gastrin, but whether these are physiologic actions is unknown.

There is evidence for the presence of cholinergic mechanisms that both stimulate and inhibit gastrin release. Vagal stimulation by electrical current, insulin hypoglycemia, or injection of 2-deoxyglucose releases gastrin. However, cholinergic blockade with atropine enhances meal-stimulated gastrin release independently of gastric pH, which suggests the presence of a cholinergic (ie, vagal) mechanism that suppresses gastrin release. One hypothesis to explain vagal inhibition of gastrin release views the G cell as under the simultaneous influence of nearby somatostatin-producing cells and bombesin-containing postganglionic neurons. The former blocks gastrin release (a paracrine effect), and the latter stimulates gastrin release. Atropine (or vagotomy) blocks meal-stimulated somatostatin release but does not affect bombesin release, which results in an exaggerated postprandial gastrin response.

Gastrin is not preferentially metabolized by the liver but appears to be removed across capillary beds in tissues throughout the body. It is metabolized by the kidneys and does not appear as an immunologically reactive peptide in the urine.

Actions

The only certain actions of gastrin that occur at physiologic levels are stimulation of gastric acid and pepsin secretion. Gastrin evokes acid secretion by several mechanisms, the most important of which is release of histamine from cells near the parietal cells. The histamine then acts directly on parietal cells to cause acid secretion. Gastrin-stimulated histamine release in gastric mucosa has been documented in vivo and in vitro. H_2 receptor antagonists completely inhibit gastrin-stimulated acid secretion in vivo, which implies that a major portion of gastrin-stimulated acid secretion is mediated through histamine. There is also evidence, however, that gastrin acts directly on parietal cells to stimulate acid secretion. For example, there are gastrin receptors on parietal cells, and gastrin induces intracellular changes that do not occur in response to histamine. Furthermore, gastrin potentiates the action of histamine on acid secretion.

Increased gastric mucosal blood flow may be caused directly by gastrin or may be secondary to increased acid secretion. Gastrin also has a trophic effect on gastric mucosa and pancreas. Several other actions have been ascribed to gastrin, such as contraction of the lower esophageal sphincter and secretion of water and electrolytes by the jejunum, but they are not seen at physiologic concentrations. Excess amounts of gastrin secreted by pancreatic tumors (gastrinoma) cause acid hypersecretion and severe peptic ulcer disease.

CHOLECYSTOKININ

In 1928, Ivy and Oldberg observed that instillation of fat into the small intestine caused the gallbladder to contract. They postulated a hormonal mechanism and named the mediator cholecystokinin (CCK). In the early 1940s, Harper and Raper discovered a substance in extracts of duodenal mucosa that stimulated the secretion of enzyme-rich juice by the pancreas and called the substance pancreozymin. In 1964, Jorpes et al found that increasing purification of a single extract from small intestine proportionately increased its potency for gallbladder contraction and pancreatic enzyme secretion, indicating that the 2 actions were properties of a single hormone. Previously, the term cholecystokinin had been used for the gallbladder effects and pancreozymin for the pancreatic effects; but because the former were discovered first, the hormone is now referred to simply as cholecystokinin, or CCK. In 1971, Mutt and Jorpes reported the amino acid sequence of CCK.

Biochemistry & Distribution

CCK exists in several molecular forms. Peptides containing 58, 39, 33, and 8 amino acids have been isolated and studied and are called CCK58, CCK39, CCK33, and CCK8, respectively. The carboxy-terminal octapeptide sequences are identical for all molecular forms of CCK. The CCK33 molecule is susceptible to tryptic digestion at positions 1, 6, 11, 21, and 25. Tryptic digestion at position 25 produces CCK8.

Like gastrin, CCK is probably synthesized as a precursor, with CCK39 and CCK33 representing progressive steps in the creation of CCK8. All of the biologic actions are contained in the terminal octapeptide, which is 4–6 times more potent than CCK33 on a molar basis. Sulfation of the tyrosine moiety in position 7 from the carboxyl terminus is necessary for full biologic potency.

CCK is located in the duodenum and proximal jejunum within the mucosal I cell. It is also found in the central nervous system, in the myenteric plexus of the intestine, and in nerves supplying the urinary bladder and uterus.

Measurement & Release

Development of a radioimmunoassay for CCK has been difficult, principally because iodination alters the CCK molecule. Several investigators have reported the ability to measure serum levels of CCK by radioimmunoassay. The serum levels increase within 10 minutes after eating and remain elevated for at least 2 hours. Fasting CCK levels vary from 0 to 20 pmol/L and postprandial levels from 20 to 100 pmol/L, depending on the immunoassay used.

Like gastrin, CCK circulates in several forms. Since CCK8 is 5–6 times more potent than CCK33, it will be necessary to measure these 2 forms separately in order to interpret the significance of the concentration of CCK in blood.

The half-life of CCK in blood is 2.5–7 minutes. CCK is taken up and degraded in the capillary beds of most organs (eg, lung, spleen, liver, intestine, stomach, and kidney). It is released by intraduodenal food, amino acids, fatty acids, calcium, and acid. Cholinergic neural mechanisms enhance CCK release in response to luminal stimulants. Phenylalanine and tryptophan are the most potent amino acids for release of CCK. For fatty acids to be effective, they must be more than 9 carbons long, and potency increases up to a chain length of 18 carbons. The magnitude of the CCK response to amino acids and fatty acids is also proportionate to the length of intestine perfused. The presence of increasing concentrations of bile acids in the intestine progressively inhibits the CCK-like effects of luminal stimuli but has no effect on the response to intravenous CCK. This suggests that bile acids block the release of endogenous CCK and that this constitutes a mechanism which allows the gallbladder to relax again in the late stages after a meal.

Postprandial increases in blood levels of CCK have been reported by several investigators. However, large discrepancies exist between different immunoassays, and it is presently unclear whether CCK8 or CCK33 is the major circulating form.

An in vitro bioassay for CCK using dispersed pancreatic acini has recently been employed by some investigators. Levels measured by bioassay are lower than those measured by radioimmunoassay.

Actions

Gallbladder contraction and pancreatic enzyme secretion are the only actions of CCK presently accepted as physiologic. CCK also affects motor function of the gastrointestinal tract; has a trophic effect on the pancreas; and induces satiety in several species, including humans. Intact vagal innervation is necessary for the latter effect. The presence of CCK in gut neurons as well as endocrine cells suggests that CCK acts in a neurocrine or paracrine manner in addition to its endocrine function.

The actions of CCK on smooth muscle include contraction of the gallbladder and stimulation of antral and intestinal motility to produce delayed gastric emptying. CCK has been shown to both relax and contract the lower esophageal sphincter and the sphincter of Oddi. A possible explanation for this apparent conflict is that CCK acts as a neurotransmitter to stimulate postganglionic inhibitory neurons to cause sphincter relaxation and also acts directly on the smooth muscle to produce contraction. The observed effect (relaxation or contraction) would depend upon which system predominates. CCK acts directly on the smooth muscle of gallbladder and sphincter of Oddi and indirectly through cholinergic nerves on the smooth muscle of the small intestine.

The secretory actions of CCK include stimulation of pancreatic enzyme secretion, hepatic bile secretion, and Brunner's gland secretion. CCK also stimulates release of insulin and pancreatic polypeptide from the pancreas and calcitonin from the thyroid. Intraperitoneal injections of CCK33 or CCK8 cause early satiety in rats.

Hypertrophy of the pancreas is produced by intraperitoneal injections of CCK8. The number of acinar, ductal, and B cells (of the islets of Langerhans) is increased. The effect entails both cellular hypertrophy and hyperplasia. While there is good evidence that the effect of CCK on gallbladder contraction, sphincter of Oddi relaxation, pancreatic enzyme secretion, and gastric smooth muscle contraction occurs under physiologic conditions, it remains to be seen whether other effects occur at physiologic levels of CCK.

SECRETIN

Secretin was the first hormone discovered when Bayliss and Starling demonstrated that intravenous injection of acid extracts of jejunum stimulated secretion of water and bicarbonate from the pancreas. Secretin was purified by Jorpes and Mutt in 1961, and its amino acid sequence was identified in 1966.

Biochemistry & Distribution

Unlike most other hormones, secretin has been identified in only one form. It is a basic 27-amino-acid polypeptide containing 4 arginine residues and one histidine residue. Fourteen of the 27 amino acids in secretin occupy the same position as in glucagon. Secretin also shows structural similarities to GIP and VIP, and these 4 peptides are known as the secretin-glucagon family. The entire molecule of secretin is necessary for biologic activity. Secretin is found in S cells in the duodenum and proximal jejunum and in the central nervous system.

Measurement & Release

Secretin is difficult to label with radioactive iodine, because the molecule lacks a tyrosine residue. This problem has been solved by iodination under conditions that label histidine or by using a synthetic secretin analog in which tyrosine has been substituted for one of the other amino acids. Most immunoassays for secretin are too insensitive to measure changes in serum levels. Furthermore, secretin is relatively unstable in solution, so that special measures must be taken to protect against degradation. The most sensitive immunoassays for secretin have reported fasting serum values of 1–5 pmol/L, but it has not been possible to measure changes after a meal.

The only known stimulus for secretin release is duodenal acidification, which causes an increase in serum levels within minutes. Small increments follow rapid drops in duodenal pH. The threshold for secretin release is a duodenal pH of less than 4.5. Infusion of bile salt into the duodenum also causes a small increase in serum levels of secretin. Other substances such as fats, alcohols, glucose, and amino acids do not release secretin if the pH of the duodenum is kept constant. Neither vagotomy nor atropinization alters the secretin response to intraduodenal acid. Vagotomy may indirectly affect secretin release by elevating duodenal pH. The half-life of secretin in blood is 3–7.5 minutes.

Actions

Secretin stimulates pancreatic bicarbonate and water secretion at physiologic levels. Because serum levels are so low, there is some question about whether circulating secretin can account for the postprandial increase in pancreatic bicarbonate and water secretion. Nevertheless, small increases in serum secretin do correlate positively with increases in the output of pancreatic bicarbonate and water. Furthermore, small amounts of secretin infused intravenously to mimic the physiologic changes in serum levels produce a corresponding increase in pancreatic water and bicarbonate secretion. Therefore, it is probably correct to conclude that secretin has a physiologic effect on pancreatic water and bicarbonate secretion. CCK markedly potentiates the effect of secretin on pancreatic secretion. In physiologic circumstances (ie, after a meal), CCK would be released in amounts sufficient to enhance the effect of secretin. Although infusion of secretin can inhibit meal-stimulated gastrin release and gastric acid secretion, these effects are not seen with physiologic amounts of secretin.

Clinical Uses

Secretin is used clinically to evaluate pancreatic function, to obtain specimens of pancreatic juice for cytologic study, and as a provocative agent for the release of gastrin from gastrinomas. When used for clinical tests, secretin is measured in clinical units (4000 clinical units = 1 mg).

To evaluate **pancreatic function,** a Dreiling tube is placed in the duodenum to aspirate pancreatic secretions, and secretin (1 clinical unit/kg body weight) is injected intravenously. Duodenal juice is collected over eight 10-minute periods, and volume and bicarbonate concentration are measured. A maximal bicarbonate concentration of less than 90 meq/L and a flow of less than 2 mL/kg body weight over 80 minutes are diagnostic of impaired pancreatic function. Secretin may also be used to stimulate secretion of pancreatic juice for examination for malignant cells. The juice may be collected through a duodenal tube or by direct endoscopic cannulation of the pancreatic duct. A description of the use of secretin in the diagnosis of gastrinoma appears in the section on gastrinoma.

GASTRIC INHIBITORY POLYPEPTIDE

Biochemistry & Distribution

Gastric inhibitory polypeptide (GIP) was first isolated in 1971, and it has subsequently been synthesized. GIP is a 43-amino-acid polypeptide with a structure similar to those of secretin, glucagon, and VIP. GIP has been found in serum in larger molecular forms that may represent precursors of the 43-amino-acid hormone. GIP is found in mucosal cells in the duodenum, jejunum, and ileum; the highest concentrations are in the jejunum.

Measurement & Release

Basal levels of GIP are in the range of 250 pg/mL (50 pmol/L). GIP release is stimulated by ingestion of food, with a peak of approximately 1000 pg/mL occurring 60 minutes postprandially. GIP remains elevated for about 3 hours. The most potent stimuli for release of GIP are intraluminal glucose and triglyceride, and the magnitude of the response is dose-dependent. Ingestion of glucose produces an increase within 60 minutes, while ingestion of fat produces an increase within 120–150 minutes. The response to glucose is dependent on glucose absorption. The half-life of GIP in plasma is about 20 minutes.

Actions

Physiologic doses of GIP given intravenously increase the insulin response to glucose, but the effect is dependent on the presence of elevated blood glucose levels. This has prompted some to suggest that GIP be renamed **glucose-dependent insulin-releasing polypeptide.** GIP also inhibits gastrin release and gastric acid secretion, but it is unlikely that these effects occur at physiologic levels of the hormone. The amino-terminal portion of the molecule is essential for the effect on insulin, and the carboxy-terminal portion is essential for the gastric effect. GIP in physiologic doses causes secretion of fluid and electrolytes by the ileal mucosa, but the importance of this is not known.

VASOACTIVE INTESTINAL POLYPEPTIDE

Vasoactive intestinal polypeptide (VIP) was isolated from porcine small intestine in 1970 by Said and Mutt. Three years later, its structure was determined, and it was synthesized. VIP exhibits many biologic actions, but its physiologic role is still only vaguely defined. VIP has been detected in nerve cells, and it is probably not present in endocrine cells.

Biochemistry & Distribution

VIP is a basic 28-amino-acid polypeptide. Although some fragments of the molecule possess biologic activity, potency increases with increasing length, and the entire molecule is more potent than any fragment.

VIP is present in nerves in the myenteric and submucosal plexuses and in nerve fibers in the core of the intestinal villi (close to mucosal cells), around blood vessels and sphincters, and in the wall of the gallbladder. VIP is also found in the central nervous system and in nerves in male and female reproductive organs.

Measurement & Release

Fasting levels of VIP in serum are low (< 7 pmol/L) and do not increase postprandially. The half-life of VIP in blood is 1–3 minutes. These characteristics suggest that VIP does not function as a circulating hormone but probably has only paracrine and neurotransmitter actions.

Actions

When infused intravenously, VIP inhibits pentagastrin and histamine-stimulated gastric acid and pepsin secretion. It stimulates lipolysis, glycogenolysis, and secretion by the small intestine and pancreas. VIP relaxes smooth muscle in many gastrointestinal sphincters and causes vasodilatation, hypotension, and flushing. The presence of nerves containing VIP in blood vessel walls, sphincter muscles, and mucosa suggests that VIP released from nerves acts locally to regulate gut motility, sphincter relaxation, local blood flow, mucosal secretion, and pancreatic bicarbonate secretion.

Abnormally large amounts of VIP produced by islet cell tumors of the pancreas are at least partly responsible for the manifestations of the pancreatic cholera (WDHA) syndrome (discussed in a subsequent section). The diarrhea in this condition is due to secretion of voluminous amounts of fluid by the small intestine.

SUBSTANCE P

Substance P was discovered by Von Euler and Gaddum in 1931 and was the first peptide found in both brain and gut. Little further research was done on substance P until 1970, when Chang and Leeman isolated and purified it from the brain. The amino acid sequence is known, and it has been synthesized.

Biochemistry & Distribution

Substance P is an 11-amino-acid polypeptide, of which the 5 carboxy-terminal amino acids are required for biologic action. There appear to be larger precursor forms in serum.

Substance P is distributed throughout the body, with the highest concentrations occurring in the gut and nervous system. High concentrations are also found in structures along the brain stem (eg, hypothalamus, substantia nigra). In the spinal cord, it is concentrated mainly in sensory areas. In the gut, substance P has been found in nerve plexuses and enterochromaffin cells.

Measurement & Release

Serum concentrations of substance P measured by immunoassay range from 40 to 300 pg/mL. Substance P is not released into the blood except in disease states (eg, carcinoid syndrome). It probably acts through neurocrine or paracrine mechanisms.

Actions

The function of substance P is not known. Experimentally, it is a potent stimulant of smooth muscle contraction of the gut. Part of the contraction is tetrodotoxin-sensitive, which suggests that substance P acts through a neural reflex. Since contraction is not completely blocked by tetrodotoxin, substance P is also thought to act directly on the muscle. Intravenous infusion of substance P increases intestinal motility and stimulates pancreatic exocrine and salivary gland secretion and gallbladder contraction. Cell bodies of substance P–containing nerves are located in the myenteric plexus, and the axons are scattered throughout the smooth muscle, suggesting that it may have an effect on intestinal motility. Because it is present in plexuses, substance P may also serve as an excitatory transmitter in afferent neurons of the gut. It also causes vasodilatation and the release of histamine from mast cells. Elevated levels of substance P have been reported in carcinoid syndrome, where it may be partially responsible for the flushing and diarrhea.

Substance P is thought to act as a neurotransmitter or modulator of sensory input in the spinal cord and specifically to have a role in the central transmission of pain impulses. In the brain, substance P stimulates secretion of prolactin (PRL) and growth hormone (GH).

ENKEPHALINS

The enkephalin peptides are fragments of larger molecules, the α- and β-endorphins. The endorphins and enkephalins are opiate peptides, molecules that bind to opiate receptors and have actions similar to those of opiates. Opiate receptors are found in brain and gut.

Biochemistry & Distribution

Each of the 2 enkephalins in the gastrointestinal tract, met-enkephalin and leu-enkephalin, contains 5 amino acids and differs only at the terminal –COOH residue, which is either methionine or leucine.

Enkephalins are located in cells in the stomach, duodenum, and gallbladder as well as in nerves. Enkephalin-containing cells are numerous in the gastrointestinal tract, and their distribution in nerves is similar to that of substance P.

Measurement & Release

Enkephalins have not been detected in plasma or serum. They are rapidly destroyed in blood, which makes it unlikely that they act as circulating hormones.

Actions

When infused intravenously, enkephalins have the same actions as morphine. In the central nervous system, they cause analgesia, sedation, respiratory depression, muscular rigidity, and emesis. In the gastrointestinal tract, the most prominent manifestation of intravenous enkephalin infusion is constipation. However, motor activity in all parts of the gut is affected. In stomach, duodenum, and jejunum, enkephalins initially cause increased contractions, followed by distention and atony. In the colon, they produce segmental areas of contraction without peristalsis and sustained contraction of the anal sphincter.

Infusion of enkephalins increases histamine-stimulated gastric acid and pepsin secretion and inhibits secretin-stimulated bicarbonate secretion from the pancreas. Enkephalins also decrease mesenteric vascular resistance and increase intestinal blood flow.

NEUROTENSIN

Neurotensin was discovered accidentally during isolation of substance P from the hypothalamus when a fraction of the extract was found to produce vasodilatation and hypotension. The term neurotensin originated from its neurologic origin and its hypotensive properties.

Biochemistry & Distribution

Neurotensin is a 13-amino-acid polypeptide that has been synthesized. It is found extensively in nerve cells in the central nervous system. In the gut, it is located in the N cells of the ileum and is almost absent from nerve fibers. The carboxy-terminal segment of the molecule is responsible for the biologic activity of neurotensin.

Measurement & Release

Release after a meal has been documented, but the half-life in serum is very short. Immunoassay for neurotensin is available in only a few laboratories.

Actions

The physiologic actions of neurotensin are not

known. Neurotensin is a kinin and causes hypotension and vasodilatation and contraction of various smooth muscle groups. It decreases gastric acid secretion and peristaltic activity in the gastrointestinal tract. Because gastric acid secretion can be blocked by vagal denervation, it is probably mediated through the vagi. Neurotensin binds to mast cells, and since many of its effects are histaminelike (ie, hypotension, hypoglycemia, increased vascular permeability, smooth muscle contraction), neurotensin may act by releasing histamine. An exaggerated postprandial release of neurotensin has been reported to occur in patients with dumping syndrome. Experimentally, intravenous infusion of neurotensin inhibits gastrin-stimulated but not histamine-stimulated acid secretion. It also delays gastric emptying.

MOTILIN

The existence of motilin was postulated by Brown et al in 1966, when they observed that alkalinization of the duodenum in dogs produced contractions in denervated pouches of the body of the stomach. Similar contractions followed injection of an impure preparation of CCK but not of pure CCK. Subsequently, motilin was isolated from the crude CCK extract, purified, and identified.

Biochemistry & Distribution
Motilin is a 22-amino-acid polypeptide. It has been synthesized, and ample quantities are available for immunoassays and physiologic studies. There is at least one larger form of motilin.

Motilin is located in endocrine cells in the mucosa of the duodenum, proximal jejunum, antrum, and fundus. It is often seen with serotonin in enterochromaffin cells. It is also present in nerves throughout the gut.

Measurement & Release
The concentration of motilin in blood ranges from 4 to 350 pmol/L, with a median of about 60 pmol/L. Motilin is released into blood in cyclic fashion in fasting dogs; if the same is true in humans, it would explain the variations reported in basal levels.

Serum motilin concentrations do not rise postprandially. In fact, a protein meal depresses serum levels.

Actions
Intravenous infusion of motilin stimulates pepsin secretion from the stomach and increases the rate of intestinal transit. In vitro, motilin causes contraction of duodenal, ileal, colonic, and gallbladder smooth muscle. Its actions are most pronounced on duodenal smooth muscle, where it is 100 times as potent as acetylcholine. The actions of motilin on smooth muscle are not blocked by atropine, phentolamine, propranolol, cimetidine, or chlorpheniramine; this suggests that the hormone acts directly on motilin receptors in the muscle. Smooth muscle other than from

the gut does not respond to motilin.

In the fasting state, the smooth muscle of the stomach and small bowel displays electrical activity termed the **interdigestive migrating myoelectric complex.** There are 4 phases (I–IV), and muscular contraction occurs in phases III and IV. In fasting dogs, phase III and IV myoelectric activity occurs at 90- to 120-minute intervals, beginning in the duodenum and propagating over 60–80 minutes to the distal ileum. Phase III and IV myoelectric activity coincides with a peristaltic wave, which propels enteric contents distally during fasting. The cyclic occurrence of phase III and IV myoelectric activity coincides with increases in serum motilin levels. Conversely, intravenous infusion of motilin produces phase III myoelectric activity in the duodenum. These observations implicate motilin in the cyclic peristalsis that occurs between meals.

Motilin has been shown to be about as potent as CCK in stimulation of gallbladder contraction, and because an effect is seen with serum levels within the physiologic range, motilin may participate in the control of gallbladder emptying, particularly in the fasting state.

SOMATOSTATIN

Somatostatin was first isolated from the hypothalamus, where it was found to inhibit the release of GH. Somatostatin was subsequently found in large amounts in endocrine cells of the stomach and pancreas and in nerve fibers in the gut mucosa.

Biochemistry & Distribution
Somatostatin is a 14-amino-acid polypeptide that exists in straight and cyclic forms. It has been synthesized, and antisomatostatin antibodies have been generated. Somatostatin also occurs in at least one larger form containing 28 amino acids, which is probably a precursor of the 14-amino-acid molecule.

Somatostatin is found in the central nervous system as well as in the gastrointestinal tract, where it is present in both endocrine and nerve cells. In the gastrointestinal tract, somatostatin is most prominent in endocrine cells within the mucosa of the gastric antrum and in the D cells of the pancreatic islets.

Measurement & Release
While antibodies have proved useful in localizing somatostatin in the gastrointestinal tract, it is difficult to measure this hormone in blood because of the presence of nonspecific interfering substances. Although some of these problems have been partially resolved by extraction procedures, there is still little information on the physiologic release of somatostatin into the circulation. By selective cannulation of the venous drainage of the gastric fundus, antrum, and pancreas, somatostatin release has been demonstrated in anesthetized dogs following intragastric instillation of fat, glucose, and amino acids.

Actions

The principal actions of somatostatin are inhibitory. It inhibits the release of gastrin, secretin, motilin, CCK, GIP, insulin, and glucagon as well as of GH. It also inhibits gastric acid and pancreatic exocrine secretion; gallbladder contraction; gastric emptying; small bowel absorption of amino acids, glucose, and triglycerides; and the release of acetylcholine from cholinergic nerves.

Because its inhibitory effects are so diffuse, somatostatin is unlikely to act as a circulating hormone. However, in physiologic levels, circulating somatostatin delays gallbladder and gastric emptying, decreases glucose uptake from the gut, and decreases gastric acid secretion. The evidence for a paracrine function for somatostatin is indirect and is based on the location of somatostatin-containing cells and the actions of somatostatin. For example, somatostatin is found near parietal cells and antral G cells and is a potent inhibitor of gastrin release and gastric acid secretion. Somatostatin is contained in the D cells of the pancreatic islets and inhibits the release of insulin and glucagon from the islets. (See also Chapter 3.)

PEPTIDE YY

Peptide YY (PYY) was so named because it has tyrosine residues at the amino and carboxyl ends of the molecule, and the symbol for tyrosine is Y.

Biochemistry & Distribution

PYY is a 36-amino-acid peptide that contains 5 tyrosine molecules and has several sequence similarities to pancreatic polypeptide (PP). PYY is present in mucosal endocrine cells in the small bowel and colon, with highest concentrations in the ileum and colon.

Measurement & Release

Information on the release of PYY is meager. Serum levels of PYY increase to 200–300 pg/mL postprandially in dogs.

Actions

Intravenous infusion of PYY (10–20 pmol/kg) inhibits pancreatic secretion of bicarbonate and enzymes. The inhibition occurs at low doses, but it is not yet known whether the action is physiologic.

BOMBESIN & GASTRIN-RELEASING PEPTIDE

Bombesin belongs to a group of peptides found in the skin of frogs. Bombesinlike immunoreactivity (BLI) has been detected in mammalian brain and gut, but the actual molecule in mammals is probably gastrin-releasing peptide (GRP). The 10 carboxy-terminal peptides are nearly identical in GRP and bombesin, and these 10 peptides are responsible for their biologic activity.

Biochemistry & Distribution

Bombesin obtained from frog skin is a 14-amino-acid polypeptide. It belongs to a group of homologous peptides (litorin, ranatensin, and alytensin) obtained from the same source. It bears no similarity to other mammalian hormones. GRP is a 27-amino-acid polypeptide isolated from mammalian gut. It has a carboxy-terminal decapeptide almost identical to that of bombesin.

BLI is seen throughout the gut in nerves and endocrine cells. It is most concentrated in the antral and duodenal mucosa and is present also in fine nerve fibers in the gut wall. The distribution of GRP in mammals is similar to that of bombesin.

Measurement & Release

Antibodies have been generated against bombesin. The hormone has been localized by immunocytochemistry to cells in the gastrointestinal tract and brain, but it has not been measured in blood.

Actions

The physiologic actions of bombesin are not definitely known. When infused intravenously, bombesin stimulates release of gastrin and CCK and inhibits release of VIP. It also causes pancreatic secretion of amylase, which occurs independently of CCK release. Finally, it contracts smooth muscle of the gallbladder, duodenum, and stomach.

Because BLI is present in the antrum and duodenum and because bombesin given experimentally releases gastrin and CCK, bombesin has been postulated to act as a paracrine messenger that releases these hormones. In the brain, it may play a role in thermoregulation and pain perception.

PANCREATIC POLYPEPTIDE

Pancreatic polypeptide (PP) was discovered in 1968 as a contaminant during isolation of chicken insulin. It has subsequently been isolated from bovine, porcine, and human pancreas.

Biochemistry & Distribution

PP is a 36-amino-acid polypeptide. The human, bovine, and porcine types differ by only a few amino acids. PP cells are located in pancreatic islets and near pancreatic acini.

Measurement & Release

Fasting levels of PP in blood are 50–200 pg/mL (high normal range in older people). The half-life of PP in blood is 5–10 minutes.

Blood levels of PP rise sharply after ingestion of just about any food. Ground beef and fish are the most potent stimuli. The release is marked and biphasic, the first phase occurring minutes after eating and the second phase 1–2 hours later. The initial phase is blocked by vagotomy and anticholinergic drugs. The second phase is at least partly augmented by vagal activity.

Actions

At physiologic levels, PP inhibits pancreatic secretion of bicarbonate and protein. It also causes relaxation of the gallbladder and a decrease in hepatic bile secretion. Intravenous infusion of PP does not affect acid secretion, carbohydrate or lipid metabolism, or the release of other hormones. PP levels may be elevated in patients with several kinds of hormone-secreting tumors (eg, gastrinoma, VIPoma). This is not a consistent finding, however, and thus the value of PP as a tumor marker is limited.

GLUCAGONLIKE IMMUNOREACTIVITY

Glucagon antibodies are of 2 general types: those that react with the carboxyl end of pancreatic glucagon and those that react with the amino end. In addition to pancreatic glucagon, there are other gut peptides referred to as glucagonlike immunoreactivity (GLI). Most of the gut GLI reacts with the amino-terminal but not the carboxy-terminal antibodies. The GLI that reacts with amino-terminal antibodies is found in highest concentration in the ileal mucosa, but it is also present throughout most of the intestine.

Biochemistry & Distribution

The major component of GLI is a peptide called **glicentin,** which contains 100 amino acids and has a molecular weight of 11,650. The amino acid sequence of pancreatic glucagon is contained within the glicentin molecule.

GLI is found in highest concentrations in L cells in the ileum and colon. In the dog stomach, GLI has been detected in cells morphologically indistinguishable from the A cell of the pancreas.

Measurement & Release

Measurement of GLI requires immunoassay with 2 antibodies. An antibody that cross-reacts with pancreatic and gut glucagon is used to measure total glucagon content. Another antibody directed at the –COOH terminus is used to measure pancreatic glucagon alone. GLI is then calculated by subtracting pancreatic glucagon content from total glucagon content. Because of difficulties in measuring GLI, little is known about its release. It is probably released by food, including carbohydrates.

Actions

Although little is known of its physiologic function, there is some evidence that GLI may release insulin and stimulate glucose production in the liver. Because constipation and mucosal hypertrophy were found in one patient with a GLI-producing tumor, it

has been suggested that GLI may affect intestinal motility and mucosal growth.

HORMONAL ABNORMALITIES IN DISEASES OF THE GASTROINTESTINAL TRACT

Because gastrointestinal peptides influence most aspects of digestion, it is important to search for abnormalities in hormone secretion or end-organ response in gastrointestinal disease. Research in this new field is hampered by difficulties in measuring serum levels of the hormones and documenting local hormone release.

DUODENAL ULCER

Patients with duodenal ulcer deliver excess acid and pepsin into the duodenum and secrete more acid in response to gastrin or histamine than do subjects without duodenal ulcer. Consequently, the search for hormonal abnormalities in duodenal ulcer has centered around mechanisms that control gastric acid secretion, neutralization of gastric acid in the duodenum, and the rate of gastric emptying (ie, the rate of delivery of gastric acid into the duodenum). Hormones that may affect acid secretion or duodenal pH are listed in Table 18–4.

The role of gastrin in duodenal ulcer disease has been the most extensively investigated. Neither basal serum levels of gastrin nor the individual components (G17 and G34) are elevated in patients with duodenal ulcer, and the number of G (gastrin-secreting) cells in the antrum is normal. However, the gastrin response to a meal and to hypoglycemia is greater than normal and more prolonged in these patients. Furthermore, inhibition of gastrin release following antral acidifi-

Table 18–4. Hormones that may affect acid secretion or duodenal pH.

Action	Stimulation	Inhibition
Acid secretion	Gastrin CCK	VIP GIP Somatostatin Secretin
Gastrin release	Bombesin	Secretin Somatostatin VIP GIP Glucagon
Pancreatic bicarbonate secretion	CCK Secretin VIP	PP
Delay of gastric emptying of acid into duodenum	CCK	

cation is less effective in these patients. In fact, the exaggerated gastrin response in duodenal ulcer disease may be explained by a blunted negative feedback response to antral acidification.

Acid secretion is greater than normal at any given dose of gastrin in ulcer patients; ie, the parietal cells have a heightened sensitivity to stimulation. In summary, most patients with duodenal ulcer have 2 abnormalities in gastrin metabolism: (1) increased gastrin response to a meal and (2) increased sensitivity of the parietal cells to stimulation by gastrin.

Basal Hypergastrinemia

There are 7 uncommon causes of basal hypergastrinemia associated with duodenal ulcer: gastrinoma, hypercalcemia, massive small bowel resection, renal failure, gastric outlet obstruction, antral G cell hyperplasia, and antral exclusion. In the evaluation of a patient with duodenal ulcer, one should measure gastrin levels, and if hypergastrinemia is present, these conditions should be considered.

A. Gastrinoma: Patients with gastrinoma have autogenous production of large amounts of gastrin by a tumor. The result is excessive acid secretion and severe ulcer disease. Treatment, as discussed in detail later in this chapter, consists of administering H_2 receptor antagonists or performing tumor resection or total gastrectomy.

B. Hypercalcemia: Patients with hypercalcemia may secrete increased amounts of gastrin and gastric acid. In patients with hyperparathyroidism, removal of a parathyroid adenoma with return of the serum calcium level to normal usually also allows the serum gastrin and gastric acid secretion to become normal. However, the relationship between hypercalcemia and duodenal ulcer disease is not close, and in general, if severe duodenal ulcer disease is present in a patient with hyperparathyroidism, the cause is more likely to be gastrinoma (as part of multiple endocrine neoplasia [MEN] syndrome type I) than a direct effect of hypercalcemia.

C. Extensive Small Bowel Resection: People who have had extensive small bowel resections often secrete increased amounts of gastric acid and have elevated gastrin levels. Although this could be a result of decreased degradation of gastrin, it more likely reflects loss of an enterogastrone (a hormone from the intestine that inhibits gastrin release and gastric acid secretion). The increased acid secretion that follows enterectomy usually subsides within a few months, so that treatment with H_2 blocking agents is usually sufficient.

D. Renal Failure: Renal failure may be accompanied by hypergastrinemia and gastric hyperacidity, probably because of decreased catabolism of the large molecular forms of gastrin by the diseased kidneys. Treatment consists of antacids and H_2 blocking agents.

E. Gastric Outlet Obstruction: Hypergastrinemia in association with gastric outlet obstruction is probably caused by antral distention. Tube decompression of the stomach usually results in a return of the gastrin levels to normal.

F. Antral G Cell Hyperplasia: Rare patients have hypergastrinemia from hyperactivity of the G cells, a condition referred to as antral G cell hyperplasia. Treatment consists of H_2 blocking agents or antrectomy.

G. Excluded Antrum Syndrome: In the past, surgeons would occasionally divide the antrum proximal to the pylorus in an attempt to simplify surgical treatment of duodenal ulcer disease. The proximal stomach was reconstructed as a Billroth II gastrojejunostomy, and the divided end of the antrum was oversewn, leaving it excluded from the influence of acid secreted by the parietal cell mucosa in the remaining body and fundus. The isolated antrum would occasionally produce large amounts of gastrin, resulting in a syndrome similar to gastrinoma. Since surgeons long ago abandoned this operation and since the phenomenon does not occur if only a small amount of antral mucosa is accidentally left attached to the duodenum, the excluded antrum syndrome is exceedingly rare nowadays.

Effects of Other Hormones

Bombesin or **GRP** releases gastrin and is not inhibited by antral acidification. GRP is present in the antral mucosa and may serve as a physiologic stimulus for gastrin release. Theoretically, excess GRP could produce the effects that characterize duodenal ulcer disease, ie, the exaggerated gastrin response to a meal and the diminished inhibition of gastrin release by acid.

CCK is a weak agonist of acid secretion, but it has a strong potentiating influence on pancreatic bicarbonate secretion and delays gastric emptying. Pancreatic bicarbonate neutralizes acid in the duodenum, and the rate of gastric emptying governs delivery of acid to the duodenum. It is unlikely that CCK could contribute to ulcer formation by directly stimulating acid secretion. However, low CCK levels could be involved by allowing more rapid emptying of acid into the duodenum and decreasing bicarbonate secretion.

Secretin inhibits meal-stimulated gastrin release and gastric acid secretion in pharmacologic doses, but secretin is liberated in such small quantities that it could have little effect on the stomach. Secretin does, however, stimulate pancreatic bicarbonate secretion, and duodenal acidification stimulates secretin release. Although abnormalities in secretin could contribute to ulcer formation, studies comparing secretin release in patients with ulcer and in normal subjects have given conflicting results. In fact, excessive duodenal acidification is usually associated with increased secretin levels.

GIP inhibits acid secretion in response to many stimuli, and GIP levels increase after a meal. However, postprandial GIP levels are higher in patients with ulcer than in controls.

VIP inhibits gastric acid secretion and stimulates pancreatic secretion, but the serum levels are low and do not change after a meal.

Somatostatin inhibits gastrin release and gastric acid secretion in response to virtually all stimuli. The location of somatostatin in antral cells near the G cells suggests that it may serve as a paracrine inhibitor of gastric acid secretion. It is possible that decreased somatostatin activity contributes to duodenal ulcer formation, but experiments testing this possibility have not yet been performed.

CELIAC SPRUE DISEASE

In sprue, the villi of the proximal small intestine are fewer, shortened, and blunted—changes that substantially decrease the absorptive area. Malabsorption of protein, carbohydrate, and fat is the result. Fat malabsorption may be aggravated by hormonal abnormalities. Postprandial gallbladder contraction is delayed and incomplete in sprue, and pancreatic exocrine function in response to intraluminal stimuli is decreased. Exogenous administration of CCK or secretin in patients with sprue evokes normal responses in the gallbladder and pancreas, suggesting that the defect is in the release of these hormones. One report has documented decreased postprandial CCK levels in patients with sprue.

The abnormal gallbladder contraction results in decreased bile flow and bile salt concentrations in the intestine, and decreased stimulation of the pancreas lowers pancreatic enzyme concentrations. The end result is impaired micelle formation and fat absorption. While decreased intestinal surface area is probably the principal cause of malabsorption in sprue, these hormonal abnormalities enhance the malabsorption defect.

MOTILITY DISORDERS OF THE GASTROINTESTINAL TRACT

Stimulation of sympathetic nerves normally relaxes the gut, and stimulation of parasympathetic nerves causes it to contract. If both adrenergic and cholinergic receptors are blocked, nerve stimulation causes muscle relaxation.

Hirschsprung's disease is characterized by absence of neurons in a segment of distal colon. The affected colon is contracted, the muscular coat is hypertrophied, and the lumen is narrow. The colon proximally is dilated as a consequence of chronic partial obstruction. The concentrations of VIP and substance P as well as the numbers of nerves containing VIP and substance P are greatly decreased in the contracted segment. The present view is that the neurologic abnormality responsible for Hirschsprung's disease consists of loss of the relaxing influences of peptidergic VIP and substance P neurons.

Conceivably, other abnormalities of peptidergic neurons could contribute to other motility disorders such as pyloric stenosis and achalasia.

APUDOMAS

Apudoma is the general term for tumors of gut endocrine cells that secrete peptide hormones. The tumors may be very small and difficult to detect even at laparotomy.

Most apudomas are found in the pancreas, but a few occur in the wall of the duodenum or the retroperitoneum. Apudomas probably arise from pleuripotential stem cells (nesidioblasts) present in pancreatic ducts. Origin in such a cell could explain why many apudomas contain more than one type of endocrine cell and secrete more than one hormone. For example, VIPomas often secrete PP in addition to VIP. Insulin, gastrin, serotonin, substance P, PP, VIP, glucagon, enteroglucagon, and somatostatin have been found to be synthesized and secreted by different apudomas.

Although apudomas often secrete more than one peptide, they are usually named after the one most responsible for the clinical manifestations. Thus, a gastrin-secreting tumor is a gastrinoma and a VIP-secreting tumor a VIPoma. The incidence of other endocrine tumors in patients with gastrinoma is about 10–20%; in patients with insulinoma, 4%.

Wermer's syndrome is an autosomal dominant inherited condition in which 2 or more endocrine glands become hyperplastic or undergo tumor formation. Wermer's syndrome is also called multiple endocrine neoplasia (MEN) type I. In MEN type I, the pancreas, pituitary, and parathyroid glands are most often involved, and the most common pancreatic tumors are gastrinoma, insulinoma, and VIPoma. MEN type IIa, also known as **Sipple's syndrome,** consists of medullary carcinoma of the thyroid, pheochromocytoma, and hyperparathyroidism (see Chapter 25). The tumors are always multiple and diffuse in both MEN type I and MEN type IIa.

The diagnosis of apudoma is most often made by finding an elevated level of a hormone in the blood, and the usual conclusion is that the patient has a hormone-secreting tumor, most probably in the pancreas. Because the tumor is often difficult to find at laparotomy, preoperative localization is helpful. Pancreatic arteriography is occasionally useful in locating insulinomas but rarely so with gastrinomas. Ultrasonography and CT scanning have been disappointing. Selective sampling of hormone levels in venous outflow from the pancreas is now being studied to determine its value. The technique entails percutaneous puncture of the liver and threading a catheter into the splanchnic tributaries of the portal vein. Hormone levels in blood draining the tail, body, and head of the pancreas can be measured, and the point where a sharp increase in concentration is detected indicates where the tumor is located.

Tumor resection is the preferred treatment for apudomas, but many of them are malignant or multifocal and cannot be cured in this way. When resection is not possible, gastrinoma may be treated by gastrectomy (removing the target organ) or with H_2 blocking agents. However, for other hormone-producing tumors (eg, insulinoma or VIPoma), it is not possible to direct therapy at the target organ, and antitumor drugs are the only alternative to resection.

Fifty percent of apudomas found at operation are malignant, and most of these are unresectable. The chemotherapeutic agent most often used to treat malignant islet cell tumors is streptozocin, a nitrosourea derivative that inhibits DNA synthesis. The drug is usually given intravenously, but for treating hepatic metastases it may be infused directly into the hepatic artery. Streptozocin has been used to treat malignant gastrinomas, VIPomas, and glucagonomas. It produces a favorable response in about 50% of patients.

ZOLLINGER-ELLISON SYNDROME (Gastrinoma)

Zollinger-Ellison syndrome consists of gastric acid hypersecretion caused by a gastrin-producing tumor (gastrinoma). Although the normal pancreas does not contain appreciable amounts of gastrin, most gastrinomas occur in the pancreas; others are found submucosally in the duodenum and rarely in the antrum. The gastrin-producing lesions in the pancreas are non–B islet cell carcinomas (60%), solitary adenomas (25%), and hyperplasia or microadenomas (10%); the remaining cases (5%) are due to solitary submucosal gastrinomas in the first or second portion of the duodenum. The tumors, which may be as small as 2–3 mm, are often difficult to find. In about one-third of cases, the tumor cannot be located at laparotomy.

The diagnosis of cancer can be made only by finding metastases or blood vessel invasion, because the histologic pattern is similar for benign and malignant tumors. In most patients with malignant gastrinomas, the manifestations of hypergastrinemia (ie, severe peptic ulcer disease) are a far greater threat to health than are those of malignant growth and spread.

About a third of patients have other endocrine tumors—most commonly of the parathyroid and pituitary glands. When associated with tumors in other endocrine organs, the condition is known as MEN type I.

Clinical Findings

The symptoms in patients with gastrinoma are principally due to acid hypersecretion, and most of them are manifestations of peptic ulcer disease. Some patients with gastrinoma have severe diarrhea from the large amounts of acid entering the duodenum that may (1) destroy pancreatic lipase and produce steatorrhea, (2) damage the small bowel mucosa, and (3) overload the intestine with gastric and pancreatic secretions. About 5% of patients present with diarrhea only.

Ulcer symptoms are often refractory to large doses of antacids. Hemorrhage, perforation, and obstruction are common complications. Marginal ulcers often appear after surgical procedures that would cure the ordinary ulcer diathesis.

Diagnosis

Hypergastrinemia in the presence of acid hypersecretion is almost pathognomonic of gastrinoma. Because gastrin levels are normally inversely proportionate to gastric acid levels, many conditions that result in an increased gastric pH will allow the serum gastrin concentration to rise. Examples are pernicious anemia, atrophic gastritis, gastric ulcer, and postvagotomy state. In addition, use of H_2 blocking agents or antacids may increase the serum gastrin concentration, and these agents should be avoided for 24 hours before making gastrin measurements. It is often helpful to measure gastric acid secretion to rule out H^+ hyposecretion as a cause of hypergastrinemia.

A. Measurement of Serum Gastrin: Serum gastrin levels should be measured in any patient suspected of harboring a gastrinoma and in any patient whose ulcer disease is severe enough to warrant consideration of surgical treatment. In most laboratories, the normal gastrin value is less than 200 pg/mL. Patients with gastrinoma have levels that usually exceed 500 pg/mL, and they may reach 10,000 pg/mL or more. Patients with borderline gastrin values (200–500 pg/mL) whose acid secretion is in the range associated with ordinary duodenal ulcer disease should have a secretin provocative test. After administration of secretin, 2 units/kg as a bolus, a rise in the gastrin level of 150 pg/mL within 15 minutes is diagnostic (Table 18–5). Calcium given intravenously has also been used for this purpose, but secretin is both safer and more reliable. Postprandially, the serum gastrin levels do not change appreciably in patients with gastrinoma, whereas in normal subjects they double within 30 minutes.

Marked basal acid hypersecretion (> 15 meq H^+ per hour) occurs in most patients with Zollinger-Ellison syndrome who have an intact stomach. In a patient with a previous gastrectomy, a basal acid output of 5 meq/h or more would be highly suggestive. Since the parietal cells are already under near-maximal stimulation from hypergastrinemia, there is little increase in acid secretion following an injection of betazole (Histalog) or pentagastrin, and the ratio of basal

Table 18–5. Provocative tests for gastrin release.*

Syndrome or Illness	Secretin Test	Calcium Test	Standard Meal
Duodenal ulcer without gastrinoma	Negative	Negative	Positive
Gastric outlet obstruction	Negative	Negative	
Retained antrum	Negative	±	±
Antral gastrin cell hyperactivity	Negative	Positive	Positive
Gastrinoma	Positive	Positive	Negative

*For secretin test, positive = increase in gastrin > 150 pg/mL; for calcium test, positive = increase in gastrin > 300 pg/mL; for standard meal, positive = change in gastrin > 80% of basal.

to maximal acid output (BAO/MAO) characteristically exceeds 0.6.

Hypergastrinemia and gastric acid hypersecretion may be seen in gastric outlet obstruction, retained antrum after Billroth II gastrojejunostomy, and antral gastrin cell hyperactivity (hyperplasia). These conditions may be differentiated from gastrinoma by use of the calcium, secretin, and standard meal provocative tests. Large increases in serum gastrin levels after calcium or secretin and little change after a meal are characteristic of gastrinoma (Table 18–5). Because associated hyperparathyroidism is so common, all patients with gastrinoma should have their serum calcium concentration measured.

B. X-Ray Findings: An upper gastrointestinal series usually shows ulceration in the duodenal bulb, although ulcers sometimes appear in the distal duodenum or proximal jejunum. The presence of ulcers in these distal ("ectopic") locations is nearly diagnostic of gastrinoma. The stomach contains prominent rugal folds, and secretions are present in the lumen despite the overnight fast. The duodenum may be dilated and exhibit hyperactive peristalsis. Edema may be detected in the small bowel mucosa. The barium flocculates in the intestine, and transit time is accelerated. Selective angiography or CT scanning can sometimes demonstrate the pancreatic tumor, but misleading results are common with each. Experience with transhepatic portal vein blood sampling to find hot spots of gastrin production is too meager to justify any statement about whether this technique will help in tumor localization.

Treatment

A. Medical Treatment: All patients should be given cimetidine (Tagamet), 300–600 mg 4 times daily, or ranitidine (Zantac), 300–450 mg twice daily. Although this usually brings the acute ulcer under control, even larger doses may be required. If the response to treatment with an H_2 blocking agent is incomplete, the addition of anticholinergic drugs may be of benefit. Although treatment with cimetidine or ranitidine improves the ulcer disease acutely in most patients, the failure rate of prolonged therapy is high.

There is a tendency in most patients for treatment with H_2 blocking agents to become less effective with time, and an upward adjustment of the dose is usually necessary. Treatment with these drugs should aim to keep H^+ secretion below 5 meq/h.

B. Operative Treatment: Although complete removal of the gastrinoma would be ideal, the lesions are so often multiple that resection for cure is possible in only 10–20% of patients. Before the routine use of H_2 blocking agents, the patient often came to surgery with rampant ulcer disease, and if resection resulted in incomplete removal of all gastrin-producing lesions, serious complications of the ulcer disease, such as bleeding or perforation, often developed postoperatively. This was one argument in favor of total gastrectomy in preference to tumor resection. Now,

however, most patients are under reasonably good control preoperatively.

Total gastrectomy is the most thoroughly tested treatment for Zollinger-Ellison syndrome, and the results are excellent. Nutrition after total gastrectomy is rarely a problem even in children—who follow normal curves for growth and development after total gastrectomy. The good result with this procedure must be used as the standard for comparison with the new approaches to therapy now undergoing trial.

One recommended approach is to perform laparotomy after first controlling the ulcer disease with an H_2 blocking agent. At operation, the pancreas and duodenum are inspected, and if a solitary lesion is found, it is resected. Then, regardless of whether a tumor has been removed, a parietal cell vagotomy is performed. The reasoning is that definitive therapy will be provided early for patients with a curable tumor and that if the tumor cannot be completely resected, the parietal cell vagotomy will enhance the effectiveness of H_2 blocking agents.

Total gastrectomy remains the treatment of choice for patients with complications of the ulcer disease and for those whose disease is unsatisfactorily controlled by H_2 blockers. Whether prolonged treatment with cimetidine or ranitidine is preferable to elective total gastrectomy is as yet unknown. In time, the relative merits of each should become apparent. Nevertheless, any patient whose ulcer disease remains active during treatment with H_2 blocking agents should be treated by total gastrectomy or resection of the tumor.

Prognosis

H_2 blocking agents control acid secretion in the majority of patients. However, if total gastrectomy is required, the patient can expect to lead a relatively normal life after surgery. Weight loss and dumping are rarely severe. Although 50% of gastrinomas are malignant, they generally tend to be dormant after total gastrectomy and, in the absence of a source of acid secretion, are of less significance. A few malignant gastrinomas grow, metastasize, and ultimately kill the patient. Lifelong oral iron and parenteral vitamin B_{12} replacement (100 μg/month) is required after total gastrectomy.

PANCREATIC CHOLERA
(WDHA Syndrome: Watery Diarrhea, Hypokalemia, & Achlorhydria; VIPoma, or Verner-Morrison Syndrome)

Pancreatic cholera is characterized by profuse watery diarrhea, massive fecal loss of potassium, low serum potassium concentration, and extreme weakness. Gastric acid secretion is usually low or absent even after stimulation with betazole or pentagastrin. Stool volume averages about 5 L/d during acute episodes and contains over 300 meq of potassium (20 times normal). Severe metabolic acidosis frequently results from loss of bicarbonate in the stool. Many patients are hypercalcemic, possibly from secretion by the tumor of a PTH-like substance. Abnormal glucose tolerance may result from hypokalemia and altered sensitivity to insulin. Patients who complain of severe diarrhea must be carefully studied for other causes before the diagnosis of WDHA syndrome is seriously entertained. Chronic laxative abuse is a frequent explanation.

Pathogenesis

WDHA syndrome is characterized by enormous jejunal secretion (instead of absorption) of water and electrolytes. The colon and ileum appear to function normally, but they are overwhelmed by the fluid load.

The hormone most often associated with WDHA syndrome is vasoactive intestinal polypeptide (VIP). In addition to VIP, 5-hydroxytryptamine (serotonin), substance P, calcitonin, PP, and some of the prostaglandins may cause diarrhea when present in high concentrations in the blood. High prostaglandin E_2 levels have been reported in some patients with WDHA syndrome, and in one patient all symptoms were abolished by indomethacin, a prostaglandin inhibitor.

Because about 80% of patients have high serum VIP levels, VIP is considered to be the principal mediator of this syndrome. In these patients, successful treatment is accompanied by a fall in serum VIP levels to normal. An intravenous infusion of VIP produces diarrhea in pigs when the blood concentration reaches levels similar to those in patients with this syndrome.

Diagnosis

The presence of severe watery diarrhea and hypokalemia with normal or low gastric acid secretion should lead one to suspect this disease. Other causes of diarrhea such as malabsorption, infection, and surreptitious laxative use should be ruled out.

The presence of hypercalcemia and abnormal results in the oral glucose test tend to reinforce the diagnosis. A high VIP level is essentially diagnostic, but a normal level does not exclude WDHA syndrome.

The diagnosis may be confirmed at operation by finding a pancreatic islet cell tumor or a retroperitoneal neural tumor. In a substantial number of patients, no tumor is found.

Treatment

Complete removal of the tumor is curative and can be accomplished in 40–50% of patients. About half of these tumors are malignant and cannot be removed. Streptozocin may produce a remission of the diarrhea if surgery is unsuccessful. Other agents that occasionally elicit a clinical response are corticosteroids and indomethacin. If no tumor is found, it is reasonable to remove the tail and body of the pancreas to look for islet cell hyperplasia. In many patients, the diarrhea improves after subtotal pancreatectomy.

GLUCAGONOMA

Glucagonoma syndrome is characterized by a migratory necrolytic dermatitis (usually involving the legs and perineum), weight loss, stomatitis, hypoaminoacidemia, anemia, and mild diabetes mellitus. Visual scotomas and changes in visual acuity have been reported in some cases. The age range is 20–70 years, and the condition is more common in women. The diagnosis may be suspected from the distinctive skin lesion; in fact, the presence of a prominent rash in a patient with diabetes mellitus should be enough to raise suspicions. Confirmation of the diagnosis depends on demonstration of elevated serum glucagon levels. It may be possible to demonstrate the tumor by arteriography or CT scanning.

Glucagonomas arise from A_2 cells in the pancreatic islets. About 25% are benign and confined to the pancreas. The remainder have metastasized by the time of diagnosis, most often to the liver, lymph nodes, adrenal glands, or vertebrae. A few cases have been the result of islet cell hyperplasia.

Surgical removal of the primary lesion and resectable secondaries is indicated if technically feasible. Even if it is not possible to remove all of the tumor deposits, considerable palliation may result from subtotal removal. Oral zinc supplements may improve the dermatitis. Streptozocin and dacarbazine are effective chemotherapeutic agents for unresectable lesions. The clinical course generally parallels changes in serum levels of glucagon in response to therapy.

SOMATOSTATINOMA

Somatostatinomas are characterized by diabetes mellitus (usually mild), diarrhea and malabsorption, and dilatation of the gallbladder (usually with cholelithiasis). High levels of calcitonin and IgM have been present in the serum in some patients. The syndrome results from secretion of somatostatin by an islet cell tumor of the pancreas, which in most cases is malignant and accompanied by hepatic metastases. The diagnosis may be made by recognizing the clinical syndrome and measuring increased concentrations of somatostatin in the serum. In most cases, however, the somatostatin syndrome has been unsuspected until histologic evidence of metastatic islet cell carcinoma has been obtained. Surgery may be indicated if the disease is localized. More often, chemotherapy with streptozocin, dacarbazine, doxorubicin, etc, is the only treatment possible.

PANCREATIC POLYPEPTIDE-PRODUCING TUMORS (PPomas)

A few tumors of the pancreas have been found to produce pancreatic polypeptide (PP). Since PP produces few (if any) symptoms, the clinical manifestations in patients with PPomas have been chiefly due to direct effects of the tumor (eg, abdominal pain, weight loss). The tumor is malignant in 50% of cases. Treatment consists of tumor resection.

CARCINOID TUMORS & CARCINOID SYNDROME

Carcinoid tumors arise from enterochromaffin cells. They are often multiple and may appear anywhere in the gut from the gastroesophageal junction to the anus. In general, carcinoid tumors less than 1 cm in diameter are benign, and those greater than 1 cm in diameter are malignant. In the gastrointestinal tract, their propensity for malignant change depends upon their location. For example, fewer than 10% of appendiceal or rectal carcinoids are malignant, whereas 30% of ileal and 60% of colonic (excluding rectal) carcinoids are malignant. Carcinoid tumors may also occur in the bronchi or ovaries. Local resection is adequate treatment for benign lesions, and wide excision including the lymphatic drainage is recommended for malignant ones.

Because carcinoids in different locations behave differently and probably have different secretory products, it is appropriate to categorize them as foregut (bronchus and stomach), midgut (small intestine and colon), or hindgut (rectum) tumors. Hindgut carcinoids synthesize no specific by-products, and they do not stain with silver salts (ie, they are argentaffin- and argyrophil-negative). Foregut carcinoids secrete 5-hydroxytryptophan and are argentaffin-negative and argyrophil-positive. Midgut tumors secrete 5-hydroxytryptamine and are both argentaffin- and argyrophil-positive.

Carcinoid syndrome is caused by release of 5-hydroxytryptamine (serotonin) and other substances from enterochromaffin tumors. The syndrome is also occasionally caused by other tumors, such as oat cell carcinoma and medullary carcinoma of the thyroid. Because the humoral substances liberated by carcinoids are deactivated during one passage through the liver, the presence of the syndrome implies either a primary lesion draining into the systemic circulation or hepatic metastasis from a gastrointestinal lesion. Fortunately, only 1% of patients with a gastrointestinal carcinoid manifest the carcinoid syndrome.

Etiology

The symptoms of carcinoid syndrome are probably caused by more than one substance, though serotonin is the most firmly established one. Carcinoid tumors contain large amounts of serotonin, and serum levels are markedly elevated in patients with this syndrome. When given intravenously, serotonin produces diarrhea and hypotension but not flushing. Kallikrein, an enzyme that promotes the formation of bradykinin from globulin, is found in some carcinoid tumors, and serum bradykinin levels are high in some patients with carcinoid syndrome. Infusion of bradykinin produces

diarrhea and flushing. Prostaglandin E and substance P are also found in carcinoid tumors, and both cause flushing and diarrhea.

Clinical Findings

The most common symptoms are flushing of the head and neck and diarrhea. The flushing attacks last a few minutes and may be accompanied by hypotension. The attacks may be provoked by emotional stress, ingestion of particular foods, straining at stool, etc. Diarrhea is often severe and may be debilitating. Both flushing and diarrhea occur in the majority of patients. About 50% of patients develop endocardial fibrosis of the tricuspid and pulmonary valves. Retroperitoneal fibrosis, arthritis, and bronchial asthma also occur but less frequently.

Diagnosis

The most useful diagnostic test for carcinoid tumors is measurement of urinary 5-hydroxyindoleacetic acid (5-HIAA), a breakdown product of serotonin. Measurement of serotonin, histamine, prostaglandin, and bradykinin levels in blood may also be of use, but these tests are difficult to perform and are not available in most laboratories.

Once the diagnosis is established, it is important to localize the tumor. If it is outside the gastrointestinal tract, it may be benign. If the syndrome is secondary to a gastrointestinal carcinoid, 60% of patients have a tumor of the ileum or jejunum with metastases to the liver. Small bowel contrast studies and arteriography help to localize these tumors.

Treatment

A. Operative Treatment: Even though systemic symptoms usually imply the presence of hepatic metastases and an incurable lesion, patients with carcinoid syndrome should be surgically explored to confirm that a gastrointestinal carcinoid is the cause of the syndrome. To prevent future bleeding and bowel obstruction, all primary tumor that can be resected safely should be removed. In selected cases, hepatic metastases may be treated by hepatic artery ligation or a limited hepatic resection (ie, lobectomy) to reduce symptoms.

B. Symptomatic Measures: Pharmacologic treatment should be aimed at minimizing diarrhea and flushing. Diarrhea can often be controlled by diphenoxylate with atropine (Lomotil), paregoric, or codeine. Specific antiserotonin agents such as methysergide and cyproheptadine are also used, but flushing is usually not meliorated by these drugs. Phenoxybenzamine (Dibenzyline) (an alpha-adrenergic blocker), glucocorticoids, methyldopa (a decarboxylase inhibitor), and phenothiazines have all been used with some success to control flushing.

C. Antitumor Chemotherapy: Because these tumors are slow-growing and may produce minimal symptoms, cytotoxic drugs are not given for early disease that is minimally symptomatic. Remissions can be achieved in about 20–70% of patients by use of cancer chemotherapeutic agents. The most successful regimen consists of streptozocin plus fluorouracil. Doxorubicin and dacarbazine are being evaluated in ongoing clinical trials. In the future, chemotherapy for hepatic metastases may be improved by delivery of the agent into a surgically placed hepatic artery catheter. A catheter is placed in the right or left hepatic artery at operation and connected to a subcutaneously placed pump. The chemotherapeutic agent is then placed in the pump, whence it is slowly delivered to the selected artery.

Prognosis

The 5-year survival rate for patients with metastases is 20%. However, the cure rate with surgical resection is relatively good for cancers that have not metastasized distantly. If only regional nodes are involved, the 5-year survival rate is 65%; if the tumor is locally invasive without lymph node involvement, the 5-year survival rate is 95%. The 5-year survival rates associated with different tumor sites are 99% for appendix, 87% for lung, 50% for small intestine and colon, and 83% for rectum and rectosigmoid.

MISCELLANEOUS GASTROINTESTINAL TUMORS

Other islet cell tumors have been reported that produce neurotensin, CCK, vasopressin, a GH-releasing factor, ACTH, and MSH.

REFERENCES

General

Bishop AE et al: Peptidergic nerves. *Scand J Gastroenterol* 1982;**17(Suppl 71)**:43.

Buchanan KD: Gastrointestinal hormones: General concepts. *Clin Endocrinol Metab* 1979;**8**:249.

Furness JB et al: Detection and characterisation of neurotransmitters, particularly peptides, in the gastrointestinal tract. *Scand J Gastroenterol* 1982;**17(Suppl 71)**:61.

Gershon MD, Erde SM: The nervous system of the gut. *Gastroenterology* 1981;**80**:1571.

Krieger D: Brain peptides: What, where and why? *Science* 1983;**222**:975.

Larsson LI: Pathology of gastrointestinal endocrine cells. *Scand J Gastroenterol* 1979;**14(Suppl 53)**:1.

Pearse AGE: The APUD concept: Embryology, cytochemistry, and ultrastructure of the diffuse neuroendocrine system. Chapter 2 in: *Surgical Endocrinology*. Friesen SR (editor). Lippincott, 1978.

Polak JM, Bloom SR: Regulatory peptides: Key factors in the control of bodily function. *Br Med J* 1983;**286**:1461.

Rehfeld JF: Gastrointestinal hormones. Pages 291–321 in: *International Review of Physiology III*. Vol 19. University Press, 1979.

Solcia E et al: The diffuse endocrine-paracrine system of the gut in health and disease: Ultrastructural features. *Scand J Gastroenterol* 1981;**16(Suppl 70)**:11.

Strauss E: Radioimmunoassay of gastrointestinal hormones. *Gastroenterology* 1978;**74**:141.

Sundler F et al: Peptidergic nervous systems in the gut. *Clin Gastroenterol* 1980;**9**:517.

Thompson J, Marx M: Gastrointestinal hormones. *Curr Probl Surg* 1984;**12**:1.

Walsh JH: Nature of gut peptides and their possible functions. In: *Cellular Basis of Chemical Messengers in the Digestive System*. Academic Press, 1981.

Weinbeck M, Erckenbrecht J: The control of gastrointestinal motility in GI hormones. *Clin Gastroenterol* 1982;**11**:523.

Welbourn RB et al: Tumors of the neuroendocrine system (APUD cell tumors—apudomas). *Curr Probl Surg* 1984;**11**:1.

Gastrin

Chew CS, Hersey S: Gastrin stimulation of isolated gastric glands. *Am J Physiol* 1982;**242**:G504.

Nilsson G: Gastrin: Isolation, characterization and functions. In: *Gastrointestinal Hormones*. Glass GBJ (editor). Raven Press, 1980.

Soll A et al: Gastrin receptors on isolated canine parietal cells. *J Clin Invest* 1984;**73**:1434.

Walsh JH, Lam SK: Physiology and pathology of gastrin. *Clin Gastroenterol* 1980;**9**:567.

Cholecystokinin

Anika SM et al: Cholecystokinin and satiety in pigs. *Am J Physiol* 1981;**240**:310.

Calam J, Ellis A, Dockray GJ: Identification and measurement of molecular variants of cholecystokinin in duodenal mucosa and plasma. *J Clin Invest* 1982;**169**:218.

Dockray GJ: The physiology of cholecystokinin. *Brain Gut* 1982;**38**:253.

Gosnell B, Hsiao S: Cholecystokinin satiety and orosensory feedback. *Physiol Behav* 1981;**27**:153.

Rehfeld JF: Cholecystokinin. *Clin Gastroenterol* 1980;**9**:593.

Wiener I et al: Release of cholecystokinin in man: Correlation of blood levels with gallbladder function. *Ann Surg* 1981;**194**:321.

Secretin

Gyr K et al: Plasma secretin and pancreatic response to various stimulants including a meal. *Am J Physiol* 1984;**246**:G535.

Hacki WH: Secretin. *Clin Gastroenterol* 1980;**9**:609.

Kleibeuker J et al: Role of endogenous secretin on acid-induced inhibition of human gastrin function. *J Clin Invest* 1984;**73**:526.

Gastric Inhibitory Polypeptide

Brown JC: Gastric inhibitory polypeptide. *Monogr Endocrinol* 1982;**24**:1.

Cataland S: Physiology of GIP in man. In: *Gut Hormones*, 2nd ed. Bloom SR (editor). Churchill Livingstone, 1981.

Sarson D, Hayter R, Blood S: The pharmacokinetics of porcine glucose-dependent insulinotropic polypeptide (GIP) in man. *Eur J Clin Invest* 1982;**12**:457.

Vasoactive Intestinal Polypeptide

Biancani P, Walsh J, Behar J: Vasoactive intestinal polypeptide: A neurotransmitter for esophageal sphincter relaxation. *J Clin Invest* 1984;**73**:963.

Fahrenkrug J: Vasoactive intestinal polypeptide: Functional aspects. *Br Med Bull* 1982;**38**:265.

Krejs G et al: Effect of VIP infusion in water and ion transport in the human jejunum. *Gastroenterology* 1980;**78**:722.

Said SI: Vasoactive intestinal polypeptide (VIP): Current status. *Peptides* 1984;**5**:145.

Said SI (editor): *Vasoactive Intestinal Peptide*. Raven Press, 1982.

Substance P

Couture R, Regori D: Mini review: Smooth muscle pharmacology of substance P. *Pharmacology* 1982;**24**:1.

Pearse AGE, Polak JM: Immunocytochemical localization of substance P in mammalian intestine. *Histochemistry* 1975; **41**:373.

Reynolds J, Ouyang A, Cohen S: A lower esophageal sphincter reflex involving substance P. *Am J Physiol* 1984; **246**:G346.

Enkephalins

Ambinder RF, Schuster MM: Endorphins: New gut peptides with a familiar face. *Gastroenterology* 1979;**77**:1132.

Polak J et al: Enkaphalin-like immunoreactivity in the human gastrointestinal tract. *Lancet* 1972;**1**:972.

Neurotensin

Brown DR, Miller RJ: Neurotensin. *Br Med Bull* 1982;**38**:239.

Miller RJ: Neurotensin as a gastrointestinal hormone. *Med Biol* 1981;**59**:65.

Motilin

Adachi H et al: Mechanism of the excitatory action of motilin on isolated rabbit intestine. *Gastroenterology* 1981;**80**:783.

Chey W, Lee KY: Motilin. *Clin Gastroenterol* 1980;**9**:645.

Poitros P et al: Motilin-independent ectopic fronts of the interdigestive myoelectric complex in dogs. *Am J Physiol* 1980;**239**:215.

Somatostatin

Armiuro A et al: Somatostatin: Abundance of immunoreactive hormone in rat stomach and pancreas. *Science* 1975; **189**:1007.

Arnold R, Lankisch PG: Somatostatin and the gastrointestinal tract. *Clin Gastroenterol* 1980;**9**:733.

Reichlin S: Somatostatin. (2 parts.) *N Engl J Med* 1983; **309**:1495, 1556.

Peptide YY

Tatemoto K: Isolation and characterization of peptide YY (PYY), a candidate gut hormone that inhibits pancreatic exocrine secretion. *Proc Natl Acad Sci USA* 1982;**79**:2514.

Bombesin & Gastrin-Releasing Peptide

Erspamer V et al: Occurrence and polymorphism of bombesin-like peptides in the gastrointestinal tract of birds and mammals. *Gut* 1979;**20**:1047.

Inoue K et al: Effect of gastrin-releasing peptide on the release of gastrointestinal hormones in dogs. *Physiologist* 1982; **25**:218.

McDonald T et al: Characterization of a gastrin-releasing peptide from porcine non-antral gastric tissue. *Biochem Biophys Res Commun* 1979;**90**:227.

McDonald T et al: A qualitative comparison of canine plasma gastroenterohepatic hormone responses to bombesin and the porcine gastrin-releasing peptide (GRP). *Regul Pept* 1981;**2**:293.

Walsh JH et al: Bombesin-like peptides in mammals. *Fed Proc* 1979;**38**:2315.

Pancreatic Polypeptide

Adrian TE et al: Inhibition of secretin-stimulated pancreatic secretion by pancreatic polypeptide. *Gut* 1979;**20**:37.

Lonovics J et al: Pancreatic polypeptide: A review. *Arch Surg* 1981;**116**:1256.

Taylor IL et al: Pancreatic polypeptide metabolism and effect on pancreatic secretion in dogs. *Gastroenterology* 1979; **76**:524.

Glucagonlike Immunoreactivity

Holst JJ: Gut glucagon, enteroglucagon, gut glucagonlike immunoreactivity, glicentin: Current status. *Gastroenterology* 1983;**84**:1602.

Hormonal Abnormalities in Diseases of the Gastrointestinal Tract

Besterman HS et al: Gut hormone profile in coeliac disease. *Lancet* 1978;**1**:785.

Chajvialle JAP et al: Somatostatin in mucosa of stomach and duodenum in gastroduodenal disease. *Gastroenterology* 1978;**75**:13.

Creutzfeld W, Arnold R: Endocrinology of duodenal ulcer. *World J Surg* 1979;**5**:605.

Low-Beer TS et al: Abnormalities of cholecystokinin and gallbladder contraction in coeliac disease. *N Engl J Med* 1975;**292**:961.

O'Connor FA et al: Impaired immunoreactive secretin release in coeliac disease. *Br Med J* 1977;**1**:811.

Taylor IL: Gastrointestinal hormones in the pathogenesis of peptic ulcer disease. *Clin Gastroenterol* 1984;**13**:355.

Zollinger-Ellison Syndrome

Bonfils S et al: Results of surgical management of 92 consecutive patients with Zollinger-Ellison syndrome. *Ann Surg* 1981;**194**:692.

Brennan MF et al: The role of surgery in patients with Zollinger-Ellison syndrome (ZES) managed medically. *Ann Surg* 1982;**196**:239.

Deveney CW, Stein S, Way LW: Cimetidine as primary treatment for gastrinoma: Long-term follow-up. *Am J Surg* 1983;**146**:116.

Deveney CW et al: The Zollinger-Ellison syndrome: 23 years later. *Ann Surg* 1978;**188**:384.

Glowniak JV et al: Percutaneous transhepatic venous sampling of gastrin: Value in sporadic and familial islet-cell tumors and G-cell hyperfunction. *N Engl J Med* 1982; **307**:293.

Harmon JW et al: Removal of gastrinomas for control of Zollinger-Ellison syndrome. *Ann Surg* 1984;**199**:396.

Jensen R: Basis for failure of cimetidine in patients with Zollinger-Ellison syndrome. *Dig Dis Sci* 1984;**29**:363.

Jensen R et al: Zollinger-Ellison syndrome: Current concepts and management. (NIH Combined Clinical Staff Conference.) *Ann Intern Med* 1983;**98**:59.

Raufman JP et al: Reliability of symptoms in assessing control of gastric acid secretion in patients with Zollinger-Ellison syndrome. *Gastroenterology* 1983;**84**:108.

Pancreatic Cholera

Field M, Chang E: Pancreatic cholera: Is the diarrhea due to VIP? *N Engl J Med* 1983;**309**:1513.

Jaffe BM, Condon S: Prostaglandins E and F in endocrine diarrheagenic syndromes. *Ann Surg* 1976;**184**:516.

Kahn CR et al: Pancreatic cholera: Beneficial effects of treatment with streptozotocin. *N Engl J Med* 1975;**292**:941.

Kane M, O'Dorisio T, Krejs G: Production of secretory diarrhea by intravenous infusion of vasoactive intestinal polypeptide. *N Engl J Med* 1983;**309**:1482.

Krejs GJ et al: Effect of VIP infusion on water and ion transport in the human jejunum. *Gastroenterology* 1980; **78**:722.

Long RG et al: Clinicopathological study of pancreatic and ganglioneuroma tumors secreting vasoactive intestinal polypeptide. *Br Med J* 1981;**282**:1767.

Read NW et al: Chronic diarrhea of unknown origin. *Gastroenterology* 1980;**78**:264.

Yamaguchi K et al: The WDHA syndrome: Clinical and laboratory data on 28 Japanese cases. *Peptides* 1984;**5**:415.

Glucagonoma

Leichter SB: Clinical and metabolic aspects of glucagonoma. *Medicine* 1980;**59**:100.

Montenegro-Rodas F, Samaan NA: Glucagonoma tumors and syndrome. *Curr Probl Cancer* 1981;**6**:3.

Nankervis A et al: The metabolic effects of chronic hyperglucagonaemia. *Clin Endocrinol* 1981;**15**:325.

Prinz RA et al: Operative and chemotherapeutic management of malignant glucagon-producing tumors. *Surgery* 1981; **90**:713.

Stacpoole PW: The glucagonoma syndrome: Clinical features, diagnosis, and treatment. *Endocr Rev* 1981;**76**:125.

Pancreatic Polypeptide–Producing Tumors (PPomas)

Strodel WE et al: Pancreatic polypeptide–producing tumors: Silent lesions of the pancreas? *Arch Surg* 1984;**119**:508.

Somatostatinoma

Axelrod L et al: Malignant somatostatinoma: Clinical features and metabolic studies. *J Clin Endocrinol Metab* 1981; **52**:886.

Sakazaki S et al: Pancreatic somatostatinoma. *Am J Surg* 1983;**146**:674.

Carcinoid Tumors & Carcinoid Syndrome

Beaton H et al: Gastrointestinal carcinoids and the malignant carcinoid syndrome. *Surg Gynecol Obstet* 1981;**152**:268.

Brandt B, Heintz SE, Rose EF: Bronchial carcinoid tumors. *Ann Thorac Surg* 1984;**38**:63.

Feldman JM: Serotonin metabolism in patients with carcinoid tumors: Incidence of 5-hydroxytryptophan-secreting tumors. *Gastroenterology* 1978;**75**:1109.

Johnson LA et al: Carcinoids: The association of histologic growth pattern and survival. *Cancer* 1981;**51**:882.

Moertel CG: Treatment of the carcinoid tumor and the malignant carcinoid syndrome. *J Clin Oncol* 1983;**1**:727.

Naunheim KS et al: Rectal carcinoid tumors: Treatment and prognosis. *Surgery* 1983;**94**:670.

Peck JJ et al: Carcinoid tumors of the ileum. *Am J Surg* 1983;**146**:124.

Sareing T, Sawyers JL: Carcinoids and the carcinoid syndrome. *Am J Surg* 1983;**145**:769.

Strodel WE et al: Surgical therapy for small-bowel carcinoid tumors. *Arch Surg* 1983;**118**:391.

Weidner FA, Ziter FJ Jr: Carcinoid tumors of the gastrointestinal tract. *JAMA* 1981;**245**:1153.

Wilkin JK: Flushing reactions: Consequences and mechanisms. *Ann Intern Med* 1981;**95**:468.

Pancreatic Hormones & Diabetes Mellitus

19

John H. Karam, MD, Patricia R. Salber, MD, & Peter H. Forsham, MD

I. THE ENDOCRINE PANCREAS

The pancreas is made up of 2 functionally different organs: the **exocrine pancreas,** the major digestive gland of the body; and the **endocrine pancreas,** the source of insulin, glucagon, and other hormones. Whereas the major role of the products of the exocrine pancreas (the digestive enzymes) is the processing of ingested foodstuffs so that they become available for absorption, the hormones of the endocrine pancreas modulate every other aspect of cellular nutrition from rate of absorption of foodstuffs to cellular storage or metabolism of nutrients. Dysfunction of the endocrine pancreas or abnormal responses to its hormones by target tissues result in serious disturbances in nutrient homeostasis, including the important clinical syndromes grouped under the name of **diabetes mellitus.**

ANATOMY & HISTOLOGY

The endocrine pancreas consists of hundreds of thousands of small endocrine glands—the islets of Langerhans—scattered within the glandular substance of the exocrine pancreas. The islet volume comprises about 2–3% of the total mass of the pancreas and weighs about 1–2 g in adult humans.

At least 4 cell types—A, B, D, and F—have been identified in the islets (Table 19–1). These cell types are not distributed uniformly throughout the islets. The F cell, which secretes pancreatic polypeptide (PP), has been found only in islets in the posterior

Acronyms Used in This Chapter

ADA	American Diabetes Association
ADH	Antidiuretic hormone (vasopressin)
ADP	Adenosine diphosphate
ATP	Adenosine triphosphate
cAMP	Cyclic adenosine monophosphate
CCK	Cholecystokinin
cGMP	Cyclic guanosine monophosphate
DNA	Deoxyribonucleic acid
FDA	Food and Drug Administration
GH	Growth hormone
GI	Glycemic index
GIP	Gastric inhibitory polypeptide
HDL	High-density lipoprotein(s)
5-HIAA	5-Hydroxyindoleacetic acid
HLA	Human leukocyte antigen
IDDM	Insulin-dependent diabetes mellitus
MODY	Maturity-onset diabetes of the young
NIDDM	Non-insulin-dependent diabetes mellitus
NPH	Neutral protamine Hagedorn
PFK	Phosphofructokinase
PP	Pancreatic polypeptide
PZI	Protamine zinc insulin
RNA	Ribonucleic acid
UGDP	University Group Diabetes Program
VLDL	Very low density lipoprotein(s)

portion of the head, a discrete lobe of the pancreas separated from the anterior portion of the head by a fascial partition. This lobe originates in the primordial ventral bud as opposed to the dorsal bud, and islets in this area consist of 80% F cells, 17–20% B cells, and less than 0.5% glucagon-producing A cells.

In contrast, the PP-poor islets located in the tail, body, and *anterior* portion of the head of the pancreas, arising from the embryonic dorsal bud, contain predominantly insulin-secreting B cells (75% of the islet cells), with approximately 20% of the cells being glucagon-secreting A cells and about 3–5% D cells that produce somatostatin. A typical islet from this part of the pancreas is depicted in Fig 19–1.

Table 19–1. Cell types in pancreatic islets of Langerhans.

Cell Types	Approximate % of Islet Mass	Secretory Products
A cell (α)	20%	Glucagon, proglucagon
B cell (β)	75%	Insulin, C peptide, proinsulin
D cell (δ)	3–5%	Somatostatin
F cell (PP cell)	< 2%	Pancreatic polypeptide

Figure 19–1. Photomicrograph of a section of the pancreas. In the islet of Langerhans, A cells appear mainly in the periphery as large cells with dark cytoplasm. Some D cells are also present in the periphery, while the central core is composed chiefly of B cells. (Reproduced, with permission, from Junqueira LC, Carneiro J, Long JA: *Basic Histology,* 5th ed. Lange, 1986.)

Figure 19–2. Structural components of the pancreatic B cell involved in glucose-induced biosynthesis and release. Schematic representation of secretory granular alignment on microfilament "tracks" that contract in response to calcium. (Based on data presented by Orci L: A portrait of the pancreatic B cell. *Diabetologia* 1974;**10**:163.) (Modified and reproduced, with permission, from Junqueira LC, Carneiro J, Long JA: *Basic Histology,* 5th ed. Lange, 1986.)

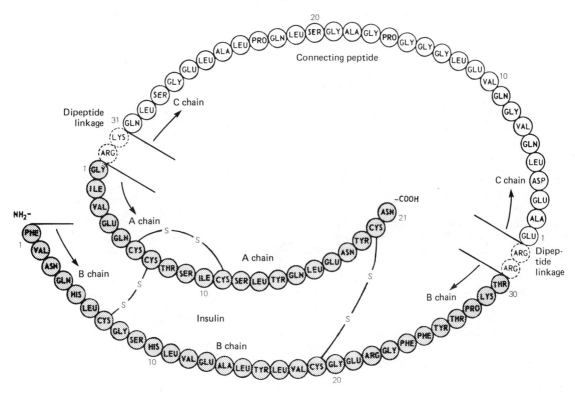

Figure 19–3. Structure of human proinsulin C peptides and insulin molecules connected at 2 sites by dipeptide links.

HORMONES OF
THE ENDOCRINE PANCREAS

1. INSULIN

Biosynthesis

Insulin, the major secretory product of the endocrine pancreas, is synthesized in the pancreatic B cell (Fig 19–2). A precursor molecule, **preproinsulin,** a long-chain peptide of MW 12,000, is produced by DNA/RNA-directed synthesis in the rough endoplasmic reticulum of these cells. It is cleaved by microsomal enzymes to **proinsulin** (MW about 9000) almost immediately after synthesis (Fig 19–3). Proinsulin is then converted to **insulin** and a smaller connecting peptide, or **C peptide**, by proteolytic cleavage at 2 sites along the peptide chain. Two different intermediate molecules are produced when proinsulin transiently retains one of its connecting terminals between C peptide and the insulin molecule. Cleavage of proinsulin occurs either before or after its transport to the Golgi apparatus, where packaging into granules occurs. Normal mature secretory granules contain insulin and C peptide in equimolar amounts and small quantities of proinsulin.

Biochemistry

Insulin is a protein hormone consisting of 51 amino acids contained within 2 peptide chains: an A chain, with 21 amino acids; and a B chain, with 30 amino acids. The chains are connected by 2 disulfide bridges as shown in Fig 19–3. In addition, there is an intrachain disulfide bridge that links positions 6 and 11 in the A chain. The molecular weight of human insulin is 5808, and that of bovine insulin is 5734.

Human insulin differs only slightly in amino acid composition from the 2 mammalian insulins presently used for therapeutic insulin replacement. Pork insulin differs from human by only one amino acid—alanine instead of threonine at the carboxyl terminus of the B chain (position B 30). Beef insulin differs by 3 amino acids—alanine instead of threonine at A 8 as well as the B 30 position and valine instead of isoleucine at A 10.

Endogenous insulin has a circulatory half-life of 3–5 minutes. It is catabolized chiefly by insulinases in liver and kidney.

Proinsulin (Fig 19–3) consists of a single chain of 86 amino acids, which includes the A and B chains of the insulin molecule plus a connecting segment of 35 amino acids. As noted above, this connecting segment is removed by as yet uncharacterized proteolytic enzymes. In the process of separating the connecting segment from proinsulin, 4 basic amino acids (one lysine and 3 arginines) are cleaved, leaving a 31-amino-acid residue, the C peptide, and the 51-amino-acid insulin molecule.

A small amount of proinsulin produced by the pancreas escapes cleavage and is secreted intact into the bloodstream. Most anti-insulin sera used in the standard immunoassay for insulin cross-react with proinsulin; about 3–5% of immunoreactive insulin extracted from human pancreas is actually proinsulin. Because proinsulin is not removed by the liver, it has a half-life 3–4 times that of insulin. This allows proinsulin to accumulate in the blood, where it accounts for 12–20% of the circulating immunoreactive "insulin" in the basal state in humans. Human proinsulin has about 7–8% of the biologic activity of insulin. There is evidence that some proinsulin is converted to insulin by the liver. The kidney is the principal site of proinsulin degradation.

Partially cleaved proinsulin molecules probably do not gain access to the bloodstream in significant quantity. Recently, however, families with such abnormal circulating insulins have been described.

C peptide, the 31-amino-acid residue (MW 3000) formed during cleavage of insulin from proinsulin, has no known biologic activity. It is released from the B cells in equimolar amounts with insulin. It is not removed by the liver but is degraded or excreted chiefly by the kidney. It has a half-life 3–4 times that of insulin. In the basal state after an overnight fast, the average concentration of C peptide may be as high as 1000 pmol/L.

Secretion

The basal concentration of insulin in the blood of fasting humans averages 10 μU/mL (0.4 ng/mL, or 69 pmol/L). In normal control subjects, insulin seldom rises above 100 μU/mL (690 pmol/L) after standard meals. There is an increase in peripheral insulin concentration beginning 8–10 minutes after ingestion of food and reaching peak concentration in peripheral blood by 30–45 minutes. This is followed by a rapid decline in postprandial plasma glucose concentration, which returns to baseline values by 90–120 minutes (Fig 19–4).

Because of the difficulties of obtaining adequate data on insulin secretion in humans (inability to administer rapid stimuli to the pancreatic artery and difficulty in obtaining samples from the portal vein), much of what is currently known about insulin secretion is inferred from models using the perfused rat pancreas or isolated rodent islets. Surprisingly, there have been only minor discrepancies between the data obtained in rodents and the general characteristics of insulin release observed in humans.

There are 2 aspects of insulin secretion that must be examined: basal secretion and stimulated secretion. **Basal insulin secretion,** which occurs in the absence of exogenous stimuli, is the quantity of insulin secreted in the fasting state. Although it is known that plasma glucose levels below about 100 mg/dL do not stimulate insulin release, it has also been demonstrated that the presence of glucose is necessary (in in vitro systems) for other known regulators of insulin secretion to be effective.

Figure 19–4. Plasma glucose and insulin response to a standard 530-kcal breakfast in normal subjects.

Stimulated insulin secretion is that which occurs in response to exogenous stimuli. In vivo, this is the response of the B cell to ingested meals. Glucose is the most potent stimulant of insulin release. The exact mechanism of action of glucose on the B cell remains to be clarified. The perfused rat pancreas has demonstrated a biphasic release of insulin in response to glucose (Fig 19–5). When the glucose concentration in the system is increased suddenly, an initial short-lived burst of insulin release occurs (the **early phase**); if the glucose concentration is held at this level, the insulin release gradually falls off and then begins to rise again to a steady level (the **late phase**).

Currently, the mechanism of action of glucose-stimulated insulin release is not well understood. There is evidence that glucose may act through a membrane-bound glucose receptor; however, despite extensive research in this area, no such glucose receptor has been identified on the B cell. There is a greater body of data suggesting that *metabolism* of glucose is essential in stimulating insulin release. Indeed, agents such as 2-deoxyglucose that inhibit the metabolism of glucose interfere with release of insulin.

Insulin release has been shown to require calcium. It has been proposed that mature insulin-containing granules in the B cell attach linearly to microtubules that contract after exposure to high intracellular calcium, thereby ejecting the granules (Fig 19–2). The following effects of glucose on calcium ion movement have been demonstrated: (1) Calcium uptake is increased by glucose stimulation of the B cell. (2) Calcium efflux from the cell is retarded by some action of glucose. (3) Mobilization of calcium from mitochondrial compartments occurs secondary to cAMP induction by glucose.

cAMP is another important modulator of insulin release. As mentioned above, glucose has been shown to directly induce cAMP formation. Furthermore, many nonglucose stimuli to insulin release are known

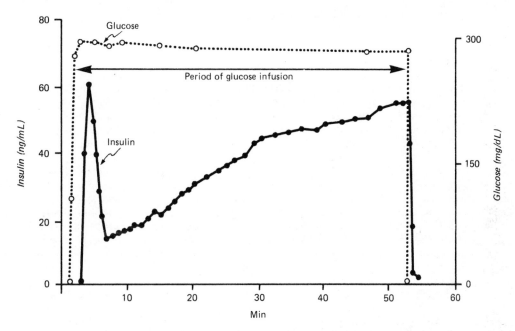

Figure 19–5. Multiphasic response of the in vitro perfused pancreas during constant stimulation with glucose. (Modified from Grodsky GM et al: Further studies on the dynamic aspects of insulin release in vitro with evidence for a 2-compartmental storage system. *Acta Diabetol Lat* 1969;**6**[Suppl 1]:554.)

to increase intracellular cAMP. Elevations of cAMP, however, will not stimulate insulin release in the absence of glucose.

Other factors involved in the regulation of insulin secretion are summarized in Table 19– 2. These factors can be divided into 3 categories: **direct stimulants,** which are known to stimulate insulin release directly; **amplifiers,** which appear to potentiate the response of the B cell to glucose; and **inhibitors.** The action of the amplifier substances, many of which are gastrointestinal hormones stimulated by ingestion of meals, explains the observation that insulin response

Table 19–2. Regulation of insulin release in humans.

Stimulants of insulin release
  Glucose, mannose
  Leucine
  Vagal stimulation
  Sulfonylureas
Amplifiers of glucose-induced insulin release
  1. Enteric hormones:
     Gastrin inhibitory polypeptide
     Cholecystokinin
     Secretin, gastrin
  2. Neural amplifiers: Beta-adrenergic stimulation
  3. Amino acids: Arginine
Inhibitors of insulin release
  Neural: Alpha-adrenergic effect of catecholamines
  Humoral: Somatostatin
  Drugs: Diazoxide, phenytoin, vinblastine, colchicine

to an ingested meal is greater than the response of intravenously administered substrates.

Insulin Receptors

Insulin action begins with binding of insulin to a receptor on the surface of the target cell membrane. Many cells of the body appear to have specific cell surface insulin receptors. In fat, liver, and muscle cells, binding of insulin to these receptors is associated with the biologic response of these tissues to the hormone. Because of the ease of obtaining them, blood cells are commonly used for studies of the insulin receptor. These receptors bind insulin rapidly, with high specificity and with an affinity high enough to bind picomolar amounts. It is thought that a "second messenger" is then generated that initiates the cell's response to insulin. Preliminary reports suggested that a fall in intracellular cAMP might represent the "second message" directing insulin's action. However, although this response occurs to some degree in hepatocytes, in other insulin target tissues neither cAMP nor cGMP concentration seems to be correlated with the cellular effects of insulin.

Because of inability to identify a second messenger for insulin, other explanations for mediation of its action have been sought, including changes in calcium flux, intracellular pH, and even changes in the cell membrane itself. It has recently been demonstrated that insulin receptors are composed of 2 subunits, a larger alpha subunit involved in binding the insulin molecule and a smaller beta subunit containing a kinase that becomes activated during insulin binding and initiates a cascade of phosphorylations of the beta subunit itself as well as of other intracellular peptides. After insulin is bound to its receptor, a number of insulin-receptor complexes are internalized. It remains controversial, however, whether this internalization contributes to the intracellular actions of insulin or merely to cellular regulation of insulin's action by removing both insulin and its receptor via scavenger lysosomes. Currently, the exact mechanism of post-receptor events is not well understood, although increased translocation of a pool of glucose transporter proteins from the Golgi region to the cell membrane has been shown to be a factor in increasing glucose transport in muscle and fat cells exposed to insulin.

Abnormalities of insulin receptors—in concentration, affinity, or both—will affect insulin action. **"Down-regulation"** is a phenomenon in which the number of insulin receptors is decreased in response to chronically elevated circulating insulin levels. When insulin levels are low, on the other hand, receptor binding is up-regulated. Conditions associated with high insulin levels and lowered insulin binding to the receptor include obesity, high intake of carbohydrates, and (perhaps) chronic exogenous overinsulinization. Conditions associated with low insulin levels and increased insulin binding include exercise and fasting. The presence of excess amounts of cortisol decreases insulin binding to the receptor, although it is not clear if this is a direct effect of the hormone itself or one that is mediated through accompanying increases in the insulin level.

Action of Insulin

The major function of insulin is to promote **storage of ingested nutrients.** Although insulin directly or indirectly affects the function of almost every tissue in the body, the discussion here will be limited to a brief overview of the effects of insulin on the 3 major tissues specialized for energy storage: liver, muscle, and fat. In addition, the **paracrine effects** of insulin will be discussed briefly. The section on hormonal control of nutrient metabolism (see below) presents a detailed discussion of the effects of insulin and glucagon on the regulation of intermediary metabolism.

A. Paracrine Effects: The effects of the products of endocrine cells on surrounding cells are termed "paracrine" effects, in contrast to actions that take place at sites distant from the secreting cells, which are termed "endocrine" effects (see Fig 3–1). Paracrine effects of the B and D cells on the close-lying A cells (Fig 19–1) are of considerable importance in the endocrine pancreas. The first target cells reached by insulin are the pancreatic A cells at the periphery of the pancreatic islets. In the presence of insulin, A cell secretion of glucagon is reduced. In addition, somatostatin, which is released from D cells in response to most of the same stimuli that provoke insulin release, also acts to inhibit glucagon secretion (Table 19–1).

Because glucose stimulates only B and D cells (whose products then inhibit A cells) whereas amino acids stimulate glucagon as well as insulin, the type and amounts of islet hormones released during a meal depend on the ratio of ingested carbohydrate to protein. The higher the carbohydrate content of a meal, the less glucagon will be released by any amino acids absorbed. In contrast, a predominantly protein meal will result in relatively greater glucagon secretion, because amino acids are less effective at stimulating insulin release in the absence of concurrent hyperglycemia but are potent stimulators of A cells.

B. Endocrine Effects: (Table 19–3.)

1. Liver–The first major organ reached by insulin via the bloodstream is the liver. Insulin exerts its action on the liver in 2 major ways:

a. Insulin promotes anabolism–Insulin promotes glycogen synthesis and storage (Fig 19–6) at the same time it inhibits glycogen breakdown. These effects are mediated by changes in the activity of enzymes in the glycogen synthesis pathway (see below). The liver has a maximum storage capacity of 100–110 g of glycogen, or approximately 440 kcal of energy.

Insulin increases triglyceride synthesis and VLDL formation by the liver. It also inhibits gluconeogenesis and promotes glycolysis through its effects on enzymes of the glycolytic pathway.

b. Insulin inhibits catabolism–Insulin acts to reverse the catabolic events of the postabsorptive state by inhibiting hepatic glycogenolysis, ketogenesis, and gluconeogenesis.

2. Muscle–Insulin promotes protein synthesis in muscle (Fig 19–6) by increasing amino acid transport as well as by stimulating ribosomal protein synthesis.

Table 19–3. Endocrine effects of insulin.

Effects on liver

Anabolic effects:

Promotes glycogen storage.

Increases synthesis of triglycerides, cholesterol, and VLDL.

Promotes glycolysis.

Anticatabolic effects:

Inhibits glycogenolysis.

Inhibits ketogenesis.

Inhibits gluconeogenesis.

Effects on muscle

Promotes protein synthesis:

Increases amino acid transport.

Stimulates ribosomal protein synthesis.

Promotes glycogen synthesis:

Increases glucose transport.

Enhances activity of glycogen synthetase.

Inhibits activity of glycogen phosphorylase.

Effects on fat

Promotes triglyceride storage:

Induces lipoprotein lipase, making fatty acids available for absorption into fat cells.

Increases glucose transport into fat cells, thus increasing availability of α-glycerol phosphate for triglyceride synthesis.

Inhibits intracellular lipolysis.

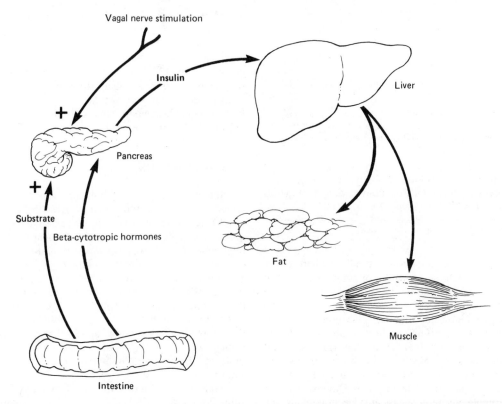

Figure 19–6. Insulin promotes synthesis (from circulating nutrients) and storage of glycogen, triglycerides, and protein in its major target tissues: liver, fat, and muscle. The release of insulin from the pancreas is stimulated by increased blood glucose, vagal nerve stimulation, and other factors (see text). (Reproduced, with permission, from Katzung BG [editor]: *Basic & Clinical Pharmacology,* 2nd ed. Lange, 1984.)

In addition, insulin promotes glycogen synthesis to replace glycogen stores expended by muscle activity. This is accomplished by increasing glucose transport into the muscle cell, enhancing the activity of glycogen synthetase, and inhibiting the activity of glycogen phosphorylase. Approximately 500–600 g of glycogen is stored in the muscle tissue of a 70-kg man, but because of the lack of glucose 6-phosphatase in this tissue, it cannot be used as a source of blood glucose (see below).

3. Fat–Fat, in the form of triglyceride, is the most efficient means of storing energy. It provides 9 kcal per gram of stored substrate, as opposed to the 4 kcal/ g generally provided by protein or carbohydrate. In the typical 70-kg man, the energy content of adipose tissue is about 100,000 kcal.

Insulin acts to promote triglyceride storage (Fig 19–6) in adipocytes by a number of mechanisms: (1) It induces the production of lipoprotein lipase (this is the lipoprotein lipase that is bound to endothelial cells in adipose tissue and other vascular beds), which leads to the active hydrolysis of triglycerides from circulating lipoproteins. (2) By increasing glucose transport into fat cells, insulin increases the availability of α-glycerol phosphate, a substance used in the ester-

ification of free fatty acids into triglycerides. (3) Insulin inhibits intracellular lipolysis of stored triglyceride by inhibiting intracellular lipase (also called "hormone-sensitive lipoprotein lipase").

2. GLUCAGON

Biochemistry

Pancreatic glucagon is a single-chain polypeptide consisting of 29 amino acids with a molecular weight of 3485 (Fig 19–7). It is synthesized in the A cells of the islets of Langerhans. In healthy humans, the average fasting plasma immunoreactive glucagon level is 75 pg/mL (25 pmol/L). Only 30–40% of this is actually pancreatic glucagon, the remainder being a biologically inactive large-molecular-weight (> 40,000 MW) precursor molecule. The circulation half-life of pancreatic glucagon is 3–6 minutes. Glucagon is mainly removed by the liver and kidney.

Secretion

Glucagon secretion is inhibited by glucose—in contrast to the effect of glucose on insulin secretion. There are conflicting data about whether the effect of

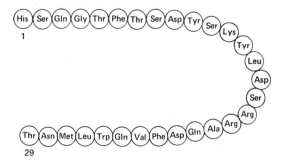

Figure 19–7. Amino acid sequence of glucagon polypeptide. (Reproduced, with permission, from Katzung BG [editor]: *Basic & Clinical Pharmacology*, 2nd ed. Lange, 1984.)

glucose is a direct one on the A cell or whether it is mediated via release of insulin or somatostatin, both of which are known to inhibit the A cell directly (see above).

Many amino acids stimulate glucagon release, although there are differences in their ability to do so. Some, such as arginine, release both glucagon and insulin; others (eg, alanine) stimulate primarily glucagon release. Leucine, a good stimulant for insulin release, does not stimulate glucagon. Other substances that promote glucagon release are catecholamines, the gastrointestinal hormones (cholecystokinin [CCK], gastrin, and gastric inhibitory polypeptide [GIP]), and glucocorticoids. Both sympathetic and parasympathetic (vagal) stimulation promote glucagon release; this is especially important in augmenting the response of the A cell to hypoglycemia. High levels of circulating fatty acid are associated with suppression of glucagon secretion.

Action of Glucagon

In contrast to insulin, which promotes energy storage in a variety of tissues, glucagon is a humoral mechanism for making energy available to the tissues between meals, when ingested food is not available for absorption. Glucagon stimulates the breakdown of stored glycogen, maintains hepatic output of glucose from amino acid precursors (gluconeogenesis), and promotes hepatic output of ketone bodies from fatty acid precursors (ketogenesis). The liver, because of its geographic proximity to the pancreas, represents the major target organ for glucagon, with portal vein glucagon concentrations reaching as high as 300–500

pg/mL. Binding of glucagon to its receptor on hepatocytes results in activation of adenylate cyclase and generation of cAMP, which both promotes glycogenolysis and stimulates gluconeogenesis. Uptake of alanine by liver cells is facilitated by glucagon, and fatty acids are directed away from reesterification to triglycerides and toward ketogenic pathways (see below). It is unclear whether physiologic levels of glucagon affect tissues other than the liver.

3. SOMATOSTATIN

Somatostatin is a cyclic polypeptide containing 14 amino acids with a molecular weight of 1640 (Fig 19–8). It is present in D cells at the periphery of the human islet (Fig 19–1). It was first identified in the hypothalamus and owes its name to its ability to inhibit release of growth hormone (pituitary somatotropin). Since that time, somatostatin has been identified in a number of tissues, including many areas of the brain, the gastrointestinal tract, and the pancreas. Not much is known about the biosynthesis of this hormone, though preliminary reports suggest that it is initially synthesized as a high-molecular-weight precursor molecule containing 28 amino acids (prosomatostatin).

Almost every known stimulator of release of insulin from pancreatic B cells also promotes somatostatin release from D cells. This includes glucose, arginine, gastrointestinal hormones, and tolbutamide. Preliminary reports suggest that physiologic levels of somatostatin in humans seldom exceed 80 pg/mL. The importance of circulating somatostatin is unclear, since a major role of this peptide may be as a paracrine regulator of the pancreatic islet and the tissues of the gastrointestinal tract (see Chapter 18). The metabolic clearance of exogenously infused somatostatin in humans is extremely rapid; the half-life of the hormone is less than 2 minutes.

Somatostatin acts in several ways to restrain the movement of nutrients from the intestinal tract into the circulation. It prolongs gastric emptying time, decreases gastric acid and gastrin production, diminishes pancreatic exocrine secretion, decreases splanchnic blood flow, and retards xylose absorption. Neutralization of circulating somatostatin with anti-somatostatin serum is associated with enhanced nutrient absorption in dogs. This implies that at least some of the effects of somatostatin are truly endocrine, as opposed to the paracrine effects discussed earlier.

Figure 19–8. Amino acid sequence of somatostatin.

4. PANCREATIC POLYPEPTIDE

Pancreatic polypeptide (PP) is found in F cells located chiefly in islets in the posterior portion of the head of the pancreas. PP is a 36-amino-acid peptide with a molecular weight of 4200. Little is known about its biosynthesis. Circulating levels of the peptide increase in response to a mixed meal; however, intravenous infusion of glucose or triglyceride does not produce such a rise, and intravenous amino acids cause only a small increase. Vagotomy abolishes the response to an ingested meal.

The physiologic action of PP is unknown. It is discussed further in Chapter 18.

HORMONAL CONTROL OF NUTRIENT METABOLISM

Hormones are important in every aspect of nutrient flux, from ingestion of foodstuffs to the ultimate assimilation of nutrients through biochemical processes at the intracellular level.

Hormones are important in regulating appetite and thus food-seeking behavior. Somatostatin, insulin, glucagon, CCK, cortisol, thyroid hormones, and estrogens have all been shown to play roles in regulating appetite in animal studies. Somatostatin and the gastrointestinal hormones are important modulators of rates of digestion and absorption, both by direct effects on the gut itself and by their effects on the exocrine pancreas and gallbladder (see Chapter 18). Once absorption of nutrients has taken place, insulin plays a crucial role in promoting movement of these circulating nutrients into target cells. Insulin enhances entry of glucose into skeletal muscle, cardiac muscle, and adipose tissue but does not appear to be necessary for glucose transport into liver or brain cells. Transport of certain amino acids, fatty acids, potassium, and magnesium is also stimulated in the presence of insulin. Gut hormones, particularly GIP, as well as vagally mediated neural signals act to potentiate the release of insulin in response to absorbed nutrients. The effects of a meal on the release of glucagon depend on the summation of a number of factors: (1) stimulation of glucagon release by absorbed amino acids, gastrointestinal hormones, and vagal stimulation, versus (2) inhibition of glucagon by postprandial hyperglycemia and concomitant insulin and somatostatin release. Circulating plasma glucagon usually shows little change after a mixed meal because of these opposing factors.

The ultimate fate of the 3 major classes of absorbed nutrients—carbohydrates (especially glucose), amino acids, and triglycerides—depends on the hormonal milieu of the individual. This hormonal milieu, in turn, is dependent on the nutrient status of the person (fed versus short-term fast). In simplified terms, the fed state is characterized by a relatively high insulin:glucagon ratio, whereas the preprandial or fasted state is characterized by a relatively lower insulin:glucagon ratio. The starving state has a number of unique features that are beyond the scope of this discussion.

EFFECT OF INSULIN & GLUCAGON ON INTERMEDIARY METABOLISM

A summary of the key steps in intermediary metabolism of nutrients is presented in Fig 19–9. After glucose enters the hepatic cell, it may be converted to glycogen for storage or it may enter the glycolytic pathway and be broken down to pyruvate, with production of a readily available form of energy, ATP. In the presence of adequate intracellular oxygenation, pyruvate enters the mitochondria and participates in the tricarboxylic acid cycle, with the ultimate production of even larger quantities of ATP. Fats enter cells as free fatty acids and may then be stored as triglycerides or broken down by beta oxidation into acetyl-CoA, which can then enter the tricarboxylic acid cycle and be used to produce ATP. Amino acids can be used to synthesize necessary structural and secreted proteins after entry into cells—or, conversely, proteins in cells can be broken down, and some of the amino acids can enter the glycolytic pathway and tricarboxylic acid cycle, where they can be broken down for the production of energy.

Insulin and glucagon affect many different steps in intermediary metabolism. Their diverse roles can best be understood by clarifying a few general principles. First, insulin is primarily an **anabolic** hormone. It enhances storage of nutrients such as glycogen, triglycerides, and protein by promoting glycogenesis, fatty acid synthesis, protein synthesis, and glycolysis (which makes available building blocks for fat and protein synthesis). Glucagon, on the other hand, functions primarily to **protect the organism from hypoglycemia** by stimulating gluconeogenesis and glycogenolysis.

The second general principle is that there are **2 types of control** of metabolism by these hormones. One type is rapid (minutes to hours) and is mediated by hormone-induced changes in the catalytic properties of key enzymes by phosphorylation-dephosphorylation. The other type of control is slower (hours to days) and involves induction of the synthesis of key enzymes by the hormone. The first type of control involves a change in enzyme kinetics; the second involves a change in the amount of enzyme without a change in the kinetics.

1. HORMONE-INDUCED CHANGES IN ENZYME KINETICS

The enzymes affected by hormone-induced changes in phosphorylation-dephosphorylation belong to a class

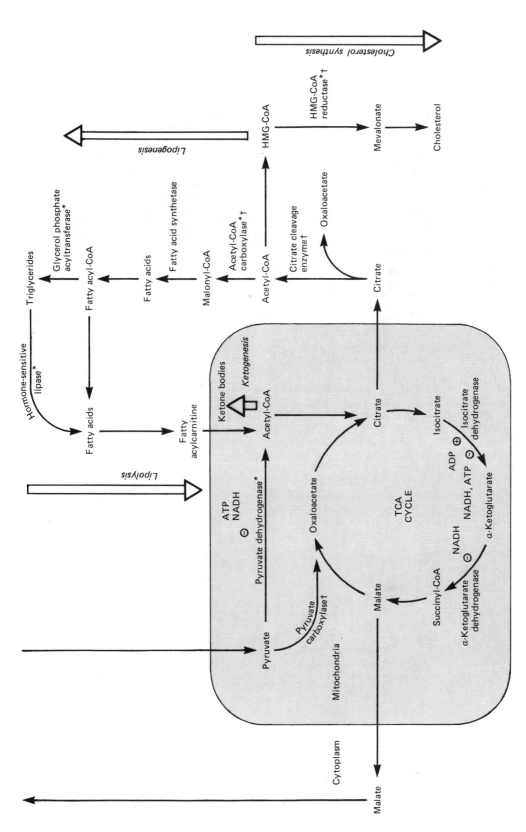

Figure 19–9. Interrelationship of fat and carbohydrate metabolism in normal energy homeostasis in the liver. Major functional pathways depicted by hollow arrows. Enzymes with asterisks are the interconvertible enzymes that are phosphorylated or dephosphorylated depending on the ratio of insulin to glucagon. Enzymes with daggers are induced or repressed depending on the ratio of insulin to glucagon. UDP, uridine diphosphate; HMG-CoA, hydroxymethylglutaryl-CoA; ATP, adenosine triphosphate; NADH, nicotinamide adenine dinucleotide (reduced form); TCA, tricarboxylic acid; ADP, adenosine diphosphate.

Table 19–4. Interconvertible enzymes important in intermediary metabolism.

Phosphofructokinase
Pyruvate kinase
Pyruvate dehydrogenase
Acetyl-CoA carboxylase
Glycerol phosphate acyltransferase
HMG-CoA reductase
Glycogen synthetase
*Glycogen phosphorylase
*Hormone-sensitive lipoprotein lipase of adipose cells

*All of these enzymes except the 2 labeled with an asterisk are **active** in the dephosphorylated form and **inactive** in the phosphorylated form. Glucagon promotes phosphorylation of these enzymes; insulin promotes their dephosphorylation.

of enzymes called **interconvertible enzymes.** The interconvertible enzymes that are important in intermediary metabolism are listed in Table 19–4. Insulin stimulates the **dephosphorylation** of these enzymes, whereas glucagon stimulates the **phosphorylation** of the same enzymes. All but 2 of the en-

zymes listed are active in the dephosphorylated form. The 2 exceptions are **glycogen phosphorylase** and **hormone-sensitive lipoprotein lipase** of adipose cells.

The mechanism of phosphorylation-dephosphorylation of glycogen phosphorylase (Fig 19–10) has been well studied and will be described in detail. It is important to remember in this example that glycogen phosphorylase is one of the 2 enzymes that are active (rather than inactive) in the phosphorylated form. Glucagon binds to a specific receptor on the outer side of the liver cell membrane. The hormone-receptor interaction leads to activation of adenylate cyclase, an enzyme bound to the cytoplasmic side of the plasma membrane. Adenylate cyclase then utilizes intracellular ATP to produce the ''second messenger'' cAMP. This cyclic nucleotide activates a cAMP-dependent protein kinase, an enzyme whose function is to phosphorylate other proteins. (This enzyme is also called phosphorylase kinase kinase, since it phosphorylates the enzyme phosphorylase kinase.) Phosphorylase kinase is activated when it is phosphorylated and inactivated when it is dephosphorylated. In its active

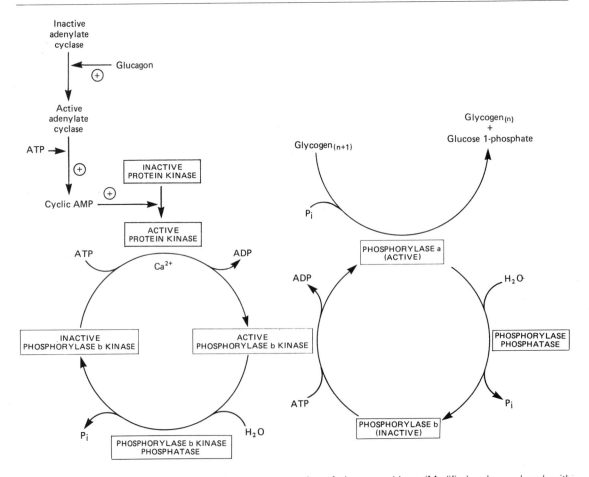

Figure 19–10. Control of phosphorylase by glucagon. n = number of glucose residues. (Modified and reproduced, with permission, from Martin DW Jr, Mayes PA, Rodwell VW: *Harper's Review of Biochemistry*, 20th ed. Lange, 1985.)

(phosphorylated) form, it phosphorylates the enzyme glycogen phosphorylase (phosphorylase b in Fig 19–10). As stated above, this enzyme is also active in its phosphorylated form, catalyzing the breakdown of glycogen into glucose 1-phosphate.

Insulin, probably via an intracellular messenger, promotes the dephosphorylation of the interconvertible enzymes; in the above example, insulin acts by opposing the action of cAMP. In addition, insulin probably increases the activity of specific phosphatases that directly catalyze dephosphorylation of the phosphorylated interconvertible enzymes. Glycogen synthetase, glycogen phosphorylase (via phosphorylase kinase), and pyruvate kinase are all known to be regulated via a cAMP-dependent protein kinase. The mechanism of regulation of the other interconvertible enzymes is still unknown.

An example of a hormone-induced change in enzyme kinetics that is important in the control of intermediary metabolism is the regulation of an enzyme known as 6-phosphofructo 2-kinase (PFK-2). PFK-2 is a remarkable enzyme in that it can act either as a kinase or as a phosphatase, depending on its own state of phosphorylation. When PFK-2 is *dephosphorylated,* it acts as a kinase; when it is *phosphorylated,* it acts as a phosphatase. This enzyme controls the level of fructose 2,6-diphosphate, a powerful regulator of both phosphofructokinase (PFK-1) and fructose 1,6-diphosphatase (Fig 19– 9).

High levels of fructose 2,6-diphosphate are associated with activation of PFK-1 and inhibition of fructose 1,6-diphosphatase, thus promoting glycolysis. Low levels of fructose 2,6-diphosphate are associated with inhibition of PFK-1 and stimulation of fructose 1,6-diphosphatase, thus promoting gluconeogenesis. The phosphorylation or dephosphorylation of PFK-2 is controlled by changes in the insulin:glucagon ratio, which affect the level of cAMP in a manner similar to that described for glycogen phosphorylase.

2. HORMONE-INDUCED CHANGES IN ENZYME QUANTITY

Table 19– 5 lists the enzymes shown to be affected by alterations in the ratio of insulin to glucagon.

Glucokinase, phosphofructokinase, and pyruvate kinase (all enzymes that promote breakdown of glucose) are induced in the presence of high insulin:glucagon ratios and repressed when the ratio is low. Glucose 6-phosphatase, fructose 1,6-diphosphatase, phosphoenolpyruvate carboxykinase, and pyruvate carboxylase (the enzymes that promote gluconeogenesis), on the other hand, are repressed in the presence of high circulating insulin and low circulating glucagon and induced when the levels of glucagon are relatively increased in comparison with insulin levels. The significance of these effects is discussed in the following section.

Table 19–5. Enzymes induced or repressed by insulin or glucagon.

Enzymes induced by a high insulin:glucagon ratio and repressed by a low insulin:glucagon ratio:
  Glucokinase
  Phosphofructokinase
  Citrate cleavage enzyme
  Acetyl-CoA carboxylase
  HMG-CoA reductase
  Pyruvate kinase
Enzymes induced by a low insulin:glucagon ratio and repressed by a high insulin:glucagon ratio:
  Glucose 6-phosphatase
  Fructose 1,6-diphosphatase
  Phosphoenolpyruvate carboxykinase
  Pyruvate carboxylase

3. INSULIN & GLUCAGON CONTROL OF INTERMEDIARY METABOLISM

The details of hormonal control of nutrient metabolism vary depending on the tissue involved. The differences between tissues arise because of differences in the hormone sensitivity of enzymes involved or because of the presence or absence of the enzyme system or insulin receptors in a particular tissue. A complete discussion of intermediary metabolism is beyond the scope of this text, and only a review of events in key tissues will be offered. Enzymes discussed below are indicated by asterisks and daggers in Fig 19– 9.

Well-Fed State

A. Liver: In the well-fed state, the insulin:glucagon ratio is relatively high, and the liver is both glycogenic and lipogenic.

Glycogenesis (glycogen formation) is enhanced by the activation of glycogen synthetase through its hormone-induced dephosphorylation. On the other hand, the simultaneous dephosphorylation of glycogen phosphorylase inactivates the enzyme, thus inhibiting glycogen breakdown. Concurrent inhibition of breakdown and stimulation of glycogen formation avoids a glycogenesis-glycogenolysis "futile cycle" and leads to glycogen storage.

Insulin promotes **lipogenesis** indirectly, by stimulation of glycolysis (which makes available precursors of fatty acid synthesis); and directly, by stimulation of enzymes in the pathway of fatty acid and cholesterol synthesis. Glycolysis is stimulated by the **dephosphorylation** of phosphofructokinase, pyruvate kinase, and pyruvate dehydrogenase as well as induction of glucokinase, phosphofructokinase, and pyruvate kinase. All of the above tend to increase the utilization of glucose in the glycolytic pathway, which leads to an accumulation of acetyl-CoA. In the well-fed state, there is a high ratio of ATP to ADP + AMP, which tends to slow down the tricarboxylic acid cycle (Fig 19– 9), and acetyl-CoA leaves the mitochondria via citrate and participates in the synthesis of fats and cholesterol rather than entering the tricarboxylic acid cycle for the production of more ATP. The fat and cholesterol synthetic activities are directly accelerated by the dephosphorylation (activation) of acetyl-CoA carboxylase and glycerol phosphate acyltransferase and by HMG-CoA reductase, respectively.

The high insulin:glucagon ratio is also associated with repression of the gluconeogenic enzymes (pyruvate carboxylase, phosphoenolpyruvate carboxykinase, fructose 1,6-diphosphatase, and glucose 6-phosphatase), which inhibits glucose production via reversal of the glycolytic pathway and thus prevents a gluconeogenic-glycolytic "futile cycle." (This is analogous to the situation described above for glycogen synthesis.)

The net effect, then, of the elevated insulin:glucagon ratio in the well-fed state is storage of nutrient energy as glycogen and fats.

B. Adipose Tissue: In the well-fed state, lipogenesis is favored in adipose tissue because pyruvate kinase, pyruvate dehydrogenase, acetyl-CoA carboxylase, and glycerol phosphate acyltransferase are in their dephosphorylated state and thus active. In addition, an enzyme that is specific to adipose tissue, **hormone-sensitive lipoprotein lipase,** is (like glycogen phosphorylase; see above) inactive in the dephosphorylated state, thereby reinforcing the lipogenic state and inhibiting the lipolytic pathway.

Fasted State

A. Liver: In the postabsorptive or fasting state and in starvation, the ratio of insulin to glucagon is low, which results in production of the phosphorylated form of the interconvertible enzymes. As noted above, all of these liver enzymes except glycogen phosphorylase are inactive in the phosphorylated state. Hence, glycolysis, glycogenesis, lipogenesis, and cholesterol synthesis are inhibited. On the other hand, **glycogenolysis** is enhanced.

The increase in glucagon and decrease in insulin levels also result in induction of the gluconeogenic enzymes pyruvate carboxylase, phosphoenolpyruvate carboxykinase, fructose 1,6-diphosphatase, and glucose 6-phosphatase. The glycolytic enzymes—glucokinase, phosphofructokinase, and pyruvate kinase—are repressed. This serves the dual purpose of inhibiting the glycolytic pathway and increasing gluconeogenesis, thereby ensuring a continuous supply of glucose by the liver to the blood and peripheral tissues.

B. Adipose Tissue: Phosphorylation of the interconvertible enzymes of fat and cholesterol synthesis (acetyl-CoA carboxylase, glycerol phosphate acyltransferase, and HMG-CoA reductase) also leads to their inactivation, thereby favoring fatty acid oxidation (beta oxidation) to acetyl-CoA and the availability of this intermediate for ketogenesis. Furthermore, beta oxidation of fatty acids leads to the production of NADH, which suppresses the tricarboxylic acid cycle (Fig 19–9) and thus promotes the production of ketone bodies as the end product of fatty acid breakdown.

Again, in the starved state, the reduced insu-

lin:glucagon ratio results in the phosphorylation (inactivation) of the interconvertible enzymes of glycolysis and fat and cholesterol synthesis and the activation of hormone-sensitive lipoprotein lipase, shutting down lipogenesis and cholesterol synthesis and promoting lipolysis and fatty acid oxidation. Adipose tissue lacks the enzymes that mediate glycogenesis, glycogenolysis, and gluconeogenesis.

C. Muscle: The same events occur as in liver in the fasted state, except that muscle lacks gluconeogenic enzymes and has no glucose 6-phosphatase and therefore cannot produce free glucose. The liver is the main source of free glucose in the postabsorptive state, with the kidney playing a minor role.

II. DIABETES MELLITUS

Clinical diabetes mellitus is a syndrome of disordered metabolism with inappropriate hyperglycemia due either to an absolute deficiency of insulin secretion or a reduction in the biologic effectiveness of insulin (or both).

CLASSIFICATION

Traditionally, diabetes has been classified according to the patient's age at onset of symptoms (juvenile-onset versus adult-onset). In 1979, the NIH Diabetes Data Group recommended that diabetes mellitus be classified into one of 2 major types according to dependence on exogenous insulin. Most patients with diabetes fall into one of 2 major categories: **insulin-dependent** (type I) or **non–insulin-dependent** (type II) diabetes mellitus (Table 19–6).

TYPE I: INSULIN-DEPENDENT DIABETES MELLITUS (IDDM)

Type I is a severe form of diabetes mellitus and is associated with ketosis in the untreated state. About 10–20% of diabetics in North America and Europe are of the insulin-dependent type. It is most common in young individuals but occurs occasionally in nonobese adults. It is a catabolic disorder in which circulating insulin is virtually absent, plasma glucagon is elevated, and the pancreatic B cells fail to respond to all known insulinogenic stimuli. In the absence of insulin, the 3 main target tissues of insulin (liver, muscle, and fat) not only fail to appropriately take up absorbed nutrients but continue to deliver glucose, amino acids, and fatty acids into the bloodstream from their respective storage depots. Furthermore, alterations in fat metabolism lead to the production and

Table 19–6. Clinical classification of diabetes mellitus.

	Ketosis	Islet Cell Antibodies	HLA Association	Estimated Prevalence (% of All Diabetics)	Treatment
Insulin-dependent diabetes (IDDM, type I)	Marked	Usually present at onset.	Yes	10–20%	1. Insulin. 2. Diet.
Non–insulin-dependent diabetes (NIDDM, type II)	Absent	Absent	No	80–90%	
Nonobese NIDDM				15% of NIDDM patients	Eucaloric diet alone or diet plus sulfonylurea or insulin.
Obese NIDDM				85% of NIDDM patients	1. Weight reduction. 2. Hypocaloric diet plus sulfonylureas or insulin *for symptomatic control only.*
Gestational diabetes					See Chapter 17.
Diabetes mellitus and impaired glucose tolerance secondary to or associated with other conditions: Pancreatic disease, drug toxicity, endocrine disorders, genetic disease, insulin receptor abnormalities with acanthosis nigricans.					Treatment varies according to the specific condition. In general, removal or correction of offending agent if possible, diet, and insulin are the foundation of treatment. See text for details.

accumulation of ketones. This inappropriate persistence of the fasted state postprandially can be reversed by the administration of insulin.

Genetics of Type I Diabetes

Studies in monozygotic twins suggest that genetic influences are less marked in type I diabetes than in type II diabetes. Only 50% of identical twins of type I diabetic patients will develop the disease. This also suggests that an environmental factor is required for induction of diabetes in these cases. In contrast, the identical twin of a type II diabetic will usually develop diabetes within a year of onset of the disease in the sibling.

Type I diabetes is believed to result from an infectious or toxic environmental insult to the pancreatic B cells in genetically predisposed persons. Environmental factors that have been associated with altered pancreatic islet cell function include viruses (mumps, rubella, coxsackievirus B4), toxic chemical agents such as Vacor (a nitrophenylurea rat poison), and other destructive cytotoxins such as hydrogen cyanide from spoiled tapioca.

Type I diabetes is strongly associated with an increased frequency of certain HLA antigens. These antigens are glycoproteins found on cell surfaces of all cells except red blood cells and sperm. They allow the immune system to recognize homologous tissues and to detect foreign antigens. The predominant HLA antigens associated with type I diabetes vary in different racial groups. Thus, HLA-B8, -B15, -B18, -Cw3, -Dw3, -DR3, and -DR4 occur with increased frequency on leukocytes of Caucasian diabetics, whereas only HLA-Dw3, -DRw3, and -DRw4 appear to be correlated with type I diabetes in Asians, Africans, and Latin-Americans.

A plausible theory that explains the association of HLA types with type I diabetes is as follows: The HLA antigens are located close to the immune response genes on chromosome 6; there may be a functional link. An initial viral infection of the B cells is aggravated by an immune deficiency that leads to a lower than normal antibody response. This in turn leads to a greater infiltration and destruction of the B cells by the virus, which then enhances the release of sensitizing proteins from the B cells with the consequent production of autoantibodies and excessive B cell destruction (''autoaggression''). Thus, it is possible that the HLA marker denotes either a hypoimmune or hyperimmune response (or a mixture of both) whose ultimate outcome is excessive loss of pancreatic B cells. Alternatively, rather than a functional link, a ''diabetes gene'' may be in linkage disequilibrium with certain subtypes of the HLA-DR3 and -DR4 regions of chromosome 6.

Circulating islet cell autoantibodies, virtually absent in nondiabetics, have been detected in as many as 85% of type I diabetics tested in the first few weeks of onset of diabetes. The high prevalence of these autoantibodies supports the concept that autoimmune mechanisms may contribute significantly to progressive B cell destruction.

In 1984, Bell et al reported a genetic link to chromosome 11 in type I diabetes. Comparison of the size of a polymorphic DNA locus flanking the 5′ region of the insulin gene on chromosome 11 revealed that 88% of the alleles in a Caucasian population of type I diabetics were in a ''small'' class of about 570 base pairs, while 12% of the alleles were in a larger class (averaging 2470 base pairs). In contrast, only 67% of the alleles in nondiabetic Caucasian controls were in the ''small'' class, and 33% were in the larger class of alleles. This polymorphic locus does not seem either to encode a protein or to affect insulin gene expression, but it may represent a marker for a linked gene that influences susceptibility to type I diabetes.

Subgroups of Type I Diabetes

In Britain, a subclassification of type I diabetes has been suggested. One subgroup, termed Ia, accounts for 80% of type I diabetics. These patients have islet cell autoantibodies only transiently, at the onset of their disease; they seldom have any other associated autoimmune phenomena. The most common HLA types in this subgroup are B15 and DR4. A viral infection appears to be mainly responsible for the B cell destruction in these patients.

Subgroup Ib accounts for the remainder of insulin-dependent diabetic patients. These patients have islet cell autoantibodies that tend to persist in high titers. Associated autoimmune disorders of the thyroid and adrenal cortex occur frequently; hypogonadism and pernicious anemia are also found. Immune destruction of pancreatic B cells appears to be responsible for the development of the disease (see Chapter 25). Most of these patients are female, and the most frequent HLA types are HLA-B8 and HLA-DR3.

TYPE II: NON–INSULIN-DEPENDENT DIABETES MELLITUS (NIDDM)

Type II diabetes, which comprises a heterogeneous group of the milder forms of diabetes, occurs predominantly in adults but may occasionally have its onset in childhood.

Type II diabetes is defined mainly in *negative* terms. It is a *non*ketotic form of diabetes which is *not* linked to HLA markers on the sixth chromosome and is *not* associated with islet cell autoantibodies. The patients are *not* dependent on exogenous insulin therapy to sustain life—thus the name, *non*–insulin-dependent diabetes mellitus. An element of tissue insensitivity to insulin has been noted in most NIDDM patients. Possible mechanisms for this are shown in Table 19–7.

Table 19–7. Factors reducing response to insulin.*

Prereceptor inhibitors: Insulin antibodies
Receptor inhibitors:
Insulin receptor autoantibodies
"Down-regulation" of receptors by hyperinsulinism:
Primary hyperinsulinism (B cell adenoma)
Hyperinsulinism secondary to a postreceptor defect
(obesity, Cushing's syndrome, acromegaly, pregnancy)
or prolonged hyperglycemia (diabetes mellitus, post–
glucose tolerance test)
Postreceptor influences:
Poor responsiveness of principal target organs; obesity;
hepatic disease; muscle inactivity
Hormonal excess: glucocorticoids, growth hormone, oral con-
traceptive agents, progesterone, human chorionic somato-
mammotropin, catecholamines, thyroxine

*Reproduced, with permission, from Krupp MA, Chatton MJ, Tierney LM Jr (editors): *Current Medical Diagnosis & Treatment 1986.* Lange, 1986.

Subgroups of Type II Diabetes

Type II diabetics can be distributed on the basis of body weight into obese or nonobese subtypes. Currently, it is impossible to identify diagnostic characteristics that allow further clear-cut separation into more specific subtypes. Circulating insulin levels are presently considered too variable to be of use in classification.

Among this ''non–type I'' group are a wide assortment of heterogeneous disorders. These include several rare instances in which a defective insulin gene produces a biologically inadequate abnormal insulin or a proinsulin that is not transformed to insulin in the B cell. Receptor and postreceptor blocks to insulin action have been demonstrated in some cases. In most patients with type II diabetes, however, the cause of the disorder is presently undefined.

Obese NIDDM

Up to 85% of type II diabetics are obese. These patients have an insensitivity to endogenous insulin that is positively correlated with the presence of distended adipocytes. In addition, overnourished liver and muscle cells may also resist the deposition of additional glycogen and triglycerides in their storage depots. Hyperplasia of pancreatic B cells is often present and probably accounts for the normal or exaggerated insulin responses to glucose and other stimuli seen in the milder forms of this disease.

Two major mechanisms have been proposed to account for the observed tissue insensitivity to insulin in obesity: (1) Chronic overfeeding may lead to sustained B cell stimulation and hyperinsulinism, and this in turn causes down-regulation of insulin receptors with resultant decreased sensitivity to insulin. (2) A postreceptor defect in insulin action, which is associated with reduced ability to clear nutrients from the circulation, may occur in overfilled storage depots. This in turn would lead to hyperinsulinism that would induce down-regulation of insulin receptors and a receptor-mediated insensitivity to insulin as well.

Regardless of the mechanism, a reduction in overfeeding can interrupt the cycle. In accordance with the first hypothesis, restricted diet would reduce B cell stimulation, leading to lower insulin levels; the lower insulin levels would then allow restoration of insulin receptor sites and improved tissue sensitivity to insulin. In the second situation, normal tissue sensitivity would return as storage depots decrease and fat cells become less distended. Accumulating evidence seems to favor this latter model of a postreceptor defect to account for the insensitivity to insulin developing in tissues of obese patients.

Nonobese NIDDM

Approximately 15% of patients with NIDDM are nonobese diabetics. In many of these patients, an absent or delayed early phase of insulin release in response to glucose can be demonstrated. This abnormal response incriminates a defective B cell as a factor in altered carbohydrate homeostasis. On the other hand, other insulinogenic stimuli, such as acute infusion of amino acids, intravenous tolbutamide, or intramuscular glucagon, often remain effective in eliciting acute insulin release.

The hyperglycemia in patients with nonobese NIDDM often responds to dietary therapy or to oral hypoglycemic agents. Occasionally, insulin therapy is required to achieve satisfactory glycemic control even though it is not needed to prevent ketoacidosis.

While most nonobese NIDDM patients cannot be subclassified, several discrete subtypes are suggested in a small proportion of patients on the basis of genetic characteristics:

A. Autosomal Dominant Nonobese NIDDM: A specific subclass of nonobese NIDDM includes patients with "maturity-onset diabetes of the young" (MODY, or Mason type). These patients have mild hyperglycemia with onset in late childhood or young adulthood. Their strong family history of a mild form of diabetes suggests an autosomal dominant transmission.

B. Mutant Insulins: Recently, 6 families have been identified as having abnormal circulating forms of insulin. In 3 of these families, there is impaired cleavage of the proinsulin molecule; in the other 3 families, abnormalities of the insulin molecule itself have been reported.

Analysis of the insulin gene, circulating insulin, and clinical features of family members in these cases indicates that individuals with mutant insulin are heterozygous for this defect, with both a normal and an abnormal insulin molecule being equally expressed. However, because the abnormal insulin binds to receptors poorly, it has very low biologic activity and accumulates in the blood to exceed the concentration of the normal insulin. This decreased removal rate of mutant insulin results in hyperinsulinemia after overnight fasting and a subnormal molar ratio of C peptide to immunoreactive insulin. Diabetes mellitus may or may not be present in association with mutant insulin, depending on the concentration and bioactivity of circulating normal and abnormal insulins and on the insulin responsiveness of peripheral tissues. Since there is no obvious resistance to insulin in any of these cases, it appears that abnormal insulin does not interfere with binding of normal insulin to receptors; therefore, a feature of this syndrome is the normal response to exogenously administered insulin.

1. Abnormalities of the proinsulin molecule– A partially cleaved intermediate of proinsulin comprising up to 90% of circulating insulin immunoreactivity has been described in 2 families, one from Japan and one from Boston. Both families seem to have similar defects, with the arginine in position 65 being replaced by another amino acid and thereby interfering with cleavage of the C peptide from the A chain of insulin. However, mild diabetes mellitus was present only in the 3 affected members of the family from Japan; it was not present in 17 affected members of the large kindred in Boston, despite a similar mutation of the insulin gene.

In a third family, hyperproinsulinemia was reported in 5 members. Although one of the 5 members (a 12-year-old girl) had borderline glucose intolerance, the other 4 had normal blood glucose levels. As much as 66% of the total immunoreactive insulin appeared to be normal proinsulin molecules, indicating a defect in the conversion of proinsulin to insulin.

2. Abnormalities of the insulin molecule– Genetic defects in insulin synthesis have resulted in substitutions of leucine for phenylalanine at position B 25 ("insulin Chicago") and serine for phenylalanine at position B 24 ("insulin Los Angeles"). (See Fig 19–3.) The observation that there was loss of a normal restriction endonuclease cleavage site in the area of the insulin gene coding for B 24 and B 25 phenylalanine was used in conjunction with results of high-performance liquid chromatographic analysis of circulating insulin to establish the nature of the mutant insulin in affected family members. Glucose tolerance ranged from normal to overtly diabetic in affected individuals, who were generally nonobese and had subnormal molar ratios of C peptide to immunoreactive insulin.

"NIDDM" Diabetics Who May Be Type I Diabetics in Remission

The current classification of diabetes mellitus has been widely accepted throughout the world, but its deficiencies are apparent in many cases. A subgroup that has been difficult to place in the current "therapeutic" classification is made up of those type I diabetics who remain in temporary remission for up to 2 years. A history of ketoacidosis with the finding of islet cell autoantibodies at the onset of the diabetes—and an HLA pattern that includes HLA-B8, -B15, -DR3, or -DR4—would indicate that these patients have type I diabetes from an etiologic standpoint even though they may be temporarily not "insulin-dependent."

SECONDARY DIABETES

As noted in Table 19–6, there is a diverse group of disorders characterized by the association of diabetes with another condition. Only a few of the many types of secondary diabetes will be discussed here.

Pancreatic Disease

Surgical removal of the pancreas, pancreatic disease due to chronic alcoholism, and other forms of pancreatitis are associated with many of the clinical characteristics of insulin-dependent diabetes mellitus, because the primary abnormality is insulin deficiency. There is, however, a greater tendency to develop insulin-induced hypoglycemia, probably because of the concomitant lack of the counterregulatory hormone glucagon. At least two-thirds of the pancreas must be destroyed to develop the clinical syndrome. It is usually associated with exocrine pancreatic insufficiency as well.

Drug Toxicity

Many drugs are associated with carbohydrate intolerance or frank diabetes mellitus. Some act by interfering with insulin release from the B cells (thiazides, phenytoin, beta-adrenergic blockers such as propranolol, and calcium channel blockers), some by inducing insulin resistance (glucocorticoids and oral contraceptive pills), and some by causing B cell destruction (pentamidine).

Endocrine Disorders

Excess production of certain hormones (GH [acromegaly], glucocorticoids [Cushing's syndrome or disease], catecholamines [pheochromocytoma], glucagon [glucagonoma], or pancreatic somatostatin [somatostatinoma]) can produce the syndrome of NIDDM by a number of mechanisms. In all but the last instance (somatostatinoma), peripheral responsiveness to insulin is impaired. In addition, excess of catecholamines or somatostatin decreases insulin release from B cells.

Insulin-Resistant Diabetes
With Acanthosis Nigricans

Patients with the rare syndrome of extreme insulin resistance associated with acanthosis nigricans can be divided into 2 groups on the basis of clinical and laboratory manifestations. **Group A** consists of younger women with androgenic features (hirsutism, amenorrhea, polycystic ovaries) in whom insulin receptors are deficient in number. **Group B** consists of older people, mostly women, in whom immunologic disease is suspected. They have a high erythrocyte sedimentation rate, DNA autoantibodies, and a circulating immunoglobulin that binds to insulin receptors, thereby reducing their affinity for insulin.

In both of the above groups, ketoacidosis does not develop despite severe insulin resistance. Occasionally, spontaneous remission of insulin resistance and diabetes occurs, particularly in the group A patients. In neither of the above groups is insulin therapy very effective.

Other Forms of Secondary Diabetes

Other rare diseases associated with insulin receptor or postreceptor abnormalities include leprechaunism, ataxia-telangiectasia, Prader-Willi syndrome, and certain forms of myotonic dystrophy.

CLINICAL FEATURES OF
DIABETES MELLITUS

The principal clinical features of the 2 major types of diabetes mellitus are listed for comparison in Table 19–8.

Table 19–8. Clinical features of diabetes.[*]

	Diabetes Type I (IDDM)	Diabetes Type II (NIDDM)
Polyuria and thirst	++	+
Weakness or fatigue	++	+
Polyphagia with weight loss	++	−
Recurrent blurred vision	+	++
Vulvovaginitis or pruritus	+	++
Peripheral neuropathy	+	++
Nocturnal enuresis	++	−
Often asymptomatic	−	++

[*]Reproduced, with permission, from Krupp MA, Chatton MJ, Tierney LM Jr (editors): *Current Medical Diagnosis & Treatment 1986.* Lange, 1986.

TYPE I DIABETES (IDDM)

IDDM patients present with a characteristic symptom complex, as outlined below. An absolute deficiency of insulin results in excessive accumulation of circulating glucose and fatty acids, with consequent hyperosmolality and hyperketonemia. The severity of the insulin deficiency and the acuteness with which the catabolic state develops determine the intensity of the osmotic and ketotic excess.

Clinical Features

A. Symptoms: Increased urination is a consequence of osmotic diuresis secondary to sustained hyperglycemia. This results in a loss of glucose as well as free water and electrolytes in the urine. Nocturnal enuresis due to polyuria may signal the onset of diabetes in very young children. Thirst is a consequence of the hyperosmolar state, as is blurred vision, which often develops as the lenses and retinas are exposed to hyperosmolar fluids.

Weight loss despite normal or increased appetite is a common feature of IDDM when it develops subacutely over a period of weeks. The weight loss is initially due to depletion of water, glycogen, and triglyceride stores. Chronic weight loss due to reduced muscle mass occurs as amino acids are diverted to form glucose and ketone bodies.

Lowered plasma volume produces dizziness and weakness due to postural hypotension when sitting or standing. Total body potassium loss and the general catabolism of muscle protein contribute to the weakness.

Paresthesias may be present at the time of diagnosis of type I diabetes, particularly when the onset is subacute. They reflect a temporary dysfunction of peripheral sensory nerves and usually clear as insulin replacement restores glycemic levels closer to normal; thus, their presence suggests neurotoxicity from sustained hyperglycemia.

When insulin deficiency is severe and of acute onset, the above symptoms progress in an accelerated manner. Ketoacidosis exacerbates the dehydration and hyperosmolality by producing anorexia, nausea, and vomiting, thus interfering with oral fluid replacement. As plasma osmolality exceeds 330 mosm/L (normal, 285–295 mosm/L), impaired consciousness ensues. With progression of acidosis to a pH of 7.1 or less, deep breathing with a rapid ventilatory rate (Kussmaul respiration) occurs as the body attempts to eliminate carbonic acid. With worsening acidosis (to pH 7 or less), the cardiovascular system may be unable to maintain compensatory vasoconstriction; severe circulatory collapse may result.

B. Signs: The patient's level of consciousness can vary depending on the degree of hyperosmolality. When insulin deficiency develops relatively slowly and sufficient water intake is maintained to permit renal excretion of glucose and appropriate dilution of extracellular sodium chloride concentration, patients remain relatively alert and physical findings may be minimal. When vomiting occurs in response to worsening ketoacidosis, dehydration progresses and compensatory mechanisms become inadequate to keep plasma osmolality below 320 mosm/L. Under these circumstances, stupor or even coma may occur. Evidence of dehydration in a stuporous patient, with rapid deep breathing and the fruity breath odor of acetone, suggests the diagnosis of diabetic ketoacidosis.

Postural hypotension indicates a depleted plasma volume; hypotension in the recumbent position is a serious prognostic sign. Loss of subcutaneous fat and muscle wasting are features of more slowly developing insulin deficiency. In occasional patients with slow, insidious onset of insulin deficiency, subcutaneous fat may be considerably depleted. An enlarged liver, eruptive xanthomas on the flexor surface of the limbs and on the buttocks, and lipemia retinalis indicate that chronic insulin deficiency has resulted in chylomicronemia, with circulating triglycerides elevated usually to over 2000 mg/dL (see Chapter 21).

TYPE II DIABETES (NIDDM)

NIDDM patients also present with characteristic signs and symptoms. The presence of obesity or a strongly positive family history of mild diabetes also suggests a high risk for the development of type II diabetes.

Clinical Features

A. Symptoms: The classic symptoms of polyuria, thirst, recurrent blurred vision, paresthesias, and fatigue are manifestations of hyperglycemia and osmotic diuresis and are therefore common to both forms of diabetes. However, many patients with type II diabetes have an insidious onset of hyperglycemia and may be relatively asymptomatic initially. This is particularly true in obese patients, whose diabetes may be detected only after glycosuria or hyperglycemia is noted during routine laboratory studies. Chronic skin infections are common. Generalized pruritus and symptoms of vaginitis are frequently the initial complaints of women with NIDDM. Diabetes should be suspected in women with chronic candidal vulvovaginitis as well as in those who have delivered large infants (> 9 lb, or 4.1 kg) or have had polyhydramnios, preeclampsia, or unexplained fetal losses. Occasionally, a man with previously undiagnosed diabetes may present with impotence.

B. Signs: Nonobese patients with this mild form of diabetes often have no characteristic physical findings at the time of diagnosis. Obese diabetics may have any variety of fat distribution; however, diabetes seems to be more often associated in both men and women with localization of fat deposits on the upper part of the body (particularly the abdomen, chest, neck, and face) and relatively less fat on the appendages, which may be quite muscular. This centripetal fat distribution has been termed "android." It differs from the more centrifugal "gynecoid" form of obesity, in which fat is localized more in the hips and thighs and less in the upper parts of the trunk. Mild hypertension may be present in obese diabetics, particularly when the "android" form of obesity is predominant. In women, candidal vaginitis with a reddened, inflamed vulvar area and a profuse whitish discharge may herald the presence of diabetes.

LABORATORY FINDINGS IN DIABETES MELLITUS

Tests of urine glucose and ketone bodies as well as whole blood or plasma glucose measured in samples obtained under basal conditions and after glucose administration are very important in evaluation of the diabetic patient. Recently developed tests for glycosylated hemoglobin have proved useful in both initial evaluation and in assessment of the effectiveness of therapeutic management. In certain circumstances, measurements of insulin levels and levels of other hormones involved in carbohydrate homeostasis (eg, glucagon, GH) may be useful. In view of the increased risk of atherosclerosis in diabetics, estimates of serum cholesterol, including its beneficial HDL fraction (HDL$_2$), and triglycerides may be helpful.

URINALYSIS

Glycosuria

Several problems are associated with using urine glucose as an index of blood glucose, regardless of the method employed. First of all, the glucose concentration in bladder urine reflects the blood glucose at the time the urine was formed. Therefore, the first voided specimen in the morning contains glucose that was excreted throughout the night and does not reflect the morning blood glucose at all. Some improvement in the correlation of urine glucose to blood glucose can be obtained if the patient "double voids"—that is, empties the bladder completely, discards that sample, and then urinates again about one-half hour later, testing only the second specimen for glucose content. However, difficulty in completely emptying the bladder (large residual volumes), problems in understanding the instructions, and the inconvenience impair the usefulness of this test. Self-monitoring of blood glucose will replace urine glucose testing in most patients with IDDM and in many patients with NIDDM (particularly those receiving insulin therapy).

Several commercial products are available for determining the presence and amount of glucose in urine.

A. Clinitest: A Clinitest tablet placed in 5 drops of urine with 10 drops of water provides a semiquantitative estimate of the degree of glycosuria. A glucose level of 0.25% (250 mg/dL) in the urine is required to show a trace reaction (green), and colors progress from yellow to orange until a brick-red color indicates a glucose content greater than 2% (2 g/dL). The Clinitest has poor specificity (a number of substances cause a false-positive reaction) and is inconvenient to perform; thus, urine dipstick tests and home blood glucose monitoring are generally preferred.

B. Dipstick Methods: A rapid and convenient glucose-specific method consists of paper strips (Clinistix, Diastix, Tes-Tape) impregnated with enzymes (glucose oxidase and hydrogen peroxidase) and a chromogenic dye. The dye forms variable color tints depending on the amount of glucose in the urine. These dipsticks are sensitive to as little as 0.1% glucose (100 mg/dL) but do not react with the small amounts of glucose normally present in urine. The strips are subject to deterioration if exposed to air, moisture, and extreme heat and must be kept in tightly closed containers except when in use. False-negative results may be obtained when certain materials are ingested in excess (Table 19–9) and in the presence of alkaptonuria. All of these false-negative results occur because of the interference of strong reducing agents with oxidation of the chromogen.

Differential Diagnosis of Glycosuria (Sugar in the Urine)

Although glycosuria reflects hyperglycemia in over 90% of patients, 2 major classes of nondiabetic glycosuria must be considered:

A. Nondiabetic Glycosuria Due to Glucose: This occurs when glucose appears in the urine despite a normal amount of glucose in the blood. Disorders associated with abnormalities in renal glucose han-

dling include Fanconi's syndrome (an autosomal dominant genetic disorder), dysfunction of the proximal renal tubule, chronic renal failure, and a benign familial disorder of the renal tubule manifest only by a defect in renal glucose reabsorption (occurs predominantly in males).

In addition, glycosuria is relatively common in pregnancy as a consequence of the increased load of glucose presented to the tubules by the elevated glomerular filtration rate during pregnancy. As many as 50% of pregnant women normally have demonstrable sugar in the urine, especially after the first trimester. This sugar is almost always glucose except during the late weeks of pregnancy, when lactose may be present (see below).

B. Nondiabetic Glycosuria Due to Sugars Other Than Glucose: Occasionally, a sugar other than glucose is excreted in the urine. Lactosuria during the late stages of pregnancy and the period of lactation is the most common example. Much rarer are other conditions in which inborn errors of metabolism allow fructose, galactose, or a pentose (1-xylose) to be excreted in the urine. Testing the urine with glucose-specific strips will help differentiate true glucosuria from other glycosurias.

Ketonuria

In the absence of adequate insulin, 3 major "ketone bodies" are formed and excreted into the urine: β-hydroxybutyric acid, acetoacetic acid, and acetone (see also Serum Ketone Determinations, below). Commercial products are available to test for the presence of ketones in the urine. Acetest tablets, Ketostix, and Keto-Diastix utilize a nitroprusside reaction that measures only acetone and acetoacetate. Therefore, these tests can be misleading if β-hydroxybutyric acid is the predominant ketone present. Ketostix and Keto-Diastix have short shelf-lives once the containers are opened and thus may give false-negative results.

Other conditions besides diabetic ketoacidosis may cause ketone bodies to appear in the urine; these include starvation, high-fat diets, alcoholic ketoacidosis, fever, and other conditions in which metabolic requirements are increased.

Proteinuria

Proteinuria as noted on a routine dipstick examination of the urine is often the first sign of renal complications of diabetes. If proteinuria is detected, a 24-hour urine collection should be analyzed to quantify the degree of proteinuria (normal individuals excrete < 150 mg of protein per day) and the rate of urinary creatinine excretion; at the same time, serum creatinine levels should be determined so that the creatinine clearance (an estimate of the glomerular filtration rate) can be calculated. In some cases, heavy proteinuria (3.5 g/d) develops later, along with other features of nephrotic syndrome such as edema, hypoalbuminemia, and hypercholesterolemia. Recently, it has been suggested that excretion of more than 30 μg of albumin per minute (microalbuminuria) may be

Table 19–9. Substances that cause false-negative urine dipstick tests.

Ascorbic acid
Salicylic acid
Levodopa
5-Hydroxyindoleacetic acid (5-HIAA)
β-Hydroxybutyric acid

an early predictor of the development of diabetic nephropathy.

BLOOD GLUCOSE TESTING

Normal Values

The normal fasting *whole blood* glucose varies from 60 to 110 mg/dL. Plasma or serum levels are 10–15% higher because structural components of blood cells are absent, so that more glucose is present per unit volume. Thus, the normal range of fasting plasma or serum glucose is 70–120 mg/dL. Plasma or serum glucose measurements are more frequently used clinically because they are independent of the hematocrit, more closely approach the glucose level in the interstitial tissue spaces, and lend themselves to automated analytic procedures. Whole blood glucose determinations are used in spot testing of glucose in emergency situations and also in the procedures for self-monitoring of capillary blood glucose, a technique that has become widely accepted in the management of diabetes mellitus (see below).

The accepted normal range of blood or plasma glucose requires a correction for age of 1 mg/dL per year of age past 60. Thus, fasting plasma glucose in elderly nondiabetics will range from 80 to 150 mg/dL.

Venous Blood Samples

Samples should be collected in tubes containing sodium fluoride, which prevents glycolysis in the blood sample that would artifactually lower the measured glucose level. If such tubes are not available, samples must be centrifuged within 30 minutes of collection and the plasma stored at 4 °C.

The laboratory methods regularly used for determining plasma glucose utilize enzymatic methods (such as glucose oxidase or hexokinase), colorimetric methods (such as *o*-toluidine), or automated methods. The automated methods utilize reduction of copper or iron compounds by the reducing sugars in dialyzed serum. They are convenient but are not specific for glucose, since they react with other reducing substances (which are elevated in azotemia or with high ascorbic acid intake).

Capillary Blood Samples

There are several paper strip (glucose oxidase) methods for measuring capillary whole blood glucose. These include Dextrostix, Chemstrip bG, and Visidex. The latter 2 may be read visually by comparison with a color chart, or all 3 may be interpreted by an appropriate machine with a digital readout (Glucometer, Glucoscan, and others). These methods are useful in the emergency department when a rapid estimation of glucose is required or in long-term management of certain diabetic patients (see below).

SERUM KETONE DETERMINATIONS

As noted above in the section on ketonuria, there are 3 major ketone bodies: β-hydroxybutyrate (often the most prevalent ketone in diabetic ketoacidosis), acetoacetate, and acetone. The same testing materials used for determining urine ketones may be used to measure serum (or plasma) ketones. When a few drops of serum are placed on a crushed Acetest tablet, the appearance of a purple color indicates the presence of ketones. A strongly positive reaction in undiluted serum correlates with a serum ketone concentration of at least 4 mmol/L. It must be kept in mind that Acetest tablets (as well as Ketostix and Keto-Diastix) utilize the nitroprusside reaction, which measures only acetoacetate and acetone. Specific enzymatic techniques are available to quantitate each of the ketone acids, but these techniques are cumbersome and not necessary in most clinical situations.

GLYCOSYLATED HEMOGLOBIN ASSAYS

Glycohemoglobin is produced by a ketoamine reaction between glucose and the N-terminal amino acid of both beta chains of the hemoglobin molecule. The major form of glycohemoglobin is hemoglobin A_{1c}, which normally comprises only 4–6% of total hemoglobin. The remaining glycohemoglobins (2–4% of total hemoglobin) contain phosphorylated glucose or fructose and are termed hemoglobin A_{1a} and A_{1b}, respectively. The hemoglobin A_{1c} fraction is abnormally elevated in diabetics with chronic hyperglycemia and appears to correlate positively with metabolic control. Specific assays for hemoglobin A_{1c} are technically less convenient than assays for total glycohemoglobin and offer little advantage for clinical purposes. Therefore, most laboratories measure the sum of these 3 glycohemoglobins and report it simply as hemoglobin A_1 or "glycohemoglobin."

The glycosylation of hemoglobin is dependent on the concentration of blood glucose. The reaction is not reversible, so that the half-life of glycosylated hemoglobin relates to the life span of red cells (which normally circulate for up to 120 days). Thus, glycohemoglobin generally reflects the state of glycemia over the preceding 8–12 weeks, thus providing a method of assessing chronic diabetic control. A glycosylated hemoglobin close to the normal range (5–8%) would reflect good control during the preceding 2–3 months, whereas a glycosylated hemoglobin in the range of 12–15% would reflect poor control during the same period.

Although measurements of glycosylation of serum proteins or serum albumin have been reported to reflect short-term glycemia occurring over the preceding several days or weeks, their usefulness in management of diabetes has not been proved.

Table 19–10. Factors interfering with chromatographic measurement of glycohemoglobins.

Substances causing falsely high values
  Prehemoglobin A_{1c} (reversible aldimine intermediate)
  Carbamoylated hemoglobin (uremia)
  Hemoglobin F
Conditions causing falsely low values
  Hemoglobinopathies (hemoglobin C, D, and S)
  Reduced life span of erythrocytes
    Hemorrhage or therapeutic phlebotomies
    Hemolytic disorders

Conditions Interfering With Glycohemoglobin Measurements (Table 19–10)

The most common laboratory error in measuring glycohemoglobins occurs when chromatographic methods measure an acutely generated intermediary aldimine in blood (prehemoglobin A_{1c}), which fluctuates directly with the prevailing blood glucose level. This artifact can falsely elevate glycohemoglobin by as much as 1–2% during an episode of acute hyperglycemia. It can be eliminated either by washing the red blood cells with saline prior to assay or by dialyzing the hemolysate prior to chromatography. Other substances that falsely elevate "glycohemoglobin" are carbamoylated hemoglobin and hemoglobin F; the former is seen in association with uremia, and the latter circulates in some adults with genetic or hematologic disorders. In these cases, more intricate methodology such as thiobarbituric acid colorimetry or isoelectric focusing is required to distinguish hemoglobin A_{1c} from the interfering substance.

Hemoglobinopathies such as those associated with hemoglobin C, D, and S will cause falsely low values, since their glycosylated products elute only partially from chromatographic columns. In addition, these hemoglobinopathies are often associated with hemolytic anemias that shorten the life span of red blood cells. Falsely low values are seen also in patients with chronic or acute blood loss from hemorrhage or phlebotomies and in diabetic patients with hemochromatosis; in the latter group, measurements of glycohemoglobin are therefore not valid for assessment of diabetic therapy.

Glycohemoglobin assays suffer from the lack of universally available reference standards. However, in a reliable laboratory where reversible aldimines (prehemoglobin A_{1c}) are routinely removed prior to chromatography, they are useful in assessing the effectiveness of diabetic therapy and particularly helpful in evaluating the reliability of a patient's self-monitoring records of urine or blood glucose values. A glycosylated hemoglobin test is presently being evaluated for diagnostic screening purposes, and while the test is generally too insensitive to rule out impaired glucose tolerance, a value above the normal range is generally a specific indicator of diabetes mellitus.

CAPILLARY MORPHOMETRY

The basement membrane of capillaries from skeletal muscle tissue of the quadriceps area is abnormally thickened in adults with overt spontaneous diabetes (fasting hyperglycemia of 140 mg/dL or more). Capillary morphometry appears to be less discriminatory in diabetic children, being normal in as many as 60% of those below age 18. Evidence of the reversibility of capillary basement membrane thickening after near-normalization of glycemia with intensive therapy suggests that this thickening in diabetes is a consequence of long-term hyperglycemia, although the rapidity and severity of its progression may vary according to an individual's genetic predisposition.

DIAGNOSIS OF DIABETES MELLITUS

SIMPLE DIAGNOSTIC TEST BY FASTING PLASMA GLUCOSE

A fasting plasma glucose value above 140 mg/dL on more than one occasion establishes the diagnosis of diabetes mellitus. The sample for fasting plasma glucose is best drawn in the morning after the night's fast.

ORAL GLUCOSE TOLERANCE TEST

An oral glucose tolerance test is only rarely indicated, since the criteria for a positive test are still poor, being based on a nonhospitalized group of active young people who are not really comparable to any bedridden, ill, or aging population. In the past, oral glucose tolerance testing led to the overdiagnosis of diabetes. The much more rigid criteria currently recommended (see interpretation, below) should alleviate this tendency for overdiagnosis and improve the utility of the test.

If the fasting plasma glucose is between 120 and 140 mg/dL, an oral glucose tolerance test may be considered, especially in men with impotence or women who have delivered infants above 9 lb (4.1 kg) birth weight or have had recurrent vaginal yeast infections.

Preparation for Test

In order to optimize insulin secretion and effectiveness, especially when patients have been on a low-carbohydrate diet, a minimum of 150–200 g of carbohydrate per day should be included in the diet for 3 days preceding the test. The patient should eat nothing after midnight prior to the test day.

Testing Procedure

Adults are given 75 g of glucose in 300 mL of water; children are given 1.75 g of glucose per kilogram of ideal body weight. The glucose load is consumed within 5 minutes. Blood samples for plasma glucose are obtained at 0, 30, 60, 90, and 120 minutes after ingestion of glucose.

Interpretation

An oral glucose tolerance test is normal if the fasting venous plasma glucose value is less than 115 mg/dL, the 2-hour value falls below 140 mg/dL, and the value in none of the samples exceeds 200 mg/dL. A 2-hour value of greater than 200 mg/dL in addition to one other value greater than 200 mg/dL is diagnostic of diabetes mellitus. The diagnosis of "impaired glucose tolerance" is reserved for values between the upper limits of normal and those values diagnostic for diabetes. False-positive results may occur in patients who are malnourished at test time, bedridden, or afflicted with an infection or severe emotional stress. Diuretics, oral contraceptives, glucocorticoids, excess thyroxine, phenytoin, nicotinic acid, and some of the psychotropic drugs may also cause false-positive results.

INSULIN LEVELS

To measure insulin levels during the glucose tolerance test, serum or plasma must be separated within 30 minutes after collection of the specimen and frozen prior to assay. Normal immunoreactive insulin levels range from 10 to 25 μU/mL (or less) in the fasting state, reach 50–130 μU/mL at 1 hour, and usually return to levels below 30 μU/mL by 2 hours. Insulin levels are rarely of clinical usefulness during glucose tolerance testing for the following reasons: When fasting glucose levels exceed 120 mg/dL, B cells generally have reduced responsiveness to further degrees of hyperglycemia regardless of the type of diabetes. When fasting glucose levels are below 120 mg/dL, late hyperinsulinism may occur as a result of insulin resistance in type II diabetes; however, it also may occur even in mild forms or in the early phases of type I diabetes when sluggish early insulin release results in late hyperglycemia that may stimulate excessive insulin secretion at 2 hours.

INTRAVENOUS GLUCOSE TOLERANCE TEST

The intravenous glucose tolerance test is performed by giving a rapid infusion of glucose followed by serial plasma glucose measurements to determine the disappearance rate of glucose per minute. The disappearance rate reflects the patient's ability to dispose of a glucose load. This test is generally used to evaluate glucose tolerance in patients with gastrointestinal abnormalities (such as malabsorption). Caution should be used in interpreting the results, because the test bypasses normal glucose absorption and associated changes in gastrointestinal hormones that are important in carbohydrate metabolism. Furthermore, the test is relatively insensitive, and adequate criteria for diagnosis of diabetes have not been established for the various age groups.

Preparation for Test

Preparation is the same as for the oral glucose tolerance test (see above).

Testing Procedure

Intravenous access is established, and the patient is given a bolus of 50 g of glucose per 1.7 m^2 body surface area (or 0.5 g/kg of ideal body weight) as a 25% or 50% solution over 2–3 minutes. Timing begins with injection. Samples for plasma glucose determination are obtained from an indwelling needle in the opposite arm at 0, 10, 15, 20, and 30 minutes. The plasma glucose values are plotted on semilogarithmic paper against time. K, a rate constant that reflects the rate of fall of blood glucose in percent per minute, is calculated by determining the time necessary for the glucose concentration to fall by one-half ($t_{1/2}$) and using the following equation:

$$K_{(glucose)} = \frac{0.693}{t_{1/2}} \times 100$$

The average K value for a nondiabetic patient is approximately 1.72% per minute; this value declines with age but remains above 1.3% per minute. Diabetic patients almost always have a K value of less than 1% per minute.

TREATMENT OF DIABETES

Rational therapy of diabetes requires the application of principles derived from current knowledge concerning both the nature of the particular type of diabetes and the mechanism of action, efficacy, and safety of the available treatment regimens: diet, oral hypoglycemic drugs, and insulin. Controversy continues about what constitutes the best therapeutic regimen. Fundamental to this controversy is the still conflicting evidence about whether microangiopathy is related exclusively to the existence and duration of hyperglycemia or whether it reflects a separate coexisting genetic disorder. The weight of current evidence tends to favor the former view, though a genetic predisposition may potentiate glucotoxic manifestations.

The recommendations of the Executive Committee of the American Diabetes Association are to try to restore known metabolic derangements to normal in an attempt to retard (if not prevent) the progression of microvascular disease. One should aim at simulating a normal physiologic status by administering insulin in such a manner as to provide a continuous low basal level of circulating insulin and produce an 8- to 10-fold rise in plasma insulin concentration with the average meal. Care should be taken to avoid administration of excessive insulin that might downregulate the insulin receptors in target tissues or induce hypoglycemia that will then call forth insulin antagonists which would reduce subsequent insulin activity. To achieve these goals, the patient, in cooperation with the physician, must make adjustments in diet, exercise, and, if indicated, hypoglycemic agents.

AVAILABLE TREATMENT REGIMENS

1. DIET

A proper diet remains a fundamental element of therapy in all patients with diabetes. However, in over half of cases, diabetic patients fail to follow their diet. The reasons include unnecessary complexity of dietary instructions and poor understanding of the goals of dietary control by the patient and physician.

Exchange lists for meal planning can be obtained from the American Diabetes Association (ADA) and its affiliate associations or from the American Dietetic Association (430 North Michigan Avenue, Chicago 60611). The ADA diet stresses caloric restriction as the major method of achieving or maintaining ideal weight, with a fat intake of 35% or less of total calories. Furthermore, it is recommended that saturated fat be reduced to only one-third of this amount by substitution of unsaturated fats for saturated fats and by substitution of poultry, veal, and fish for red meats as the major protein source. At the same time, cholesterol is restricted to less than 300 mg daily. Complex carbohydrates may be consumed liberally (as much as 45–50% of total calories) as long as refined and simple sugars are limited.

Prescribing the Diet

A. Type I Diabetes (IDDM): In type I diabetes, total calories are calculated to maintain ideal body weight. In the typical patient, insulin is administered at least twice a day, often as a mixture of a short-acting and an intermediate-acting insulin. Meals should be adjusted accordingly in an effort to match food intake with insulin action. Breakfast should be eaten within ½–1 hour of the morning insulin dose (especially if short-acting insulin is administered at this time). A carbohydrate snack should be eaten 3 hours after and lunch no later than 5 hours after the morning insulin dose. A midafternoon carbohydrate snack is given 7–8 hours after the morning insulin. Dinner should follow the second insulin injection by ½–1½ hours, depending on whether a short-acting insulin is administered at this time. A bedtime snack high in

protein and low in carbohydrate should be given 3 hours after the evening insulin in order to provide a slow influx of carbohydrate from metabolized protein during most of the night.

B. Type II Diabetes (NIDDM): In type II diabetes, patients are often at least mildly obese. Treatment requires a vigorous program to achieve weight reduction. A fall in fasting blood sugar may follow caloric restriction prior to any significant weight loss. Weight reduction is an elusive goal that can be achieved and maintained only by close supervision of the obese patient and a supervised exercise program. The total amount of calories prescribed must take into account the patient's ideal body weight, life-style, and activity level. A diet consisting of no more than 600 kcal daily may be appropriate for a sedentary patient who is overweight, but a mildly active person can lose weight on a diet of up to 1400 kcal.

Special Considerations in Dietary Control

A. Dietary Fiber and "Glycemic Index": It has been demonstrated that when indigestible plant components such as cellulose, gum, and pectin are ingested with meals, glucose absorption is slowed and both hyperglycemia and hyperlipidemia are diminished. Although the ADA diet does not include fiber supplements such as bran, it recommends foods with a relatively high fiber content as staple components of the diet of diabetics.

Ingestion of beans and lentils, which contain a high content of leguminous fiber such as guar, produces lower glycemic responses than ingestion of comparable amounts of glucose. Jenkins et al have attempted to quantitate the relative glycemic contribution of different carbohydrate foods and have suggested the use of a "glycemic index" (GI) in which the area of blood glucose (plotted on a graph) generated over a 3-hour period following ingestion of a test food containing 50 g of carbohydrate is compared with the area plotted after giving a similar quantity of reference food such as glucose or white bread:

$$GI = \frac{\text{Blood glucose area of test food}}{\text{Blood glucose area of reference food}} \times 100$$

White bread is preferred to glucose as a reference standard because it is more palatable and has less tendency to slow gastric emptying by high tonicity, as happens when glucose solution is used.

Differences in GI were noted in normal subjects and diabetics when various foods were compared. In comparison to white bread, which was assigned an index of 100, the mean GI for other foods was as follows: baked potato, 135; table sugar (sucrose), 86; spaghetti, 66; kidney beans, 54; ice cream, 52; and lentils, 43. Some investigators have questioned whether the GI for a food ingested alone is meaningful, since the GI may become altered considerably by the presence of fats and protein when the food is consumed in a mixed meal.

Further studies of the reproducibility of the GI in the same person and the relation of a particular food's GI to its insulinotropic action on pancreatic B cells are needed before the utility of the GI in prescribing diabetic diets can be appropriately assessed. At present, however, it appears that small amounts of sucrose—particularly when taken with high-fiber substances such as cereals or whole-grain breads—may have no greater glycemic effects than comparable portions of starch from potatoes, rice, or bread.

B. Sweeteners: The nonnutritive sweetener **saccharin** continues to be available in certain foods and beverages despite recent warnings by the FDA about its potential long-term bladder carcinogenicity. Recently, a committee of the National Academy of Sciences recommended restrictions in the use of saccharin in children and pregnant women. The panel felt that physicians might be best suited to determine on an individual basis its comparative benefit versus risk for patients with diabetes or obesity.

Aspartame may prove to be the safest sweetener for use in diabetics; it consists of 2 major amino acids: aspartic acid and phenylalanine.

Other sweeteners such as sorbitol and fructose have recently gained popularity. Except for acute diarrhea induced by ingestion of large amounts of sorbitol-containing foods, their relative risk has yet to be established. **Fructose** represents a "natural" sugar substance that is a highly effective sweetener which induces only slight increases in plasma glucose levels and does not require insulin for its utilization.

C. Starch Blockers: The FDA has decided that enzymatic antagonists of amylase and sucrase (alpha-glucosidase inhibitors) can no longer be classified as "foods" but must be classified as drugs. At present, clinical trials are in progress to ascertain the efficacy and safety of these substances in reducing postprandial hyperglycemia in diabetes. They have not proved effective as an adjunct to weight reduction in the management of obesity.

2. ORAL HYPOGLYCEMIC DRUGS (Sulfonylureas & Biguanides)

There are 2 major types of oral hypoglycemic drugs: the sulfonylureas and the biguanides. The modes of action of the 2 types are quite different. Considerable controversy exists over their exact mechanisms of action, therapeutic indications, and safety for long-term use. In 1977, the United States Department of Health, Education, and Welfare recommended discontinuing general use of phenformin, the only biguanide available in the USA. It was considered to be a health hazard because of its reported association with the development of lactic acidosis.

Sulfonylureas

Currently, the sulfonylureas are the only oral hypoglycemic drugs available in the USA. This group of drugs contains a sulfonic acid–urea nucleus that can be modified by chemical substitutions to produce agents that have similar qualitative actions but differ widely in potency. The proposed mechanisms of action of the sulfonylureas include (1) augmentation of insulin release from pancreatic B cells and (2) increased insulin binding to insulin receptors.

A. Indications: Sulfonylureas are not indicated in ketosis-prone type I diabetic patients, since these drugs depend at least in part on functioning pancreatic B cells to produce their effect on blood glucose. In a well-designed prospective clinical trial, Goldman et al found that the effect of insulin on long-term glycemic control was not potentiated when sulfonylureas were added to the treatment regimen during insulin therapy of type I diabetes. Most nonobese type II patients as well as obese diabetics with moderately severe fasting hyperglycemia (> 180 mg/dL) are candidates for sulfonylurea therapy. Use of these agents is probably not justified in the obese, asymptomatic mild diabetic patient (fasting glucose of < 150 mg/dL) who has peripheral insulin insensitivity and levels of circulating insulin that are already elevated. Primary emphasis should be on weight reduction in these patients.

B. Sulfonylureas Currently Available in the USA: (See Table 19–11.)

1. Tolbutamide (Orinase)–Tolbutamide is supplied in tablets of 250 and 500 mg. It is rapidly oxidized in the liver to an inactive form. Because its duration of effect is short (6–12 hours), it is usually administered in divided doses (eg, 500 mg before each meal and at bedtime). The usual daily dose is 1.5–3 g; some patients, however, require only 250–500 mg daily. Acute toxic reactions are rare, with skin rashes occurring most commonly. Prolonged hypoglycemia has been reported rarely, mainly in elderly people or in patients receiving certain drugs (eg, dicumarol, phenylbutazone, or sulfonamides) that compete with sulfonylureas for hepatic oxidation, resulting in maintenance of high levels of unmetabolized active sulfonylureas in the body.

2. Chlorpropamide (Diabinese)–This drug is supplied in tablets of 100 and 250 mg. It has a half-life of 36 hours and a duration of action of up to 60 hours. It is slowly metabolized by the liver, with approximately 20–30% excreted unchanged in the urine. It can also interact with the drugs cited above that depend on hepatic oxidative catabolism.

Chlorpropamide is contraindicated in patients with hepatic or renal insufficiency. The average maintenance dose is 250 mg daily (range, 100–500 mg), given as a single dose in the morning. A potential hazard in the use of this drug is development of prolonged hypoglycemia, which occurs more commonly with the use of chlorpropamide than with the shorter-acting oral hypoglycemic agents. Elderly patients, especially those with reduced renal function, are at greatest risk for development of hypoglycemia with chlorpropamide, and the drug should probably not be used in this group of patients. About 15% of patients

Table 19—11. Sulfonylureas.*

	Chemical Structure	Daily Dose	Duration of Action (hours)
Tolbutamide (Orinase)		1500–3000 mg in divided doses	6–12
Tolazamide (Tolinase)		200–1000 mg as single dose or in divided doses	12–24
Acetohexamide (Dymelor)		250–1500 mg as single dose or in divided doses	12–24
Chlorpropamide (Diabinese)		100–500 as single dose	Up to 60
Glyburide (glibenclamide; DiaBeta, Micronase)		2.5–30 mg	10–24
Glipizide (glydiazinamide; Glucotrol)		2.5–40 mg	3–8

*Modified slightly and reproduced, with permission, from Katzung BG (editor): *Basic & Clinical Pharmacology,* 2nd ed. Lange, 1984.

taking chlorpropamide develop a facial flush when they drink alcohol, and occasionally they may develop a full-blown disulfiramlike reaction, with nausea, vomiting, weakness, and even syncope. There appears to be a genetic predisposition to the development of this reaction.

Other side effects of chlorpropamide include water retention and the development of hyponatremia, effects that are mediated through an ADH mechanism. The hyponatremia is generally a benign condition with sodium values between 125 and 130 meq/L, but occasional cases of symptomatic hyponatremia with sodium concentrations below 125 meq/L have been reported, particularly when concomitant diuretic therapy is being used. Chlorpropamide stimulates ADH secretion and also potentiates its action at the renal tubule. Its antidiuretic effect is somewhat unusual, since 3 other sulfonylureas (acetohexamide, tolazamide, and glyburide) appear to facilitate water excretion in humans.

3. Acetohexamide (Dymelor)–This agent is supplied in tablets of 250 and 500 mg. Its duration of action is about 12–24 hours (intermediate in duration of action between tolbutamide and chlorpropamide). The usual daily dose is 250–1500 mg given in one or 2 doses. Liver metabolism is rapid, but an active metabolite is produced and excreted by the kidney.

4. Tolazamide (Tolinase)–Tolazamide is supplied in tablets of 100, 250, and 500 mg. The average daily dose is 200–1000 mg, given in one or 2 doses. It is comparable to chlorpropamide in potency but is devoid of disulfiramlike or water-retaining effects. It has a duration of action similar to that of acetohexamide and, like acetohexamide, is metabolized to partially active metabolites by the liver; these metabolites are then excreted by the kidney.

5. Second-generation sulfonylureas–In April, 1984, the FDA approved 2 potent sulfonylurea compounds, glyburide and glipizide. These agents have similar chemical structures, with cyclic carbon rings at each end of the sulfonylurea nucleus; this causes them to be highly potent (100-fold more potent than tolbutamide). Initial use of these drugs in other countries (glyburide in 1969, glipizide in 1971) was associated with a high rate of severe hypoglycemic reactions and even some deaths. This probably resulted from overdosage due to lack of familiarity with the potent effects of the agents. The drugs should be used with caution in patients with cardiovascular disease as well as in elderly patients, in whom hypoglycemia would be especially dangerous. Neither glyburide nor glipizide should be prescribed to patients with hepatic or renal impairment, since a reduced clearance of these drugs from the blood would greatly increase the risk of hypoglycemia.

Occasionally, diabetic patients who have not responded to the more potent first-generation sulfonylureas such as chlorpropamide have responded to second-generation sulfonylureas. Unfortunately, substantial benefit has not always resulted when a maximum therapeutic dose of chlorpropamide or tolazamide has been replaced with that of a second-generation drug.

a. Glyburide (glibenclamide; DiaBeta, Micronase)–Glyburide is supplied in tablets containing 1.25, 2.5, and 5 mg. The usual starting dose is 2.5 mg/d, and the average maintenance dose is 5–10 mg/d given as a single morning dose; maintenance doses higher than 30 mg/d are not recommended. Glyburide is metabolized in the liver into products with such low hypoglycemic activity that they are considered clinically unimportant. Although assays specific for the unmetabolized compound suggest a plasma half-life of only 1–2 hours, the biologic effects of glyburide clearly persist for 24 hours after a single morning dose in diabetic patients.

Glyburide has few adverse effects other than its potential for causing hypoglycemia. Flushing has been reported to occur after ethanol ingestion, but this side effect is rare. Glyburide does not cause water retention, as chlorpropamide does, but it slightly enhances free water clearance.

b. Glipizide (glydiazinamide; Glucotrol)–Glipizide is supplied in tablets containing 5 and 10 mg. For maximum effect in reducing postprandial hyperglycemia, this agent should be ingested 30 minutes before breakfast, since rapid absorption is delayed when the drug is taken with food. The recommended starting dose is 5 mg/d, with up to 15 mg/d given as a single daily dose. When higher daily doses are required, they should be divided and given before meals. The maximum recommended dose is 40 mg/d.

At least 90% of glipizide is metabolized in the liver to inactive products, and 10% is excreted unchanged in the urine. Glipizide therapy is thus contraindicated in patients who have hepatic or renal impairment and who would therefore be at high risk for hypoglycemia.

Biguanides

Unlike sulfonylureas, the biguanides (Table 19–12) do not require functioning pancreatic B cells for reduction of hyperglycemia. They are believed to act by retarding absorption of nutrients from the intestine, decreasing hepatic gluconeogenesis, and facilitating insulin binding to receptors on insulin target tissues. Use of **phenformin** was discontinued in the USA because of its association with the development of lactic acidosis in patients with coexisting liver or kidney disease. Also of note was lack of documentation of any long-term efficacy of this drug in treating diabetes. Phenformin continues to be used in many countries throughout the world, although in some of these countries the indications for biguanide therapy

in diabetics are being reevaluated. **Metformin,** another biguanide, is reported to be less likely to produce lactic acidosis.

Efficacy & Safety of Oral Hypoglycemic Agents

The University Group Diabetes Program (UGDP) reported that the number of deaths due to cardiovascular disease in diabetic patients treated with tolbutamide or phenformin was excessive when compared to either insulin-treated patients or to patients receiving placebos. Controversy persists about the validity of the conclusions reached by the UGDP because of the heterogeneity of the population studied, its preponderance of obese subjects, and certain features of the experimental design, such as the use of a fixed dose of oral drug and lack of control for cigarette smoking.

The original data of the UGDP study were reexamined by Kilo and Williamson. As a result of these published recommendations, the ADA in 1979 withdrew its earlier (1970) endorsement of the UGDP findings and suggested that the choice of therapy be left to the judgment of the physician after discussion with the patient. They postponed a more formal recommendation until complete evaluation of all new data relating to the UGDP has been completed. The United States Supreme Court rejected attempts by the UGDP critics to prevent the FDA from requiring a special package insert warning regarding use of oral hypoglycemic agents. In April 1984, an FDA directive required the use of a special package insert warning that treatment with sulfonylureas has been reported to be associated with a higher cardiovascular mortality rate than treatment with diet alone or diet plus insulin. The insert acknowledges that controversy exists over the conclusions of the UGDP study upon which the warning is based.

3. INSULIN

Insulin is indicated for type I diabetics as well as for those type II diabetics whose hyperglycemia does not respond to diet therapy alone or combined with oral hypoglycemic drugs.

Table 19–12. Biguanides in clinical use outside the USA.*

	$R-\underset{\underset{NH}{\|\|}}{C}\quad\underset{\underset{NH}{\|\|}}{C}-NH_2$ (with $\overset{H}{\underset{\|}{N}}$)	Daily Dose	Duration of Action (hours)
Phenformin	⟨benzene ring⟩–$(CH_2)_2$–NH–	0.05–0.1 g as single dose or in divided doses as timed disintegration capsules	8–14
Buformin	$CH_3-(CH_2)_3-NH-$	0.05–0.3 g in divided doses	...
Metformin	$(CH_3)_2-N-$	1–3 g in divided doses	...

*Reproduced, with permission, from Katzung BG (editor): *Basic & Clinical Pharmacology,* 2nd ed. Lange, 1984.

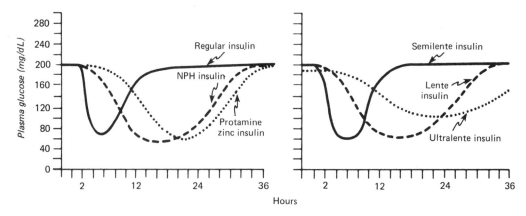

Figure 19–11. Extent and duration of action of various types of insulin (in a fasting diabetic). (Reproduced, with permission, from Katzung BG [editor]: *Basic & Clinical Pharmacology,* 2nd ed. Lange, 1984.)

Insulin replacement in patients with type I diabetes has been less than optimal because it is not possible to completely reproduce the normal physiologic pattern of insulin secretion into the portal vein. The problem of achieving optimal insulin delivery remains unsolved with the present state of technology. Subcutaneous injections do not reproduce the physiologic patterns of insulin secretion; however, with the help of appropriate modifications of diet and exercise, acceptable control may be achieved by using multiple injections of mixtures of short- and intermediate-acting insulins. In some patients, a single injection of a long-acting insulin combined with multiple injections of a short-acting insulin may be required for optimal control.

An additional problem with currently available modes of insulin therapy is that impurities in most animal insulin preparations enhance their immunogenicity. The development of highly purified porcine insulin preparations, however, has markedly reduced immunogenicity, and this problem might well be eliminated now that human insulin is available.

Characteristics of Currently Available Insulin Preparations

Commercial insulin preparations differ with regard to the animal species from which they are obtained; their purity, concentration, and solubility; and their time of onset and duration of biologic action (Tables 19–13 and 19–14; Fig 19–11).

A. Species of Insulin: Because the supply of pork insulin is too limited to satisfy the demand for insulin in the USA, most commercial insulins are composed of beef insulin or mixtures of beef and pork insulin. Beef insulin, which differs by 3 amino acids from human insulin, is more antigenic than pork insulin, which differs from human insulin by just one amino acid. The standard preparation of Iletin I (Lilly) is a mixture of 70% beef and 30% pork insulin, whereas the highly purified Iletin II insulins are available as either beef or pork insulin. With the production of highly purified pork insulins (Table 19–14), a considerable increase in the availability of porcine insulin has resulted. Furthermore, methods for mass production of human insulin—either by recombinant DNA techniques (Humulin, Lilly) or by chemical transformation of porcine to human insulin (Squibb-Novo)—have become available. Human insulin prepared by these methods has been approved by the FDA for clinical use.

B. Purity of Insulin: (Table 19–14.) Improvements in purification techniques with Sephadex gel columns have reduced or eliminated contamination with proteins having molecular weights greater than that of insulin (eg, proinsulin). Although these contaminants were biologically inactive, they were capable of inducing anti-insulin antibodies. The degree of purification in which proinsulin contamination is greater than 10 ppm but less than 25 ppm justifies their present labeling as "new improved single peak

Table 19–13. Summary of bioavailability characteristics of the insulins.

	Insulin Type	Onset	Peak Action	Duration
Short-acting	Regular, Actrapid, Velosulin	15–30 minutes	1–3 hours	5–7 hours
	Semilente, Semitard	30–60 minutes	4–6 hours	12–16 hours
Intermediate-acting	Lente, Lentard, Monotard	2–4 hours	8–10 hours	18–24 hours
	NPH, Insulatard, Protaphane			
Long-acting	Ultralente, Ultratard, PZI	4–5 hours	8–14 hours	25–36 hours

Table 19–14. Insulin preparations available in the USA.*

	Species Source	Concentration
Short-acting		
Standard†		
Regular Iletin I (Lilly)	Beef and pork	U40, U100
Regular (Squibb-Novo)	Pork	U40, U100
Semilente Iletin I (Lilly)	Beef and pork	U40, U100
Semilente (Squibb-Novo)	Beef	U40, U100
"Purified"‡		
Regular Humulin (Lilly)	Human	U100
Regular Iletin II (Lilly)	Pork or beef	U100, U500§
Actrapid (Squibb-Novo)	Pork or human	U100
Velosulin (Nordisk)	Pork	U100
Semitard (Squibb-Novo)	Pork	U100
Intermediate-acting		
Standard†		
NPH Iletin I (Lilly)	Beef and pork	U40, U100
Lente Iletin I (Lilly)	Beef and pork	U40, U100
Isophane NPH (Squibb-Novo)	Beef and pork	U40, U100
Lente (Squibb-Novo)	Beef	U40, U100
"Purified"‡		
NPH Humulin (Lilly)	Human	U100
NPH Iletin II (Lilly)	Pork or beef	U100
Lente Humulin (Lilly)	Human	U100
Lente Iletin II (Lilly)	Pork or beef	U100
Protaphane NPH (Squibb-Novo)	Pork or human	U100
Lentard (Squibb-Novo)	Beef and pork	U100
Monotard (Squibb-Novo)	Pork or human	U100
Insulatard NPH (Nordisk)	Pork	U100
Mixtard (Nordisk)	Pork	U100
Long-acting		
Standard†		
Ultralente Iletin I (Lilly)	Beef and pork	U40, U100
PZI Iletin I (Lilly)	Beef and pork	U40, U100
Ultralente (Squibb-Novo)	Beef	U100
PZI (Squibb-Novo)	Beef and pork	U40, U100
"Purified"‡		
PZI Iletin II (Lilly)	Pork or beef	U100
Ultratard (Squibb-Novo)	Beef	U100

*Modified and reproduced, with permission, from Krupp MA, Chatton MJ, Tierney LM Jr (editors): *Current Medical Diagnosis & Treatment 1986.* Lange, 1986.
†Greater than 10 but less than 25 ppm proinsulin.
‡Less than 10 ppm proinsulin.
§U500 available only as pork insulin.

insulin." This is currently the principal form of insulin used commercially in the USA (Iletin I, Lilly). When the proinsulin content is reduced to less than 10 ppm, manufacturers are entitled by FDA regulations to label the insulin **"purified."** These "purified" insulins are generally available as a monospecies of pork or beef or human insulin (Table 19–14); however, a monocomponent beef and pork mixture is also available (Lentard, Squibb-Novo).

The more highly purified insulins currently in use preserve their potency quite well; therefore, refrigeration while in use is not necessary. During travel, reserve supplies of insulin can be readily transported for weeks without significant loss of potency provided they are protected from extremes of heat or cold.

Concentrations of Insulin

At present, most insulins in the USA are available in a concentration of 100 units/mL (U100); all are dispensed in 10-mL vials. To accommodate children and the occasional adult who may require small quantities of insulin, a U40 (40 units/mL) insulin continues to be available. However, with the popularity of the "low-dose" (0.5-mL) disposable insulin syringes, there is less need for U40 insulin, since U100 can now be measured accurately in doses as low as 1 or 2 units. For use in rare cases of severe insulin resistance in which large quantities of insulin are required, a limited supply of U500 (500 units/mL) regular insulin is available from Lilly (pork, Iletin II).

Bioavailability Characteristics

Three principal types of insulins are available: (1) short-acting insulin, with rapid onset of action; (2) intermediate-acting; and (3) long-acting, with slow onset of action (Table 19–13; Fig 19–11). Short-acting (unmodified) insulin is a crystalline zinc insulin with a neutral pH in soluble form; it is dispensed as a *clear* solution. All other commercial insulins have been specifically modified to obtain more prolonged action. They are dispensed as opaque suspensions at neutral pH with either protamine (derived from fish sperm) in phosphate buffer (protamine zinc insulin and NPH) or varying concentrations of zinc in acetate buffer (ultralente, semilente, and lente insulins), rendering the insulin insoluble.

As noted above, conventional insulin therapy relies on combinations of short-acting and either intermediate-acting or long-acting insulin. The characteristics of these various insulins are discussed below and summarized in Table 19–13. It is important to recognize that values given for time of onset of action, peak effect, and duration of action are only approximate ones and that there is great variability in these parameters from patient to patient and even in a given patient depending on the size of the dose, the site of injection, the degree of exercise, the avidity of circulating anti-insulin antibodies, and other less well defined variables.

A. Short-Acting Insulins:

1. Regular insulin–(Regular insulin [Lilly], Actrapid [Squibb-Novo], Velosulin [Nordisk], Insulin Injection [Squibb-Novo].) Regular insulins are short-acting soluble crystalline zinc insulins whose hypoglycemic effect appears within 15 minutes after subcutaneous injection, peaks at 1–3 hours, and lasts for about 5–7 hours. Regular insulin is the only type of insulin that can be administered *intravenously* or used in continuous subcutaneous infusion pumps. When mixed with less than 50% of an intermediate form in the same syringe, it apparently retains enough of its rapid action to provide a rising insulin level during breakfast and dinner, if administered before these meals.

2. Semilente insulin–(Semilente [Lilly], Semitard [Squibb-Novo].) These insulins are an amorphous (or microcrystalline) form of insulin and zinc in acetate buffer. The onset of action is 30–60 minutes, peak action is reached at 6 hours, and the duration of action is 12–16 hours.

B. Intermediate-Acting Insulins:

1. Lente insulin–This is a mixture of 30% semilente with 70% ultralente insulin (Lente Iletin I and II [Lilly], Monotard [pork, Squibb-Novo], Lentard [beef-pork, Squibb-Novo]). Its onset of action is delayed to 2–4 hours, and its peak response is generally reached in about 8–10 hours. Because its duration of action is often less than 24 hours (with a range of 18–24 hours), most patients require at least 2 injections daily to maintain a sustained insulin effect.

2. NPH (neutral protamine Hagedorn, or isophane) insulin–(NPH Iletin I and II [Lilly], NPH Insulin [Squibb-Novo], Insulatard [Nordisk], Protaphane [Squibb-Novo].) NPH is an intermediate-acting insulin in which the onset of action is delayed by combining 2 parts of soluble crystalline zinc insulin with one part protamine zinc insulin. The mixture is reported to have equivalent concentrations of protamine and insulin, so that neither is in excess ("isophane"). The peak action and duration of action of NPH insulin are similar to those of lente insulin.

C. Long-Acting Insulins:

1. Ultralente–(Iletin I Ultralente [Lilly], Ultratard [Squibb-Novo].) Ultralente is a long-acting crystalline suspension of insulin whose onset of action is quite delayed, with peak effects at 8–14 hours and a duration of action of up to 36 hours. Beef insulin is less soluble than pork insulin, producing larger crystals and thus assuring a prolonged action. Beef insulin has thus been preferred in producing the ultralente insulins. Ultratard (Squibb-Novo) is a pure beef insulin, whereas Ultralente Iletin I is 70% beef and 30% pork. Recently, a limited quantity of pork Iletin II Ultralente has become available for clinical trials.

2. Protamine zinc insulin (PZI)–This modified insulin was the first long-acting insulin available. The addition of protamine to insulin produced an insulin with poor solubility and therefore slow absorption. The very long duration of action of PZI limits its usefulness. In addition, it contains an excess of protamine, which binds to any crystalline insulin added to the same syringe and thus converts the short-acting insulin to long-acting protamine insulin. Because of these problems, PZI is seldom used in the USA.

Methods of Insulin Administration

A. Insulin Syringes and Needles: Disposable plastic syringes have essentially replaced the more cumbersome glass syringes. Their finely honed 27- or 28-gauge attached needles have greatly reduced the pain of injections. They are lighter, less susceptible to damage, and much more convenient when traveling. Moreover, their clearer markings and tighter plungers allow more accurate measurement of insulin dosage. In cases where very low insulin doses are prescribed, a specially calibrated 0.5-mL disposable syringe is available to facilitate accurate measurement of U100 insulin in doses up to 50 units. These "low-dose" syringes have become increasingly popular because it is now recommended that diabetics not take more than 50 units of insulin in a single injection except in the rare instance of extreme insulin resistance. Several recent reports indicate that "disposable" syringes may be reused until blunting of the needle occurs (usually after 3–5 injections). Wiping the needle with a clean alcohol swab, reapplying the needle guard, and refrigeration after use appear to maintain adequate sterility to avoid infection.

B. Mixing Insulin: When mixing insulin, it is necessary to inject into both bottles a quantity of air equivalent to the volume of insulin being withdrawn. Traditionally, regular insulin is withdrawn first, and the longer-action insulin is then added to the syringe. Care must be taken to avoid contaminating either insulin bottle with insulin of the different type. No attempt should be made to mix the insulins in the syringe. The injection is preferably given immediately after loading the syringe, since the proportion of short-acting to long-acting insulin will decrease with prolonged mixing, particularly when the lente insulins are used.

C. Sites for Injection: Any part of the body covered by loose skin can be used as an injection site, including the abdomen, thighs, upper arms, flanks, and upper outer quadrants of the buttocks. With the use of the newer purified insulins, which reduce or eliminate scarring and fibrosis at the injection site, the previous emphasis on rotation of sites of injection may be less important. It has been shown, for example, that subcutaneous infusion of soluble purified neutral regular insulin for periods up to several weeks through a fixed, indwelling catheter attached to a syringe pump does not result in scarring, fibrosis, or lipoatrophy. Exercise appears to mobilize insulin more rapidly when the injection site is adjacent to the exercising muscle. This would argue against indiscriminate rotation of injection sites, which could lead to variable absorption. It is possible that some of the stability of glycemic control achieved by infusion pumps may be related to the constancy of the site of infusion from day to day. For patients who exercise a great deal, subcutaneous injection into the abdominal skin may yield greater stability of glycemic control than intramuscular injection.

D. Insulin Delivery Systems: Efforts to administer insulin by **"closed loop"** systems (glucose-controlled insulin infusion systems [Biostator]) have recently been successful in acute situations such as diabetic ketoacidosis or during surgery. However, chronic use is precluded by the bulkiness of the computerized pump and by the need for continuous aspiration of blood for the external glucose sensor that activates the appropriate insulin or glucose infusion.

Many small portable **"open loop" devices** for the delivery of insulin are on the market. These devices contain an insulin reservoir and a pump programmed to deliver regular insulin (by either a subcutaneous, intravenous, or intraperitoneal route) at a previously determined rate; they do not contain a glucose sensor. With improved methods for self-monitoring of *blood* glucose at home (see below), these pump systems have become very useful for managing some diabetic patients. However, there have been reports of numerous acute complications, such as infection at the catheter site and ketoacidosis due to kinking of the tube attached to the insulin reservoir. At present, conventional methods of insulin administration, with multiple subcutaneous injections of mixtures of a rapid and either an intermediate-acting or long-acting insulin, can provide glycemic control almost as effectively as the open loop systems in most patients with IDDM who self-monitor their blood glucose levels accurately and regularly.

Intranasally administered soluble insulin is rapidly adsorbed when given along with a detergent substance to facilitate adsorption. Preliminary clinical trials have demonstrated its efficacy in reducing postprandial hyperglycemia in insulin-dependent diabetics. Further studies are in progress to assess its usefulness as an insulin delivery system in treating diabetic patients.

Pancreatic islet cells have been successfully transplanted in genetically similar strains of rodents with experimental diabetes; however, this approach has not yet been successful in humans because of immunologic rejection of the tissue. Similarly, **whole pancreas transplants** have generally proved unsatisfactory in treating the insulin-dependent (type I) patient because of the necessity for prolonged antirejection therapy.

STEPS IN THE MANAGEMENT OF THE DIABETIC PATIENT

Diagnostic Examination

A. History and Physical Examination: A complete history is taken and physical examination is performed for diagnostic purposes and to rule out the presence of coexisting or complicating disease. Nutritional status should be noted, particularly if catabolic features such as progressive weight loss are present despite a normal or increased food intake. The family history should include not only the incidence but also the age at onset of diabetes in other members of the family, and it should be noted whether affected family members were obese and whether they required insulin. Other factors that increase cardiovascular risk, such as a smoking history, presence of hypertension or hyperlipidemia, or oral contraceptive pill use should be documented.

A careful physical examination should include baseline weight, pulse rate, and blood pressure. All peripheral arterial pulses should be examined, noting whether bruits or other signs of atherosclerotic disease are present. Neurologic and ophthalmologic examinations should be performed, with emphasis on investigation of abnormalities that may be related to

diabetes, such as neovascularization of the retina or stocking/glove sensory loss in the extremities.

B. Laboratory Diagnosis: (See also Laboratory Findings in Diabetes Mellitus, above.) Laboratory diagnosis should include documentation of the presence of fasting hyperglycemia (plasma glucose > 140 mg/dL) or postprandial (post–glucose tolerance test) values consistently above 200 mg/dL. An attempt should be made to characterize the diabetes as IDDM or NIDDM, based on the clinical features present and on whether or not ketonuria accompanies the glycosuria. With current emphasis on home blood glucose monitoring, laborious attempts to document the renal threshold for glucose are no longer necessary in the initial evaluation of diabetic patients, particularly since "double-voided" urine specimens are difficult to obtain and since acceptable control of glycemia now allows only rare episodes of glycosuria.

Other baseline laboratory measurements that should be made part of the record include either glycohemoglobin or hemoglobin A_{1c}, total and HDL cholesterol, plasma triglycerides, electrocardiogram, chest x-ray, complete blood count, complete urinalysis, and renal function studies (serum creatinine, blood urea nitrogen, and, if possible, creatinine clearance).

Patient Education

Education is the most important task of the physician who provides care to diabetic patients. It must be remembered that education is necessary not only for newly diagnosed diabetic patients and their families but also for patients with diabetes of any duration who may never have been properly educated about their disorder or who may not be aware of advances in diabetes management. The "teaching curriculum" should include explanations of the nature of diabetes, its potential acute and chronic complications, and information on how these complications can be prevented or at least recognized and treated early. Patients must be helped to accept the fact that they have diabetes; until this difficult adjustment has been made, efforts to cope with the disorder are likely to be futile.

A. Diet Instruction: All diabetic patients should receive individual instruction on diet, as described earlier in this chapter. Unrestricted diets are not advised for insulin-requiring diabetics. Until new methods of insulin replacement are available to provide more normal patterns of insulin delivery in response to metabolic demands, multiple small feedings restricted in simple sugars will continue to be recommended.

B. Insulin: Give the patient an understanding of the actions of the various insulins and the methods of administration of insulin. Patients and their families or friends should also be taught to recognize signs and symptoms of hypoglycemia and how to institute appropriate therapy for hypoglycemic reactions (see Acute Complications of Diabetes Mellitus, below). All patients should be made aware of community agencies (Diabetes Association chapters, etc) that serve as resources for continuing education.

Instructions in the Care of the Feet for Persons With Diabetes Mellitus or Vascular Disturbances*

Hygiene of the Feet

(1) Wash feet daily with mild soap and lukewarm water. Dry thoroughly between the toes by pressure. Do not rub vigorously, as this is apt to break the delicate skin.

(2) When feet are thoroughly dry, rub well with vegetable oil to keep them soft, prevent excess friction, remove scales, and prevent dryness. Care must be taken to prevent foot tenderness.

(3) If the feet become too soft and tender, rub them with alcohol about once a week.

(4) When rubbing the feet, always rub upward from the tips of the toes. If varicose veins are present, massage the feet very gently; never massage the legs.

(5) If the toenails are brittle and dry, soften them by soaking for one-half hour each night in lukewarm water containing 1 tbsp of powdered sodium borate (borax) per quart. Follow this by rubbing around the nails with vegetable oil. Clean around the nails with an orangewood stick. If the nails become too long, file them with an emery board. File them straight across and no shorter than the underlying soft tissues of the toe. Never cut the corners of the nails. (The podiatrist should be informed if a patient has diabetes.)

(6) Wear low-heeled shoes of soft leather that fit the shape of the feet correctly. The shoes should have wide toes that will cause no pressure, fit close in the arch, and grip the heels snugly. Wear new shoes one-half hour only on the first day and increase by 1 hour each day following. Wear thick, warm, loose stockings.

Treatment of Corns & Calluses

(1) Corns and calluses are due to friction and pressure, most often from improperly fitted shoes and stockings. Wear shoes that fit properly and cause no friction or pressure.

(2) To remove excess calluses or corns, soak the feet in lukewarm (not hot) water, using a mild soap, for about 10 minutes and then rub off the excess tissue with a towel or file. Do not tear it off. Under no circumstances must the skin become irritated.

(3) Do not cut corns or calluses. If they need attention, it is safer to see a podiatrist.

(4) Prevent callus formation under the ball of the foot (a) by exercises, such as curling and stretching the toes several times a day; (b) by finishing each step on the toes and not on the ball of the foot; and (c) by wearing shoes that are not too short and that do not have high heels.

Aids in Treatment of Impaired Circulation (Cold Feet)

(1) Never use tobacco in any form. Tobacco contracts blood vessels and so reduces circulation.

(2) Keep warm. Wear warm stockings and other clothing. Cold contracts blood vessels and reduces circulation.

(3) Do not wear circular garters, which compress blood vessels and reduce blood flow.

(4) Do not sit with the legs crossed. This may compress the leg arteries and shut off the blood supply to the feet.

(5) If the weight of the bedclothes is uncomfortable, place a pillow under the covers at the foot of the bed.

(6) Do not apply any medication to the feet without directions from a physician. Some medicines are too strong for feet with poor circulation.

(7) Do not apply heat in the form of hot water, hot water bottles, or heating pads without a physician's consent. Even moderate heat can injure the skin if circulation is poor.

(8) If the feet are moist or the patient has a tendency to develop athlete's foot, a prophylactic dusting powder should be used on the feet and in shoes and stockings daily. Change shoes and stockings at least daily or oftener.

Treatment of Abrasions of the Skin

(1) Proper first-aid treatment is of the utmost importance even in apparently minor injuries. Consult a physician immediately for any redness, blistering, pain, or swelling. Any break in the skin may become ulcerous or gangrenous unless properly treated by a physician.

(2) Dermatophytosis (athlete's foot), which begins with peeling and itching between the toes or discoloration or thickening of the toenails, should be treated immediately by a physician or podiatrist.

(3) Avoid strong irritating antiseptics such as tincture of iodine.

(4) As soon as possible after any injury, cover the area with sterile gauze, which may be purchased at drugstores. Only fine paper tape or cellulose tape (Scotch Tape) should be used on the skin if adhesive retention of the gauze is required.

(5) Elevate and, as much as possible until recovery, avoid using the foot.

*Reproduced, with permission, from Krupp MA, Chatton MJ, Tierney LM Jr (editors): *Current Medical Diagnosis & Treatment 1986*. Lange, 1986.

C. Hypoglycemic Agents: Information must be provided on the principles of hypoglycemic therapy (including information about time of onset, peak action, and duration of action of any pharmacologic agent being used).

D. Effect of Exercise: Exercise increases the effectiveness of insulin, and regular daily moderate exercise is an excellent means of improving utilization of fats and carbohydrates in diabetic patients. A judicious balance of the size and frequency of meals with moderate regular exercise can often stabilize the insulin dosage in diabetics who tend to slip out of control easily. Strenuous exercise, however, can precipitate hypoglycemia in an unprepared patient, and diabetics must therefore be taught to reduce their insulin dosage or take supplemental carbohydrate in anticipation of strenuous activity. Injection of insulin into a site farthest away from the muscles most involved in exercise may help meliorate exercise-induced hypoglycemia, since insulin injected to exercising muscle is much more rapidly mobilized. With more knowledge regarding the relationship between caloric intake and expenditure and insulin requirements, the patient can become liberated from much of the regimentation imposed by the disorder.

E. Good Hygiene: All diabetic patients must receive adequate instruction on personal hygiene, especially with regard to care of the feet (see p 554), skin, and teeth.

F. Infections: Infections with fever and severe illness provoke the release of high levels of insulin antagonists that will bring about a marked increase in insulin requirements. It is essential to limit the period of infection, since infection raises the blood glucose level and this, in turn, immobilizes the general defense mechanisms that the body uses against bacterial and even viral organisms. Thus, the early and sufficient use of bactericidal antibiotics is imperative. Type I diabetics must be taught how to supplement the regimen with regular insulin if persistent glycosuria and ketonuria occur—especially if associated with infection. Patients must understand that insulin therapy should never be withheld in the presence of gastric upset and vomiting if glycosuria with ketonuria is present. When food intake is limited by nausea or vomiting, the patient should take ginger ale, apple juice, or grape juice in small sips and should notify the physician in case supplemental intravenous fluids might be required.

G. Self-Monitoring: Patients in whom labile diabetes is difficult to control should receive instructions on techniques for self-monitoring of blood glucose (see below). They should be encouraged to keep careful records of their glucose measurements and instructed on appropriate measures to correct for emerging patterns of hyperglycemia as well as to prevent recurrent episodes of hypoglycemia. Self-monitoring allows for greater flexibility in life-style, instructs patients on the glycemic effects of specific foods and exercise, and alleviates the likelihood of unexpected episodes of severe hypoglycemia.

H. Identification Bracelet: All patients receiving hypoglycemic therapy should wear a Medic-Alert bracelet or necklace that clearly states that insulin or an oral sulfonylurea drug is being taken. A card in the wallet or purse is less useful, since legal problems may arise if a victim's person and belongings are searched without permission. (Information on how to obtain a Medic-Alert identification device can be obtained from the Medic-Alert Foundation, PO Box 1009, Turlock, CA 95380.)

I. Restrictions on Occupation: Certain occupations potentially hazardous to the diabetic patient or others will continue to be prohibited (eg, piloting airplanes, crane operating).

Avoidance of Stress & Emotional Turmoil

Prevention of psychologic turmoil is of great importance in the control of diabetes, particularly when the disease is difficult to stabilize. One reason blood glucose control in diabetics may be particularly sensitive to emotional upset is that their pancreatic A cells are hyperresponsive to physiologic levels of epinephrine, producing excessive levels of glucagon with consequent hyperglycemia.

Specific Therapy

Treatment must be individualized depending on the specific needs of each patient. Certain general principles of management pertaining to each type of diabetes will be outlined below.

A. Type I Diabetes (IDDM): IDDM patients require replacement therapy with exogenous insulin. This should be instituted under conditions of an individualized diabetic diet with multiple feedings and normal daily activities so that an appropriate dosage regimen can be developed.

At the onset of diabetes, many type I patients recover some pancreatic B cell function and may temporarily need only low doses of exogenous insulin to supplement their own endogenous insulin secretion. This is known as the "honeymoon period." Within 2 years, however, most of these patients show either absent or negligible pancreatic B cell function. At this point, these patients should be instructed to take 2 injections of insulin mixtures (a short-acting combined with either an intermediate-acting or a long-acting insulin). In the past, these insulin injections were regulated on the basis of measurements of glucose in double-voided urines at least 4 times a day, as well as with random and fasting plasma glucose levels, until a stable therapeutic regimen was established. At present, however, self-monitoring of blood glucose levels is the recommended means of determining the adjustment of insulin dosage and the need for other therapeutic interventions in type I diabetes.

1. Conventional insulin therapy (split doses of insulin mixtures)—A conventional insulin regimen in a 70-kg patient taking 2200 kcal divided into 6 feedings might be 10 units of regular and 10 units of NPH insulin in the morning and 8 units of regular and 8 units of NPH insulin in the evening. The morning blood glucose level gives a measure of the effectiveness of NPH insulin administered the previous evening; the noon level reflects the effects of the morning regular insulin; and the 5 PM and 9 PM levels represent the effects of the morning NPH and the evening regular insulins, respectively. A properly educated patient can be taught to adjust insulin dosage by observing the pattern of recorded self-monitored blood glucose levels and correlating it with the approximate duration of action and the time of peak effect after injection of the various insulin preparations (Table 19–13). Adjustments should be made gradually, preferably not more often than every 2 or 3 days if possible.

2. Intensive multiple-dose insulin therapy–While split doses of insulin mixtures daily have improved the quality of glycemic control as compared to single injections of intermediate insulin in type I diabetics, blood glucose values throughout the day are often not optimal, and nocturnal hypoglycemia may result from attempts to achieve euglycemia. In cases in which conventional split doses of insulin mixtures cannot maintain near-normalization of blood glucose without hypoglycemia (particularly at night), multiple injections of insulin may be required. An increasingly popular regimen consists of reducing or omitting the evening dose of intermediate insulin and adding a portion of it at bedtime. In some cases, a regimen consisting of 10 units of regular insulin mixed with 10 units of NPH insulin in the morning, 8–10 units of regular insulin before the evening meal, and 6 units of NPH at bedtime might be more efficacious than the conventional regimen of split doses mentioned above because it counteracts the "dawn phenomenon," ie, a rise in fasting blood glucose level caused by a nocturnal rise in growth hormone secretion.

In cases in which hypoglycemia occurs unexpectedly and at inconsistent times in the day or night, variable or delayed insulin absorption from large subcutaneous depots containing regular and NPH insulin may be a contributing factor. Reducing the size and character of the depots by administering small doses of regular insulin more frequently (eg, 4 times a day) and giving one injection of a long-acting insulin at bedtime (eg, ultralente insulin) has often been most helpful in reducing the frequency and severity of hypoglycemia in patients attempting near-normalization of blood glucose. This regimen also gives greater flexibility regarding meal patterns and content than conventional therapy with split doses of insulin mixtures.

3. Intensive insulin therapy using insulin pumps–Several types of portable battery-operated "open loop" devices have been marketed to deliver insulin continuously (see Methods of Insulin Administration, above). These generally infuse insulin through a needle or catheter implanted subcutaneously in the abdomen. A basal infusion rate of regular insulin is provided over a 24-hour period, and this is augmented by a bolus of regular insulin prior to meals. In addition, since insulin requirements appear to increase slightly in the early dawn period in the majority of patients with type I diabetes, most pumps also have adjustable basal rates that can be programmed to rise automatically at 6 AM.

The use of pumps requires knowledgeable and compliant patients who can be depended on to monitor their blood glucose levels as often as 4 times daily. The indwelling needle or catheter should be changed every 48 hours to reduce the risk of infection, and patients should be alert for symptoms of sudden deterioration of glycemic control, due to pump blockage, pump failure, or leakage of insulin from the tubing. The selection of dosage is usually based on providing 40–50% of the estimated daily dose of insulin as the basal infusion rate and the remaining amount divided as intermittent boluses given prior to meals to control postprandial metabolism. For example, in a 70-kg patient requiring 40–45 units of insulin a day, 20 units of regular insulin would be administered as a basal infusion of 0.8 unit/h, with the remaining units administered as follows: 7–8 units before breakfast, 5–6 units before lunch, 6–8 units before supper, and 0–2 units prior to a bedtime snack. The results of blood glucose monitoring as well as the extent of physical activity and dietary intake will all contribute to fine-tuning the proper dosage of insulin administered at various meals and basally.

4. Selection of patients for intensive insulin therapy–Patient selection is difficult, and exact criteria are controversial. Patients should be highly motivated and willing to monitor their blood glucose levels several times daily and record the results. They should not have impaired adrenergic responses to hypoglycemia, as is often seen with autonomic neuropathy, since this increases the risk of severe hypoglycemic episodes. Finally, if nonproliferative ("background") or proliferative retinopathy is present, intensive insulin therapy should be initiated slowly and with careful attention to possible progression of retinal disease (see Ophthalmologic Complications, below).

5. Self-monitoring of blood glucose levels–Monitoring of capillary glucose levels has greatly improved glycemic control by enabling patients to alter their dietary intake or insulin dose to maintain glycemic ranges below the renal threshold for glycosuria. This has been particularly helpful at bedtime to determine whether supplementary feedings are required to avoid nocturnal hypoglycemia.

Self-monitoring of blood glucose levels is particularly helpful in managing diabetes in the following groups: patients with brittle diabetes; patients who are attempting ideal glycemic control, such as during pregnancy; patients with impaired or absent early warning of hypoglycemic episodes; and patients in whom urine glucose levels are misleading, ie, those with an abnormally functioning bladder or an altered renal threshold for glucose. Self-monitoring is useful in educating patients about the glycemic effects of specific foods in their diet and reduces the likelihood of unexpected episodes of severe hypoglycemia in insulin-treated diabetics. It has proved to be an effective and safe clinical tool that is a valuable adjunct to therapy in compliant patients.

There are 3 essential elements to self-monitoring of blood glucose: (1) obtaining the blood specimen, (2) applying the specimen to enzyme-impregnated strips capable of discriminating the glucose level, and (3) reading the glucose level from the test strip. Each of these will be discussed briefly.

The patient may obtain a capillary blood sample from the fingertip by means of a lancet designed for this purpose. The patient should be taught how to clean the site and how to rapidly pierce the skin to obtain a drop of blood. Automatic spring-loaded devices such as the Autolet or Penlet are useful in simplifying the finger-pricking technique and ensuring an adequate blood sample.

The drop of blood is then applied to the appropriate area of an enzyme-impregnated strip such as the Dextrostix, Chemstrip bG, or Visidex. It is important to follow the instructions for each type of strip. The strips vary with respect to the area necessary to cover with the blood drop, washing technique, and timing of the procedure.

Chemstrip bG and Visidex results can be visually interpreted by comparing the color or colors obtained on the strip with the color chart supplied by the manufacturer. For patients who have difficulty with color discrimination or who have frank visual impairment, devices with automated digital readouts are available to quantitate the color changes of Dextrostix (Glucometer, Glucoscan) or of Chemstrip bG (Accu-Chek bG). These devices vary in cost, ease of use, portability, and strip compatibility. The physician should learn the advantages and disadvantages of these devices and help the patient make an appropriate choice.

Initially, blood glucose levels should be checked at least 4 times a day in patients with type I diabetes. Generally, these measurements are taken before each meal and at bedtime. Once these levels are brought into an acceptable range, the patient should continue to check blood glucose levels twice daily and occasionally measure blood glucose after meals. In addition, patients should be taught to check their blood glucose level whenever they develop symptoms that could represent a hypoglycemic episode. All blood glucose levels and their timing and corresponding insulin doses should be recorded in an organized fashion and brought with the patient for physician review during regularly scheduled check-ups; such personal blood glucose logs are commercially available.

6. Management of early morning hyperglycemia in IDDM patients–One of the more difficult therapeutic problems in managing patients with IDDM is determining the proper adjustment of insulin dose when the early morning blood glucose level is high before breakfast. Prebreakfast hyperglycemia is sometimes due to the Somogyi effect, in which nocturnal hypoglycemia evokes a surge of counterregulatory hormones to produce high blood glucose levels by 7 AM. If this is the case, lowering the evening dose of intermediate insulin is indicated. However, a possibly more common cause of prebreakfast hyperglycemia is the waning of circulating insulin levels, which would suggest use of more (rather than less) intermediate insulin in the evening. These 2 phenomena are not mutually exclusive and can occur together to produce a greater magnitude of hyperglycemia in affected patients with IDDM. A third phenomenon—the recently described "dawn phenomenon"—has been reported to occur in as many as 75% of IDDM patients and in the majority of NIDDM patients and normal subjects as well. It is characterized by a reduced tissue sensitivity to insulin between 5 AM and 8 AM (dawn), and recent evidence (see Bolli and Gerich, 1984; Bolli et al, 1984) suggests that it is evoked by spikes of growth hormone released hours before, at onset of sleep. When the "dawn phenomenon" occurs alone, it may produce only mild hyperglycemia in the early morning; however, when it is associated with either or both of the other phenomena, it can further aggravate the hyperglycemia (Table 19–15). Diagnosis of the cause of prebreakfast hyperglycemia can be facilitated by asking the patient to self-monitor blood glucose levels at 3 AM in addition to monitoring at the usual times, bedtime and 7 AM. In insulin-treated patients, serum levels of free immunoreactive insulin (particularly in the basal or low ranges) are difficult to quantitate accurately because of technical interference. In specialized research laboratories, however, these levels have been measured in hospitalized patients with prebreakfast hyperglycemia (Table 19–15).

Table 19–15. Typical patterns of overnight blood glucose levels and serum free immunoreactive insulin levels in prebreakfast hyperglycemia due to various causes in patients with IDDM.

	Blood Glucose Levels (mg/dL)			Serum Free Immunoreactive Insulin Levels (μU/mL)		
	10 PM	3 AM	7 AM	10 PM	3 AM	7 AM
Somogyi effect	90	40	200	High	Slightly high	Normal
"Dawn phenomenon"	110	110	150	Normal	Normal	Normal
Waning of circulating insulin levels plus "dawn phenomenon"	110	190	220	Normal	Low	Low
Waning of circulating insulin levels plus "dawn phenomenon" plus Somogyi effect	110	40	380	High	Normal	Low

When a particular pattern emerges from monitoring blood glucose levels at 10 PM, 3 AM, and 7 AM, appropriate therapeutic measures can be taken. Prebreakfast hyperglycemia due to the Somogyi effect can be treated by either reducing the dose of intermediate insulin, giving a portion of it at bedtime, or supplying more food at bedtime. When the ''dawn phenomenon'' alone is present, shifting a portion of the intermediate insulin from dinnertime to bedtime often suffices; or when insulin pumps are used, the basal infusion rate can be stepped up appropriately (eg, from 0.8 unit/h to 1 unit/h) from 6 AM until breakfast. Finally, in cases in which the circulating insulin level is waning, either increasing the evening insulin dose or shifting it from dinnertime to bedtime (or both) may be efficacious.

B. Type II Diabetes (NIDDM): The principles of therapy are less well defined in this heterogeneous group of diabetic patients than is the case with type I diabetes. Therapeutic recommendations are based upon the relative contributions of B cell insufficiency and insulin insensitivity in individual patients.

1. The obese patient–The most common type of diabetic patient is the obese diabetic with insulin insensitivity. Characteristically, these patients have normal or increased basal levels of circulating insulin, and in the presence of mild hyperglycemia they are capable of responding to a glucose load with insulin secretion. However, as hyperglycemia progresses, the insulin response to a glucose load decreases. This refractoriness of the B cell is primarily related to the hyperglycemic stimulation, since other B cell–stimulating agents such as sulfonylureas, arginine, and glucagon still provoke rapid insulin release.

a. Weight reduction–One of the primary modes of therapy in the obese type II diabetic patient is weight reduction. Normalization of glycemia can be achieved by reducing adipose stores, with consequent restoration of tissue sensitivity to insulin. A combination of caloric restriction, increased exercise, modification of behavior, and consistent reinforcement of good eating habits is required if a weight reduction program is to be successful. Knowledge of the symptoms of diabetes and an understanding of the risks and complications of diabetes often increase the patient's motivation for weight reduction. Even so, significant weight loss is seldom achieved in the morbidly obese patient; there is a variable effectiveness in moderately obese patients depending on the enthusiasm of the therapist and the motivation of the patient.

b. Hypoglycemic agents–Hypoglycemic agents, including insulin as well as the oral hypoglycemic drugs, are generally *not* indicated for long-term use in the obese patient with mild diabetes. A weight reduction program can be disrupted by real or imagined hypoglycemic reactions when insulin therapy is used. It is also possible that administration of insulin to an obese patient who already has excessive circulating levels may maintain insulin insensitivity through down-regulation of receptor sites and by interference with catabolic mechanisms during caloric

deprivation. The obese diabetic who has been previously treated with insulin, often in high doses and in an interrupted fashion, may develop immune insulin resistance (see below). This not only increases the requirements for exogenous insulin but may further impair the effectiveness of endogenous insulin because of cross-reacting antibodies; on occasion, this can even precipitate ketoacidosis.

Oral sulfonylureas, therefore, are more appropriate than insulin for *symptomatic* moderately severe diabetes in an obese patient. If sulfonylurea therapy (combined with a weight reduction regimen) is inadequate to control symptoms and reduce hyperglycemia, insulin therapy may be necessary, directed at elimination of symptoms rather than restoration of euglycemia. Use of a sulfonylurea agent or insulin to supplement a weight reduction program should be for a limited period (weeks or months) to meliorate hyperglycemic symptoms until sufficient weight reduction has occurred to keep the patient symptom-free.

2. The nonobese patient–In the nonobese NIDDM diabetic with moderately severe hyperglycemia, pancreatic B cells are refractory to glucose stimulation. Peripheral insulin resistance is detectable but is considerably less intense than in obese diabetics who have a comparable degree of hyperglycemia; it is also of less therapeutic import.

a. Diet–If hyperglycemia is mild (fasting blood glucose levels of < 200 mg/dL), normal metabolic control can occasionally be restored by a diet devoid of simple sugars and with calories calculated to maintain ideal body weight. Restriction of saturated fats and cholesterol is also strongly advised. The standard ADA diet with its recommended exchange list should be prescribed for these nonobese NIDDM patients.

b. Oral hypoglycemic agents–When diet therapy alone is not sufficient to correct hyperglycemia, a trial of sulfonylurea drugs is indicated to supplement the dietary regimen. The controversies raised by the UGDP (see Efficacy and Safety of Oral Hypoglycemic Agents, above) apply mainly to obese patients with relatively mild diabetes (who represented the great majority of patients in that study), and there are few data on which to base an assessment of the risk-benefit ratio of sulfonylureas in nonobese patients with fasting hyperglycemia above 140 mg/dL. Therefore, because of their proved efficacy in these patients and the absence of evidence suggesting harm to them, it seems reasonable to continue the use of sulfonylureas as long as they remain effective in controlling hyperglycemia. The degree of control to aim for remains arbitrary at present; however, data from the United Kingdom and from studies of Pima Indians suggest that maintaining postprandial plasma glucose levels below 200 mg/dL seems to spare NIDDM patients from increased risk of severe retinopathy or vascular complications. Once the dosage of sulfonylurea reaches the upper recommended limit in a compliant patient without maintaining plasma glucose below 200 mg/dL throughout the day, insulin therapy is indicated.

c. Insulin–A single dose of intermediate-acting

insulin may suffice to supplement endogenous insulin secretion in nonobese NIDDM patients who require insulin therapy. This is in contrast to type I diabetics, who can seldom be rendered euglycemic unless multiple injections or a continuous infusion of insulin is employed. Many nonobese patients with mild insulinopenia can have their glycohemoglobin levels brought into the normal range with relatively small doses of insulin and with no suggestion of nocturnal hypoglycemia. Occasional patients with more severe insulinopenia may require split doses of insulin.

Immunopathology of Insulin Therapy

At least 5 molecular classes of insulin antibodies are produced during the course of insulin therapy: IgA, IgD, IgE, IgG, and IgM. Even though the use of highly purified pork insulins has considerably reduced the immunogenicity of insulin, most diabetics continue to be treated with mixed beef-pork insulins (Table 19– 14). These beef-containing insulins usually induce antibodies to insulin after about 2– 3 weeks of therapy.

A. Insulin Allergy: Insulin allergy, a hypersensitivity reaction of the immediate type, is a rare condition in which local or systemic urticaria occurs immediately after insulin injection. This reaction is due to histamine release from tissue mast cells sensitized by adherence of IgE antibodies to insulin. In severe cases, anaphylaxis can occur. The appearance of a subcutaneous nodule at the site of insulin injection, occurring several hours after the injection and lasting for up to 24 hours, has been attributed to an IgG-mediated complement-binding Arthus reaction. Because sensitivity is often to noninsulin protein contaminants, the highly purified insulins have markedly reduced the incidence of insulin allergy, especially of the local variety. When allergy to beef insulin is present, a species change (eg, to pure pork insulin or to human insulin) may correct the problem. Antihistamines, corticosteroids, and even desensitization may be required, especially for systemic hypersensitivity in an insulin-dependent patient. A commercial kit containing various dilutions of pure beef or pure pork insulin for allergy testing and insulin desensitization is distributed by the Eli Lilly Company on request.

B. Immune Insulin Resistance: Except for some patients initially treated with highly purified pork or human insulin, all patients who receive insulin develop a low titer of circulating IgG antibodies to insulin, and this neutralizes to a small extent the rapid action of insulin. In some diabetic patients with a history of intermittent exposure to insulin therapy—and especially those with some degree of tissue insensitivity to insulin (such as obese NIDDM patients)—a high titer of circulating IgG antibodies to insulin develops. This results in extremely high insulin requirements, often to more than 200 units/d. This frequently is a self-limited condition and may clear spontaneously after several months. However, in cases where the circulating antibody is specifically more reactive to beef insulin, switching to a less antigenic highly pu-

rified pork insulin or human insulin may make possible a dramatic reduction in insulin dosage or at least may shorten the duration of immune resistance. In immune resistance that responds poorly to a change of insulin species, other forms of therapy include use of sulfated beef insulin (a chemically modified form of beef insulin containing an average of 6 sulfate groups per molecule) and immunosuppression with corticosteroids. In NIDDM patients, whose excessive circulating insulin antibodies do not completely neutralize endogenous (human) insulin, the foreign insulin can be discontinued and the patient maintained on oral sulfonylureas combined with diet therapy.

C. Lipodystrophy at Injection Sites: Rarely, a disfiguring atrophy of subcutaneous fatty tissue occurs at the site of insulin injection. Although the cause of this complication is obscure, it seems to represent a form of immune reaction, particularly since it occurs predominantly in females and is associated with lymphocyte infiltration in the lipoatrophic area. This complication has become even less common since the development of highly purified insulin preparations of neutral pH. Injection of highly purified preparations of insulin directly into the atrophic area often results in restoration of normal contours.

Lipohypertrophy, on the other hand, is not a consequence of immune responses; rather, it seems to be due to the pharmacologic effects of depositing insulin in the same location repeatedly. It can occur with purified insulins and is best treated by avoiding the hypertrophic areas. It is prevented by rotation of injection sites.

ACUTE COMPLICATIONS OF DIABETES MELLITUS

HYPOGLYCEMIA

Hypoglycemic reactions (see below and Chapter 20) are the most common complications that occur in insulin-treated diabetic patients. They may also occur in patients taking oral sulfonylureas, especially older patients or those with impaired liver or kidney function treated with long-acting agents such as chlorpropamide. Hypoglycemia may result from delay in taking a meal or from unusual physical exertion without supplemental calories or a decrease in insulin dose.

Clinical Features

Signs and symptoms of hypoglycemia may be divided into those resulting from neuroglycopenia (insufficient glucose for normal central nervous system function leading to confusion and coma) and those resulting from stimulation of the autonomic nervous system. There is great variation in the pattern of hypoglycemic signs and symptoms from patient to patient; however, individual patients tend to experience the same pattern from episode to episode. In older diabetics, autonomic responses are less frequent, so that hypoglycemia may be manifested only by signs and symptoms of neuroglycopenia. The gradual onset of hypoglycemia with intermediate-acting or long-acting insulin also makes recognition more difficult in older patients.

A. Neuroglycopenia: Signs and symptoms of neuroglycopenia include mental confusion with impaired abstract and, later, concrete thought processes; this may be followed by bizarre antagonistic behavior. Stupor, coma, and even death may occur with profound hypoglycemia. Full recovery of central nervous system function does not always occur if treatment is delayed.

B. Autonomic Hyperactivity: Signs and symptoms of autonomic hyperactivity can be both adrenergic (tachycardia, palpitations, sweating, tremulousness) and parasympathetic (nausea, hunger).

Treatment

All of the manifestations of hypoglycemia are rapidly relieved by glucose administration. Because of the danger of insulin reactions, diabetic patients should carry packets of table sugar or a candy roll at all times for use at the onset of hypoglycemic symptoms. Family members or friends of the patient should be provided with a 1-mg ampule of glucagon that can be injected intramuscularly if the patient is found unconscious; the ampules are available by prescription and can be injected with an insulin syringe. Detailed instructions in the use of glucagon are an essential part of the diabetic education program.

A. The Conscious Patient: Patients with symptoms of hypoglycemia who are conscious and able to swallow should eat or drink orange juice, glucose, or any sugar-containing beverage or food except pure fructose (which does not cross the blood-brain barrier).

B. The Unconscious Patient: In general, oral feeding is contraindicated in stuporous or unconscious patients. If trained personnel are not available to administer intravenous glucose, the treatment of choice is for a family member or friend to administer 1 mg of glucagon intramuscularly (see above), which will usually restore the patient to consciousness within 15 minutes; the patient should then be given an oral form of sugar to ingest. If glucagon is not available, small amounts of honey, syrup, or glucose gel (Glutose) can be rubbed into the buccal mucosa. Rectal administration of syrup or honey (30 mL per 500 mL of warm water) has also been used effectively.

COMA

Coma is a *medical emergency* calling for immediate evaluation to determine its cause so that proper therapy can be started. There are several causes of coma that result directly from diabetes mellitus or its treatment. When evaluating a comatose diabetic patient, these must be considered *in addition* to the myriad causes included in the differential diagnosis of coma (cerebrovascular accidents, head trauma, intoxication with alcohol or other drugs, etc).

Etiologic Classification of Diabetic Coma

The causes of coma resulting directly from diabetes mellitus or its treatment include the following:

A. Hyperglycemic Coma: Hyperglycemic coma may be associated with either severe insulin deficiency (diabetic ketoacidosis) or with mild to moderate insulin deficiency (hyperglycemic, hyperosmolar, nonketotic coma).

B. Hypoglycemic Coma: This results from excessive doses of insulin or oral hypoglycemic agents (see above).

C. Lactic Acidosis: Lactic acidosis in diabetics is particularly apt to occur in association with severe tissue anoxia, sepsis, or cardiovascular collapse.

Emergency Management of Coma

The standard approach to *any comatose patient* is outlined below. Prompt action is required.

(1) Establish an airway.

(2) Establish intravenous access. About 30 mL of blood should be drawn and sent for complete blood count, serum electrolyte determinations, renal function and liver function tests, and blood glucose measurements.

(3) Administer 50 mL of 50% dextrose in water to *all comatose patients*. This will rapidly reverse hypoglycemic coma and will not significantly alter the ultimate course of the mildly hyperglycemic patient. Since hypoglycemic blood left on an enzyme-impregnated glucose oxidase strip for longer than 1 minute (which can occur in the hectic atmosphere of an emergency situation) will give falsely elevated values, it is probably best not to withhold administration of intravenous dextrose to undiagnosed comatose patients.

(4) Administer 1 ampule (0.4 mg) of naloxone intravenously and 100 mg of thiamine intravenously.

Diagnosis of Coma

After emergency measures have been instituted, a careful history (from family, friends, paramedics, etc), physical examination, and laboratory evaluation are required to resolve the differential diagnosis. Patients in deep coma from a hyperosmolar nonketotic state or from hypoglycemia are generally flaccid and have quiet breathing—in contrast to patients with acidosis, whose respirations are rapid and deep if the pH of arterial blood has dropped to 7.1 or below. When hypoglycemia is a cause of the coma, hypothermia is usually present and the state of hydration is usually normal. Although the clinical laboratory remains the final arbiter in confirming the diagnosis, a rapid *estimation* of blood glucose and ketones can be obtained by the use of enzyme-impregnated glucose oxidase

Table 19–16. Summary of some laboratory abnormalities in patients with coma directly attributable to diabetes or its treatment.

	Urine		Plasma			
	Glucose	Acetone	Glucose	Bicarbonate	Acetone	Osmolality
Hyperglycemic, hyperosmolar coma						
Diabetic ketoacidosis	++ to ++++	++++	High	Low	++++	+++
Hyperglycemic nonketotic coma	++ to ++++	0 or +*	High	Normal or slightly low†	0	++++
Hypoglycemia	0‡	0 or +	Low	Normal	0	Normal
Lactic acidosis	0 or +	0 or +	Normal, low, or high	Low	0 or +	Normal

*A small degree of ketonuria may be present if the patient is severely stressed or has not been eating because of illness.
†Patient may be acidotic if there is severe volume depletion with cardiovascular collapse or if sepsis is present.
‡Leftover urine in bladder might still contain sugar from earlier hyperglycemia.

strips and crushed Acetest tablets (see Laboratory Findings in Diabetes Mellitus, above). Table 19–16 is a summary of some laboratory abnormalities found in diabetic patients with coma attributable to diabetes or its treatment. The individual clinical syndromes are discussed in detail on the following pages.

1. DIABETIC KETOACIDOSIS

This acute complication of diabetes mellitus may be the first manifestation of previously undiagnosed diabetes, or it may be the result of failure of a known diabetic to take adequate exogenous insulin. In either case, precipitating factors, such as infection, should be searched for and treated appropriately. In juveniles with type I diabetes, particularly in the teen years, recurrent episodes of severe ketoacidosis often indicate the need for counseling to alter this behavior.

Pathogenesis

Acute insulin deficiency results in rapid mobilization of energy from stores in muscle and fat depots, leading to an increased flux of amino acids to the liver for conversion to glucose and of fatty acids for conversion to ketones (acetoacetate, β-hydroxybutyrate, and acetone). In addition to this increased availability of precursor, there is a direct effect of the low insulin:glucagon ratio on the liver that promotes increased production of ketones. In response to both the acute insulin deficiency and the metabolic stress of ketosis, the levels of insulin-antagonistic hormones (corticosteroids, catecholamines, glucagon, and GH) are consistently elevated. Furthermore, in the absence of insulin, peripheral utilization of glucose and ketones is reduced. The combination of increased production and decreased utilization leads to an accumulation of these substances in blood, with plasma glucose levels reaching 500 mg/dL or more and plasma ketones reaching levels of 8–15 mmol/L or more.

The hyperglycemia causes osmotic diuresis leading to depletion of intravascular volume. As this progresses, impaired renal blood flow reduces the kidney's ability to excrete glucose, and hyperosmolality is worsened. Severe hyperosmolality (> 330 mosm) correlates closely with central nervous system depression and coma.

In a similar manner, impaired renal excretion of hydrogen ions aggravates the metabolic acidosis that occurs as a result of the accumulation of the ketone acids, β-hydroxybutyrate and acetoacetate. The accumulation of ketones may cause vomiting, which exacerbates the intravascular volume depletion. In addition, prolonged acidosis can compromise cardiac output and reduce vascular tone. The result may be severe cardiovascular collapse with generation of lactic acid, which then adds to the already existent metabolic acidosis.

Clinical Findings

A. Symptoms and Signs: As opposed to the *acute* onset of hypoglycemic coma, the appearance of diabetic ketoacidosis is usually preceded by a day or more of polyuria and polydipsia associated with marked fatigue, nausea, and vomiting. Eventually, mental stupor ensues and can progress to frank coma. On physical examination, evidence of dehydration in a stuporous patient with rapid and deep respirations and the "fruity" breath odor of acetone would strongly suggest the diagnosis. Postural hypotension with tachycardia indicates profound dehydration and salt depletion.

B. Laboratory Findings: Four-plus glycosuria, strong ketonuria, hyperglycemia, ketonemia, low arterial blood pH, and low plasma bicarbonate are typical laboratory findings in diabetic ketoacidosis. Serum potassium is usually normal or slightly elevated (5–8 meq/L) despite total body potassium depletion, because of the shift of potassium from the intra- to extracellular spaces that occurs in systemic acidosis. The average total body potassium deficit resulting from osmotic diuresis, acidosis, and gastrointestinal losses is about 5–10 meq/kg body weight. Similarly, serum phosphate is elevated (6–7 mg/dL), but total body phosphate is generally depleted. Serum sodium may be slightly reduced (to about 125–130 meq/L) because of expansion of plasma volume by glucose. (For every 100 mg/dL of plasma glucose above normal, serum sodium decreases by 1.6 meq/L.) Blood urea nitrogen and serum creatinine are invariably elevated because of dehydration. In the presence of keto acids, values from multichannel chemical analysis of serum creatinine are falsely elevated and therefore quite unreliable. However, most laboratories can correct for these interfering chromogens by using a more specific method if asked to do so.

In about 90% of cases, serum amylase is elevated. However, this often represents salivary as well as pancreatic amylase and correlates poorly with symptoms of pancreatitis, such as pain and vomiting. Therefore, in patients with diabetic ketoacidosis, an elevated serum amylase does not justify a diagnosis of acute pancreatitis; serum lipase may be useful if the diagnosis of pancreatitis is being seriously considered.

C. Data Recording on a Flow Sheet: The need for frequent evaluation of the patient's status cannot be overemphasized. Patients with moderately severe diabetic ketoacidosis (pH < 7.2) are best managed in an intensive care unit. Essential baseline blood chemistries include glucose, ketones, electrolytes, arterial blood gases, blood urea nitrogen, and serum creatinine. Typically, the patient with moderately severe diabetic ketoacidosis will have a plasma glucose of 350–900 mg/dL, the presence of serum ketones at a dilution of 1:8 or greater, slight hyponatremia of 130 meq/L, hyperkalemia of 5–8 meq/L, hyperphosphatemia of 6–7 mg/dL, and an elevated blood urea nitrogen and creatinine. Acidosis may be severe (pH ranging from 6.9 to 7.2 and bicarbonate ranging from 5 to 10 meq/L); P_{CO_2} is low (15–20 mm Hg) from hyperventilation.

A comprehensive flow sheet that includes vital signs, serial laboratory data, and therapeutic interventions should be meticulously maintained by the physician responsible for the patient's care. Plasma glucose should be recorded hourly and electrolytes and pH at least every 2–3 hours during the initial treatment period. Insulin therapy is greatly facilitated when plasma glucose results are available within a few minutes of sampling. This can be achieved by the use of such instruments as the Beckman or Yellow Springs glucose analyzers. Recently developed instruments designed for bedside glucose measurements such as the Glucometer (Ames), Glucoscan (Lifescan), or Accu Chek bG (Bio-Dynamics/BMC) are also sufficiently accurate for use in this situation. Fluid intake and output as well as details of insulin therapy and the administration of other medications should also be carefully recorded on the flow sheet.

Treatment

A. Immediate Resuscitation and Emergency Measures: If the patient is stuporous or comatose, immediately institute the emergency measures outlined in the section on coma (see above). Once the diagnosis of diabetic ketoacidosis is established, a rapid intravenous bolus of 0.3 unit of regular insulin per kilogram of body weight should be given. This will inhibit both gluconeogenesis and ketogenesis while promoting utilization of glucose and ketoacids. Administration of at least 1 L of normal saline (in an adult patient) in the first 1–2 hours is recommended initially to help restore plasma volume and stabilize blood pressure while acutely reducing the hyperos-

molar state. In addition, by improving renal plasma flow, fluid replacement also restores the renal capacity to excrete hydrogen ions, thereby meliorating the acidosis as well. If arterial blood pH is less than 7.1, intravenous bicarbonate should be administered (details of administration are outlined below). Gastric intubation is recommended in the comatose patient to prevent vomiting and aspiration that may occur as a result of gastric atony, a common complication of diabetic ketoacidosis. An indwelling bladder catheter is required in all comatose patients but should be avoided, if possible, in a fully cooperative diabetic patient because of the risk of bladder infection. In patients with preexisting cardiac or renal failure or those in severe cardiovascular collapse, a central venous pressure catheter or a Swan-Ganz catheter should be inserted to evaluate the degree of hypovolemia and to monitor subsequent fluid administration.

B. Specific Measures: Each case must be managed individually depending on the specific abnormalities present and subsequent response to initial therapy.

1. Insulin–Only regular insulin should be used in the management of diabetic ketoacidosis. As noted above, a "loading" dose of 0.3 unit/kg body weight of regular insulin is given initially as an intravenous bolus. This should be followed by 0.15 unit/kg/h, administered either as a continuous infusion or as intramuscular injections. If continuous infusion of insulin is used, the tubing should first be flushed with insulin-containing fluid. If the plasma glucose level fails to fall by at least 10% in the first hour, a repeat bolus of 0.3 unit/kg of regular insulin should be given. Rarely, a patient with insulin resistance is encountered; this requires doubling the insulin dose every 2–4 hours if hyperglycemia does not improve after the first 2 doses of insulin.

Insulin therapy, either as a continuous infusion or as injections given every 1–2 hours, should be continued until arterial pH has normalized.

2. Fluid replacement–In most adult patients, the fluid deficit is 5–10 L. Initially, normal saline is preferred for restoration of plasma volume and, as noted above, should be infused rapidly to provide 1 L/h over the first 1–2 hours. After the first 2 L of fluid have been given, the fluid should be changed to 0.45% saline solution given at a rate of 300–400 mL/h; this is because water loss exceeds sodium loss in uncontrolled diabetes with osmotic diuresis. When blood glucose falls to approximately 250 mg/dL, the fluids should be changed to a 5% glucose solution to maintain plasma glucose in the range of 250–300 mg/dL. This will prevent the development of hypoglycemia and reduce the likelihood of cerebral edema, which could result from too rapid decline of blood glucose. Intensive insulin therapy should be continued until metabolic acidosis is corrected.

3. Sodium bicarbonate–The use of sodium bicarbonate in management of diabetic ketoacidosis has been questioned by some because of the following potential consequences: (1) development of hypokalemia from rapid shift of potassium into cells; (2) tissue anoxia from reduced dissociation of oxygen from hemoglobin when acidosis is rapidly reversed (leftward shift of the oxygen dissociation curve); and (3) cerebral acidosis resulting from lowering of cerebrospinal fluid pH. It must be emphasized, however, that these considerations are less important when severe acidosis exists. It is therefore recommended that bicarbonate be administered to diabetic patients in ketoacidosis if the arterial blood pH is less than 7.1 or if hypotension, arrhythmia, or coma is present along with an arterial blood pH of less than 7.1.

One to 2 ampules of sodium bicarbonate (one ampule contains 44 meq/50 mL) should be added to 1 L of 0.45% saline. (*Note:* Addition of sodium bicarbonate to 0.9% saline would produce a markedly hypertonic solution that could aggravate the hyperosmolar state already present.) This should be administered rapidly (over the first hour). It can be repeated until the arterial pH reaches 7.1 but should not be given if pH is greater than 7.1. As noted earlier, serious consideration should be given to placement of a central venous or Swan-Ganz catheter when administering fluids to severely ill patients with cardiovascular compromise.

4. Potassium–Total body potassium loss from polyuria and vomiting may be as high as 200–300 meq. However, because of shifts of potassium from cells into the extracellular space as a consequence of acidosis, serum potassium is usually normal to slightly elevated prior to institution of treatment. As the acidosis is corrected, potassium flows back into the cells, and hypokalemia can develop if potassium replacement is not instituted. If the patient is not uremic and has an adequate urine output, potassium chloride in doses of 10–30 meq/h should be infused during the second and third hours after beginning therapy as soon as the acidosis starts to resolve. Replacement should be started sooner if the initial serum potassium is inappropriately normal or low. Cooperative patients with only mild ketoacidosis may receive part or all of their potassium replacement orally.

An ECG can be of help in monitoring the patient's potassium status: high peaked T waves are a sign of hyperkalemia, and flattened T waves with U waves are a sign of hypokalemia.

5. Phosphate–Because severe hypophosphatemia also develops during insulin therapy of diabetic ketoacidosis, some of the potassium can be replaced as the phosphate salt. Correction of hypophosphatemia helps to restore the buffering capacity of the plasma, thereby facilitating renal excretion of hydrogen. It also corrects the impaired oxygen dissociation from hemoglobin by regenerating 2,3-diphosphoglycerate. However, a recent randomized study in which phosphate was replaced in only half of a group of 18 patients with diabetic ketoacidosis did not show any apparent clinical benefit from phosphate administration. Moreover, attempts to use the phosphate salt of potassium as the sole means of replacing potassium have led to a number of reported cases of severe hypocalcemia

with tetany. To minimize the risk of inducing tetany from too rapid replacement of phosphate, the average deficit of 40–50 mmol of phosphate should be replaced intravenously at a rate *no greater than 3–4 mmol/h* in a 60- to 70-kg person. A stock solution (Abbott) provides a mixture of 1.12 g KH_2PO_4 and 1.18 g K_2HPO_4 in a 5-mL single-dose vial (this equals 22 mmol of potassium and 15 mmol of phosphate). One-half of this vial (2.5 mL) should be added to 1 L of either 0.45% saline or 5% dextrose in water. Two liters of this solution, infused at a rate of 400 mL/h, will correct the phosphate deficit at the optimal rate of 3 mmol/h while providing 4.4 meq of potassium per hour. (Additional potassium should be administered as potassium chloride to provide a total of 10–30 meq of potassium per hour, as noted above.) If the serum phosphate remains below 2.5 mg/dL after this infusion, a repeat 5-hour infusion can be given.

It remains controversial whether phosphate replacement is beneficial. Several clinics prohibit its use in the routine treatment of diabetic ketoacidosis, since the risk of inducing hypocalcemia is thought to outweigh its potential benefits. However, potential hazards of phosphate replacement can be greatly reduced by administering phosphate at a rate no greater than 3–4 mmol/h. To prevent errors of overreplacement, phosphate should be administered separately rather than included as a component of potassium replacement.

Prognosis

Insulin and fluid and electrolyte replacement combined with careful monitoring of patients' clinical and laboratory responses to therapy have dramatically reduced the morbidity and mortality rates of diabetic ketoacidosis. However, this complication still represents a potential threat to survival, especially in older people with cardiovascular disease. Even in specialized centers, the mortality rate may approach 5–10%. Therefore, physicians treating diabetic ketoacidosis must not be lured into adopting "cookbook" approaches that lessen their attentiveness to changes in the patient's condition. Signs to be watched for include failure of improvement in mental status after a period of treatment, continued hypotension with minimal urine flow, or prolonged ileus (which may suggest bowel infarction). Laboratory abnormalities to be watched include failure of blood glucose to fall by 80–100 mg/dL during the initial therapeutic period, failure to increase serum bicarbonate or arterial pH appropriately, serum potassium above 6 or below 2.8 meq/L, and electrocardiographic evidence of cardiac arrhythmias. Any of these signs call for a careful search for the cause of the abnormality and prompt specific therapy.

Disposition

After recovery and stabilization, the patient should receive intensive detailed instructions about how to avoid this potentially disastrous complication of diabetes mellitus.

2. HYPERGLYCEMIC, HYPEROSMOLAR, NONKETOTIC STATE

This form of hyperglycemic coma is characterized by severe hyperglycemia, hyperosmolality, and dehydration in the absence of significant ketosis. It occurs in patients with mild or occult diabetes, who are usually middle-aged to elderly. Underlying renal insufficiency or congestive heart failure is common, and the presence of either worsens the prognosis. A precipitating event such as pneumonia, cerebrovascular accident, myocardial infarction, burns, or recent operation can often be identified. Certain drugs, such as phenytoin, diazoxide, glucocorticoids, and thiazide diuretics, may also be related to its development.

Pathogenesis

A partial or relative insulin deficiency may initiate the syndrome by reducing glucose utilization by muscle, fat, and the liver while at the same time inducing hyperglucagonemia and increasing hepatic glucose output. The result is hyperglycemia that leads to glycosuria and osmotic diuresis with obligatory water loss. The presence of even small amounts of insulin is believed to prevent the development of ketosis by inhibiting lipolysis in the adipose stores. Therefore even though a low insulin:glucagon ratio promotes ketogenesis in the liver, the limited availability of precursor free fatty acids from the periphery restricts the rate at which ketones are formed. If a patient is unable to maintain adequate fluid intake because of an associated acute or chronic illness or has suffered excessive fluid loss (eg, from burns or therapy with diuretics), marked dehydration results. As plasma volume contracts, renal insufficiency develops; this, then, limits renal glucose excretion and contributes markedly to the rise in serum glucose and osmolality. Hyperosmolality causes mental confusion, and when the serum osmolality reaches approximately 330 mosm/L, coma may ensue.

Clinical Findings

A. Symptoms and Signs: The onset of the hyperglycemic, hyperosmolar, nonketotic state may be insidious, preceded for days or weeks by symptoms of weakness, polyuria, and polydipsia. A history of reduced fluid intake is common, whether due to inappropriate absence of thirst, gastrointestinal upset, or, in the case of elderly or bedridden patients, lack of access to water. A history of ingestion of large quantities of glucose-containing fluids, such as soft drinks or orange juice, can occasionally be obtained; these patients are usually less hyperosmolar than those in whom fluid intake was restricted. The absence of toxic features of ketoacidosis may retard recognition of the syndrome and thus delay institution of therapy until dehydration is profound. Because of this delay in diagnosis, the hyperglycemia, hyperosmolality, and dehydration in hyperglycemic, hyperosmolar, nonketotic coma is often more severe than in diabetic ketoacidosis.

Physical examination will reveal the presence of profound dehydration (orthostatic fall in blood pressure and rise in pulse, supine tachycardia or even frank shock, dry mucous membranes, decreased skin turgor). The patient may be lethargic, confused, or comatose. Kussmaul respirations are absent unless the precipitating event for the hyperosmolar state has also led to the development of metabolic acidosis (eg, sepsis or myocardial infarction with shock).

B. Laboratory Findings: Severe hyperglycemia is present, with blood glucose values ranging from 800 to as high as 2400 mg/dL. In mild cases, where dehydration is less severe, dilutional hyponatremia as well as urinary sodium losses may reduce serum sodium to about 120–125 meq/L*—this protects, to some extent, against extreme hyperosmolality. Once dehydration progresses further, however, serum sodium can exceed 140 meq/L, producing serum osmolalities of 330–440 mosm/L† (normal, 280–295 mosm/L). Ketosis is usually absent or mild; however, a small degree of ketonuria may be present if the patient has not been eating because of illness. Acidosis is not a part of the hyperglycemic, hyperosmolar state, but it may be present (usually lactic acidosis) because of other acute underlying conditions (sepsis, acute renal failure, myocardial infarction, etc). (See Lactic Acidosis, below.)

Treatment

There are some differences in fluid, insulin, and electrolyte replacement in this disorder, as compared to diabetic ketoacidosis. However, in common with the treatment of ketoacidotic patients, careful monitoring of the patient's clinical and laboratory response to therapy is essential.

A. Fluid Replacement: Fluid replacement is of paramount importance in treating nonketotic hyperglycemic coma. If circulatory collapse is present, fluid therapy should be initiated with isotonic saline. In all other cases, initial replacement with hypotonic (usually 0.45%) saline is preferable, because these patients are hyperosmolar with excess solute in the vascular compartment. As much as 4–6 L of fluid may be required in the first 8–10 hours. Careful monitoring of fluid quantity and type, urine output, blood pressure, and pulse is essential. Placement of a central venous pressure or Swan-Ganz catheter should be strongly considered to guide replacement of fluid, especially if the patient is elderly or has underlying renal or cardiac disease. Because insulin therapy will decrease plasma glucose and therefore serum osmolality, a change to isotonic saline may be necessary at some time during treatment in order to maintain an

---

*See p 561 for formula used in correcting hyponatremia due to hyperglycemia.

†A convenient method for estimating serum osmolality is as follows:

$$\text{Serum osmolality} \atop (\text{mosm/L}) = 2 \ (Na^+) \ (\text{mmol/L}) + \frac{\text{Glucose (mg/dL)}}{18} + \frac{\text{BUN (mg/dL)}}{2.8}$$

adequate blood pressure and urine output. Once blood glucose reaches 250 mg/dL, 5% dextrose in 0.45% or 0.9% saline solution should be substituted for the sugar-free fluids. When consciousness returns, oral fluids should be encouraged.

B. Electrolyte Replacement: Hyperkalemia is less marked and much less potassium is lost in the urine during the osmotic diuresis of hyperglycemic, hyperosmolar, nonketotic coma than in diabetic ketoacidosis. There is, therefore, less severe total potassium depletion, and less potassium replacement is needed to restore potassium stores to normal. However, because the initial serum potassium usually is not elevated and because it declines rapidly as insulin therapy allows glucose and potassium to enter cells, it is recommended that potassium replacement be initiated earlier than in ketotic patients: 10 meq/L of potassium chloride can be added to the *initial* bottle of fluid administered if the initial serum potassium is not elevated and if the patient is making urine. When hypophosphatemia develops during insulin therapy, phosphate replacement can be given intravenously with the same precautions as those outlined for ketoacidotic patients (see above). If the patient is awake and cooperative, part or all of the potassium and phosphate replacement can be given orally.

C. Insulin Therapy: In general, less insulin is required to reduce the hyperglycemia of nonketotic patients than is the case for patients in diabetic ketoacidosis. In fact, fluid replacement alone can decrease glucose levels considerably. An initial dose of 15 units of regular insulin given intravenously and 15 units given intramuscularly is usually quite effective in lowering blood glucose. In most cases, subsequent doses need not be greater than 10–25 units every 4 hours. (Insulin should be given intramuscularly or intravenously until the patient has stabilized; it may then be given subcutaneously.) Some patients—especially those who are severely ill because of other underlying diseases—may require continuous intravenous administration of insulin (in a manner similar to that described for ketoacidosis) with careful monitoring, preferably in an intensive care setting.

D. Search for the Precipitating Event: The physician must initiate a careful search for the event that precipitated the episode of hyperglycemic, hyperosmolar, nonketotic coma if it is not obvious after the initial history and physical examination. Chest x-rays and cultures of blood, urine, and other body fluids should be obtained to look for occult sources of sepsis; empiric antibiotic coverage should be considered in the seriously ill patient. Cardiac enzymes and serial ECGs can be ordered to look for evidence of "silent" myocardial infarction.

Prognosis

The overall mortality rate of hyperglycemic, hyperosmolar, nonketotic coma is over 10 times that of diabetic ketoacidosis, chiefly because of its higher incidence in older patients, who may have compromised cardiovascular systems or associated major ill-

nesses. (When patients are matched for age, the prognoses of these 2 forms of hyperosmolar coma are reasonably comparable.)

Disposition

After the patient is stabilized, the appropriate form of long-term management of the diabetes must be determined. This must include patient education on how to recognize situations (gastrointestinal upset, infection) that will predispose to recurrence of hyperglycemic, hyperosmolar, nonketotic coma as well as detailed information on how to prevent the escalating dehydration (small sips of sugar-free liquids, increase in usual hypoglycemic therapy, or early contact with the physician) that culminates in hyperosmolar coma. For a detailed discussion of therapeutic alternatives for type II diabetic patients, see Steps in the Management of the Diabetic Patient (above).

3. HYPOGLYCEMIC COMA

Hypoglycemia is a common complication of insulin replacement therapy in diabetic patients. In most cases, it is detected and treated by patients or their families before coma results. However, it remains the most frequent cause of coma in the insulin-treated diabetic patient. In addition, it can occur in any patient taking oral sulfonylurea drugs, particularly if the patient is elderly, has renal or liver disease, or is taking certain other medications that alter metabolism of the sulfonylureas (eg, phenylbutazone, sulfonamides, or coumarin derivatives). It occurs more frequently with the use of long-acting sulfonylureas than when shorter-acting agents are used.

Clinical Findings & Treatment

The clinical findings and emergency treatment of hypoglycemia are discussed above.

Prognosis

Many patients who arrive at emergency rooms in hypoglycemic coma appear to recover fully; however, profound hypoglycemia or delays in therapy can result in permanent neurologic deficit or even death. Furthermore, repeated episodes of hypoglycemia may have a cumulative adverse effect on intellectual functioning.

Disposition

The physician should carefully review with the patient the events leading up to the hypoglycemic episode. Associated use of other medications, as well as alcohol or narcotics, should be noted. Careful attention should be paid to diet, exercise pattern, insulin or sulfonylurea dosage, and general compliance with the prescribed diabetes treatment regimen. Any factors thought to have contributed to the development of the episode should be identified and recommendations made in order to prevent recurrences of this potentially disastrous complication of diabetes therapy.

If the patient is hypoglycemic from use of a long-acting oral hypoglycemic agent (eg, chlorpropamide) or a long-acting insulin, admission to hospital for treatment with continuous intravenous glucose and careful monitoring of blood glucose is indicated.

4. LACTIC ACIDOSIS

When severely ill diabetic patients present with profound acidosis but relatively low or undetectable levels of ketoacids in plasma, the presence of excessive plasma lactate (> 6 mmol/L) should be considered, especially if other causes of acidosis such as uremia are not present.

Pathogenesis

Lactic acid is the end product of anaerobic metabolism of glucose. Normally, the principal sources of this acid are the erythrocytes (which lack the enzymes for aerobic oxidation), skeletal muscle, skin, and brain. The chief pathway for removal of lactic acid is by hepatic (and to some degree renal) uptake for conversion first to pyruvate and eventually back to glucose, a process that requires oxygen. Lactic acidosis occurs when excess lactic acid accumulates in the blood. This can be the result of overproduction (tissue hypoxia), deficient removal (hepatic failure), or both (circulatory collapse). Patients with lactic acidosis are usually severely ill, with problems such as myocardial infarction with shock, sepsis, hemorrhage, severe anemia, carbon monoxide poisoning, severe pulmonary disease, severe liver disease, or cyanide poisoning. Phenformin, an oral hypoglycemic agent no longer available in the USA, has been reported to cause lactic acidosis, especially in patients with altered lactate or phenformin metabolism. In addition, lactic acidosis has been reported after the use of salicylates, sodium nitroprusside, intravenous fructose, sorbitol, ethanol, and other substances.

Clinical Findings

A. Symptoms and Signs: The main clinical features of lactic acidosis are marked hyperventilation and mental confusion, which may progress to stupor or coma. When lactic acidosis is secondary to tissue hypoxia or vascular collapse, the clinical presentation is variable, being that of the prevailing catastrophic illness. In the rare instance of idiopathic or spontaneous lactic acidosis, the onset is rapid (usually over a few hours), the cardiopulmonary status is stable, and mentation may be relatively normal.

B. Laboratory Findings: Plasma glucose can be low, normal, or high in diabetic patients with lactic acidosis, but usually it is moderately elevated. Plasma bicarbonate and arterial pH are quite low. An anion gap will be present (calculated by subtracting the sum of the plasma bicarbonate and chloride from the plasma sodium; normal is $12-16$). Ketones are usually absent from plasma, but small amounts may be present in urine if the patient has not been eating recently. Other causes of "anion gap" metabolic acidosis should be excluded—eg, uremia, diabetic or alcoholic ketoacidosis, and salicylate, methanol, ethylene glycol, or paraldehyde intoxication. In the absence of azotemia, hyperphosphatemia may be a clue to the presence of lactic acidosis.

The diagnosis is confirmed by demonstrating, in a sample of blood that is promptly chilled and separated, a plasma lactate concentration of 6 mmol/L or higher (normal is about 1 mmol/L). Failure to rapidly chill the sample and separate the plasma can lead to falsely high plasma lactate values as a result of continued glycolysis by the red blood cells. Frozen plasma remains stable for subsequent assay.

Treatment

The cornerstone of therapy is aggressive treatment of the precipitating cause. An adequate airway and good oxygenation should be ensured. If hypotension is present, fluids and, if appropriate, pressor agents must be given to restore tissue perfusion. Appropriate cultures and empiric antibiotic coverage should be instituted in any seriously ill patient with lactic acidosis in whom the cause is not immediately apparent. If the arterial pH is less than 7.1 (or 7.2 in the presence of circulatory collapse), intravenous bicarbonate should be administered. One or 2 ampules of sodium bicarbonate (44 meq of bicarbonate per ampule) can be added to 1 L of 0.45% saline and administered rapidly over 1 hour. Bolus injections of bicarbonate should be reserved for patients requiring cardiopulmonary resuscitation. Intravenous bicarbonate should be continued until the pH reaches 7.2. Therapy should be monitored with frequent arterial blood gases to prevent inadvertent development of metabolic alkalosis. Occasionally, it is necessary to treat a patient with severe refractory lactic acidosis with hemodialysis, especially if congestive heart failure or hypernatremia interferes with further bicarbonate therapy. Dialysis is also useful for phenformin-induced lactic acidosis, since phenformin is dialyzable. Dichloroacetate, an anion that facilitates pyruvate removal by activating pyruvate dehydrogenase, reverses certain types of lactic acidosis in animals and may prove useful in some cases of lactic acidosis in humans. Methylene blue, a redox dye, has not been as useful as early reports gave reason to hope.

CHRONIC COMPLICATIONS OF DIABETES MELLITUS
(Table 19–17)

In most patients with diabetes, a number of pathologic changes occur at variable intervals during the course of the disease. Although they are termed com-

Table 19–17. Chronic complications of diabetes mellitus.

Eyes
Diabetic retinopathy
Nonproliferative (background)
Proliferative
Cataracts
Subcapsular (snowflake)
Nuclear (senile)

Kidneys
Intracapillary glomerulosclerosis
Diffuse
Nodular
Infection
Pyelonephritis
Perinephric abscess
Renal papillary necrosis
Renal tubular necrosis
Following dye studies (urograms, arteriograms)

Nervous system
Peripheral neuropathy
Distal, symmetric sensory loss
Motor neuropathy
Foot drop, wrist drop
Mononeuropathy multiplex (diabetic amyotrophy)
Cranial neuropathy
Cranial nerves III, IV, VI, VII
Autonomic neuropathy
Postural hypotension
Resting tachycardia
Loss of sweating
Gastrointestinal neuropathy
Gastroparesis.
Diabetic diarrhea
Urinary bladder atony
Impotence (may also be secondary to pelvic vascular disease)

Skin
Diabetic dermopathy (shin spots)
Necrobiosis lipoidica diabeticorum
Candidiasis
Foot and leg ulcers
Neurotropic
Ischemic

Cardiovascular system
Heart disease
Myocardial infarction
Cardiomyopathy
Gangrene of the feet
Ischemic ulcers
Osteomyelitis

Bones and joints
Diabetic cheirarthropathy
Dupuytren's contracture
Charcot's joint

Unusual infections
Necrotizing fasciitis
Necrotizing myositis
Mucor meningitis
Emphysematous cholecystitis
Malignant otitis externa

plications, this is really a misnomer, because these changes are really parts of the diabetic state, ie, its late clinical manifestations. These changes involve the vascular system for the most part; however, they also occur in the nerves, the skin, and the lens. Abnormalities in lipoprotein metabolism are also common.

Classifications of Diabetic Vascular Disease

Diabetic vascular disease is conveniently divided into 2 main categories: microvascular disease and macrovascular disease.

A. Microvascular Disease: Disease of the smallest blood vessels, the capillary and the precapillary arterioles, is manifested mainly by thickening of the capillary basement membrane. Microvascular disease involving the retina leads to diabetic retinopathy, and disease involving the kidney causes diabetic nephropathy. Small vessel disease may also involve the heart; recently, cardiomegaly with heart failure has been described in diabetic patients with patent coronary arteries.

B. Macrovascular Disease: Large vessel disease in diabetes is essentially an accelerated form of atherosclerosis. It accounts for the increased incidence of myocardial infarction, stroke, and peripheral gangrene in diabetic patients. Just as in the case of atherosclerosis in the general population, the exact cause of accelerated atherosclerosis in the diabetic population remains unclear. Abnormalities in vessel walls, platelets and other components of the clotting system, red blood cells, and lipid metabolism have all been postulated to play a role. In addition, there is evidence that coexistent risk factors such as cigarette smoking and hypertension may be important in determining the course of the disease.

In addition to the above complications, diabetic patients have an increased incidence of certain types of infections and may handle their infections less well than the general population.

Prevalence of Chronic Complications by Type of Diabetes

Although all of the known chronic complications of diabetes can be found in both types of the disease, some are more common in one type than in the other. Renal failure due to severe microvascular nephropathy is the major cause of death in patients with type I diabetes, whereas macrovascular disease is the leading cause in type II. Although blindness occurs in both types, it occurs more commonly as a result of severe proliferative retinopathy, vitreous hemorrhages, and retinal detachment in type I disease, whereas macular edema and ischemia or cataracts are the usual cause in type II. Similarly, although diabetic neuropathy is common in both type I and type II diabetes, severe autonomic neuropathy with gastroparesis, diabetic diarrhea, resting tachycardia, and postural hypotension is much more common in type I.

Relationship of Glycemic Control to Development of Chronic Complications

There is still uncertainty about whether strict blood glucose control significantly alters the incidence of diabetic complications. There are 2 main reasons for this uncertainty: (1) past inability to safely achieve glycemic control that approaches normality and (2) present inability to accurately assess the degree of glycemic control being achieved. The use of improved delivery systems and highly purified insulins has now made "tight" glycemic control a possibility. Combined with newer methods for evaluating control, such as glycohemoglobin and self-monitoring of blood glucose, these developments may soon allow resolution of this important issue.

A prospective randomized trial involving 21 clinical centers (the Diabetes Control and Complications Trial) has recently been initiated by the National Institutes of Health to determine if tight glycemic control over a period of 7–10 years can prevent or delay the development of diabetic retinopathy or nephropathy in patients with IDDM.

In addition to this "prevention" trial, 2 short-term "intervention" trials in 95 IDDM patients with established nonproliferative retinopathy have been initiated. Preliminary results of these intervention trials show that tight control of glycemia was achieved by patients using insulin pumps for 1 year, while only fair control was achieved by patients receiving conventional treatment. Both the Steno Study Group (in Denmark) and the Kroc Collaborative Study Group (in the USA) agreed that intensified metabolic control does not retard the progression of mild nonproliferative retinopathy. Of concern was the observation in both studies that tight glycemic control appeared to even accelerate the progression of retinopathy. Although retinal deterioration was only transient in some patients and in no case was visual acuity reduced by the accelerated progression of retinopathy, these results suggest that caution should be exercised in restoring euglycemia rapidly in patients with established retinopathy.

The Kroc Collaborative Study Group reported that in patients with established diabetic nephropathy, tight glycemic control did not retard the progression of renal disease, even though in earlier stages of renal involvement microalbuminuria was reduced considerably by near-normalization of blood glucose levels. This evidence of functional (but not structural) improvement was also noted by the Steno Study Group, which reported that patients with tight glycemic control showed reduced retinal leakage of fluorescein despite the fact that their diabetic retinopathy continued to worsen.

An encouraging finding in regard to therapeutic intervention, as reported by Raskin et al, is that the thickness of the quadriceps capillary basement membrane was significantly reduced in IDDM patients whose glycemia was tightly controlled by intensive insulin therapy, whereas no significant change in thickness was seen in conventionally treated IDDM patients with only fair control of glycemia.

SPECIFIC CHRONIC COMPLICATIONS OF DIABETES MELLITUS (Table 19–17)

1. OPHTHALMOLOGIC COMPLICATIONS

Diabetic Retinopathy

For early detection of diabetic retinopathy, patients who have had type I diabetes for more than 5 years and *all* non–insulin dependent diabetic patients should be referred to an ophthalmologist for examination and follow-up. When hypertension is present in a patient with diabetes, it should be treated vigorously, since hypertension is associated with an increased incidence and accelerated progression of diabetic retinopathy.

A. Pathogenesis and Clinical Findings: Two main categories of diabetic retinopathy exist: nonproliferative and proliferative.

Nonproliferative ("background") retinopathy represents the earliest stage of retinal involvement by diabetes and is characterized by such changes as microaneurysms, dot hemorrhages, exudates, and retinal edema. During this stage, the retinal capillaries leak proteins, lipids, or red cells into the retina. When this process occurs in the macula, the area of greatest concentration of visual cells, there will be interference with visual acuity; this is the most common cause of visual impairment in type II diabetes.

Proliferative retinopathy involves the growth of new capillaries and fibrous tissue within the retina and into the vitreous chamber. It is a consequence of small vessel occlusion, which causes retinal hypoxia; this in turn stimulates new vessel growth. Proliferative retinopathy can occur in both types of diabetes but is more common in type I, developing about 7–10 years after onset of symptoms. Vision is usually normal until vitreous hemorrhage or retinal detachment occurs.

B. Treatment: Once maculopathy or proliferative changes are detected, panretinal xenon or argon laser photocoagulation therapy is indicated. Destroying retinal tissue with photocoagulation means that surviving tissue receives a greater share of the available oxygen supply, thereby abolishing hypoxic stimulation of new vessel growth. Results of a large-scale clinical trial (the Diabetic Retinopathy Study) have verified the effectiveness of photocoagulation, particularly when recent vitreous hemorrhages have occurred or when extensive new vessels are located near the optic disk.

The best results with photocoagulation are achieved if proliferative retinopathy is detected early. This is best done by obtaining a baseline fluorescein angiogram within 5–10 years after onset of type I diabetes and then repeating this study at intervals of 1–5 years, depending on the severity of the retinal involvement found.

Pituitary ablation, which has been associated with delay in progression of severe retinopathy in the past, is rarely used today because photocoagulation therapy is just as effective and avoids the risks associated with destruction of the pituitary. Occasional cases of rapidly progressive ("florid") proliferative retinopathy in type I adolescent diabetics have been reported in which photocoagulation was less effective than pituitary ablation in preventing blindness. While further studies are needed to confirm this observation, transsphenoidal hypophysectomy remains a choice of therapy for the adolescent with severe progressive retinopathy.

Cataracts

Two types of cataracts occur in diabetic patients: subcapsular and senile. **Subcapsular cataract** occurs predominantly in type I diabetics, may come on fairly rapidly, and has a significant correlation with the hyperglycemia of uncontrolled diabetes. This type of cataract has a flocculent or "snowflake" appearance and develops just below the lens capsule.

Senile cataract represents a sclerotic change of the lens nucleus. It is by far the most common type of cataract found in either diabetic or nondiabetic adults and tends to occur at a younger age in diabetic patients.

Two separate abnormalities found in diabetic patients, both of which are related to elevated blood glucose levels, may contribute to the formation of cataracts: (1) glycosylation of the lens protein and (2) an excess of sorbitol, which is formed from the increased quantities of glucose found in the insulin-independent lens. Accumulation of sorbitol leads to osmotic changes in the lens that ultimately result in fibrosis and cataract formation.

2. RENAL COMPLICATIONS

Diabetic Nephropathy

A. Pathogenesis and Clinical Findings: Diabetic nephropathy is a disease of the microvasculature of the kidney. It is characterized by thickening of the basement membrane of the capillaries of the glomeruli and mesangial deposits of glycoproteins (classic Kimmelstiel-Wilson lesions). Clinically, diabetic renal disease is heralded by the onset of proteinuria, which can sometimes progress to a full-blown nephrotic syndrome, with hypoalbuminemia, hypertension, edema, and an increase in circulating beta-lipoproteins. This is followed by the development of progressive renal failure, usually within 5 years after onset of proteinuria.

About 4000 cases of end-stage renal disease occur annually among diabetic patients in the USA. Retrospective studies of the evolution of end-stage renal failure suggest that microalbuminuria (albumin overnight excretion rate of > 30 μg/min) is associated with a markedly increased risk of subsequently developing clinical diabetic nephropathy. Unlike all other renal disorders, the proteinuria of diabetic nephropathy does not diminish as renal failure progresses. It is important to remember that there is an elevation in the tubular maximum of glucose reabsorption (and, therefore, of the threshold at which glycosuria appears) with advancing renal failure.

B. Treatment: Hemodialysis has been of limited success in the treatment of renal failure due to diabetic nephropathy, primarily because of progression of large-vessel disease with resultant death and disability from stroke and myocardial infarction. Growing experience with chronic ambulatory peritoneal dialysis suggests that it may be a more convenient method of providing adequate dialysis with a lower incidence of complications.

Renal transplantation, especially from related donors, is often successful. For certain patients with compatible donors and no contraindications (such as severe cardiovascular disease), it is the treatment of choice.

Necrotizing Papillitis

This unusual complication of pyelonephritis occurs primarily in diabetic patients. It is characterized by fever, flank pain, pyuria, and sloughing of renal papillae in the urine. It is treated by intravenous administration of appropriate antibiotics.

Renal Decompensation After Radiographic Dyes

The use of radiographic contrast dyes in diabetic patients with reduced creatinine clearance has been associated with the development of acute renal failure. If a contrast study is considered essential, the patient should be adequately hydrated before the procedure, and other nephrotoxic agents should be avoided. After the procedure, serum creatinine should be followed closely. These agents should not be used in a patient with a serum creatinine greater than 3 mg/dL.

3. NEUROLOGIC COMPLICATIONS (Diabetic Neuropathy)

Peripheral and autonomic neuropathies are frequent complications of both types of diabetes. Their pathogenesis is poorly understood. Some lesions, such as the acute cranial nerve palsies, have been attributed to ischemic infarction of the involved peripheral nerve. The much more common symmetric sensory and motor peripheral neuropathies and autonomic neuropathy are felt to be due to metabolic or osmotic toxicity somehow related to hyperglycemia.

Unfortunately, there is no consistently effective treatment for any of the neuropathies. It remains to be demonstrated definitively whether normalization of blood glucose levels can prevent development and progression of this devastating complication.

Sensory Neuropathy

A. Pathogenesis and Clinical Findings: Sensory loss is commonly preceded by months or years of paresthesias such as tingling, itching, and increasing pain. The pains can vary from mild paresthesias to severe shooting pains and may be more severe at night. Radicular pains in the chest and the abdominal area can at times be extremely difficult to distinguish from pain due to an intrathoracic or intra-abdominal source. Eventually, patients develop numbness, and tactile sensations decrease. The sensory loss is symmetric and can involve both the hands and the feet. Because all of these sensory disturbances are made worse by pressure applied to the involved nerves, symptoms may appear first in nerves that are entrapped, such as the median nerve in carpal tunnel syndrome or the nerves around the ankle.

Characteristic syndromes that develop in diabetic patients with sensory neuropathy and are related to their failure to perceive trauma include osteopathy of the distal hand and foot, deformity of the knee or ankle (so-called Charcot joint), and neuropathic ulceration of the foot.

B. Treatment: A combination of fluphenazine (1 mg 3 times daily) and amitriptyline (75 mg at bedtime) has occasionally produced remarkable improvement in the lower extremity pain in some patients with sensory neuropathy. A short therapeutic trial with this recently described regimen can therefore be recommended for patients with painful diabetic neuropathy.

It is essential that diabetic patients with peripheral neuropathy receive detailed instructions in foot care (see p 554).

Motor Neuropathy

Symmetric motor neuropathy occurs much less frequently than sensory neuropathy. Its pathogenesis is presumed to be similar to that of sensory loss. Mononeuropathy develops when there is vascular occlusion of a specific nerve trunk; if more than one nerve trunk is involved, the syndrome of **mononeuritis multiplex** occurs. Motor neuropathy is manifested by an abrupt onset of weakness in a distribution that reflects the nerve involved (eg, peroneal nerve involvement produces foot drop). A surprising number of these neuropathies improve after 6–8 weeks. Reversible **cranial nerve palsies** can occur and may present as lid ptosis (cranial nerve III), lateral deviation of the eye (IV), inability to move the eye laterally (VI), or facial paralysis (Bell's palsy) (VII). Even cranial nerve VIII (the auditory nerve) can be affected, and early deafness is observed in many poorly controlled diabetics. Again, the prognosis is good, with recovery of motor function over weeks to months.

Autonomic Neuropathy

Neuropathy of the autonomic nervous system is common in patients with diabetes of long duration and can be a very disconcerting clinical problem. It can affect many diverse visceral functions. Early signs include tachycardia at rest, fixation of pupillary diameter, and progressive loss of sweating. Postural hypotension may become extreme. Involvement of the gastrointestinal system may be manifested by nausea, vomiting, and postprandial fullness (from gastric atony); symptoms of reflux or dysphagia (from esophageal involvement); constipation and recurrent diarrhea, especially at night (from involvement of the small bowel and colon); and fecal incontinence (from anal sphincter dysfunction). Gallbladder function is altered, and this enhances stone formation. Impotence, urinary incontinence, large volumes of residual urine, and retrograde ejaculation can result from urogenital involvement.

Therapy is difficult and must be directed specifically at each abnormality. Use of Jobst fitted stockings, tilting the head of the bed, and arising slowly from the supine position are useful in minimizing symptoms of **orthostatic hypotension.** Some patients may require the addition of a mineralocorticoid such as fludrocortisone acetate (0.05–0.2 mg twice daily). Metoclopramide (10 mg 3 or 4 times daily) may increase gastric emptying and provide some relief from symptoms of **gastric atony** and **esophageal reflux.** Bethanechol (Urecholine) has also been used in this setting. An occasional patient may require gastrojejunal anastomosis.

Diabetic diarrhea is occasionally due to bacterial overgrowth from stasis in the small intestine, and a trial of broad-spectrum antibiotics may give relief. If this does not help, symptomatic relief can sometimes be achieved with cholinergic drugs or antidiarrheal agents such as diphenoxylate with atropine (Lomotil) or loperamide (Imodium). Bethanechol has occasionally improved emptying of the **atonic urinary bladder.** When **impotence** is due to neuropathy, penile implants can be considered (see Chapter 13).

4. CARDIOVASCULAR COMPLICATIONS

Heart Disease

Microangiopathy has recently been recognized to occur in the heart and may explain the existence of congestive cardiomyopathies found in diabetic patients without demonstrable coronary artery disease. Much more commonly, however, heart failure in the diabetic is a consequence of coronary atherosclerosis. Myocardial infarction is 3–5 times more common in diabetic patients than in age-matched controls and is the leading cause of death in patients with type II diabetes. A loss of the protection against myocardial infarction usually present in women during the age of childbearing is particularly evident in diabetic women. The exact reason for the increased incidence of atherosclerosis in diabetics is not clear. It may be a consequence of hyperlipidemia; abnormalities of platelet adhesiveness or coagulation factors (or both); or hypertension.

Peripheral Vascular Disease

Atherosclerosis is markedly accelerated in the

larger arteries. It is often diffuse, with localized enhancement in certain areas of turbulent blood flow, such as at the bifurcation of the aorta or other large vessels. Clinical manifestations of peripheral vascular disease include ischemia of the lower extremities, impotence, and intestinal angina.

The incidence of **gangrene of the feet** in diabetics is 30 times that in age-matched controls. The factors responsible for its development, in addition to peripheral vascular disease, are small vessel disease, peripheral neuropathy, and secondary infection. In two-thirds of patients with ischemic gangrene, pedal pulses are not palpable. In the remaining one-third who have palpable pulses, reduced blood flow through these vessels can be demonstrated by plethysmographic or Doppler ultrasound examination. Prevention of foot injury is imperative, and certain principles that should be emphasized are outlined on p 554. Agents that reduce peripheral blood flow such as tobacco and propranolol should be avoided. Control of other risk factors such as hypertension is essential. Patients should be advised to seek immediate medical care if a diabetic foot ulcer develops. Improvement in peripheral blood flow with endarterectomy and bypass operations is possible in certain patients.

5. SKIN CHANGES

Diabetic dermopathy is characterized by atrophic brown spots on the skin, usually in the pretibial area ("shin spots"). These changes may be a consequence of increased glycosylation of tissue proteins or vasculopathy. Eruptive xanthomas may develop in some poorly controlled diabetics who have marked hypertriglyceridemia. A rare skin complication, necrobiosis lipoidica diabeticorum, occurs predominantly on the shins and is characterized by marked thinning of the skin which allows the subcutaneous vessels to be seen as though through tissue paper. An element of vascular occlusion is generally present.

6. BONE & JOINT COMPLICATIONS

Bone and joint complications are generally attributed to metabolic or vascular sequelae of diabetes of long standing.

Juvenile Diabetic "Cheirarthropathy"
This is a syndrome of chronic progressive stiffness of the hand secondary to contracture and tightening of the skin over the joints. It is characterized by inability to flatten the palms against a flat surface. It usually occurs within 5–6 years after onset of type I diabetes. It is believed to be due to glycosylation of collagen and perhaps other proteins in connective tissue.

Dupuytren's Contracture
This consists of nodular thickening of the palmar fascia of the hand, producing a clawlike deformity. Although not specific to diabetes, when it occurs in a diabetic patient it may be the result of ischemic necrosis and secondary scarring of connective tissue as a consequence of diabetic microangiopathy.

Bone Demineralization
Bone demineralization has been reported to occur with increased frequency in diabetic patients. Bone density, as measured by photon absorption in the forearms, is 10–20% below normal in diabetics as compared to appropriately matched controls. Diabetes mellitus, however, does not seem to be associated with clinically important osteopenia, since there is no increase in the occurrence of skeletal fractures.

Joint Abnormalities
Bursitis, particularly of the shoulders and hips, occurs more frequently than expected in patients with diabetes. Gout also has a higher than expected incidence, especially in obese diabetics.

7. INFECTION

Certain types of infection, such as bacteriuria, candidal esophagitis, and candidal vaginitis, occur more frequently in diabetic patients than in nondiabetic matched controls. There are also several unusual infections that occur almost exclusively in diabetics (eg, emphysematous cholecystitis, mucormycosis, malignant otitis externa). As noted above, atherosclerosis with peripheral vascular disease is very common in the diabetic population, and the resultant ischemia undoubtedly plays a role in the frequent lower extremity infections seen in these patients.

SURGERY IN THE DIABETIC PATIENT

Surgery represents a stress situation during which most of the insulin antagonists (catecholamines, GH, corticosteroids) are mobilized. In the diabetic patient, this can lead to a worsening of hyperglycemia and perhaps even ketoacidosis. The aim of medical management of diabetics during the perioperative period is to minimize these stress-induced changes. Recommendations for management depend both on the patient's usual diabetic regimen and on the type of surgery (major or minor) to be done.

DIABETICS REGULATED BY DIET ALONE

No special precautions must be taken unless diabetic control is markedly disturbed by the procedure.

If this occurs, small amounts of regular insulin twice a day will establish euglycemia in a patient whose food intake is adequate. Human insulin is recommended, since it sensitizes the patient least—ie, anaphylactic complications are very rare, and patients are less likely to be sensitized to the future use of insulin.

DIABETICS TAKING ORAL HYPOGLYCEMIC AGENTS

When oral medications are allowed, these agents should be administered in the usual doses in the perioperative period. Carbohydrates should be supplied orally or by intravenous infusion of dextrose in water, with careful monitoring of blood glucose levels to avoid hypoglycemia or extremes of hyperglycemia. As in the case of diet-controlled diabetes, human insulin can be substituted if symptomatic hyperglycemia or ketosis develops.

DIABETICS TAKING INSULIN

Patients taking insulin represent the only serious challenge to management of diabetes when surgery is necessary. However, with careful attention to changes in the clinical or laboratory picture, most diabetic patients can be managed successfully.

Minor Surgery

For minor surgery requiring only local or spinal anesthesia or intravenous administration of a very transient anesthetic, half of the usual dose of insulin should be given in the morning. The patient should be placed early on the operating room schedule. A constant drip of 5% dextrose in water (at a rate of approximately 5 g of glucose per hour) should be infused if delays are necessary. Blood glucose levels should be checked at regular intervals.

Major Surgery

The night before major surgery, a 9 PM bedtime snack is given. Thereafter, the patient should receive nothing by mouth. On the morning of surgery, the usual morning subcutaneous insulin dose is omitted; instead, 10 units of regular insulin is added to 1 L of 5% dextrose in water, and this is infused intravenously at a rate of 100–180 mL/h. This will give the patient 1–1.8 units of insulin per hour, which, except in the most severe cases, will generally keep the blood glucose within the range of 100–250 mg/dL. The infusion may be continued for several days if necessary. Plasma glucose or blood glucose should be determined at least 4 times a day to be sure metabolic control is adequate. If it is not, adjustments in the ratio of insulin to dextrose in the intravenous solution can be made.

After surgery, when the patient has resumed an adequate oral intake, intravenous administration of insulin and dextrose can be stopped. Two hours after discontinuing the intravenous insulin, subcutaneous administration of insulin can be resumed. Insulin needs may vary in the first several days after surgery because of continuing postoperative stresses and because of variable caloric intake. In this situation, multiple doses of regular insulin guided by blood glucose determinations can keep the patient in acceptable metabolic control. Routine "sliding scale" insulin orders based on urine glucose should be avoided in this setting.

PROGNOSIS FOR PATIENTS WITH DIABETES MELLITUS

The period between 10 and 20 years after the onset of diabetes seems to be a critical one. If the patient survives this period without fulminating microvascular complications, there is a strong likelihood that reasonably good health will continue. Currently, the prospect for retarding the progression of diabetic complications is good. Newer methods for delivering purified insulins and for monitoring blood glucose at home have improved the overall outlook for patients with diabetes mellitus; however, it is clear that the diabetic patient's intelligence, motivation, and awareness of potential complications of the disease are major factors contributing to a successful outcome.

REFERENCES

The Endocrine Pancreas
Adrian TE et al: Mechanism of pancreatic polypeptide release in man. *Lancet* 1977;**1**:161.
Hellerström C: The life story of the pancreatic B cell. *Diabetologia* 1984;**26**:393.
Hermensen K: Secretion of somatostatin from the normal and diabetic pancreas. *Diabetologia* 1980;**19**:492.
Howell SL: The mechanism of insulin secretion. *Diabetologia* 1984;**26**:319.

Malaisse-Lagae F et al: Identification of a lobe in the adult human pancreas rich in pancreatic polypeptide. *Diabetologia* 1979;**17**:361.
McCullough AJ et al: Effect of graded intraduodenal glucose infusions on the release and physiological actions of gastric inhibitory polypeptide. *J Clin Endocrinol Metab* 1983; **56**:234.
Reichlin S: Somatostatin. (2 parts.) *N Engl J Med* 1983; **309**:1495, 1556.

Unger RH, Orci L: Glucagon and the A cell. *N Engl J Med* 1981;**304**:1518.

Williams JA, Goldfine ID: The insulin-pancreatic acinar axis: A review. *Diabetes* 1985;**34**:980.

Diagnosis, Classification, & Pathophysiology of Diabetes Mellitus

Bell GI, Horita S, Karam JH: A polymorphic locus near the human insulin gene is associated with insulin-dependent diabetes mellitus. *Diabetes* 1984;**33**:176.

Bennett PH: The diagnosis of diabetes: New international classification and diagnostic criteria. *Annu Rev Med* 1983;**34**:295.

Cahill GF, McDevitt HO: Insulin-dependent diabetes mellitus: The initial lesion. *N Engl J Med* 1981;**304**:1454.

Defronzo RA, Ferrannini E, Kovisto V: New concepts in the pathogenesis and treatment of NIDDM. *Am J Med* 1983;**74(Suppl 1A):**52.

Flier JS: Insulin receptors and insulin resistance. *Annu Rev Med* 1983;**34**:145.

Gerich JE: Assessment of insulin resistance and its role in non–insulin-dependent diabetes mellitus. *J Lab Clin Med* 1984;**103**:497.

Hall PM et al: Glycosylated hemoglobins and glycosylated plasma proteins in the diagnosis of diabetes mellitus and impaired glucose tolerance. *Diabetes Care* 1984;**7**:147.

Lernmark A: Molecular biology of type I (insulin-dependent) diabetes mellitus. *Diabetologia* 1985;**28**:195.

National Diabetes Data Group: Classification and diagnosis of diabetes mellitus and other categories of glucose intolerance. *Diabetes* 1979;**28**:1039.

Olefsky JM: Pathogenesis of insulin resistance and hyperglycemia in non–insulin-dependent diabetes mellitus. *Am J Med* 1985;**79(Suppl 3B):**1.

Permutt MA et al: Insulin gene structure and function: A review of studies using recombinant DNA methodology. *Diabetes Care* 1984;**7**:386.

Rotter JI, Rimoin DL: The genetics of the glucose intolerance disorders. *Am J Med* 1981;**70**:116.

Schade DS et al: The etiology of incapacitating, brittle diabetes. *Diabetes Care* 1985;**8**:12.

Srikanta S et al: First-degree relatives of patients with type I diabetes mellitus: Islet cell antibodies and abnormal insulin secretion. *N Engl J Med* 1985;**313**:461.

Tager HS: Abnormal products of the human insulin gene. *Diabetes* 1984;**33**:693.

Ulrich A et al: Human insulin receptor and its relationship to the tyrosine kinase family of oncogenes. *Nature* 1985;**313**:756.

Ward WK et al: Pathophysiology of insulin secretion in non–insulin-dependent diabetes mellitus. *Diabetes Care* 1984;**7**:491.

Treatment of Diabetes Mellitus

Bantle JP et al: Postprandial glucose and insulin responses to meals containing different carbohydrates in normal and diabetic subjects. *N Engl J Med* 1983;**309**:7.

Berger M et al: Absorption kinetics and biologic effects of subcutaneously injected insulin preparations. *Diabetes Care* 1982;**5**:77.

Binder C et al: Insulin pharmacokinetics. *Diabetes Care* 1984;**7**:188.

Bolli GB, Gerich JE: The "dawn phenomenon": A common occurrence in both non–insulin-dependent and insulin-dependent diabetes mellitus. *N Engl J Med* 1984;**310**:746.

Bolli GB et al: Glucose counterregulation and waning of insulin in the Somogyi phenomenon (posthypoglycemic hyperglycemia). *N Engl J Med* 1984;**311**:1214.

Cryer PE, Gerich JE: Glucose counterregulation, hypoglycemia, and intensive insulin therapy in diabetes mellitus. *N Engl J Med* 1985;**313**:232.

Deckert T: Intermediate-acting insulin preparations: NPH and lente. *Diabetes Care* 1980;**3**:623.

Fineberg SE et al: Effects of species of origin, purification levels, and formulation on insulin immunogenicity. *Diabetes* 1983;**32**:592.

Galloway JA: Insulin treatment for the early 80s: Facts and questions about old and new insulins and their usage. *Diabetes Care* 1980;**3**:615.

Garvey WT et al: The effect of insulin treatment on insulin secretion and insulin action in type II diabetes mellitus. *Diabetes* 1985;**34**:222.

Goldman J et al: Effect of glyburide on metabolic control and insulin binding in insulin-dependent diabetes mellitus. *Diabetes Care* 1984;**7(Suppl 1):**106.

Hansen B et al: New approaches to therapy and diagnosis of diabetes. *Diabetologia* 1982;**22**:61.

Health and Public Policy Committee, American College of Physicians: Glycosylated hemoglobin assays in the management and diagnosis of diabetes mellitus. *Ann Intern Med* 1984;**101**:710.

Kadowaki T et al: Chlorpropamide-induced hyponatremia: Incidence and risk factors. *Diabetes Care* 1983;**6**:468.

Karam JH, Etzwiler DD (editors): International Symposium on Human Insulin. *Diabetes Care* 1983;**6(Suppl 1):**1.

Kolterman OG et al: The acute and chronic effects of sulfonylurea therapy in type II diabetic subjects. *Diabetes* 1984;**33**:346.

The Kroc Collaborative Study Group: Blood glucose control and the evolution of diabetic retinopathy and albuminuria: A multicenter trial. *N Engl J Med* 1984;**311**:365.

Lauritzen T et al: Effect of 1 year of near-normal blood glucose levels on retinopathy in insulin-dependent diabetics. *Lancet* 1983;**1**:200.

Lockwood DH, Gerich JE, Goldfine I: Symposium on effects of oral hypoglycemic agents on receptor and postreceptor actions of insulin. *Diabetes Care* 1984;**7(Suppl 1):**1.

Lord JM et al: Effect of metformin on insulin receptor binding and glycaemic control in type II diabetes. *Br Med J* 1983;**286**:830.

Marliss EB et al: Present and future expectations regarding insulin infusion systems. *Diabetes Care* 1981;**4**:325.

Mazze RS et al: Reliability of blood glucose monitoring by patients with diabetes mellitus. *Am J Med* 1984;**77**:211.

Mecklenburg RS et al: Acute complications associated with insulin infusion pump therapy: Report of experience with 161 patients. *JAMA* 1984;**252**:3265.

Mecklenburg RS et al: Long-term metabolic control with insulin pump therapy: Report of experience with 127 patients. *N Engl J Med* 1985;**313**:465.

Mirouze J: Insulin treatment: A non-stop revolution. *Diabetologia* 1983;**25**:209.

Murphy J et al: Conservative management of pregnancy in diabetic women. *Br Med J* 1984;**288**:1203.

Nathan DM et al: The clinical information value of the glycosylated hemoglobin assay. *N Engl J Med* 1984;**310**:341.

Nolte MS et al: Reduced solubility of short-acting soluble insulins when mixed with longer-acting insulins. *Diabetes* 1983;**32**:1177.

Nuttal FQ: Diet and the diabetic patient. *Diabetes Care* 1983;**6**:197.

Owens DR: Effects of oral sulfonylureas on the spectrum of defects in non–insulin-dependent diabetes mellitus. *Am J Med* 1985;**79(Suppl 2B):**27.

Pfeifer MA et al: Acute and chronic effects of sulfonylurea drugs on pancreatic islet function in man. *Diabetes Care* 1984;**7(Suppl 1):**25.

Raskin P et al: The effect of diabetic control on the width of skeletal-muscle capillary basement membrane in patients with type I diabetes mellitus. *N Engl J Med* 1983;**309:**1546.

Richter EA, Ruderman NB, Schneider SH: Diabetes and exercise. *Am J Med* 1981;**70:**201.

Skyler JS (editor): Symposium on human insulin of recombinant DNA origin. *Diabetes Care* 1982;**5(Suppl 2):**186.

Sutherland D, Kendall D: Pancreas transplantation. *West J Med* 1985;**143:**845.

Teutsch SM et al: Mortality among diabetic patients using continuous subcutaneous insulin-infusion pumps. *N Engl J Med* 1984;**310:**361.

Young CW: Rationale for glycemic control. *Am J Med* 1985;**79(Suppl 3B):**8.

Acute Complications of Diabetes Mellitus

Adrogué HJ et al: Plasma acid-base patterns in diabetic ketoacidosis. *N Engl J Med* 1982;**307:**1603.

Bending JJ, Pickup JC, Keen H: Frequency of diabetic ketoacidosis and hypoglycemic coma during treatment with continuous subcutaneous insulin infusion. *Am J Med* 1985;**79:**685.

Brown RH et al: Caveat on fluid replacement in hyperglycemic hyperosmolar nonketotic coma. *Diabetes Care* 1978; **1:**305.

Casparie AF, Elving LD: Severe hypoglycemia in diabetic patients: Frequency, causes, prevention. *Diabetes Care* 1985;**8:**141.

Clements RS, Bell DSH: Complications of diabetes: Prevalence, detection, current treatment, and prognosis. *Am J Med* 1985;**79(Suppl 5A):**2.

Clements RS, Vourganti B: Fatal diabetic ketoacidosis: Major causes and approaches to their prevention. *Diabetes Care* 1978;**1:**314.

Cohen RD, Woods HF: Lactic acidosis revisited. *Diabetes* 1983;**32:**181.

Fisher JN, Kitabchi AE: A randomized study of phosphate therapy in the treatment of diabetic ketoacidosis. *J Clin Endocrinol Metab* 1983;**57:**177.

Flexner CW et al: Repeated hospitalization for diabetic ketoacidosis: The game of "Sartoris." *Am J Med* 1984; **76:**691.

Foster DW, McGarry JD: The metabolic derangements and treatment of diabetic ketoacidosis. *N Engl J Med* 1983;**309:**159.

Fulop M: The treatment of severely uncontrolled diabetes mellitus. *Adv Intern Med* 1984;**29:**327.

Keller U, Berger W: Prevention of hypophosphatemia by phosphate infusion during treatment of diabetic ketoacidosis and hyperosmolar coma. *Diabetes* 1980;**29:**87.

Krane EJ et al: Subclinical brain swelling in children during treatment of diabetic ketoacidosis. *N Engl J Med* 1985;**312:**1147.

Kreisberg RA: Pathogenesis and management of lactic acidosis. *Annu Rev Med* 1984;**35:**181.

Lever E, Jaspan JB: Sodium bicarbonate therapy in severe diabetic ketoacidosis. *Am J Med* 1983;**75:**263.

Park R, Arieff AI: Lactic acidosis: Current concepts. *Clin Endocrinol Metab* 1983;**12:**339.

Peterson CM, Javanovic L: *The Diabetes Self-Care Method.* Simon & Schuster, 1984.

Salzman R et al: Intranasal aerosolized insulin: Mixed-meal studies and long-term use in type I diabetes. *N Engl J Med* 1985;**312:**1078.

Schade DS, Eaton RP: Diabetic ketoacidosis: Pathogenesis, prevention and therapy. *Clin Endocrinol Metab* 1983; **13:**332.

Sutherland DE, Goetz FC, Najarian JS: Pancreas transplants from related donors. *Transplantation* 1984;**38:**625.

Chronic Complications of Diabetes Mellitus

American Diabetes Association: *The Physician Guide to Type 2 Diabetes (NIDDM): Diagnosis and Treatment.* American Diabetes Association, 1984.

Bradley WE (editor): Aspects of diabetic autonomic neuropathy. (Symposium.) *Ann Intern Med* 1980;**92:**289.

Brownlee M, Vlassara H, Cerami A: Nonenzymatic glycosylation and the pathogenesis of diabetic complications. *Ann Intern Med* 1984;**101:**527.

Christlieb AR: The hypertensions of diabetes. *Diabetes Care* 1982;**5:**50.

Cogan DG et al: Aldose reductase and complications of diabetes. *Ann Intern Med* 1984;**101:**82.

Dunn FL: Hyperlipidemia and diabetes. *Med Clin North Am* 1982;**66:**1347.

Ganda OP: Pathogenesis of macrovascular disease in the human diabetic. *Diabetes* 1980;**29:**931.

Greene DA et al: Glucose-induced alterations in nerve metabolism: Current perspective on the pathogenesis of diabetic neuropathy and future directions for research and therapy. *Diabetes Care* 1985;**8:**290.

Herman WH et al: An approach to the prevention of blindness in diabetes. *Diabetes Care* 1983;**6:**608.

Jervell J et al: Clinical results of renal transplantation in diabetic patients. *Transplant Proc* 1984;**16:**599.

LoGerfo FW, Coffman D: Vascular and microvascular disease of the foot in diabetes: Implications for foot care. *N Engl J Med* 1984;**311:**1615.

Mauer SM et al: Structural functional relationships in diabetic nephropathy. *J Clin Invest* 1984;**74:**1143.

McCulloch DK et al: The prevalence of diabetic impotence. *Diabetologia* 1980;**18:**279.

National Diabetes Advisory Board, US Department of Health and Human Services: *The Prevention and Treatment of Five Complications of Diabetes.* Centers for Disease Control, 1984.

Rand LI: Recent advances in diabetic retinopathy. *Am J Med* 1981;**70:**595.

Rosenbloom AL et al: Limited joint mobility in childhood diabetes: Family studies. *Diabetes Care* 1983;**6:**370.

Sidenius P: The axonopathy of diabetic neuropathy. *Diabetes* 1982;**31:**356.

Viberti G, Keen H: The patterns of proteinuria in diabetes mellitus: Relevance to pathogenesis and prevention of diabetic nephropathy. *Diabetes* 1984;**33:**686.

Ward JD: The diabetic leg. *Diabetologia* 1982;**22:**141.

Wheat LJ: Infection and diabetes mellitus. *Diabetes Care* 1980;**3:**187.

Wiseman MJ et al: Effect of blood glucose on increased glomerular filtration rate and kidney size in insulin-dependent diabetes. *N Engl J Med* 1985;**312:**617.

Zatz R et al: Predominance of hemodynamic rather than metabolic factors in the pathogenesis of diabetic glomerulopathy. *Proc Natl Acad Sci USA* 1985;**82:**5963.

Hypoglycemic Disorders

20

Clinton W. Young, MD, & John H. Karam, MD

Circulating plasma glucose concentrations are kept within a relatively narrow range by a complex system of interrelated neural, humoral, and cellular controls. Under the usual metabolic conditions, the central nervous system is wholly dependent on plasma glucose and counteracts declining blood glucose concentrations with a carefully programmed response. This is often associated with a sensation of hunger; and, as the brain receives insufficient glucose to meet its metabolic needs (neuroglycopenia), an autonomic response is triggered to mobilize storage depots of glycogen and fat. Hepatic glycogen reserves directly supply the central nervous system with glucose, which is carried across the blood-brain barrier by a specific glucose transport system, while the mobilization of fatty acids from triglyceride depots provides energy for the large mass of skeletal and cardiac muscle, renal cortex, liver, and other tissues that utilize fatty acids as their basic fuel, thus sparing glucose for use by the tissues of the central nervous system.

PATHOPHYSIOLOGY OF THE COUNTERREGULATORY RESPONSE TO NEUROGLYCOPENIA

The plasma concentration of glucose that will signal the need by the central nervous system to mobilize energy reserves depends on a number of factors, such as the status of blood flow to the brain, the integrity of cerebral tissue, the prevailing arterial level of plasma

Table 20–1. Sympathetic nervous system response to hypoglycemia.

Alpha-Adrenergic Effects
  Inhibition of endogenous insulin release.
  Increase in cerebral blood flow (peripheral vasoconstriction).
Beta-Adrenergic Effects
  Hepatic and muscle glycogenolysis.
  Stimulation of plasma glucagon release.
  Lipolysis to raise plasma free fatty acids.
  Impairment of glucose uptake by muscle tissue.
  Increase in cerebral blood flow (increase in cardiac output).
Adrenomedullary Discharge of Catecholamines
  Augmentation of all of the above alpha- and beta-adrenergic effects.

---

glucose, the rapidity with which plasma glucose concentration falls, and the availability of alternative metabolic fuels. In most healthy people, hypoglycemic symptoms occur at plasma glucose levels below 45 mg/dL (blood glucose < 40 mg/dL). However, in elderly people with compromised cerebral blood supply, neuroglycopenic manifestations may be provoked at slightly higher plasma glucose levels.

Restoring and maintaining an adequate supply of glucose for cerebral function proceeds by a series of neurogenic events that act directly to raise the plasma glucose concentration and to stimulate hormonal responses that augment the adrenergic mobilization of energy stores (Table 20–1).

Hormonal Response to Hypoglycemia

A. Insulin: Endogenous insulin secretion is lowered both by reduced glucose stimulation to the pancreatic B cell and by sympathetic nervous system inhibition from a combination of alpha-adrenergic neural effects and increased circulating catecholamine levels. This reactive insulinopenia facilitates the mobilization of energy from existing energy stores (glycogenolysis and lipolysis), increases hepatic enzymes involved in gluconeogenesis and ketogenesis, and at the same time prevents muscle tissue from consuming the blood glucose being released from the liver (see Chapter 19).

B. Catecholamines: Circulating catecholamines and norepinephrine produced at sympathetic nerve endings provide muscle tissue with alternative sources of fuel by activating beta-adrenergic receptors—resulting in mobilization of muscle glycogen—and by providing increased plasma free fatty acids from lipolysis of adipocyte triglyceride.

C. Glucagon: Plasma glucagon is released by the beta-adrenergic effects of both sympathetic innervation and circulating catecholamines on pancreatic A cells as well as by the direct stimulation of A cells by the low plasma glucose concentration itself. This glucagon release increases hepatic output of glucose by direct glycogenolysis as well as by facilitating the activity of gluconeogenic enzymes. As shown in Fig 20–1, plasma glucagon appears to be the key counterregulatory hormone affecting recovery from acute hypoglycemia in humans, with the adrenergic-catecholamine response representing a major backup system.

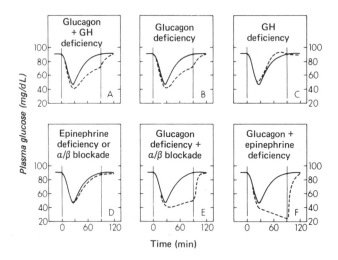

Figure 20–1. Solid lines show changes in plasma glucose that occur in normal subjects in response to insulin administration. Note the rapid recovery of glucose levels mediated by intact counterregulatory mechanisms. The dashed lines show the response to insulin-induced hypoglycemia in patients with deficiencies of the counterregulatory mechanisms induced as follows: *A:* Somatostatin infusion (inhibits both glucagon and growth hormone [GH] release). *B:* Somatostatin infusion plus GH infusion (now with functional isolated glucagon deficiency). *C:* Somatostatin infusion plus glucagon infusion (isolated GH deficiency). Note return of glucose response to normal, implying that glucagon is the main counterregulatory hormone. *D:* Bilateral adrenalectomy, leading to epinephrine deficiency, or infusion of phentolamine plus propranolol (alpha and beta blockers, respectively). Note that such deficiencies cause no major abnormality in response to induced hypoglycemia when glucagon is present. *E and F:* Sympathetic modulation (by phentolamine plus propranolol in E and by bilateral adrenalectomy in F), which seriously impairs the ability to respond to hypoglycemia in the patient made glucagon-deficient by somatostatin infusion. (Reproduced, with permission, from Cryer PE: Glucose counterregulation in man. *Diabetes* 1981;**30:**261.)

D. Corticotropin and Hydrocortisone: Pituitary ACTH is released in association with the sympathetic nervous system stimulation by neuroglycopenia. This results in elevation of plasma cortisol levels, which permissively facilitates lipolysis and actively promotes protein catabolism and conversion of amino acids to glucose by the liver.

E. Growth Hormone: Pituitary growth hormone is also released in response to falling plasma glucose levels. Its role in counteracting hypoglycemia is less well defined, but it is known to antagonize the action of insulin on glucose utilization in muscle cells and to directly activate lipolysis by adipocytes.

Maintenance of Euglycemia in the Postabsorptive State

Glucose absorption from the gastrointestinal tract ceases by 5–8 hours after a meal. During the "postabsorptive state" immediately following, glucose must be produced endogenously from previously stored nutrients to meet the requirements of the central nervous system. The liver is the central organ involved in this process, producing the 125 mg of glucose per minute required by the brain as well as an additional 25 mg/min for other glucose-dependent tissues—predominantly blood cell elements. This is initially provided by the breakdown of stored hepatic glycogen. How-

ever, because these reserves are limited to 80–100 g, they begin to be depleted several hours into the postabsorptive state. Thereafter, hepatic glucose production is augmented by gluconeogenesis—the formation of glucose from amino acids, lactate, and glycerol. These substrates are delivered to the liver from peripheral stores: Muscle and other structural tissues supply amino acids, mainly alanine; blood cell elements supply lactate, the end product of glycolytic metabolism; and adipose tissue supplies glycerol from lipolysis of triglyceride. In addition, oxidation of the free fatty acids released from adipose cells during lipolysis supplies the energy required for gluconeogenesis and provides ketone bodies, acetoacetate, and β-hydroxybutyrate, which can serve as alternative metabolic fuels for the central nervous system during periods of prolonged fasting.

Hormonal changes that begin early in the postabsorptive state regulate the enzymatic steps necessary for hepatic glycogenolysis and gluconeogenesis and ensure the delivery of the necessary substrate (Table 20–2). An appropriate fall in circulating insulin levels is most important; elevations in the counterregulatory hormones glucagon, cortisol, and growth hormone are less critical.

In summary, numerous endocrine and metabolic events interact to provide a continuous source of fuel for proper functioning of the central nervous system.

Table 20—2. Hormonal changes to maintain euglycemia in the postabsorptive state.

Decreased Insulin Secretion
  Increases hepatic glycogenolysis.
  Increases lipolysis.
  Increases hepatic gluconeogenesis.
  Decreases muscle uptake of glucose.
Increased Glucagon Secretion
  Increases hepatic glycogenolysis.
  Facilitates hepatic gluconeogenesis.
Increased Cortisol Secretion
  Facilitates lipolysis.
  Increases protein catabolism.
  Augments hepatic gluconeogenesis.

Malfunction of any of these mechanisms can lead to symptomatic hypoglycemia.

CLASSIFICATION OF HYPOGLYCEMIC DISORDERS

Symptomatic Hypoglycemia

A clinical classification of the more common causes of symptomatic hypoglycemia in adults is presented in Table 20– 3. (The inborn errors of metabolism that produce hypoglycemia in infants and children are mentioned but will not be discussed in detail in this chapter.) This classification is useful in directing diagnostic considerations.

Table 20—3. Common causes of symptomatic hypoglycemia.

Fasting
  A. With Hyperinsulinism:
    Insulin reaction.
    Sulfonylurea overdose.
    Surreptitious insulin or sulfonylurea administration.
    Autoimmune hypoglycemia (idiopathic insulin antibodies, insulin receptor autoantibodies).
    Pentamidine-induced hypoglycemia.
    Pancreatic B cell tumors.
  B. Without Hyperinsulinism:
    Severe hepatic dysfunction.
    Chronic renal insufficiency.
    Inanition, ketotic hypoglycemia of childhood.
    Hypocortisolism.
    Alcohol use.
    Nonpancreatic tumors.
    Inborn errors of carbohydrate metabolism (glycogen storage disease, gluconeogenic enzyme deficiencies).
Nonfasting
  Alimentary.
  Functional.
  Occult diabetes.
  Ethanol.
  Leucine sensitivity.
  Hereditary fructose intolerance.
  Galactosemia.
  Newborn infant of diabetic mother.

Symptomatic **fasting hypoglycemia** is a serious and potentially life-threatening problem warranting thorough evaluation. Conditions that produce inappropriate fasting hyperinsulinism are the most common cause of fasting hypoglycemia in otherwise healthy adults. These include insulin-secreting pancreatic B cell tumors and iatrogenic or surreptitious administration of insulin or sulfonylureas. In patients with illnesses that produce symptomatic fasting hypoglycemia despite appropriately suppressed insulin levels, the clinical picture is dominated by the signs and symptoms of the primary disease, with hypoglycemia often only a late or associated manifestation. This is in contrast to patients with inappropriate hyperinsulinism, who usually appear healthy between hypoglycemic episodes.

Symptoms of **nonfasting hypoglycemia** in adults, although distressing to the patient, do not imply serious illness or warrant extensive evaluation. Overstimulation of the B cells postprandially as a result of accelerated glucose absorption after rapid gastric emptying may result in too rapid disposal of glucose, with resulting symptoms of sympathetic nervous system hyperactivity. Other than in patients who have had gastric surgery, this sequence may be difficult to establish for diagnosis.

Asymptomatic Hypoglycemia

Hypoglycemia may be seen during prolonged fasting, strenuous exercise, or pregnancy or may occur as a laboratory artifact. In normal men, plasma glucose does not fall below 55 mg/dL during a 72-hour fast. However, for reasons that are not clear, normal women may experience a fall to levels as low as 30 mg/dL despite a marked suppression of circulating insulin to less than 6 μU/mL. They remain asymptomatic in spite of this degree of hypoglycemia, presumably because ketogenesis is able to satisfy the energy needs of the central nervous system. Basal plasma glucose declines progressively during normal pregnancy, and hypoglycemic levels may be reached during prolonged fasting. This may be a consequence of a continuous fetal consumption of glucose and diminished availability of the gluconeogenic substrate alanine. The cause of these diminished alanine levels in pregnancy is unclear, and it is not known whether the hypoglycemia ever produces symptoms. The greatly increased glucose consumption by skeletal muscle that occurs during prolonged strenuous exercise may lead to hypoglycemia despite increases in hepatic glucose production. Whether the hypoglycemia in this circumstance contributes to fatigue or other symptoms in distance runners is unknown.

In vitro consumption of glucose by blood cell elements may give rise to laboratory values in the hypoglycemic range. This is most commonly seen when an insufficient amount of the metabolic inhibitor sodium fluoride is added to specimens containing increased numbers of leukocytes (as in leukemia and leukemoid reactions).

CLINICAL PRESENTATION OF HYPOGLYCEMIA

Regardless of the cause, hypoglycemia presents certain common features characterized by **Whipple's triad:** (1) symptoms and signs of hypoglycemia, (2) an associated plasma glucose level of 45 mg/dL or less, and (3) reversibility of symptoms upon administration of glucose.

The symptoms and signs of hypoglycemia are the consequences of neuroglycopenia. They vary depending on the degree of hypoglycemia, the age of the patient, and, in diabetics, the plasma glucose level prevailing before the fall. The manifestations also depend on the rapidity of the decline, so that symptoms and signs are different depending on whether acute or subacute and chronic hypoglycemia occurs.

A. Acute Hypoglycemia: A precipitous fall in plasma glucose ($>$ 1 mg/dL/min) to low levels often accompanies conditions associated with arterial hyperinsulinism—a condition that leads to increased peripheral glucose uptake and decreased hepatic glucose output. In diabetics, excessive absorption of exogenous insulin either from overtreatment or from rapid mobilization from an injection site during exercise may be responsible. In nondiabetics, reactive hypersecretion may be the cause, as in postgastrectomy patients with rapid gastric emptying time. The symptoms include anxiety, tremulousness, and feelings of unnaturalness or detachment. These are usually accompanied by palpitations, tachycardia, sweating, and hunger and can progress to neurologic sequelae of ataxia, coma, or convulsions.

B. Subacute and Chronic Hypoglycemia: A relatively slow fall in plasma glucose accompanies conditions caused primarily by a reduction in hepatic glucose output in response to hyperinsulinism (predominantly within the portal vein [insulinoma]), to the inappropriately sustained effects of long-acting insulin preparations on the liver in the postabsorptive state, or to metabolic derangements of liver functions (eg, alcohol hypoglycemia). Symptoms due to hypoglycemia in patients with these conditions may be less apparent, particularly because symptoms of sympathetic overactivity are usually absent. These patients develop progressive confusion, inappropriate behavior, lethargy, and drowsiness. If the patient does not eat, seizures or coma may develop, although this is not inevitable, and spontaneous recovery can occur. Because these patients are seldom aware of their degree of functional impairment, a history should be obtained from relatives or friends who have observed the episode. Except for hypothermia (often seen during hypoglycemic coma), there are no identifying characteristics on physical examination. Hypoglycemia will often be misdiagnosed as a seizure disorder, transient ischemic attack, or personality disorder.

Documentation of Low Plasma Glucose Values

With the specific laboratory methods now available, it has been arbitrarily decided that fasting hyperglycemia is present when plasma glucose is 45 mg/dL or less after an overnight fast (corresponding to a blood glucose level of 40 mg/dL or less). In the fasting state, there is no substantial difference between arterial, venous, or capillary blood samples (in contrast to nonfasting hyperglycemia, in which arteriovenous glucose differences may be considerable because of arterial hyperinsulinism and consequent increases in glucose uptake across capillary beds).

The development of glucose oxidase–hydrogen peroxidase paper strips has been of great value for a rapid estimate of blood glucose levels, particularly for insulin-treated diabetics undergoing home monitoring. In emergency room or hospital settings, the paper strips are helpful in the differential diagnosis of coma, but a laboratory sample should also be obtained for definitive diagnosis. Although therapeutic decisions to administer glucose can be based on the paper strip results alone in an emergency situation, variability due to exposure to air or aging makes them less dependable as the sole laboratory indicator for a definitive diagnosis of hypoglycemia.

Reversibility of Clinical Manifestations of Hypoglycemia With Treatment

Because prolonged hypoglycemia may cause permanent brain damage and death, prompt recognition and treatment are mandatory. (It is prudent to consider the possibility of hypoglycemic coma in most unconscious patients.)

The goal of therapy is to restore normal levels of plasma glucose as rapidly as possible. If the patient is conscious and able to swallow, glucose-containing foods such as candy, orange juice with added sugar, and cookies should be quickly ingested. Fructose, found in many nutrient low-calorie sweeteners for diabetics, should not be used, because although it can be metabolized by neurons, it lacks a transport system and therefore does not cross the blood-brain barrier.

If the patient is unconscious, rapid restoration of plasma glucose must be accomplished by giving 20–50 mL of 50% dextrose intravenously over 1–3 minutes (the treatment of choice) or, when intravenous glucose is not available, 1 mg of glucagon intramuscularly or intravenously. Families or friends of insulin-treated diabetics should be instructed in the administration of glucagon intramuscularly for emergency treatment at home. Attempts to feed the patient or to apply glucose-containing jelly to the oral mucosa should be avoided because of the danger of aspiration.

When consciousness is restored, oral feedings should begin immediately. Periodic blood glucose surveillance after a hypoglycemic episode may be needed for 12–24 hours to ensure maintenance of euglycemia. Prevention of recurrent hypoglycemic attacks depends upon proper diagnosis and management of the specific underlying disorder.

SPECIFIC HYPOGLYCEMIC DISORDERS

SYMPTOMATIC FASTING HYPOGLYCEMIA WITH HYPERINSULINISM

1. INSULIN REACTION

It is not surprising that insulin-treated diabetics make up the bulk of the patient population with symptomatic hypoglycemia. Present methods of insulin delivery rely upon subcutaneous depots of mixtures of soluble and insoluble insulin whose absorption varies with the site of injection and the degree of exercise in surrounding muscles. Variations in physical and emotional stresses can alter the response of patients to insulin, as can the cyclic hormonal changes relating to menstruation. A deficient glucagon response to hypoglycemia in diabetes compounds the problem, as does the lack of awareness of hypoglycemic symptoms in older patients and in those with neuropathy, which reduces or obliterates the autonomic responses to hypoglycemia.

Once the patient's acute hypoglycemic episode is managed, the physician should carefully examine possible correctable factors that may have contributed to the insulin reaction:

Inadequate Food Intake

An insufficient quantity of food or a missed meal is one of the commonest causes of hypoglycemia in insulin-treated diabetics. Until improved insulin delivery systems are available, patients attempting to achieve satisfactory glycemic control should self-monitor their blood glucose levels and eat 3 regular meals as well as small midmorning, midafternoon, and bedtime snacks, particularly when they are receiving 2 or more injections of insulin mixtures daily.

Exercise

The insulin-treated diabetic is especially prone to exercise-induced hypoglycemia. In nondiabetics, the enhancement of skeletal muscle glucose uptake (a 20- to 30-fold increase over basal uptake) is compensated for by enhanced hepatic glucose production. This is mediated primarily by a fall in circulating insulin levels consequent to an exercise-induced catecholamine discharge, which inhibits B cell secretion. Such regulation is impossible in the insulin-treated diabetic, whose subcutaneous depot not only continues to release insulin during exercise but also shows an accelerated absorption rate when the injection site is in close proximity to the muscles being exercised. When this occurs, increased levels of circulating insulin compromise the hepatic output of glucose. To prevent hypoglycemia, insulin-treated diabetics must be advised to avoid injections into areas adjacent to muscles most involved in the particular exercise and either to eat supplementary carbohydrate before exercising or to reduce their insulin dose appropriately.

Impaired Glucose Counterregulation in Diabetics

Most patients with insulin-dependent diabetes have a deficient glucagon response to hypoglycemia. They are thus solely dependent on epinephrine to recover from hypoglycemia. Some patients, especially those with long-standing diabetes or autonomic neuropathy, lack both a glucagon and an epinephrine response and are virtually defenseless against insulin-induced hypoglycemia. Insulin infusion tests can be used to identify these alterations in glucose counterregulation; however, at present these tests are cumbersome, and their ability to accurately predict which patients will suffer frequent severe and prolonged hypoglycemic episodes is yet to be established. Easier and more reliable methods of identifying such patients are needed. The ability of a patient to recover from hypoglycemia may determine whether or not aggressive attempts to maintain euglycemia are associated with undue risk.

Inadvertent or Deliberate Insulin Overdosage in Diabetics

Excessive insulin may be administered inadvertently by patients with poor vision or inadequate instruction or understanding of dosage and injection technique. The widespread use of highly concentrated U100 insulin enhances the likelihood of overdosage with relatively small excesses of administered insulin.

Deliberate overdosage may occur in certain maladjusted patients, particularly adolescents, who wish to gain special attention from their families or escape tensions at school or work.

Miscellaneous Causes of Hypoglycemia in Insulin-Treated Diabetics

A. Stress: Physical stresses, such as intercurrent illnesses, infection, and surgery, or psychic stresses often require an increased insulin dosage to control hyperglycemia. Reduction to prestress doses is necessary to avoid subsequent hypoglycemia when the stresses have abated.

B. Hypocortisolism: In patients with insulin-dependent diabetes who have otherwise unexplained hypoglycemic attacks, reduced insulin requirements may indicate unusual causes (eg, Addison's disease).

C. Pregnancy: Pregnancy, with high fetal glucose consumption, decreases insulin requirements in the first trimester.

D. Renal Insufficiency: Renal insufficiency, through impairment of insulin degradation while hepatic gluconeogenesis and food intake are often reduced, also requires a reduction in insulin dosage.

E. Drugs: Numerous pharmacologic agents may potentiate the effects of insulin and predispose to hypoglycemia. Common offenders include ethanol, salicylates, and beta-adrenergic blocking drugs.

Beta blockade inhibits fatty acid and gluconeogenic substrate release and reduces plasma glucagon levels; furthermore, the symptomatic response is altered, because tachycardia is blocked while hazardous elevations of blood pressure may result during hypoglycemia in response to the unopposed alpha-adrenergic stimulation from circulating catecholamines and neurogenic sympathetic discharge. However, symptoms of sweating, hunger, and uneasiness are not masked by beta-blocking drugs and remain indicators of hypoglycemia in the aware patient.

2. SULFONYLUREA OVERDOSE

Any of the sulfonylureas may produce hypoglycemia. Chlorpropamide (Diabinese), with its prolonged half-life (35 hours), is a common offender. Older patients, especially those with impaired hepatic or renal function, are particularly susceptible to sulfonylurea-induced hypoglycemia: Liver dysfunction prolongs the hypoglycemic activity of tolbutamide (Orinase), acetohexamide (Dymelor), and tolazamide (Tolinase), as well as that of the second-generation compounds, glyburide (DiaBeta, Micronase) and glipizide (Glucotrol); renal insufficiency perpetuates the blood glucose–lowering effects of chlorpropamide, acetohexamide, tolazamide, glyburide, and glipizide. In the presence of other pharmacologic agents such as dicumarol, phenylbutazone, or certain sulfonamides, the hypoglycemic effects of sulfonylureas may be markedly prolonged.

3. SURREPTITIOUS INSULIN OR SULFONYLUREA ADMINISTRATION (Factitious Hypoglycemia)

Factitious hypoglycemia should be suspected in any patient with access to insulin or sulfonylurea drugs. It is most commonly seen in health professionals and diabetic patients or their relatives. The reasons for self-induced hypoglycemia vary, with many patients having severe psychiatric disturbances or a need for attention.

When insulin is used to induce hypoglycemia, an elevated serum insulin level often raises suspicion of an insulin-producing pancreatic B cell tumor. It may be difficult to prove that the insulin is of exogenous origin. The triad of hypoglycemia, high immunoreactive insulin levels, and suppressed plasma C-peptide immunoreactivity* is pathognomonic of exogenous insulin administration. Technical difficulties in measuring immunoreactive insulin, caused by the in-

*C peptide, a major portion of the connecting chain in amino acids in proinsulin, remains intact during the conversion of proinsulin to insulin in the B cell and is secreted in equimolar amounts with insulin (see Chapter 19).

appropriate presence of circulating antibodies (usually seen only in insulin-treated individuals) will generally support the diagnosis of factitious hypoglycemia. However, the absence of detectable insulin antibodies does not rule out the possibility of exogenous insulin administration, especially with the advent of new highly purified pork and human insulins with low immunogenicity in humans.

When sulfonylurea abuse is suspected, plasma and urine should be screened for its presence. Hyperinsulinism may not persist despite sustained hypoglycemia from a sulfonylurea overdose.

Treatment of factitious hypoglycemia involves psychiatric therapy and social counseling.

4. AUTOIMMUNE HYPOGLYCEMIA

In recent years, a rare autoimmune disorder has been reported in which patients have circulating insulin antibodies and the paradoxic feature of hypoglycemia. While many of these patients may be surreptitiously administering insulin, an increasing number of case reports have not been able to document exogenous insulin as the inducer of the insulin antibodies. Hypoglycemia results from sudden dissociation of insulin antibody immune complexes.

Hypoglycemia due to insulin receptor autoantibodies is also an extremely rare syndrome, reported in only 6 patients. All of these patients have also had episodes of insulin-resistant diabetes and acanthosis nigricans. Their hypoglycemia is attributed to an agonistic action of the antibody on the insulin receptor. Balance between the antagonistic and agonistic effects of the antibody determines whether insulin-resistant diabetes or hypoglycemia occurs. Hypoglycemia was found to respond to glucocorticoid therapy but not to plasmapheresis or immunosuppression.

5. PENTAMIDINE-INDUCED HYPOGLYCEMIA

Pentamidine, an investigational drug in the USA, is available through the Centers for Disease Control. With the increasing use of this agent for treatment of *Pneumocystis carinii* infection in patients with acquired immunodeficiency syndrome (AIDS), more reports of pentamidine-induced hypoglycemia are appearing. The cause of acute hyperglycemia appears to be the drug's lytic effect on B cells, which produces acute hyperinsulinemia followed by insulinopenia and diabetes. Physicians treating patients with pentamidine should be aware of the potential complication of acute hypoglycemia.

6. PANCREATIC B CELL TUMORS

Spontaneous fasting hypoglycemia in an otherwise healthy adult is most commonly due to **insulinoma,** an insulin-secreting tumor of the islets of Langerhans. Eighty percent of these tumors are single and benign; 10% are malignant (if metastases are identified); and the remaining 10% are multiple, with scattered micro- or macroadenomas interspersed within normal islet tissue. (As with some other endocrine tumors, histologic differentiation between benign and malignant cells is difficult, and close follow-up is necessary to ensure the absence of metastases.) Diffuse B cell hyperplasia has rarely been documented as a cause of hypoglycemia in adults.

These adenomas may be familial and have been found in conjunction with tumors of the parathyroid glands and the pituitary (multiple endocrine neoplasia type I). (See Chapter 25.) Ninety-nine percent of them are located within the pancreas and less than 1% in ectopic pancreatic tissue.

These tumors may appear at any age, although they are most common in the fourth to sixth decades. There is no sex predilection.

Clinical Findings

The signs and symptoms are predominantly those of subacute neuroglycopenia rather than adrenergic discharge. The typical picture is that of recurrent central nervous system dysfunction at times of exercise or fasting. The preponderance of neurologic symptoms rather than those commonly associated with hypoglycemia (adrenergic symptoms) often leads to delayed diagnosis following prolonged psychiatric care or treatment for seizure disorders or transient ischemic attacks. Some patients learn to relieve or prevent their symptoms by taking frequent feedings. Obesity may be the result; however, obesity is seen in less than 30% of patients with insulin-secreting tumors.

Diagnosis of Insulinoma

B cell tumors do not reduce secretion in the presence of hypoglycemia, and a serum insulin level of 10 μU/mL or more with concomitant plasma glucose values below 45 mg/dL suggests an insulinoma. Other causes of hyperinsulinemic hypoglycemia must be considered, however, such as surreptitious administration of insulin or sulfonylureas.

A. Insulin Assay: Because the insulin radioimmunoassay is crucial in diagnosing insulin-secreting tumors, it is important to be aware of certain limitations in its use. It detects not only human but also beef and pork insulins, and a high level may therefore indicate either endogenous or exogenous insulin. (C-peptide measurements are necessary to make this distinction.) In addition, the assay is of no value in patients who have ever taken insulin, as virtually all will have developed low-titer insulin antibodies that will interfere. Falsely low or elevated values will result, depending on the method used. Collection of samples is also important: If they are not frozen immediately, falsely low values will result, because the insulin molecule will undergo proteolytic digestion.

B. Suppression Tests: Failure of endogenous insulin secretion to be suppressed in the presence of

hypoglycemia is the hallmark of an insulin-secreting tumor. The most reliable suppression test is the prolonged supervised fast in hospitalized subjects, and this remains the preferred diagnostic maneuver in the workup of suspected insulinomas.

1. Prolonged fasting–In normal men, the blood glucose value will not fall below 55 mg/dL during a 72-hour fast, while insulin levels fall below 10 μU/mL; in some normal women, however, plasma glucose may fall below 30 mg/dL (lower limits have not been established), while serum insulin levels also fall appropriately. (These women remain asymptomatic despite this degree of hypoglycemia, presumably because ketogenesis is able to provide sufficient fuel for the central nervous system.) Calculation of ratios of insulin (in μU/mL) to plasma glucose (in mg/dL) is useful diagnostically. Nonobese normal subjects maintain a ratio of less than 0.25; obese subjects may have an elevated ratio, but hypoglycemia does not occur with fasting. Virtually all patients with insulin-secreting islet cell tumors will have an abnormal insulin:glucose ratio at some time during a 72-hour fast. The majority of these will experience progressive and symptomatic fasting hypoglycemia with associated elevated insulin levels within 24– 36 hours and no evidence of ketonuria. However, an occasional patient will not demonstrate hypoglycemia until 72 hours have elapsed. Brisk exercise during the fast may help precipitate hypoglycemia. Once symptoms of hypoglycemia occur, plasma glucose should be obtained and the fast immediately terminated if plasma glucose is below 45 mg/dL.

2. Acute B cell suppression with exogenous insulin–Whereas normal subjects will suppress C-peptide levels to 50% of baseline or less during hypoglycemia (induced by infusing 0.1 unit of insulin per kilogram of body weight per hour), absence of suppression suggests the presence of an autonomous insulin-secreting tumor. However, the lower limits of this assay are often not reliable, and a diagnosis should not be made solely on the basis of failure of C-peptide suppression during this test.

C. Stimulation Tests: A variety of stimulation tests with intravenous tolbutamide, glucagon, or calcium have been devised to demonstrate exaggerated and prolonged insulin secretion. However, because insulin-secreting tumors have a wide range of granular content and degrees of differentiation, they are variably responsive to these secretagogues. Thus, absence of an excessive insulin secretory response during any of these stimulation tests does not rule out the presence of an insulinoma. In addition, the tests may be extremely hazardous to patients with responsive tumors by inducing prolonged and refractory hypoglycemia. (None of these secretagogues should be given to a patient when hypoglycemia is present.) The following stimulation tests should be reserved for the difficult case in which results of a prolonged fast are equivocal. They can also be useful for screening when the index of suspicion for an insulin-secreting tumor is low.

1. Tolbutamide stimulation test–One gram of

sodium tolbutamide dissolved in 20 mL of distilled water is infused intravenously over 2 minutes. Serum insulin is measured every 5 minutes for 15 minutes; a level exceeding 195 μU/mL during this time suggests an insulin-secreting tumor. However, this response is seen in only 60% or less of patients with insulinomas, and false-positive results may occur (eg, with obesity or hepatic disease). Continuation of the test beyond 15 minutes will uncover additional patients with insulinomas by demonstrating prolonged elevations of insulin; however, hazardous hypoglycemia may result.

2. Glucagon stimulation test–One milligram of glucagon is given intravenously, and serum insulin levels are measured every 5 minutes for 15 minutes. A level exceeding 135 μU/mL suggests an insulin-secreting tumor. However, only approximately 50% of patients with insulinomas will demonstrate this hyperinsulinism, and false-positive results may occur. When an exaggerated increase in serum insulin occurs, the hyperglycemic effect of glucagon may be subnormal, and profound hypoglycemia may subsequently develop by 60 minutes.

3. Calcium infusion test–Calcium gluconate (10 mg/kg body weight administered intravenously over a 2-hour period) stimulates hypersecretion of insulin in some patients with insulinomas, but false-negative results limit its usefulness. Also, one must consider possible toxic cardiac arrhythmias, which could result from provoking hypoglycemia in the presence of hypercalcemia.

D. Oral Glucose Tolerance Test: The oral glucose tolerance test is of no value in the diagnosis of insulin-secreting tumors.

A common misconception is that patients with insulinomas will have flat glucose tolerance curves, because the tumor will discharge insulin in response to oral glucose. In fact, most insulinomas respond poorly, and curves typical of diabetes are more common. In those rare tumors that do release insulin in response to glucose, a flat curve may result; however, this is also seen in normal subjects.

E. Euglycemic Clamp: Continuous blood glucose monitoring with feedback-controlled dextrose infusion by an artificial pancreas has been used to demonstrate excessive dextrose requirements to maintain fasting euglycemia in insulinoma patients. This test remains experimental; however, it has the advantage of avoiding hypoglycemia during a supervised fast.

F. Proinsulin Measurements: Normally, less than 20% of fasting plasma insulin immunoreactivity is due to proinsulin released directly into the bloodstream from the pancreatic B cell. Insulin-secreting pancreatic tumors often secrete an excessive amount of proinsulin. However, hyperproinsulinemia is not specific for insulinomas, since familial hyperproinsulinemia (without hypoglycemia or hyperglycemia) has been reported. Furthermore, proinsulin assays are not readily available, and—although the results may have academic interest—the tests are seldom diagnostic.

G. Glycohemoglobin Measurements: Low gly-cohemoglobin values have been reported in occasional cases of insulinoma, reflecting the presence of chronic hypoglycemia. However, the diagnostic usefulness of glycohemoglobin measurements is limited by the relatively low sensitivity of this test as well as poor accuracy at the lower range of normal in many of the assays. In addition, it is nonspecific for hypoglycemia, with low levels being found in certain hemoglobin-opathies and hemolytic states.

H. Tumor Localization Studies:

1. Imaging studies–The diagnosis of an insulin-secreting tumor is dependent on biochemical testing. Since most tumors are too small (80% are < 2 cm) to localize by current ultrasonography and CT scanning, a negative result will not be conclusive.

Arteriography is presently the most effective method for preoperative localization of small tumors, particularly if catheterization of small arterial branches and subbranches of the celiac artery (selective and subselective arteriography) is combined with subtraction and magnification methods. However, even with these advances, arteriography is seldom helpful enough to outweigh its disadvantages, and it remains a painful and relatively imprecise procedure that exposes insulinoma patients to the risk of hypoglycemia and the discomfort of several hours of invasive and expensive radiography. In most cases, a tumor mass large enough to "blush" on arteriography is large enough for an experienced surgeon to identify by direct visualization or palpation. In addition, false-positive and false-negative results are so common that reliance on operative localization by an experienced surgeon has preempted the use of arteriography in a growing number of medical centers.

2. Transhepatic portal vein sampling–Demonstration of insulin gradients or "step-ups" in insulin concentration in the pancreatic venous effluent is becoming the method of choice in localizing small insulin-secreting tumors. The procedure entails percutaneous transhepatic portal vein catheterization under local anesthesia with subsequent cannulation of the splenic vein. Samples for insulin are obtained along the splenic and portal venous systems in an attempt to show a gradient of 300 μU/mL or more of insulin concentration that would evidence a tumor. Results may be equivocal, however, because of the high rate of blood flow in these venous systems and the consequent dilution of insulin values. In addition, this uncomfortable procedure is not without complications; bile leakage, intraperitoneal hemorrhage, and infection have been reported. Since diazoxide would interfere with this test, it should be discontinued for at least 48–72 hours before sampling. An infusion of dextrose may be required, therefore, and patients should be closely monitored during the procedure to avoid hypoglycemia (as well as hyperglycemia, which could affect insulin gradients). Venous sampling is indicated for cases in which hypoglycemia does not respond to diazoxide (see below), so that surgical removal of the insulinoma is therefore mandated. In this instance, only an angiographer with extensive experience in the technique should perform the procedure.

Treatment of Insulinoma

The treatment of choice for insulin-secreting tumors is surgical resection. A flow diagram for the approach to these patients is shown in Fig 20–2.

A. Surgical Treatment: Tumor resection should be performed only by surgeons with extensive experience with islet cell tumors, since these tumors may be small and difficult to recognize. An 85% success rate has been reported without localization procedures if surgeons have prior experience with insulinomas.

1. Preoperative management–

a. Trial of diazoxide–Oral diazoxide (Proglycem), a potent inhibitor of insulin secretion, will maintain euglycemia in most patients with insulin-secreting tumors. Doses of 200–400 mg/d (divided) will usually suffice, but an occasional patient will require up to 1 g/d. Side effects include edema due to sodium retention (which generally necessitates concomitant thiazide administration), gastric irritation, and mild hirsutism.

b. Selection of patients–Patients who remain euglycemic on diazoxide may be operated on by an experienced surgeon, without attempts at preoperative tumor localization. Patients who do not respond to diazoxide or cannot tolerate its side effects are candidates for venous sampling studies in an attempt to localize the tumor preoperatively.

2. Treatment during surgery–

a. Glucose need during surgery–To estimate glucose needs during surgery, 5 or 10% dextrose should be infused a day or so before surgery to determine the approximate rate of glucose administration needed to maintain euglycemia. This amount can then be prescribed on the day of surgery; counterregulatory stress responses during surgery should ensure that additional glucose will probably not be required. However, plasma glucose should be monitored frequently to regulate glucose replacement during surgery, especially during manipulation of the pancreas. The recently developed ''closed loop'' artificial B cell system can aid in this regard. It is capable of monitoring blood glucose continuously and infusing sufficient dextrose to maintain euglycemia. It not only ensures maintenance of protective euglycemia; it can also provide evidence of complete removal of insulin-secreting tumor tissue by demonstrating a prompt fall in dextrose requirements and a prompt rise in blood glucose.

b. Diazoxide–Diazoxide should be administered preoperatively as well as on the day of surgery in patients who are responsive to it, since the drug greatly reduces the need for glucose supplements and the risk of hypoglycemia during surgery while not masking the glycemic rise indicative of surgical cure.

3. Postoperative hyperglycemia–Postoperatively, several days of hyperglycemia may ensue. This is due to a combination of factors, including edema and inflammation of the pancreas after surgery, high

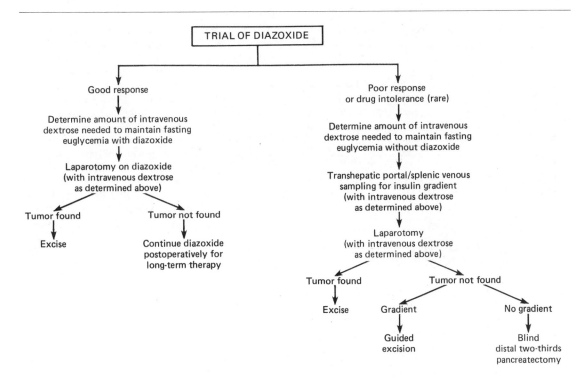

Figure 20–2. Management of patients with confirmed diagnosis of insulinoma.

levels of counterregulatory hormones induced by the procedure, chronic down-regulation of insulin receptors by the previously high circulating insulin levels in the tumor, and perhaps suppression of normal pancreatic B cells by long-standing hypoglycemia. Small subcutaneous doses of regular insulin may be prescribed every 4–6 hours if plasma glucose exceeds 300 mg/dL, but in most cases pancreatic insulin secretion recovers after 48–72 hours and very little insulin replacement is required.

4. Failure to find the tumor at operation–In approximately 10% of patients with biochemically demonstrated autonomous insulin secretion, no tumor can be found at exploratory laparotomy. The tumor will most likely be in the head of the pancreas, as this is the most difficult area for the surgeon to mobilize and explore; therefore, blind distal two-thirds pancreatectomy is seldom successful. Rather than subject a patient to the increased risk of partial pancreatectomy in such cases, it is best to let the prior response to diazoxide therapy dictate the proper procedure (Fig 20–2). If the patient has responded to diazoxide, this can be continued indefinitely. If the patient has not responded or is intolerant of diazoxide therapy, and if preoperative venous sampling has not been helpful in localizing a tumor, then—and only then—a blind distal two-thirds pancreatectomy should be performed. This procedure has a success rate of only 25%.

B. Medical Treatment: Diazoxide therapy is the treatment of choice in patients with inoperable functioning islet cell carcinomas and in those who are poor candidates for operation. Many patients have been maintained on long-term (> 10 years) diazoxide therapy without apparent ill effects. Frequent carbohydrate feedings (every 2–3 hours) can also be helpful in maintaining euglycemia, although obesity may become a problem.

Streptozocin has proved beneficial in patients with islet cell carcinomas, and effective doses have been achieved without the undue renal toxicity that characterized early experience. Benign tumors appear to respond poorly, if at all.

SYMPTOMATIC FASTING HYPOGLYCEMIA WITHOUT HYPERINSULINISM

1. DISORDERS ASSOCIATED WITH LOW HEPATIC GLUCOSE OUTPUT

Reduced hepatic gluconeogenesis can result from a direct loss of hepatic tissue (acute yellow atrophy from fulminating viral or toxic damage); from disorders reducing amino acid supply to hepatic parenchyma (severe muscle wasting and inanition from anorexia nervosa, chronic starvation, uremia, and glucocorticoid deficit from adrenocortical deficiency); or from inborn errors of carbohydrate metabolism affecting glycogenolytic or gluconeogenic enzymes.

2. ETHANOL HYPOGLYCEMIA

Ethanol impairs hepatic gluconeogenesis but has no effect on hepatic glycogenolysis. In the patient who is imbibing ethanol but not eating, fasting hypoglycemia may occur after hepatic glycogen stores have been depleted (within 8–12 hours of a fast). No correlation exists between the blood ethanol levels and the degree of hypoglycemia, which may occur while blood ethanol levels are declining. (It should be noted that ethanol-induced fasting hypoglycemia may occur at ethanol levels as low as 45 mg/dL—considerably below most states' legal standards [100 mg/dL] for being "under the influence.") Most patients present with neuroglycopenic symptoms, which may be difficult to differentiate from the neurotoxic effects of the alcohol. These symptoms in a patient whose breath smells of alcohol may be mistaken for alcoholic stupor. Intravenous dextrose should be administered promptly to all such stuporous or comatose patients. Because hepatic glycogen stores have been depleted by the time hypoglycemia occurs, parenteral glucagon or epinephrine will not be effective. Adequate food intake during alcohol ingestion will prevent this type of hypoglycemia.

3. NONPANCREATIC TUMORS

A variety of nonpancreatic tumors have been found to cause fasting hypoglycemia. Most are large and mesenchymal in origin, retroperitoneal fibrosarcoma being the classic prototype. However, hepatocellular carcinomas, adrenal cortical carcinomas, hypernephromas, gastrointestinal tumors, lymphomas and leukemias, and a variety of other tumors have also been reported. The mechanisms by which these tumors produce hypoglycemia are not entirely clear. None has been unequivocally shown to secrete insulin; thus, true ectopic hyperinsulinemia probably does not exist. Up to 50% of these tumors have been reported to secrete low-molecular-weight peptides with insulin-like activity. These NSILA peptides (so-called because of their nonsuppressible insulinlike activity) include human insulinlike growth factors and some of the somatomedins. Whether further refinement in the assays for these peptides will allow the demonstration of NSILA in all cases of nonpancreatic tumors that are associated with hypoglycemia remains to be seen. Treatment is aimed toward the primary tumor, with supportive therapy using frequent feedings. Diazoxide is ineffective in reversing the hypoglycemia caused by these tumors.

NONFASTING HYPOGLYCEMIA
(Reactive Hypoglycemia)

Reactive hypoglycemia may be classified as early (within 2– 3 hours of a meal) or late (at 3– 5 hours). Early (alimentary) hypoglycemia occurs when there is a rapid discharge of ingested carbohydrate into the small bowel followed by rapid glucose absorption and hyperinsulinism. It may be seen after gastrointestinal surgery and is notably associated with the "dumping syndrome" after gastrectomy; occasionally, it is functional and may result from overactivity of the parasympathetic nervous system mediated via the vagus nerve. Late hypoglycemia (occult diabetes) is caused by a delay in early insulin release, which then results in exaggeration of initial hyperglycemia during a glucose tolerance test. As a consequence, an exaggerated insulin response produces late hypoglycemia. Early or late hypoglycemia may also occur as a consequence of ethanol's potentiation of the insulin-secretory response to glucose, as when sugar-containing soft drinks are used as mixers to dilute alcohol in beverages (gin and tonic, rum and cola).

1. POSTGASTRECTOMY ALIMENTARY HYPOGLYCEMIA

Reactive hypoglycemia after gastrectomy is a consequence of hyperinsulinism. This results from rapid gastric emptying of ingested food, which produces overstimulation of vagal reflexes and overproduction of beta-cytotrophic gastrointestinal hormones, causing arterial hyperinsulinism and consequent acute hypoglycemia. The symptoms are caused by adrenergic hyperactivity in response to the rapidly falling plasma glucose. Treatment is properly directed at avoiding this sequence of events by more frequent feedings with smaller portions of less rapidly assimilated carbohydrate and more slowly absorbed fat or protein. Occasionally, anticholinergic drugs such as propantheline (15 mg orally 4 times daily) may be useful in reducing vagal overactivity.

2. FUNCTIONAL ALIMENTARY HYPOGLYCEMIA

Early alimentary-type reactive hypoglycemia in a patient who has not undergone surgery is classified as functional. It is most often associated with chronic fatigue, anxiety, irritability, weakness, poor concentration, decreased libido, headaches, hunger after meals, and tremulousness. Whether or not hypoglycemia actually accounts for these symptoms or actually occurs at all is difficult to prove.

The usual sequence of events is that the patient presents with a number of nonspecific complaints. Normal laboratory findings and a normal physical examination confirm the initial impression that organic disease is not present, and the symptoms are then attributed to the stresses of modern living. The only form of therapy usually given is reassurance or a mild tranquilizer. When this fails to be of benefit, the patient seeks help elsewhere. Inevitably, the question of hypoglycemia is raised—frequently by the patient, who has heard of the diagnosis from friends or relatives with similar symptoms or has read of it in the lay press. The diagnosis is often supported by the demonstration of hypoglycemia with symptoms during a 5-hour oral glucose tolerance test.

Unfortunately, the precipitation of hypoglycemia with or without symptoms during oral glucose tolerance testing does not distinguish between normal and "hypoglycemic" patients. As many as one-third or more of normal subjects who have never had any symptoms will develop hypoglycemia with or without symptoms during a 5-hour glucose tolerance test. In addition, many patients will develop symptoms in the absence of hypoglycemia. Thus, the test's nonspecificity makes it a highly unreliable tool that is no longer recommended for evaluating patients with suspected episodes of postprandial hypoglycemia. In 1983, Hogan et al reported that ingestion of a mixed meal did not produce hypoglycemia in 33 patients who had been diagnosed as having reactive hypoglycemia on the basis of oral glucose tolerance testing; this attempt to increase specificity for the diagnosis of reactive hypoglycemia resulted in loss of sensitivity. For increased diagnostic reliability, hypoglycemia should be documented during a spontaneous symptomatic episode in routine daily activity. However, attempts to demonstrate this are almost never successful. Patients should be instructed in the proper use of Chemstrip bG, whose color development is stable enough to allow test strips to be saved and brought to the physician's office for documentation up to 72 hours after the measurement was made. Personality evaluation suggestive of hyperkinetic compulsive behavior in thin, anxious patients is often found.

The foregoing discussion should not be taken to imply that functional reactive hypoglycemia does not occur—merely that at present we have no reliable means of diagnosing it. There is no harm (and there is occasional benefit) in reducing or eliminating the content of refined sugars in the patient's diet while increasing the frequency and reducing the size of meals. However, it should not be expected that these maneuvers will cure the asthenia, since the reflex response to hypoglycemia is only a possibly aggravating feature of a generalized primary hyperactivity. Counseling and support and mild sedation should be the mainstays in therapy, with dietary manipulation only an adjunct.

3. LATE HYPOGLYCEMIA
(Occult Diabetes)

This condition is characterized by delay in early insulin release from pancreatic B cells, resulting in initial exaggeration of hyperglycemia during a glucose tolerance test. In response to this hyperglycemia, an exaggerated insulin release produces late hypoglycemia 4– 5 hours after ingestion of glucose. These patients are usually quite different from those with early hypoglycemia, being more phlegmatic and often obese and frequently having a family history of diabetes mellitus. In the obese, treatment is directed at reduction to ideal weight. These patients often respond to reduced intake of refined sugars with multiple, spaced small feedings high in dietary fiber. They should be considered early diabetics and advised to have periodic medical evaluations.

REFERENCES

Berger M et al: Functional and morphological characterization of human insulinomas. *Diabetes* 1983;**32**:921.

Bouchard T et al: Diabetes mellitus following pentamidine-induced hypoglycemia in humans. *Diabetes* 1982;**31**:40.

Cryer PE: Glucose counterregulation in man. *Diabetes* 1981;**30**:261.

Cryer PE, Gerich JE: Relevance of glucose counterregulatory systems to patients with diabetes: Critical roles of glucagon and epinephrine. *Diabetes Care* 1983;**6**:95.

Daggett PR et al: Is preoperative localization of insulinomas necessary? *Lancet* 1981;**1**:483.

Feingold KR: Hypoglycemia: A pitfall of insulin therapy. *West J Med* 1983;**139**:688.

Hogan MJ et al: Oral glucose tolerance test compared with a mixed meal in the diagnosis of reactive hypoglycemia. *Mayo Clin Proc* 1983;**58**:491.

Johnson DD et al: Reactive hypoglycemia. *JAMA* 1980;**243**:1151.

Kahn CR: The riddle of tumor hypoglycemia revisited. *Clin Endocrinol Metab* 1980;**9**:335.

Service FJ (editor): *Hypoglycemia Disorders: Pathogenesis, Diagnosis and Treatment.* G. K. Hall, 1983.

Taylor SI et al: Hypoglycemia associated with antibodies to the insulin receptor. *N Engl J Med* 1982;**307**:1422.

Williams HE: Alcoholic hypoglycemia and ketoacidosis. *Med Clin North Am* 1984;**68**:33.

Disorders of Lipoprotein Metabolism

21

John P. Kane, MD, PhD, & Mary J. Malloy, MD

The clinical importance of hyperlipoproteinemia derives chiefly from the role of lipoproteins in atherogenesis. However, the greatly increased risk of acute pancreatitis associated with severe hypertriglyceridemia is an additional indication for intervention. Detection and characterization of hyperlipoproteinemia is important for selection of appropriate treatment and may provide clues to underlying primary clinical disorders.

Arteriosclerosis

Arteriosclerosis is the leading cause of death in the USA. Abundant epidemiologic evidence establishes the multifactorial character of this disease and indicates that the effects of the multiple risk factors are at least additive. Risk factors that have been convincingly identified for atherosclerosis of the coronary arteries are hyperlipidemia, arterial hypertension, cigarette smoking, diabetes mellitus, physical inactivity, and decreased levels of high-density lipoproteins (HDL) in plasma. Coronary atheromas are complex lesions containing cellular elements, collagen, and lipids. It is clear, however, that the progression of the lesion is chiefly attributable to its content of unesterified cholesterol and cholesteryl esters. It is now firmly established that the cholesterol in the atheroma is delivered to the site by circulating lipoproteins. Epidemiologic evidence indicates that the atherogenic lipoproteins are the low-density (LDL), intermediate-density (IDL), and very low density (VLDL) species, all of which contain the B-100 apoprotein. Interaction between this apoprotein and a mucopolysaccharide (chondroitin sulfate B) of the artery wall may play an important role in the degradation of lipoproteins in situ. In animal models, hypertension is associated with increased access of lipoprotein to the subintimal region. Smoking may accelerate the process of atherogenesis chiefly through its influence on blood platelets, though it is also associated with decreased levels of HDL in plasma. Increased platelet interaction at sites of damaged endothelium leads to release of platelet-derived growth factor (PDGF), which stimulates migration of cells of smooth muscle origin into the lesion, where they proliferate. Cholesteryl esters appear in macrophages in the atheroma. Along with free cholesterol, they also appear in the extracellular matrix, where they induce the production of collagen by fibroblasts. The inverse relationship between plasma

Acronyms Used in This Chapter

ACAT	Acyl-CoA:cholesterol acyltransferase
Apo-	Apolipoprotein or apoprotein
CoA	Coenzyme A
FFA	Free fatty acids
HDL	High-density lipoprotein(s)
HMG-CoA	Hydroxymethylglutaryl-CoA
IDDM	Insulin-dependent diabetes mellitus
IDL	Intermediate-density lipoprotein(s)
LCAT	Lecithin:cholesterol acyltransferase
LDL	Low-density lipoprotein(s)
LPL	Lipoprotein lipase
NIDDM	Non–insulin-dependent diabetes mellitus
PDGF	Platelet-derived growth factor
VLDL	Very low density lipoprotein(s)

HDL levels and the rate of atherogenesis probably reflects the involvement of at least certain species of HDL in the movement of cholesterol away from the atheroma.

Reversal of Atherosclerosis

A number of studies in animals, including higher primates, indicate that atherosclerotic coronary disease resulting from diet-induced hyperlipidemia is reversible when levels of lipoproteins in plasma are restored to normal. These findings support the concept that the atheroma is a dynamic lesion. The striking similarity of the lesions induced in primates to early lesions occurring in human coronary arteries suggests that the progression of human lesions could also be retarded or perhaps that regression could occur if hyperlipidemia were controlled. The results of several recent intervention studies in humans indicate that the progression of atheromas in coronary and femoral arteries can indeed be retarded by moderate reductions of levels of atherogenic lipoproteins in serum. More effective treatments that are emerging may be capable of at least partial reversal of atheromas.

It should be noted that average levels of LDL in plasma in the United States population are considerably higher than in many other nations, where the levels appear to approach the biologic norm for humans. This probably accounts in large part for the markedly higher incidence of coronary vascular disease in industrialized Western nations and suggests that dietary changes that reduce lipoprotein levels toward normal would be beneficial.

OVERVIEW OF LIPID TRANSPORT

The Plasma Lipoproteins

Because all the lipids of plasma are relatively insoluble in water, they are transported in association with proteins. The simplest complexes are those formed between unesterified, or free, fatty acids (FFA) and albumin, which serve to carry the FFA from peripheral adipocytes to other tissues. Similarly, lysolecithins (phospholipids formed when 1 mol of fatty acid is removed from lecithin) are bound to albumin.

The remainder of the plasma lipids are transported in lipoprotein complexes (Table 21–1). All of the major lipoproteins of plasma are spherical, and each has a core region containing hydrophobic lipids. The principal core lipids are cholesteryl esters and triglycerides (Fig 21–1). Triglycerides predominate in the cores of the chylomicrons, which transport newly absorbed lipids from the intestine, and in the cores of the very low density lipoproteins, which originate in the liver. The relative content of cholesteryl ester is increased in remnants derived from these 2 classes of lipoproteins, and cholesteryl esters predominate in the cores of low-density and high-density lipoproteins. Surrounding the core in each type of lipoprotein is a stabilizing monolayer containing amphiphilic (detergentlike) lipids, chiefly phospholipids and unesterified cholesterol (frequently termed free cholesterol). Amphiphilic (or amphipathic) lipids are characterized by having a polar or charged region that associates readily with the aqueous environment surrounding the lipoprotein particle and a hydrophobic region that preferentially interacts with hydrophobic core lipids. Proteins called apoproteins (also called apolipoproteins), which are noncovalently bound to the lipids, are mostly located in or on this surface monolayer.

B Apoproteins

Several of the lipoproteins contain proteins of very high molecular weight known as the B apoproteins, which behave like intrinsic proteins of cell membranes. Unlike the smaller apoproteins, the B apoproteins do not migrate from one lipoprotein particle to another. The B apoproteins of intestinal and hepatic origin are different. They are now described by numbers in a centile system based on the relative apparent molecular weights of the different species. Thus, VLDL contain the B-100 protein, which is retained in the formation of LDL from VLDL remnants by the liver. The intestinal B protein, B-48, is found in chylomicrons and their remnant particles but is completely absent from LDL.

Other Apoproteins

In addition to the B apoproteins, the following apoproteins are present in lipoproteins. (The distribution of these proteins in the different lipoproteins is shown in Table 21–1.)

(1) C apoproteins: These are low-molecular-weight (7000–10,000) proteins that equilibrate rapidly among the lipoproteins. There are 3 distinct species with unique amino acid sequences, designated C-I, C-II, and C-III. Apoproteins C-II and C-III each have several subspecies with slightly differing electrostatic charges. Apoprotein C-II has been identified as a requisite cofactor for lipoprotein lipase.

(2) E apoproteins: At least 2 normal isoforms (E-3 and E-4) of this MW-35,000 protein appear to be the products of allelic genes. Normal individuals thus may have either or both isoforms, which share with B-100 protein the property of interacting with certain high-affinity receptors (B-100-E receptors) on cell membranes. Another isoform (E-2), which lacks this property, contains one more mole of cysteine than E-3 and 2 more than E-4. About 15% of individuals are heterozygous for this isoform.

(3) Apoprotein A-I: This protein of MW 28,300 is the major apoprotein of HDL; it is also present in chylomicrons and is the most abundant of the apoproteins of human serum (about 125 mg/dL). It is a cofactor for lecithin:cholesterol acyltransferase (LCAT).

(4) Apoprotein A-II: This protein of MW 17,400 is an important constituent of HDL. It contains cysteine, which permits the formation of disulfide-bridged oligomers with apo-E.

Table 21–1. Major lipoproteins of human serum.

Lipoprotein	Electrophoretic Mobility in Agarose Gel	Density Interval g/cm³	Predominant Core Lipids	Diameter	Apolipoproteins in Order of Quantitative Importance
High-density (HDL)	Alpha	1.21–1.063	Cholesteryl ester	7.5–10.5 nm	A-I, A-II, C, E, D
Low-density (LDL)	Beta	1.063–1.019	Cholesteryl ester	~21.5 nm	B-100, B-74, B-26
Intermediate-density (IDL)	Beta	1.019–1.006	Cholesteryl ester, triglyceride	25–30 nm	B-100, some C and E
Very low density (VLDL)	Prebeta; some "slow prebeta"	< 1.006	Triglyceride	30–100 nm	B-100, C, E
Chylomicrons	Remain at origin	< 1.006	Triglyceride	80–500 nm	B-48, C, E, A-I, A-II, A-IV, proline-rich apoprotein

Figure 21–1. Major lipids of plasma lipoproteins. R = hydrocarbon chain of a fatty acid.

(5) D apoprotein: This protein of MW 35,000 catalyzes the transfer of cholesteryl ester to acceptor lipoproteins from the lipoprotein subspecies of HDL that contain LCAT.

(6) Apoprotein A-IV: This protein of MW 46,000 is chiefly associated with chylomicrons.

(7) Proline-rich protein: This protein of MW 74,000 is associated with chylomicrons and occurs also as a multimer in plasma that is not associated with lipoproteins.

An additional apoprotein, the Lp(a) protein, is found in association with a minor species of lipoprotein, the Lp(a) lipoprotein that occurs in the density interval 1.030–1.090 g/cm³.

Absorption of Dietary Fat; Secretion of Chylomicrons

Dietary triglycerides are largely hydrolyzed in the intestine to β-monoglyceride and fatty acids by pancreatic lipase. This enzyme requires activation by bile acids and a protein cofactor. The partial glycerides and fatty acids form micelles that are absorbed by intestinal epithelial cells. Within these cells, the fatty acids are reesterified with the monoglyceride to form triglycerides. Some dietary cholesterol absorbed with the micelles is esterified by the acyl-CoA:cholesterol acyltransferase (ACAT) system, and some appears as free cholesterol in the surface monolayers of the chylomicrons. Droplets of triglyceride containing small amounts of cholesteryl esters form in the vesicles of the Golgi apparatus. Phospholipids and free cholesterol form a surface monolayer. Some of the phospholipid originates in bile, some is from dietary sources, and some is synthesized by the intestine. Newly synthesized apoprotein B-48, apoprotein A-I, and apoprotein A-II are added, and the nascent chylomicron emerges into the extracellular lymph space (Fig 21–2). Chylomicrons have diameters ranging from about 80 nm to 500 nm. Once in the lymph spaces, the new chylomicron begins to exchange surface components with HDL, acquiring C apoproteins and apo-E and losing phospholipids. This process continues as the chylomicron is carried via the intestinal lymphatics to the thoracic duct and thence into the bloodstream. Increased triglyceride transport from the intestine results chiefly in an increase of particle diameter of chylomicrons rather than increased numbers of particles.

Formation of Very Low Density Lipoproteins

The liver exports triglycerides to peripheral tissues in the cores of very low density lipoproteins (Fig 21–3). These triglycerides are synthesized in liver from free fatty acids abstracted from plasma and from fatty acids synthesized de novo. Acetyl-CoA for de novo synthesis is derived from the catabolism of carbohydrate, certain amino acids, and acetate formed

Figure 21–2. Metabolism of chylomicrons. TG = triglyceride; CE = cholesteryl esters; A-I, A-II, B-48, and C proteins = apoproteins. See text for details.

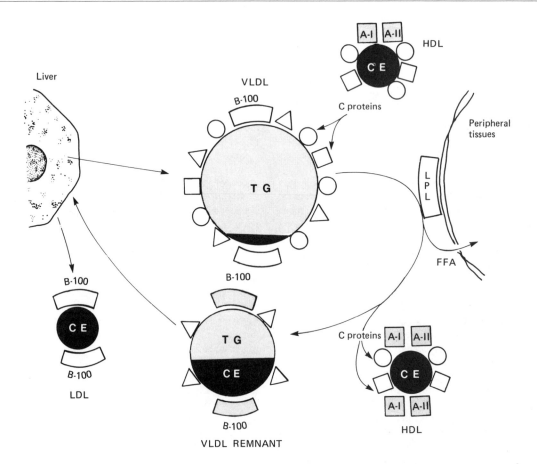

Figure 21–3. Metabolism of VLDL. TG = triglyceride; CE = cholesteryl esters; A-I, A-II, B-48, and C proteins = apoproteins. See text for details.

by oxidation of ethanol. Several major features distinguish VLDL from chylomicrons. The only B apoprotein of VLDL is B-100, and VLDL contain none of the major apoproteins of HDL. Whereas the intestine produces only very limited amounts of C apoproteins, the liver secretes the bulk of these proteins with newly formed VLDL. Upon reaching the plasma, the VLDL acquire still more C proteins from HDL and yield phospholipid in exchange. Release of VLDL by liver is increased by any condition that results in increased flux of FFA to liver in the absence of increased ketogenesis. Increased caloric intake, ingestion of ethanol, and the administration of estrogens all greatly stimulate release of VLDL from liver and are important causative factors in clinical disorders resulting in elevated levels of triglycerides in plasma.

Metabolism of Triglyceride-Rich Lipoproteins in Plasma

A. Hydrolysis by Lipoprotein Lipases: Fatty acids derived from the triglycerides of chylomicrons and VLDL are delivered to tissues predominantly through a common pathway involving hydrolysis by the lipoprotein lipase (LPL) system. Alternative pathways of low efficiency also degrade triglyceride-rich lipoproteins in peripheral tissues. These pathways can account for a larger than normal fraction of the degradation of VLDL and chylomicrons in patients with hypertriglyceridemia. Over three-fourths of the FFA derived during hydrolysis of triglycerides by LPL enters tissue directly. The remainder enters the pool of plasma FFA. Lipoprotein lipase enzymes are bound to capillary endothelium in heart, skeletal muscle, adipose tissue, mammary gland, and other tissues. The hydrolysis of triglycerides thus takes place within the vascular compartment. Removal of the first 2 fatty acids from the triglyceride appears to be mediated by LPL (triglyceridase and diglyceridase activities), whereas a separate monoglyceridase enzyme system is required for the last step.

B. Biologic Regulators of Lipoprotein Lipases: When glucose levels in plasma are elevated and the release of insulin is stimulated, LPL activity in adipose tissue increases, and fatty acids derived from triglycerides of circulating lipoproteins are stored. During prolonged fasting, however, LPL activity of adipose tissue falls to undetectable levels, completely preventing storage of fatty acids from VLDL and chylomicrons. The LPL activity of mammary gland is increased by the administration of estrogens and during lactation. Heparin, a mucopolysaccharide, is a cofactor for LPL. When heparin is given intravenously in doses of 0.1–0.2 mg/kg, LPL activity is displaced into plasma. This permits the in vitro measurement of LPL activity. An additional obligatory cofactor is one of the C apoproteins, C-II. Normally, the content of this apoprotein in plasma is far in excess of that required for activation of the LPL system.

C. Formation of Lipoprotein Remnants: Hydrolysis by LPL results in progressive depletion of the content of triglyceride in the hydrophobic core regions of chylomicrons and VLDL, producing a progressive decrease in particle diameter. Amphiphilic lipids from the surface monolayer are transported to HDL directly and also indirectly via membranes of cells, principally erythrocytes. This maintains an appropriate core:monolayer relationship for spheres of smaller diameters. During this process, C apoproteins—and, to a lesser extent, apo-E—are transferred to HDL. The product of this series of events is a "remnant" lipoprotein containing its original complement of apo-B, a portion of the original amount of apo-E, and little apo-C. In the case of chylomicrons, apoproteins A-I and A-II also leave the particles and become part of the circulating mass of HDL. The remnant particles of VLDL are 25–30 nm in diameter, and those of chylomicrons are up to 80 nm in diameter. Remnant particles are found both in the d < 1.006 g/cm³ fraction of plasma and in the IDL fraction (1.006 < d < 1.019 g/cm³). They have lost about 70% of their original complement of triglyceride but are enriched in cholesteryl esters.

D. Fate of Lipoprotein Remnants: Chylomicron remnants are removed from blood quantitatively by high-affinity, receptor-mediated endocytosis in the liver. The receptors appear to interact with apo-E on the lipoproteins. The lipid constituents enter hepatic pools, and the B-48 protein appears to be degraded completely. The cholesterol derived from chylomicron remnants is the major mediator of feedback control of cholesterol biosynthesis in liver. Some VLDL remnants are removed from blood via the B-100-E receptors (see below) and are degraded. Those which escape uptake are transformed into LDL. Thus, the rate of removal of VLDL remnants by liver is a determinant of LDL production. The process of formation of LDL involves the removal of essentially all of the residual triglyceride and a portion of the cholesteryl esters and amphipathic lipids. The LDL particles contain chiefly cholesteryl esters in their core regions. They retain virtually all of the original complement of the B-100 protein but only traces of other apoproteins. In normal individuals, a major fraction of VLDL is converted to LDL, and all of the LDL apo-B comes from VLDL. In certain hypertriglyceridemic states, conversion of VLDL to LDL is decreased.

The fact that LDL originates from the metabolism of VLDL remnants suggests that increases of LDL in plasma can arise from an increased rate of secretion of precursor VLDL as well as from decreased catabolism of LDL. The formation of LDL from VLDL may also contribute to the clinical phenomenon referred to as the "beta shift." This is an increase of LDL (beta-lipoprotein) as hypertriglyceridemia is resolving. A classic example of the beta shift occurs following institution of adequate insulin treatment in ketoacidotic diabetes with lipemia. Insulin induces increased lipoprotein lipase activity, resulting in rapid conversion of VLDL to LDL. Because of its longer half-life, the LDL accumulates in plasma. Elevated levels of LDL may persist beyond the time when levels of triglyceride-rich lipoproteins have returned to normal.

E. Half-Lives of Lipoproteins: Normally, the half-life of chylomicron apo-B in plasma is 5–20 minutes; that of the apo-B in VLDL is 1–3 hours; and that of LDL is about 2½ days. At triglyceride levels of 800–1000 mg/dL, the lipoprotein lipase mechanism is at kinetic saturation; therefore, increases in the input of triglyceride-rich lipoproteins into plasma at those levels rapidly result in much higher levels.

F. Effect of Dietary Fat Restriction: Individuals consuming a typical North American diet (with about 45% of calories as fat) transport 75–100 g or more of triglyceride per day into plasma in chylomicrons, whereas the liver exports 10–30 g of triglyceride in VLDL. Thus, the flux of triglyceride into plasma can be influenced most acutely by restriction of dietary fat. When the removal mechanisms involving lipoprotein lipase are saturated and plasma triglyceride levels are measured in thousands of milligrams per deciliter, acute restriction of dietary triglyceride intake will usually produce a significant reduction in triglyceride levels. This intervention is important in the lipemic patient with impending pancreatitis. If symptoms suggest that an attack of pancreatitis is imminent, all oral intake should be eliminated and the patient should be maintained on parenteral glucose until the symptoms subside and triglyceride levels decrease to less than 1000 mg/dL.

Catabolism of
Low-Density Lipoproteins

A. Endocytosis via Specific High-Affinity Receptors: The catabolism of LDL appears to proceed by several mechanisms. The best-understood of these is a regulated adsorptive endocytosis mediated by high-affinity receptors on the cell membranes of virtually all types of cells. The receptors bind the apo-B protein of LDL. Because they also bind apo-E, they are called B-100-E receptors. The receptor region invaginates into the cell, forming an endocytotic vesicle that fuses with a lysosome. The apo-B of the LDL is degraded to amino acids, and the receptor returns to the cell membrane. The cholesteryl esters of the LDL core are hydrolyzed by a lysosomal hydrolase to yield free cholesterol, which passes to the cytosol, where it is utilized in the production of cell membrane bilayers. The free cholesterol suppresses the activity of hydroxymethylglutaryl-CoA (HMG-CoA) reductase, a rate-limiting enzyme in the biosynthetic pathway for cholesterol. Thus, the intake of cholesterol by this pathway decreases the formation of new cholesterol in the cell. Cholesterol entering the cell by this pathway in excess of need for membrane synthesis is esterified by the acyl-CoA:cholesterol acyltransferase (ACAT) system, chiefly forming cholesteryl oleate, which is stored in the cell. In addition to suppression of cholesterol biosynthesis, the entry of cholesterol via the LDL pathway leads to down-regulation of LDL receptors expressed on the cell surface, resulting in decreased uptake and catabolism of LDL.

B. Other Pathways: In addition to the high-affinity receptor-mediated pathway of degradation, LDL appears to be catabolized by at least 2 additional pathways. Macrophages take up chemically altered LDL by a high-capacity mechanism that is apparently not subject to feedback control. This mechanism resembles the uptake of other altered serum proteins. The biologic significance of this pathway remains unclear, because the chemical alterations of LDL that may occur in vivo have not yet been determined. LDL are also taken up by many types of cells by a low-affinity process.

Metabolism of
High-Density Lipoproteins

High-density lipoproteins, like the other major lipoproteins, have cholesteryl ester–filled core regions. On the basis of their flotation properties, there appear to be 2 major subclasses of HDL: HDL_3, of density 1.21–1.125, are about 7.5–10.5 nm in diameter; and HDL_2, of density 1.125–1.063, are about 9.5–10.5 nm in diameter. HDL_3 predominate in human serum. Males and females have nearly equal amounts of HDL_3 in their serum (about 300 mg/dL of total lipid and protein mass). Women, however, have greater amounts of HDL_2 than do men (about 80 mg/dL versus about 36 mg/dL). There is epidemiologic evidence that the inverse relationship between coronary risk and HDL levels is chiefly dependent upon the content of HDL_2 in plasma. Other evidence indicates that a number of subspecies of HDL exist which may have individual roles in lipid metabolism.

A. Sources of HDL: HDL arise from 2 sources. The liver secretes a form of nascent HDL that is a bilayer disk composed of phospholipid and unesterified cholesterol. Apoproteins E, A-I, and possibly A-II are associated with this nascent particle. It has a bilayer structure, because it contains essentially no hydrophobic lipid (Fig 21–4). It is rapidly transformed into spherical HDL particles by the action of LCAT. This enzyme transfers 1 mol of fatty acid from a lecithin molecule to the hydroxyl group of unesterified cholesterol, forming cholesteryl ester, which then enters the hydrophobic region between the lamellae of the bilayer. Lysolecithin, formed by transfer of the fatty acid from lecithin, leaves the lipoprotein complex, binds to albumin, and is transported to various tissues, where it is reacylated to form lecithin. The process of transesterification by LCAT rapidly forms sufficient cholesteryl ester to fill the hydrophobic core region to a spherical shape.

LCAT enzyme is secreted by liver. In severe hepatic parenchymal disease, levels of this enzyme in plasma are low and esterification of cholesterol is impeded, leading to the accumulation of free cholesterol in lipoproteins and in membranes of erythrocytes and other cells. Excess free cholesterol in the membranes of erythrocytes transforms them into the target cells classically associated with hepatic parenchymal disease.

Figure 21–4. Schematic diagram depicting conversion of hepatic discoidal HDL to spherical plasma HDL.

HDL also originate from the catabolism of chylomicrons. Nascent chylomicrons contain apoproteins A-I and A-II, the principal apoproteins of plasma HDL. As the triglycerides of chylomicrons are removed by hydrolysis by LPL in plasma, lipids of the surface monolayer and apoproteins A-I and A-II dissociate from the complex to form new HDL molecules. VLDL do not contain the major apoproteins found in HDL; however, phospholipids and cholesterol derived from their monolayers, released during intravascular hydrolysis of these lipoproteins, contribute to the lipid moiety of HDL.

B. Metabolic Roles for HDL: Several metabolic roles for HDL are now recognized. These lipoproteins serve as carriers for the C apoproteins, transferring them to nascent VLDL and chylomicrons. Whereas one of these, apoprotein C-II, serves as a requisite cofactor in the process of intravascular lipolysis, roles for the other C proteins remain undetermined. The relative concentrations of these apoproteins in triglyceride-rich lipoproteins and in HDL are apparently determined by their individual association constants. Apoprotein C-I, for example, comprises a much larger fraction of the C proteins in HDL than in VLDL. HDL as well as LDL deliver cholesterol to the adrenal cortex and gonads in support of steroidogenesis. HDL play a major role in the centripetal transport of cholesterol—ie, the transport of surplus cholesterol away from peripheral tissues. Although this process is not fully understood, it appears that several subspecies of HDL are involved. Unesterified cholesterol is acquired from the membranes of peripheral tissues and is esterified by LCAT. The resulting cholesteryl esters, predominantly cholesteryl linoleate, are then transferred to LDL and to triglyceride-rich lipoproteins. Remnants of VLDL and chylomicrons are taken up by liver very quickly, providing for rapid transport of the newly formed cholesteryl esters to the liver. Recently, it has been discovered that the processes of esterification and transfer are both mediated by a spe-

cies of lipoprotein that comprises but a small fraction of total HDL mass. In addition to lipids, this particle contains apoprotein A-I, LCAT, and apo-D. The apoprotein A-I is a cofactor for LCAT, and apo-D is required for transfer of the cholesteryl esters to recipient lipoproteins. At least one subspecies of HDL is involved in transferring free cholesterol from tissues to the esterification transfer particle.

HDL appear to play a major role in the degradation of bacterial endotoxins in plasma. They also apparently exert a potent inhibitory effect against certain species of trypanosomes.

C. Catabolism of HDL: The pathways of catabolism of HDL are not yet known. Radiochemical studies indicate that apoproteins A-I and A-II are removed from plasma synchronously and that a portion of the degradation occurs in liver. Because degradation by perfused rat livers is slower than for the intact animal, it must be presumed that peripheral tissues contribute substantially to the catabolism of HDL.

The Cholesterol Economy

Cholesterol is an essential constituent of the plasma membranes of mammalian cells and of the myelin sheath. It is also required for adrenal and gonadal steroidogenesis and for the production of bile acids by the liver. Virtually all nucleated mammalian cells can synthesize cholesterol, commencing with acetyl-CoA. Formation of HMG-CoA is the initial step. The first committed step, mediated by HMG-CoA reductase, is the formation of mevalonic acid from HMG-CoA. Mevalonic acid is then metabolized via a series of isoprenoid intermediaries to squalene, which cyclizes to form a series of sterols leading to cholesterol. A small amount of the mevalonate is converted eventually to the important isoprenoid substances ubiquinone, dolichol, and isopentenyl pyrophosphate. The portion of the pathway leading to cholesterol synthesis is tightly regulated by cholesterol, or some metabolite of cholesterol, which suppresses the activity of HMG-

CoA reductase. Thus, the cells have the ability to produce cholesterol to the extent that their requirements are not met by that derived from circulating lipoproteins. Cholesteryl esters stored in cells serve as an immediate reserve of cholesterol. Large requirements for cholesterol result from rapid proliferation of cells with attendant need for elaboration of cell membranes. Hepatocytes and intestinal epithelial cells require large amounts of cholesterol for secretion of lipoproteins. In addition to these requirements, cells appear to be constantly transferring cholesterol to circulating lipoproteins, chiefly HDL. A relatively small amount of cholesterol is lost from the body in desquamated skin and through the loss of intestinal epithelial cells in the stool. The net daily loss of cholesterol from the gut, derived both from biliary cholesterol and from desquamated epithelial cells, is about 500 mg. In addition, about 2% of the mass of bile acids secreted into the intestine are lost in the stool, equivalent to about 250 mg of cholesterol.

Cholesterol is acquired from the diet as well as from endogenous synthesis. Humans, unlike many other species, do not absorb dietary cholesterol quantitatively; however, at normal levels of intake, about one-third of the amount ingested reaches the bloodstream. Most of this cholesterol is transported to liver in chylomicron remnants, leading to suppression of hepatic cholesterogenesis. Recent evidence suggests that individuals may differ substantially in the effect of dietary cholesterol on serum lipoproteins, reflecting in part differences in the efficiency of absorption of cholesterol. The range of cholesterol content in the usual North American diet is 0.4–2 g/d or more. In many parts of the world, the average daily intake of cholesterol is below 0.2 g.

About 1.5 g of cholesterol per day passes through LDL. Approximately one-fourth of this is unesterified, and the remainder largely represents cholesterol esterified by the LCAT mechanism in plasma.

DIFFERENTIATION OF DISORDERS OF LIPOPROTEIN METABOLISM

Laboratory Analyses of Lipids & Lipoproteins

Because chylomicrons normally may be present in plasma up to 14 hours after a meal, they contribute triglyceride to the total measured during that period, raising the triglyceride concentration to as much as 600 mg/dL. For this reason, it is conventional to measure serum lipids and lipoproteins after a 14-hour fast. If blood glucose is not to be measured, patients may have fruit juice and black coffee with sugar (which provide no triglyceride) for breakfast.

A. Inspection: Much useful information is gained from inspection of the serum, especially before and after overnight refrigeration. As a screening technique, this will identify sera in which triglycerides need to be measured. Opalescence is due to light scattering by large triglyceride-rich lipoproteins. Serum begins to appear hazy when the level of triglycerides reaches 200 mg/dL, about the point at which clinical significance begins. The presence of chylomicrons is readily detected, because they form a white supernatant layer overnight. A marked increase in opalescence with chilling suggests familial dysbetalipoproteinemia, in which there is an increased tendency of the abnormal lipoproteins to aggregate in the cold. A further observation made on serum, which is critical to the detection of the uncommon cases in which binding of immunoglobulins to lipoproteins takes place, is the formation of a curdlike lipoprotein aggregate or a snowy precipitate as serum cools. If one of these disorders is suspected, blood should be drawn, allowed to clot, and serum separated at 37 °C, because the critical temperatures for precipitation of the cryoglobulin complex may be so high that precipitation will have occurred at room temperature before the serum and clot are separated.

B. Laboratory Techniques: The cholesterol and triglyceride contents of serum can be measured by several chemical techniques that provide reliable results. These measurements are an essential minimum for differentiation of disorders of lipoprotein metabolism. The usual methods determine unesterified and esterified cholesterol together, so that the reported value is the total content of cholesterol in serum. In most cases, electrophoresis of lipoproteins contributes little additional information; thus, this technique is not a necessary part of the routine laboratory examination. The exception is the identification of lipoproteins found in familial dysbetalipoproteinemia. The best electrophoretic separation of lipoproteins is made in agarose gel. The most complete characterization of a patient's lipoproteins is achieved by measurement of the cholesterol and triglyceride contents and electrophoretic behavior of individual lipoprotein fractions, separated by sequential preparative ultracentrifugation, a technique usually available only in research laboratories. However, the content of high-density lipoproteins can be measured in many laboratories using a technique in which HDL are the only lipoproteins that remain in solution after treatment of the serum with heparin and manganese. The cholesterol content of the solution is taken as HDL cholesterol. Albeit rapid, the results of this technique tend to be unacceptably variable unless rigid quality control is exercised. The prognostic implications of small changes in HDL cholesterol make such controls necessary.

An important determinant of the content of cholesteryl esters in HDL is the amount of triglyceride-rich lipoproteins to which the HDL is exposed in plasma. Triglycerides from these lipoproteins exchange into the core regions of HDL, displacing cholesteryl esters and leading to an inverse logarithmic dependence of HDL cholesterol level upon the plasma triglycerides. Thus, the HDL cholesterol value cannot be interpreted without knowledge of the level of serum triglycerides. For example, a level of HDL that would normally contain 45 mg/dL of cholesterol would contain 37 mg/

dL when the triglycerides were 200 mg/dL and 30 mg/dL when they reach 500 mg/dL. In certain forms of hypertriglyceridemia, there may also be a moderate decrease in the protein-phospholipid vehicle of HDL, but the principal effect on the measurement of HDL cholesterol levels remains the exchange of triglyceride for cholesteryl esters.

More sophisticated tests of composition of isolated lipoprotein fractions are of use in certain instances. The most important of these is analysis of the ratio of cholesterol to triglycerides by chemical techniques and of the apoproteins of VLDL by isoelectric focusing. The latter allows the identification of deficiency of the normal isoforms of apo-E, the apparent underlying molecular defect in familial dysbetalipoproteinemia. In this disorder, there is an unusually high content of cholesterol in the VLDL. Quantitative measurement of the apoproteins of VLDL can be made by electrophoresis in agarose gel (following delipidation by tetramethylurea) or by immunochemical analysis. A number of immunoassays for various apolipoproteins are available.

Clinical Differentiation of Abnormal Patterns of Plasma Lipoproteins

A. Preliminary Screening: The first step in the diagnosis of hyperlipidemia is the determination that levels of lipids in serum are abnormal. Serum cholesterol and triglyceride levels are both continuously distributed in the population; therefore, some arbitrary levels must be established to define significant hyperlipidemia. In general, the greater the departure from these norms, the greater will be the clinical importance of the hyperlipidemia. Selection of these arbitrary values should not imply that the levels of circulating lipids prevalent in most of the population in Western countries are without risk. As indicated in the introductory paragraphs, average levels of LDL in these populations appear to be well above the biologic ideal and may be a major etiologic factor underlying the increased incidence of atherosclerotic vascular disease in Western societies. Epidemiologic studies in Europe and the USA have shown that there is a progressive increase in risk of coronary artery disease as levels of serum cholesterol increase above 180 mg/dL. Present evidence would indicate that physicians should at least encourage patients at risk to eat diets low in saturated fats and cholesterol in order to minimize the burden of LDL in plasma.

In general, levels of serum cholesterol above 260 mg/dL and serum triglycerides above 190 mg/dL merit investigation. One abnormality associated with increased risk of coronary artery disease that will not be detected if only cases with hyperlipidemia are studied is hypoalphalipoproteinemia, or deficiency of HDL. Many of the affected individuals have normal levels of both cholesterol and triglycerides in serum and no clinical stigmas to draw the attention of the physician. The argument has been offered that detection of these individuals is unavailing, because there is little that can currently be done to modify levels of HDL in serum. Appreciation that hypoalphalipoproteinemia is present, however, is important if for no other reason than to underscore the importance of controlling other risk factors and perhaps the avoidance of drugs that reduce HDL levels in serum. The recent demonstrations that cigarette smoking is associated with lower levels of HDL and that heavy exercise, at least in normal subjects, may be associated with increased levels suggest further that some modulation of HDL levels may be possible.

B. Identification of Abnormal Patterns: The second step in investigation of hyperlipidemia is determination of the species of lipoproteins that account for the increased content of lipids in serum. In some cases, multiple species may be involved; in others, qualitative properties of the lipoproteins are of diagnostic importance. After identifying the pattern of the lipoprotein abnormality, the physician must search for underlying disorders that cause secondary hyperlipidemias of similar pattern. Such disorders may be the sole cause of the lipoprotein abnormality or may aggravate primary disorders of lipoprotein metabolism. The differentiation of specific primary disorders usually requires additional clinical and genetic information.

The following diagnostic protocol, based upon initial measurement of cholesterol and triglycerides in serum after a 14-hour fast, supplemented by observation of serum and by additional laboratory measurements where essential, will serve as a practical guide in identifying abnormal patterns of lipoprotein distribution. The term "hyperlipidemia" denotes high levels of any class of lipoprotein; "hyperlipemia" denotes high levels of any of the triglyceride-rich lipoproteins.

Case 1. Serum Cholesterol Levels Increased; Triglycerides Normal:

(a) If the serum cholesterol level is only modestly elevated (up to 290 mg/dL), the HDL cholesterol level should be measured. Hyperalphalipoproteinemia (elevated levels of HDL in serum) may account for the observed increase in serum cholesterol level. Hyperalphalipoproteinemia is not associated with disease processes. The LDL cholesterol level in serum may be estimated by subtracting the HDL cholesterol level and the estimated cholesterol contribution of VLDL from the total serum cholesterol level. The VLDL cholesterol is approximated as one-fifth of the serum triglyceride level.

$$\text{LDL cholesterol} = \text{Total cholesterol} - (\frac{TG}{5} + \text{HDL cholesterol})$$

Calculated values of LDL cholesterol over 180 mg/dL are clinically significant.

(b) Because HDL almost never contribute more than 120 mg/dL of cholesterol, serum cholesterol levels in excess of 290 mg/dL always represent significant hyperlipidemia. Unless the patient has obstructive hepatic disease, the abnormality may be assumed to be due to an increase in low-density lipoproteins. The abnormal lipoprotein of cholestasis, like LDL, is selectively rich in cholesterol. It can be differentiated because it has gamma mobility on electrophoresis in agarose gel and because it stains metachromatically with Sudan black in agarose gel.

Case 2. Predominant Increase of Triglycerides in Serum; Moderate Increase in Cholesterol Level May Be Present: Here it is apparent that the primary abnormality is an increase in the triglyceride-rich VLDL (hyperprebetalipoproteinemia) or chylomicrons (chylomicronemia), or both (mixed lipemia). Because both VLDL and chylomicrons contain free cholesterol in their surface monolayers and a small amount of cholesteryl ester in their cores, the total cholesterol level in serum may be increased, though to a much smaller extent than is the serum triglyceride level. The contribution of cholesterol in these lipoproteins to the total in serum is about 8–15% of the triglyceride content. Low levels of LDL cholesterol often seen in hypertriglyceridemia may largely offset the increase in cholesterol due to the triglyceride-rich lipoproteins, especially in primary chylomicronemia. A white supernatant layer in serum refrigerated overnight reveals the presence of chylomicrons. Because VLDL and chylomicrons compete as substrates in a common removal pathway, chylomicrons will nearly always be present when triglyceride levels exceed 1000 mg/dL.

Case 3. Cholesterol and Triglyceride Levels in Serum Both Elevated: This pattern can be the result of either of 2 abnormal lipoprotein distributions. One of these is a combined increase of VLDL (prebetalipoproteins), which provide most of the increase in triglycerides, and LDL (beta-lipoproteins), which account for the bulk of the increase in cholesterol in serum. This pattern is termed combined hyperlipidemia and is one of the 3 phenotypic patterns encountered in kindreds with the disorder termed familial multiple lipoprotein-type hyperlipidemia. The second distribution is an increase of remnant lipoproteins derived from VLDL and chylomicrons. These lipoprotein particles have been partially depleted of triglyceride by lipoprotein lipase and have been enriched with cholesteryl esters by the LCAT system, such that the total content of cholesterol in serum is similar to that of triglycerides. This pattern is almost always an expression of familial dysbetalipoproteinemia. Differentiation of these 2 patterns requires application of additional diagnostic tests. Presumptive differentiation can be made with high-quality agarose gel electrophoresis. In combined hyperlipidemia, the prebeta- and beta-lipoprotein bands are both increased in staining intensity, but each has its typical electrophoretic mobility, and they are well resolved from one another. Preparative ultracentrifugation of serum in this disorder shows elevated levels of both VLDL and LDL. In contrast, the remnant particles in dysbetalipoproteinemia are distributed in a "broad beta" pattern that obscures the resolution of beta- and prebeta-lipoprotein bands. A substantial portion of the triglyceride-rich lipoproteins shows beta-electrophoretic mobility after separation from serum in the ultracentrifuge (at a density of 1.006 g/cm^3), and they have an increased content of cholesterol. Dysbetalipoproteinemia is confirmed by the absence or severe deficiency of the E-3 and E-4 isoforms of apoprotein E when the triglyceride-rich fraction of serum is analyzed by isoelectric focusing.

CLINICAL DESCRIPTIONS OF PRIMARY & SECONDARY DISORDERS OF LIPOPROTEIN METABOLISM

THE HYPERTRIGLYCERIDEMIAS

Atherogenicity

In addition to LDL, certain triglyceride-rich lipoproteins appear to be atherogenic. There is ample clinical evidence that the remnant lipoproteins of dysbetalipoproteinemia are associated with accelerated atherosclerosis in coronary and peripheral vessels. The atherogenicity of other triglyceride-rich lipoproteins is probably dependent upon particle diameter and perhaps on other properties as well. For example, patients with primary chylomicronemia do not appear to have accelerated atherosclerosis despite extremely high levels of triglycerides in serum, whereas there is some clinical evidence in support of the atherogenicity of VLDL of small to moderate particle diameter. Impaired capacity of the VLDL of some individuals to accept cholesteryl esters from the LCAT reaction may also contribute to atherogenesis by impeding centripetal transport of cholesterol.

Cause of Pancreatitis

Very high levels of triglycerides in plasma are associated with risk of acute pancreatitis, probably from the local release of amphipathic free fatty acids and perhaps lysolecithin from lipoprotein substrates in the capillary bed of the pancreas. If the concentrations of these lipids exceed the binding capacity of albumin, they could lyse membranes of parenchymal cells, initiating a chemical pancreatitis. Patients who have had previous attacks of pancreatitis appear to be at higher risk. Many patients with lipemia have intermittent episodes of epigastric pain during which serum amylase does not reach levels commonly considered diagnostic for pancreatitis. This is especially true in patients who have had previous attacks. The observation that these episodes frequently evolve into classic pancreatitis suggests that they represent incipient pancreatic inflammation. The progression of pancreatitis can be prevented by rapid reduction of triglyceride levels in serum, which can usually be accomplished by rigorous restriction of dietary fat and institution of other corrective measures. In more threatening cases, parenteral feeding with glucose may be required for a few days. The clinical course of pancreatitis in patients with lipemia is typical of the general experience with this disease. Fatal hemorrhagic pancreatitis occurs in a few; many develop pseudocysts; and some progress to pancreatic exocrine insufficiency or compromised insulinogenic capacity.

Clinical Signs

When triglyceride levels in serum exceed 3000–4000 mg/dL, light scattering by these particles in the blood lends a whitish cast to the venous vascular bed of the retina, a sign known as **lipemia retinalis.** Markedly elevated levels of VLDL (and perhaps small chylomicrons) in plasma may be associated with the appearance of eruptive cutaneous xanthomas. These lesions, filled with foam cells, appear as yellow morbilliform eruptions 2–5 mm in diameter, often with erythematous areolae. They usually occur in clusters on extensor surfaces such as the elbows, knees, and buttocks. They are transient and usually disappear within a few weeks after triglyceride levels are reduced below 2000–3000 mg/dL.

Effects of Hypertriglyceridemia on Laboratory Measurements

Very high levels of triglyceride-rich lipoproteins may introduce several important errors in clinical laboratory measurements. Light scattering from these large particles can cause erroneous results in most chemical determinations involving photometric measurements in spite of corrections for blank values. Amylase activity in serum may be inhibited by triglyceride-rich lipoproteins; hence, lipemic specimens should be diluted for measurement of this enzyme. Because the lipoproteins are not permeable to ionic or polar small molecules, their hydrophobic regions constitute a second phase in plasma. When the volume of this phase becomes appreciable, electrolytes (measured by flame photometry) and other hydrophilic species in serum will be underestimated with respect to their true concentration in plasma water. A practical rule for correcting these values is as follows: for each 1000 mg/dL of triglyceride in serum, the concentrations of all hydrophilic molecules and ions should be increased by 1%.

1. PRIMARY HYPERTRIGLYCERIDEMIA

Deficiency of Lipoprotein Lipase or Its Cofactor

A. Clinical Findings: Because the clinical expressions of these defects are identical, they will be considered together. Both appear to be transmitted as autosomal recessive traits. On a typical North American diet, lipemia is usually severe (serum triglyceride levels of 2000–25,000 mg/dL). Lipemia retinalis is

apparent if triglyceride levels exceed 3000–4000 mg/dL. Hepatomegaly and splenomegaly are frequently present. Foam cells laden with lipid are found in liver, spleen, and bone marrow. Splenic infarct has been described and may be a source of abdominal pain. Hypersplenism with anemia, granulocytopenia, and thrombocytopenia can occur. Recurrent epigastric pain and overt pancreatitis are frequently encountered. Patients may have eruptive xanthomas, though many do not despite very high levels of triglycerides in serum. These disorders are present from birth and may be recognized in early infancy or may go unnoticed until an attack of acute pancreatitis occurs or lipemic serum is noted on blood sampling. Thus, diagnosis may be delayed until as late as middle age. Patients with these disorders are classically not obese and have normal carbohydrate metabolism, unless pancreatitis impairs insulinogenic capacity. Estrogens intensify the lipemia by stimulating production of VLDL by liver. Therefore, in pregnancy and lactation or during the administration of estrogenic steroids, triglyceride levels in serum rise and the risk of pancreatitis increases. There is no apparent increase in the risk of atherosclerosis, which suggests that chylomicrons are not an atherogenic lipoprotein species.

B. Laboratory Findings: These patients have a preponderance of chylomicrons over VLDL in serum such that the infranatant layer of serum refrigerated overnight may be nearly clear. Many have a moderate increase in VLDL, however, and in pregnant women or those receiving estrogens, a pattern of mixed lipemia is usually present. Levels of low-density lipoproteins in serum are decreased, probably representing the predominant catabolism of VLDL by pathways that do not involve the production of LDL. Levels of HDL are also decreased. A presumptive diagnosis of these disorders can be made by restricting the oral intake of fat to 10–15 g/d for 3–5 days. The triglyceride level of plasma drops precipitously, usually reaching 200–600 mg/dL within 3–4 days. Confirmation of deficiency of lipoprotein lipase is obtained by measurement in vitro of the lipolytic activity of plasma prepared from blood drawn 10 minutes after heparin, 0.2 mg/kg, is injected intravenously. Analysis of lipolysis is carried out with and without 0.5 M sodium chloride, which inhibits lipoprotein lipase but does not suppress the activity of other plasma lipases, including a hepatic lipase. Classically, the lipolytic activity of plasma is very low and is similar in the saline-inhibited and saline-uninhibited incubates. Recent findings suggest that several forms of LPL deficiency can be differentiated by prolonged infusions of heparin. These findings are compatible either with selective deficiencies of the LPL species in different tissues or with the existence of a form of the disorder in which binding to endothelium is abnormal. The latter is supported by heterogeneity in levels of another heparin-releasable enzyme, histaminase, in sera of patients with LPL deficiency. Absence of the cofactor protein of LPL, apoprotein C-II, is the counterpart of deficiency of LPL and can be demonstrated most readily by electrophoresis or isoelectric focusing of the proteins of VLDL.

C. Treatment: Treatment of primary chylomicronemia is entirely dietary. Intake of fat should be reduced to 10% or less of total calories. In an adult, this represents 15–30 g/d. Because the defect involves lipolysis, both saturated and unsaturated fats must be curtailed. Medium-chain triglycerides may be added to increase palatability, since their fatty acids are transported to liver in portal vein blood, bypassing transport in chylomicrons. The diet should contain at least 5 g of polyunsaturated fat as a source of essential fatty acids, and an ample supply of fat-soluble vitamins must be provided. Careful adherence to this diet will invariably maintain serum triglyceride levels below 1000 mg/dL in the absence of pregnancy, lactation, or the administration of exogenous estrogens. Because this is below the level at which pancreatitis usually occurs, compliant patients with these disorders are at low risk.

Endogenous & Mixed Lipemias

A. Etiology and Pathogenesis: Endogenous lipemia (primary hyperprebetalipoproteinemia) and mixed lipemia probably both result from several genetically determined disorders. The occurrence of multiple cases in a kindred is the basis for considering them primary. Thus, a number of "sporadic cases" may be similar, only lacking evidence of familial occurrence. Because VLDL and chylomicrons are competing substrates in the intravascular lipolytic pathway, saturating levels of VLDL will cause an impedance in the removal of chylomicrons. Therefore, as the severity of endogenous lipemia increases, a pattern of mixed lipemia may supervene. In other cases, the pattern of mixed lipemia appears to be present continuously. Though specific pathophysiologic mechanisms remain obscure, certain familial patterns are known. In all forms, however, factors that increase the rate of secretion of VLDL from liver aggravate the hypertriglyceridemia—ie, obesity with insulin resistance, or the appearance of fully developed non–insulin-dependent diabetes mellitus (NIDDM); ethanol ingestion; and the use of exogenous estrogens. Studies of VLDL turnover indicate that either increased production or impaired removal of VLDL may be operative in different individuals. It appears that a substantial number of patients with mixed lipemia have partial defects in catabolism of triglyceride-rich lipoproteins. Increases in production rates of VLDL secondary to excess caloric intake, ethanol, or estrogens tend not to be accompanied by increased removal, as in normal individuals, but rather result in increased levels of circulating triglycerides. Some patients with mixed lipemia have decreased levels of lipoprotein lipase in plasma after a heparin stimulus, which may be of importance in this regard. Most patients with significant endogenous or mixed lipemia have the hypertrophic form of obesity, in which there is a reduced population of insulin receptors on cell membranes associated with impaired effectiveness of insulin. Mobilization of free fatty acids is maintained at a higher than normal rate, providing an increased flux of fatty acids to the liver, in turn increasing the secretion of triglyceride-rich VLDL. Recent studies also suggest that the removal of triglycerides from circulating chylomicrons is decreased in obesity. This factor would be expected to be important in obese subjects with hypertriglyceridemia.

B. Clinical Findings: Clinical features of these forms of hypertriglyceridemia depend upon severity and include eruptive xanthomas, lipemia retinalis, recurrent epigastric pain, and acute pancreatitis (described above). One constellation of clinical features that may be monogenic is endogenous lipemia with obesity, insulin resistance, elevated baseline levels of insulin, hyperglycemia, and hyperuricemia. There is also a tendency toward the development of hypertension in patients with this syndrome. In some kindreds in which this constellation of symptoms is present, some individuals will be more severely affected than others and will have a mixed lipemia, as though they had a double dose of the involved gene or a compound genetic state, including an aggravating trait. Many of the clinical features described above are associated with endogenous lipemia that does not present a clearly monogenic pattern of inheritance, suggesting that several mechanisms may be operative and that endogenous lipemia and mixed lipemia may also be polygenic.

C. Treatment: The primary mode of treatment is dietary. In the short term, severe restriction of total fat intake will usually result in a rapid decline of serum triglyceride levels to 1000–3000 mg/dL, averting pancreatitis. The objective of long-term dietary management is reduction to ideal body weight. Because ethanol causes significant augmentation of VLDL production, abstinence is important.

If weight loss is achieved, the serum triglycerides almost always show a marked response, often approaching normal values. In cases of endogenous lipemia, where the fall in triglyceride levels is not satisfactory, clofibrate, gemfibrozil, or nicotinic acid will usually produce further reductions. In mixed lipemia, gemfibrozil and clofibrate are less likely to be of value, but nicotinic acid is often capable of effecting substantial reductions in serum triglyceride levels. (See Treatment of Hyperlipidemia, below.) Certain synthetic androgenic steroids that increase the activity of heparin-releasable hepatic triglyceridase may be very effective in reducing triglyceride levels in severe mixed lipemia.

Multiple Lipoprotein-Type Hyperlipidemia (Combined Hyperlipidemia)

A. Etiology: Epidemiologic studies of the kindreds of survivors of myocardial infarction revealed this common heredofamilial disorder. Some of the affected individuals have increased levels of both VLDL and LDL in serum (combined hyperlipidemia); some have increased levels of VLDL only; and others have increased levels of LDL. Without family studies, the latter 2 patterns would not be identified as belonging with this syndrome. Patterns in the serum of an individual patient may change with time. It is known that a mating of an individual having any one of the 3 phenotypic patterns with a normal individual can result in the appearance of one of the other patterns. The hypertriglyceridemia and hypercholesterolemia are both relatively mild. Obese children in these kindreds may have hyperlipemia, but hypercholesterolemia tends not to become apparent until adulthood. The underlying process in this disorder is overproduction of VLDL.

B. Clinical Findings: Neither tendinous nor cutaneous xanthomas occur. Available data suggest that this disorder is inherited as a mendelian dominant trait. It appears that the factors that increase the severity of hypertriglyceridemia in other disorders aggravate the lipemia in this syndrome as well.

C. Treatment: The risk of coronary vascular disease is increased in these patients. Therefore, dietary measures are indicated, and drugs are usually given. Clinical experience indicates that reduction of body weight and restriction of saturated fat and cholesterol are only partially effective. Lipemia responds to clofibrate or gemfibrozil, but these agents may increase LDL levels (beta shift). Hence, nicotinic acid may be a better choice. Patients with increased LDL levels respond to bile acid–binding resins but may then have increases in VLDL. Therefore, the combination of a resin and nicotinic acid is frequently required. (See Treatment of Hyperlipidemia, below.)

Familial Dysbetalipoproteinemia (Broad Beta Disease, Type III Hyperlipoproteinemia)

A. Etiology and Pathogenesis: A permissive genetic constitution for this form of familial hyperlipoproteinemia occurs commonly, but expression of hyperlipemia apparently requires additional genetic or environmental determinants. The molecular basis of this disorder is the presence of mutant forms of apo-E that cannot interact normally with high-affinity receptors. In its fully expressed form, the lipoprotein pattern is dominated by the accumulation of remnants of VLDL and chylomicrons. These particles are normally removed very rapidly from serum, principally by the liver. In familial dysbetalipoproteinemia, 2 populations of VLDL are usually present: normal pre-beta-lipoproteins and remnants with beta-electrophoretic mobility. Remnant particles of intermediate density are also present. Characteristically, levels of LDL in serum are decreased, probably reflecting interruption of the normal transformation of VLDL remnants to LDL. Thus, the primary defect appears to involve the uptake of remnants of triglyceride-rich lipoproteins from plasma. Chylomicron remnants are frequently present in serum obtained after a 14-hour fast even when total serum triglycerides are only 300– 600 mg/dL. All the remnant particles are enriched in choles-

teryl esters such that the level of cholesterol in serum is often as high as the level of triglycerides. The ''broad beta'' electrophoretic pattern of VLDL is highly suggestive of familial dysbetalipoproteinemia. However, this pattern is seen also in hypothyroidism, resolving lipemias of other origins, and certain disorders involving immunoglobulin-lipoprotein complexes. Virtual absence of the E-3 and E-4 isoforms of apo-E, detected on isoelectric focusing of VLDL proteins, confirms the diagnosis of genetic dysbetalipoproteinemia. Heterozygosity for apo-E-2, which may be associated with intensification of hyperlipemia from other causes, occurs in about 15% of the white population. Whereas homozygosity is present in about 1% of the population, the incidence of clinical hyperlipidemia among these patients is much smaller. Additional mutations of apo-E that cannot be distinguished from E-3 by isoelectric focusing are now known to result in dysbetalipoproteinemia.

B. Clinical Findings: Hyperlipidemia and clinical stigmas are not usually evident before age 20. In younger patients with hyperlipidemia, hypothyroidism or obesity is likely to be present. Adults with dysbetalipoproteinemia frequently have tuberous or tuberoeruptive xanthomas. Both tend to occur on extensor surfaces, especially elbows and knees. Tuberoeruptive xanthomas are pink or yellowish skin nodules 3– 8 mm in diameter that often become confluent. Tuberous xanthomas—reddish or orange, often shiny nodules up to 3 cm in diameter—are usually moveable and nontender. Another type, planar xanthomas of the palmar creases, strongly suggests dysbetalipoproteinemia. The skin creases assume an orange color from deposition of carotenoids in addition to other lipids. They occasionally are raised above the level of adjacent skin and are not tender. (Planar xanthomas can also be observed in cholestatic disease.) Xanthelasma—yellowish plaques on the canthus—may also occur in dysbetalipoproteinemia.

Some patients have impaired glucose tolerance, which is usually associated with higher levels of blood lipids. Obesity is commonly present and tends to aggravate the lipemia. Patients with the genetic constitution for dysbetalipoproteinemia often develop severe hyperlipidemia if they are hypothyroid.

Atherosclerotic vascular disease of the coronary and peripheral vessels occurs with increased frequency in hyperlipidemic subjects with dysbetalipoproteinemia. The prevalence of atherosclerotic disease of the iliac and femoral vessels appears to be especially high in this disorder.

C. Treatment: Management should begin with institution of a weight reduction diet providing a reduced intake of cholesterol. The use of alcohol should be minimized. Patients who achieve ideal body weight seldom require drug treatment. When the hyperlipidemia does not respond satisfactorily, clofibrate, even in doses as low as 0.5– 1 g/d, is usually effective. Similar results can be obtained with nicotinic acid in moderate doses (1– 2 g/d). (See Treatment of Hyperlipidemia, below.)

2. SECONDARY HYPERTRIGLYCERIDEMIA

Diabetes Mellitus

In patients with insulin-dependent diabetes mellitus (IDDM), levels of VLDL in plasma are frequently elevated despite the regular use of insulin, reflecting the difficulty of control of carbohydrate metabolism in this disorder.

A. Clinical Findings: Lipemia may be very severe, with elevated levels of both VLDL and chylomicrons when control is poor. Lipemic patients usually have ketoacidosis, but lipemia can occur in its absence. Patients with IDDM who have been chronically undertreated with insulin may have mobilized most of the triglyceride from peripheral adipose tissue, so that they no longer have sufficient substrate for significant ketogenesis. These emaciated individuals may have severe lipemia and striking hepatomegaly.

B. Pathogenesis: The severe lipemia associated with absence or marked insufficiency of insulin is attributable to deficiency of LPL activity, reflecting the fact that this enzyme is induced by insulin. The administration of insulin in such cases usually restores triglyceride levels to normal within a few days. However, if massive fatty liver is present, weeks may be required for the VLDL levels to return to normal while the liver secretes its triglyceride into plasma. Conversion of massive amounts of VLDL to LDL, as the impedance of VLDL catabolism is relieved, leads to marked accumulation of LDL that may persist for weeks. This "beta shift" phenomenon may lead to a spurious diagnosis of hypercholesterolemia.

The moderately high levels of VLDL seen in diabetes under average control probably reflect chiefly an increased flux of FFA to liver that stimulates production of triglycerides and their secretion in VLDL. In addition to VLDL, LDL levels are also somewhat increased in insulin-dependent diabetics under poor control, probably accounting in part for their increased risk of coronary heart disease. Mild increases in VLDL and in FFA occur in many individuals with non–insulin-dependent diabetes mellitus (NIDDM). Some have much higher levels of VLDL, suggesting that an additional genetic factor predisposing to lipemia is present. Still another cause of lipemic diabetes is the compromised insulinogenic capacity that can result from acute pancreatitis in individuals with severe primary lipemias. The deficiency may be severe enough to require exogenous insulin, often only in small doses. In diabetics who develop nephrosis as a consequence of their microvascular disease, the secondary lipemia of nephrosis compounds their hypertriglyceridemia.

C. Treatment: The rigid control of blood glucose levels, which can be attained with continuous subcutaneous insulin infusion, is associated with sustained normalization of levels of both LDL and VLDL. HDL cholesterol levels usually rise to the normal range over a period of several months on this treatment.

The lipemia of IDDM responds well to control of the underlying disorder of carbohydrate metabolism.

In obese, insulin-resistant individuals, weight loss is the key to treatment. Diets containing a large fraction of calories as carbohydrates are actually well tolerated, allowing a decrease in the burden of chylomicron triglycerides in plasma.

Uremia

Uremia is associated with modest isolated increases in VLDL. The most important underlying mechanisms are probably insulin resistance and impairment of catabolism of VLDL. Many uremic patients are also nephrotic. The additional effects of nephrosis upon lipoprotein metabolism may produce a combined hyperlipoproteinemia. Patients who have had renal transplants may be receiving glucocorticoids, which also induce a combined hyperlipidemia.

Corticosteroid Excess

In endogenous Cushing's syndrome, there is insulin resistance, and levels of both LDL and VLDL are increased. It appears that the combined hyperlipidemia is primarily due to increased secretion of VLDL, which is then catabolized to LDL. More severe lipemia ensues when steroidogenic diabetes appears. When this occurs, catabolism of triglyceride-rich lipoproteins via the LPL pathway is reduced.

Estrogens

When estrogens are administered to normal premenopausal women, triglyceride levels may increase by as much as 15%. This is believed to reflect chiefly increased hepatic production of VLDL, though other mechanisms may be operative. Paradoxically, estrogens increase the efficiency of catabolism of triglyceride-rich lipoproteins. Whereas estrogens tend to induce insulin resistance, it is not clear that this is an important mechanism, because certain nortestosterone derivatives decrease plasma triglyceride levels despite the induction of appreciable insulin resistance.

Certain individuals, usually with preexisting mild lipemia, show marked hypertriglyceridemia when receiving estrogens even in relatively small doses. Thus, the triglyceride level of serum should be measured in any woman receiving exogenous estrogens. Contraceptive combinations with predominant progestational effects produce less hypertriglyceridemia than purely estrogenic compounds.

Certain synthetic androgenic steroids that increase the activity of heparin-releasable hepatic triglyceridase may be very effective in reducing triglyceride levels in severe mixed lipemia.

Alcohol Ingestion

Ingestion of appreciable amounts of alcohol may not necessarily result in significantly elevated levels of triglycerides in serum, but many alcoholics are lipemic. Furthermore, alcohol profoundly increases triglyceride levels in patients with primary and secondary hyperlipemias. In Zieve's syndrome, the lipemia is associated with hemolytic anemia and hyperbilirubinemia. Because LCAT originates in liver, severe hepatic parenchymal dysfunction may lead to deficiency in the activity of this enzyme. A resultant accumulation of unesterified cholesterol in erythrocyte membranes may account for the hemolysis seen in Zieve's syndrome.

Ethanol is converted to acetate, exerting a sparing effect on the oxidation of fatty acids. The fatty acids are incorporated into triglyceride in liver, resulting in hepatomegaly due to fatty infiltration and in marked enhancement of secretion of VLDL. In many individuals, there is sufficient adaptive increase in the removal capacity for triglycerides from plasma that triglyceride levels tend to return toward normal if alcohol intake is continued over a period of weeks. In individuals in whom the adaptive response is impaired, marked lipemia may ensue. Increased levels of HDL in plasma associated with ethanol ingestion may be coupled to the increased secretion of VLDL.

Nephrosis

The hyperlipidemia of nephrosis is biphasic. Before serum albumin levels fall below 2 g/dL, levels of LDL increase selectively. This is probably a result of increased secretion of albumin by liver to compensate for that lost in the urine. The synthesis of VLDL in the Golgi apparatus of liver appears to be coupled to that of albumin. The increased flux of VLDL from liver would be expected to increase the production of its daughter particles, LDL; however, altered surface properties of LDL, functional hypothyroidism, and even changes in capillary perfusion may contribute to increased levels of LDL. As albumin levels fall below 1–2 g/dL, lipemia ensues. Impaired hydrolysis of triglycerides by LPL may be due in large part to lack of albumin as an FFA receptor. Free fatty acids, which normally circulate complexed to albumin, bind to lipoproteins when albumin levels are low. The ability of these altered lipoproteins to undergo hydrolysis is thus impaired. Lysolecithin and bile acids that normally bind to albumin also associate with lipoproteins. In nephrosis, VLDL contain abundant cholesteryl esters, probably reflecting an increased rate of synthesis of these lipids.

Because coronary vascular disease is quite prevalent in patients with long-standing nephrotic syndrome, treatment of the hyperlipidemia appears to be indicated, though no studies of the effect of treatment have been reported. The hyperlipidemia is relatively resistant to diet. Clofibrate or gemfibrozil may precipitate myopathy even in relatively small doses. Bile acid–binding resins and nicotinic acid appear to be the drugs of choice. Nephrotic patients may be deficient in tryptophan, and oral administration of this amino acid has been reported to ameliorate the hypertriglyceridemia.

Glycogen Storage Disease

In type I glycogenosis, insulin secretion is decreased, leading to an increased flux of FFA to liver, where a substantial fraction is converted to triglycerides, leading to increased secretion of VLDL. The

low levels of insulin in plasma also are the probable cause of reduced activity of LPL, which may cause impaired removal of triglycerides from serum. The fatty liver in these patients tends to progress to cirrhosis.

Frequent small feedings help to maintain blood glucose levels and ameliorate the lipemia. A program of nocturnal nasogastric drip feeding may be of considerable benefit in this disease. In less tractable cases, portacaval shunting may be of considerable benefit, both in maintaining blood glucose levels and in reducing the hypertriglyceridemia. Other forms of hepatic glycogen storage disease may be associated with elevated levels of VLDL and even LDL in serum.

Hypopituitarism & Acromegaly

Part of the hyperlipidemia of hypopituitarism is attributable to secondary hypothyroidism, but hypertriglyceridemia persists even in the face of thyroxine replacement therapy. Dwarfism due to isolated deficiency of growth hormone is associated with higher than normal levels of both LDL and VLDL. Decreased insulin levels may be the major underlying defect; however, deficiency of growth hormone may impair the disposal of FFA by oxidation and ketogenesis in liver, favoring synthesis of triglycerides. Mild hypertriglyceridemia is often associated with acromegaly, probably resulting from insulin resistance. Though growth hormone acutely stimulates lipolysis in adipose tissue, FFA levels are normal in acromegaly.

Hypothyroidism

Whereas significant hypothyroidism tends to produce elevated levels of LDL in serum in nearly all individuals, only a fraction will develop hypertriglyceridemia. The increase in LDL levels results at least in part from decreased numbers of B-100-E receptors on cell membranes, although decreased conversion of cholesterol to bile acids may also contribute. Lipemia is usually mild, though serum triglyceride levels in excess of 3000 mg/dL can occur. The underlying mechanisms are not fully understood, though it is probable that impaired removal of triglycerides from blood is involved. Increased content of cholesteryl esters and apo-E in the triglyceride-rich lipoproteins suggests that accumulation of remnant particles occurs. Hypothyroidism, even of very mild degree, causes expression of hyperlipidemia in otherwise latent carriers of familial dysbetalipoproteinemia.

Immunoglobulin-Lipoprotein Complex Disorders

Both polyclonal and monoclonal hypergammaglobulinemias may cause hypertriglyceridemia. IgG, IgM, and IgA have each been involved. Of the underlying monoclonal disorders causing hypertriglyceridemia, myeloma and macroglobulinemia are the most important, but lymphomas and lymphocytic leukemias have also been implicated. Lupus erythematosus and other collagen vascular disorders have been associated with the polyclonal type. Binding of heparin by immunoglobulin, with resulting inhibition of LPL, can cause severe mixed lipemia. More commonly, the triglyceride-rich lipoproteins have an abnormally high density, probably as a result of bound immunoglobulin, though some may be remnantlike particles. These complexes, which bind lipophilic stains, usually have gamma mobility on electrophoresis in agarose gel.

Xanthomatosis associated with immunoglobulin complex disease includes tuberous or eruptive xanthomas and xanthelasma. Planar xanthomas of large areas of skin are associated with immunoglobulin-lipoprotein complexes. These xanthomas are otherwise seen only in patients with cholestasis. Deposits of lipid-rich hyaline material can occur in the lamina propria of the intestine, causing malabsorption and protein-losing enteropathy. Circulating immunoglobulin-lipoprotein complexes can fix complement, leading to hypocomplementemia.

Treatment is directed at the underlying disorder. Because the critical temperature of cryoprecipitation of some of these complexes is close to body temperature, plasmapheresis should be done at a temperature above the critical temperature measured in the serum of individual patients.

THE HYPERCHOLESTEROLEMIAS

1. PRIMARY HYPERCHOLESTEROLEMIA

Familial Hypercholesterolemia

A. Etiology and Pathogenesis: This disorder, which in its heterozygous form occurs in approximately one in 500 individuals in the USA, is transmitted as a mendelian dominant trait with very high penetrance. Because nearly half of first-degree relatives are affected, including children, all members of an affected individual's family should be screened for this disorder. Hypercholesterolemia, representing a selective increase in LDL, exists from birth. Levels of LDL tend to increase during childhood and adolescence such that average levels of serum cholesterol in adult heterozygotes are about 425 mg/dL. VLDL levels are usually normal, though some individuals, especially those in kindreds in which hypertriglyceridemia is present, may have higher than normal levels of both VLDL and LDL. Aside from an increase in content of cholesteryl esters, the LDL is normal in structure.

The underlying defect appears to be a deficiency of normal high-affinity receptor sites for LDL on cell membranes. Thus, heterozygotes have approximately half of the normal population of such receptors, and homozygotes have none. Three types of receptor defects are now recognized: receptors with no binding capacity; those with impaired binding capacity; and, rarely, a defect of internalization of bound LDL into cells. Clinically and biochemically, it is apparent that some individuals may have combined heterozygosity; ie, they may have a typical gene for absent receptor

activity coupled with an allele for kinetically defective binding, or perhaps some other allele affecting LDL metabolism. Such individuals are more severely affected than heterozygotes, with serum cholesterol levels in the range of 500–800 mg/dL. They usually have aggressive coronary disease. Production rates for LDL appear to be nearly normal in heterozygotes but are increased in the homozygous state, perhaps largely owing to increased conversion of VLDL to LDL. In the heterozygote, a greater fraction of LDL is removed by non–receptor-dependent mechanisms than in normal subjects. In homozygotes, all removal of LDL proceeds through such pathways.

B. Clinical Findings: One of the most striking clinical features that may be present is tendinous xanthomatosis. The xanthomas, which usually appear in early adulthood, cause a broadening or fusiform mass in the tendon. They can occur in almost any tendon but are most readily detected in the Achilles and patellar tendons and in the extensor tendons of the hands (Fig 21–5). Affected adolescents or older patients who are physically active may complain of achillodynia. Arcus corneae (Fig 21–5B) may occur as early as the third decade. Xanthelasma (Fig 21–5A) may also be present. Both arcus and xanthelasma are seen in individuals who do not have hyperlipidemia, however. Coronary atherosclerosis tends to occur prematurely in heterozygotes. The median age at onset of overt coronary disease is 42 years for men and 48 for women. Eighty-five percent of the men will have had a myocardial infarction before age 60, compared with 15% of unaffected men. Coronary artery disease is particularly prominent in individuals who are relatively deficient in HDL. It is probable that this represents a coincident inheritance of both traits. The homozygous form of familial hypercholesterolemia is catastrophic. Levels of cholesterol in serum may exceed 1000 mg/dL, and xanthomatosis progresses rapidly. Patients may have tuberous xanthomas (Fig 21–5C) and elevated plaquelike xanthomas of the extremities, buttocks, and especially the interdigital webs. Many homozygotes have overt coronary disease in the first decade of life, and many do not survive through the second decade.

Homozygous familial hypercholesterolemia is easily diagnosed. Differentiation of the heterozygous disorder from other forms of primary hypercholesterolemia is more difficult; however, the presence of a serum cholesterol level in excess of 350 mg/dL in the absence of significant hypertriglyceridemia makes the diagnosis of heterozygous familial hypercholesterolemia likely. The presence of affected first-degree relatives is supportive of this diagnosis, especially if no other types of hyperlipidemia are present in the family that would suggest combined or multiple lipoprotein-type disease. The presence of affected children is typical of familial hypercholesterolemia but is not associated with multiple lipoprotein-type disease. The presence of tendon xanthomas is nearly pathognomonic—betasitosterolemia and cerebrotendinous xanthomatosis (cholestanolosis) excepted. Although the cholesterol

Figure 21–5. Clinical manifestations of hyperlipidemias. *A:* Xanthelasma involving medial and lateral canthi. *B:* Severe xanthelasma and arcus corneae. *C:* Tuberous xanthomas. *D:* Large tuberous xanthoma of elbow. *E:* Eruptive xanthomas, singly and in rosettes. *F:* Xanthomas of extensor tendons of the hands. *G:* Xeroradiogram of Achilles tendon xanthoma. *H:* Xanthoma of Achilles tendon. (Normal Achilles tendons do not exceed 7 mm in diameter in the region between the calcaneus and the point at which the tendon fibers begin to radiate toward their origins.)

content of serum from umbilical cord blood is usually elevated in patients with this disorder, the diagnosis is most easily established by measuring serum cholesterol levels after the first year of life.

C. Treatment: Treatment with various single drug regimens is of moderate benefit in decreasing LDL levels in serum. However, complete normalization of LDL levels can be achieved in most compliant heterozygotes with a combination of a bile acid–binding resin and nicotinic acid, when they are eating a diet low in saturated fat and cholesterol. Treatment of homozygotes is extremely difficult. Partial control may be achieved with portacaval shunt or repeated plasmapheresis in conjunction with combined drug regimens. Recently, immunopheresis has been reported to be of considerable value. (See Treatment of Hyperlipidemia, below.)

Multiple Lipoprotein-Type Hyperlipidemia (Combined Hyperlipidemia)

In some individuals in kindreds in which this disorder is present (see Primary Hypertriglyceridemia, above), LDL will be the only lipoprotein that is elevated. This pattern may vary within an individual over time, and elevated VLDL alone or combined elevations of LDL and VLDL may be observed in the patient or the patient's relatives. In contrast to most cases of familial hypercholesterolemia, the serum cholesterol level will usually be lower than 350 mg/dL, and neither tendinous nor tuberous xanthomas occur. Few children in these kindreds show hyperlipidemia, but, if present, it is usually VLDL levels that are increased. Studies of kindreds suggest a mendelian dominant mechanism of transmission. Coronary atherosclerosis appears to be accelerated in this disorder, which is sufficiently prevalent to be observed in about 10% of survivors of myocardial infarction. The underlying biochemical mechanism appears to involve increased synthesis of apo-B-100.

Treatment of the hypercholesterolemia should begin with diet and a bile acid–binding resin; however, it may be necessary to add nicotinic acid to control rising levels of triglyceride or to normalize levels of LDL.

Lp(a) Hyperlipidemia

A lipoprotein that normally comprises a very minor fraction of circulating lipoproteins, Lp(a), is present in high concentrations in some individuals. Upon ultracentrifugation, this lipoprotein ranges on both sides of the density that discriminates LDL from HDL. It contains apo-B-100 and a specific glycoprotein. It is identified in LDL or HDL fractions obtained by ultracentrifugation by its prebeta-electrophoretic mobility. It appears to be an atherogenic lipoprotein. Little is known about its response to diet or drug therapy.

Poorly Defined Types of Hypercholesterolemia

Kindreds have been found in which there are sev-

eral individuals with higher than normal levels of LDL who respond dramatically to diets low in cholesterol and saturated fats. There are also kindreds in which multiple genetic factors that lead to higher levels of LDL appear to aggregate in individuals (polygenic hypercholesterolemia). The incidence of hyperlipidemia is smaller in the latter kindreds than in those with monogenic disorders, and the LDL increase is not great. There is also a group of recessive types of hypercholesterolemia that show marked responsiveness to dietary restriction of saturated fat and cholesterol. Tuberous or raised planar xanthomas may be present, and in some individuals serum cholesterol levels may reach 600 mg/dL. Retrospective examination in some of these patients has revealed the presence of beta-sitosterol in the LDL; therefore, at least some of these disorders may be variants of betasitosterolemia.

2. SECONDARY HYPERCHOLESTEROLEMIA

Hypothyroidism

The most consistent disorder of lipoproteins associated with hypothyroidism is high LDL and IDL concentrations. Increased content of apo-E in the VLDL and IDL is consistent with an increase in remnant particles in plasma. In addition to elevated LDL, some patients may have lipemia as described in the section on secondary hyperlipemia. The hyperlipidemia of hypothyroidism may occur in individuals with no overt signs or symptoms of decreased thyroid function. Biliary excretion of cholesterol and bile acids is depressed; however, cholesterol biosynthesis is also decreased. Absorption of cholesterol from the intestine is unchanged. Cholesterol stores in tissues appear to be increased, although the number of B-100-E receptors on cells appears to be decreased. Activity of hepatic lipase is also markedly decreased. Atherogenesis is accelerated by myxedema. The hyperlipidemia responds dramatically to treatment with thyroxine.

Nephrosis

As described in the section on secondary hypertriglyceridemias, nephrosis produces a biphasic hyperlipoproteinemia. The earliest alteration of lipoproteins in nephrosis is elevated LDL. The underlying mechanisms are not clearly identified, but increased secretion of VLDL by liver is probably involved. Because the lipids of the lipoprotein surfaces are altered by enrichment with sphingomyelin, lysolecithin, and FFA, the catabolism of LDL could be impaired. Perhaps the low metabolic rate in affected patients introduces metabolic changes similar to those associated with hypothyroidism. The hyperlipidemia may be an important element in the markedly increased risk of atherosclerotic heart disease in these patients. The treatment of choice appears to be bile acid–binding resins with nicotinic acid.

Immunoglobulin Disorders

One of the lipoprotein abnormalities that can be associated with monoclonal gammopathy is elevated LDL. A "gamma lipoprotein" that is a stable complex of immunoglobulin and lipoprotein may be observed in agarose gel electrophoretograms of the sera of some patients. Cryoprecipitation, often in the temperature range encountered in peripheral tissues when the environmental temperature is low, may occur. Patients may have symptoms from the vascular effect of complement fixation resulting from complex formation and may have hyperviscosity syndrome from the elevated immunoglobulins per se.

Treatment is directed at the underlying process. Plasmapheresis is often effective; however, if cryoprecipitation occurs at critical temperatures near or above room temperature, the procedure must be carried out in a special warm environment. Transfusion of whole blood or serum may be dangerous in these patients because of rapid production of anaphylatoxins from complement in the serum, resulting from interaction with circulating antibody-antigen complexes. This risk can be minimized by the use of packed red blood cells and albumin in place of whole blood.

Anorexia Nervosa

About 40% of patients with anorexia nervosa have elevated LDL in serum, and levels of cholesterol in serum may reach 400–600 mg/dL. The hyperlipidemia, which persists despite correction of hypothyroidism, is probably a result of decreased fecal excretion of bile acids and cholesterol.

Serum lipoproteins return to normal when proper nutrition is restored.

Cholestasis

The hyperlipidemia associated with the obstruction of biliary flow is complex. It occurs either with extrahepatic or intrahepatic obstruction, though it tends to be more severe with the former. Levels of cholesterol in serum exceeding 400 mg/dL usually are associated with extrahepatic obstruction or with intrahepatic tumor. At least 3 types of abnormal lipoproteins are present in plasma. The most abundant, termed LP-X, is a bilayer vesicle about 40 nm in diameter. It is composed of unesterified cholesterol and lecithin, with associated apoproteins but not apo-B. Certain other plasma proteins are also associated with this particle, some of which may be trapped within the vesicle. LP-X is apparent on electrophoresis of lipoproteins in agarose gel as a band of zero to gamma mobility which shows metachromatic staining with Sudan black. It is these vesicular particles that cause the serum phospholipid content to be extremely high. In addition to LP-X, there is another abnormal species called LP-Y, which is also about 40 nm in diameter. It contains appreciable amounts of triglycerides and carries apo-B. It may represent a remnant particle derived from chylomicrons. The LDL in cholestasis also contain an unusually large amount of triglycerides.

Patients with cholestasis may have planar xanthomas of the skin, especially at sites of minor trauma, and may have xanthomas of the palmar creases. Occasionally, eruptive xanthomas are present. Xanthomatous involvement of nerves may lead to symptoms of peripheral neuropathy, and the abnormal lipoproteins may be atherogenic. Whereas bilirubin levels in serum may be nearly normal in some patients with chronic cholestasis, all have elevated serum alkaline phosphatase activity.

Neuropathy is the chief indication for treatment of the hyperlipidemia. Bile acid–binding resins may be of some value, whereas clofibrate causes an increase in serum cholesterol levels. Plasmapheresis is the most effective treatment.

THE HYPOLIPIDEMIAS

Although the clinician is confronted infrequently by the problem of a striking deficiency in plasma lipids, it is important to recognize the primary and secondary hypolipidemias. A serum cholesterol level less than 110 mg/dL in an adult patient is noteworthy. Since levels of triglycerides in normal fasting serum may be as low as 25 mg/dL, significance is limited to cases in which triglycerides are virtually absent.

1. PRIMARY HYPOLIPIDEMIA

DEFICIENCY OF HIGH-DENSITY LIPOPROTEINS

Tangier Disease

A. Etiology and Pathogenesis: Severe deficiency of HDL occurs in the primary disorder known as Tangier disease. Heterozygotes lack clinical signs but have about half the normal complement of HDL and of apoprotein A-I in plasma. Homozygotes lack normal plasma HDL, and apoproteins A-I and A-II are present at extremely low levels. Serum cholesterol levels are usually below 120 mg/dL and may be half that value. Mild hypertriglyceridemia is usually present. The genetic defect probably involves alteration of catabolism of apoprotein A-I.

Several biochemical defects in the metabolism of triglyceride-rich lipoproteins are probably the result of the deficiency of HDL. The chylomicrons and VLDL are deficient in C proteins, which may account for the mild hypertriglyceridemia. Abnormal oblate (oval) lipoproteins in the HDL density interval that contain cholesteryl esters are probably remnant particles derived largely from chylomicrons. The LDL also are abnormal; they are greatly enriched in triglycerides at the expense of cholesteryl esters.

The mechanism that accounts for accumulation of lipid in reticuloendothelial cells is incompletely understood; however, it appears likely that they phagocytose abnormal lipoproteins, probably chiefly the abnormal chylomicron remnants, though impaired centripetal transport of cholesterol may be involved.

B. Clinical Findings: The clinical features of this rare autosomal recessive disease include large, orange-colored, lipid-filled tonsils, accumulation of cholesteryl esters in the reticuloendothelial system, and an episodic and recurrent peripheral neuropathy with predominant motor weakness in the later stages. The course of the disease is benign in early childhood, but the neuropathy may appear as early as age 8. Cholesteryl ester accumulates most prominently in peripheral nerve sheaths. Carotenoid coloration may be apparent in pharyngeal and rectal mucous membranes. Splenomegaly and corneal infiltration may also be present.

C. Treatment: Because much of the lamellar lipoprotein material in plasma is believed to originate in chylomicrons, restriction of dietary fats should be of benefit. Restriction of dietary cholesterol is also indicated.

Familial Hypoalphalipoproteinemia

A. Etiology and Pathogenesis: This recently recognized pattern involves partial deficiency of HDL in serum and may involve heterogeneous mechanisms. These presumed constitutional disorders must be differentiated from the condition in which moderately low levels of HDL cholesterol are seen in individuals consuming a diet very low in fat, perhaps reflecting decreased generation of HDL from chylomicrons. For example, white and Asian men on such diets usually have HDL cholesterol levels of 38–44 mg/dL by ultracentrifugal analysis, in contrast with a median value of 49 mg/dL when consuming a typical North American diet. Such levels are commonplace, for example, in Asiatic populations and among vegetarians, where risk of coronary disease is small. The physician must further interpret HDL cholesterol levels in the light of the amount of triglyceride-rich lipoproteins in plasma. Because triglyceride is progressively substituted for cholesteryl esters in the core of HDL as the plasma triglyceride level rises, the HDL cholesterol will decrease as an inverse logarithmic function of the triglyceride level, causing an apparent decrease in HDL levels, since cholesterol is the component of HDL that is commonly measured. In severe forms of hypertriglyceridemia, there is an additional absolute decrease in levels of the HDL vehicle in the serum of many individuals.

B. Etiologic Factor in Coronary Disease: It appears that familial hypoalphalipoproteinemia is fairly common and an important risk factor in coronary vascular disease. Clinical experience already indicates that this abnormality may be the only apparent risk factor in many cases of premature coronary atherosclerosis. Furthermore, it may accelerate the appearance of coronary disease in patients with familial hypercholesterolemia or other hyperlipidemias. Several investigators have reported low levels of HDL cholesterol or total HDL mass in individuals with heterozygous familial hypercholesterolemia; however, because such kindreds are frequently brought to the attention of physicians by reason of having premature coronary disease, the associated hypoalphalipoproteinemia may merely reflect this preselection bias. Hypoalphalipoproteinemia shows a strong familial incidence. Although several mechanisms and modes of transmission may be involved, many kindreds show distributions consistent with mendelian dominance.

C. Treatment: To date, there has been no demonstration that increasing total HDL levels will decrease the risk of progression of arteriosclerotic disease. Furthermore, only limited means of raising HDL levels are at hand. Recent findings that HDL exist in as many as 8 discrete species further complicate this problem. It is not yet known which of these species may be involved in protecting against arteriosclerosis or whether levels of those species can be increased. Thus, though alcohol ingestion can increase total HDL levels in some individuals, it appears that the effect is primarily on the HDL$_3$ ultracentrifugal fraction, which correlates poorly with decreased risk in epidemiologic studies. Therefore, no recommendation for increased alcohol consumption should be made on this account. Heavy exercise is associated with increases in HDL in some individuals, but exercise must be approached with caution in patients who may have coronary disease. Niacin increases total HDL levels in many subjects, chiefly in the HDL$_2$ ultracentrifugal fraction. Its effects on individual subspecies of HDL remain to be determined.

Perhaps the most important reason at present for measuring HDL cholesterol levels is to identify patients who are at increased risk. Thus, just as with patients who have premature vascular disease or a family history of early arteriosclerosis, patients with low HDL levels should be treated more aggressively for elevated levels of lipoproteins that appear to be atherogenic (LDL, IDL, and VLDL). Furthermore, vigorous efforts should be directed at the control of other risk factors, such as hypertension and smoking. Because the latter is known to decrease HDL cholesterol levels significantly, smoking should be strongly interdicted.

Reports of substantial decreases of HDL cholesterol in plasma of patients treated with the drug probucol would appear to be a general contraindication to its use. Modest lowering of HDL cholesterol levels by beta-adrenergic blocking agents must be weighed against the need for their cardiovascular effects in individual cases.

Deficiency of LCAT

A third genetic disorder associated with low serum levels of HDL is LCAT deficiency. This rare autosomal recessive disorder is not expressed in clinical or biochemical form in the heterozygote. In the homozygote, clinical characteristics are variable. The diagnosis is usually made in adult life, although corneal opacities may begin in childhood. Proteinuria may be an early sign. Deposits of unesterified cholesterol and phospholipid in the renal microvasculature, leading to progressive loss of nephrons and ultimate renal failure, have been a frequent cause of death. Many patients have mild to moderate normochromic anemia with target cells. Hyperbilirubinemia or peripheral neuropathy may be present. Red blood cell lipid composition is abnormal, with increased content of unesterified cholesterol and lecithin. Most have elevated plasma triglycerides (200–1000 mg/dL), and levels of serum cholesterol vary from low normal to 500 mg/dL, only a small fraction of which is esterified. The large triglyceride-rich lipoproteins, presumably derived from VLDL and chylomicrons, are unusually rich in unesterified cholesterol and appear to have abnormal surface monolayers. The LDL are rich in triglycerides, and abnormal vesicular lipoproteins are present in the LDL density interval. Two abnormal HDL species are present: bilayer disks and small spherical particles. Because restriction of dietary fat results in a decrease of VLDL-like particles and lamellar LDL in plasma, it is the recommended treatment.

DEFICIENCY OF LOW-DENSITY LIPOPROTEINS

Recessive Abetalipoproteinemia & Familial Hypobetalipoproteinemia

A. Etiology and Pathogenesis: Previously recognized forms of genetic hypolipidemia involving deficiency of LDL are recessive abetalipoproteinemia and familial hypobetalipoproteinemia. The latter is inherited as an autosomal dominant. Affected heterozygotes with familial hypobetalipoproteinemia are usually asymptomatic but have moderately low levels of total plasma cholesterol (55–146 mg/dL), LDL cholesterol levels about 50% of normal (50–90 mg/dL), and normal HDL cholesterol levels. Individuals homozygous for this disorder share features in common with those who have recessive abetalipoproteinemia. In serum of patients homozygous for either disorder, all forms of apoprotein B are absent. No chylomicrons, VLDL, or LDL are found in plasma, leaving only HDL. Plasma triglyceride levels are usually less than 10 mg/dL and fail to rise after a fat load. The plasma cholesterol, essentially all of which is found in HDL, is usually less than 90 mg/dL. There is a defect in the incorporation of newly synthesized triglycerides into chylomicron particles. However, at low levels of fat intake, about 80% of the ingested triglycerides are absorbed, probably by direct absorption of fatty acids via the portal vein.

B. Clinical Findings: Clinical features include a paucity of adipose tissue, associated with malabsorption of long-chain fatty acids due to failure of the intestine to secrete chylomicrons; red blood cells that may be acanthocytic, with a high cholesterol:phospholipid ratio; progressive degeneration of the central nervous system, including cerebellar degeneration and posterior and lateral spinal tract disease; retinal degeneration, which may be severe; and, usually, very low levels of fat-soluble vitamins in plasma. The neurologic defects may be related to deficiency of vitamin E (normally transported largely in LDL). Patients are apparently normal at birth and develop steatorrhea with impaired growth in infancy. The neuromuscular disorder often appears in late childhood with ataxia, night blindness, decreased visual acuity, and nystagmus. Cardiomyopathy with arrhythmias has been reported and may be a cause of death.

C. Treatment: Treatment includes administration of fat-soluble vitamins. Very large doses of tocopherols (1000–5000 IU/d) appear to limit the progressive central nervous system degeneration. Although vitamin A seems to correct the night blindness, it does not alter the course of the retinitis pigmentosa. Vitamins D and K may also be indicated. Restriction of long-chain triglycerides and use of medium-chain triglycerides, whose fatty acids are absorbed via the portal vein, help to increase needed caloric intake and minimize steatorrhea.

Normotriglyceridemic Abetalipoproteinemia

A newly recognized form of primary hypolipoproteinemia is normotriglyceridemic abetalipoproteinemia, a disorder in which LDL is absent from plasma but fat absorption proceeds normally. The underlying defect appears to be deletion of the B-100 apoprotein, which is essential for formation of VLDL and its daughter particle LDL, whereas secretion of the B apoprotein of chylomicrons, B-48, is intact. Clinical features may include ataxia, minimal stomatocytosis of erythrocytes, and profound deficiency of tocopherols. Tocopherol levels in plasma can be significantly increased by supplementation with this vitamin.

2. SECONDARY HYPOLIPIDEMIA

Hypolipidemia may be secondary to a number of diseases characterized by chronic cachexia, eg, advanced cancer. Myeloproliferative disorders can lead to extremely low levels of LDL, probably owing to increased uptake related to rapid proliferation and membrane synthesis. A wide variety of conditions leading to intestinal malabsorption produce hypolipidemia. In both of these situations, levels of chylomicrons, VLDL, and LDL in serum are low, but these lipoproteins are never absent. Because most of the lipoprotein mass of fasting serum is of hepatic origin, massive parenchymal liver failure can cause severe hypolipidemia. In Reye's syndrome, there appears to be a contravention of the normal production of VLDL by liver, leading to near absence of both VLDL and LDL from serum. Reye's syndrome is a disorder usually associated with influenza B or varicella virus infection in which there is some anatomic disturbance of the mitochondrion attributable to the virus. There is often interference with the Krebs urea cycle resulting in hyperammonemia.

The hypolipidemias associated with immunoglobulin disorders result from diverse mechanisms. Affected patients usually have myeloma or macroglobulinemia, but disturbances of lipoprotein metabolism have also been described with some lymphomas and lymphocytic leukemia. Any of the major classes of immunoglobulins may be involved. In many cases, the immunoglobulins are cryoprecipitins; thus, the diagnosis may be missed if blood is not drawn and serum prepared at 37 °C and observed for cryoprecipitation as it cools. Complexes between immunoglobulins and lipoproteins may circulate in plasma and fix complement, leading to hypocomplementemia and the risk of anaphylaxis on transfusion with whole blood or plasma. The complexes may precipitate in various tissues. When this occurs in the lamina propria of the intestine, a syndrome of malabsorption and protein-losing enteropathy may result. Monoclonal IgA in myeloma may precipitate with lipoproteins, causing xanthomas of the gingiva and cervix. Lesions in the skin are usually planar and xanthomatous and may involve intracutaneous hemorrhage, producing a classic purple xanthoma. Planar xanthomas occurring in cholestasis may be confused with this condition, because the abnormal lipoprotein of cholestasis (LP-X), like the circulating lipoprotein complex of immunoglobulin and lipoprotein, has gamma mobility on electrophoresis.

OTHER DISORDERS OF LIPOPROTEIN METABOLISM

THE LIPODYSTROPHIES

Classification

Current classification of the lipodystrophies is based on their familial or acquired origin and the regional or generalized nature of the fat loss. Among the associated metabolic abnormalities, insulin resistance is the common finding. Two of these disorders are known to be inherited.

Familial generalized lipodystrophy (Seip-Berardinelli syndrome), a rare recessive trait, may be diagnosed at birth and is associated with macrosomia. Genital hypertrophy, hypertrichosis, acanthosis nigricans, hepatomegaly, insulin resistance, hypertriglyceridemia, and glucose intolerance are regularly observed.

Familial lipodystrophy of limbs and trunk (Köbberling-Dunningan syndrome) appears to be transmitted as a dominant gene, affects women predominantly, and is not evident until puberty. The face, neck, and upper trunk are usually spared. Growth is normal, but otherwise this syndrome shares features of the generalized form noted above. It is frequently associated with Stein-Leventhal syndrome.

Acquired forms of lipodystrophy, generalized (Lawrence's syndrome) and partial (Barraquer-Simmons syndrome), usually begin in childhood, affect females predominantly, and often follow an acute febrile illness. The generalized type commonly shares the features described above, invariably involving the trunk and extremities but sometimes sparing the face. A sclerosing panniculitis, as seen in Weber-Christian syndrome, may appear at the outset. The partial type usually begins in the face and then involves the neck, upper limbs, and trunk. In this disorder, reduced levels of C3 complement are frequently encountered. This appears to be due to the presence of C3-splitting factor. Most patients have proteinuria, and some develop overt vascular nephritis.

Associated Disorders

Because a number of patients with disorders resembling both familial and acquired types of lipodystrophy have tumors or other lesions of the hypothalamus, appropriate neurologic evaluation should be obtained. Similarly, the physician should be alert to the association of collagen vascular disorders, including scleroderma and dermatomyositis, with some cases of acquired lipodystrophy.

RARE DISORDERS

Werner's Syndrome, Progeria, Infantile Hypercalcemia, & Sphingolipidoses

These rare disorders may be associated with hypercholesterolemia, but levels of triglycerides are usually normal. Some patients with Niemann-Pick disease have hypercholesterolemia, but most have hypertriglyceridemia, as do many patients with Gaucher's disease.

Wolman's Disease & Cholesteryl Ester Storage Disease

These rare, recessive lipid storage disorders involve the absence and partial deficiency, respectively, of lysosomal acid lipase, resulting in abnormal cholesteryl ester and triglyceride stores in the liver, spleen, adrenal glands, the small intestine, and the bone marrow. Most patients have elevated levels of both LDL and VLDL in plasma. Wolman's disease is fatal in infancy.

Cerebrotendinous Xanthomatosis

In this rare disorder, cholesterol and cholestanol, which are synthesized at increased rates, accumulate in body tissues, but plasma levels of cholesterol and triglyceride are normal. Cataracts, tendon xanthomas, progressive neurologic dysfunction, and premature coronary atherosclerosis are hallmarks of this disease. Its central nervous system effects include dementia, spasticity, and ataxia. Death usually ensues before age 50 from neurologic degeneration or coronary disease. There is no known treatment.

Betasitosterolemia

This rare disorder is distinguished by normal or elevated plasma cholesterol levels; high concentrations of plant sterols in serum, adipose tissue, and skin; and prominent xanthomas of both the tendinous and tuberous types. Individuals with this disorder absorb a substantially larger fraction of phytosterols and cholesterol from the intestine than do normal individuals. Restricting intake of foods rich in sterols is effective treatment. A more severe form apparently exists in which serum cholesterol levels may be as high as 700 mg/dL, reflecting an increase in LDL that contain sitosterol esters in addition to cholesteryl esters. Premature coronary arteriosclerosis may be present.

TREATMENT OF HYPERLIPIDEMIA

The first therapeutic measure in all forms of hyperlipidemia is institution of an appropriate diet. In most forms of hyperlipidemia, a single "universal" diet is indicated. In many subjects with lipemia or with hypercholesterolemia of mild to moderate severity, compliance with this diet will be sufficient to control lipoprotein levels. However, many patients with severe hypercholesterolemia or lipemia will require drug therapy. In all of these individuals, the prescribed diet must be continued to achieve the full potential of drug treatment.

Caution Regarding Drug Therapy

There are insufficient data to evaluate the effects on the fetus of drugs used in treatment of hyperlipoproteinemia. Therefore, women of childbearing age should be advised of the potential risk and should be given these agents only if pregnancy is being actively avoided. If a contraceptive strategy is elected, estrogens should not be used in patients with hypertriglyceridemia.

In children, hyperlipidemias other than familial hypercholesterolemia rarely require drug treatment. Children with heterozygous familial hypercholesterolemia should probably not be treated with drugs until after myelination of the central nervous system is complete (about 6 years of age), because data are lacking on the effects of lowering serum cholesterol levels on the myelination process. After 6 years, children with serum cholesterol levels exceeding 300 mg/dL might reasonably be treated with bile acid–binding resins. However, other factors such as the severity and age at onset of symptomatic coronary disease in the child's family and psychologic considerations should be evaluated in deciding when drug treatment should be started. Dietary treatment is indicated for all children with familial hypercholesterolemia and should be started after the first year.

DIETARY FACTORS IN THE MANAGEMENT OF LIPOPROTEIN DISORDERS

Restriction of Caloric Intake

The secretion of VLDL by liver is greatly stimulated by caloric intake in excess of requirements for physical activity and basal metabolism. Therefore, the total caloric content of the diet is of greater importance than its specific composition in treating endogenous hyperlipemia. There is a positive correlation between serum levels of VLDL triglyceride and various measures of obesity, but many obese patients have normal serum lipids. On the other hand, most patients with hypertriglyceridemia are obese. This association is more consistently observed in persons whose weight gain occurred in later childhood or adulthood and who have adipocyte hypertrophy with relative insulin resistance. As obese patients lose weight, plasma VLDL stabilizes at lower levels. In theory, reduction of output of VLDL by the liver should reduce the production rate of its daughter particle, LDL. In fact, there is a modest correlation of LDL levels with body weight in the general population.

Restriction of Fat Intake

In primary chylomicronemia, saturated and polyunsaturated fats both must be restricted rigidly, because the underlying defect is in lipolysis. Similarly, in the acute management of mixed lipemia with impending pancreatitis, elimination of dietary fat leads to a rapid decrease in chylomicron-borne triglycerides in plasma.

The cholesterol-lowering effect of a significant reduction in total fat content of the diet is well known. It has also been shown that a 15–20% fall in serum cholesterol levels is achieved when individuals who have been consuming a typical North American diet restrict their intake of saturated fats to 8% of total calories. The mechanism for these effects remains unclear, but increased bile acid and perhaps also neutral sterol excretion are known to occur at least transiently until a new steady state with lower levels of LDL and VLDL is established. This is accompanied by a decrease in the flux of the apoprotein of LDL, suggesting that production of the precursor lipoprotein, VLDL, is decreased. Substitution of polyunsaturated fats for saturates also reduces LDL cholesterol levels. The safety of diets containing large amounts of polyunsaturates has not been established, however. Diets very rich in these fatty acids may lower HDL levels and might lead to increased generation of free radicals as a result of hydroperoxidation. In obese subjects, increased intake of polyunsaturates may induce lithogenicity of bile.

Recently, it has become apparent that the omega-3 fatty acids found in fish oils have special properties relevant to the treatment of hypertriglyceridemia. Substantial decreases in triglyceride levels can be induced in patients with severe endogenous or mixed lipemia at doses of 10–15 g/d. Certain members of this class of fatty acids, such as eicosapentaenoic acid, are potent inhibitors of platelet reactivity.

Reduction of Cholesterol Intake

The amount of cholesterol in the diet affects serum cholesterol levels, but individual responses vary. Restriction of dietary cholesterol to less than 200 mg/d in normal individuals usually results in a decrease of 10–15% in serum cholesterol. This apparently in part reflects the fact that increased cholesterol intake in humans is not completely balanced by reduced cholesterogenesis in the liver. The ingestion of cholesterol is generally reflected in increased LDL content of serum. Some individuals whose serum levels increase very little with increased dietary intake may have greatly increased tissue stores of cholesterol. Excessive intake of dietary cholesterol can also lead to the production of HDL_c lipoproteins, which are large HDL complexes rich in cholesteryl esters that contain apo-E. Cholesteryl ester–laden VLDL of beta-electrophoretic mobility also appear. The dietary cholesterol content and saturated fat content have independent effects on levels of serum cholesterol. A decrease in the amount of saturated fat in the diet has also been shown to lower levels of triglyceride in serum, reflecting a reduction in VLDL.

Role of Carbohydrate in Diet

The role of dietary carbohydrate in lipid metabolism is still being investigated, but certain effects seem to have been uniformly observed. There is, however, great individual variation in these responses. When a high-carbohydrate diet is fed, serum triglyceride levels fall and remain lower for about 10 hours. If this diet is continued, hypertriglyceridemia then develops within 48–72 hours, and levels of triglyceride in serum rise to a maximum in 1–5 weeks. Persons with higher basal triglyceride levels and those consuming hypercaloric diets show the greatest effect. After 1–8 months on a high-carbohydrate diet, triglycerides fall to basal levels, with only an occasional subject showing sustained hypertriglyceridemia. Similar induction of lipemia by carbohydrate is seen in patients with endogenous and mixed lipemia, but the increases in serum triglycerides are not proportionately greater than in normal subjects. Thus, there is apparently no type of hyperlipemia that is particularly "carbohydrate-sensitive." It must be emphasized, however, that both of these patterns of lipemia are extremely sensitive to excess total caloric intake. Levels of HDL in serum are lower on a high-carbohydrate intake, but the observed differences are small.

Alcohol Ingestion

Ingestion of alcohol is a common cause of secondary hypertriglyceridemia, owing to overproduction of VLDL. Some individuals with endogenous hypertriglyceridemia on a familial basis are particularly sensitive to the effects of alcohol on triglyceride levels in serum, and abstinence may normalize their triglyceride levels. Chronic alcohol intake may also be associated with hypercholesterolemia. Increased cholesterol synthesis and decreased conversion to bile acids have been observed. Alcohol ingestion may account for alimentary lipemia persisting beyond 12–14 hours. This possibility should be excluded by the history or a repeat lipid analysis before further diagnostic studies are undertaken. In population studies, a positive correlation has been found between alcohol intake and HDL cholesterol levels; however, increased HDL levels are not observed in all individuals when alcohol is added to the diet. Because alcohol-induced changes in HDL appear primarily to involve the HDL_3 subfraction, there does not seem to be an indication for the use of alcohol to increase the "protective effect" of HDL against arteriosclerosis.

Fiber in Diet

Although much attention has been devoted to the possible role of fiber in the development of coronary heart disease and levels of triglyceride and cholesterol in serum, there is little evidence that plasma lipids can be significantly affected by intake of most forms of fiber.

Other Dietary Substances

Several other nutrients have been studied in relation to atherosclerotic heart disease, including calcium, magnesium, trace elements, vitamins D, E, and C, and pyridoxine. The results of these studies are generally equivocal, and the observed effects on serum lipid levels are small. Caffeine and sucrose have negligible effects on serum lipids, and their statistical relationship to coronary heart disease is generally unimpressive when data are corrected for cigarette smoking. Ingestion of large amounts of zinc appears to be associated with decreased levels of HDL.

The "Universal Diet"

Dietary treatment is an important aspect of the management of all forms of lipoprotein disorders and may in some cases be all that is required. Knowledge of the dietary factors reviewed above allows the physician to select appropriate modifications for an individual patient. However, a basic diet, termed the universal diet, is useful in the treatment of most patients with hyperlipoproteinemia. The elements of this diet are as follows:

(1) Ideal body weight should be achieved and maintained.

(2) Total fat calories should be reduced by substantial reduction in saturated fat. The latter should be less than 8% of total calories.

(3) Cholesterol should be reduced to less than 250 mg/d.

(4) Caloric difference should be made up with carbohydrate.

(5) Alcohol should be avoided in any patient with hypertriglyceridemia.

Caloric restriction and reduction of adipose tissue mass are particularly important for patients with increased levels of VLDL and IDL. Diets of 800–1200 kcal are usually appropriate for weight reduction in adults.

Patients with familial hypercholesterolemia are usually of normal weight. When such an individual is obese, losing weight may achieve modest reduction in serum cholesterol levels, but effects are variable. All patients who have hypercholesterolemia should eat only foods low in cholesterol and saturated fat. Serum cholesterol concentration usually decreases only about 10% on this fat-modified diet. Patients with the highest initial levels of cholesterol in serum usually have the poorest response. Since some hypertriglyceridemic patients on the fat-modified diet also achieve some lipid-lowering effect, the diet is generally employed after weight reduction in all hyperlipidemic subjects. The exception to this is the patient who has primary chylomicronemia due to deficiency of LPL or its cofactor apoprotein C-II and whose diet must contain extremely low levels of total fat, usually 10–20 g/d. At least 5 g of the total fat intake in these patients should be a vegetable oil, such as safflower, rich in essential fatty acids.

Patients on low-fat diets should be given fat-soluble vitamin supplementation.

Sources of Dietetic Information

Dietary management must be started early, as soon as the diagnosis of hyperlipidemia is made. Referral to a local American Heart Association office or other source of dietetic consultation is often helpful in ensuring compliance. Several recipe books have been published, and food manufacturers are developing products that add variety and palatability to the restricted diet. Since the prudent diet, as proposed by the American Heart Association and others, is generally recommended, it is helpful to urge the entire family of a hyperlipidemic patient to eat a modified diet, providing greater ease of preparation and an added measure of psychologic support.

DRUGS USED IN TREATMENT OF HYPERLIPOPROTEINEMIA

BILE ACID SEQUESTRANTS

Mechanism of Action

Cholestyramine and colestipol are cationic resins that bind bile acids in the intestinal lumen. The resin particles are not absorbed by the bowel and therefore increase the excretion of bile acids in the stool. Normally, 98% of the bile acid secreted in bile is reabsorbed. However, excretion of bile acids can be increased up to 10-fold when bile acid–binding resins are given. There is a large attendant increase in the synthesis of cholesterol by the liver, but the pool of cholesterol in circulating LDL is also tapped for bile

acid synthesis by increased expression of high-affinity receptors on cell membranes of the liver and other tissues. These agents are useful only in disorders involving elevated LDL. In fact, patients who have increased levels of VLDL may have further increases in serum triglyceride levels during treatment with resins. Thus, in combined hyperlipidemia, where the resins may be given because of high LDL levels, a second agent such as nicotinic acid may be required to control the hypertriglyceridemia. Levels of LDL will fall approximately 20% in compliant patients with heterozygous familial hypercholesterolemia who are receiving maximal doses of the resins. Larger decrements of LDL cholesterol may be seen in patients with other, less severe forms of hyperbetalipoproteinemia; and in some, levels of LDL will be normalized completely.

Drug Dosage

In disorders involving moderately high levels of LDL, 20 g of cholestyramine (Questran) or colestipol (Colestid) daily may lower cholesterol levels effectively. The maximum dose of 30 g daily is required in more severe cases. In familial hypercholesterolemia and combined hyperlipidemia, the resins may be used in combination with nicotinic acid (see below).

Side Effects

Because the resins are confined to the lumen of the intestine, few systemic side effects are observed. Patients frequently complain of a bloated sensation and constipation, both of which are readily relieved by adding concentrated sources of bran to the diet. Malabsorption of fat or fat-soluble vitamins with a daily dose of resin of up to 30 g occurs only in individuals with preexisting bowel disease or with cholestasis. Hypoprothrombinemia has been observed in patients with malabsorption due to these causes. The resins bind thyroxine, digitalis glycosides, and warfarin and impair the absorption of iron and perhaps other drugs. Absorption of all of these substances is ensured if they are administered 1 hour before the resin. During long-term treatment with the resins, some patients may complain of dry, flaking skin, perhaps reflecting some effect on cutaneous sterols. This minor symptom responds to local application of lanolin. Because they change the composition of bile micelles, bile acid sequestrants theoretically may increase the risk of cholelithiasis, particularly in obese subjects. In practice, this risk appears to be very small.

NICOTINIC ACID (Niacin)

Mechanism of Action

Nicotinic acid (but not its amide) is able to effect major reductions in LDL and triglyceride-rich lipoproteins, including chylomicrons. It has been postulated that this is due to decreased flux to liver of free fatty acids, which are normally an important source of VLDL triglyceride fatty acids. Nicotinic acid is a potent inhibitor of the mobilization of free fatty acids from adipose tissue, at least in the short term; its ability to inhibit intracellular lipolysis chronically has not been established. Nicotinic acid inhibits the secretion of VLDL by liver. Incorporation of amino acids into the protein moiety of VLDL is inhibited, and turnover of the lipoprotein is decreased. Nicotinic acid also appears to increase the efficiency of removal of VLDL triglyceride via the LPL pathway. Nicotinic acid has several effects on cholesterol metabolism. It increases sterol excretion acutely and mobilizes cholesterol from tissue pools until a new steady state is established. Although it has no effect on the conversion of cholesterol to bile acids, it decreases cholesterol biosynthesis. That it can cause a continued decrease in cholesterol production even when given with bile acid–binding resins is probably an important feature of the complementary action of these agents. Because nicotinic acid does not change the turnover of LDL per se, it appears that the reduction of levels of LDL associated with its use must reflect decreased production of LDL resulting from decreased secretion of its precursor, VLDL, from liver. Levels of HDL in plasma, particularly HDL_2, are significantly increased by nicotinic acid, reflecting a decrease in the fractional catabolic rate of these lipoproteins. Nicotinic acid stimulates production of tissue plasminogen activator, an effect that may be of value in preventing thrombotic events.

Drug Dosage

The dose of nicotinic acid required for effective treatment varies with the diagnosis. Complete normalization of LDL levels in heterozygous familial hypercholesterolemia is only achieved when a bile acid–binding resin is combined with 4.5–7.5 g of nicotinic acid daily (in 3 doses). For other forms of hyperbetalipoproteinemia and for various types of hypertriglyceridemia, a dose of 1.5–3.5 g/d usually has a dramatic effect. Because nicotinic acid causes a flushing sensation, it is usually started at a dosage of 100 mg 3 times daily and increased slowly. Tachyphylaxis to the flushing occurs within a few days at any dose, allowing stepwise increases. Most patients have no flushing or only occasional minimal flushing when stabilized on a given dose. Because the flushing sensation is prostaglandin-mediated, 0.3 g of aspirin given 20–30 minutes before each dose of nicotinic acid will mitigate this symptom in unusually susceptible individuals. It is important to counsel the patient beforehand that the flushing is a harmless cutaneous vasodilatation.

Side Effects

Moderate elevations of transaminases are often observed if the dosage of nicotinic acid is increased too rapidly. If a daily dose of 2.5 g is not exceeded by the end of the first month, 5 g after the second month, and 7.5 g after the third month, such abnormalities are uncommon. A daily dose of 7.5 g is the maximum under any circumstances. Some patients have mild abnormalities of serum glutamic aminotransferase or alkaline phosphatase activities that do not appear to be clinically significant and revert to normal if the medication is discontinued. In a group of patients treated continuously with nicotinic acid for up to 10 years, no significant liver disease developed despite such mild enzyme abnormalities. About one-fifth of patients have mild hyperuricemia, which is almost invariably asymptomatic unless the patient has previously had gout. In such cases, a uricosuric agent can be added to the regimen. A few patients will have moderate elevations of blood glucose during treatment. Again, this is reversible except possibly in some patients who have latent diabetes. A more common side effect is gastric irritation, which responds well to antacids. Rarely, patients develop acanthosis nigricans, which clears if the drug is discontinued. Some patients can have cardiac arrhythmias while taking nicotinic acid. Reversible retinopathy involving macular degeneration has been described rarely.

CLOFIBRATE
(Ethyl Chlorphenoxyisobutyrate)

Mechanism of Action

A number of effects are attributed to clofibrate. It appears to act chiefly by increasing the activity of the lipolytic pathway in plasma, specifically increasing levels of LPL activity. It may also increase oxidation of fatty acids by liver and decrease VLDL production modestly. Inhibition of cholesterol biosynthesis in liver during treatment with clofibrate may be secondary to changes in VLDL secretion and catabolism. Since decreases in VLDL levels are frequently attended by increased levels of LDL (the so-called beta shift), serum cholesterol levels of some patients may not change despite reductions in triglyceride levels.

Drug Dosage

Clofibrate (Atromid-S) is most useful in treating familial dysbetalipoproteinemia and moderate endogenous hypertriglyceridemia. It is also of value in some patients with mild elevations of LDL. The usual dose is 1 g twice daily, though patients with dysbetalipoproteinemia may respond well to half this dose or less. Clofibrate is usually without benefit in familial hypercholesterolemia and has limited effect when severe chylomicronemia is present. In the latter case, nicotinic acid is usually more effective.

Side Effects

Side effects include nausea, diarrhea, skin eruptions, leukopenia, and moderate elevations of serum glutamic aminotransferase activity. Impotence has also been reported. Muscle pain or cramps associated with elevated muscle creatine phosphokinase activity have been noted. Because this syndrome is most likely to occur when serum albumin levels are low, clofibrate should not be given to patients with nephrosis. Clofibrate potentiates the activities of coumarin and indanedione anticoagulants, and the hypoglycemic effects of sulfonylureas may be enhanced. It also increases the lithogenicity of bile, particularly in obese patients. Results of a recent multicenter study indicate that clofibrate may have a modest carcinogenic potential for tissues of the gastrointestinal tract.

GEMFIBROZIL

Mechanism of Action

Gemfibrozil, a congener of clofibrate, is bound tightly to plasma proteins and is ultimately excreted chiefly by the kidney. It decreases lipolysis in adipose tissue, reduces levels of circulating triglycerides, and causes modest reductions in LDL cholesterol levels. It causes moderate increases in levels of HDL, including the protein moiety. In general, the indications are the same as for clofibrate. It is not yet clear whether the increases in HDL with this drug are greater than those resulting from clofibrate.

Drug Dosage

Gemfibrozil (Lopid) is supplied in 300-mg capsules. The usual dose is 600 mg twice daily. Patients with familial dysbetalipoproteinemia may be managed with smaller doses.

Side Effects

Skin eruptions and gastrointestinal and muscular symptoms similar to those associated with clofibrate have been described, as well as blood dyscrasias and elevated plasma levels of transaminases and alkaline phosphatase. It is likely that most of the toxic effects associated with clofibrate will be observed as experience with this drug increases. Like clofibrate, it enhances the effects of the coumarin and indanedione anticoagulants.

NEOMYCIN

Neomycin is of some usefulness in treating hypercholesterolemia. It apparently acts by inhibiting absorption of cholesterol and bile acids. The dosage required for this effect is 0.5–2 g/d. Even in this dosage range, some patients develop diarrhea that persists as long as the drug is taken. Patients should be observed for ototoxicity and nephrotoxicity.

DEXTROTHYROXINE
(D-Thyroxine)

Dextrothyroxine is isomeric to the normal thyroid hormone, L-thyroxine. It acts in a fashion similar to L-thyroxine on lipid metabolism, increasing conversion of cholesterol to bile acids. Preparations available in the USA have had hypercalorigenic activity, how-

ever, either because of residual L-thyroxine or because of inherent effects of the D-isomer on oxidative phosphorylation, and this activity causes increased cardiac work and may induce angina. Dextrothyroxine is no longer indicated, because it has only limited effectiveness in treating hyperlipidemia and because its use may increase the risk of fatal cardiac arrhythmias.

HMG-CoA REDUCTASE INHIBITORS

HMG-CoA reductase mediates a key step in cholesterol biosynthesis. Several potent inhibitors of this enzyme which have been isolated from fungi are now under investigation. Preliminary studies have shown that 2 of these, compactin and mevinolin, cause significant reduction in levels of LDL in plasma. In heterozygous familial hypercholesterolemia, mevinolin alone is about as effective as bile acid sequestrants alone. When these agents are given together, reductions in LDL levels are comparable to reduction achieved with combinations of a resin and nicotinic acid. However, the mevinolin-resin combination does not increase levels of HDL.

PROBUCOL

Probucol differs structurally from the other hypolipidemic agents, and its mechanism of action remains unclear. It causes only small decreases in LDL levels. Because considerable evidence indicates that it lowers HDL levels, its usefulness is in doubt. The observation that it causes fatal ventricular arrhythmias in animals suggests that it could do so in humans as well under some circumstances.

Probucol (Lorelco) is available as 250-mg tablets.

COMBINED DRUG THERAPY

Combinations of drugs are indicated (1) when LDL and VLDL levels are both elevated; (2) in cases of hypercholesterolemia in which significant increases of VLDL occur during treatment with bile acid–binding resins; and (3) where a complementary effect is required to normalize LDL levels, as in familial hypercholesterolemia.

Clofibrate & Resins

Whereas clofibrate has some effectiveness in decreasing levels of VLDL in plasma in conjunction with bile acid–binding resins, it usually does not complement the effect of the resins on plasma LDL levels in familial hypercholesterolemia. The effectiveness of clofibrate is thus generally limited to disorders in which moderate elevations in levels of plasma VLDL occur. Theoretically, clofibrate should increase the lithogenicity of bile, which may already be increased by bile acid–binding resins.

Nicotinic Acid & Resins

Nicotinic acid alone generally has a more potent effect on levels of triglyceride-rich lipoproteins than does clofibrate and also decreases levels of LDL. Nicotinic acid usually normalizes the triglyceride levels in individuals who have increased levels of VLDL while taking resins. Furthermore, the combination of resin and nicotinic acid is the only currently available regimen that will completely normalize levels of LDL in heterozygous familial hypercholesterolemia. This complementarity of action on LDL presumably results from the additive effects of increased catabolism of LDL due to the resin and decreased production of the precursor lipoprotein, VLDL, induced by nicotinic acid. No additional toxicity or side effects have been described with this regimen beyond those encountered when the agents are used individually. The median daily dose of nicotinic acid required for complete normalization of LDL levels in familial hypercholesterolemia is 6.5 g in conjunction with 24–30 g of resin daily. Levels of HDL cholesterol are significantly elevated on this regimen, reflecting the effect of nicotinic acid. In view of the inverse relationship of HDL levels to the risk of coronary vascular disease, this latter effect might possibly add benefit to the reduction of levels of the atherogenic species, LDL. That this combined regimen is capable of mobilizing cholesterol from tissue sites is supported by the finding that the diameters of tendinous xanthomas, measured by a xeroradiographic technique, are reduced significantly even over a period of only a few months. It appears that this regimen can be used in the long-term treatment of heterozygous familial hypercholesterolemia. Patients who have been treated with this regimen for 10 years show evidence of a sustained effect on lipoprotein levels and have not developed additional side effects or toxicity.

In treating disorders in which levels of VLDL and LDL are both increased, doses of nicotinic acid used in conjunction with bile acid–binding resins are usually much smaller, 1.5–3 g/d. Despite the fact that nicotinic acid is an anion, it does not bind to the resin in vitro. Its absorption from the intestine is unimpeded by the presence of resin; the 2 medications may therefore be taken together for convenience. Because colestipol has potent acid-neutralizing properties, there is further reason to give the 2 medications together when a patient complains of the gastric irritation that sometimes occurs as an adverse effect of nicotinic acid.

Neomycin & Resins

Another combination reported to have some effectiveness in familial hypercholesterolemia is neomycin plus bile acid resin. Though not normalized, serum cholesterol levels are reduced about 35%.

SURGICAL TREATMENT OF HYPERLIPIDEMIA

The operation that has received the most study in the treatment of hyperlipidemia is ileal bypass. This procedure is intended to impede the reabsorption of bile acids and not to cause malabsorption of triglycerides. Evidence supporting impeded absorption of cholesterol is weak. The procedure appears merely to mimic the effect of bile acid–binding resins. Serum cholesterol levels are apparently decreased in a variety of disorders, but, as with bile acid sequestrants, levels of triglycerides in serum may be significantly elevated. Thus, the procedure is not indicated in hypertriglyceridemia. Furthermore, in a series of well-documented cases of heterozygous familial hypercholesterolemia, levels of cholesterol in serum were reduced by only 33%. Clearly, ileal bypass is less effective in that disorder than is treatment with bile acid–binding resins and nicotinic acid. A significant number of patients develop diarrhea, which may be difficult to control, and if the procedure is not performed correctly there may be steatorrhea. Absorption of vitamin B_{12} is impaired in all patients, and this necessitates lifelong parenteral administration of the vitamin. The results obtained from ileal bypass can certainly be duplicated or exceeded in compliant patients with proper diet and drug regimens. This surgical procedure would appear to be indicated only for patients who refuse drug therapy. Ironically, those who develop diarrhea may require treatment with bile acid–binding resins.

In patients with homozygous familial hypercholesterolemia, ileal bypass, even augmented by aggressive multiple drug therapy, has had only a modest effect on the massively expanded pool of circulating LDL. End-to-side portacaval shunts have ameliorated but not normalized LDL levels in some of these patients.

REFERENCES

GENERAL

Goldstein JL, Brown MS: Familial hypercholesterolemia. Pages 672–712 in: *The Metabolic Basis of Inherited Disease*, 5th ed. Stanbury JB et al (editors). McGraw-Hill, 1983.

Havel RJ (editor): Lipid disorders. *Med Clin North Am* 1982; **66:**317. [Entire issue.]

Havel RJ, Goldstein JL, Brown MS: Page 393 in: *Metabolic Control and Disease*, 8th ed. Bondy PK, Rosenberg LE (editors). Saunders, 1980.

Rifkind BM, Segal P: Lipid Research Clinics Program reference values for hyperlipidemia and hypolipidemia. *JAMA* 1983;**250:**1869.

RELATIONSHIP OF CORONARY HEART DISEASE TO DISORDERS OF LIPOPROTEIN METABOLISM

Arteriosclerosis

Berg K, Borresen A-L, Dahlén G: Serum high density–lipoprotein and atherosclerotic heart disease. *Lancet* 1976; **1:**499.

Castelli WF: Epidemiology of coronary heart disease: The Framingham Study. *Am J Med* 1984;**76:**4.

Goldstein JL, Kita T, Brown MS: Mechanisms of disease: Defective lipoprotein receptors and atherosclerosis: Lessons from an animal counterpart of familial hypercholesterolemia. *N Engl J Med* 1983;**309:**288.

Goldstein JL et al: Hyperlipidemia in coronary heart disease. (2 parts.) *J Clin Invest* 1973;**52:**1533, 1544.

Gordon T et al: High density lipoprotein as a protective factor against coronary heart disease: The Framingham Study. *Am J Med* 1977;**62:**707.

Havel RJ: Role of the liver in atherosclerosis. *Arteriosclerosis* 1985;**5:**569.

Miller GJ, Miller NE: Plasma high density lipoprotein concentration and development of ischaemic heart-disease. *Lancet* 1975;**1:**16.

Ostrander LD Jr et al: Biochemical precursor of atherosclerosis: Studies in apparently healthy men in a general population, Tecumseh, Michigan. *Arch Intern Med* 1974; **134:**224.

Rhoads GG, Gulbrandson CL, Kagan A: Serum lipoproteins and coronary heart disease in a population study of Hawaii Japanese men. *N Engl J Med* 1976;**294:**293.

Modification of Atherosclerosis

Lipid Research Clinics Program: The Lipid Research Clinics Coronary Primary Prevention Trial Results. (2 parts.) *JAMA* 1984;**251:**351, 365.

Mahley RW: Dietary fat, cholesterol, and accelerated atherosclerosis. Page 1 in: *Atherosclerosis Reviews*. Vol 5. Paoletti R, Gotto AM Jr (editors). Raven Press, 1979.

Ross R, Glomset JA: The pathogenesis of atherosclerosis. (2 parts.) *N Engl J Med* 1976;**295:**369, 420.

Smith EB: The relationship between plasma and tissue lipids in human atherosclerosis. *Adv Lipid Res* 1974;**12:**1.

LIPOPROTEIN METABOLISM

Brown MS, Faust JR, Goldstein JL: Role of the low density lipoprotein receptor in regulating the content of free and esterified cholesterol in human fibroblasts. *J Clin Invest* 1975;**55:**783.

Fielding CJ, Havel RJ: Lipoprotein lipase. *Arch Pathol Lab Med* 1977;**101:**225.

Havel RJ: The formation of LDL: Mechanisms and regulation. *J Lipid Res* 1984;**25:**1570.

Havel RJ: Lipoprotein biosynthesis and metabolism. *Ann NY Acad Sci* 1980;**348:**16.

Kane JP: Apolipoprotein B: Structural and metabolic heterogeneity. *Annu Rev Physiol* 1983;**45:**637.

PRIMARY HYPERLIPIDEMIAS

Hyperlipemia

Brunzell JD et al: Evidence for a common, saturable triglyceride removal mechanism for chylomicrons and very low density lipoproteins in man. *J Clin Invest* 1973;**52:**1578.

Cox DW, Breckenridge WC, Little JA: Inheritance of apolipoprotein CII deficiency with hypertriglyceridemia and pancreatitis. *N Engl J Med* 1978;**299:**1421.

Havel RJ, Goldstein JL, Brown MS: Pages 415 and 440 in: *Metabolic Control and Disease*, 8th ed. Bondy PK, Rosenberg LE (editors). Saunders, 1980.

Nikkila EA: Page 622 in: *The Metabolic Basis of Inherited Disease*, 5th ed. Stanbury JB et al (editors). McGraw-Hill, 1983.

Multiple Lipoprotein-Type Hyperlipidemia

Goldstein JL et al: Hyperlipidemia in coronary heart disease. 2. Genetic analysis of lipid levels in 176 families and delineation of a new inherited disorder, combined hyperlipidemia. *J Clin Invest* 1973;**52:**1544.

Rose HG et al: Inheritance of combined hyperlipoproteinemia: Evidence for a new lipoprotein phenotype. *Am J Med* 1973;**54:**148.

Familial Dysbetalipoproteinemia

Brown MS, Goldstein JL, Fredrickson DS: Page 655 in: *The Metabolic Basis of Inherited Disease*, 5th ed. Stanbury JB et al (editors). McGraw-Hill, 1983.

Havel RJ: Familial dysbetalipoproteinemia. *Med Clin North Am* 1982;**66:**441.

Havel RJ, Goldstein JL, Brown MS: Page 422 in: *Metabolic Control and Disease*, 8th ed. Bondy PK, Rosenberg LE (editors). Saunders, 1980.

Kane JP et al: Remnants of lipoproteins of intestinal and hepatic origin in familial dysbetalipoproteinemia. *Arteriosclerosis* 1983;**3:**47.

Pagnan A et al: Characterization of very low density lipoproteins containing two electrophoretic populations: Double prebeta lipoproteinemia and primary dysbetalipoproteinemia. *J Lipid Res* 1977;**18:**613.

Familial Hypercholesterolemia

Brown MS, Goldstein JL: Expression of the familial hypercholesterolemia gene in heterozygotes: Mechanism for a dominant disorder in man. *Science* 1974;**185:**61.

Goldstein JL, Brown MS: Familial hypercholesterolemia: A genetic regulatory defect in cholesterol metabolism. *Am J Med* 1975;**58:**147.

Goldstein JL, Brown MS: Page 672 in: *The Metabolic Basis of Inherited Disease*, 5th ed. Stanbury JB et al (editors). McGraw-Hill, 1983.

SECONDARY HYPERLIPIDEMIAS

Havel RJ, Goldstein JL, Brown MS: Page 393 in: *Metabolic Control and Disease,* 8th ed. Bondy PK, Rosenberg LE (editors). Saunders, 1980.

HYPOLIPIDEMIAS

Glomset JA, Norum KR, Gjone E: Page 643 in: *The Metabolic Basis of Inherited Disease,* 5th ed. Stanbury JB et al (editors). McGraw-Hill, 1983.

Herbert PN et al: Abetalipoproteinemia, hypobetalipoproteinemia, and Tangier disease. Pages 589– 621 in: *The Metabolic Basis of Inherited Disease,* 5th ed. Stanbury JB et al (editors). McGraw-Hill, 1983.

Malloy MJ, Kane JP: Hypolipidemia. *Med Clin North Am* 1982;**66:**469.

Malloy MJ et al: Normotriglyceridemic abetalipoproteinemia: Absence of the B100 apolipoprotein. *J Clin Invest* 1981;**67:**1441.

TREATMENT OF HYPERLIPIDEMIA WITH DIET

Belfrage P et al: Alterations of lipid metabolism in healthy volunteers during long-term ethanol intake. *Eur J Clin Invest* 1977;**7:**127.

Connor WE, Connor SL: The dietary treatment of hyperlipidemia. *Med Clin North Am* 1982;**66:**485.

Keys A: Coronary heart disease, serum cholesterol, and the diet. *Acta Med Scand* 1980;**207:**153.

Lewis B: Influence of diet, energy balance and hormones on serum lipids. Page 131 in: *The Hyperlipidemias: Clinical and Laboratory Practice.* Blackwell, 1976.

Mahley RW: Dietary fat, cholesterol, and accelerated atherosclerosis. Page 1 in: *Atherosclerosis Reviews.* Vol 5. Paoletti R, Gotto AM Jr (editors). Raven Press, 1979.

Nutrition Committee and the Council on Arteriosclerosis of the American Heart Association: Recommendations for the treatment of hyperlipidemia in adults. *Circulation* 1984;**69:**443A.

Olefsky J, Reaven GR, Farquhar JW: Effects of weight reduction in obesity: Studies of lipid and carbohydrate metabolism in normal and hyperlipoproteinemic subjects. *J Clin Invest* 1974;**53:**64.

TREATMENT OF HYPERLIPOPROTEINEMIA WITH DRUGS

General

Brensike JF et al: Effects of therapy with cholestyramine on progress of coronary arteriosclerosis: Results of the NHLBI Type II Coronary Intervention Study. *Circulation* 1984;**69:**313.

Grundy SM: Hypertriglyceridemia: Mechanisms, clinical significance, and treatment. *Med Clin North Am* 1982;**66:**519.

Havel RJ, Kane JP: Drugs and lipid metabolism. *Annu Rev Pharmacol* 1973;**13:**287.

Kane JP, Havel RJ: Treatment of hypercholesterolemia. *Annu Rev Med* 1986. [In press.]

Kane JP, Malloy MJ: Treatment of hypercholesterolemia. *Med Clin North Am* 1982;**66:**537.

Levy RI et al: The influence of changes in lipid values induced by cholestyramine and diet on progression of coronary artery disease: Results of the NHLBI Type II Coronary Intervention Study. *Circulation* 1984;**69:**325.

Lipid Research Clinics Program: The Lipid Research Clinics Coronary Primary Prevention Trial Results. (2 parts.) *JAMA* 1984;**251:**351, 365.

Bile Acid Sequestrants

Grundy SM, Ahrens EH Jr, Salem G: Interruption of the enterohepatic circulation of bile acids in man: Comparative effects of cholestyramine and ileal exclusion on cholesterol metabolism. *J Lab Clin Med* 1971;**78:**94.

Levy RI et al: Dietary and drug treatment of primary hyperlipoproteinemia. *Ann Intern Med* 1972;**77:**267.

Miettinen TA, Lempinen M: Cholestyramine and ileal bypass in the treatment of familial hypercholesterolemia. *J Clin Invest* 1977;**7:**509.

Miller NE, Clifton-Bigh P, Nestel PJ: Effects of colestipol, a new bile-acid-sequestering resin, on cholesterol metabolism in man. *J Lab Clin Med* 1973;**82:**876.

Shepherd J et al: Cholestyramine promotes receptor-mediated low-density lipoprotein catabolism. *N Engl J Med* 1980;**302:**1219.

Nicotinic Acid

Carlson LA: Nicotinic acid and inhibition of fat mobilizing lipolysis: Present status of effects on lipid metabolism. *Adv Exp Med Biol* 1978;**109:**225.

Grundy SM et al: Influence of nicotinic acid on metabolism of triglycerides and cholesterol in man. *J Lipid Res* 1981;**22:**24.

Kudchodkar BJ et al: Mechanism of hypolipidemic action of nicotinic acid. *Clin Pharmacol Ther* 1978;**24:**354.

Shepherd J et al: Effects of nicotinic acid therapy on plasma high density lipoprotein subfraction distribution and composition and on apolipoprotein A metabolism. *J Clin Invest* 1979;**63:**858.

Clofibrate & Gemfibrozil

Bridgeman JF, Rosen SM, Thorp JM: Complications during clofibrate treatment of nephrotic syndrome. *Lancet* 1972;**2:**506.

Coronary Drug Project Research Group: Clofibrate and niacin in coronary heart disease. *JAMA* 1975;**231:**360.

Ditzel J, Bang HO: Clofibrate in type II hyperlipoproteinemia. *Acta Med Scand* 1976;**200:**55.

Kesaniemi YA, Grundy SM: Influence of gemfibrozil on metabolism of cholesterol and plasma triglycerides in man. *JAMA* 1986. [In press.]

Langer T, Levy RI: Acute muscular syndrome associated with administration of clofibrate. *N Engl J Med* 1968;**279:**856.

Oliver MF, Roberts SD, Hayes D: Effects of atromid and ethylchlorophenoxyisobutyrate on anticoagulant requirements. *Lancet* 1963;**1:**143.

Wolfe BM et al: Mechanism of the hypolipidemic effect of clofibrate in postabsorptive man. *J Clin Invest* 1973;**52:**2146.

Neomycin

Sedaghat A et al: Effects of neomycin on absorption, synthesis and/or flux of cholesterol in man. *J Clin Invest* 1975;**55:**12.

Combined Drug Therapy

Faergeman O: Effects and side effects of treatment of hypercholesterolemia with cholestyramine and neomycin. *Acta Med Scand* 1973;**194:**165.

Grundy SM, Mok HYI: Colestipol, clofibrate and phytosterols in combined therapy of hyperlipidemia. *J Lab Clin Med* 1977;**89**:354.

Hoeg JM et al: Normalization of plasma lipoprotein concentrations in patients with type II hyperlipoproteinemia by combined use of neomycin and niacin. *Circulation* 1984; **70**:1004.

Illingworth DR: Mevinolin plus colestipol in therapy for severe heterozygous familial hypercholesterolemia. *Ann Intern Med* 1984:**101**:598.

Kane JP et al: Normalization of low-density lipoprotein levels in heterozygous familial hypercholesterolemia with a combined drug regimen. *N Engl J Med* 1981;**304**:251.

Miettinen TA: Effects of neomycin alone and in combination with cholestyramine on serum cholesterol and fecal steroids in hypercholesterolemic subjects. *J Clin Invest* 1979; **64**:1485.

22

Obesity

Mary J. Malloy, MD, & John P. Kane, MD, PhD

Adipose tissue is an organ of metabolism that serves as a capacitor for energy-rich fatty acids. In comparison with glycogen stored in hydrated form in liver and muscle, the unhydrated triglycerides stored in adipose tissue contain over twice the available energy per unit mass. Triglycerides are laid down during times when the supply of circulating energy substrates exceeds the need; in periods of caloric deficit, their constituent fatty acids and glycerol are yielded to the plasma for catabolism at distant tissue sites. Regulation of triglyceride storage involves both neural and endocrine factors but, as would be expected, primarily reflects the net surplus of caloric substrate available to the organism. Obesity, the state of excess storage of triglyceride,* in turn exerts important effects on metabolic processes in adipose tissue and in other organs. The metabolic and pathologic consequences of obesity increase continuously with the extent of deviation above ideal weight.

*The triglycerides are now called triacylglycerols in some current texts.

Acronyms Used in This Chapter

ACTH	Adrenocorticotropic hormone
ATP	Adenosine triphosphate
cAMP	Cyclic adenosine monophosphate
CCK	Cholecystokinin
FFA	Free fatty acids
LPL	Lipoprotein lipase
SHBG	Sex hormone–binding globulin
VLDL	Very low density lipoprotein(s)

METABOLISM OF ADIPOSE TISSUE

The preponderant mass of the fatty acids stored in adipose tissue appears to come from circulating triglyceride-rich lipoproteins. The triglycerides of very low density lipoproteins (VLDL) and chylomicrons are hydrolyzed by lipoprotein lipase (LPL) located on the capillary endothelium, yielding fatty acids, most of which are transported into adipocytes (Fig 22–1).

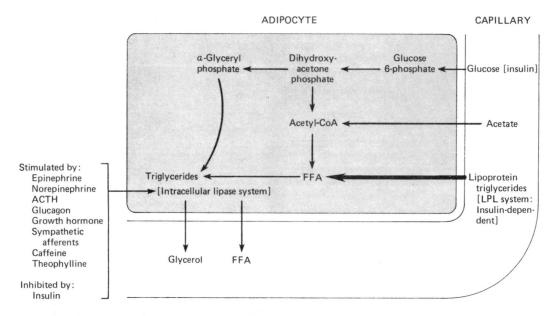

Figure 22–1. Metabolism of adipocytes.

Insulin, which induces LPL activity, also facilitates the entry of glucose into adipocytes, where it is largely converted to α-glyceryl phosphate. This compound provides the glyceryl moiety for esterification of free fatty acids to triglycerides. Adipose tissue is capable of forming fatty acids from acetate derived from ethanol. Glucose also contributes to the synthesis of fatty acids to a limited extent.

Free fatty acids and glycerol are mobilized from adipose tissue into plasma by the hydrolysis of stored triglycerides, a process mediated by an intracellular hormone-sensitive lipase system. The first steps of hydrolysis, which are rate-limiting, release 2 mol of fatty acid. The process is rapidly completed by a monoglyceridase. Hormones that stimulate the hydrolysis of triglycerides are epinephrine, norepinephrine, ACTH, glucagon, and growth hormone. Afferent autonomics serving adipose tissue, which also mediate fatty acid mobilization, represent an important pathway by which the central nervous system exerts control over the mobilization of fatty acids. Many of these stimuli increase the activity of adenylate cyclase. The resulting increase in cAMP activates a protein kinase that phosphorylates inactive triglyceridase to its active form. The phosphorylation is reversible via a phosphatase enzyme, allowing tonic control of the lipolytic process. A phosphodiesterase damps the cAMP signal by hydrolysis of the cyclic nucleotide. Inhibition of phosphodiesterase by caffeine and theophylline potentiates the hormonal stimulation of lipolysis. Thyroxine and cortisol have a permissive effect on lipolysis. The hormonal and neural stimuli are opposed by insulin. Thus, when blood glucose and triglyceride levels increase after a meal, insulin promotes storage of fat and inhibits lipolysis, whereas fasting and exercise promote lipolysis relatively unopposed by insulin.

PROLIFERATION OF ADIPOCYTES

Although evidence for proliferation of adipocytes at other times has been adduced, it appears that such proliferation normally occurs predominantly during early infancy and perhaps again around puberty. If excess calories are provided during the stage of proliferation, it is thought that an increased number of adipocytes develops, to remain throughout life. This early determination of adipocyte number highlights the importance of obesity in infancy and childhood as a predisposing factor in the subsequent development of lifelong obesity. Patients with this type of obesity, then, have increased numbers of fat cells, and the cells are usually also hypertrophic. These individuals may become grossly obese, often exceeding 150% of ideal weight. Their obesity tends to be uniformly distributed centrally and peripherally. Prognosis for weight loss is very poor.

Adult-onset obesity is characterized by a normal number of adipocytes of large size with increased content of triglycerides. This form of obesity is much more common, and environmental etiologic factors are more obvious. The obesity tends to be centrally distributed, and response to various therapeutic measures is—though still only fair—much better than in the patient with lifelong obesity. A consequence of hypertrophy of adipocytes is insulin resistance and reduction in the number of cellular insulin receptors. The severity of these consequences generally correlates positively with the degree of cellular hypertrophy. Patients with adipocyte hypertrophy tend to be relatively resistant to the development of ketosis during a fast.

OBESITY

Adipose tissue comprises about 10% of the body mass of normal infants at birth. In early adulthood, slender males also have about 10% of body mass as fat, whereas in normal slender females, adipose mass is about 15%. Because body weight and quantity of fat are continuously distributed in populations, the definition of obesity must be arbitrary. However, some guides are useful in identifying individuals who are significantly obese. A principal problem in defining obesity is the great variation in lean body mass among individuals of the same stature. Persons of mesomorphic body build, with heavy bone structure and musculature, may easily exceed the tabular norms of weight for height without being obese.

Indices of Obesity

Several indices have been developed to express the relationship of height to weight: weight/height ratio; weight divided by the square of height, called the body mass index; and height divided by the cube root of weight, called the ponderal index. These indices have been used mostly in research. More practical guides for adults are the height and weight tables of the Metropolitan Life Insurance Company, which are divided into 3 arbitrary classes of frame size, permitting a rough accommodation for the effect of lean body mass on total weight. Allowing for frame, patients must be considered obese if their weight exceeds the average by 20% or more.* Another factor that must be considered is that lean body mass decreases somewhat with age. Not only the percent of fat in the body but also its distribution differs between the sexes. In men, fat tends to be distributed about the trunk; in women, more adipose mass is present over the limbs and gluteal region. Departures from these patterns are of some importance in differentiating certain disorders associated with obesity. Skinfold thickness, another measure of obesity, has the advantage that the distribution of adipose mass can

---

*A simple rule that does not allow for differences in body frame but is useful as a screening test is as follows: Beginning with a body weight of 100 lb for women and 105 lb for men at 60 inches, an increment of 6 lb per inch for men and 5 lb per inch for women is permissible.

be set out in quantitative terms when measured at the proper sites with constant tension calipers. In general, adults may be considered obese if skinfolds exceed 19 mm for men and 30 mm for women at the mid-triceps level or 22 mm for men and 27 mm for women at the subscapular level. These figures represent the upper 20% in a United States population survey.

ETIOLOGIC FACTORS IN OBESITY

Genetic Factors

A number of genetic forms of obesity are well known in animals. Perhaps the best-studied of these is the obese (ob/ob) mouse, which appears to have a constitutional defect in thermogenesis. When these mice are exposed to cold, they do not increase their heat production as do normal mice. The defect in thermogenesis appears to involve reduced levels of sodium/potassium ATPase in muscle and liver. The resulting decreased energy expenditure apparently leads to accumulation of energy stores in adipose tissue in the form of triglycerides.

A similar defect involving both a decrease in the number of ouabain-binding sodium/potassium ATPase sites and the activity of this enzyme has been described in the erythrocytes of some obese humans. The observation that these abnormalities did not change after weight loss suggests that it may be a constitutional defect associated with obesity. Because other investigators have failed to confirm this finding, such a conclusion must await further understanding of the technical aspects of measurement of ATPase activity.

Recent investigations suggest that cholecystokinin octapeptide (CCK8) inhibits appetite in mammals when infused into the cerebral ventricles. This polypeptide, which corresponds to the 8 C-terminal amino acids of intestinal cholecystokinin (CCK33), is found in higher concentrations in the central nervous system than in plasma. Deficiencies in levels of CCK8 and of its central nervous system receptors have been postulated to exist in genetic animal models of obesity.

Obesity in humans is frequently familial, but separation of genetic from environmental effects is difficult. Much of the observed familial aggregation of obesity may be related to family eating patterns, especially as they affect nutrition in infancy and early childhood. Nevertheless, studies of identical twins reared apart provide convincing evidence for substantial genetic determinacy of adipose mass.

Endocrine Factors

There is no established endocrine cause for most cases of obesity. However, several uncommon endocrine disorders do include obesity as one of the clinical features. Cushing's syndrome is characterized by centripetal redistribution of adipose tissue and is readily recognized by other prominent stigmas. Hyperinsulinism associated with insulinoma can lead to marked obesity, presumably by stimulating hyperphagia as well as by adipotropic metabolic effects.

Some individuals with hypothyroidism become obese, probably largely because of diminished catabolic activity, although the permissive role of thyroxine in lipolysis may also be important. It should be remembered, however, that most excess gain with hypothyroidism is due to myxedema. Obesity may also be associated with Klinefelter's and Turner's syndromes, male hypogonadism, and castration.

It is well established that insulin resistance accompanies obesity, often with elevated levels of insulin in plasma and increased rates of insulin secretion. The concentration of insulin receptors in monocytes, fibroblasts, and adipocytes from obese individuals is reduced, probably owing in large part to the hyperinsulinemia per se. This phenomenon is accompanied by decreased insulin-induced glucose transport, glucose oxidation, and lipogenesis by adipocytes. The sensitivity of the inhibition of lipolysis in isolated fat cells from obese subjects appears to be increased. This could result in impaired hydrolysis of stored triglycerides during fasting when insulin levels are relatively low and thus may be significant in the etiology of obesity.

Another metabolic feature of hypertrophic obesity is increased activity of lipoprotein lipase in adipose tissue, a phenomenon that persists with weight reduction.

Neurologic Factors

Lesions of the ventromedial hypothalamus in animals regularly produce hyperinsulinism, hyperphagia, and obesity. Diverse structural or functional lesions of this region in humans, including tumors, trauma, and inflammation, have produced a similar type of hypertrophic obesity. Hypothalamic dysfunction is also postulated in certain rare heredofamilial syndromes of obesity.

Psychologic Factors

Psychologic determinants are of great importance in both the etiology of obesity and its management. Individuals reared in a kindred of obese people tend to regard obesity as the norm. Overeating may represent disturbed family dynamics and involve the whole family. Parents may overfeed children in an attempt to deal with guilt, as an expression of their own unmet emotional needs, or as a distorted expression of love. Such a child often becomes passive, overdependent, and immature in later childhood and as an adult. Overeating and decreased activity leading to obesity may occur as a response to some environmental or emotional stress such as death of a loved one, disruption of a family unit, or school or job pressures or failures. Eating patterns in some obese patients ("night-eating syndrome," "eating binge syndrome") have been associated with periods of psychologic stress. Food may become a substitute for other gratifications or may serve to relieve boredom, loneliness, or anxiety. Eating may help to stave off uncomfortable feelings of anger or depression. Obesity may serve to protect an individual from normal social interaction, sexual conflicts, and exposure to the possibility of failure in such interpersonal relationships.

Habit and environmental factors appear to influence appetite regulation. Thin individuals tend to eat only when hungry, whereas obese people eat in response to such stimuli as time of day, flavor, odors, etc. Another important factor is the Old World cultural view that obesity is a sign of health and prosperity. But in a society such as ours, which favors an image of youthful slimness, obesity can cause serious psychologic problems as well as originate from them.

SYNDROMES ASSOCIATED WITH OBESITY

Prader-Willi Syndrome

This syndrome is not clearly genetic, but several cases have been reported in some kindreds. Clinical features include mental retardation, hypotonia, small hands and feet, and hypogonadism. Obesity begins at age 2–5 and is progressive into adulthood.

Laurence-Moon-Biedl Syndrome

Consanguinity is common in this disorder, which is characterized by retinal degeneration, mental retardation, polydactyly, and hypogenitalism, especially of males, who have small testes and gynecomastia. Obesity begins in childhood.

Alström-Hallgren Syndrome

The obesity in this syndrome also begins before puberty. Clinical features include retinal degeneration and nerve deafness. Diabetes frequently occurs, and acanthosis nigricans and male hypogonadism are occasionally present.

Fröhlich's Syndrome (Adiposogenital Dystrophy)

Obesity in this disorder is truncal in distribution. There is hypogenitalism with absence of secondary sex characteristics. Short stature, decreased visual acuity, diabetes insipidus, and mental retardation may be associated findings.

Hyperostosis Frontalis Interna

This syndrome of women may begin as late as the sixth decade. It includes hyperostosis of the frontal bones, with mental obtundation, headache, and occasionally virilism and impaired equilibrium or seizure.

Multiple Lipomatosis

Several syndromes of lipomatosis are recognized. The lipomas are usually distributed in a bilaterally symmetric fashion. Often they enlarge when the patient is consuming alcohol and may regress with abstinence. One variety, **Madelung's disease,** selectively involves lipomatosis of the neck.

EFFECT OF OBESITY ON DISEASE

Hyperlipoproteinemia

Obesity chiefly affects the metabolism of triglyceride-rich lipoproteins and is almost a prerequisite for the appearance of primary hyperprebetalipoproteinemia. Levels of VLDL in plasma fall as soon as body weight begins to decrease and can usually be maintained near normal if ideal body weight can be achieved. Likewise, in primary and secondary mixed lipemias, obesity profoundly amplifies the expression of the underlying defect. In familial dysbetalipoproteinemia, where remnant lipoprotein particles accumulate in blood, obesity is also a major determinant of expression of the metabolic defect. In all forms of lipemia, reduction of adipose mass to normal is an important element of therapy. There is an independent inverse relationship of adipose mass with the levels of plasma high-density lipoproteins.

Diabetes

Hypertrophic obesity is an essential element in the development of maturity-onset diabetes, in which insulin resistance, hyperinsulinism, and resistance to ketosis are prominent features. With the exception of those patients who develop severely compromised insulinogenic capacity, reduction of adipose mass to normal is attended by amelioration or even normalization of blood glucose and insulin levels.

Cardiopulmonary Disease

Obesity is associated with a moderate increase in risk of atherosclerotic heart disease, probably mediated at least in part by its effects on circulating lipoproteins and perhaps also by its association with hypertension. Obesity increases cardiac work as a result of the expanded requirement for blood transport, thus increasing the risk of underlying valvular or cardiomyopathic disease, where load is important. Cardiac failure is the cause of death in most morbidly obese patients. Hypoventilation with decreased arterial oxygen content, with or without hypercapnia, is encountered in grossly obese persons. The fully developed **pickwickian syndrome** may include somnolence, cyanosis, and muscle twitching.

Complications of Pregnancy, Labor, & Puerperium

Obese women are at significantly increased risk of preeclampsia-eclampsia. Labor tends to be difficult and prolonged, and the incidence of postpartum hemorrhage is increased.

Cholelithiasis

Lithogenic bile, commonly seen in obese patients and largely resulting from increased cholesterol synthesis and excretion, increases the risk of cholelithiasis severalfold, especially in women.

Other Consequences of Obesity

An enlarged, fatty liver is often seen in association with obesity. Nonspecific gastrointestinal symptoms such as bloating and dyspepsia may be reported, and osteoarthritis may appear in its most severe form in obese patients.

A number of effects of obesity on endocrine function are now recognized. The production of cortisol by the adrenal cortex is increased in proportion to body mass. The conversion of androstenedione to estrone is increased up to 5-fold in obese women. In addition, the sex hormone–binding capacity attributable to sex hormone–binding globulin (SHBG) is low in obese individuals, leading to a higher level of unbound estradiol in plasma. Amenorrhea and oligomenorrhea are associated findings in some obese women. However, menarche tends to occur early in obese girls. Plasma levels of progesterone, pregnenolone, androsterone, and dehydroepiandrosterone are elevated in obese prepubertal girls, whereas their levels of 17β-estradiol are much lower than those seen in slender girls. There is a significant association of obesity, impaired glucose tolerance, and endometrial carcinoma.

TREATMENT OF OBESITY

Efforts to reduce body weight in hyperplastic obesity—ie, in patients with increased adipose cellularity resulting from early proliferation of adipocytes—are almost uniformly unsuccessful. These patients often have no insulin resistance, and the significance of their obesity with respect to carbohydrate and lipid metabolism is therefore probably less than in the case of patients with adult-onset obesity. Management of any obese patient must be individualized and based on information obtained from a complete history of family and environmental factors, eating habits, appetite, and physical activity patterns. The patient's attitude toward and desire for weight loss must be assessed. Causes of secondary obesity that may require specific treatment must be identified by physical examination or appropriate laboratory studies.

Drug Therapy

Because of the addiction potential of appetite suppressant drugs and the rapid tachyphylaxis that occurs during their use, there is no reasonable role for these agents in the management of obesity. In the absence of hypothyroidism, thyroid hormone is not helpful, and it may actually be dangerous if given in truly hypercalorigenic doses. No other hormonal substances, including chorionic gonadotropin, are of any demonstrated value.

Diet & Exercise

To reduce caloric intake below the level of expenditure, the patient's physical activity must be considered. An exercise regimen, when cardiovascular status permits, is a useful adjunct to diet. A consistent deficit of 1000 kcal/d will achieve a weight loss of approximately 1 kg (2.2 lb) per week. Patients should be counseled not to expect daily loss of weight, because some water-soluble cell constituents may be retained along with water for brief periods as triglycerides are removed. Ideally, the calories should be distributed over at least 3 meals. Patients should be advised to prepare their food attractively and to eat slowly. Careful dietary counseling should be given to ensure adequate intake of protein, vitamins, and minerals. Claims have been made for various extreme dietary regimens. One of these, total fasting, leads to substantial ketosis that induces anorexia. A variation of this diet involves severe restriction of carbohydrate; another involves feeding of protein with essentially no carbohydrate or fat. In all of these diets, hyperuricemia, hypercholesterolemia, and cholelithiasis may occur. Prolonged metabolic acidosis may lead to demineralization of bone. Certainly, patients with insulin-dependent diabetes, liver disease, renal disease, or gout should not be given these diets.

A number of cases of sudden death have been reported in patients eating only liquid formulas in which protein is the major source of calories. These deaths are attributed to ventricular arrhythmias resulting from electrolyte disturbances. Supplementation with potassium is not sufficient to prevent arrhythmias, however, and other micronutrients appear to be involved. Because of their intermittence, there is no way of anticipating the appearance of the arrhythmias, which can occur as early as 10 days after commencement of the diet. For this reason, such diets should never be used. However, substitution of a balanced fixed-composition liquid formula for one meal a day may facilitate successful initiation of weight loss.

In general, consistent application of a nutritionally balanced reducing diet appears to be the most judicious course. In patients with severe chylomicronemia, fat should be restricted specifically to achieve the greatest reduction in plasma triglycerides. Alcohol should be avoided by patients with hypertriglyceridemia, and all patients on a reducing diet should be counseled that alcohol provides nearly twice as many calories as carbohydrate per unit mass. Patients must be seen frequently for nutritional monitoring and psychologic support if success is to be achieved.

Psychologic Interventions

In patients who prove refractory to the initial dietary intervention, it is important to evaluate underlying psychologic mechanisms more thoroughly. Psychotherapy, group therapy, and behavior modification are all of potential benefit. In a seriously disturbed patient, rapid reduction may lead to severe depression or even psychosis. Goals in weight loss must be individualized and realistic. Reduction to ideal body weight is not realistic for the patient with the lifelong type of obesity. Supportive therapy, building on the patient's strengths, should be the goal in such cases rather than persistent striving for the unattainable. Physicians must be aware of the importance of their relationship with the obese patient and the patient's need for help in achieving a sense of personal worth.

Surgical Treatment

Jejunoileal bypass has been employed to induce intestinal malabsorption in patients with morbid obesity. Loss of weight is achieved at the expense of diverse local and systemic symptoms resulting from bacterial overgrowth in the lower bowel. Patients have persistent, often severe diarrhea, which frequently causes significant disturbances in fluid and electrolyte balance. Deficiencies of iron, vitamin B_{12}, and folate occur frequently. Osteomalacia may occur, perhaps secondary to abnormal absorption of vitamin D. Hepatic parenchymal function may be severely affected, leading to death in some patients. Nephritis, arthritis, angiopathic skin lesions, and autohemolysis have been

described and appear to be immune complex disorders secondary to bacterial overgrowth. Another significant consequence of jejunoileal bypass is hyperoxaluria with nephrolithiasis. Recently, a syndrome involving intermittent episodes of bizarre behavior, confusion, ataxia, and acidosis has been noted in patients with jejunoileal bypass. It is associated with production of D-lactic acid by intestinal bacteria. Because the overall mortality rate associated with the operation may exceed 10%, it should be considered a method to be used, if at all, only in cases of extreme, life-threatening obesity. Close monitoring in such patients is essential.

Gastric stapling is another surgical procedure currently being evaluated for the treatment of morbid obesity. Insufficient information is available about the safety of this technique, and it should be regarded as experimental at this time.

REFERENCES

Alpers DH: Surgical therapy for obesity. *N Engl J Med* 1983; **308**:1026.

Amer P et al: Influence of obesity on the antilipolytic effect of insulin in isolated human fat cells obtained before and after glucose ingestion. *J Clin Invest* 1984;**73**:873.

Bray GA: *The Obese Patient*. Vol 9 in: *Major Problems in Internal Medicine*. Smith LH Jr (editor). Saunders, 1976.

Bray GA (editor): *Obesity in Perspective*. Publication No. 75-711. Vol 2, part 2. US Department of Health, Education, and Welfare, 1973.

Bray GA, Kral JG, Björntorp P: Hepatic sodium-potassium–dependent ATPase in obesity. *N Engl J Med* 1981; **304**:1580.

Della-Fera MA, Baile CA: Cholecystokinin octapeptide: Continuous picomole injections into the cerebral ventricles of sheep suppress feeding. *Science* 1979;**206**:471.

DeLuise M, Blackburn GL, Flier JS: Reduced activity of the red-cell sodium-potassium pump in human obesity. *N Engl J Med* 1980;**303**:1017.

Edman CD, MacDonald PC: Effect of obesity on conversion of plasma androstenedione to estrone in ovulatory and anovulatory young women. *Am J Obstet Gynecol* 1978;**130**:456.

Flier JS: Insulin receptors and insulin resistance. *Annu Rev Med* 1983;**34**:145.

Foster WR, Burton BT (editors): Health implications of obesity. (National Institutes of Health Consensus Development Conference.) *Ann Intern Med* 1985;**103(6-Part 2 Suppl)**: 981. [Entire issue.]

Harrison LC, Martin IR, Melick RA: Correlation between insulin receptor binding in isolated fat cells and insulin sensitivity in obese human subjects. *J Clin Invest* 1976;**58**:1435.

Hirsch J, Batchelor B: Adipose tissue cellularity in human obesity. *Clin Endocrinol Metab* 1976;**5**:299.

Hirsch J, Knittle JL: Cellularity of obese and nonobese human adipose tissue. *Fed Proc* 1970;**29**:1516.

Kannel WB, Gordon T: Page 125 in: *Physiological and Medical Concomitants of Obesity: The Framingham Study*. Publication No. (NIH) 79-359. Bray GA (editor). US Department of Health, Education, and Welfare, 1975.

Keill N (editor): *Psychology of Obesity*. Thomas, 1973.

Mir MA et al: Erythrocyte sodium-potassium-ATPase and sodium transport in obesity. *N Engl J Med* 1981;**305**:1264.

Mott DM et al: Altered insulin binding to monocytes and diploid fibroblasts from obese donors. *J Clin Endocrinol Metab* 1983;**57**:1.

Pedersen O, Hjollund E, Sorensen NS: Insulin receptor binding and insulin action in human fat cells: Effects of obesity and fasting. *Metabolism* 1982;**31**:884.

Salans LB: Obesity of the adipose cell. Chap 8, pp 495–521, in: *Metabolic Control and Disease*, 8th ed. Bondy PK, Rosenberg LE (editors). Saunders, 1980.

Siiteri PK: Extraglandular estrogen formation and serum binding of estradiol: Relationship to cancer. *J Endocrinol* 1981;**89**:119.

Simat BM et al: Is the erythrocyte sodium pump altered in human obesity? *J Clin Endocrinol Metab* 1983;**56**:925.

Straus E, Yallow RS: Cholecystokinin in the brain of obese and nonobese mice. *Science* 1979;**203**:68.

Stunkard AJ et al: An adoption study of human obesity. *N Engl J Med* 1986;**314**:193.

US National Center for Health Statistics: *Preliminary Findings of the First Health and Nutrition Examination Survey, United States 1971–1972: Anthropometric and Clinical Findings*. Publication No. (HRA) 75-1229. US Department of Health, Education, and Welfare, 1975.

York DA, Bray GA, Yukimura Y: An enzymatic defect in the obese (ob/ob) mouse: Loss of thyroid-induced sodium- and potassium-dependent adenosinetriphosphatase. *Proc Natl Acad Sci USA* 1978;**75**:477.

23

Hormones & Cancer

Christopher C. Benz, MD, & Brian J. Lewis, MD

HORMONAL EFFECTS ON TUMORS

GROWTH-PROMOTING HORMONES

It would be logical to suppose that hormones which support normal growth might also promote tumorigenesis. However, although a great deal is known about endocrine factors regulating normal pre- and postnatal growth, very little from that body of information can be applied to our current understanding of tumorigenesis. Growth hormone (GH), thyroid hormone, insulin, and sex and adrenal steroids have permissive roles in prenatal growth. Of these hormones, only the sex steroids directly stimulate tissue growth during the postnatal period: genetic rather than endocrine factors play the major role in determining body stature. Gigantism results from excessive secretion of GH by a pituitary tumor; however, the end-organ tropic responses to GH as well as the responses to thyroxine and insulin are mediated by mitogenic factors called somatomedins (see Chapter 4). These polypeptides are structurally homologous to proinsulin, and their serum concentrations are hormonally regulated. Acting via membrane receptors, somatomedins directly stimulate the cellular proliferation of normal and neoplastic cells.

INDUCTION OF NEOPLASIA

It has been shown that human tumors, including fibrosarcomas and breast cancers, actively secrete somatomedinlike peptides that act as mitogenic autocrine factors. Of further significance is the finding that cellular expression of somatomedin receptors requires stimulation by epidermal, fibroblast, or platelet-derived growth factors (EGF, FGF, or PDGF). These factors and the larger group of structurally related transforming growth factors can be isolated from human tumor specimens as well as cell lines derived from chemically or virally transformed nonmalignant cells.

Transforming growth factors have been broadly characterized as protein kinases, and they are coded for by cellular transforming genes that have also been identified in a wide variety of rodent, avian, and human cancers (including endocrine-sensitive human breast cancers). Activation of transforming genes and the subsequent expression of the malignant phenotype can be induced by chemical carcinogens (including steroidal and nonsteroidal estrogens) and by regional integration of viral DNA into the genome of a normal cell. Long-term or in utero exposure to exogenous estrogens is now believed to be associated with an increased incidence of human breast and endometrial carcinomas as well as clear cell adenocarcinoma of the vagina.

Murine mammary tumor virus (MMTV) is a weakly oncogenic type B retrovirus that may also serve as an important example for the development of endocrine-sensitive cancers. Regionally inserted DNA sequences from MMTV activate transforming gene sequences in normal rodent epithelial cells, and this can result in mammary cancer. In addition, MMTV-induced effects are subject to transcriptional regulation by steroids, particularly glucocorticoids. The steroid regulatory sequences in MMTV have been unambiguously identified within the long terminal repeat (LTR) segments of genomically inserted virus. These data collectively support the view that hormones play an important role in the development of tumors and the expression of their characteristic behavior.

STEROIDS & CANCER

The early studies of Bittner, Huggins, Furth, and others established the concept that sex steroids can cause or at least promote tumor growth. Until recently, the only cancers believed to be promoted by sex steroids included the common tumors arising from breast (male and female), endometrial, and prostatic tissue (Table 23–1).

It may be generally true that endocrine dependency can develop as an associated trait of tumors derived from any tissue whose normal growth is stimulated by a hormone. Recent studies in fact have demonstrated associations between sex steroids (especially estrogens) and vaginal, ovarian, and laryngeal carcinomas as well as hepatomas. It has been suggested that sex steroids alone may play a pathogenic role in almost 30% of all cancer cases in the USA. Thyroid, testicular, and ovarian tumors occur in glands under the tropic influences of TSH, FSH, and LH and may also be putatively included in the list of endocrine-dependent cancers. With increasing epidemiologic data, it is likely that this list will increase. For example, the incidence of osteosarcoma closely parallels the different age-specific growth patterns of men and women, implicating pubertal hormonal changes in the etiology of this tumor. Meningiomas and thyroid and

Table 23–1. Endocrine-responsive tumors.

Primary treatment involves endocrine therapy
    Breast carcinoma
    Endometrial carcinoma
    Prostatic carcinoma
    Leukemia
    Lymphoma
Tumor treatment may include endocrine therapy
    Renal cell carcinoma
    Thyroid carcinoma
    Ovarian carcinoma
    Pituitary adenoma
Tumor subsets may be endocrine-dependent
    Vaginal carcinoma
    Meningioma
    Melanoma and apudoma
    Gastrointestinal carcinoma
    Sarcoma

renal cell carcinomas show a marked discrepancy in male-female incidence (and prognosis), also suggesting tropic sex hormone influences on tumor growth.

In contrast to the tropic sex steroids, glucocorticoids are capable of cytolytic responses mediated by steroid-induced enzymatic pathways. Since the realization nearly 15 years ago that glucocorticoids could lyse human lymphoblasts, these steroids have been extensively employed in the treatment of leukemia and lymphoma.

TUMORS AFFECTING ENDOCRINE STATUS

Tumors that are not hormone-responsive (or amenable to endocrine therapy) may still affect endocrine status, and these tumor-induced endocrine effects are important for clinical diagnosis and management.

NONSECRETORY TUMORS

Nonsecretory primary or metastatic tumors may invade and replace normal glandular tissue and thereby cause loss of endocrine function. The most common syndrome in this category is hypopituitarism due to pressure necrosis that occurs gradually during tumor growth or that occurs abruptly from tumor infarction and bleeding (Sheehan's syndrome). Tumors such as breast cancer, leukemia, or lymphoma may be metastatic to the sella; may directly invade, as with a craniopharyngioma or hypothalamic glioma; or may originate from a primary adenoma in the anterior pituitary. Rarely, infarction of the posterior pituitary and the clinical development of diabetes insipidus may be the presenting sign of metastatic cancer. Adrenal insufficiency can also occur with metastatic infiltration of both glands by a variety of epithelial cancers (eg, lung cancer, breast cancer, melanoma). However, this is a rare event clinically, especially considering the high overall incidence of adrenal metastases from these and other malignant tumors found at autopsy. Although extensive pancreatic or ovarian replacement can occur with metastatic retroperitoneal tumor spread, diabetes mellitus or ovarian failure virtually never results. Ovarian failure may develop in association with a primary ovarian carcinoma that secretes steroid precursors which in turn inhibit pituitary gonadotropin production.

SECRETORY TUMORS

Several types of benign and malignant tumors secrete hormones or hormonelike substances. When these chemicals are produced ectopically or "inappro-

Table 23–2. Secretory tumors of endocrine glands.

Tumor Origin	Secretory Product(s)
Anterior pituitary	GH, PRL, ACTH, TSH, FSH, LH
Adrenal	
Cortex	Aldosterone, glucocorticoids, androgens, estrogens (rare)
Medulla	Catecholamines
Kidney	Erythropoietin
Gonads	
Germ cell, trophoblast	hCG
Stroma	Estrogens, androgens, progestins
Pancreas and gut (APUD cells)	Serotonin, kallikrein, prostaglandins, somatostatin, gastrin, glucagon, insulin, VIP, CCK, vasopressin, ACTH, neurotensin
Parathyroids	Parathyroid hormone
Thyroid	
Parafollicular (medullary) cells	Calcitonin
Follicular cells	Thyroglobulin, T_3 and T_4 (rare)

priately'' (by a tumor arising in a tissue not normally associated with the hormone), the resulting paraneoplastic syndrome may provide a diagnostic clue or may signify recurrence of an otherwise undetectable lesion (see Chapter 24). For example, gynecomastia associated with an elevated titer of human chorionic gonadotropin (hCG) strongly suggests an underlying testicular carcinoma that can be cured with chemotherapy. "Appropriate" hormone production by secretory tumors arising within endocrine tissue may also produce symptoms leading to early tumor detection and cure, as is occasionally observed with insulinomas. On the other hand, endocrine symptoms from secretory tumors may develop in association with advanced disease and result in life-threatening or debilitating clinical complications. The difficulty in palliating symptoms from carcinoid or one of the other apudomas (see Chapter 18) can actually become of greater clinical concern than controlling the tumor

itself, and symptomatic control of these unresectable lesions can only be achieved with chemotherapeutic agents. These secretory tumors are usually well differentiated and may occur in genetic patterns (eg, Klinefelter's syndrome associated with a breast or pituitary tumor) or in familial patterns involving multiple endocrine glands (eg, multiple endocrine neoplasia type I, IIa, or IIb; see Chapter 25). Table 23–2 lists the origin of commonly occurring secretory tumors and their associated secretory products.

TREATMENT-INDUCED ENDOCRINOPATHY

With the improved prognosis of patients with leukemia, lymphoma, stage II breast cancer, and germ cell neoplasms treated with irradiation and chemotherapy, there is a growing awareness of the long-term endocrine complications of treatment. The glands associated with treatment-induced endocrinopathy include the hypothalamus, pituitary, thyroid, parathyroids, and gonads. As shown in Table 23–3, local or regional effects from radiation therapy and the systemic effects of radiomimetic drugs (alkylating agents) produce the greatest clinical problems.

BRAIN & PITUITARY

Children receiving cranial irradiation either to prevent leukemia of the central nervous system or to treat a curable brain tumor have blunted GH responses, impaired growth rates, and some impairment of intellectual function. Less commonly, they may have reduced secretion of TSH, ACTH, FSH, and LH. In adults, apart from the use of hormonal agents, anti-

Table 23–3. Treatment-induced endocrinopathy.

	Hormone Abnormality	Clinical Abnormality
Radiation therapy		
Brain	↓GH; less commonly, ↓TSH, ACTH, FSH, LH	Growth retardation.
Head and neck		
Low-dose (≤750 rads)	↑Parathyroid hormone	Hyperparathyroidism, thyroid cancer.
High-dose (≥1400 rads)	↓Thyroxine; ↑TSH	Hypothyroidism, thyroid cancer.
Abdomen and pelvis (including gonads)	↓Estrogen; ↑FSH, LH	Sterility, menopause, azoospermia.
Chemotherapy		
Alkylating agents, vinblastine, others	↓Estrogen; ↑FSH, LH (normal testosterone, adrenal steroids)	Sterility, menopause, azoospermia.
Vincristine	↑Vasopressin	SIADH*
Cyclophosphamide	(Normal vasopressin)	SIADH*
Mitotane	↓Adrenal steroids	Primary adrenal insufficiency.
Aminoglutethimide	↓Estrogens, adrenal steroids	Primary adrenal insufficiency.
	↓Thyroxine; ↑TSH	Hypothyroidism.

*Syndrome of inappropriate secretion of vasopressin (antidiuretic hormone).

tumor therapy results in very few abnormalities in the hypothalamic-pituitary-neuroendocrine axis. Adjuvant chemotherapy for breast cancer has been reported to lower serum PRL levels, but the underlying mechanism is unclear. Vincristine and cyclophosphamide have both been associated with a syndrome of inappropriate secretion of vasopressin (antidiuretic hormone), or SIADH. While a direct effect on renal tubules is believed to be the cause of the antidiuresis that occurs with cyclophosphamide, vincristine may increase vasopressin release by disrupting microtubules within the neurohypophysis.

THYROID

One-third of patients with cervical lymphomas or carcinomas of the pharynx or larynx treated with curative doses of radiation (which includes the thyroid) develop increased TSH levels, and most of these also develop decreased thyroxine levels. A few become clinically hypothyroid. Both low-dose and (less frequently) high-dose irradiation increase the incidence of thyroid carcinomas occurring 10 or more years after treatment.

ADRENALS

Adrenal gland function appears resistant to the toxic effects of conventional doses of radiation or chemotherapy. However, prolonged busulfan administration for chronic granulocytic leukemia results in a clinical syndrome resembling adrenocortical insufficiency. Some investigators believe that pituitary secretion of ACTH—rather than adrenocortical function—is damaged by the drug. This mechanism could be similar to that resulting in impaired PRL secretion, mentioned above.

GONADS

Perhaps the most frequently encountered endocrinopathy resulting from antitumor therapy is gonadal failure. Radiation therapy and chemotherapy can cause infertility in both men and women. In women, amenorrhea (or oligomenorrhea), dyspareunia, decreased libido, and hot flushes may follow either form of therapy. These symptoms are associated with reduced plasma estradiol and increased levels of FSH and LH. In fact, ovarian failure occurs so frequently after adjuvant chemotherapy for breast cancer that some have suggested that the effectiveness of adjuvant therapy results from "chemical oophorectomy." In younger women, there is a greater probability that gonadal function will return to normal. In men, azoospermia (or oligospermia) occurs in association with reduced testicular size, increased FSH, and (occasionally) gynecomastia. Leydig cells are much more resistant to toxic therapy, and serum testosterone levels therefore usually remain normal, although there may be evidence for partial Leydig cell failure compensated for by higher levels of LH. Depending on radiation or drug dosage, male gonadal function and fertility may recover. With the aggressive drug combinations used to cure lymphomas, however, gonadal recovery is unlikely, and men should be offered the opportunity for sperm storage before chemotherapy begins. Recent successes with in vitro fertilization and cryopreservation suggest that a similar option may become available for women. GnRH analogs, which decrease serum gonadotropin levels, are currently being investigated for their ability to protect the gonads during cytotoxic therapy. The use of birth control pills to reversibly suppress gonadotropins and suspend ovarian function has reportedly been successful in sparing women from gonadal toxicity during chemotherapy.

ENDOCRINE THERAPY FOR CANCER

STEROID RECEPTORS & TREATMENT

At present, endocrine treatment is of major therapeutic value in breast, endometrial, and prostatic cancers. The specific applications of endocrine therapy in these diseases will be discussed later. However, the measurement of steroid receptors has added a further refinement to the technology of determining which tumors are endocrine-sensitive. Estrogen receptors (ER), useful for predicting the endocrine responsiveness of breast cancer, are now being detected in a variety of other human tumors, including hepatomas, sarcomas, meningiomas, and renal cell and ovarian carcinomas as well as melanomas and colorectal and pancreatic carcinomas. On average, these tumors probably have a much lower frequency of ER positivity and lower receptor level than breast cancer; thus, it is not surprising that early clinical studies have failed to detect any significant role for endocrine therapy in their management.

The mere presence of a steroid receptor does not ensure either a functioning receptor mechanism or a cytostatic or cytolytic response when endocrine treatment is employed. For example, glucocorticoids are known to alter liver metabolism, but they do not produce the cytolytic effects on hepatocytes that are observed with lymphocytes, although both cell types contain high levels of glucocorticoid receptor. Similarly, it appears that breast tumors possessing ER capable of inducing synthesis of progesterone receptor (PgR) are the tumors most responsive to endocrine treatment. In short, the therapeutic importance of receptors depends on both a functioning receptor mechanism and a growth-regulating receptor response.

One additional comment should be made in reference to tumor treatment and receptor status. It is recognized that hormone therapy can reduce tumor ER and PgR levels to about 25% of their pretreatment values, and it is recommended that at least 2 months elapse after treatment before the tumor is sampled for receptor analysis. Treatment with radiation therapy or chemotherapy may similarly result in falsely low or falsely negative receptor levels that may persist for 12–24 months of treatment before they return to pretreatment levels. Thus, the results of a receptor assay performed during or within a few weeks after therapy should be interpreted with great caution.

RECEPTOR AGONISTS & ANTAGONISTS

Surgeons in the late 19th century first observed the regression of breast cancer following bilateral oophorectomy, thus marking the beginning of endocrine therapy and the awareness of endocrine-dependent tumors. Surgical ablation has only recently been challenged by drugs that can chemically ablate selected endocrine organs. Unfortunately, the long-standing empiricism surrounding endocrine therapy has not yet been totally supplanted by scientific rationale. Although the biology and biochemistry of ER and PgR are of primary importance in predicting breast cancer treatment response and prognosis, at present there is insufficient experience on which to base any recommendations about using receptor data in deciding upon the clinical management of prostatic and endometrial cancers, leukemia, or lymphoma. In the near future, histochemical detection of steroid receptors will probably emerge as an important diagnostic tool, improving our ability to predict endocrine responses in individual patients and perhaps expanding our list of endocrine-dependent tumors.

The empiricism of endocrine therapy is also evident from recent trials showing few differences in response rates when receptor agonists or antagonists are compared with surgical ablative therapy. For example, premenopausal breast cancer patients respond to either oophorectomy, tamoxifen, or medroxyprogesterone acetate. Similarly, patients with prostatic carcinoma respond equally well to orchiectomy or diethylstilbestrol (DES). These generalities seem puzzling only because of our limited understanding of receptor function and the mechanisms resulting in either cytostatic or cytolytic tumor control and of the effect of treatment on hypothalamic and pituitary factors that also modify tumor growth. How do we explain that when hormone agonists bind to cellular receptors in tumors, they can trigger either a complete or a partial response? Prolonged agonist binding may exhaust the cellular response or down-regulate the receptor (tachyphylaxis). We also know for a certainty that individual tumors are heterogeneous—they may contain subpopulations of cells with and without receptor proteins and with quantitative and qualitative variations in receptor function.

Apart from the commonly administered steroid agonists (estrogens, androgens, progestins, and glucocorticoids), there are also analogs of nonsteroid hormones currently being tested for antitumor potential. For example, bromocriptine and other tight-binding dopamine agonists are capable of shrinking pituitary adenomas. Agonists and antagonists of GnRH that reduce serum PRL and gonadotropin levels can produce clinical responses in breast and prostatic cancers.

The classic concept has been that hormone antagonists bind to receptors and block the subsequent steps to hormonal response, including the signals to undergo cell division and synthesize proteins. However, clinically effective steroid antagonists such as tamoxifen, clomiphene, cyproterone, and flutamide may or may not share the steroid ring structure of the hormones they antagonize and may bind with high affinity to nonreceptor sites within the cytoplasm. Some, in addition to blocking hormonal response, also induce synthesis of unique proteins with as yet unknown functions. Flow cytometric studies comparing the cell cycle responses of tumors to either antiestrogen administration or estrogen deprivation have shown different points of cell cycle arrest, again suggesting dissimilar mechanisms of antitumor activity. Equally disconcerting to investigators is the therapeutic significance of "spillover" among steroid hormones: the potential cross-reactivity of androgens for ER, progestins for ER and glucocorticoid receptors, and glucocorticoids for androgen receptors.

ENZYME INHIBITORS

Within the subcellular microsome system of endocrine-responsive cells are enzymes necessary for interconverting steroids to more active hormonal derivatives. These enzymes have become the targets of a new family of synthetic agents used to treat breast and prostatic cancers. Aminoglutethimide was the first of such agents released for use; it was initially introduced as an anticonvulsant in 1960 but then was found to inhibit adrenal steroidogenesis, resulting in "medical adrenalectomy." This drug is now used to treat breast cancer in postmenopausal women and has subsequently been found to be a potent inhibitor of aromatase activity. Aromatase is actually a complex of enzymes found in many extra-adrenal tissues, including breast cancers, that converts circulating androgens to estrogens (see Fig 14–4). The estrogen products (estrone and estradiol) can then bind to intracellular ER and produce estrogen-specific responses.

The predominant circulating estrogen in postmenopausal women is estrone sulfate, which is derived from adrenal steroid synthesis, peripheral aromatization, and hepatic conjugation. To be reutilized in ER-positive tissues, estrone sulfate must first be reactivated by another microsomal enzyme, sulfatase.

Active investigation is under way to develop inhibitors of sulfatase which could be used clinically in ovariectomized or postmenopausal women with breast cancer.

Estrogen responsiveness is also related to the activity of a catabolic enzyme, estradiol 17β-dehydrogenase. High-dose medroxyprogesterone acetate exerts part of its antitumor effect by increasing 17β-dehydrogenase levels and internally depriving the breast tumor cells of active estrogens.

COMBINATION ENDOCRINE THERAPY

Medroxyprogesterone acetate and other steroid agonists and antagonists are now being combined with enzyme inhibitors to try to increase endocrine response rates. There can be multiple mechanisms at work when such combinations are employed; for instance, besides increasing 17β-dehydrogenase activity, medroxyprogesterone acetate is also known to suppress adrenal production of androstenedione and thereby deplete cells of their androgenic substrate for aromatase and reduce conversion to estrogen. Thus, combining medroxyprogesterone acetate with aminoglutethimide brings into play at least 2 mechanisms of interaction that could result in enhanced inhibition of ER-positive tumors. Furthermore, higher doses of medroxyprogesterone acetate can bind (spill over) to glucocorticoid receptors, and this obviates the need for administering exogenous cortisol to patients receiving aminoglutethimide.

In benign and malignant prostatic tissues, it is believed that ER-positive stromal cells provide the tropic androgens required by the androgen receptor–containing epithelial cells. In the stromal cells, 5α-reductase converts testosterone to the most active androgen, dihydrotestosterone. Strategy for the endocrine treatment of prostatic cancers has focused on androgen ablation, either by surgical or medical means. Because of the hormonal interdependence between epithelial and stromal cells and the overall dependence of prostatic tissue on pituitary factors (FSH, LH, and PRL), medical ablation can be accomplished using estrogen agonists and antagonists, GnRH analogs, or inhibitors of 5α-reductase. All of these nonsurgical modalities are under clinical investigation, and preliminary studies suggest that combining some of these agents may vastly improve response rates in prostatic carcinoma.

CHEMO-ENDOCRINE THERAPY

Combining chemotherapy and endocrine therapy is emerging as a popular treatment approach for endocrine-sensitive tumors (especially breast cancer) despite an almost complete lack of supporting preclinical studies. Estramustine and prednimustine are 2 chemically similar steroid alkylating agents designed to be selectively toxic against receptor-positive cells. At present, it appears that these derivatives are no more effective than their parent compounds, suggesting that impaired receptor binding or systemic drug metabolism is limiting their cytotoxic potential. Simultaneous administration of tamoxifen with drug combinations such as CMF (cyclophosphamide, methotrexate, fluorouracil) may indeed increase response rates in selected groups of breast cancer patients; however, such additive effectiveness has not generally been observed in all patients, in all endocrine-sensitive tumors, or with other drug-hormone combinations. In fact, the potential for adverse therapeutic effects with chemoendocrine combinations has also been pointed out, and this form of treatment must still be considered investigative. Specifically, by suppressing tumor cell growth, hormonal therapy may protect the tumor from chemotherapeutic agents most effective against replicating cells.

In summary, endocrine therapy has a long and established history of empiric usefulness, although at present it must be considered palliative rather than curative. With the recent emergence of some biochemical understanding of the mechanisms underlying endocrine response and hormonal growth promotion, we are now witnessing the advent of more scientifically based applications. The hope is that this new understanding will lead to better tumor control.

CLINICAL PROBLEMS

BREAST CANCER IN WOMEN

Epidemiology

Breast cancer is a common tumor in the USA. There are over 100,000 new cases annually, and a woman in the USA has roughly a 7–8% lifetime risk of developing the disease. The cause of breast cancer is unknown. Associated risk factors are listed in Table 23–4.

Table 23–4. Associated risk factors for breast cancer in women.

Family history
Menstrual history
Parity
Population differences
Endogenous hormones
Exogenous hormones
Benign breast disease
Obesity
Ionizing radiation
Prior breast cancer
Prior endometrial or ovarian cancer

A. Family History: It is well established that the daughters of women with breast cancer are at higher risk of developing the disease than other women in the general population. The highest lifetime risk, 50%, is borne by women whose mothers had bilateral breast cancer with onset before menopause.

B. Menstrual History: Early age at menarche and late age at menopause increase the risk of breast cancer. Conversely, late age at menarche or early menopause (natural or surgical) reduces the risk.

C. Parity: Younger age of the mother at the time of her first pregnancy and a history of full-term pregnancy lower the subsequent risk of breast cancer.

D. Population Differences: There are striking variations across cultures in the incidence of breast cancer. Oriental women have a much lower risk than women in Western countries. Women of Japanese descent who grow up in the USA have a higher incidence of breast cancer than those who grow up in Japan. Within the USA, the probability of developing breast cancer by age 75 shows significant ethnic variation: 8.2% for whites, 7% for blacks, 4.8% for Hispanics, 2.5% for Native Americans, 5.4% for Japanese-Americans, and 6.1% for Chinese-Americans.

E. Endogenous Hormones: The data on menstrual function and parity in women—and experimental work in animals, where estrogen is clearly permissive or even carcinogenic in the induction of breast cancer—strongly implicate estrogen exposure as an important factor in the development of breast cancer. Many case control studies have examined estrogen profiles as well as PRL levels, but no clear pattern or association has emerged. There is also no linkage with androgens or thyroid hormone levels. An inherent flaw in these studies is that the induction of breast cancer is a long-term process, and if the estrogen profile of a patient or a control were to be related to cancer, it is probable that a short-term analysis of hormones—a snapshot, as it were—when the cancer was detected would not tell enough of the story. One would need instead a longitudinal, integrated profile starting at least at the menarche in a large cohort of women in order to reliably detect differences in endocrine physiology and relate them to the development of cancer.

F. Exogenous Hormones: Retrospective analyses of users of birth control pills or of postmenopausal women who take estrogen are inconclusive. There is, however, some suggestion that increased duration of exposure may increase the risk of breast cancer. Prospective studies of birth control pill usage do not indicate an increased risk, and there might even be a slight reduction in risk in some studies; but because of the considerable latent period for induction of breast cancer—presumably decades—further observation will be necessary to resolve the issue. The data certainly do not justify withholding birth control pills, but it would be prudent to limit the overall period of use as much as possible. The administration of estrogen to postmenopausal patients is a hotly debated issue, especially because estrogen use is associated with endometrial cancer. The possibility that prolonged use or high doses can increase the risk of breast cancer warrants further caution. One should keep the dose and duration of exposure to exogenous estrogen to a minimum.

G. Benign Breast Disease: "Fibrocystic disease" is not a very specific term and usually refers to painful breast nodules that may wax and wane during the menstrual cycle. This commonly diagnosed condition occurs in up to 50% of women and reflects variability in end-organ response to fluctuations in endogenous hormone levels. The condition is less frequent in users of birth control pills and may also respond to the elimination of caffeine from the diet. Histologically, one can see macrocysts, microcysts, adenosis, apocrine change, fibrosis, fibroadenomas, or ductal hyperplasias. These conditions are not found with higher frequency in patients who develop breast cancer, but it has been noted that having had a previous biopsy for benign breast disease increases the relative risk (from 1.86 to 2.13) of developing breast cancer compared to the general population.

Retrospective analysis of a large group of patients was recently performed to better define who within the benign breast disease category had an increased relative risk for subsequent breast cancer. The presence of a proliferative lesion without atypical hyperplasia (atypia) increased the risk to 1.9 relative to the presence of a nonproliferative lesion. Atypia increased the risk to 5.3, and patients with atypia plus a family history of breast cancer had a relative risk of 11. It should be noted that the majority of patients (70%) who underwent biopsy for benign breast disease did not have lesions associated with an increased risk of breast cancer.

H. Other Factors: Obese habitus may correlate positively with an increased risk of breast cancer. Ionizing radiation is an established carcinogen. Atomic bomb survivors, patients who received therapeutic radiation for mastitis, and those who had repeated chest fluoroscopy for tuberculosis show increased rates of breast cancer. Cancer in one breast is associated with a 10–20% lifetime chance of developing primary cancer in the opposite breast. A history of endometrial or ovarian cancer also increases the chances for developing breast cancer.

It appears from the above data that the hormonal milieu is a critical element in the development of breast cancer. Estrogen seems to be the most important factor. There may be a dose-response effect, as suggested by the correlation with an increased duration of ovulatory cycling or with obesity. In the latter instance, there may be added estrogen contributed by peripheral conversion of sex steroids in adipose tissue. Early pregnancy may cause subtle changes in the set points for estrogen and PRL levels, or it may induce a protective change at a critical time in the breast tissue itself. In women with a strong family history, endogenous estrogen may enhance some inherent genetic susceptibility to carcinogens in the breast. Radiation is clearly a carcinogen for the breast, but other exogenous factors (eg, diet) that might account for population differences in the attack rate of breast cancer are less easy to document. Diet could be influential through specific elements such as fat or fiber content, or it could have a more complex interaction. The overall calorie content and balance of foodstuffs could produce variations in growth, hormone profiles (anterior pituitary hormones such as GH as well as sex steroids), age at menarche, and the like, and these could influence susceptibility to breast cancer later in life.

Treatment of Metastatic Breast Cancer

A. Steroid Receptors and Other Considerations: Hormonal therapy is a main feature in the treatment of advanced breast cancer. A fairly straightforward algorithm to guide the selection of treatment utilizes the patient's menopausal status and the ER and PgR profile of the tumor (Fig 23– 1). The chance of responding to endocrine therapy increases directly with tumor concentrations of ER and PgR. Table 23– 5 shows how breast cancer response rates vary with receptor status. These data also indicate that postmenopausal patients are more apt to have receptor-positive tumors than premenopausal patients and, by implication, to respond better to endocrine therapy.

Important ancillary data include the performance status of the patient, the tempo of tumor growth, the extent of visceral involvement, and the prior treatment

Table 23–5. Rates of response to endocrine therapy according to estrogen and progesterone receptors (ER, PgR) in women with breast cancer.*

Tumor Receptor Status	Frequency Distribution		Rate of Response to Endocrine Therapy
	Premeno-pausal Women	Postmeno-pausal Women	
ER−, PgR−	30%	19%	11%
ER−, PgR+	9%	3%	46%
ER+, PgR−	12%	23%	27%
ER+, PgR+	49%	55%	77%

*Modified and reproduced, with permission, from McGuire WL: Steroid hormone receptors in breast cancer treatment strategy. *Recent Prog Horm Res* 1980;**36**:135.

history. The better the general condition of the patient and the lower the tumor burden, the more likely that an appropriately chosen hormonal treatment will be effective. Since the response to hormonal treatment is often not evident for several weeks and it can take 6– 8 weeks for maximum response to occur, patients who are critically ill from breast cancer and require an immediate antitumor effect should receive chemotherapy. Likewise, patients with explosive tumor growth or with a short interval between mastectomy and the development of metastases are less likely to benefit from hormonal therapy than those with more indolent tumor growth. Skin, soft tissue, lymph nodes,

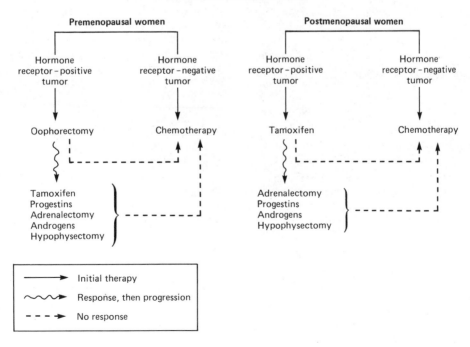

Figure 23 –1. Treatment algorithm for advanced breast cancer in women.

and bone are the metastatic sites most responsive to endocrine maneuvers. Significant lung or liver involvement and brain metastases require chemotherapy and radiation therapy, respectively. Limited lung or liver infiltration may well respond to hormone treatment. The patient who has responded favorably to a prior hormonal maneuver has an increased likelihood of responding to subsequent endocrine treatment. Conversely, if a patient's tumor is refractory to one form of endocrine therapy, subsequent hormone treatments are usually of little value, and it is better to consider starting chemotherapy.

B. Premenopausal Endocrine Therapy: For premenopausal patients with ER-positive tumors, ablative treatment with oophorectomy is the first-line hormonal maneuver. Preliminary data suggest that the antiestrogen tamoxifen may be effective in this role. However, because it can lead to increased circulating estrogens and gonadotropins—and because (by mass action effect) it may not adequately block these higher endogenous estrogen levels—tamoxifen is not generally considered first-line treatment in premenopausal patients. The response rate to either oophorectomy or tamoxifen as initial treatment ranges from 30 to 60%, depending upon the level of ER protein and the sites of metastatic disease. Responses average 12–15 months in duration.

In premenopausal patients who respond to oophorectomy but whose tumors progress, several options are available. Tamoxifen may induce a further response in 20–40% of patients. Responders whose tumors progress can next receive a trial of progestational agents or androgens. The former have few side effects, can increase appetite and the sense of well-being, and produce responses in 15–30% of patients when used as third-line treatment. Response rates for progestins may be higher when they are used as second-line treatment. Androgens are effective 10–20% of the time but cause masculinizing effects. Attempts to develop less virilizing analogs of testosterone have been only moderately successful, and it is argued that the frequency of virilization may not be all that different between various congeners at equipotent antitumor doses. Another ablative maneuver, adrenalectomy—either surgical or medical using aminoglutethimide—can be employed as either second- or third-line treatment, with a response rate in the range of 15–30%. Medical adrenalectomy appears equal to surgical ablation in antitumor effect, but its effects are reversible once the drug is stopped. However, like surgical adrenalectomy, it also requires the administration of replacement hydrocortisone. In addition to maintaining vital functions, this replacement therapy also prevents increased pituitary ACTH production and overriding of the adrenal blockade. Since dexamethasone metabolism is augmented by aminoglutethimide, it should not be used as the replacement steroid during treatment. Up to 30% of patients receiving aminoglutethimide will initially experience somnolence or rash, side effects that usually subside with continued treatment.

Finally, the development of transsphenoidal surgery has made hypophysectomy a more feasible ablative maneuver. Before the advent of receptor analyses, hypophysectomy was used as palliative treatment in end-stage patients, especially those with extensive and painful bone metastases. Patients who were responders would awaken from anesthesia with dramatic pain relief. That it occasionally benefits hormone-refractory cases suggests that its palliative effects are not mediated via sex steroid mechanisms. When compared to adrenalectomy in ER-positive tumors as second- or third-line treatment, hypophysectomy is equally effective and may have a slightly longer duration of action. However, the availability of aminoglutethimide, the operative risk, and the requirement for permanent adrenal replacement make hypophysectomy a less desirable option.

Premenopausal patients with ER-negative tumors would immediately be placed on a chemotherapy protocol.

C. Postmenopausal Endocrine Therapy: The initial endocrine maneuver in postmenopausal patients with ER-positive tumors is the administration of the antiestrogen tamoxifen. Five to 10 years ago, additive therapy with diethylstilbestrol (DES) was used; but this agent is associated with many more side effects than tamoxifen and has now largely been abandoned. Response rates to tamoxifen or DES range from 30 to 60%, again in proportion to the disease-free interval, metastatic sites, and the ER content of the tumor. Response durations are similar to those for oophorectomy. Once the breast cancer of a patient who has responded to tamoxifen progresses, second-line endocrine therapy is either medical adrenalectomy or administration of progestins, with response rates ranging from 15 to 40%. It should be noted that 10–20% of patients initially failing to respond to tamoxifen may have a clinical response to adrenalectomy. Thus, if the tempo of the disease and the clinical status of the patient permit, one can offer a trial of adrenalectomy before proceeding to chemotherapy.

When DES was in wider use, induction of therapy in patients with skeletal metastases would occasionally be accompanied by a "flare" with exacerbation of bone pain and hypercalcemia. This phenomenon usually heralded a clinical response and did not necessarily require prolonged interruption of treatment. When the cancer of patients who had responded to DES progressed, drug withdrawal was frequently followed by another clinical remission in up to 30% of patients, and this could last for several months. The flare phenomenon and the response to withdrawal are rarely seen with tamoxifen, although the flare has been noted to occur with androgen therapy.

Postmenopausal patients with ER-negative tumors would immediately be placed on a chemotherapy protocol.

BREAST CANCER IN MEN

Cancer of the male breast is extremely rare, occurring with a frequency of about 1% of that of cancer of the female breast. There is an association with Klinefelter's syndrome and with exogenous estrogen exposure (eg, in transsexuals), emphasizing the importance of hormonal factors, especially estrogen.

Up to 80% of tumors in men are ER-positive. Sixty to 70% of patients with metastatic tumors will respond to orchiectomy, and adrenalectomy and hypophysectomy are effective as second-line hormonal treatments. More recently, tamoxifen has shown activity as primary treatment and may eventually supplant orchiectomy. As in female patients with breast cancer, male patients whose tumors become refractory to hormone therapy go on to receive chemotherapy. Androgens are contraindicated because of their potential for facilitating tumor growth.

ENDOMETRIAL CANCER

Epidemiology

There are approximately 30,000 new cases of endometrial cancer annually in the USA. In contrast to the somewhat equivocal role of estrogen in the induction of breast cancer, its place in the causation of endometrial cancer appears more certain.

At the clinical level, as shown in Table 23–6, a variety of conditions have been associated with an increased risk of developing endometrial cancer. Their common denominator is unopposed or increased estrogen stimulation of the endometrium. This produces endometrial hyperplasia, a condition that can in turn progress to frank cancer. Progesterone antagonizes this effect of estrogen and induces the endometrium to mature or differentiate to a secretory state. Its action may be mediated by augmentation of enzymes in endometrial cells that metabolize estrogen and by decreasing levels of ER in this same tissue. There is a more frequent history of irregular menses in patients who develop endometrial cancer, and while combination birth control pills may have no influence on or may even decrease the risk of uterine cancer, sequential birth control pills may impart an increased risk, possibly because of the days of therapy where only estrogen is being administered.

Table 23–6. Conditions associated with an increased risk of developing endometrial cancer.

Prolonged or unopposed estrogen effect on the uterus
    Exogenous estrogen administration
    Late menopause
    Obesity (increased peripheral conversion of precursors to estrogen)
    Polycystic ovary syndrome
    Ovarian cortical stromal hyperplasia
    Estrogen-secreting ovarian tumors

At the population level, an upsurge in the incidence of endometrial cancer was noted in the USA in the early 1970s. This followed and paralleled an increase in the number of prescriptions written over the preceding years for replacement estrogen therapy in postmenopausal women. Case control studies of this phenomenon have clearly shown that exogenous estrogen use imparts a 3- to 8-fold increase in the risk of developing uterine cancer. The higher the dose and the longer the duration of estrogen use, the greater the risk. One follow-up study from the late 1970s reported that a decline in the number of estrogen prescriptions (after the initial recognition of their association with endometrial cancer) was accompanied by a decline in the incidence of endometrial cancer in the same population base.

Taken together, the above observations strongly support a conservative approach to the use of exogenous estrogens. They should be given in the smallest possible dose, for the shortest duration feasible, and on an intermittent schedule, with consideration given to adding a progestin to the treatment regimen. (See also Chapter 8 for a discussion of estrogens in the treatment of osteoporosis.)

Treatment of Metastatic Endometrial Cancer

A. Steroid Receptors: As is true in breast cancer, hormonal therapy is a primary therapeutic modality for advanced endometrial cancer. Unlike the situation in breast cancer, receptor profiles are not used to guide treatment selection in cases of endometrial cancer, although it was from uterine tissue that Jensen first isolated and characterized estrogen receptors in the 1960s. Uterine estrogen receptors increase during the proliferative phase of the menstrual cycle and fall in the presence of exogenous progesterone or with the rise of endogenous progesterone during the luteal phase. Progesterone receptors are induced by estrogen, and their level peaks coincident with the estradiol peak in the menstrual cycle. Most endometrial carcinomas contain ER, and, in contrast to breast cancer, levels are higher and inversely proportionate to the degree of histologic differentiation of the tumor. Progesterone receptors are also present in endometrial cancer, and their presence correlates directly with the degree of differentiation. As yet, ER and PgR have no practical application in the management of patients, probably because of the difficulty in distinguishing tumor from receptor-positive normal tissue.

B. Endocrine Therapy: Approximately one-third of metastatic tumors will respond to progestins. The probability of response is highest in patients with the most differentiated tumors and in those with the longest interval between primary treatment and the appearance of metastases. Responders live an average of 2 years after treatment is started, while nonresponding patients survive only about 6 months. Until recently, parenteral preparations such as hydroxyprogesterone and medroxyprogesterone were used. An orally effective compound, megestrol, has simplified treatment and appears to be as potent as the earlier parenteral formulations. Potential side effects of these compounds include salt retention and an increased predisposition to thrombophlebitis.

In patients who progress on progestational therapy or who do not respond initially, disease may be palliated with chemotherapy. However, in many patients, advanced disease stage, poor general health, and a history of pelvic irradiation limit tolerance to the most effective agents, ie, doxorubicin, cyclophosphamide, fluorouracil, and cisplatin.

PROSTATIC CANCER

Epidemiology

There are approximately 55,000 new cases annually of prostatic cancer in the USA. Prostatic cancer is essentially a disease of men in their 60s and 70s, and autopsy series have shown occult carcinoma in over one-third of cases in men over age 70.

Several lines of evidence support the idea that testosterone plays a role in the development of prostatic cancer. Testosterone can induce adenocarcinoma of the prostate in rats; castrated men do not develop prostatic cancer; and the disease is less frequent in patients with cirrhosis. Cirrhotic patients tend to be in a stage of relative estrogen excess from decreased hepatic estrogen metabolism, and they frequently exhibit testicular atrophy and gynecomastia.

Less clearly understood are racial and geographic differences. American blacks have a much higher incidence of prostatic cancer than Nigerian blacks, and Japanese-Americans who live in Hawaii have an attack rate intermediate between the low rate seen in Japan and the higher rates seen in whites in the USA. There are inconclusive data suggesting that patients may have higher testosterone production than controls; that viruses with oncogenic potential may play a permissive role; and that the number of sexual partners and a history of sexually transmitted disease also influence the incidence of prostatic cancer.

Treatment of Metastatic Prostatic Cancer

A. Steroid Receptors: Cytosol receptors for androgen have been isolated from prostatic cancers, and while they may predict for response, they are not presently integrated into clinical use. This is because (1) initial response rates to standard endocrine therapy are high, and alternative choices are far less promising (ie, second-line hormonal maneuvers or chemotherapy); (2) androgen receptor assays are technically difficult and often unreliable; and (3) the volume of tumor specimens from primary sites or metastatic sites (eg, bone) is not usually adequate for receptor determination.

B. Endocrine Therapy: It is difficult to compare the response data and therapies from different treatment centers. Typically, a patient with metastatic disease will complain of bone pain and manifest abnormalities on bone scan or plain x-ray. The acid phosphatase level may be specifically elevated in prostatic cancer, along with increased levels of the relatively nonspecific enzyme alkaline phosphatase. Response to therapy is hard to quantitate, since subjective complaints are difficult to measure, bone lesions resolve slowly, and the acid phosphatase does not always correlate reliably with variation in tumor volume. Only in less common instances of discrete lung, lymph node, or liver metastases is it possible to objectively and directly measure antitumor response.

Within these limitations, it appears that one-half to three-fourths of patients will benefit from treatment. Initial therapy is hormonal and is based upon the pioneering work of Huggins, showing that prostatic cancer is a testosterone-dependent tissue. Therapy consists of lowering testosterone levels either by orchiectomy or by the administration of DES. Since DES may have direct suppressive effects on the tumor and may inhibit pituitary gonadotropin secretion, some advocate the use of both DES and orchiectomy. However, the response rates with all 3 maneuvers—DES, orchiectomy, or DES plus orchiectomy—are essentially the same. Disease that progresses after initially responding to orchiectomy or to DES rarely responds to crossover treatment with the other maneuver.

A large Veterans Administration study established that 1 mg of DES daily orally was as effective as 5 mg but imposed less risk of cardiovascular complications. Since a 1-mg dose may lead to submaximal reduction in testosterone levels, a 3-mg dose is frequently employed. Patients who take DES may be troubled by painful gynecomastia; this can be prevented by low-dose breast irradiation prior to initiation of treatment. The average response duration to orchiectomy or DES is 15 months.

The presence of low levels of circulating androgens after orchiectomy has led to trials of adrenalectomy or hypophysectomy in patients with progressive disease. However, subsequent response rates to these ablative therapies are quite low, and responses are short-lived. More recently, alternative methods of depriving prostatic cancer of the tropic stimulus of testosterone have been tested. Androgen antagonists such as cyproterone or flutamide appear to be potent agents in previously untreated patients, but they are not effective in patients who have been treated by orchiectomy. Most recently, GnRH analogs have been quite effective in reducing testosterone to castrate levels and producing response rates equivalent to those achieved with DES or orchiectomy. The side effects from these analogs are virtually nil. GnRH analogs alone—or in combination with antiandrogens—may become the frontline agents for treatment of prostatic cancer.

MISCELLANEOUS TUMORS

Steroid hormone receptors have been isolated from tumors arising from organs not usually considered to be under primary endocrine control. Corticosteroid receptor protein is present in leukemia and lymphoma cells. It shows some correlation with response to steroid therapy, but levels are not used prospectively to guide treatment.

As mentioned earlier, there are reports of low but reproducible levels of ER or ER-like proteins in human renal, ovarian, hepatic, and pancreatic tumors and in melanomas. Progestational agents produce regression in 10% of hypernephromas; there are case reports that tamoxifen and progestins have caused regressions in ovarian cancer; and there are also reports that tamoxifen can cause regressions in melanomas that contain ER, though follow-up studies have failed to confirm this antitumor activity. Hepatomas have responded to

progestins on occasion, and trials are in progress to determine whether hormonal agents can produce regressions in pancreatic cancer.

In summary, it can be said that endocrine treatments for these tumor types do not appear promising at present. This reservation relates to the observation that traditional targets of endocrine therapy (eg, breast cancer) arise from a physiologic "target" tissue, and the probability of response appears to increase with increasing concentration of steroid receptor protein. The miscellaneous tumors just mentioned are not from obvious physiologic target tissues and contain low levels of steroid receptors; it is not surprising that they have shown no more than a glimmer of response to the endocrine modalities tested to date.

REFERENCES

Bittner JJ: The causes of mammary cancer in mice. *Harvey Lect* 1947;**42**:221.

Breciani F et al (editors): *Hormones and Cancer 2*. Vol 31 of: *Progress in Cancer Research and Therapy*. Raven Press, 1984.

Dupont WD, Page DL: Risk factors for breast cancer in women with proliferative breast disease. *N Engl J Med* 1985; **312**:146.

Furth J: Hormones as etiological agents in neoplasia. Pages 75–120 in: *Cancer, A Comprehensive Treatise*. Vol 1. Becker FF (editor). Plenum Press, 1975.

Henderson BE et al: Endocrine hormones as a major factor in human cancer. *Cancer Res* 1982;**42**:3232.

Huggins C: Endocrine-induced regression of cancers. *Science* 1967;**156**:1050.

King RJB: Oestrogen and progestin receptors as markers for the behavior of human breast tumors. Pages 357–370 in: *Bio-

chemical and Biological Markers of Neoplastic Transformation*. Chandra P (editor). Plenum Press, 1983.

Lane MA, Sainten A, Cooper GM: Activation of related transforming genes in mouse and human mammary carcinomas. *Proc Natl Acad Sci USA* 1981;**78**:5185.

Leclercq G et al (editors): *Clinical Interest of Steroid Hormone Receptors in Breast Cancer*. Vol 91 of: *Recent Results in Cancer Research*. Springer-Verlag, 1984.

Lippman ME: Endocrine responsive cancers of man. In: *Textbook of Endocrinology*, 7th ed. Williams RH (editor). Saunders, 1985.

May FEB et al: Mouse mammary tumor virus–related sequences are present in human DNA. *Nucleic Acids Res* 1983;**11**:4127.

Salomon DS et al: Presence of transforming growth factors in human breast cancer cells. *Cancer Res* 1984;**44**:4069.

Shalet SM: Disorders of the endocrine system due to radiation and cytotoxic chemotherapy. *Clin Endocrinol* 1983;**18**:637.

24 Ectopic Hormone Production

Betty S. Roof, MD, & Gilbert S. Gordan, MD, PhD

GENERAL CONCEPT OF ECTOPIC HORMONE PRODUCTION

Tumors of the endocrine glands and some tumors of nonendocrine organs secrete many types of hormones, enzymes, and other protein substances called tumor markers. In some cases, laboratory identification of such a substance may be the earliest clue to the presence of neoplastic disease. When a hormone or marker protein is produced by a tumor arising in a tissue not normally associated with the indicator, the substance is characterized as **ectopic** or **inappropriate.** A great many ectopic hormones have been studied, some of which appear to be identical in structure, immunoreactivity, and biologic action with "true" hormones, whereas others differ from usual hormones in some significant respect.

Although "humors from tumors" are fairly common phenomena, not all tumors produce all ectopic hormones or other protein markers. Even in cases where a paraneoplastic syndrome could arise ectopically, the nature of the marker may enable the clinician to identify the actual source of the hormone. For example, a woman with breast cancer may have hypercalcemia, hypophosphatemia, low tubular reabsorption of phosphate, and measurable immunoreactive parathyroid hormone in her serum. In this case, the elevated parathyroid hormone cannot be attributed to ectopic production by the breast cancer, because breast cancers do not produce parathyroid hormone. This patient almost certainly has a coexisting parathyroid adenoma. Very rarely, she could also have another primary tumor, such as carcinoma of the lung, kidney, ovary, or colon, any one of which can produce ectopic parathyroid hormone.

Tumors may affect the host by altering the function of the tissue in which they arise, by pressure on neighboring tissues, and, in the case of malignant tumors, by magnifying their effect through distant metastases. In addition, tumors that secrete one or more ectopic hormones may impose a further metabolic derangement on the existing disease. On rare occasions, the humor is the only early manifestation of a tumor, since many tumor hormones do not produce the expected endocrinopathy. This is an important generalization in our understanding of ectopic hormone production and host-cancer relationships. For example, elevated

Acronyms Used in This Chapter

ACTH	Adrenocorticotropic hormone
ADH	Antidiuretic hormone (vasopressin)
AFP	Alpha-fetoprotein
APUD	Amine precursor uptake and decarboxylation
cAMP	Cyclic adenosine monophosphate
CEA	Carcinoembryonic antigen
CGRP	Calcitonin gene–related peptide
CRH	Corticotropin-releasing hormone
FSH	Follicle-stimulating hormone
GRH	Growth hormone–releasing hormone
hCG	Human chorionic gonadotropin
hGH	Human growth hormone
hpGRH	Human pancreatic growth hormone-releasing hormone
LH	Luteinizing hormone
LPH	Lipotropin
mRNA	Messenger ribonucleic acid
MSH	Melanocyte-stimulating hormone
NSILA	Nonsuppressible insulinlike activity
OAF	Osteoclast-activating factor
PRL	Prolactin
PTH	Parathyroid hormone
SIADH	Syndrome of inappropriate secretion of vasopressin (antidiuretic hormone)
TSH	Thyroid-stimulating hormone (thyrotropin)

serum ACTH levels are found in a great many patients with bronchogenic carcinomas of all histologic patterns, but few of these patients have the full clinical manifestation of Cushing's syndrome. (Interestingly, ectopic Cushing's syndrome was reported* in a woman with bronchogenic carcinoma in 1928, 4 years before Harvey Cushing's classic description of the syndrome that now bears his name.) Many cancer patients have elevated serum parathyroid hormone levels without hypercalcemia, just as many male patients with lung cancer have elevated chorionic gonadotropin (hCG) levels without gynecomastia. The probable reason for this apparent hormonal failure is that tumor-associated peptides are often precursor molecules or lack carbohydrate and so have little or no hormonal activity. The concept that some tumor peptides are not "nor-

*By W. Hurst Brown.

Table 24—1. Direct and indirect evidence of ectopic secretion by nonendocrine tumors.

Clinical Observations	Molecular Basis	Tumor Sites or Tumor Types
Molecular basis known		
Cushing's syndrome (usually incomplete)	ACTH, big ACTH, β-MSH, LPH, CRH.	Lung, thymus, pancreas, cervix, adrenal medulla.
Hyperparathyroidism (or nothing)	PTH-like peptide.	Lung, kidney, colon, ovary, liver, esophagus, urogenital tract.
Hyponatremia (SIADH)	ADH, neurophysin.	Lung, pancreas.
Erythrocytosis	Erythropoietin.	Cerebellar hemangioblastoma.
Precocious puberty (boys), gynecomastia (men) (or nothing)	hCG, a-chain, β-chain.	Liver, adrenal, lung, esophagus, pancreas, gonads.
Galactorrhea	Prolactin.	Lung, kidney.
Neuroma	Nerve growth factor (? insulin).	Sarcoma.
Acromegaly (or nothing)	Growth hormone or GRH.	Lung, endometrium, pancreas.
Migratory necrolytic erythema	Enteroglucagon.	Kidney.
Cause unknown		
Hypoglycemia	Not insulin (NSILA), insulinlike growth factor IGF-II (? somatomedin). Other growth factors are not identified.	Liver, fibroma, sarcoma, adrenal, ovary.
Hypercalcemia without hypophosphatemia	Prostaglandin E_1 or E_2, phytosterol esters, prostacyclin (PGI_2), osteoclast-activating factor, growth factors.	Breast, ovary, blood vessels, kidney, lung.
Vitamin D resistance, hypophosphatemia, perhaps hypocalcemia	?	Benign tumors of bone and blood vessels, prostate.
Erythrocytosis	Not erythropoietin.	Liver, uterine fibroids, sarcoma.
Central nervous system disease: multifocal leukoencephalopathy, myasthenia, peripheral neuropathy	? Virus.	Lung, lymphoma.
Skin disease: dermatomyositis, acanthosis nigricans, hirsutism	?	Breast, ovary, lung, stomach, lymphoma.
Blood disease: bleeding, clotting	?	Pancreas, liver.
Tumor molecules without clinical manifestations		
None known	Growth hormone or GRH.	Lung, endometrium, pancreas.
	Somatostatin.	Medullary carcinoma of thyroid, lung.
	Calcitonin, CGRP.	Lung, breast, bronchial carcinoid.
	Bombesin.	Lung.
	Placental alkaline phosphatase (Regan isoenzyme).	Lung, breast, colon, ovary, pancreas, stomach, cervix, lymphomas.
	Carcinoembryonic antigen (CEA).	Bowel, breast, lung, liver, pancreas.
	Alpha-fetoprotein (AFP).	Liver, teratoma, metastasis to liver.
	Polyamines (eg, cadaverine).	Ubiquitous.

mal'' is fundamental to our understanding of these ectopic hormones and other tumor markers, since their presence can provide us with an important clue to early diagnosis of certain neoplasms.

It is now clear, as outlined in Table 24–1, that many nonendocrine tumors can manufacture hormonal peptides and that a single tumor can produce many hormones.

NATURE OF ECTOPIC PEPTIDES

Several important peptides have been sufficiently well characterized to demonstrate significant differences between them and their ''parent'' hormones. These ectopic hormones have been differentiated from the normal circulating hormone by the suffix -*like*— eg, PTH-like, ACTH-like, and insulinlike hormones. Insulinlike hormone cannot be suppressed by insulin antibody (NSILA) and is sufficiently different in structure from true insulin that it is not recognized by the specific radioimmunoassay for insulin. For these reasons, ectopically produced insulinlike hormone is thought to be a form of somatomedin. Tumors that produce ACTH-like and PTH-like hormones are in fact, for the most part, manufacturing *large* precursor molecules that possess only a fraction of the biologic activity of ''true'' hormones. Tumor calcitonin is also a large precursor molecule. On the other hand, tumor chorionic gonadotropin (hCG) is often characterized by a discordant synthesis of *small* precursor subchains or by a lack of glucose residues.

The number of peptides that can be produced by a single tumor is widely variable, and their identification probably depends on the sensitivity of available tests. The most versatile nonendocrine tumor in secreting ectopic hormones is apparently bronchogenic carcinoma, particularly the small or oat cell type. The

Table 24–2. Relative frequency of hormones, peptides, and tumor markers in untreated lung cancer.

Molecule	Incidence
Hormones	
Pro-opiomelanocortin (including ACTH, MSH, and β-LPH)	45–95%
Calcitonin	61%
ADH	40%
Bombesin	24%
β-hCG	6–11%
Parathyroid hormone	0–35%
Growth hormone	4–39%
Peptides and tumor markers	
CEA	70%
Prostaglandins E_2 and F_{2a}	69%
Placental alkaline phosphatase (Regan isoenzyme)	14%

relative frequency of ectopic hormones in the serum of patients with established lung cancer is set forth in Table 24–2.

CALCIOTROPIC SUBSTANCES & THEIR EFFECTS

Disorders of calcium and phosphate metabolism are common complications of neoplastic disease. In some cases, they represent the systemic effects of tumor-associated PTH-like peptides and may result in severe metabolic disturbances, including fatal hypercalcemia. However, many cancer patients whose tumors manufacture PTH-like humors or calcitonin have normal serum calcium levels.

1. ECTOPIC PARATHYROID HORMONE PRODUCTION

PTH-like peptides can be differentiated from parathyroid hormone found in normal, adenomatous, or hyperplastic parathyroid glands by differential immunoreactivity or by molecular sieving. In 1970, we first showed that ectopic hormones are disparate as determined by 2 antisera derived from chicken and guinea pig. Both antisera reacted with the biologically active one- to 34-amino-acid terminal sequence of the parathyroid hormone molecule, the intact molecule, and the carboxy-terminal fragment, and one antiserum reacted with a larger molecule, presumably proPTH. However, normal circulating hormones were equally immunoreactive with both antisera. In the serum of a patient with renal cell cancer that was the source of ectopic hyperparathyroidism, both the prohormone and the 84-amino-acid parathyroid hormone were present, but there were no C-terminal or N-terminal fragments (see Fig 8–7). The probable mechanism, according to the Jacob-Monod hypothesis, is deletion of re-

pressors for synthesis of parathyroid hormone. It would be a great coincidence if there were simultaneous repression of the enzyme that cleaves parathyroid hormone to C-terminal and N-terminal fragments. *Accordingly, antisera that recognize the large precursor molecules are essential for diagnosis of ectopic parathyroid hormone syndrome.* Antisera specific for the C-terminal fragment, which are most widely used these days, will probably *not* recognize the ectopic syndrome.

Tumor extracts contain water-soluble substances that have similarities to parathyroid hormone. Peptides include those which have immunoreactivity recognized in some radioimmunoassays but not in others (a function of the antiserum as described above) and bind to parathyroid hormone receptors in renal membranes sufficiently to activate adenylate cyclase and to increase the content of glucose 6-phosphate dehydrogenase in renal tubular cells. The effects of these extracts can be inhibited by the 3–34 analog of parathyroid hormone. The factor may have a molecular weight of 30,000–40,000 instead of 8400. Possible evidence that the effective agent is not parathyroid hormone is the reported failure of some tumors producing hypercalcemia to synthesize mRNA of parathyroid hormone. Unfortunately, in this last report, no tumor from a patient exhibiting both hypercalcemia and hypophosphatemia characteristic of hyperparathyroidism was examined.

Differential diagnosis in apparent hyperparathyroidism can be a difficult problem. High levels of ectopically produced parathyroid hormone may result in the identical syndrome produced by parathyroid hormone from a parathyroid adenoma, and parathyroid adenomas commonly coexist with cancer. The following may suggest an ectopic origin for hyperparathyroidism: (1) high serum alkaline phosphatase levels without x-ray evidence of subperiosteal resorption of cortex; (2) low serum chloride (< 102 meq/L) and elevated serum bicarbonate; (3) positive response of hypercalcemia to corticosteroids; and (4) rapid weight loss and anemia. Any or all of the above should suggest the possibility of an ectopic source for the elevated parathyroid hormone concentration, though only the first is pathognomonic. Urinary cAMP and nephrogenous cAMP are elevated both in primary hyperparathyroidism and in ectopic hyperparathyroidism, as well as in some cancer-associated hypercalcemias due to other causes.

Immunoreactive serum parathyroid hormone with or without hypercalcemia is common in many cancers. This phenomenon may prove to be a useful marker for early detection of cancers that tend to metastasize early and rapidly and which are often not diagnosed until they are no longer amenable to treatment—eg, cancers of the lung, colon, rectum, ovary, and kidney.

2. ECTOPIC ALKALINE PHOSPHATASE PRODUCTION

High serum alkaline phosphatase levels may occur in many cancers, either because of hepatic or osseous metastases or because of the presence of an ectopically produced phosphatase—the Regan isoenzyme. The latter is easily identified because, like placental alkaline phosphatase, it is heat-stable. Unfortunately, it is highly nonspecific, occurring not only in many tumors but also in some precancerous conditions, eg, ulcerative colitis and polyposis of the colon.

Still another form of alkaline phosphatase has been identified in myocardial tumors. This type differs from the enzyme that normally occurs in bone, liver, and intestine and also from the Regan isoenzyme.

3. ECTOPIC PROSTAGLANDIN PRODUCTION

The prostaglandins comprise a family of lipid-soluble derivatives of arachidonic acid and have a variety of activities, including bone resorption. Ectopic secretion of prostaglandin E_2 (PGE_2) associated with hypercalcemia has been demonstrated in fibrosarcomas, in lung cancers, and in medullary carcinoma of the thyroid. A metabolite of PGE_2 (prostaglandin E_m) has been identified in the urine of patients with solid tumors associated with hypercalcemia. Serum and urinary prostaglandin levels are suppressed in most cases by indomethacin or aspirin, and normocalcemia can be restored usually within 48 hours. Whether PGE_2 actually causes hypercalcemia, however, is quite doubtful. It is difficult to elevate serum calcium in test animals by prostaglandin infusion, probably because of rapid inactivation of PGE_2 by the lung. Prostacyclin (PGI_2) survives passage through the pulmonary circulation and is almost as potent as PGE_2 in resorbing bone.

4. ONCOGENIC HYPERCALCEMIA

Hypercalcemia is a grave and potentially fatal complication of so many cancers that it warrants special attention and immediate treatment. Hypercalcemia may result from metastatic lytic lesions of bones, coincidental primary hyperparathyroidism, or ectopic production of PTH or prostaglandins and osteoclast-activating factor (OAF) in patients with hematologic cancers. (OAF, a protein of MW 20,000, is normally produced by leukocytes.) In addition, hypercalcemia can dangerously complicate an otherwise indolent underlying tumor. The earliest symptoms of hypercalcemia are usually nocturia and anorexia, leading to hyposthenuria, polyuria, thirst, and eventually a diabetes insipidus–like syndrome resulting from refractoriness to antidiuretic hormone (ADH) produced by high concentrations of serum calcium. Renal tubular damage may quickly ensue, causing wasting of sodium and potassium and resulting in profound hyponatremia and hypokalemia. Gastrointestinal symptoms may be severe, ranging from anorexia and nausea to vomiting, paralytic ileus, and severe abdominal pain of unknown cause. Central nervous system involvement usually occurs late and is manifested by weakness, somnolence, coma, or psychosis. When the serum calcium rises rapidly, psychosis may be the first and only sign. Hypercalcemia is usually reversible even in advanced disease and with rare exceptions warrants vigorous therapy because a vicious cycle can easily be established when dehydration aggravates the hypercalcemia. When recognized early enough, the syndrome can be reversed with oral hydration or vigorous use of intravenous saline infusions. Later, corticosteroids or cytotoxic agents such as methotrexate or mithramycin in low doses are very effective. Calcitonin has also been used to control hypercalcemia.

5. ECTOPIC CALCITONIN PRODUCTION

The hypocalcemic peptide calcitonin is appropriately produced by thyroid C cells in medullary carcinoma of the thyroid, where elevated levels of calcitonin often identify asymptomatic familial cases. Calcitonin is also frequently produced ectopically by bronchial carcinoids and by cancers of the lung and breast. Calcitonin is *not* present in detectable amounts in extracts of benign breast tumors, normal lung, or normal breast tissue. Therefore, ectopic calcitonin provides a useful tumor marker, particularly for lung and breast cancer. Calcitonin gene–related peptide (CGRP), a peptide encoded by alternative splicing of mRNA for calcitonin, also serves as a tumor marker for medullary carcinoma of the thyroid and for some cases of bronchogenic carcinoma.

The normal action of calcitonin is to inhibit osteolysis and thereby lower serum calcium and phosphate. In calcium homeostasis, there is an intimate link between parathyroid hormone and calcitonin in that the latter provides fine control of the feedback mechanism. Thus, the principal effect of calcitonin is to counteract the hypercalcemia overshoot when parathyroid hormone mobilizes calcium from the skeleton. Because the normal action of calcitonin is weak and of brief duration, normocalcemia can be maintained. In contrast, ectopic calcitonin associated with tumors is a large precursor molecule lacking this biologic activity, so that hypocalcemia, dense bones, and evidence of vasoactivity have not been found even in patients with medullary carcinoma of the thyroid and astronomically high levels of calcitonin and CGRP.

The presence of immunoreactive calcitonin in sporadic pheochromocytomas has recently raised a question about whether this calcitonin is ectopically produced. The incidence of elevated serum calcitonin in patients with lung or breast cancer varies with the laboratory and antiserum used and depends upon antigen recognition of the antiserum, with those that detect carboxy-terminal fragments showing higher levels than those requiring the intact molecule.

6. ONCOGENIC OSTEOMALACIA

The nature of the substance presumed to originate most commonly in benign bone and blood vessel tumors—and which is responsible for acquired vitamin D resistance (oncogenic osteomalacia)—is under investigation. Fragmentary data suggest that this resistance may occur because of failure of renal 1α-hydroxylation of vitamin D, so that the most active form of the vitamin hormone, 1,25-dihydroxycholecalciferol, is not formed. Patients with this syndrome have osteomalacia in adulthood, or rickets as children, despite normal vitamin D intake as evidenced by normal 25-hydroxycholecalciferol levels. They often also have low serum phosphate levels and normal or low serum calcium levels. When the tumor is removed, 1,25-dihydroxycholecalciferol levels become normal within a few days. Hypocalcemia is found in about one-sixth of all cancer patients, especially in patients with carcinoma of the prostate, in whom abnormal vitamin D metabolism and osteomalacia have been reported.

ECTOPIC ACTH & CRH PRODUCTION

As noted in Chapters 4 and 9, the complete form of Cushing's syndrome is a rare complication of cancer; incomplete Cushing's syndrome, manifested by diabetes mellitus, hypertension, and hypokalemia, is more often seen. Even more common is no clinical manifestation at all despite the presence of ectopic big ACTH. Yalow and Berson were the first to recognize the heterogeneity of peptide hormones, and they observed that although the small intact molecule is the most common circulating form of ACTH—and in fact predominates in most pathologic states, eg, Addison's disease and Nelson's syndrome—it is the larger molecule, "big ACTH," that commonly characterizes bronchogenic carcinoma and pancreatic tumors (both islet and acinar). There is evidence that big ACTH is pro-opiomelanocortin. Both big ACTH and pro-opiomelanocortin can be converted by treatment with trypsin to fragments containing ACTH, melanocyte-stimulating hormone, and lipotropin. All of these fragments have been consistently found in tumors with ectopic ACTH production.

Ectopic production of ACTH is found in a wide variety of tumors, most commonly cancers of the lung, thymus, and pancreas. ACTH also occurs in some medullary cancers of the thyroid along with calcitonin, the latter being deemed an appropriate secretion from the neural crest–derived C cells. ACTH is also occasionally found in similarly derived pheochromocytomas, together with excess catecholamine elaboration, and—here again—the latter is deemed appropriate for this tissue. These combinations have led to the hypothesis that production of ACTH under such circumstances may not be truly ectopic but rather a characteristic of the amine precursor uptake and decarboxylation (APUD) system. This concept considerably enlarges our understanding of the common central nervous system and gastrointestinal origin of some tumors and hormones, though a number of ectopic secretions cannot presently be explained in this manner.

Variations in molecular structure probably best explain the disparity between immunologic and biologic activity in ACTH-like and MSH-like peptides. Heightened immunoreactivity in some ACTH-like peptides is probably due in part to excess quantities of both the N-terminal (one- to 13-amino-acid sequence) and the C-terminal (25- to 34-amino-acid sequence) fragments. These fragments of ACTH and large amounts of proACTH have been extracted from some cancers. Although the prohormone possesses all of the immunoreactivity of the 1–34 sequence of normally produced ACTH, it has only about 10% of its biologic activity and ability to bind to receptors, but it can be converted to biologically active ACTH by treatment with trypsin. The C-terminal fragment of ACTH is biologically inactive and can be separated by Sephadex sieving. Ectopic melanocyte-stimulating hormone (MSH) is usually found in the same tumors that produce ectopic ACTH. β-MSH may be an artifact of extraction, since its sequence is contained in the larger lipotropin (LPH) precursors; biologic activity is restricted to the lipotropin fragment, probably β-LPH (see Fig 4–3).

The N-terminal fragment of human ACTH–β lipotropin precursor protein is glycosylated. Both ACTH and α-MSH from plasma of patients with ectopic ACTH syndrome have little to about half of the expected polysaccharide moieties.

Unfortunately, big ACTH is not pathognomonic of cancer, since it also occurs commonly in heavy smokers. These individuals probably harbor an earlier form of bronchogenic neoplasia than is usually considered to be a true invasive lung cancer, since they also have cellular atypia in their sputum and have low serum levels of carcinoembryonic antigen (CEA). All of these features are reversible upon cessation of smoking.

Ectopic hormones with biologic actions similar to those of corticotropin-releasing hormone (CRH) have been reported. Ovine and rat CRH has been isolated and found to be a 41-amino-acid polypeptide. The amino acid sequence has been determined; it is likely that it is very similar if not identical to human CRH, both normal and ectopic. It is not known whether tumor peptides are present in the blood before other clinical evidence is manifest, but the possibility is important because the cancers most often affected (lung and pancreas) are not usually diagnosed until very late, when cure is rarely feasible.

ECTOPIC ADH & NEUROPHYSIN PRODUCTION

Some bronchogenic carcinomas appear to manufacture a vasopressinlike (ADH-like) hormone that can produce dilutional hyponatremia with inappropriately high urine osmolality, also known as the Schwartz-Bartter syndrome of inappropriate antidiuretic hormone (or SIADH). Cytotoxic chemotherapy has reversed these electrolyte imbalances in some cases, but in others the syndrome has been intensified perhaps through increased secretion of ADH from the posterior pituitary in response to dehydration secondary to vomiting induced by the chemotherapy. Radioimmunoassays have shown that some of these tumors associated with the symptoms of inappropriate ADH secretion have significant levels of neurophysin as well. Neurophysins are polypeptides that act as binding proteins for vasopressin and oxytocin but may be precursors of ADH. It is suggested that the presence of neurophysin in tumors that also elaborate ectopic ADH-like hormones is further evidence for genetic depression, since synthesis, storage, and secretion of neurophysin and of both vasopressin and oxytocin appear to share a common basic control.

ONCOGENIC ERYTHROCYTOSIS

Erythrocytosis may result from erythropoietin ectopically produced by cerebellar hemangioblastomas. When erythrocytosis accompanies hypernephroma, this is not considered "ectopically produced," since the kidney normally produces erythropoietin. In other tumors with erythrocytosis such as hepatomas, uterine fibroids, and sarcomas, erythropoietin has not been demonstrated.

ECTOPIC CHORIONIC GONADOTROPIN PRODUCTION

Ectopic chorionic gonadotropin (hCG) may be produced in nontrophoblastic cancers, resulting in precocious puberty in boys with certain hepatomas or pronounced gynecomastia in some men with tumors of the adrenal cortex. Ectopic hCG is elaborated by many other tumors, notably some cancers of the bronchus and of the gastrointestinal tract—particularly the esophagus. In most of these tumors, hormone-induced signs and symptoms are rare although several bronchogenic carcinomas have been diagnosed with gynecomastia as the first symptom. When hCG is produced by trophoblastic tumors such as choriocarcinomas, hydatidiform moles, or embryonal cancers of the testis, this secretion is deemed appropriate and provides a valuable marker in early detection and in evaluation of the efficacy of treatment of these cancers. The urine of males with significant levels of hCG gives a positive pregnancy test.

The glycopeptide hormones, including hCG, are composed of both alpha and beta chains of amino acids. While the alpha chains are similar in structure in this entire group of hormones (hCG, LH, FSH, and TSH), the beta chains are unique for each one, despite some remarkable similarities in a few, eg, β-hCG and β-LH, which are so similar that until recently it was virtually impossible to distinguish them. The unique biochemical properties of the beta chains have permitted development of specific antisera, so that each glycopeptide hormone can now be identified by radioimmunoassay. Placental hCG and about 30% of the hCG produced by cancers contain a carbohydrate component, while hCG *without carbohydrate* has been identified in many types of normal tissue from males and females and in about 70% of the hCG produced by tumors. The latter form is more rapidly cleared from the circulation and has no biologic activity in vivo, but it does retain both immunologic and receptor-binding properties in vitro. These apparently conflicting properties have raised the question whether hCG produced by tumors is appropriate or inappropriate.

ONCOGENIC HYPOGLYCEMIA

A number of nonpancreatic tumors have been associated with severe symptomatic hypoglycemia. Most common are large retroperitoneal fibromas and fibrosarcomas, some hepatomas, and some tumors of the adrenal cortex. The metabolic consequences in affected patients are profound; however, despite many attempts, immunoreactive insulin has only occasionally been recovered from these tumors, their metastases, or the sera of patients with tumors of the cervix or ovary. A substance with insulinlike activity as assayed on the epididymal fat pad of the rat has been recovered from some tumor extracts, but this cannot be suppressed by an insulin antibody. Nonsuppressible insulinlike activity (NSILA) is presently thought to be a somatomedin.

The mechanism by which some tumors produce hypoglycemia is not known. Starvation of the patient as a consequence of the immense size of some of these tumors has been postulated, but the serum free fatty acid level was not elevated in patients who were tested, so it appears unlikely that the mechanism is simply an excessive consumption of serum glucose by the tumor. The metabolic consequences of the hypoglycemia—though very severe—often provide the first clue to diagnosis. Symptoms vary from coma to an unexplained increase in appetite. Oncogenic hypoglycemia is easily induced by fasting; is substantiated by blood glucose concentrations less than 40 mg/dL; and is reversed by administration of oral or intravenous glucose. The serum and tumor levels of immunoreactive insulin in oncogenic hypoglycemia are low or undetectable. Many of these tumors are large, well-differentiated, slow-growing, and benign. The prognosis of the tumor is made substantially worse by the potentially fatal complication of hypoglycemia; early recognition and treatment are essential in all patients to prevent irreversible brain damage. Treatment includes total or, if this is not possible, partial surgical extirpation (or irradiation) of the tumor, with simultaneous correction of the hypoglycemia by frequent feedings, sustained intravenous infusion of hypertonic glucose, and, sometimes, corticosteroids. Chemotherapy has not been very effective in controlling oncogenic hypoglycemia, although some apparent tumor regression has been reported. (See also Chapter 20.)

ECTOPIC GROWTH HORMONE PRODUCTION

Ectopic secretion of growth hormone (hGH) or of growth hormone–releasing hormone (GRH) by some bronchial carcinoids and pancreatic islet tumors has produced acromegaly. Human pancreatic growth hormone–releasing hormones (hpGRH) recently isolated from 2 pancreatic tumors were found to be peptides of 40– 44 amino acids with close structural homology to peptides of the glucagon-secreting family and were indistinguishable from human hypothalamic GRH on high-performance liquid chromatography peptide maps. By radioimmunoassay, hpGRH can be measured in the peripheral circulation of patients with ectopic production of GRH but not in patients with pituitary acromegaly or in normal subjects. The biologic activity appears to reside in amino acids 1– 29. Conversely, hGH has been found in a number of other tumors, notably cancers of the lung and endometrium, without any clinical manifestations. The hypothesis that pulmonary hypertrophic osteodystrophy in lung cancer might be the result of hGH secretion has been discarded.

ECTOPIC PRODUCTION OF OTHER HORMONES

Prolactin & Secretin

Ectopic PRL secretion by tumors has rarely been demonstrated. In one hypernephroma, clear-cut secretion of biologically active PRL was reported with appropriate blocking of the activity by specific antiserum. Many lung cancers synthesize PRL but do not secrete it. The elevated serum levels in patients with tumors are the result of therapy with antidepressant drugs or with opiates or may result from radiotherapy to the chest wall. Secretin has also been demonstrated in 2 lung cancers.

Bombesin

Bombesin, a tetradecapeptide first isolated from frog skin, can release prolactin and growth hormone from pituitary cells in tissue culture. A larger form of bombesin known as gastrin-releasing peptide has also been identified in tumor and plasma from patients with lung cancers. Assays were negative for chole-

cystokinin, gastrin, vasoactive intestinal polypeptide, and substance P. Bombesin has been found in all lung cancers of the small cell lines that have been tested but not in those of non–small cell lines.

Somatostatin

Somatostatin 14 and somatostatin 28 have been found in medullary carcinoma of the thyroid, oat cell carcinoma, and bronchial carcinoids. Both forms of somatostatin have biologic activity; however, no clinical effect has been evidenced in patients with these tumors.

ONCOGENIC DISEASES IN WHICH THE MOLECULAR BASIS IS UNKNOWN

Other instances in which the molecular basis for the clinically observed phenomenon is unknown include central nervous system diseases, skin diseases, and either clotting or bleeding accompanying tumors.

Cancers of the lung or lymphoma may present initially as central nervous system diseases (eg, multifocal leukoencephalopathy, myasthenia gravis) or as peripheral neuropathy. Similarly, skin diseases such as dermatomyositis, acanthosis nigricans, or hirsutism (excess lanugo type hair) may herald cancers of the breast, ovary, lung, stomach, or lymphoma. Bleeding or clotting (or both) may be the initial presentation of diffuse intravascular coagulation in patients with cancer of the pancreas or liver; and marrow suppression, particularly of leukocyte and platelet formation, has been noted with pancreatic islet cell cancer.

NONHORMONAL TUMOR MARKERS

There are many nonhormonal tumor markers. Some of the most useful are the oncofetal antigens. Alphafetoprotein (AFP) and carcinoembryonic antigen (CEA) have been widely studied and are now well established as chemically useful in diagnosis and in early detection of recurrence. CEA in particular often rises when a precancerous lesion such as ulcerative colitis or ''C'' cell hyperplasia becomes cancerous. Conversely, the CEA level falls after removal of the tumor and rises again with recurrence of cancer. CEA is not specific for intestinal neoplasms, since it has also been found to be elevated in patients with lung cancer, breast cancer, medullary carcinoma of the thyroid, and cirrhosis. Low levels are also found in the serum of smokers. A promising recent advance is the use of radiolabeled monoclonal antisera to CEA to localize tumors in patients.

SUMMARY

Knowledge about specific peptide hormones, enzymes, and other indicators in certain tumors can be exploited for disease detection and evaluation of treatment. In some cases, the metabolic consequences are reversible when accurate diagnosis of the underlying tumor leads to appropriate treatment, eg, ectopic Cushing's syndrome from thymoma. In others, the absence of metabolic effects is a function of the precursor nature of the immunoreactive peptide with little or no hormonal activity. This area offers great potential for early detection of tumors that are often diagnosed too late for cure—eg, tumors of the lung, ovary, colon, and pancreas.

REFERENCES

Baylin SB, Mendelsohn G: Ectopic (inappropriate) hormone production by tumors: Mechanisms involved and the biological and clinical implications. *Endocr Rev* 1980;**1**:45.

Bower BF, Gordan GS: Hormonal effects of nonendocrine tumors. *Annu Rev Med* 1965;**16**:83.

Carey RM et al: Ectopic secretion of corticotropin-releasing factor as a cause of Cushing's syndrome. *N Engl J Med* 1984;**311**:13.

Daughaday WH, Trivedi B, Kapadia M: Measurement of insulin-like growth factor II by a specific radioreceptor assay in serum of normal individuals, patients with abnormal growth hormone secretion and patients with tumor associated hypoglycemia. *J Clin Endocrinol Metab* 1981;**53**:289.

Edbroke MR et al: Expression of human calcitonin/CGRP gene in lung and thyroid carcinoma. *EMBO J* 1985;**4**:715.

Feibusch J et al: Tumor-associated nephrogenic diabetes insipidus. *Ann Intern Med* 1980;**92**:797.

Frohman LA et al: Partial purification and characterization of a peptide with growth hormone–releasing activity from extrapituitary tumors in patients with acromegaly. *J Clin Invest* 1980;**65**:43.

Guillemin R et al: Growth hormone–releasing factor from a human pancreatic tumor that caused acromegaly. *Science* 1982;**218**:585.

Hall TC (editor): Paraneoplastic syndromes. *Ann NY Acad Sci* 1974;**230**:1.

Hershman JM: Hyperthyroidism caused by trophoblastic tumor. *Thyroid Today* 1981;**4**:1.

Hussa RO: Biosynthesis of human chorionic gonadotropin. *Endocr Rev* 1980;**1**:268.

LoGerfo P, Krupey J, Hansen HJ: Demonstration of an antigen common to several varieties of neoplasia. *N Engl J Med* 1971;**285**:138.

McFadzean AJS, Yeung RTT: Further observations on hypoglycemia in hepatocellular carcinoma. *Am J Med* 1969;**47**:220.

Megyesi V et al: Hypoglycemia in association with extra-pancreatic tumor: Demonstration of elevated NSILA-S by a new radioreceptor assay. *J Clin Endocrinol Metab* 1974;**38**:931.

Mundy GR et al: The hypercalcemia of cancer. *N Engl J Med* 1984;**310**:1718.

Nathanson L, Fishman WH: New observations on the Regan isoenzyme of alkaline phosphatase in cancer patients. *Cancer* 1971;**27**:1388.

Odell WD, Wolfsen AR: Humoral syndromes associated with cancer: Ectopic hormone production. *Prog Clin Cancer* 1982;**8**:57.

Roof BS et al: Immunoheterogeneity of the calcitonin of hypercalcemia, breast and lung cancers and medullary carcinoma of the thyroid. *Biomedicine* 1979;**30**:82.

Roof BS et al: Some thoughts on the nature of the ectopic parathyroid hormones. *Am J Med* 1971;**50**:686.

Simpson EL et al: Absence of parathyroid hormone messenger RNA in nonparathyroid tumors associated with hypercalcemia. *N Engl J Med* 1983;**309**:325.

Spiess J et al: Sequence analysis of a growth hormone–releasing factor from a human pancreatic islet tumor. *Biochemistry* 1982;**21**:6037.

Stevens RE, Moore GE: Inadequacy of APUD concept in explaining production of peptide hormones by tumors. *Lancet* 1983;**1**:118.

Stewart AF et al: Biochemical evaluation of patients with cancer associated hypercalcemia. *N Engl J Med* 1980;**303**:1377.

Stewart AF et al: Identification of adenylate cyclase stimulating activity and cytochemical glucose-6-phosphate dehydrogenase stimulating activity in extracts of tumors from patients with humoral hypercalcemia of malignancy. *Proc Natl Acad Sci USA* 1983;**80**:1454.

Strabanek P, McPartlin J, Powell D: Tumor hypercalcemia and "ectopic hyperparathyroidism." *Medicine* 1980;**59**:262.

Tashjian AH Jr et al: Evidence that the bone resorption–stimulating factor produced by mouse fibrosarcoma cells is prostaglandin E_2: A new model for the hypercalcemia of cancer. *J Exp Med* 1972;**136**:1329.

Turkington N: Ectopic production of prolactin. *N Engl J Med* 1971;**285**:1455.

Upton GV, Amatruda TT Jr: Evidence for the presence of hormone peptides with corticotropin-releasing-factor-like activity in the ectopic ACTH syndrome. *N Engl J Med* 1971;**28**:419.

Wilkinson M, Urich H, Croft PB: The remote effects of cancer on the nervous system. *Proc R Soc Med* 1967;**60**:683.

Wood SM et al: Bombesin, somatostatin and neurotensin-like immunoreactivity in bronchial carcinoma. *J Clin Endocrinol Metab* 1981;**53**:1310.

Yalow RS: Big ACTH and bronchogenic carcinoma. *Annu Rev Med* 1979;**30**:241.

Zerbe R, Stropes L, Robertson G: Vasopressin function in the syndrome of inappropriate antidiuresis. *Annu Rev Med* 1980;**31**:315.

25

Syndromes Involving Multiple Endocrine Glands

Leonard J. Deftos, MD, & Bayard D. Catherwood, MD

MULTIPLE ENDOCRINE NEOPLASIA

Decades of clinical observation have resulted in the identification of neoplastic syndromes involving multiple endocrine glands. The glands most commonly involved in such syndromes are the parathyroid, pituitary, pancreas, thyroid, and adrenal. The cell types involved in these tumors are postulated to have a common embryologic precursor in the neuroectoderm. This embryologic feature may be accompanied by the presence of the metabolic pathway for *a*mine *p*recursor *u*ptake and *d*ecarboxylation—thus the appellation APUD cells. Oncogenic mutational factors may also influence expression of these tumors. The multiple endocrine neoplasia syndromes are usually transmitted in an autosomal dominant inheritance pattern, but there may be considerable variability in penetrance and in specific tumor incidences among kindreds.

There are 3 well-defined types of multiple endocrine neoplasia (MEN) syndromes: **MEN type I** (also called Wermer's syndrome), **MEN type IIa** (also called Sipple's syndrome and MEN type II), and **MEN type IIb** (also called MEN type III). The clinical descriptions and terminology for these syndromes have evolved from 1954 to the present. The first MEN syndrome was clearly described by Wermer in 1954 and was characterized by tumors of the parathyroids, pituitary, and pancreas. Shortly afterward, Zollinger and Ellison described a syndrome that consisted of gastric hypersecretion and severe peptic disease associated with a non–insulin-producing islet cell tumor of the pancreas. This syndrome, the Zollinger-Ellison syndrome, is found in association with MEN type I in some cases but more commonly occurs by itself. In 1961, Sipple reported the association between thyroid cancer and pheochromocytoma. Through the subsequent studies of Williams and Hazard, a distinct thyroid tumor of the calcitonin-producing cells (C cells) of the thyroid—ie, medullary thyroid carcinoma—was defined. Characterization of the second MEN syndrome, consisting of medullary thyroid carcinoma, parathyroid tumors, and pheochromocytoma,

Acronyms Used in This Chapter

ACTH	Adrenocorticotropic hormone
APUD	Amine precursor uptake and decarboxylation
CGRP	Calcitonin gene–related peptide
CT	Calcitonin
GH	Growth hormone
HLA	Human leukocyte antigen
LH	Luteinizing hormone
MEN	Multiple endocrine neoplasia
MSH	Melanocyte-stimulating hormone
POEMS	Polyneuropathy, organomegaly, endocrinopathy, M protein, and skin changes
PP	Pancreatic polypeptide
PRL	Prolactin
PTH	Parathyroid hormone
TSH	Thyroid-stimulating hormone (thyrotropin)
VIP	Vasoactive intestinal polypeptide

evolved from these observations. The additional observation that there were 2 accompanying somatotypic features—ie, a marfanoid habitus and multiple mucosal neuromas—in some patients with this second type of MEN syndrome has led to the classification of a third type of MEN syndrome. In summary, the **major components** of the 3 syndromes are as follows: **MEN type I**—tumors of the parathyroids, pituitary, and pancreas, and, in some cases, components of the Zollinger-Ellison syndrome; **MEN type IIa**—medullary thyroid carcinoma, hyperparathyroidism, and pheochromocytoma; and **MEN type IIb**—medullary thyroid carcinoma, pheochromocytoma, marfanoid habitus, and multiple mucosal neuromas.

In general, the clinical and biochemical characteristics of component tumors of MEN syndromes do not differ markedly from characteristics of each tumor when it occurs by itself; therefore, those aspects are only briefly described in this chapter. For example, primary hyperparathyroidism as part of a MEN syndrome has most of the characteristics of primary hyperparathyroidism occurring alone, and the reader should consult Chapter 8 for a more detailed description of the features of primary hyperparathyroidism. However, the presence of multiple endocrinopathies presents a unique clinical picture (Table 25–1), and

Table 25—1. Abnormal hormone production by endocrine tumors of MEN syndromes. Measurement of these substances or their metabolites in blood and urine can serve as diagnostic tests.

	Pituitary	Pancreas	Parathyroid	Thyroid	Adrenal
PTH			+		
CT		+		+	
ACTH	+			+	
GH	+				
Somatostatin	+	+			
PRL	+				
VIP		+			
PP		+			
Gastrin		+			
Insulin		+			
Glucagon		+			
Catecholamines				+	+
Chromogranin A	+	+	+	+	+

the presence of multiple endocrine tumors does have specific implications for therapy.

MULTIPLE ENDOCRINE NEOPLASIA TYPE I

MEN type I is characterized by tumors of the parathyroids, pituitary, and pancreas. The most common pituitary tumor is benign chromophobe adenoma; the most common pancreatic tumor is gastrinoma; and the most common parathyroid lesion is

Table 25—2. Components of MEN type I and their approximate frequency of occurrence in patients with MEN type I.

Component	Frequency
Hyperparathyroidism	80%
Pancreatic tumors	75%
Gastrinomas	
Benign	20%
Malignant	30%
Insulinomas	
Benign	20%
Malignant	5%
Nonfunctioning tumors	
Benign	< 5%
Malignant	< 5%
Pituitary tumors	65%
Chromophobe or nonfunctioning adenomas	
Benign	40%
Malignant	< 5%
Eosinophilic tumors or acromegaly (benign)	15%
Cushing's disease, basophilic	5%
Mixed and other types (benign)	< 5%
Prolactin-secreting tumors	< 5%
Other tumors	
Carcinoid and bronchial adenomas	< 5%
Lipomas and liposarcomas	5%
Adrenocortical adenomas	10%

multiglandular primary hyperparathyroidism. Table 25–2 shows the approximate frequency of occurrence of the components of MEN type I. The actual pattern may vary among kindreds. Tumors other than the 3 principal components of the syndrome (Table 25–2) are rare, and their relationship to the genetic disorder is unclear.

Primary Hyperparathyroidism

Primary hyperthyroidism is the most common endocrine neoplasia of MEN type I. Thus, upon identifying a patient with primary hyperthyroidism, it is important to determine whether other components of the syndrome are present. The pathologic characteristics of the parathyroid glands can be best understood by recognizing the multiglandular nature of the disorder. The glands have been described in various terms ranging from adenomatous to hyperplastic. The histologic features necessary to make these classifications are not always apparent. Although chief cells are usually dominant, clear cells or a mixed picture may also be seen. The most important practical point to be derived from pathologic descriptions is the potential for all parathyroid glands to be involved in the neoplastic process, even ectopic glands. This means that aggressive surgical therapy directed toward subtotal parathyroidectomy may be necessary for effective treatment.

Pituitary Tumors

The most common pituitary tumor of MEN type I is chromophobe adenoma. This nonfunctioning tumor is usually benign by histologic criteria but can cause endocrine abnormalities by the effect of its mass on adjacent endocrine cells. Tumors producing growth hormone (GH), adrenocorticotropic hormone (ACTH), prolactin (PRL), and somatostatin have also been described in this syndrome, and their manifestations are classically related to their location and hormonal products. The incidence of pituitary microadenomas is not well defined.

Pancreatic Tumors

Gastrin-producing islet cell tumors are the most common pancreatic neoplasias of MEN type I, accounting for at least 50% of all pancreatic tumors. Gastrinomas can also occur at other sites such as the duodenal wall and stomach. Insulinomas are the next most common neoplasias. In addition, there are case reports of tumors producing vasoactive intestinal polypeptide (VIP), glucagon, pancreatic polypeptide (PP), somatostatin, and calcitonin (CT). Measurement by radioimmunoassay of these hormones in serum is an important diagnostic procedure. The "tumors" are usually composed of hyperplastic islet cells or multiple small tumors. The secretory products of these tumors can explain some of the associated findings. Examples are the peptic ulcer diathesis with gastrin, hypoglycemia with insulin, and secretory diarrhea with VIP and perhaps with PP. Glucagonomas can be associated with bullous dermatitis, but the pathogenesis of this lesion is obscure.

The production of excess gastrin leading to peptic ulceration by a pancreatic islet tumor is called **Zollinger-Ellison syndrome.** Zollinger-Ellison syndrome more commonly occurs by itself, but it can also be part of MEN type I. The ulcer diathesis of Zollinger-Ellison syndrome makes gastrointestinal symptoms a dominant clinical feature. Gastrointestinal symptoms may also be dominant in a patient with a VIP-producing islet cell tumor (VIPoma).

Other Tumors

The other tumors indicated in Table 25–2 are also found in patients with MEN type I, but their link to this disorder is not clearly established. Carcinoid tumors associated with MEN type I are more likely to be found in foregut-derived structures such as the thymus and bronchial tree than in midgut-derived structures, where sporadic carcinoid tumors usually occur. Bronchial carcinoid can produce its vasoactive symptoms without metastasizing. Adrenal and thyroid adenomas occurring in MEN type I represent predominantly the results of autopsy findings and are usually nonfunctioning. Lipomas may be present in some kindreds in MEN type I, and when cutaneous they may provide a useful sign of the syndrome.

MULTIPLE ENDOCRINE NEOPLASIA TYPES IIa & IIb

In the early reports of medullary thyroid carcinoma as part of a multiple endocrine disorder, the associated lesions were pheochromocytoma, hyperparathyroidism, and a syndrome consisting of multiple mucosal neuromas and marfanoid habitus (mucosal neuroma syndrome). It is now appreciated that 2 distinct clinical syndromes can be defined by these associated endocrinopathies: MEN type IIa (Table 25–3) and MEN type IIb (Table 25–4). MEN type IIa consists of medullary thyroid carcinoma, pheochromocytoma, and hyperparathyroidism; MEN type IIb consists of med-

Table 25–3. Components of MEN type IIa and their approximate frequency of occurrence in patients with MEN type IIa.

Component	Frequency
Medullary thyroid carcinoma	97%
Hyperparathyroidism	50%
Pheochromocytoma	30%

Table 25–4. Components of MEN type IIb and their approximate frequency of occurrence in patients with MEN type IIb.

Component	Frequency
Multiple mucosal neuromas	100%
Medullary thyroid carcinoma	90%
Marfanoid habitus	65%
Pheochromocytoma	45%

ullary thyroid carcinoma, pheochromocytoma, multiple mucosal neuromas, and marfanoid habitus. The component tumors of MEN type IIa and MEN type IIb vary in their incidence and prevalence. Since medullary thyroid carcinoma is the central tumor, it will be discussed first.

Medullary Thyroid Carcinoma

Medullary thyroid carcinoma, a tumor of the calcitonin-producing cells (C cells) of the thyroid gland, is a component of MEN type IIa and IIb. The thyroidal C cells are now generally accepted to be of neural crest origin. These cells migrate to the ultimobranchial bodies from the neural crest. In submammals, the cells form a distinct organ, the ultimobranchial organ, which harbors C cells and their secretory product, calcitonin. In mammals, C cells become incorporated into the thyroid gland and perhaps other sites. The neural crest origin of C cells offers an explanation for the association of medullary thyroid carcinoma with other tumors of neural crest origin and also appears to explain the production by these tumors of a wide variety of bioactive substances.

Medullary thyroid carcinoma is usually a firm, rounded tumor located in the middle or upper lobes of the thyroid gland. The cells usually are polyhedral or polygonal and are arranged in a variety of patterns. Calcification is commonly found in the tumor, and a characteristic calcification may be visible on x-ray. Although the presence of amyloid has long been considered to be important in the diagnosis of medullary thyroid carcinoma, the diagnosis is best established by the use of specific immunohistochemical procedures for calcitonin that demonstrate the abnormal C cells. The frank malignancy of medullary thyroid carcinoma, at least in familial cases, is preceded by a progressive hyperplasia of C cells referred to as **C cell hyperplasia.** This predecessor of medullary thyroid carcinoma can become manifest in early childhood or as late as the second decade. There may be corresponding changes in the parathyroid and adrenal glands. Several instances of **C cell adenoma** have also been reported. The natural history of medullary thyroid carcinoma can vary greatly, and this may make decisions regarding therapy difficult. The tumor is generally regarded as intermediate between the aggressive behavior of anaplastic thyroid carcinoma and the more indolent behavior of papillary and follicular thyroid carcinoma. The most common presentation is a thyroid nodule, and the most common symptom is diarrhea.

There are 2 general groups of factors that can contribute to the diarrhea commonly seen in patients with medullary thyroid carcinoma—humoral factors and anatomic ones. Many of the various bioactive substances produced by medullary thyroid carcinoma have been implicated in the pathogenesis of the diarrhea seen with this tumor. These peptide hormones include (1) calcitonin, (2) ACTH and MSH, (3) neurotensin, (4) somatostatin, (5) β-endorphin, and (6) nerve growth factor. The various anatomic abnormalities discussed subsequently that can be found in the gastrointestinal tract of patients with medullary thyroid carcinoma may also account for the diarrhea. These anatomic lesions may reflect and perhaps even produce fundamental abnormalities in gastrointestinal innervation that can produce abnormal motility.

A. Calcitonin and Related Peptides and Proteins: Since medullary thyroid carcinoma is a neoplastic disorder of the C cells of the thyroid gland, the tumor produces abnormally high amounts of calcitonin. As a result, patients with this tumor have elevated concentrations of calcitonin in peripheral blood and urine. In many patients, basal concentrations of the hormone are sufficiently elevated to be diagnostic of the presence of medullary thyroid carcinoma. However, in an increasing percentage of patients with this tumor, basal levels of calcitonin are indistinguishable from normal. Thus, **provocative tests** with calcium and pentagastrin have been developed for the diagnosis of medullary thyroid carcinoma and its histologic antecedents. These tests are based on the observation that calcium and pentagastrin are potent calcitonin secretagogues.

Opinion differs regarding the relative clinical value of pentagastrin and calcium infusion in the diagnosis of medullary thyroid carcinoma. One must remember that most tumors respond to either agent and that both infusion procedures sometimes give false-negative re-

Table 25–6. Plasma calcitonin and chromogranin A concentrations (mean ± SE) in patients with endocrine tumors.[*]

Group	Chromogranin A (ng/mL)	Calcitonin (pg/mL)
Normal controls (n = 16)	82 ± 16	60 ± 15
Pheochromocytoma (n = 11)	1614 ± 408†	...
Medullary thyroid carcinoma (n = 6)	789 ± 333†	7485 ± 3009†
Parathyroid adenoma (n = 7)	218 ± 13†	...

[*]Unpublished observations of O'Connor and Deftos.
†$p \leqslant .01$ compared to control.

sults. Therefore, either procedure can be recommended, and if one procedure gives negative results in a patient suspected of having medullary thyroid carcinoma, the alternative procedure should be considered before the diagnosis is excluded. In general, both the sensitivity and the specificity of the calcitonin immunoassay are probably just as important as the choice between calcium and pentagastrin in provocative testing of a patient suspected of having medullary thyroid carcinoma. Selective venous catheterization with measurements of calcitonin can also be useful, but its greatest value is probably not in primary diagnosis but in the location of tumor metastases (or sources of ectopic calcitonin production), since knowledge of the presence of metastatic (or ectopic) disease can greatly influence therapy. The effectiveness of therapy in patients with calcitonin-producing tumors can be monitored by serial measurements of plasma calcitonin. In addition to determining the relatively acute effects of a given treatment regimen, periodic surveillance with appropriate provocative testing can be conducted for recurrence of tumor.

It has been recently shown that the calcitonin gene encodes other peptides, among them a 37-amino-acid peptide termed CGRP (calcitonin gene–related peptide) (Table 25–5). Although the function of these peptides is unknown, they are secreted by medullary thyroid carcinoma and may thus serve as tumor markers. C cells also secrete chromogranin A, a high-molecular-weight protein originally discovered in the secretory granules of pheochromocytomas and now known to be present in other endocrine tissues, among them the parathyroid, pancreas, and pituitary (Table

Table 25–5. Calcitonin gene–related peptides and other products secreted by medullary thyroid carcinoma.

Catecholamines	Adrenocorticotropic hormone	Amyloid
Dopa decarboxylase	Melanocyte-stimulating hormone	Carcinoembryonic antigen
Histaminase	Somatostatin	Melanin
Serotonin	β-Endorphin	Neuron-specific enolase
Prostaglandins	Substance P	Chromogranin A
Kallikrein and kinins	Vasoactive intestinal polypeptide	
	Corticotropin-releasing hormone	
	Prolactin-releasing hormone	
	Nerve growth factor	

25–1). This protein could thus be a marker for each of the endocrine neoplasias encountered in any of the multiple endocrine neoplasias (Table 25–6).

B. Other Secretory Products: In addition to calcitonin, medullary thyroid carcinoma produces other substances, nonpeptides as well as peptides (Table 25–5). Their measurement in blood, eg, histaminase, may also be useful in diagnosis and management. This unusual biosynthetic capacity of medullary thyroid carcinoma may be related to the neural crest origin of C cells.

Pheochromocytoma

Pheochromocytoma is a component of MEN type IIa and IIb. Pheochromocytomas occurring in association with medullary thyroid carcinoma have several distinct features. Bilateral and multifocal pheochromocytomas are very common in this clinical setting, with an incidence of over 70%. This contrasts with a bilateral incidence of usually less than 10% for sporadic pheochromocytomas. Pheochromocytomas are much more likely to occur in patients with familial rather than sporadic medullary thyroid carcinoma. The thyroid tumor may antedate the pheochromocytoma by as much as 2 decades. Furthermore, a second pheochromocytoma may become manifest after removal of the first. Thus, there is a greater incidence of pheochromocytomas in older patients with medullary thyroid carcinoma. If hyperparathyroidism also exists, it too is likely to be diagnosed before the pheochromocytoma. **Adrenal medullary hyperplasia** may be a predecessor of the pheochromocytomas seen with medullary thyroid carcinoma, just as C cell hyperplasia may be a predecessor of medullary thyroid carcinoma and chief cell hyperplasia a predecessor of primary hyperparathyroidism in these patients. The increase in adrenal medullary mass results from diffuse or multifocal proliferation of adrenal medullary cells, primarily those found within the head and body of the glands. Diagnostic tests for pheochromocytoma should be pursued vigorously, because the biochemical as well as clinical manifestations of this tumor may be subtle.

Hyperparathyroidism

The exact incidence of hyperparathyroidism in patients with medullary thyroid carcinoma is difficult to establish. Hyperparathyroidism is much more common in MEN type IIa than in MEN type IIb. Recent research suggests that hyperplasia is more common than adenoma. Despite these uncertainties, the concurrence of hyperparathyroidism and medullary thyroid carcinoma in MEN syndromes is well established, and although it cannot be quantitated, the presence of one tumor should always make one suspect the presence of the other. Hyperparathyroidism does not easily fit into a unitary concept of embryogenesis, since parathyroid cells are not classically considered to be of neural crest origin. However, some authorities have suggested a neural crest origin for the parathyroid gland. An alternative explanation for the hyperpara-

thyroidism is a functional relationship between it and medullary thyroid carcinoma. According to this hypothesis, the abnormal concentrations of calcitonin induce hyperparathyroidism, which is secondary to the hypocalcemic actions of the calcitonin. Although this type of functional relationship between the neoplasias may exist, the most convincing evidence supports a genetic relationship between medullary thyroid carcinoma and hyperparathyroidism.

Mucosal Neuromas

The presence of neuromas with a centrofacial distribution is the most consistent component of MEN type IIb. The most common location of neuromas is the oral cavity (tongue, lips, buccal mucosa), but other sites may be involved (Table 25–7). The oral lesions (Fig 25–1) are almost invariably present by the first decade and in some cases even at birth. The most prominent microscopic feature of neuromas is an increase in the size and number of nerves.

Mucosal neuromas can be present in the eyelids, conjunctiva, and cornea. The thickened medullated corneal nerves traverse the cornea and anastomose in the pupillary area. These hypertrophied nerve fibers are readily seen with a slit lamp but occasionally may be evident even on direct ophthalmoscopic examination.

Gastrointestinal tract abnormalities are part of the multiple mucosal neuroma syndrome. The most common of these is **gastrointestinal ganglioneuromatosis.** Ganglioneuromatosis is best observed in the small and large intestine but has also been noted in the esophagus and stomach. The anatomic lesions are sometimes associated with functional difficulties in swallowing, megacolon, diarrhea, and constipation. Similar lesions may be present on other mucosal surfaces.

Table 25–7. Summary of clinical features in 41 patients with MEN type IIb.

	Number of Patients With Findings*		
	Positive	Probable	Negative
Family history of MEN type IIb	14	2	15
Neuroma (any type)	41		
Oral type	37		4
Ocular type	24		16
Other type	4		36
"Bumpy" lips	35	2	
Pheochromocytoma	19†	4	18
Medullary thyroid carcinoma	38		2
Marfanoid habitus	26	5	
Hypertrophied corneal nerves	23		
Skeletal defects	24		4
Gastrointestinal tract abnormalities	23		10

*In some cases, the status of some of the clinical features was not known.

†Unilateral in 7 patients; bilateral in 12 patients.

Figure 25–1. Mucosal neuromas on the tongue of a 12-year-old child with MEN type IIb.

Marfanoid Habitus

The term "marfanoid habitus" denotes a tall, slender body with long arms and legs, an abnormal ratio of upper to lower body segment, and poor muscle development. It is seen commonly in multiple mucosal neuroma syndrome. The extremities are thin, and there may be lax joints and hypotonic muscles. Other features associated with the marfanoid habitus may include dorsal kyphosis, pectus excavatum or pectus carinatum, pes cavus, and high-arched palate. In contrast to patients with true Marfan's syndrome, no patients with multiple mucosal neuromas have been reported to have aortic abnormalities, ectopia lentis, homocystinuria, or mucopolysaccharide abnormalities.

MANAGEMENT OF PATIENTS WITH MULTIPLE ENDOCRINE NEOPLASIA (MEN) SYNDROMES

The individual endocrine components of MEN syndromes have, in general, the same clinical and biochemical manifestations as when they occur as individual entities. The unique clinical aspect of the patient with MEN is the way in which the individual presents to the physician. The patient may be part of a kindred with well-established MEN, and the physician must then evaluate the patient for each potential component of the kindred's syndrome. Or the physician may search for the presence of MEN when a patient presents with one of the endocrine components; in this latter circumstance, the yield will not be great, but when one patient with MEN is discovered, it leads to the identification of other patients.

Surgery is the treatment of choice for the 3 neoplasias in MEN type IIa. All are potentially lethal—especially medullary thyroid carcinoma and pheochromocytoma—but all can be cured by early diagnosis followed by operation. Aggressive therapy is thus warranted, and special consideration should be given to certain aspects of the treatment, since one is dealing with a patient with 3 potential endocrine tumors.

Management of the individual components of MEN syndromes generally follows the accepted procedures for each of the neoplasias, and these are discussed in detail elsewhere in this book. Thus, the management of pituitary tumors is guided by the availability of transsphenoidal hypophysectomy and the management of mucosal neuromas by cosmetic factors. However, the clinical setting does influence the sequence and extent of surgical therapy. The sequence of treatment is guided by the presence of multiple endocrine tumors. Pheochromocytomas, which are commonly bilateral, especially in MEN type IIb, should be treated first, medically or surgically, in order to obviate their cardiovascular effects on surgical procedures. Thyroid and parathyroid surgery must be aggressive, because all glandular tissue may be involved.

An essential feature of appropriate clinical management is evaluation of family members, since MEN syndromes are transmitted in an autosomal dominant pattern. Family members must be reevaluated periodically because of the varying penetrance of the component tumors.

FAILURE OF MULTIPLE ENDOCRINE GLANDS

This section deals mainly with the syndromes involving autoimmune destruction of multiple endocrine and specific other tissues. Historically, the first of these associations was Schmidt's syndrome of nontuberculous Addison's disease and lymphocytic thyroiditis. In a 1964 review of Schmidt's syndrome, Carpenter et al found coexisting diabetes mellitus in 10 out of 15 patients with Addison's disease and thyroiditis. They broadened the definition of the syndrome to include diabetes mellitus associated with nontuberculous Addison's disease. However, multiglandular failure may also involve the parathyroids, ovaries, testes, and possibly adenohypophysis. Schmidt's syndrome (the Carpenter definition will be used in this chapter) is thus but one subset of these disorders. In addition, these endocrinopathies are frequently associated with other disorders of tissue-specific autoimmunity, notably pernicious anemia and vitiligo. This discussion will emphasize the evidence for clinical, immunologic, and possibly genetic het-

Table 25—8. Types of immunologic tissue injury.*

IgE-mediated immediate hypersensitivity
Complement-dependent direct humoral cytotoxicity
Antigen-antibody complex deposition
T cell–mediated immunity
Receptor autoantibody binding (blocking or stimulating)
Antibody-dependent cell-mediated cytotoxicity

*Modified and reproduced, with permission, from Deftos LJ, Catherwood BD, Bone HG: Multiple endocrine disorders. Chapter 28 in: *Endocrinology and Metabolism.* Felig P et al (editors). McGraw-Hill, 1981.

erogeneity among groups of patients with these disorders.

Six mechanisms of immunologic tissue injury have been described (Table 25–8). The primary effectors in autoimmune reactions are immunoglobulins, T cells (thymus-dependent lymphocytes that become sensitized to specific antigens and release soluble non-immunoglobulin mediators), and monocytes (which possess receptors for the Fc region of immunoglobulins and cytotoxic capabilities in the presence of tissue-specific antibody). The role of these mechanisms in autoimmune endocrine disease has been most extensively studied in Hashimoto's thyroiditis and Graves' disease. Although immune complexes are present in the sera of some patients with autoimmune thyroid disease, T cell–mediated immunity and antibody-dependent cell-mediated cytotoxicity have received the greatest attention as mechanisms of target organ destruction in Hashimoto's thyroiditis. Evidence for specifically sensitized T cells has been found in other autoimmune endocrinopathies as well. To explain this apparent break in the immunologically privileged status of autologous tissues, Volpe has proposed a unifying theory of pathogenesis of autoimmune thyroid disease based on a defect in immunoregulation by suppressor T cells (thymus-dependent lymphocytes that suppress immune responses, possibly including recognition of autoantigens); in vitro evidence supports this hypothesis.

Table 25—9. Methods for assessment of tissue-specific immunity.*

Cell-Mediated Immunity (Type IV)	Immunoglobulin-Dependent Immunity
Direct lymphocytotoxicity	Precipitation
Lymphocyte blast transformation	Complement fixation
Leukocyte migration inhibition	Indirect immunofluorescence
Intradermal skin testing	Direct serum cytotoxicity (type II)
	Enablement of cell-mediated cytotoxicity (type VI)

*Modified and reproduced, with permission, from Deftos LJ, Catherwood BD, Bone HG: Multiple endocrine disorders. Chapter 28 in: *Endocrinology and Metabolism.* Felig P et al (editors). McGraw-Hill, 1981.

A number of methods have been used for assessment of tissue-specific immunity in the autoimmune endocrinopathies (Table 25–9). Immunoprecipitation, latex or tanned red cell agglutination, and radioimmunoassay have been used to detect thyroglobulin autoantibodies, the last being the most sensitive method. The indirect immunofluorescence test for autoantibodies to endocrine cells in frozen tissue sections is a versatile technique that has demonstrated autoantibodies to adrenal, thyroid, islet cell, parathyroid, and gonadal ''cytoplasmic'' antigens. The thyroid cytoplasmic antigen has been localized to microsomal preparations and titered by complement fixation. With the exception of thyroglobulin and immunofluorescent thyroid epithelial autoantibody tests, the immunofluorescence tests are performed only in specialized laboratories.

PROTOTYPICAL AUTOIMMUNE ENDOCRINOPATHY: ADDISON'S DISEASE

Addison's disease plays a central role in several groups of patients with failure of multiple endocrine glands, and there is strong evidence that idiopathic Addison's disease is the end result of autoimmune adrenalitis in most cases. Addison's disease has also provided a good focus for investigation of endocrine autoimmunity (1) because few of these patients should escape medical attention and (2) because tuberculous Addison's disease has provided a natural control group for clinical and immunologic comparison.

Idiopathic Addison's disease is diagnosed when there is no evidence of tuberculosis or any other reasonable explanation for adrenal failure. Pulmonary tuberculosis and adrenal calcification justify a presumptive diagnosis of tuberculous Addison's disease; however, in patients with granulomatous disease on chest film but without adrenal calcification, the cause of adrenal failure is indeterminate. Autoantibodies to adrenal tissue can be detected by indirect immunofluorescence in a high percentage (48–74%) of patients with idiopathic Addison's disease, while the incidence of adrenal autoantibodies is essentially zero in patients with unequivocal tuberculous Addison's disease. Although comparable data are not available for patients with Addison's disease due to other causes such as histoplasmosis, this information suggests that adrenal autoantibodies are not an epiphenomenon due to tissue destruction. In vitro evidence of cell-mediated immunity to adrenal antigens is also present in many patients with idiopathic Addison's disease but not in patients with tuberculous Addison's disease. The autoimmune nature of idiopathic Addison's disease is further substantiated by its specific association with a wide variety of second endocrinopathies with in vitro evidence for tissue-specific autoimmunity. Table 25–10 shows the strikingly higher frequency of second diseases in idiopathic compared with tuberculous Addison's disease. The diseases found with

Table 25–10. Incidence of other autoimmune disorders in patients with Addison's disease.

	Idiopathic Addison's Disease (n = 419)	Tuberculous Addison's Disease (n = 114)
Diabetes mellitus	10%	...
Hyperthyroidism	8%	...
Thyroiditis and primary myxedema	9%	...
Pernicious anemia	4%	...
Hypogonadism	16%	...
Hypoparathyroidism	5%	...
One or more disorders	39%	8%

tuberculous Addison's disease have generally been diabetes mellitus and thyroid disease. These results support the conclusion that idiopathic Addison's disease is part of a larger autoimmune endocrine syndrome.

The presence of adrenal autoantibodies in the blood may be a marker for activity of the autoimmune diathesis. Adrenal autoantibodies tend to have disappeared in patients studied later than 1–5 years after the onset of Addison's disease. Table 25–11 shows the relationship of adrenal autoantibody to the sex of the patient, the age at onset of adrenal insufficiency, and the presence of a second autoimmune disorder. The higher prevalence of autoantibodies in Addison's disease associated with other disorders is particularly striking. Patients with idiopathic Addison's disease with adrenal autoantibodies have a 2- to 3-fold greater incidence of other clinically manifest endocrinopathies compared with patients without adrenal autoantibodies. Several investigators have found a higher prevalence of adrenal autoantibodies in women, although this has not been uniformly reported. The frequency of autoantibodies is much less in patients with Addison's disease alone who are male or whose onset of adrenal insufficiency was before age 20 years. Adrenal autoantibodies have been found in 13% of pa-

Table 25–11. Incidence of adrenal autoantibodies in patients with idiopathic Addison's disease according to sex, age at onset of adrenal insufficiency, and presence of other disease.*

	Sex		Age at Onset		
	Female	Male	<20	>20	Total
Addison's disease alone	14/27 (52%)	7/40 (18%)	4/26 (15%)	16/36 (44%)	21/67 (31%)
Addison's disease plus other disease	23/30 (77%)	13/21 (62%)	15/21 (71%)	20/28 (71%)	36/51 (71%)
					57/118 (48%)

*Source of data: Blizzard RM, Chee D, Davis W: *Clin Exp Immunol* 1967;2:19. Modified and reproduced, with permission, from Deftos LJ, Catherwood BD, Bone HG: Multiple endocrine disorders. Chapter 28 in: *Endocrinology and Metabolism.* Felig P et al (editors). McGraw-Hill, 1981.

tients with idiopathic hypoparathyroidism alone. They are found rarely in first-degree relatives of patients with autoimmune Addison's disease, in patients with Cushing's disease, and in patients with Hashimoto's thyroiditis or diabetes mellitus alone. The prevalence of adrenal autoantibodies in apparently normal individuals is less than one per 1000 population.

Many investigators have found an increased prevalence of subclinical autoimmunity to other tissues in patients with autoantibody-positive Addison's disease, as evidenced by autoantibodies to parathyroid, islet cell, thyroid, and gastric mucosa. Nerup found a 6-fold higher frequency of thyroid autoantibodies and a 10-fold increase in parietal cell autoantibodies in patients with adrenal autoantibody-positive Addison's disease, but patients with Addison's disease without adrenal autoantibodies showed no difference from age- and sex-matched controls. When a panel of in vitro immunologic tests was used along with clinical data, 84% of patients with Addison's disease and adrenal autoantibodies were found to have evidence of extra-adrenal autoimmune involvement.

CLINICAL & IMMUNOLOGIC HETEROGENEITY

From what has been said, we infer that idiopathic Addison's disease is not a homogeneous disorder with a random coincidence of other autoimmune endocrine disease and that patients with failure of additional glands might also be heterogeneous. Fig 25–2 supports this thesis, showing the distribution of the age at onset in 3 clinical subsets of patients with Addison's disease studied in the USA and the UK. It is clear that Addison's disease associated with hypoparathyroidism has a much earlier age at onset than Addison's disease associated with Schmidt's syndrome or without other endocrinopathy. Analyzing 182 patients from 140 families with idiopathic Addison's disease, idiopathic hypoparathyroidism, or both disorders, Spinner et al found evidence for genetic as well as clinical heterogeneity among these patients and divided their patients into 4 groups: Addison's disease with hypoparathyroidism, isolated hypoparathyroidism, isolated Addison's disease, and Schmidt's syndrome. Immunologic differences also distinguish groups of patients with autoimmune endocrine disease. Patients with Addison's disease in adulthood are predominantly female and frequently have thyroid autoantibodies. They therefore resemble the group with complete Schmidt's syndrome. However, patients with childhood-onset Addison's disease without other endocrinopathy tend to be male and have predominantly autoantibodies to parathyroid tissue, resembling more closely the patients with Addison's disease associated with clinical hypoparathyroidism. Some of these patients may represent a forme fruste of pluriglandular endocrine insufficiency. Several types of study have thus led to the concept that multiglandular autoimmune endocrinopathy is not a uniform syndrome nor

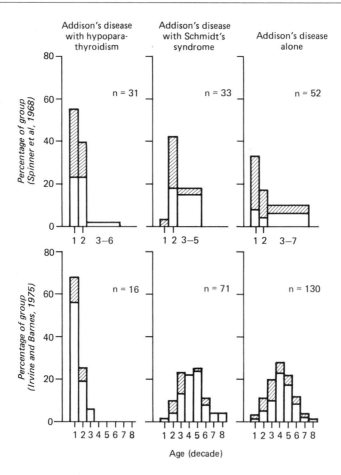

Figure 25–2. Clinical heterogeneity of Addison's disease. Distribution of age at onset (upper) or of diagnosis (lower) of Addison's disease with hypoparathyroidism, Addison's disease with Schmidt's syndrome, and Addison's disease alone. The open area represents females; the closed area represents males. Note that age is measured in decades. (Reproduced, with permission, from Deftos LJ, Catherwood BD, Bone HG: Multiple endocrine disorders. Chapter 28 in: *Endocrinology and Metabolism,* 2nd ed. Felig P et al [editors]. McGraw-Hill, 1985.)

the random coincidence of a number of individual diseases but that there are at least 2 distinct patterns of glandular involvement. These ideas are summarized as major types and variations in Fig 25–3. Besides the groups of patients with Addison's disease outlined above, there are groups in which a direct association of thyroiditis and diabetes mellitus is found in the absence of Addison's disease. In addition, other endocrine and some nonendocrine disorders occur with increased frequency in these patients.

Addison's Disease With Hypoparathyroidism

In the set of patients with Addison's disease and hypoparathyroidism, male and female patients are usually affected in childhood (Fig 25–2). Chronic mucocutaneous candidiasis frequently precedes both endocrinopathies; conversely, 84% of patients with this infection and an associated endocrinopathy have hypoparathyroidism. The typical sequence of events

is shown in Fig 24–4: Hypoparathyroidism develops in the first decade in 88% of patients. Addison's disease follows in about 2 years, and in 75% of patients it occurs within 9 years of the onset of the syndrome. These patients may be affected by a third endocrinopathy, including thyroid disease, diabetes mellitus, pernicious anemia, and ovarian failure. The probability that the sibling of an affected person will have Addison's disease or hypoparathyroidism or any one of the above-mentioned secondary disorders has been estimated to be 0.35.

Patients with idiopathic hypoparathyroidism frequently have circulating autoantibodies to parathyroid tissue; patients with Addison's disease and hypoparathyroidism also have an increased frequency of thyroid and parietal cell autoantibodies. A number of defective immune responses have been reported in patients with chronic mucocutaneous candidiasis with or without endocrinopathies. These include defective blast transformation, macrophage migration inhibi-

PLURIGLANDULAR ENDOCRINE FUNCTION

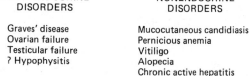

Figure 25–3. The 3 major clinical categories of pluriglandular autoimmune endocrinopathy (center column), with forme fruste variants (dashed boxes) and less frequently associated endocrine disorders and nonendocrine disorders. Graves' disease may substitute for thyroiditis. Gonadal failure is associated with a pan–steroid cell autoantibody in Addison's disease, and candidiasis is strongly associated with hypoparathyroidism. (Modified and reproduced, with permission, from Deftos LJ, Catherwood BD, Bone HG: Multiple endocrine disorders. Chapter 28 in: *Endocrinology and Metabolism,* 2nd ed. Felig P et al [editors]. McGraw-Hill, 1985.)

OTHER ENDOCRINE DISORDERS

Graves' disease
Ovarian failure
Testicular failure
? Hypophysitis

NONENDOCRINE DISORDERS

Mucocutaneous candidiasis
Pernicious anemia
Vitiligo
Alopecia
Chronic active hepatitis
Malabsorption

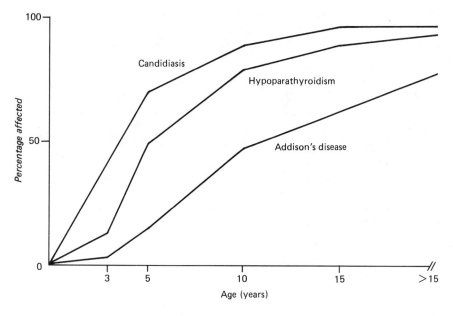

Figure 25–4. Typical sequence for childhood onset of chronic mucocutaneous candidiasis, autoimmune hypoparathyroidism, and Addison's disease. Patients with hypoparathyroidism may not develop Addison's disease, but frequent adrenal autoantibodies suggest that the polyendocrine diathesis is still present. (Source of data: Neufeld et al: *Medicine* 1981;**60**:355. Reproduced with permission, from Deftos LJ, Catherwood BD, Bone HG: Multiple endocrine disorders. Chapter 28 in: *Endocrinology and Metabolism,* 2nd ed. Felig P et al [editors]. McGraw-Hill, 1985.)

tion, and lymphocytotoxicity. The role of these abnormalities in the pathogenesis of immune sensitization to endocrine tissue is unclear.

Isolated Hypoparathyroidism

Patients with isolated hypoparathyroidism are similar to those with Addison's disease plus hypoparathyroidism in having an early onset of disease (73% in the first decade) and associated candidiasis. The frequency of parathyroid autoantibodies in this group is similar to that in the group with Addison's disease. Immunofluorescent adrenal autoantibodies are detected in 7% of patients with hypoparathyroidism, whereas in hypoparathyroidism with candidiasis, most patients have subclinical adrenal autoimmunity. The occurrence of adrenal autoantibodies and candidiasis thus indicates that this subset may represent a forme fruste of pluriglandular endocrine insufficiency.

Isolated Addison's Disease

As noted above, patients with isolated idiopathic Addison's disease still have an increased prevalence of thyroid, parathyroid, and islet cell autoantibodies when compared with control populations. These immunologic findings suggest that despite the absence of clinically evident involvement of other glands, isolated Addison's disease should be considered part of the spectrum of multiple endocrine autoimmunity, since some patients with this disorder may ultimately develop an associated endocrinopathy.

Schmidt's Syndrome

As shown in Fig 25–2, Schmidt's syndrome (defined in the introduction) is more frequent in females, and all of the components including the Addison's disease commonly have their onset in the age range from 20 to 50 years. Table 25–10 shows that the occurrence of diabetes mellitus in idiopathic Addison's disease is 10% and that of Hashimoto's thyroiditis and primary myxedema 9% overall. Although many of these patients may have onset of diabetes in young adulthood, most of them have been treated with insulin. Hashimoto's thyroiditis or diabetes develops an average of 7 years after adrenal insufficiency. Schmidt's syndrome is frequently accompanied by additional autoimmune diseases, including ovarian failure and pernicious anemia (see below).

Patients with Schmidt's syndrome have the highest rate of thyroid autoantibodies of any group with Addison's disease, which suggests that thyroid autoantibodies in Addison's disease may be predictive of thyroid failure. Islet cell autoantibodies may also be important in Schmidt's syndrome. These autoantibodies circulate in the majority of patients at the time of diagnosis of insulin-dependent diabetes mellitus, even in the absence of any other tissue-specific autoimmune disease. The incidence is substantially lower in patients not requiring insulin therapy at the time of diagnosis. In most patients, islet cell autoantibodies disappear with time; their persistence in the blood is associated with the presence of other autoimmune disorders (19%) or autoantibodies to thyroid or gastric tissue (65%). In patients without insulin dependence at the time of diagnosis of their diabetes, the presence of islet cell autoantibodies appears to predict future insulin requirement and failure of oral hypoglycemic agent therapy.

For about half of index individuals, one or more other family members can be found with autoimmune endocrinopathies. These relatives frequently have only thyroiditis and diabetes without adrenal disease. Such family members may be assigned to this syndrome on the basis of their relative with Addison's disease. Many more family members have been found to have thyroid autoantibodies in the blood.

Other Endocrinopathies Associated With Addison's Disease

Ovarian failure is common in women with idiopathic Addison's disease. In one large series, the prevalence of amenorrhea was 24%, and another 6% had oligomenorrhea. Abnormal reproductive function persists after adrenal replacement therapy and is uncommon in tuberculous Addison's disease, which leads to the conclusion that it is not related to deficiency of adrenal corticosteroids. The presumed autoimmune oophoritis is closely correlated with the onset of the patient's adrenal failure. In girls with Addison's disease and hypoparathyroidism occurring before the age of menarche, the presentation of oophoritis is that of primary amenorrhea, and in some cases streak gonads have been found at laparoscopy.

Ovarian failure in Addison's disease is closely related to a distinctive type of autoantibody against common antigens present in multiple steroid-producing cells, including theca interna, corpus luteum, Leydig cells, placenta, and adrenal cortex. These autoantibodies are cytotoxic for granulosa cells in monolayer cell culture. The presence of such autoantibodies is not only a risk factor for ovarian failure but may also be an independent risk factor for other extraadrenal endocrinopathies. Steroid cell autoantibodies are uncommon in men with Addison's disease, but several instances of testicular failure associated with Addison's disease have been reported.

Although decreased function or failure is the most common consequence of attack on the endocrine glands, Graves' disease is intimately associated with these disorders; thyrotoxicosis occurs in about 8% of patients with Addison's disease. In patients with idiopathic Addison's disease, clinical atrophic gastritis may occur with or without diabetes, thyroid disease, hypoparathyroidism, or ovarian failure. Pernicious anemia is found in approximately 4% of patients with Addison's disease (Table 25–10).

Direct Association of Thyroid Disease & Diabetes Mellitus

The general frequency of diabetes mellitus and thyroid disease makes the study of a link between these disorders difficult. Nevertheless, an increased frequency of autoimmune thyroid disease in diabetics

Table 25–12. Interrelationships of autoimmunity against islet, parietal, and thyroid cells: Representative frequencies of occurrence.

Index Disease	Associated Finding	Frequency
Diabetes mellitus	Thyroid autoantibodies	16%
	↑ TSH (males)	6%
	↑ TSH (females)	17%
	Parietal cell autoantibodies	17%
Thyroiditis	Islet cell autoantibodies	9%
	Intrinsic factor autoantibodies	2%
	Pernicious anemia	9%
Hyperthyroidism	Islet cell autoantibodies	3%
	Intrinsic factor autoantibodies	3%
	Pernicious anemia	3%
Pernicious anemia	Islet cell autoantibodies	11%
	Thyroid autoantibodies	38%
	Hypothyroidism	12%
	Hyperthyroidism	9%

*Modified and reproduced, with permission, from Deftos LJ, Catherwood BD, Bone HG: Multiple endocrine disorders. Chapter 28 in: *Endocrinology and Metabolism,* 2nd ed. Felig P et al (editors). McGraw-Hill, 1985.

has been reported by many authors; pernicious anemia is also associated. Comparison of the frequency of tissue-specific autoantibodies in unselected diabetics versus age- and sex-matched controls provides additional support for this association. Table 25–12 provides a representative summary of the interrelationships of autoimmunity against islet, parietal, and thyroid cells.

Other Disorders

A dozen cases of presumed "autoimmune hypophysitis" have been reported, and half were associated with autoimmune diseases, especially lymphocytic thyroiditis and atrophic gastritis. All of these cases have been temporally related to pregnancy and have presented as sellar masses or sudden collapse. A diagnosis of hypopituitarism has been made in life in at least one of these patients. Diabetes insipidus has been associated with autoimmune adrenalitis and hypoparathyroidism in one instance, but the pathogenesis of this defect is unclear.

Vitiligo may occur with any autoimmune endocrinopathy. This disorder probably represents tissue-specific autoimmunity to melanin-producing cells.

MANAGEMENT OF PATIENTS WITH FAILURE OF MULTIPLE ENDOCRINE GLANDS

The history, physical examination, laboratory findings, and treatment of the hormonal disorders discussed in this section are similar to those of the disorders as they occur individually and are discussed in other chapters in this book.

The most serious pitfall in diagnosis of multiple autoimmune endocrinopathy would be to confuse ad-

renal, thyroid, and ovarian failure with hypopituitarism. In every such case, the integrity of pituitary function should be proved by showing elevated blood levels of TSH, LH, or ACTH. Failure of other glands not dependent on pituitary function (hypoparathyroidism or diabetes mellitus) should be an indicator of autoimmune endocrinopathy.

Patients with Addison's disease should receive particular attention in surveillance for failure of previously uninvolved glands, as these individuals are at greater risk. The physician should be alert for signs of the insidious onset of hypothyroidism and pernicious anemia. Elevated serum TSH alone does not necessarily indicate future clinical hypothyroidism, but simultaneous observation of thyroid autoantibodies predicts an incidence of clinical hypothyroidism estimated to be 4% per year; and when autoantibody titers are markedly elevated, the incidence may be as high as 26% per year.

The implications of multiglandular endocrine failure for treatment are not well characterized. Since cortisol antagonizes the intestinal calcium transport effects of vitamin D, including vitamin D metabolites used to treat hypoparathyroidism, the development of adrenal failure can result in sudden vitamin D intoxication in affected patients.

GENETIC ASPECTS OF AUTOIMMUNE DISORDERS

Early genetic studies of autoimmune disorders have estimated probabilities of clinical involvement of 0.25–0.35 for siblings of probands with Schmidt's syndrome and Addison's disease with hypoparathyroidism.

Typing of antigens coded by the major histocompatibility (HLA) complex on chromosome 6 has provided genetic correlations with the clinical and immunopathologic findings in the individual autoimmune endocrinopathies. Antigens of the A and B loci (serologically defined) are detected by testing sera for cytotoxicity to the patient's lymphocytes. Antigens of the D locus are the most widely recognized alleles originally detected by the ability of the patient's lymphocytes to stimulate a panel of test lymphocytes (lymphocyte-defined). The immunologic defect in immune regulation resulting in autosensitization to endocrine tissue may be a gene in the HLA region genetically linked to certain HLA antigens. HLA-D an-

Table 25–13. HLA antigen associations with autoimmune diseases (Caucasians).

Addison's disease	HLA-D3
Atrophic thyroiditis	HLA-D3
Graves' disease	HLA-D3
Diabetes mellitus	HLA-D3 and HLA-D4
Hashimoto's thyroiditis	HLA-D5
Hypoparathyroidism	?

tigens are most closely associated with the endocrine disorders (Table 25– 13). Common haplotypes such as HLA-A1-B8-D3 and HLA-A2-B15-D4 occur because of linkage disequilibrium. HLA studies in type I diabetes mellitus have suggested that only the HLA-(B8)-D3–linked diabetogenic gene is associated with persistent islet cell autoantibodies and with other autoimmune disease and that homozygosity for this haplotype confers no increased risk of development of diabetes.

Although similar data are not available for Addison's disease, HLA typing of a few kindreds with pluriglandular autoimmune endocrinopathy has been reported. In some families, this type of analysis has suggested dominant inheritance with a high degree of penetrance, whereas in other kindreds the predictive value of HLA typing appeared questionable.

NONAUTOIMMUNE ENDOCRINE FAILURE

Bardwick et al have recently reviewed a syndrome, previously reported mostly from Japan, to which they give the acronym POEMS (polyneuropathy, organomegaly, endocrinopathy, M protein, and skin changes) (Table 25– 14). Gonadal failure, gynecomastia, and glucose intolerance are frequent endocrine disorders, while adrenal failure is uncommon. Seventy-five percent of affected patients are male, and they have plasma cell dyscrasias with onset in the fourth or fifth decade, usually sclerotic plasmacytomas. In one of the cases reported by Bardwick et al, insulin-dependent diabetes mellitus remitted with irradiation of the patient's plasmacytoma, returned 3 years later with the appearance of a new tumor, and disappeared again with another course of radiation treatment. Neither the polyneuropathy nor the endocrinopathy appears to be due to amyloidosis. In contrast to findings in autoimmune endocrinopathies, Bardwick et al did not find tissue-specific endocrine autoantibodies. The mechanism of this interesting syndrome needs to be elucidated.

Table 25–14. Incidence of abnormalities in patients with "POEMS" syndrome.[*]

Polyneuropathy	
Peripheral neuropathy	100%
Papilledema	68%
Increased cerebrospinal fluid	94%
Organomegaly	
Hepatomegaly	67%
Splenomegaly	37%
Lymphadenopathy	64%
Endocrinopathy	
Gynecomastia	70%
Impotence	67%
Amenorrhea	100%
Glucose intolerance	48%
Hypothyroidism	10%
M protein	61%
IgG	41%
IgA	20%
Marrow plasma cells	48%
Sclerotic bone lesions	71%
Skin changes	
Hyperpigmentation	98%
Thickening	85%
Hirsutism	78%
Hyperhidrosis	66%
Other	
Peripheral edema	92%
Ascites	68%
Pleural effusions	24%
Fever	48%

[*]Reproduced, with permission, from Bardwick PA et al: Plasma cell dyscrasia with polyneuropathy, organomegaly, endocrinopathy, M protein, and skin changes. *Medicine* 1980;**59**:311.

Pseudohypoparathyroidism type Ia is due to hereditary deficiency of the guanine nucleotide–binding regulatory protein of the cell membrane–adenylate cyclase complex and is characterized by resistance to multiple hormones besides parathyroid hormone. This disorder is discussed in Chapter 8.

REFERENCES

Multiple Endocrine Neoplasia

Austin LA, Heath H III: Calcitonin: Physiology and pathophysiology. *N Engl J Med* 1981;**304**:269.

Becker KL et al: Calcitonin heterogeneity in lung cancer and medullary thyroid carcinoma. *Acta Endocrinol* 1978;**89**:89.

Carney JA, Sizemore GW, Tyce GM: Bilateral adrenal medullary hyperplasia in MEN, type 2. *Mayo Clin Proc* 1975;**50**:3.

Catherwood BD, Deftos LJ: Presence of radioimmunoassay of a calcitonin-like substance in porcine pituitary glands. *Endocrinology* 1980;**106**:1886.

Chong GC et al: Medullary carcinoma of the thyroid gland. *Cancer* 1975;**35**:695.

Copp DH, Crockroft DW, Kueh Y: Calcitonin from ultimobranchial glands of dogfish and chickens. *Science* 1967;**158**:924.

Cushman P Jr: Familial endocrine tumors: Report of two unrelated kindred affected with pheochromocytomas, one also with multiple thyroid carcinomas. *Am J Med* 1962;**32**:352.

Deftos LJ: *Medullary Thyroid Carcinoma.* Karger, 1983.

Deftos LJ: Radioimmunoassay for calcitonin in medullary thyroid carcinoma. *JAMA* 1974;**227**:403.

Deftos LJ, Bone HG, Parthemore JG: Immunohistological studies of medullary thyroid carcinoma and C-cell hyperplasia. *J Clin Endocrinol Metab* 1980;**51**:857.

Deftos LJ et al: Demonstration by immunoperoxidase histochemistry of calcitonin in the anterior lobe of the rat pituitary. *J Clin Endocrinol Metab* 1978;**47**:457.

Gagel FR et al: Natural history of the familial medullary thyroid carcinoma–pheochromocytoma syndrome and the identification of preneoplastic stages by screening studies: A five-year report. *Trans Assoc Am Physicians* 1975; **88:**177.

Hazard JB: The C cells (parafollicular cells) of the thyroid gland and medullary thyroid carcinoma: A review. *Am J Pathol* 1977;**88:**213.

Hennessey JF et al: A comparison of pentagastrin injection and calcium infusion as provocative agents for the detection of medullary thyroid carcinoma. *J Clin Endocrinol Metab* 1974;**39:**487.

Jackson CE et al: The two-mutational-event theory in medullary thyroid carcinoma. *Am J Hum Genet* 1979;**31:**704.

Khairi MRA et al: Mucosal neuroma, pheochromocytoma and medullary thyroid carcinoma: MEN, type III. *Medicine* 1975;**54:**89.

Melvin KE, Tashjian AH Jr, Miller HH: Studies in familial (medullary) thyroid carcinoma. *Recent Prog Horm Res* 1972;**28:**399.

O'Connor DT, Burton D, Deftos LJ: Immunoreactive human chromogranin A in diverse polypeptide hormone–producing human tumors and normal endocrine tissues. *Clin Endocrinol Metab* 1983;**57:**1084.

Parthemore JG et al: A short calcium infusion in the diagnosis of medullary thyroid carcinoma. *J Clin Endocrinol Metab* 1974;**39:**108.

Pearse AGE, Ewen SEB, Polak JM: The genesis of APUD amyloid in endocrine polypeptide tumors: Histochemical distinction from immunamyloid. *Virchows Arch [Cell Pathol]* 1972;**10:**93.

Samaan NA et al: Immunoreactive calcitonin in medullary carcinoma of the thyroid and in maternal and cord serum. *J Lab Clin Med* 1973;**81:**671.

Schimke RN, Hartman WH: Familial amyloid-producing medullary thyroid carcinoma and pheochromocytoma: A distinct genetic entity. *Ann Intern Med* 1965;**63:**1027.

Sipple JH: The association of pheochromocytoma with carcinoma of the thyroid gland. *Am J Med* 1961;**31:**163.

Steiner AL, Goodman AD, Powers SR: Study of a kindred with pheochromocytoma, medullary thyroid carcinoma, hyperparathyroidism, and Cushing's disease: MEN, type II. *Medicine* 1968;**47:**371.

Wallach SR et al: Plasma calcitonin as a marker of disease activity in patients with small cell carcinoma of the lung. *J Clin Endocrinol Metab* 1981;**53:**602.

Wermer P: Genetic aspects of adenomatosis of endocrine glands. *Am J Med* 1954;**16:**363.

Williams ED: A review of 17 cases of carcinoma of the thyroid and phaeochromocytoma. *J Clin Pathol* 1965;**18:**288.

Wolfe HJ et al: C-cell hyperplasia preceding medullary thyroid carcinoma. *N Engl J Med* 1973;**289:**437.

Zollinger RM, Ellison EH: Primary peptic ulceration of the jejunum associated with the islet cell tumors of the pancreas. *Ann Surg* 1955;**142:**709.

Failure of Multiple Endocrine Glands

Asa SL et al: Lymphocytic hypophysitis of pregnancy resulting in hypopituitarism: A distinct clinicopathologic entity. *Ann Intern Med* 1981;**95:**166.

Bardwick PA et al: Plasma cell dyscrasia with polyneuropathy, organomegaly, endocrinopathy, M protein, and skin changes: The POEMS syndrome. *Medicine* 1980;**59:**311.

Blizzard RM, Chee D, Davis W: The incidence of adrenal and other antibodies in the sera of patients with idiopathic adrenal insufficiency (Addison's disease). *Clin Exp Immunol* 1967;**2:**19.

Blizzard RM, Chee D, Davis W: The incidence of parathyroid and other antibodies in the sera of patients with idiopathic hypoparathyroidism. *Clin Exp Immunol* 1966;**2:**19.

Bottazzo GF et al: Autoimmunity in juvenile diabetics and their families. *Br Med J* 1978;**2:**165.

Calder EA, Irvine WJ: Cell-mediated immunity and immune complexes in thyroid disease. *Clin Endocrinol Metab* 1975;**4:**379.

Carpenter CCJ et al: Schmidt's syndrome (thyroid and adrenal insufficiency): A review of the literature and a report of fifteen new cases including ten instances of coexistent diabetes mellitus. *Medicine* 1964;**43:**153.

Deftos LJ, Catherwood BD, Bone HG: Multiple endocrine disorders. Chapter 28 in: *Endocrinology and Metabolism,* 2nd ed. Felig P et al (editors). McGraw-Hill, 1985.

Doniach D: Humoral and genetic aspects of thyroid autoimmunity. *Clin Endocrinol Metab* 1975;**4:**287.

Dwyer JM: Chronic mucocutaneous candidiasis. *Annu Rev Med* 1981;**32:**491.

Eisenbarth GS et al: The polyglandular failure syndrome: Disease inheritance, HLA type, and immune function. *Ann Intern Med* 1979;**91:**528.

Gordin A, Lamberg BA: Spontaneous hypothyroidism in symptomless autoimmune thyroiditis: A long-term follow-up study. *Clin Endocrinol* 1981;**15:**537.

Irvine WJ, Barnes EW: Addison's disease, ovarian failure and hypoparathyroidism. *Clin Endocrinol Metab* 1975; **4:**379.

Irvine WJ et al: Immunological aspects of premature ovarian failure associated with idiopathic Addison's disease. *Lancet* 1968;**2:**883.

Irvine WJ et al: Pancreatic islet cell antibodies in diabetes mellitus correlated with the duration and type of diabetes, coexistent autoimmune disease, and HLA type. *Diabetes* 1977;**26:**138.

Irvine WJ et al: Thyroid and gastric autoimmunity in patients with diabetes mellitus. *Lancet* 1970;**2:**164.

McCarthy-Young S, Lessof MH, Maisey MN: Serum TSH and thyroid antibody studies in Addison's disease. *Clin Endocrinol* 1972;**1:**45.

Nerup J: Addison's disease. *Acta Endocrinol* 1974;**76:**127.

Okita N, Row VV, Volpe R: Suppressor T-lymphocyte deficiency in Graves' disease and Hashimoto's thyroiditis. *J Clin Endocrinol Metab* 1981;**52:**528.

Rotter J, Rimoin DL: Heterogeneity in diabetes mellitus: Update 1978. *Diabetes* 1978;**27:**599.

Spinner MW, Blizzard RM, Childs B: Clinical and genetic heterogeneity in idiopathic Addison's disease and hypoparathyroidism. *J Clin Endocrinol* 1968;**28:**795.

Spinner MW et al: Familial distribution of organ-specific antibodies in the blood of patients with Addison's disease and hypoparathyroidism and their relatives. *Clin Exp Immunol* 1969;**5:**461.

Sridama V, Pacini F, Degroot L: Decreased suppressor T-lymphocytes in autoimmune thyroid diseases detected by monoclonal antibodies. *J Clin Endocrinol Metab* 1982;**54:**316.

Volpe R: The role of autoimmunity in hypoendocrine and hyperendocrine function with special emphasis on autoimmune thyroid disease. *Ann Intern Med* 1977;**87:**86.

Wuepper KD, Wegienka LC, Fudenberg HH: Immunologic aspects of adrenocortical insufficiency. *Am J Med* 1969;**45:**206.

26 Gene Expression & Recombinant DNA in Endocrinology & Metabolism

Barry J. Gertz, MD, PhD, & John D. Baxter, MD

Over the past few decades, significant data have accumulated concerning the detailed structure and function of genes. This information is now being used to devise more sophisticated and direct means of diagnosing, preventing, and treating disease. The technology that has been developed, particularly the genetic engineering techniques of recombinant DNA, is also providing new approaches to understanding human physiology and the pathogenesis of disease.

Human insulin and growth hormone produced by recombinant DNA techniques are already available for clinical use, and numerous additional applications for recombinant DNA technology are forthcoming. Many new drugs will be developed, capabilities for predicting susceptibility to disease and for diagnosing disease will be greatly expanded, and new types of therapy (eg, gene transfer) may also become available. The physician will therefore require some understanding of this new technology in order to apply it to the management of endocrine and metabolic diseases and to assess its strengths and weaknesses. The rapid development of technology will also raise ethical issues whose consideration requires knowledge of gene function, gene regulation, and recombinant DNA techniques. The purpose of this chapter is to provide a conceptual framework for understanding gene expression and the role of recombinant DNA in endocrinology.

GENES & THEIR EXPRESSION

The modern era of molecular biology received its greatest impetus in 1953, when Watson and Crick reported the structure of deoxyribonucleic acid (DNA). This finding provided an understanding of how replication occurs (ie, through complementary base pairing) and thus how the genetic profile of an organism can be maintained from generation to generation. The discovery was followed by a series of breakthroughs revealing (1) the way in which the DNA of a cell

The material in this chapter is based on material written by the authors for a chapter entitled "Gene Expression and Recombinant DNA in Endocrinology and Metabolism" in: *Endocrinology and Metabolism*, 2nd ed. Felig P et al (editors). McGraw-Hill. [In press.]

Acronyms Used in This Chapter

ACTH	Adrenocorticotropic hormone
cDNA	Complementary DNA
CGRP	Calcitonin gene–related peptide
DNA	Deoxyribonucleic acid
GRE	Glucocorticoid regulatory element
mRNA	Messenger RNA
PTH	Parathyroid hormone
RFLP	Restriction fragment length polymorphism
RNA	Ribonucleic acid
rRNA	Ribosomal RNA
tRNA	Transfer RNA

evolves and replicates; (2) the means by which the DNA is expressed (ie, how it is transcribed into ribonucleic acid [RNA]) and how these transcripts are then either translated into protein (eg, for messenger RNA [mRNA]) or utilized in other ways (as with transfer RNA [tRNA], ribosomal RNA [rRNA], etc); and (3) the means by which gene expression is controlled. Knowledge in these areas continues to accumulate at an impressive rate.

Important aspects of the structure and function of DNA are briefly described below. For more detailed information, the reader is encouraged to consult the general references at the end of this chapter.

Structure of DNA

The structure of DNA is shown in Figs 26–1 and 26–2. The backbone of DNA is composed of deoxyribose molecules linked by connecting phosphate groups. These connections occur through the 3'-hydroxyl moiety of the first sugar and the 5'-hydroxyl moiety of the next sugar. Since the 5' moiety of the first sugar and the 3' moiety of the last sugar are free, the direction of the molecule is said to be from 5' to 3'. These designations serve as a reference for orientation. Genes are described as being transcribed from 5' to 3', since the first sugar of the RNA product contains a 5'-triphosphate group. The 5' end of a gene ordinarily refers to its transcriptional start site, or the "upstream" portion of the gene; the 3' end designates the "downstream" portion of the gene, where transcription is terminated.

Figure 26–1. Structural features of a short segment of double-stranded DNA. Shaded areas show the sugar-phosphate backbones running antiparallel to one another (one running from 5' to 3' and the other from 3' to 5'). The unshaded area shows the pyrimidines cytosine (C) and thymine (T), the purines guanine (G) and adenine (A), and the hydrogen bonding of C to G and A to T.

Figure 26–2. Highly simplified depiction of the essential features of DNA replication. The double helix unwinds, and 2 daughter strands of DNA are synthesized. Each of the resulting DNA molecules contains one strand of the original (parent) DNA molecule (semiconservative replication). Complementary base pairing directs the sequence of addition of nucleoside triphosphates by DNA polymerase (not shown). Each daughter strand of DNA is synthesized in the direction of 5' to 3', requiring one strand to be synthesized in a discontinuous fashion.

Connected to each sugar of the DNA backbone is one of 4 **bases:** adenine (A), guanine (G), cytosine (C), or thymine (T). Adenine and guanine are **purines,** whereas cytosine and thymine are **pyrimidines.** A base to which only a sugar is attached is called a **nucleoside;** a base to which both a sugar and a phosphate group are attached is called a **nucleotide.** For example, adenine (base) bound to ribose is termed adenosine (nucleoside); adenosine coupled to a phosphate group is designated adenylic acid (nucleotide). When nucleotides are linked together in a polymer, they generate a **nucleic acid.**

DNA is composed of 2 strands of nucleic acid that are antiparallel to each other (ie, running in opposite directions) such that the A moieties of one strand are hydrogen-bonded to the T moieties of the complementary strand and the C and G moieties are similarly bonded to each other. This **complementary base pairing** means that the order of the bases along one strand of DNA dictates the order along the other strand. This feature is the critical one in DNA replication and transcription for determining, respectively, the precise structures of DNA progeny and of RNA products of genes. The 2 strands are wound around each other in a configuration called a **double helix.** Within the nucleus of a cell, the DNA is packaged into chromatin, a highly ordered structure composed of DNA and proteins.

It is the order of bases along the DNA strand that can be construed as the "secret of life." This order, along with precise base pairing, permits "like to replicate like" and allows for information storage. It is in a sense the body's "computer program" for transmitting similar information to progeny, for directing cells of the developing embryo to differentiate properly into adult anatomic structures, and for directing all of the complex metabolic functions of the cell.

DNA Replication

When DNA replicates (Fig 26–2), the individual strands are separated and nucleoside triphosphates are aligned along the phosphodiester backbones by complementary base pairing. The sugar moieties are then connected enzymatically, resulting in complementary DNA strands. The many steps in this process are highly complex and outside the scope of this chapter, but the result is 2 daughter strands of DNA that are identical to the original DNA. Because one strand of each daughter DNA molecule is from the parent and the other is newly synthesized, the process is called **semiconservative replication.**

Structure & Function of RNA

The first step in gene expression is the transcription of DNA into RNA (Fig 26–3). While the structures of RNA and DNA are similar in most respects, there are several differences: (1) The sugar moiety of RNA is ribose instead of deoxyribose. (2) In RNA, the base uracil (U) replaces T, and U therefore base-pairs with A. RNA in mammalian cells is ordinarily not double-stranded, although there may be folding of the RNA on itself ("secondary structure") that causes portions of it to be double-stranded. Some of the RNA viruses, however, are double-stranded.

There are 3 major classes of RNA: mRNA, tRNA, and rRNA. (There are other minor RNA classes, but these will not be discussed here.) **mRNA** contains sequences that are translated into protein (see below). **tRNA** is involved in transferring amino acids into protein. **rRNA,** along with proteins, forms **ribosomes,** structures that also are involved in protein synthesis. As described in Chapter 1 and illustrated in Fig 1–2, mRNA binds to the ribosome along with the tRNA molecules. Each type of tRNA in the series of tRNA molecules is specific for an amino acid that can bind to the tRNA covalently. Such "charged"

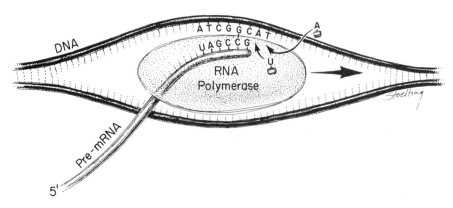

Figure 26–3. Synthesis of RNA. The DNA template is shown to open over the region where transcription of a precursor species (in this case depicted as pre-mRNA) is taking place. The enzyme RNA polymerase directs the addition of ribonucleoside triphosphates into the growing mRNA, with the actual sequence determined by complementary base pairing of purines and pyrimidines. In RNA, the pyrimidine uracil (U) base-pairs with adenine (A).

tRNA molecules participate in the incorporation of amino acids into protein through the formation of peptide bonds.

Gene Structure & Expression

In addition to the segments of DNA that are copied into RNA, there are some segments that are involved in receiving signals which either inhibit or facilitate gene transcription **(control sequences,** or **regulatory sequences).** Other regions determine where the enzymes involved in transcription (ie, the RNA polymerases) are to start and at what basal level a specific gene is to be expressed. These latter regions are called **promoters.** In the case of RNA polymerase II, involved in transcription of genes that encode mRNA molecules, the promoter is located just upstream from the starting point of transcription. The 2 strands of DNA are separated during transcription, and RNA polymerase facilitates base pairing along one of the strands and subsequent polymerization from individual ribonucleoside triphosphates that serve as building blocks (Figs 26–2 and 26–3). At the end of the gene are "stop" signals that terminate transcription; these signals have not been well defined for mammalian genes.

The structure of a mammalian gene encoding an mRNA is shown in Fig 26–4. In the initial stage of expression of this gene, a precursor **(pre-mRNA)** is formed from transcription of the DNA that consists of **exons** (sequences whose transcripts occur in mature mRNA) and **introns** (sequences that interrupt the exons). Posttranscriptional processing leads to the formation of mature mRNA and results in the removal of the intron transcripts. In most mRNA molecules, 2 other modifications occur: (1) The 3' end is cleaved, and a chain of A residues **(the poly[A] tail)** is added to the newly generated 3' end of the mRNA. (2) A **cap,** consisting of a methylated nucleotide inserted in the reverse orientation, is added to the 5' end of the mRNA. The DNA upstream from the start of transcription is called the **5'-flanking DNA,** and that downstream from the completion of transcription is called the **3'-flanking DNA,** although the latter usually refers to the DNA following the poly(A) addition site.

Introns are present in most genes that code for mRNA, but their number varies; there may be as many as 50 in exceptional cases. They are not found in bacterial genes. In a few cases, DNA structures important for regulating the expression of the gene are found in introns. For example, a structure that binds the glucocorticoid receptor and probably accounts for responsiveness to this class of hormones is found in an intron of the human growth hormone gene.

The fact that genes are split into introns and exons has in all likelihood facilitated the process of evolution

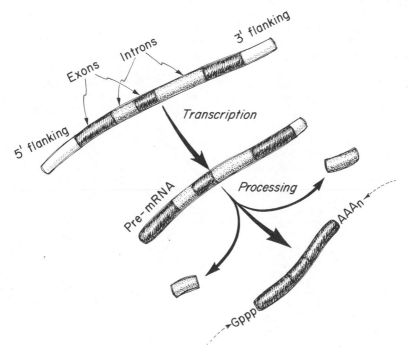

Figure 26–4. The initial steps in gene expression of a typical eukaryotic gene encoding a polypeptide. Exons (regions present in the mature transcript) and introns (regions destined to be excised from the primary transcript) are distinguished in the parent gene by shading. Both the exons and introns are transcribed into the primary gene product, or pre-mRNA. This precursor species then undergoes several processing steps, including splicing of the exons associated with removal of the introns, addition of a cap at the 5' end, and cleavage and polyadenylation at the 3' end. The mature transcript is then transported into the cytoplasm. These processing steps may occur sequentially.

of genes. It is now thought that one critical mechanism for gene evolution involves the movement of DNA segments into existing genes, in which case the inserted segment could, for example, contain (1) structures that code for additional amino acids or (2) structures that regulate the expression of the new gene in a different way. The advantage of introns for such rearrangements of DNA lies in the fact that the genetic events can be somewhat imprecise. In the first example, the inserted segment might consist of an exon flanked by 2 introns; when inserted into an intron of the existing DNA, this would result in an altered mRNA product of the gene, and the protein translated from the mRNA would have an additional segment of amino acids. For this evolutionary event to occur, all that is needed are breaks in the DNA in the middle of the intron in segments that do not contain critical control structures such as those which affect RNA processing; if introns and their removal by processing did not occur, such insertions would be more difficult to achieve without compromising the original gene.

After the mRNA is formed in the nucleus, it is transported to the cell cytoplasm, where it is translated into a protein whose amino acid sequence is determined by the codons of the mRNA according to the genetic code. Each **codon** consists of 3 nucleotides. The first codon of the mRNA that is translated is always AUG, which codes for methionine, and codons for other amino acids then follow. Individual amino acids are each covalently linked to a specific tRNA. These tRNA molecules bind to the mRNA through an **anticodon loop** containing 3 nucleotides that are complementary to the codons of the mRNA. For example, UAC on the anticodon loop pairs with AUG on the mRNA. Whereas each codon is unambiguous in terms of the amino acid specificity, the code is redundant in that more than one codon specifies a given amino acid (except in the case of tryptophan and methionine). Thus, if the nucleic acid sequence of an mRNA is known, the amino acid sequence of its protein translation product will be known with certainty. Conversely, if the amino acid sequence of a protein is known, the nucleic acid sequence of the mRNA and the gene from which it is transcribed can only be partially known. At the end of each coding segment is a "stop" codon, which is UAA, UAG, or UGA; these do not recognize tRNA, and when the ribosome reaches them as it moves along the mRNA in the process of protein synthesis, translation ceases and the ribosome dissociates from the mRNA.

As discussed in Chapter 1, many proteins result from modification of the primary translation product, or precursor protein. For example, a signal peptide sequence that can serve to target a protein for secretion may be removed from a preprotein during the process of entry of the protein into the secretory apparatus (as with preproinsulin). ACTH, a 39-amino-acid protein that is contained within a much larger protein (pro-opiomelanocortin) is released from the larger protein by specific proteolytic cleavage events. In some cases, sugars or other chemical groups may be added after translation.

REGULATION OF GENE EXPRESSION

During development of an organism, cells must differentiate in order to perform specialized functions. Furthermore, hormones, neurotransmitters, and other regulatory signals must be capable of controlling the expression of DNA in various tissues in different ways. The molecular mechanisms involved in the regulation of gene expression are just beginning to be understood. Although many of the steps in the process of gene expression are regulated, the principal control appears to be at the level of transcription of the DNA into pre-mRNA.

In most cases, the structure of genes in the germ line cells is essentially identical to that in the various differentiated or somatic cells. However, in some cases, the bases of DNA are modified such that gene expression is altered. For example, cytosine residues can be methylated, and this can inhibit expression of the gene. The methylation patterns can also be inherited. Methylation appears to contribute to the inactivation of one of the X chromosomes in cells that contain two X chromosomes. The result is transcriptional activity of only one of each pair of X chromosomes in a given cell. In other cases, DNA undergoes rearrangement or mutation (or both). This occurs, for example, with cells of the immune system, in which both rearrangement and mutation of the immunoglobulin gene regions permit millions of different immunoglobulin genes to be formed from a relatively small number of genes present in the progenitor cells.

Details are beginning to emerge about the regulation of transcription. Promoter structures for different genes (discussed in a previous section) may vary in their capacity to initiate transcription, and these affect the total level of activity of the gene. Regulatory sequences also affect the efficiency of the promoter in initiating transcription. Two examples illustrate this point. The insulin gene contains a regulatory sequence located upstream from the promoter, and this sequence is critical for efficient transcription initiation. However, the sequence functions only in the pancreatic B cells. This explains why insulin is made in pancreatic endocrine cells but not in exocrine cells. Presumably, another gene (or genes) in the islets encodes a protein that acts on the insulin gene regulatory element to facilitate initiation of transcription. A second example is the regulatory structure mediating glucocorticoid hormone action. As described in Chapter 1, glucocorticoids bind to intracellular receptors, and the steroid-receptor complex binds to DNA. The site on DNA where these receptors act is called the **glucocorticoid regulatory element** (GRE). The receptor complex binds to the GRE more tightly than to random DNA, and this binding enhances RNA polymerase action at the promoter located near the GRE (Fig 26–5). GREs found in glucocorticoid-responsive genes are usually in the 5′-flanking DNA at a distance of a few to over a thousand nucleotides away from the promoter; however, a GRE of the human growth hor-

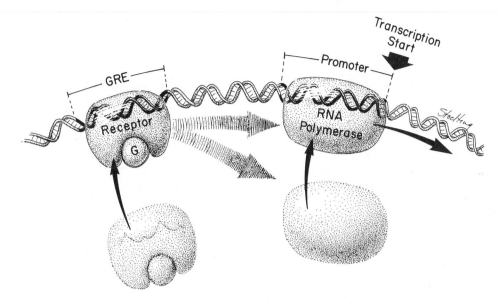

Figure 26 –5. Regulatory structure mediating glucocorticoid (G) hormone action. The steroid-receptor complex binds to a specific DNA sequence called the glucocorticoid regulatory element (GRE). This binding event, in some unknown fashion, enhances (or in some cases inhibits) the interaction of RNA polymerase with the promoter of the glucocorticoid-regulated gene. The result is stimulation (or inhibition) of transcription of the gene.

mone gene is found in an intron. Thus, these regulatory sequences can be thought of as ''cassettes'' of information inserted in the vicinity of a promoter that affect promoter action, in some cases in response to regulatory proteins.

Gene expression can also be regulated at the level of RNA processing or mRNA turnover, although this is probably a less common mechanism than transcriptional control. For example, pre-mRNA from the calcitonin gene can be processed in 2 different ways that vary in the sequences removed. In brain and certain other tissues, the result is an mRNA that encodes calcitonin gene–related peptide (CGRP). In the parafollicular cells of the thyroid gland, calcitonin mRNA is primarily made. These 2 types of mRNA have in common the sequences at the 5' end that encode the amino-terminal portion of the precursor protein molecules. They differ in the 3' sequences that encode the carboxy-terminal portions of the molecules. Thus, this mechanism allows one gene to functionally serve as 2 genes. Variable RNA processing has been described for transcripts of the growth hormone and prolactin genes, although the differences in the resulting mRNA molecules are less striking. Hormones and other factors can regulate mRNA levels (and, consequently, protein levels) by affecting mRNA stability. Estrogens, for example, cause accumulation of ovalbumin mRNA in the chicken oviduct, owing in part to a steroid-mediated decrease in the rate of ovalbumin mRNA breakdown with a consequent increase in the level of ovalbumin mRNA. The means by which this is accomplished are unknown.

There are several instances in which regulation of

the efficiency of mRNA translation is observed, although these are unusual.

Finally, it should be emphasized that the activity of proteins is extensively controlled through actions of hormones and other regulatory substances, as described in Chapter 1.

GENE EVOLUTION

Genes are generated during evolution through rearrangements, additions, or deletions of DNA segments; mutations of nucleotides; and duplications. The products of such duplication events can then evolve independently. This is the probable origin of the so-called **gene families,** which can comprise from a few to many genes. Related genes in these families can be identified through similarities in their overall organization and homologies (similarities) in their nucleotide sequences.

Examples of hormone gene families are (1) growth hormone, prolactin, and placental lactogen (chorionic somatomammotropin); (2) insulin and the somatomedins; and (3) the glycoprotein hormones (thyroid-stimulating hormone, chorionic gonadotropin, luteinizing hormone, and follicle-stimulating hormone). In this first example, the genes for growth hormone, prolactin, and placental lactogen all have a similar overall structure, with 5 exons separated by 4 introns. The sequences encoding the hormones have considerable homology, and when their exons are aligned to maximize this sequence similarity between them, the introns are found to interrupt the coding sequences at similar locations. In the case of the glycoprotein hormones, the same gene encodes the alpha subunit of the various hormones in the group, whereas the beta subunits of the hormones, although similar, are nonetheless unique for each hormone.

MECHANISMS OF GENETIC DISEASE

The precise molecular mechanisms for most of the genetic diseases encountered by endocrinologists are not known. Examples of diseases with a genetic basis are pseudohypoparathyroidism, testicular feminization, congenital adrenal hyperplasia, some forms of dwarfism, and type II diabetes mellitus. In other circumstances, the inherited defect is an increased susceptibility to developing a disease, eg, type I diabetes mellitus and the multiple endocrine neoplasia syndromes.

A number of molecular mechanisms can account for genetic disease, and these have been most clearly elucidated from nonendocrine diseases such as the thalassemias. In some cases, mutations are present—for example, a codon may be altered or a stop codon generated—and these mutations in turn alter the amino acid sequence and result in a protein that is deficient in its function. Mutations sometimes result in an RNA

product that does not accumulate in adequate quantities. Alternatively, deletion or insertion of genetic material can disrupt gene function or result in an abnormal RNA product. Mutations can also affect the processing of pre-mRNA into mRNA by occurring at sites on the gene required to specify proper processing. Finally, the entire gene can be deleted, as has been reported to occur in a rare form of growth hormone deficiency.

RECOMBINANT DNA TECHNOLOGY

The essence of recombinant DNA technology is that isolated fragments of DNA can be cut and ligated together outside of living cells. This recombinant DNA can then be inserted back into a living cell of a prokaryote (nonnucleated cell such as a bacterium) or eukaryote (nucleated cell such as yeast or a mammalian cell) in which it can be replicated. In this way, starting from a single molecule, many new molecules can be obtained. These molecules can be used to study basic biologic processes such as how cells regulate gene expression. Alternatively, the technology can be

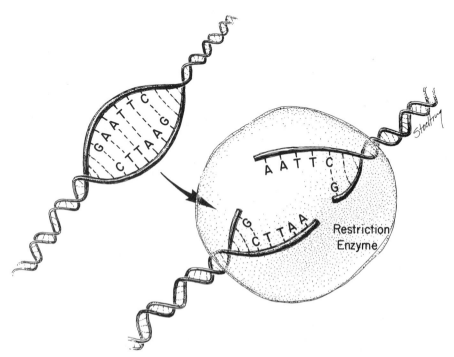

Figure 26–6. Endonucleolytic cleavage of DNA by the restriction enzyme EcoRI. The 6-base-pair sequence recognized by the restriction endonuclease is enlarged for purposes of illustration. The result of cleavage is 2 single-stranded "sticky ends," ie, ends overhanging 3 nucleotide complementary DNA segments.

put to practical uses such as the production of hormones that cannot be synthesized in adequate quantity or purity by other means. The methods available for producing recombinant DNA molecules have made it easier in many circumstances to work with DNA to yield novel protein products than to work with protein molecules themselves.

A major development that led to this new technology involved studies of the process of restriction and modification in bacteria, a process whereby bacteria destroy DNA recognized as foreign yet protect their own genetic information by appropriate modifications. These studies initially led to the discovery of a set of enzymes, called **restriction enzymes** or **restriction endonucleases,** that bind to DNA at specific sequences and cleave the DNA at these loci in a characteristic fashion. Fig 26– 6 illustrates the action of the first restriction enzyme discovered, EcoRI, which was derived from *Escherichia coli.* (The name of each subsequently discovered enzyme likewise incorporates part of the name of the bacterium from which it was derived.) By use of these enzymes, scientists are able to cleave DNA at specific sites. Thus, if a DNA fragment is incubated under appropriate conditions with EcoRI, the DNA will be cleaved at all sequences containing the structure shown in the figure. In this case, the cleavage will yield short single-stranded ends that are complementary to each other (''sticky ends''). If one of the resulting pieces is isolated and incubated with a DNA fragment from another source that has been cut with the same enzyme, the 2 ends with complementarity will base-pair. These hybrid DNA molecules can then be ligated together enzymatically to form a recombinant DNA molecule. Cleavage with some restriction enzymes yields fragments without sticky ends; these blunt-ended fragments can be ligated to other blunt-ended fragments, although this is somewhat less efficient.

Plasmids are frequently the starting material for such reconstructions. These are circular pieces of double-stranded DNA that replicate in bacteria as episomes—ie, they replicate extrachromosomally. They frequently transmit antibiotic resistance; eg, they may contain a gene for β-lactamase that cleaves the β-lactam ring of ampicillin and thus confers ampicillin resistance. A recombinant plasmid may be constructed as depicted in Fig 26– 7 and inserted into a bacterium, usually *E coli,* by a process that makes the bacterium permeable and thus able to take up foreign DNA. The plasmid can subsequently replicate within the bacterial cell, and in this way the inserted DNA is replicated and transmitted along with the other genes carried on the plasmid. If a plasmid containing an antibiotic resistance gene is used, bacteria harboring the plasmid can be enriched by culturing them in the presence of the antibiotic. The population of cells derived from a single parent cell harboring a unique piece of foreign DNA is referred to as a **clone of cells,** and the DNA contained within them is said to be cloned (Fig 26– 8). Once a clone is obtained, the bacteria can be grown in mass quantities, the plasmid DNA isolated and separated from other bacterial constituents, and the inserted DNA released from the plasmid by cleavage with the same restriction enzyme used for its initial isolation. This DNA can then be separated from the plasmid DNA by electrophoretic techniques and characterized.

HYBRIDIZATION

A fundamental property of single-stranded DNA or RNA is its propensity to anneal through base pairing (ie, hybridize) to a complementary strand of DNA or RNA. This is a very precise process based on the hydrogen bonding of A to T or U and of C to G, which permits a single-stranded nucleic acid to find its complement among millions of noncomplementary competing molecules. Recombinant DNA technology makes extensive use of this property in virtually all of its applications. For example, a homogeneous piece of DNA, after radiolabeling, can be used as a **probe** (1) to identify a complementary piece of DNA or RNA that has been size-fractionated on a gel; (2) to localize a single colony of bacteria (from among thousands) that harbors a plasmid containing complementary sequences; or (3) to quantify levels of a specific mRNA. The latter process consists of allowing the probe to hybridize to a mixture of mRNA molecules, either in solution or after the RNA has been transferred to filter paper; eliminating the nonhybridized probe; and then measuring the radioactivity in the hybrids, which reflects the amount of specific mRNA present.

DNA SEQUENCING

Another breakthrough that has facilitated the development of recombinant DNA technology was the design of methods to rapidly sequence DNA. Two methods are currently available.

The **chemical degradation technique** of Maxam and Gilbert relies on the systematic cleavage of homogeneous DNA fragments radiolabeled at one end. Reaction conditions are chosen such that the cleavage process in a given reaction occurs only at one of the 4 nucleotides (A residues, for instance) and such that on average only one of the susceptible positions in a DNA molecule is cleaved. The result is a series of radiolabeled DNA fragments extending from the labeled end to each location of the given nucleotide (ie, at each A) in the original DNA fragment. These can be visualized after size fractionation of the DNA and radioautography; the size of each band corresponds to the position of the base in the starting DNA.

The **chain termination technique** of Sanger uses a homogeneous population of single-stranded DNA molecules as templates for complementary DNA synthesis. DNA synthesis is initiated at a particular site with the use of a small ''primer'' oligonucleotide that hybridizes to a specific sequence. DNA synthesis then proceeds in the presence of radiolabeled nucleoside

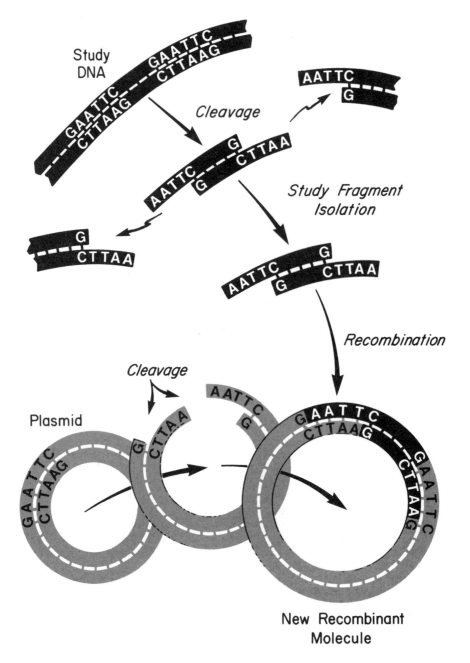

Figure 26–7. Generation of a recombinant DNA molecule. The study DNA is cleaved with a restriction enzyme (in this case, EcoRI), and the released fragment is purified (eg, separated from the parent DNA on the basis of size by agarose gel electrophoresis). A suitable plasmid containing a unique site for the same enzyme is prepared by cleavage with the enzyme and is then mixed with the purified fragment. The complementary overhanging ends anneal to one another and are then ligated together enzymatically (DNA ligase) to yield a new recombinant molecule.

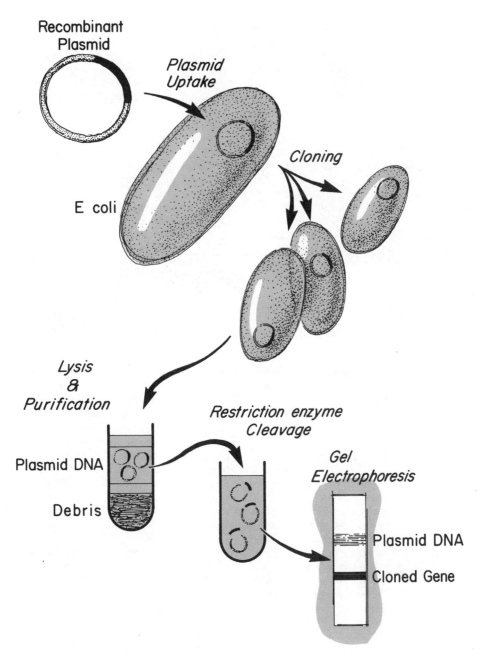

Figure 26–8. Cloning of DNA. Bacteria are treated to facilitate the uptake of recombinant plasmids containing the DNA insert of interest. Culturing in the presence of an antibiotic selects for those bacteria harboring a plasmid containing an appropriate antibiotic-resistance gene (resident on the same plasmid as the insert). Those bacteria that have failed to take up the plasmid will succumb to the antibiotic. Single colonies (a clone) of the now-resistant bacteria are selected for mass culture and are then lysed and the cloned plasmid DNA purified. Cleavage with the appropriate restriction enzyme will release the DNA insert, yielding quantities of homogeneous DNA suitable for further experimentation (eg, for sequencing or preparation of specific radiolabeled DNA probes).

triphosphate precursors. In addition, the reaction is performed in the presence of a nucleotide analog in which the 3'-OH group has been modified so that, after its incorporation, further elongation beyond the nucleotide cannot proceed. Four separate reactions are run, each reaction including a separate modified nucleotide (dideoxy ATP, for example) in addition to the 4 unmodified nucleotides. Conditions are chosen such that termination of synthesis of the complementary DNA molecule occurs at low frequency at each site of a given base (A in this example). The resulting radiolabeled fragments, terminated at each nucleotide, are then size-fractionated on gels; the size of the band corresponds to the position of the complementary base in the original template DNA.

By use of these methods, even genes that are several thousand nucleotides in length can be sequenced in a reasonable period of time. Thus, once a gene is obtained in pure form, its primary structure, or nucleotide sequence, can be determined rapidly and accurately.

SOURCES OF DNA FOR MOLECULAR CLONING

Three different sources of DNA are ordinarily utilized for molecular cloning: DNA produced by chemical synthesis, cellular mRNA transcribed into DNA by the process of reverse transcription, and chromosomal DNA.

DNA Synthesis

DNA molecules composed of as many as 70 nucleotides can now be synthesized within a reasonable time by use of mechanical synthesizers. By combining a number of oligonucleotides synthesized in this fashion, it is also possible to construct an entire gene. This approach was used for the first synthesis of human insulin by recombinant DNA techniques. At the time this was done, the structure of human insulin was known, but the sequence of the gene had not been determined. Thus, based on the known amino acids of human insulin, DNA fragments encoding the A and B chains of insulin were inserted into separate plasmids. These were used to program separate clones of bacteria to produce either the A or B chain, and the chains were then purified from the bacteria and joined chemically.

More commonly, however, smaller DNA segments are produced to facilitate the construction of genes. For example, small DNA segments containing restriction enzyme sites are frequently added to the ends of DNA fragments to facilitate the construction of recombinant DNA molecules. Other chemically synthesized fragments are used as probes to detect complementary DNA pieces in genes or in clones of bacteria. Finally, as discussed below, synthetic DNA may be used to prepare hybrid genes that are combinations of different mammalian or bacterial genes.

These may be used for protein production in the appropriate host cell.

Reverse Transcription of mRNA

Cellular mRNA encoding a particular protein can be isolated from cells that produce the specific protein product. DNA strands complementary to this mRNA (cDNA) can be produced from the mRNA template using deoxyribonucleoside triphosphates and the enzyme reverse transcriptase. This enzyme is isolated from retroviruses, which are RNA viruses with the ability to copy their RNA into DNA (reverse transcription). As discussed in a previous section, most mRNA molecules have a poly(A) tail, and this tail can be hybridized (annealed) to an oligomer of polydeoxythymidylate (oligo-dT) that serves as a required "primer" to initiate the reverse transcription. After the RNA is transcribed, it is destroyed, and the single-stranded cDNA formed through transcription is then copied into a double-stranded molecule. This latter step is facilitated either by the reverse transcriptase that can also copy DNA into DNA or by DNA polymerase.

One of several different methods can be utilized to insert the cDNA into a plasmid. For example, chemically synthesized double-stranded DNA "linker" molecules containing an appropriate restriction site can be ligated to the ends of the fragment, and the entire fragment can then be inserted into the plasmid at the same restriction enzyme site (Fig 26–7).

Since any given cell contains thousands of different mRNA molecules, reverse transcription of total cellular mRNA will yield thousands of different cDNA molecules. Thus, in order to obtain a given cDNA, the investigator must either (1) isolate the mRNA of interest from the remainder of the mRNA molecules prior to cDNA synthesis and subsequent cloning or (2) generate a large number of clones and then identify those containing the cDNA of interest. In most cases, the specific mRNA cannot be obtained in homogeneous form prior to cloning; thus, some reliance must be placed on the latter technique. However, methods can be used to "enrich" the mRNA prior to molecular cloning. These methods include (1) starting with a tissue containing a high concentration of the mRNA; (2) using physical separation techniques that may be applied to separate mRNA molecules based on size; and (3) performing immunoprecipitation of polysomes (collections of mRNA-containing ribosomes), utilizing an antiserum that recognizes the nascent peptide product of the mRNA.

In any case, all of the mRNA molecules present at the time of reverse transcription will be transcribed, thereby yielding a so-called cDNA library. After this library is cloned into the appropriate host cell, there may be anywhere from a few clones up to millions of clones, each harboring the same parent plasmid but a different cDNA insert. These must be screened to find the clone containing plasmids with the cDNA insert of interest. Screening of a cDNA library may be performed in several ways, 3 of which will be discussed.

First, if even a portion of the amino acid sequence of the protein encoded by the mRNA is known, this information can be used, through knowledge of the genetic code, to predict a partial DNA sequence for the cDNA. Small oligonucleotide DNA molecules that contain the nucleotide sequence complementary to the cDNA are then synthesized and radiolabeled. The DNA of the clones comprising the cDNA library is transferred to filter papers and hybridized to the labeled oligonucleotides. The DNA from those clones of cells carrying plasmids with the correct cDNA— but not other cDNAs—will hybridize to the oligonucleotide probes. The hybridization can be identified by radioautography. The clones can then be grown in large-scale culture for further analysis.

A second approach for screening a cDNA library is to insert the cDNA into a site in the plasmid that is somewhere in the middle of a bacterial gene, so that the codons of the cDNA will be expressed as part of a ''fusion protein'' containing bacterial and cDNA-encoded amino acid sequences. Screening this cDNA expression library with an antibody to the protein product of interest will permit identification of the clone producing the appropriate fusion protein and thus harboring the correct cDNA-containing plasmid.

One additional method for screening relies on translation of mRNA in a cell-free reaction; the mRNA is identified by assaying for its protein product, detected, for example, by immunoprecipitation. Plasmid DNA containing the cDNA of interest can then be identified, since it will hybridize exclusively to the mRNA from which it was derived and thereby block the cell-free translation of the protein encoded by that mRNA. This phenomenon, in which the correct cDNA blocks in vitro translation by the mRNA of interest, is known as **hybrid arrest.**

To rigorously establish that the cDNA isolated by screening methods is in fact the correct one, the nucleotide sequence of the cDNA is determined. This is then compared with the amino acid sequence of the protein.

Chromosomal Genes

By use of techniques analogous to those employed for cDNA cloning, it is possible to clone the portions of a chromosome that contain the gene of interest. Chromosomal DNA isolated from cell nuclei can be cleaved into fragments by use of a restriction enzyme and the resultant fragments ligated into the appropriate restriction site of bacterial virus (bacteriophage) DNA. Bacteriophages are advantageous in this case, since they can accommodate larger inserts (to several thousand nucleotides) than plasmids can. Certain classes of viruses can also be used to clone cDNA. The recombinant bacteriophage is used to infect a bacterial host in which its DNA is replicated. A radiolabeled cDNA or chemically synthesized oligonucleotide may then be used to screen for the clone of bacteria containing the bacteriophage with the chromosomal insert of interest. This is done by transferring the DNA of the phage that has infected the bacteria to a filter paper

and then hybridizing the filter-bound phage DNA to radioactive cDNA. The specificity of this hybridization allows one to identify the correct clone with the chromosomal insert. One can then produce this particular bacteriophage in large quantities to obtain sufficient chromosomal DNA for analysis.

TRANSFER OF CLONED GENES INTO MAMMALIAN CELLS

Methods for transferring cloned genes or other DNA into mammalian cells have had their greatest impact in the study of gene function, but the techniques are also being used to produce medically important proteins. DNA can be transferred into mammalian cells in several ways. For example, it can be microinjected into the cell nucleus. Alternatively, calcium phosphate precipitates of DNA can be prepared that will be phagocytosed by the cells, or bacteria that contain plasmids with inserted DNA can be stripped of their cell wall to form protoplasts that will fuse to mammalian cells. Direct electroporation of plasmid DNA into recipient cells is also sometimes used. In addition, viral vectors have been designed to deliver the DNA of interest into target cells.

Most of the ''transfected'' DNA will not become integrated into the host chromosome and be stably expressed. However, this DNA may be transiently expressed, and the function of the transfected DNA can be studied in this way (transient expression assays). In other circumstances, it is desirable to isolate those few cells in which the transfected DNA has become integrated and therefore replicated along with the host DNA. This can be achieved, for example, by ''co-transfecting'' the DNA of interest with DNA containing a ''selectable'' gene, such as the gene encoding resistance to neomycin. In this case, when the cells are then cultured in the presence of an analog of neomycin that ordinarily kills the cells, only the cells that both integrate and express the neomycin resistance gene will survive and propagate. These cells will usually have integrated the study gene as well.

Gene transfer into mammalian cells has proved to be of enormous usefulness for studying the mechanisms of gene expression and its regulation. For example, information about the glucocorticoid regulatory element shown in Fig 26–5 was derived chiefly from such gene transfer studies. Initially, these studies involved transferring a cloned glucocorticoid-responsive gene into a mammalian cell, which normally does not express that specific gene, and documenting that the transferred gene was glucocorticoid-responsive. This type of experiment demonstrates that elements responsive to the steroid reside somewhere on the cloned DNA that was transferred. Follow-up studies have included deleting the putative steroid regulatory sequences prior to gene transfer to demonstrate extinction of hormone responsiveness and splicing the putative control sequence to another gene that ordinarily is not steroid-regulated and demonstrating that the hybrid gene is glucocorticoid-responsive.

PRODUCTION OF MEDICALLY IMPORTANT PROTEINS BY RECOMBINANT DNA TECHNIQUES

A major use of recombinant DNA technology is to produce medically useful proteins. Employing genes to produce the proteins encoded by them is presently the only means available for producing moderate-sized to large proteins in quantity. Although the methods for chemically synthesizing peptides have improved considerably in recent years, they have not progressed to the point where large proteins (eg, > 100 amino acids) can be made efficiently. Whereas some proteins, such as insulin, can be obtained by isolating them from animals, this approach (even for insulin) has its limitations. The approach is impractical when large quantities of scarce proteins are needed, as is the case with interferon and erythropoietin.

As discussed earlier, genes must have regulatory sequences in order to be expressed. If mammalian DNA sequences are inserted randomly into bacteria, they will usually not be expressed efficiently. Therefore, sequences that encode the desired proteins must be inserted in the regions of plasmids downstream from bacterial regulatory sequences. The region would include a promoter; the sequences encoding a ribo-

somal binding site; and an AUG codon, which codes for methionine and is necessary in mRNA to initiate translation. The bacterial regulatory sequences are responsible for directing the synthesis of the desired proteins. By this method of direct expression, the synthesized proteins can frequently be obtained in yields that represent several percent of the total bacterial proteins. These proteins are then purified from the bacteria. An alternative approach is the synthesis of a fusion (hybrid) protein from which the desired protein can be cleaved (Fig 26–9). To do this, the DNA sequences encoding the desired protein are inserted into the middle of the coding sequences of the bacterial gene. The bacterium synthesizes a hybrid protein containing sequences of bacterial and mammalian amino acids, with the sequences joined at a site that is susceptible to proteolytic or chemical cleavage. The mammalian protein can then be released from the fusion protein with the appropriate enzymes or chemical reagent. This approach was used for the first bacterial synthesis of human insulin and β-endorphin.

In some cases, proteins are produced more efficiently by yeasts than by bacteria. These organisms have plasmids similar to those of bacteria, and the approaches used for protein synthesis are similar to those described above. One useful feature of yeasts is that they can be programmed to secrete their expressed proteins into the medium, a feature that aids in purification.

Mammalian cells are being used increasingly for

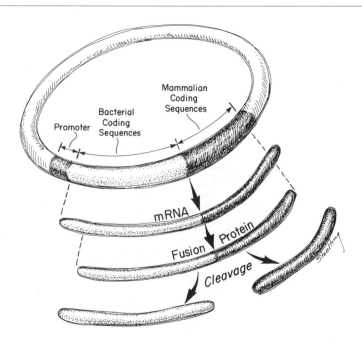

Figure 26–9. Expression of a mammalian protein as a fusion protein in bacteria. Sequences coding for a mammalian protein are linked to sequences coding for a bacterial protein. The linkage occurs in phase with respect to the genetic code. The hybrid protein gene is expressed under the control of the bacterial promoter. If engineered properly, the fusion protein can be cleaved (chemically or enzymatically) to release the mammalian protein, which can then be further purified.

the production of recombinant DNA–derived proteins. This research has been stimulated by methods that increase the production yields and allow for the use of media that are devoid of expensive animal serum. An advantage of the use of mammalian cells is that these cells can add important carbohydrate groups to the proteins when this is necessary; this may not be done correctly by yeasts and is not performed at all by bacteria. Plasminogen activators now in clinical trials are being produced by mammalian cells, and more complex proteins such as factor VIII are likely to be produced most effectively by mammalian cells.

PRODUCTS OF RECOMBINANT DNA TECHNOLOGY

The human body produces thousands of different proteins, including proteins that function as hormones or enzymes, and it is well recognized that deficiencies or excesses of many of these proteins contribute to human disease. The potential for clinical use of recombinant DNA products in this area is enormous. Technology is aimed at producing pure proteins, protein antagonists, and protein derivatives that possess a more limited and thus clinically more specific range of activities compared to the parent protein. The following is a brief review of the progress in this area related to endocrinology.

Human insulin prepared by recombinant techniques is now available, and this ensures an unlimited supply of this hormone. **Growth hormone** has recently become available to replace the cadaver-derived human growth hormone, which may in some cases be contaminated with Creutzfeldt-Jakob virus. **Erythropoietin,** currently being tested, should prove useful in the management of a number of anemias and may decrease the need for transfusion and thereby reduce the risk of transfusion-associated complications, eg, in patients with renal failure. **Atrial natriuretic factor** is being tested in humans for the treatment of hypertension, edema, and related states. This hormone directly increases the glomerular filtration rate and antagonizes the renin-angiotensin system, thereby promoting hypotension and natriuresis with relative potassium sparing. It also is a vasodilator. Recombinant DNA–produced **epidermal growth factor** and **somatomedins** may also have clinical utility.

Other products may replace hormones as therapeutic agents. The protein(s) called **macrocortin** or **lipomodulin** inhibits phospholipase A_2, a key enzyme in the generation of arachidonic acid and thus in the formation of prostaglandins, prostacyclins, and leukotrienes. This protein is induced by glucocorticoids and is thought to mediate some of the anti-inflammatory actions of these steroids. It may therefore one day supplant glucocorticoids for some uses, since it may have fewer or less severe side effects than the steroids. **Pulmonary surfactant protein** is another peptide that may replace glucocorticoid use in neonatology. This protein is also induced by glucocorticoids and is deficient in patients with neonatal respiratory distress syndrome.

Products targeted principally at nonendocrinologic diseases may also become part of the armamentarium of endocrinologists. A number of agents being tested for anticancer activity, such as the **interferons, tumor necrosis factor,** and **interleukins,** may prove useful in treating endocrine neoplasia or ectopic hormone-producing cancers. Recombinant DNA technology is also being used to develop **vaccines** that potentially could prevent viral illnesses thought to be involved in the pathogenesis of diseases such as diabetes mellitus.

Not only can naturally occurring proteins be made, but variant proteins can be produced with specific advantages. The genetic engineering methodologies lend themselves readily to altering the structure of genes and thereby producing variants of the natural compounds. In addition, hybrid molecules can theoretically be produced by linking together parts of different genes to form a protein that has, for example, greater agonist activity than the natural compound or more specificity for a particular response. Currently, major efforts are under way to test the activities of hybrid and variant immunoglobulin molecules. Molecules with antagonist activity are also being produced. For example, **parathyroid hormone (PTH) antagonists,** produced by deleting amino acids from the amino terminus of PTH, could conceivably be useful in treating certain hypercalcemic states associated with excess PTH or PTH-like activity.

DRUG DELIVERY SYSTEMS

Most of the products of recombinant DNA technology are proteins that cannot be given orally for therapy. In general, they are unstable and poorly absorbed from the gastrointestinal tract. Thus, they must be given by injection, and this limits their use. It may be possible to determine the critically active regions of these proteins and design orally active drugs that contain these essential elements. A number of drug delivery systems are also being developed to overcome this problem. In one approach, the drug is encapsulated in a liposome or a microemulsion designed to facilitate movement of the drug through and into the cell. A second approach involves the development of implantable devices that release medication at appropriate intervals during a prolonged period. Yet another type of drug delivery system involves mixing the protein with a bile salt analog and spraying the mixture into the nose. This system has been shown to be effective, at least over short periods of time, for delivering insulin to diabetics. Because the insulin is absorbed rapidly into the circulation, mimicking intravenous delivery, it is especially helpful in controlling postprandial hyperglycemia.

USE OF DNA FOR THE DIAGNOSIS OF GENETIC DISEASE

The DNA of a patient's cells obtained from blood, amniotic fluid, or biopsy material can be readily analyzed utilizing recombinant DNA technology. Rapid tests based on DNA analysis are available for diagnosis of such classic genetic diseases as the thalassemias, sickle cell anemia, and phenylketonuria. Genetic differences also contribute to many more common diseases in which the specific genetic defect has not yet been defined (eg, hypertension and type II diabetes mellitus), and the ability to analyze genes in detail may allow for the detection of DNA segments responsible for these diseases and thus provide a new means of diagnosis.

Although a gene can be isolated from an individual and its primary structure determined, this procedure at present is cumbersome and not yet adaptable for general clinical use. However, genetic defects can be detected in many cases by isolating DNA from a pa-

tient, cleaving it with restriction enzymes, running it on gels, transferring it to nitrocellulose filters, and hybridizing it with particular DNA probes. This method relies heavily on analysis of **genetic polymorphisms**—ie, analysis of differences in the primary structures of genes, such as differences between the 2 alleles of a given gene in the same individual or between the genes of 2 different individuals. Such differences can occur in the gene sequences that are transcribed or in the 5'- or 3'-flanking DNA. Polymorphisms are generated in the process of replication of the DNA, when mutations occur at low frequency. Most of these are "silent" in that they have no effect on the function of the gene or on its products. Nevertheless, these mutations are inherited and can be used as **genetic markers.**

The following is an illustration of one use of polymorphism analysis. Assume, for instance, that a mutation in one base occurs in an individual and that this results in a genetic trait—eg, susceptibility to developing a disease such as diabetes mellitus. Somewhere in or around the affected gene, this individual is likely

Figure 26–10. Use of restriction fragment length polymorphisms (RFLPs) as genetic markers of disease. In the case illustrated, a mutation resulting in a defective gene is associated with a polymorphic variation in the 5'-flanking DNA, and this results in the presence of a restriction site not present in unafflicted individuals. Cleavage with the appropriate restriction enzyme will yield a smaller fragment for the defective gene than for the normal gene. Subjecting the various fragments to size fractionation on a gel and to hybridization to a radiolabeled probe will allow identification of the aberrant fragment. This obviates the need for isolation and cloning of the genomic DNA to identify the mutation within the gene.

to have additional differences in comparison to other people. Occasionally, these differences result in the generation or loss of a restriction endonuclease cleavage site (Fig 26–10). In this case, cleavage of the affected individual's DNA with the restriction enzyme will result in DNA fragments that differ in size from those of other people. Subjecting the fragments to size fractionation on a gel, transferring them to nitrocellulose filters, and performing hybridization to a radiolabeled probe from the gene will allow identification of the aberrant fragment. Since the restriction site polymorphism will be inherited along with the mutation that results in disease susceptibility, this polymorphism can be used as a genetic marker for the disease. This type of analysis only requires an established linkage between a disease and a restriction fragment length polymorphism (RFLP) and an appropriate DNA probe; it is not necessary to know anything about the gene product.

POTENTIAL FOR GENE THERAPY

Since genes can be transferred into mammalian cells and can then function after such transfer, it follows that genes might be inserted into the cells of patients where they could function, in effect, as therapeutic agents. The advantages of such an approach are obvious. For example, if the insulin gene could be appropriately transferred into a patient with type I diabetes mellitus, this gene might be capable of delivering insulin to the patient on a continuing basis, thereby obviating the need for insulin injections. Similar considerations apply to other diseases such as the thalassemias, sickle cell anemia, and hypoparathyroidism and other hormonal deficiency states. Conversely, gene transfer therapy could also be used to treat states of pathologic excess, such as hypercholesterolemia or hypertension, by using genes that would lower cholesterol levels or blood pressure. However, the first application of such a therapeutic approach will probably involve the correction of certain immunodeficiency states.

Although most researchers now agree that this therapy will ultimately be possible, it is also true that a number of problems must be solved before it becomes generally applicable. The gene must be delivered to the right tissue—eg, globin genes to erythroid cells. The gene needs to function adequately but not excessively. For example, to ensure that the insulin gene does not overfunction and thereby produce hypoglycemia, the transferred gene must be capable of responding to blood glucose levels. Stably integrated genes can now be obtained with the use of dividing cells, but many targets for gene transfer are nondividing cells. Since the integration of genes into the chromosome results in an interruption of the cellular DNA at the site of integration, there is a potential for mutation and, consequently, a malignant transformation or death of the cell. One approach to prevent the latter from occurring may involve isolating target cells, removing them from the body, propagating them in cell culture, transferring the gene, documenting its proper function, demonstrating that the cells are normal metabolically and not malignantly transformed, and then delivering them back to appropriate locations in the body. These cells might, for instance, be inserted in a capsule so they could be removed if it became desirable to terminate treatment.

This technology should provide a powerful means for treating a number of diseases. It will also raise a number of ethical and related issues.

ETHICAL & BIOSAFETY CONSIDERATIONS

Recombinant DNA technology, like most other technologies, has the potential for misuse, either accidental or deliberate. When it first emerged in the 1970s, great concern was raised about its overall safety. It was feared, for example, that *E coli* harboring potentially toxic genes, if accidentally leaked into the environment, would propagate and cause great damage. Fortunately, most of these concerns have now been allayed; the strains of *E coli* used in the laboratory do not multiply well outside the laboratory or in the human intestine, and in general there is no environmental pressure that would favor the survival of those organisms harboring cloned genes. Nevertheless, the potential does exist for inserting genes into other organisms in ways that could produce harmful results. For these and other reasons, most agree that there should be guidelines for conducting recombinant DNA research.

IMPACT OF MOLECULAR BIOLOGY ON MEDICINE

The basic information about genes—their function, regulation, and production—has been the greatest contribution of recombinant DNA technology, notwithstanding the numerous practical applications already achieved (as discussed earlier in this chapter). These applications have, in turn, provided the means for increasing the body of knowledge. For example, now that erythropoietin is available in substantial supply, it is possible to learn much more about its actions, biologic roles, and therapeutic uses.

Recent progress in cancer research is also illustrative. The study of retrovirus genes capable of inducing neoplastic transformation (oncogenes) has generated an enormous body of information. Several potential mechanisms by which normal cellular proliferation may become neoplastic have been identified. In some cases, the tumor-promoting genes of these viruses encode proteins related to growth factors. The v-sis gene product of one class of such viruses is similar to one of the 2 subunits of platelet-derived growth factor. In other cases, these viral oncogenes encode proteins that are analogs of growth factor receptors; the v-erb B oncogene encodes a protein similar to the epidermal growth factor receptor. In addition, this group of viruses, through their insertion into the DNA, might also activate cellular genes with growth-stimulating activity. Of tremendous importance was the finding that these viral oncogenes were actually acquired from the DNA of vertebrates (the loci referred to as proto-oncogenes). The gene known as c-Ha-ras (because of its homology to the viral v-Ha-ras gene) was isolated from a bladder carcinoma and found to encode a protein that appears to be a version of the guanyl nucleotide–binding protein that activates adenylate cyclase. This gene may be involved in a significant number of human cancers.

There is much evidence to suggest that cancer is not a one-step process. For example, some genes may perform the function of converting the cell to a state that allows for continued replication; cancer would not ensue until a second gene was activated that stimulated cell growth. The requirements of a multistep process might explain why certain endocrine cancers (postirradiation thyroid cancer, the tumors of multiple endocrine neoplasia syndromes) require years to develop. Other aspects of malignant transformation may involve processes that result in inability of the tumor to be suppressed by the body's immune system. The recent availability of recombinant DNA–produced proteins, such as tumor necrosis factor, will greatly facilitate studies of these latter aspects.

Increased knowledge of the mechanisms of cancer provides the basis for developing new approaches to cancer prevention, diagnosis, and treatment. For example, if specific growth factors are involved, therapies can be designed to block their action. Likewise, knowledge of the molecular mechanisms of hormone action should further our understanding of the pathogenesis and expression of endocrinologic diseases.

REFERENCES

General

Alberts B et al: *Molecular Biology of the Cell.* Garland, 1983.

Baxter JD: Recombinant DNA and medical progress. *Hosp Pract* (Feb) 1980;**15**:57.

Gardner DG, Baxter JD: Recombinant DNA. *Am J Med* 1982;**72**:551.

Lewin B: *Genes II.* Wiley, 1985.

Steel CM: DNA in medicine: The tools. (2 parts.) *Lancet* 1984;**2**:908, 966.

Williamson R: *Genetic Engineering.* Vols 1–4. Academic Press, 1981–1983.

Wolpert L: DNA and its message. *Lancet* 1984;**2**:853.

Regulation of Gene Expression & Gene Transfer

Chandler V, Maler B, Yamamoto RK: DNA sequences bound specifically by glucocorticoid receptor in vitro render a heterologous promoter hormone responsive in vivo. *Cell* 1983;**33**:489.

Gehring WJ: The homeo box: A key to the understanding of development? *Cell* 1985;**40**:3.

Goodbourn S, Zinn K, Maniatis T: Human β-interferon gene expression is regulated by an inducible enhancer element. *Cell* 1985;**41**:509.

Johnson LK, Baxter JD: The mechanism of action of adrenocorticosteroids at the molecular level. Chapter 2 in: *Landmark Advances in Rheumatology.* Contact Associates, 1985.

Karin M et al: Activation of a heterologous promoter in response to dexamethasone and cadmium by metallothionein gene 5'-flanking DNA. *Cell* 1984;**36**:371.

Karin M et al: Characterization of DNA sequences through which cadmium and glucocorticoid hormones induce human metallothionein-IIA gene. *Nature* 1984;**308**:513.

Khoury G, Gruss P: Enhancer elements. *Cell* 1983;**33**:313.

Lan NC et al: Mechanisms of glucocorticoid hormone action. *J Steroid Biochem* 1984;**20**:77.

Nevins JR: The pathway of eukaryotic mRNA formation. *Annu Rev Biochem* 1983;**52**:441.

O'Malley BW: Steroid hormone action in eukaryotic cells. *J Clin Invest* 1984;**74**:307.

Rabbitts TH: DNA juggling in the immune system. *Lancet* 1984;**2**:1086.

Tonegawa S: The molecules of the immune system. *Sci Am* 1985;**253**:122.

Walker MD et al: Cell-specific expression controlled by the 5'-flanking region of insulin and chymotrypsin genes. *Nature* 1983;**306**:557.

Wright S et al: DNA sequences required for regulated expression of β-globin genes in murine erythroleukemia cells. *Cell* 1984;**38**:265.

Gene Evolution

Gilbert W: Genes in pieces revisited. *Science* 1985;**228**:823.

Miller WL, Baxter JD, Eberhardt NL: Peptide hormone genes: Structure and evolution. Page 15 in: *Brain Peptides.* Krieger D, Brownstein M, Martin J (editors). Wiley, 1983.

Moore DD, Conkling MA, Goodman HM: Human growth hormone: A multigene family. *Cell* 1982;**29**:285.

O'Malley BW, Means AR, Stein JP: Gene structure and evolution. Page 1 in: *Gene Regulation by Steroid Hormones II.* Roy AK, Clark JN (editors). Springer-Verlag, 1983.

Mechanisms of Genetic Disease

Busslinger M, Moschonas N, Flavell RA: β⁺-Thalassemia: Aberrant splicing results from a single point mutation in an intron. *Cell* 1981;**27**:289.

Dobkin C et al: Abnormal splice in a mutant human β-globin gene not at the site of mutation. *Proc Natl Acad Sci USA* 1983;**80**:1184.

Higgo DR et al: α-Thalassemia caused by a polyadenylation signal mutation. *Nature* 1983;**306**:398.

Kinniburgh AJ et al: mRNA-deficient β⁰-thalassemia results from a single nucleotide deletion. *Nucleic Acids Res* 1982;**10**:5421.

Orkin SH, Kazazian HH: The mutation and polymorphism of the human β-globin gene and its surrounding DNA. *Annu Rev Genet* 1984;**18**:1331.

Trecartin RF et al: β⁰-Thalassemia in Sardinia is caused by a nonsense mutation. *J Clin Invest* 1981;**68**:1012.

Treisman R, Orkin SH, Maniatis T: Specific transcription and RNA splicing defects in five cloned β-thalassemia genes. *Nature* 1983;**302**:591.

Cloning Methodology & DNA Sequencing

Gilbert W: DNA sequencing and gene structure. *Science* 1981;**214**:1305.

Glover DM (editor): *DNA Cloning*. Vols 1 and 2. IRL Press (Oxford), 1985.

Maniatis T, Fritsch EF, Sambrook J: *Molecular Cloning: A Laboratory Manual*. Cold Springs Harbor Laboratory, 1982.

Old RW, Primrose SB: *Principles of Gene Manipulation*. Vol 2 of: *Studies in Microbiology*, 3rd ed. Blackwell, 1985.

Sanger F: Determination of nucleotide sequences in DNA. *Science* 1981;**214**:1205.

Genetic Engineering

Blackwell GJ et al: Macrocortin: A polypeptide causing the anti-phospholipase effect of glucocorticoids. *Nature* 1980;**287**:147.

Collen D et al: Coronary thrombolysis with recombinant human tissue-type plasminogen activator: A prospective, randomized, placebo-controlled trial. *Circulation* 1984; **70**:1012.

Duff G: Many roles for interleukin-1. *Nature* 1985;**313**:352.

Flameng W et al: Coronary thrombolysis and infarct size reduction after intravenous infusion of recombinant tissue-type plasminogen activator in nonhuman primates. *J Clin Invest* 1985;**75**:84.

Goeddel DV et al: Direct expression in *Escherichia coli* of a DNA sequence for human growth hormone. *Nature* 1975;**281**:544.

Goeddel DV et al: Expression in *Escherichia coli* of chemically synthesized genes for human insulin. *Proc Natl Acad Sci USA* 1979;**76**:106.

Greenberg BD et al: Nucleotide sequence of the gene encoding human atrial natriuretic factor precursor. *Nature* 1984; **312**:656.

Lee-Huang S: Cloning and expression of human erythropoietin cDNA in *Escherichia coli*. *Proc Natl Acad Sci USA* 1984;**81**:2708.

Murray K: New routes to drugs, diagnostic agents, and vaccines. *Lancet* 1984;**2**:1194.

Richards AM et al: Renal, haemodynamic, and hormonal effects of human alpha atrial natriuretic peptide in healthy volunteers. *Lancet* 1985;**1**:545.

Shirai T et al: Cloning and expression in *Escherichia coli* of the gene for human tumor necrosis factor. *Nature* 1985; **313**:803.

Vane JK, Cuatracasas P: Genetic engineering and pharmaceuticals. *Nature* 1984;**312**:303.

White RT et al: Isolation and characterization of the human pulmonary surfactant apoprotein gene. *Nature*. [In press.]

Drug Delivery Systems

Gordon GS et al: Nasal absorption of insulin: Enhancement by hydrophobic bile salts. *Proc Natl Acad Sci USA* 1985;**82**:7419.

Moses AC et al: Insulin administered intranasally as an insulin−bile salt aerosol: Effectiveness and reproducibility in normal and diabetic subjects. *Diabetes* 1983;**32**:1040.

Salzman R et al: Intranasal aerosolized insulin: Mixed meal and long-term use in type I diabetes. *N Engl J Med* 1985;**312**:1078.

Diagnosis of Genetic Disease

Chang JC, Kan YW: A sensitive new prenatal test for sickle cell anemia. *N Engl J Med* 1982;**307**:30.

Engleber NC, Eisenstein BI: The impact of new cloning techniques on the diagnosis and treatment of infectious disease. *N Engl J Med* 1984;**311**:892.

Gusella JF et al: A polymorphic DNA marker genetically linked to Huntington's disease. *Nature* 1983;**306**:234.

Jackson LG: First-trimester diagnosis of fetal genetic disorders. *Hosp Pract* (March) 1985;**20**:39.

Kan YW, Dozy AM: Polymorphism of DNA sequence adjacent to human β-globin structural gene: Relationship to sickle mutation. *Proc Natl Acad Sci USA* 1978;**75**:5631.

Kidd VJ et al: α_1-Antitrypsin deficiency detection by direct analysis of the mutation in the gene. *Nature* 1983;**304**:230.

Marx JL: Putting the human genome on the map. *Science* 1985;**229**:150.

Orkin SH et al: Linkage of β-thalassemia mutations and β-globin gene polymorphisms with DNA polymorphisms in human β-globin gene cluster. *Nature* 1982;**296**:627.

Phillips JA: Genetic diagnosis: Differentiating growth disorders. *Hosp Pract* (April) 1985;**20**:85.

Pirastu M et al: Prenatal diagnosis of β-thalassemia. *N Engl J Med* 1983;**309**:284.

Saiki RK et al: Enzymatic amplification of β-globin genomic sequences and restriction site analysis for diagnosis of sickle cell anemia. *Science* 1985;**230**:1350.

Woo SLC et al: Cloned human phenylalanine hydroxylase gene allows prenatal diagnosis and carrier detection of classical phenylketonuria. *Nature* 1983;**306**:151.

Gene Therapy

Anderson WF: Prospects for human gene therapy. *Science* 1984;**226**:401.

Anderson WF, Fletcher JC: Gene therapy in human beings: When is it ethical to begin? *N Engl J Med* 1980;**303**:1293.

Cullston BJ: Gene therapy: Research in public. *Science* 1985;**227**:493.

Rose S: Human perfectibility. *Lancet* 1984;**2**:1380.

Weatherall DJ: DNA in medicine: Implications for medical practice and human biology. *Lancet* 1984;**2**:1440.

Oncogenes

Bishop JM: Cellular oncogenes and retroviruses. *Annu Rev Biochem* 1983;**52**:301.

Bishop JM: Viral oncogenes. *Cell* 1985;**42**:23.

Doolittle RF et al: Simian sarcoma virus oncogene, v-sis, is derived from the gene (or genes) encoding a platelet-derived growth factor. *Science* 1983;**221**:275.

Downward J et al: Close similarity of epidermal growth factor receptor and v-erb B oncogene protein sequences. *Nature* 1984;**307**:521.

Heldin CH, Westermark B: Growth factors: Mechanisms of action and relation to oncogenes. *Cell* 1984;**37**:9.

Kingston RE, Baldwin AS, Sharp PA: Transcription control by oncogenes. *Cell* 1985;**41**:3.

Reddy EP et al: A point mutation is responsible for the acquisition of transforming properties by the T24 human bladder carcinoma oncogene. *Nature* 1982;**300**:149.

Shih C, Weinberg RA: Isolation of a transforming sequence from a human bladder carcinoma cell line. *Cell* 1982;**29**:161.

Waterfield MD et al: Platelet-derived growth factor is structurally related to the putative transforming protein p28sis of simian sarcoma virus. *Nature* 1983;**304**:35.

Index